Essentials of General Surgery

FOURTH EDITION

About the Cover

"Portrait of Professor Gross," also called "The Gross Clinic," was painted by Thomas Eakins in 1875. Eakins had attended lectures at Jefferson Medical College during Samuel David Gross's lecture as Chairman of Surgery. Eakins's students and friends posed as spectators of the operation, and a self-portrait of Eakins himself sketching the procedure (removal of a piece of bone diseased by osteomyelitis) can be found at the center of the painting. The law at that time required the presence of a relative for surgery on a charity patient (note woman at lower left), a situation permitted by doctors who even then wished to avoid malpractice suits. This nearly life-size painting has hung at Jefferson Medical College since 1879.

(Courtesy of Jefferson Medical College, Thomas Jefferson University, Philadelphia, Pennsylvania)

Essentials of General Surgery

FOURTH EDITION

SENIOR EDITOR

PETER F. LAWRENCE, MD
Professor and Bergman Chief of Vascular Surgery
Director of the Gonda (Goldschmied) Vascular Center
David Geffen School of Medicine at UCLA
Los Angeles, California

EDITORS

RICHARD M. BELL, MD
Professor and Chairman
Department of Surgery
University of South Carolina School of Medicine
Columbia, South Carolina

MERRIL T. DAYTON, MD
Professor and Chairman
Department of Surgery
State University of New York at Buffalo
Buffalo, New York

TEXTBOOK CONTENT EDITOR

MOHAMMED I. AHMED, MBBS, MS (SURGERY)
Department of Surgery
Affiliated Institute for Medical Education
Chicago, Illinois

QUESTION BANK EDITOR

JAMES C. HEBERT, MD
Professor of Surgery
The University of Vermont College of Medicine
Burlington, Vermont

LIPPINCOTT WILLIAMS & WILKINS
A **Wolters Kluwer** Company
Philadelphia • Baltimore • New York • London
Buenos Aires • Hong Kong • Sydney • Tokyo

Editor: Betty Sun
Managing Editors: Amy Oravec and Kathleen H. Scogna
Marketing Manager: Joe Schott
Production Editor: Jennifer Ajello
Designer: Doug Smock
Compositor: Maryland Composition, Inc.
Printer: Courier-Westford

351 West Camden Street
Baltimore, MD 21201

530 Walnut Street
Philadelphia, PA 19106

Printed in the United States of America

Library of Congress Cataloging-in-Publication Data

ISBN 13: 978-0-7817-5003-5
LOC Data is available: ISBN 10: 0-7817-5003-2

06 07 08 09
3 4 5 6 7 8 9 10

Preface

The primary responsibility of medical schools is to educate medical students to become competent clinicians. Because most physicians practice medicine in a nonacademic setting, clinical training is paramount. The third year of medical school, which focuses on basic clinical training, is the foundation for most physicians' clinical training. These realities do not diminish the other critical functions of medical school, including basic science education for MD and PhD candidates, basic and clinical research, and the education of residents and practicing physicians. However, the central role of providing clinical education for medical students cannot be overemphasized.

The education of students, residents, and practicing surgeons is a continuum, although it may be fragmented at times. Because of the length of time needed to completely train surgeons, surgical residents remain "students" for 3 to 9 years beyond medical school. As a result of this extensive training period, most medical schools have large numbers of surgical residents, and resident training makes up the bulk of their educational efforts. Student education is part of the continuum that starts in the first or second year of medical school, continues through residency, and never ends, because continuing education is essential for all physicians.

This textbook and its companion volume, *Essentials of Surgical Specialties*, were produced with the goal of developing an educational program in surgery for medical students who are not planning a surgical career. The book asks the question, "What do all medical students need to know about surgery to be effective clinicians in their chosen field?" Rather than using traditional textbook-writing techniques to address this question, members of the Association for Surgical Education (ASE), an organization of surgeons dedicated to undergraduate education, have conducted extensive research to define the content and skills needed for an optimal medical education program in surgery. Somewhat surprisingly, there has been consensus among these disparate groups (including practicing surgeons, internists, and even psychiatrists) about the knowledge and skills in surgery needed by all physicians. The information from this research has become the basis for this textbook. The research process also identified technical skills, such as suturing skin, that should be mastered by all physicians.

The fourth edition of this textbook has continued the approach that has resulted in its use by many medical students in the United States and Canada: (1) We select authors who are surgeons devoted to teaching medical students; they understand the appropriate depth of knowledge for a third-year student to master. (2) We include only information that third- and fourth-year students need to know—and explain it well. We do not attempt to provide an encyclopedia of surgery. (3) We limit the length of each section, so that it can reasonably be read during the clerkship.

A companion textbook on the surgical specialties, *Essentials of Surgical Specialties*, is based on a similar approach to the specialty and subspecialty fields of surgery. This text is separate from *Essentials of General Surgery* because some medical schools teach the specialties in the third year and others teach them in the fourth year. Students who complete both the general surgery and specialty programs and multiple-choice questions will acquire the essential surgical knowledge and problem-solving skills that all physicians need.

You are entering the most exciting and dynamic phase of your professional life. This educational package is designed to help you achieve your goal of becoming an adept clinician and developing lifelong learning skills. Best wishes for success in your endeavor.

Acknowledgments

Many members of the Association for Surgical Education (ASE) provided advice and expertise in starting the first edition of this project 20 years ago. Since that time, ASE members have volunteered to assist in writing chapters and editing the textbook. At its annual meetings, the ASE provides an excellent forum to discuss and test ideas about the content of the surgical curriculum and methods to teach and evaluate what has been learned.

We would like to extend our thanks to Cathy Council, our editor in Salt Lake City, who has spent 2 years editing, revising, and coordinating all components of this project. She has been the glue that holds the project together. I also would like to thank our editors at Lippincott Williams & Wilkins, Donna Balado and Kathleen Scogna.

Contributors

Kimberly D. Anderson, PhD
Professor of Surgery
The University of Texas Medical School at Houston
Houston, Texas

David Antonenko, MD
Professor and Chair
Department of Surgery
University of North Dakota
Grand Forks, North Dakota

Lecia Apantaku, MD
Associate Professor of Surgery
The Chicago Medical School
Rosalind Franklin University
Chicago, Illinois

Richard M. Bell, MD
Professor and Chairman
Department of Surgery
University of South Carolina School of Medicine
Columbia, South Carolina

Karen R. Borman, MD
Professor of Surgery
University of Mississippi Medical Center
Jackson, Mississippi

Anthony P. Borzotta, MD
Adjunct Assistant Professor of Surgery
Division of Trauma and Critical Care
Department of Surgery
University of Cincinnati
Cincinnati, Ohio
Medical Director, Trauma Services
Bethesda North Hospital
Cincinnati, Ohio

Kenneth W. Burchard, MD
Professor of Surgery and of Anesthesiology
Dartmouth-Hitchcock Medical Center
Lebanon, New Hampshire

William C. Chapman, MD
Professor of Surgery
Chief, Section of Transplantation
Washington University School of Medicine
St. Louis, Missouri

Jeffrey G. Chipman, MD
Assistant Professor of Surgery
Division of Surgical Critical Care
University of Minnesota
Minneapolis, Minnesota

Nicholas P.W. Coe, MD
Professor of Surgery
Tufts University
Baystate Medical Center
Springfield, Massachusetts

Claudia Corwin, MD
Medical Director of Healthcare Services
Medical Director, State Hospital Disaster/Terrorism
Preparedness Program
Iowa Department of Public Health
Des Moines, Iowa

Rudolph G. Danzinger, MD
Professor of Surgery
University of Manitoba
Winnipeg, Manitoba, Canada

Debra A. DaRosa, PhD
Professor of Surgery
The Feinberg School of Medicine
Northwestern University
Chicago, Illinois

Merril T. Dayton, MD
Professor and Chairman
Department of Surgery
State University of New York at Buffalo
Buffalo, New York

Chris de Gara, MBBS, MS
Professor
Director, Division of General Surgery
Department of Surgery, University of Alberta
Director, Department of Surgical Oncology
Cross Cancer Institute, Alberta Cancer Board
Edmonton, Alberta, Canada

Matthew O. Dolich, MD
Assistant Clinical Professor of Surgery
Division of Trauma/Critical Care
UCI Medical Center
University of California, Irvine
Irvine, California

Gary L. Dunnington, MD
Professor of Surgery
Southern Illinois University School of Medicine
Springfield, Illinois

Virginia A. Eddy, MD
Clinical Associate Professor of Surgery
The University of Vermont College of Medicine
Burlington, Vermont

Donald E. Fry, MD
Professor of Surgery
The University of New Mexico Health Sciences Center
Albuquerque, New Mexico

Richard N. Garrison, MD
Professor of Surgery
University of Louisville School of Medicine
Louisville, Kentucky

Bruce L. Gewertz, MD
The Dallas B. Phemister Professor
Chairman, Department of Surgery
Chief, Section of Vascular Surgery
University of Chicago
Chicago, Illinois

Steven B. Goldin, MD, PhD
Assistant Professor of Surgery
University of South Florida
Tampa, Florida

Mitchell H. Goldman, MD
Professor and Chairman
Department of Surgery
University of Tennessee Graduate School of Medicine
Knoxville, Tennessee

Ian Gordon, MD
Associate Clinical Professor of Surgery
UCI Medical Center
University of California, Irvine
Irvine, California

Oscar H. Grandas, MD
Assistant Professor of Surgery
University of Tennessee Medical Center at Knoxville
Knoxville, Tennessee

James C. Hebert, MD
Professor of Surgery
The University of Vermont College of Medicine
Burlington, Vermont

Susan Kaiser, MD, PhD
Clinical Assistant Professor
The Mount Sinai School of Medicine
New York, New York

Nicholas P. Lang, MD
Chief of Staff, Central Arkansas Veterans Healthcare System
Associate Dean for Veterans Affairs and
Professor of Surgery
College of Medicine
University of Arkansas for Medical Sciences
Little Rock, Arkansas

Peter F. Lawrence, MD
Professor and Bergman Chief of Vascular Surgery
Director of the Gonda (Goldschmied) Vascular Center
David Geffen School of Medicine at UCLA
Los Angeles, California

Kimberly D. Lomis, MD
Assistant Professor of Surgery
Vanderbilt University Medical Center
Nashville, Tennessee

Bruce V. MacFadyen, Jr., MD
Professor of Surgery and Moretz-Mansberger Chairman
Department of Surgery
Medical College of Georgia
Augusta, Georgia

Mary C. Mancini, MD, PhD
Professor of Surgery
Louisiana State University Health Sciences Center
Shreveport, Louisiana

Barry D. Mann, MD
Executive Director
Annenberg Conference Center for Medical Education
Lankenau Hospital
Wynnewood, Pennsylvania

James A. McCoy, MD
Associate Professor of Surgery
Morehouse School of Medicine
Atlanta, Georgia

D. Byron McGregor, MD
Professor Emeritus of Surgery
University of Nevada School of Medicine
Reno, Nevada

James F. McKinsey, MD
Associate Professor and Site Chief of Vascular Surgery
Columbia University
New York, New York

John D. Mellinger, MD
Associate Professor of Surgery
General Surgery Residency Program Director
Medical College of Georgia
Augusta, Georgia

David W. Mercer, MD
Professor and Chief of Surgery, LBJ General Hospital
Vice Chairman and Chief of General Surgery Division
Department of Surgery
The University of Texas Medical School at Houston
Houston, Texas

Hollis W. Merrick, III, MD
Professor and Chief
Division of General Surgery
Medical College of Ohio
Toledo, Ohio

William Miles, MD
Clinical Associate Professor of Surgery
University of North Carolina
Chapel Hill, North Carolina

Gamal Mostafa, MD
Clinical Assistant Professor of Surgery
University of North Carolina
Chapel Hill, North Carolina

Russell Nauta, MD
Professor of Surgery
Harvard University
Cambridge, Massachusetts

Leigh Neumayer, MD, MS
Professor of Surgery
University of Utah Health Sciences Center
Salt Lake City, Utah

J. Patrick O'Leary, MD
The Isidore Cohn, Jr., Professor and Chairman
Department of Surgery
Louisiana State University School of Medicine
New Orleans, Louisiana

John Paige, MD
Assistant Professor of Clinical Surgery
Louisiana State University School of Medicine
New Orleans, Louisiana

Tina L. Palmieri, MD
Assistant Professor of Surgery
University of California, Davis
Assistant Chief of Burns
Shriners Hospitals for Children, Northern California
Sacramento, California

Jason Park, MD
R5 Resident in General Surgery
University of Toronto
Toronto, Ontario, Canada

Elizabeth Peralta, MD
Assistant Professor of Surgery
Southern Illinois University School of Medicine
Springfield, Illinois

Hiram C. Polk, Jr., MD
Ben A. Reid, Sr., Professor and Chairman of Surgery
University of Louisville School of Medicine
Louisville, Kentucky

John R. Potts, III, MD
Professor of Surgery
Vice Chair, Department of Surgery
The University of Texas Medical School at Houston
Houston, Texas

Roshni Rao, MD
Clinical Associate in Surgery
Tufts University School of Medicine
Springfield, Massachusetts

Jeffrey R. Saffle, MD
Professor of Surgery
Director, Intermountain Burn Center
University of Utah Health Sciences Center
Salt Lake City, Utah

Hilary Sanfey, MD
Associate Professor
University of Virginia Health System
Charlottesville, Virginia

Kennith H. Sartorelli, MD
Assistant Professor of Surgery
The University of Vermont College of Medicine
Burlington, Vermont

Kenneth W. Sharp, MD
Professor of Surgery
Vanderbilt University Medical Center
Nashville, Tennessee

Mary R. Smith, MD
Associate Dean for Graduate and Clinical
Undergraduate Education
Professor of Clinical Medicine and Pathology
Medical College of Ohio
Toledo, Ohio

David A. Spain, MD
Professor of Surgery
Chief, Trauma and Surgical Critical Care
Stanford University School of Medicine
Stanford, California

Michael Stone, MD
Professor of Surgery
Boston University School of Medicine
Chief of Surgical Oncology
Boston Medical Center
Boston, Massachusetts

Glenn E. Talboy, Jr., MD
Assistant Professor of Surgery
University of Missouri—Kansas City
Kansas City, Missouri

Richard B. Wait, MD, PhD
Clinical Professor of Surgery
Tufts University School of Medicine
Springfield, Massachusetts

James Warneke, MD
Associate Professor of Surgery
University of Arizona
Tucson, Arizona

Contents

1

DEBRA A. DAROSA, PHD ■ KIMBERLY D. ANDERSON, PHD
GARY L. DUNNINGTON, MD

How to Survive (and Excel!) in a Surgery Clerkship

Learning the principles of surgery is critical regardless of a student's future discipline. All physicians need to be able to recognize surgical diseases, know when to refer their patients to a surgeon, and understand enough about surgical interventions to effectively collaborate with the surgeon and patient in pre- and postoperative care. The surgery clerkship can also equip students with technical skills used by physicians in several specialties such as suturing, knot tying, and antiseptic techniques, to name a few. The purpose of this chapter is to set students up to succeed on their surgery clerkship by suggesting strategies for dealing with six common problem areas: (1) unclear expectations; (2) overwhelming reading requirements; (3) lack of feedback; (4) stress; (5) preparing for examinations; and (6) not knowing what is required to become an honors student. Reading this chapter before, or at the start of, your clerkship will maximize your enjoyment and learning and minimize your difficulties.

PROBLEM ONE: WHAT EXACTLY IS MY ROLE? WHAT ARE THE EXPECTATIONS?

Principles for Meeting Clerkship Expectations

- Be first and foremost a student rather than an "extra house officer." Even when you are busy clinically, develop and maintain a reading schedule to be well prepared for formal teaching sessions, patient care, and your exams.
- Carefully review the clerkship objectives and other information provided in your syllabus.
- Strive to know more about your patients and their diseases than anyone else on the service.
- Prepare *before* you go into the operating room. Review the diagnosis and indications for surgical intervention, the pathophysiology, the anatomy, and potential postoperative complications.
- Focus on critical thinking skills (e.g., What is the underlying patient problem? Why are we doing this procedure?) when developing patient assessments.
- Be enthusiastic, punctual, assertive in assuming responsibility, and respectful of the medical hierarchy. Also, be aware of the institution's work-hour policies so that you can plan your day within the appropriate time parameters.

Perhaps the most startling difference between the first 2 years of medical school and the clinical clerkship year is the loss of a defined daily structure and the consequent difficulty in determining what is expected of you as a student. During the surgical clerkship, the content to be learned is less well defined than in the basic sciences. Many surgery clerkship directors have outlined clinical responsibilities for the students as well as learning objectives to guide your reading and study. Whether these guidelines exist or are poorly defined, the following recommendations may be helpful:

Remember That Your Goal Is to Learn

During the surgical clerkship, the student is expected to be a student, not an extra house officer or an extra pair of hands to complete the work of the ward. Although these roles may often conflict, if you maintain your perspective as a learner, acquiring a sound knowledge base should always take precedence over learning intern survival skills.

Keep in mind that ward work (e.g., changing dressings, obtaining arterial blood gases) is not scut work when it is associated with your patients.

Your reading should focus on three areas:

- Managing the clinical problems that you encounter—read about *your* patients
- Preparing for teaching rounds, student presentations, didactic sessions, or any planned teaching sessions that your institution holds
- Preparing for the final examination (and midterm if offered)

Know Your Ward Responsibilities

During the day, the setting for your patient care activities may be the ward, the operating room, the clinic or office, or the ambulatory setting (outpatient operating room). Give yourself plenty of time to evaluate the patients assigned to you before morning rounds, including a chart review (i.e., nursing notes from the previous night, bedside chart, and a focused history and examination). You should be sensitive to patient needs in planning these early morning activities. Your morning presentation should include data from the previous 24 hours. In contrast, afternoon presentations traditionally cover only the previous 8 hours.

For typical inpatients who are recovering from surgery, your presentation format should be flexible enough to meet the demands of the service. However, you should generally include subjective and objective data as well as your assessment (supported by the data and examination findings) and a plan for care. Table 1-1 reflects a presentation format for a presentation on morning rounds for a surgical ward patient. A presentation for a patient in the intensive care unit would be more detailed and systems based. For example, the pulmonary system presentation would include ventilatory status, exam findings on lung evaluation, chest x-ray and sputum culture results, and the assessment and plan for the pulmonary system. Additional information will be included as necessary regarding extremities or other injuries or systems. Discuss the format with your resident to ensure it matches the format he or she wants used in patient presentations. Request feedback when your assessments are considered inappropriate or when the treatment plans selected differ from the ones that you proposed.

Table 1-1 Format for Morning Presentation and Progress Note for a Surgical Patient

Mrs. Schramm is a 59-year-old female who is 2 days status post–right hemicolectomy for adenocarcinoma of the ascending colon.

- Subjective data including patient complaints and pain assessment
- Current vital signs and significant changes in vital signs overnight including the maximum temperature
- Ins and outs for oral intake, intravenous fluid totals for 24 hours, and urine output. This section would also include nasogastric tube output and outputs from surgical drains
- Focused physical examination findings, that is, chest exam, abdominal exam including wound, and extremity exam to rule out deep vein thrombosis
- New laboratory or imaging results since the previous day's p.m. rounds
- Your assessment, including any new problems indicated by the above data
- Your recommendations for treatment plan for the day

For patients who have complicated cases and are being treated in the intensive care unit and for patients with multiple ongoing problems, your presentation is best delivered with an organ system approach. In this approach, subjective and objective data, assessments, and plans are presented for each area for which there are ongoing problems (e.g., neurologic, cardiovascular, pulmonary, gastrointestinal, genitourinary, infection, nutrition). In the beginning, if surgery is your first rotation, practice a presentation with an intern or a classmate.

Because most of the team must be in the operating room at an early hour, remember to keep your presentations succinct. To allow time for a thorough assessment and care plan after discussion with the ward team, plan to write your daily progress notes before or after morning rounds. These notes should be finished before you or your team goes to the operating room. Your evening presentations should focus on significant events of the day and should provide the results of diagnostic studies that were performed. Your credibility will increase if you have discussed the studies with the appropriate persons (e.g., radiology faculty member or resident for radiographic studies). Be careful to ensure that your data are accurate. For example, if you do not remember the exact numbers, it is better to say so than to estimate.

In addition to work rounds on the wards, you will probably participate in attending rounds or teaching rounds. When you are asked to present a patient, be sure to know every detail of the patient's history, initial presentation, and hospital course to date. Rehearse your presentation so that you can deliver it in a polished, succinct manner, with only minimal references to notes. Although you can use notes to refresh your memory, do not read your presentation. Most attending physicians and chief residents emphasize presentation skills in their overall student evaluations.

Know Your Operating Room Responsibilities

The key to deriving the most benefit from your operating room experience is **advance preparation.** In addition to familiarizing yourself with all aspects of your patient's presentation and hospital course to date, review an anatomy textbook to prepare for the operative dissection. Also, review the planned procedure so that you have a preliminary understanding of the technical approach. You may need to check the surgical schedule 1 to 2 days in advance to allow time to prepare adequately. Ask questions at appropriate times in the operating room if they are not answered by your observation. During the operation, do not restrain your impulse to be a helpful assistant. As the patient's assigned student, you should be one of the first to arrive in the operating room. After surgery, accompany your patient to the recovery room. Think about the postoperative orders you will write in the recovery room (e.g., type of dressing change, type of drain).

Know Your Clinic or Office Responsibilities

Most clerkships provide students with the opportunity to participate in outpatient offices. This participation is a vital aspect of surgical education. Many of the surgical problems you will face are managed in the ambulatory setting, especially if you ultimately practice primary care. If clinic participation is optional, make every effort to participate, focusing on the problems that you will not see on the inpatient service (e.g., breast lumps and mammographic abnormalities, benign perianal disease, intermittent claudication, venous insufficiency). When you are assigned to a faculty member's office, familiarize yourself with his or her patients' typical presenting complaints and disease entities, and prepare by practicing *focused* history-taking and physical exam skills.

Know Your Call Schedule Responsibilities

The call schedule is typically prepared by the first day of the rotation. It is important to be flexible and to do your share; however, it is also important to ensure that you can meet your personal and family obligations. If you have an important personal event on your calendar, be certain to notify whoever creates the schedule well in advance of the date. People who create call schedules are usually willing to accommodate special or significant events, but they also must consider the needs of many other people. If you are scheduled to be on call when you have a conflict, do not complain to the person who created the call schedule; take care of the problem yourself. If switching is permitted, trade with one of your classmates. Remember to reciprocate when classmates get into a similar bind. Complaints about the number of calls you are taking or the number of weekends you are covering are usually not well received by those who create the schedule; again, work with your peers to resolve issues, and inform those in charge of the changes. To the degree possible, try to be on call with your assigned preceptor (if attending preceptors are assigned) or with a member of your resident team. Being on call with team members enhances both your team relationships and the continuity of patient care.

Know to Whom You Are Responsible

If you will work with a variety of faculty and residents while on call, find out to whom you are accountable. Talk with this faculty member or resident before call begins to identify his or her expectations. If you have a beeper, be sure that you have given out the correct beeper number. If your institution uses an overhead paging system, make certain that the operator is informed that you are on call. You must be easily accessible to the faculty member or resident; become his or her shadow. Faculty members or residents typically make an effort to call you and inform you of ongoing developments, but if you do not respond to pages or are difficult to reach, they will not search for you. Call is often exhausting, but it can also be exhilarating and can provide you with unique learning opportunities.

At no time should you be alone in the decision-making process. However, do not simply play the role of "data gatherer." You should formulate an assessment and a plan as though you are managing the patient, and then discuss them with the faculty member or resident. These steps are important for practicing clinical reasoning and self-assessment of what you know and what else you need to know to make a sound plan or decision.

Be Realistic About Time Management

When you are scheduled to be on call, plan on being on call. Period. Do not try to find time for your scheduled reading. When you create your reading schedule (see Problem Two), allot your assignments to days when you are not on call. If your night on call affords some downtime, read to get ahead in your schedule, or use the time for review. Most important, do not try to schedule family time or promise to try to attend events when you are on call. Trying to "fit" other responsibilities into a call night sets up false expectations and often results in disappointment, frustration, and resentment among those you care about most. Plan quality time with family and friends when you have control over your time.

Maintain a Positive Attitude

In addition to the expectations outlined previously, there are six general expectations of all students on surgical clerkships:

1. Be enthusiastic, regardless of the number of patients you are assigned, your interest in surgery, or your feelings about a particular clinical encounter. Although this attitude may appear artificial, an enthusiastic approach sets a frame of mind that is conducive to optimal learning.
2. Be punctual for all assigned responsibilities. A stellar performance in any clinical setting is seldom appreciated if that performance begins late.
3. Accept additional responsibilities without referring to the inequality of caseloads among fellow students or the hour of the day. This attitude shows that you understand that the surgical clerks who have the most clinical experiences learn the most. Keep in mind, however, any policies relevant to student work hours to ensure you do not violate them and remain in compliance.

4 Show that you understand the hierarchy that exists in all of medical education. Discuss concerns about patient care (e.g., an early "scoop" about a diagnostic study) with the surgical intern, not with a more senior resident or surgical faculty member. Although it is easy to criticize this hierarchy when you first encounter it, the concept promotes a team effort and provides clear lines of responsibility and communication.

5 Admit when you do not know something. Although it is nearly impossible to anticipate every question that you will be asked, it is never acceptable to generalize data or "shoot from the hip." Admitting that you "don't know" is uncomfortable, but it is a vital element of professional growth. Following up "I'm sorry, I don't know" with "but I will find out" shows the attending physician or resident that you are concerned about the patient and about improving your knowledge base.

6 Finally, during your surgical rotation, immerse yourself in the experience, recognizing its value to you as a future physician regardless of career choice.

PROBLEM TWO: THERE IS NOT ENOUGH TIME TO READ

Principles for Managing Overload

- Develop a reading plan.
- Read actively.
- Evaluate how well you retain what you read.

A primary source of frustration is lack of time. For this reason, the ability to set priorities and manage time effectively and efficiently is critical. The following tips will help you to use your reading time wisely.

Develop a Reading Plan

Adhering to a weekly reading schedule requires both persistence and good time management skills. You can accomplish your reading goal by realistically determining at the start of the clerkship what you want to have read by the end of the clerkship and establishing a schedule that includes benchmarks or deadlines for maintaining a consistent pace and volume. You can identify what you must read by the end of your clerkship by reviewing old examinations (if they are available), reviewing the learning objectives for the clerkship, talking with students who completed the clerkship and did well, and speaking with the clerkship director or with faculty members. To avoid becoming frustrated, devise a reading plan that is realistic, allow time to take notes, review previously taken notes, and process the information. When you read text, your brain should sort, select, and link new information to related areas of knowledge. Simply running your eyes across the words does not count.

Differentiating important from nice-to-know content when reading the text is a critical skill that keeps students from becoming overwhelmed. There is an enormous volume of information, and the successful student uses the cues provided by textbook authors and publishers to help readers identify key concepts and organize information for optimal understanding and learning.

Much of your reading will center on your patients' problems. Concentrate on learning about the involved anatomy, physiology, and pathology. Then read about the clinical signs and symptoms, diagnostic options, differential diagnosis, and alternative methods of therapy. As a surgery clerk, you do not need to know the detailed operative techniques and principles. However, you should go to the operating room with an understanding of the treatment or modification of the pathologic process intended by the operation, the prognosis, and the postoperative care of the patient. You should also be aware of possible complications and how to address them.

Your patient-related reading should be done as soon as possible. Rather than waiting until evening to begin reading, try to find a place where you can do some abbreviated reading during the day. Because using information organizes and reinforces it, you are more likely to retain what you read if you use the information shortly afterward. Another idea is to carry in your pocket blank 3×5-inch index cards and each day jot two to five learning issues relevant to your patients that you want to read about later that day or evening. This way important questions you might have about your patients won't be lost and can be followed up on.

Schedule study time every day, with a minimum period of 30 minutes. You'll want to schedule some longer periods for certain days, but don't count on 8 hours of study on a Saturday when you know you have other activities.

Some students find it helpful to copy the "core reading" chapters that they are scheduled to read that day and carry them in their pockets. Students spend a significant amount of time waiting for lectures, rounds, or the OR case to begin. If you carry a book or copied pages, you can make good use of these 10 or 20 minutes by catching up on your reading.

Read Actively

Good readers remember what they read, not because they have photographic memories, but because they read to understand, not just to count pages or chapters read. As noted by Pauk,[1] understanding is essential for efficient and accurate learning, and efficient learning requires activation of prior knowledge. Memory is like a file cabinet. If you reflect on what you are reading and how it applies to what you already know, it will be better organized in your "file cabinet," which provides for more focused, efficient, and complete information retrieval. The following suggestions are included to help you read actively and retain what you read in an organized fashion for efficient retrieval.

Pre-Read

Pre-reading takes about 5 to 10 minutes and gives a sense of what the authors highlighted and how they organized the chapter information. There are three steps involved with pre-reading. First, before you begin reading a chapter, look for the "big picture" or its main points. Kelman and Straker[2] recommend you pre-read the following when provided:

- Chapter objectives
- First paragraph
- Subtitles
- Bold-faced, colored, and italicized print
- Shaded areas or boxed information
- Diagrams, charts, graphs, and tables (scan for concepts at this point, not for details!)
- Lists
- Pictures or drawings
- Glossary of new terms
- Summary
- First sentence of paragraphs

This will enable you to glean the big ideas and main subordinate details, as well as anticipate what is coming rather than just diving in and hoping some of the words will stick.

Second, reflect about what you already know on the topic presented in the chapter. State aloud what you already know about the topic, jot it down, or draw a chart, picture, or other visual.

Third, write questions that address what you don't know but believe to be important about the topic. Write these questions in an open-ended format and keep them visible while you read the chapter. This is key to active reading.

Note Taking

Note taking helps you focus your reading, but it also provides a document for repeated reviews that is critical to the learning process and to long-term memory. Notes can also be used to self-test, another practice associated with retention. Different note-taking strategies exist. Use one or a combination of the following, depending on which is most compatible with your past experiences or preferences:

- Note cards — Use note cards to write questions on one side with the answers on the other. Include questions that address important facts or concepts that might appear on an exam or be asked by a faculty member or resident.
- Charts and tables — Create your own charts or tables to compare and contrast between concepts, disease presentations, etc. For example, if reading a chapter on appendicitis, create a chart comparing the similarities and differences between how patients initially presenting with acute abdominal pain and possible appendicitis compare with those who might have other problems. How might such patients differ in history, physical exam findings, and diagnostic laboratory results if they have other problems associated with belly pain?
- Flowcharts and diagrams — These are useful for showing sequence of logically ordered information such as the flow of decision making or sequence of T-cell activation.
- Outlines — Beware of linear sequential note taking! It is not recommended that outlines be used as a note-taking strategy. Anything that you can outline you can put into charts or maps that better position you to integrate information and see relationships between concepts and information. The aim of note taking is to help search for relationships, comparisons, and contrasts. It is also difficult to self-test using outline format notes.

Taking the time to take notes and summarize information during and after reading a section or chapter helps readers reflect on what they learned. Regularly reviewing your notes is a more effective review tool than rereading an entire or highlighted text to prepare for an examination.

In summary, pre-read a chapter, reflect on what you already know about the topic and what you think you need to know, and then read actively and deliberately, taking notes in whatever forms you prefer. Ask yourself questions as you proceed (e.g., What are the key points? Now that I have read this chapter, do I know how to detect and treat a patient who has this problem?). After you read the chapter, self-test yourself.

Evaluate Your Reading Retention

To evaluate how well you retained what you read, review questions you wrote down during your pre-reading stage and the objectives at the start of the chapter as part of the self-test process. Find a good review book that contains test questions or ask interns or residents to quiz you. If your institution uses a National Board of Medical Examiners subtest, you can view the content outline on its Website (www.nbme.org) by clicking "Subject Examination" and "Surgery." Your answers to these questions can help you to determine whether you can recall important facts and concepts and use them in a clinical problem-solving situation or a multiple-choice format.

PROBLEM THREE: I AM GETTING LITTLE OR NO FEEDBACK

Principles of Feedback

- Recognize the importance of feedback for learning.
- Make constructive use of positive and negative feedback.
- To get effective feedback, be assertive and ask for it.

Good feedback is descriptive (not judgmental), timely, and specific. It is a crucial aspect of learning. Identify areas in which you need feedback, and ask for it. Most faculty and residents are pleased to see that students care enough about what they are learning to ask for feedback, and they are happy to oblige. If feedback is not a formal part of your clerkship experience, "midterm" in the clerkship is an ideal time to ask for it. Schedule a time to speak with your supervising faculty member, resident, or clerkship director in a one-on-one setting. Stopping this person in the hall is unlikely to lead to thoughtful commentary about your performance. Explain why you scheduled the meeting and what you hope to accomplish. Provide a self-evaluation of your performance, including specific areas (i.e., skills, knowledge, interpersonal qualities) in which you think you have met or exceeded expectations; areas of skill, knowledge, or behavior that you are working to improve; and your plan for improvement. Ask for specific feedback about your performance and your plan for improvement. How you phrase your request will influence what you receive. Consider asking, "Can you tell me two things I've done well and two or more things I need to work on to improve my performance?"

Typically, students assume that they are doing fine unless they hear otherwise. This assumption can be misleading! Some students who receive poor ratings do not recognize that they are performing poorly. This type of surprise can be avoided by asking for feedback.

If you do not receive feedback routinely, be sure to request it in the following areas:

- History and physical examination write-ups (e.g., Did I state the history correctly?)
- Physical examinations skills (e.g., Am I locating the spleen correctly?)
- Progress notes and preoperative and postoperative orders (e.g., Were there major omissions?)
- Presentation skills (e.g., Did I present any unnecessary data?)
- Technical skills (e.g., Are my stitches too far apart?)
- Base of knowledge (e.g., What else do I need to know about this patient's problem?)

You may need more feedback in the early part of the clerkship and less as you hone your skills. Recognize your own learning needs, and assert yourself tactfully to get specific feedback when and where you need it.

PROBLEM FOUR: I HAVE NO LIFE, AND I AM STRESSED TO THE MAX!

Stress Management Principles

- Eat sensibly.
- Take time for your family and friends.
- Commit time to exercise.
- Find a confidant.

You can do well in a surgery clerkship without compromising every other aspect of your life. In fact, you will perform better if you do not give up everything else. This section will help you manage your priorities so that you can accomplish tasks faster and with a more positive attitude.

Balancing your work-related responsibilities with your personal needs and those of others takes conscious effort. It is not always easy, and it does not occur overnight. Each day, you should take care of yourself by doing something to meet your physical, social, and emotional needs. You cannot always control how much time you spend at the hospital. The concept is the same, however, regardless of your profession or status. Sources on stress management[3,4] emphasize several common principles:

Eat Sensibly

- Eat before you go into the operating room in the morning. You cannot be certain how long you will be in there, and some students feel faint when they do not eat something beforehand.
- In case you miss a meal, keep in your pocket or locker healthy snack foods, such as dried fruit, cereal, popcorn (no butter, of course), or other nonperishables with nutritional value.
- Limit caffeine and sugar. (The number of aluminum cans disposed of by medical students over a few days could probably be recycled to yield enough money for one person's tuition for a semester.)

Take Time for Your Family and Friends

- Talk openly with the people in your life who will be affected by your being busy in a clerkship. Discuss your needs and their needs, and come to an agreement. Some flexibility will be needed on both sides.
- When you take time for others, give them your full attention. Try to leave your troubles and pressures at the hospital.
- Do not expect others always to play second fiddle to your student-related responsibilities. Yes, you need their support, but they have needs too, and if these needs are consistently ignored, resentment will build and problems will occur.

Commit Time to Exercise

A study of medical students showed a significant relation between stress and attitudes toward leisure. Those who did not feel guilty when taking time to exercise reported fewer symptoms of stress and anxiety and an overall more positive attitude toward school.[5] Schedule time to exercise!

Find a Confidant

Choose someone to be your sounding board, and be prepared to reciprocate. Air your complaints to a trusted confidant who will maintain your confidences, will not give advice unless asked, and will empathize with you.

PROBLEM FIVE: HOW CAN I DO WELL ON THE EXAMINATION?

Principles for Examination Preparation and Administration

- Do not procrastinate or deviate from your study schedule.
- Use multiple methods to retain the material (e.g., answer study questions, take practice examinations, teach your peers the material).
- Relate your reading to patients you have encountered.
- Ask yourself, "Why is this important?"

Assisting in the operating room or emergency department or doing procedures is often more interesting (and fun) than reading. Regardless of your specialty preference, the activity of a surgery clerkship can be invigorating, even if it means being up all night. Although being an active member of the surgical team clearly enhances your clinical performance evaluation and your enjoyment of the clerkship, it does not necessarily prepare you for the rigors of the final written examination. Your success in the clerkship will depend in part on your ability to manage the time you spend on clinical activities, to adhere to a steady reading schedule, and to relate your reading material to patients you have encountered.

Whether you take the National Board of Medical Examiners (NBME) self-examination or an internally generated departmental examination, and whether the test items assess the ability to apply knowledge framed within the context of patient vignettes or written objectives of the clerkship or lectures, you will be held accountable for a basic fund of knowledge that reflects the fundamental principles of surgery. The guidelines for managing reading overload (see Problem Two) will keep you on track throughout your clerkship.

Students who have problems with the final examination typically fall into two categories: (1) those who did not keep up with their reading and (2) those who kept up with their reading superficially but did not process the information. Students who say, "I didn't keep up with my reading because I was too busy on the service," pose significant problems for surgical educators. Faculty and residents praise their work ethic, interest, and enthusiasm. They reward them by letting them take a more active role in the operating room or clinic. They may tell them that they are among the best students they have ever had and that they have a good working fund of knowledge. What they do not tell them is that they jeopardize their grade in the clerkship because they cannot state what percentage of patients is likely to get a certain disease, what medical and surgical alternatives exist, what percentage of these people will get well because of the treatment, and what percentage will die. You will be held accountable for this type of information on the final written examination, and these are the types of questions in every surgeon's examination-writing armamentarium. Faculty and residents appropriately recognize students who demonstrate a strong work ethic and show personal and professional maturity with patients and the team. However, you must pass the written examination to complete the clerkship, and that means keeping up with reading and reviewing. The following tips may help you with your written exam:

Pace Yourself

Find out how many items are on the test, or count them once it is received, and calculate how long you have to answer each one. Leave sufficient time to review your answers. Use your watch to keep yourself properly paced. Most examinations allow 1 minute per item. Easier items will take less time, yielding more time for long or difficult questions. Do not spend too much time on one item, however, or you will not have enough time to complete the examination. Needless mistakes are made as a result of poor pacing when students rush through the final items. Even if the test does not have time limits, students often grow fatigued and make mistakes at the end of the examination. To avoid these mistakes, check your pacing quarterly during the examination.

Analyze the Questions in Whole and in Part

Preview the questions and immediately answer those you are confident that you know. Then go back to the beginning and complete those that you did not automatically know during the first run-through. Answer the questions that are mostly guesses last. Some students find it helpful to cover the distractors (they are designed to do just that—distract) and mentally answer the question, then uncover the distractors and select the corresponding option. Some students use shorthand in the margins, such as the example below:

L = You are satisfied with your answer and consider the item *low priority* for reconsideration.

S = You are not entirely confident with your answer, but consider the item *second priority* for reconsideration.

H = You are completely unsure of the answer and consider the item *high priority* for reconsideration.

After you complete the examination, check your answers. Make sure that you did not skip any questions or double-mark any items. If you answered questions out of order, verify that you recorded the answers in the correct spaces.

When you read a question, circle the most important words as well as any words that alter the meaning substantially or offer cues for finding the answer (e.g., except, most common, least common, must).

Thorough preparation for an examination is the best way to reduce panic and anxiety; however, pacing, analyzing, and checking can help reduce unnecessary errors.

PROBLEM SIX: WHAT DOES IT TAKE TO BE AN HONORS STUDENT?

Principles for Achieving Honors

- The honors student understands the criteria that are used to determine honors level performance.
- The honors student uses frequent self-assessment to test his or her fund of knowledge.
- The honors student: (1) demonstrates intellectual curiosity; (2) understands the role of a team player; (3) exhibits polished presentation skills; (4) provides the team with information from recent literature; (5) shadows the house officer on call at night; and (6) looks for opportunities to work one-on-one with faculty.

It is safe to assume that every student who is beginning a surgical clerkship is capable of receiving honors as a final grade.

Identify the Criteria for Honors

Understand the emphasis that the clerkship places on test performance versus ward performance. This understanding will help you allocate your time between reading and involvement in ward activities. Typically, examinations carry significant weight when separating many would-be honors students from honors students. It is important to understand the nature of the final examination and the weight placed on general surgery with respect to the other specialties.

Self-Assess Frequently

If the final examination is a multiple-choice test, your chances for success will be improved by frequently self-testing your knowledge with your notes as well as books that contain multiple-choice questions and board review type questions.

Display the Characteristics of Honors Students

The assessment of student ward performance is subjective. However, attending physicians look for certain characteristics in an honors student. These characteristics are described by comparing them with characteristics that are found in the average, or passing, student on the clerkship:

- The passing student reads about his or her patients' problems and is prepared to answer questions during rounds. The honors student demonstrates intellectual curiosity by asking pertinent, probing questions (e.g., after rounds, during breaks) about the etiology, pathophysiology, and natural history of the disease process. These questions can come only from an effort to read for comprehension (i.e., active reading) rather than for memorization.
- The passing student follows through on assigned tasks and enthusiastically provides assistance in the care of his or her assigned patients. The honors student understands the importance of being a team player. In addition to providing excellent care for his or her own patients, the honors student is willing to help with any patient as long as there is an opportunity to learn. This attitude involves avoiding actions that make others (especially other students) look bad. Think in terms of the good of the team and that of every member. Help others, but do not be fawning or obsequious.
- The average, or passing, student makes certain that all pertinent data are presented on rounds and makes logical and thoughtful assessments based on the data. The honors student does this as well, but also presents the material in a fluent, dynamic, and succinct manner that paints a visual picture for the rest of the team. You can polish your presentation skills by rehearsing, either aloud or mentally, on the way to the hospital, in front of a mirror, or elsewhere. An honors level of presentation results from a great deal of practice and a focus on presentation skills during those early morning hours.
- The average student reads enough from basic texts to achieve a knowledge base that is sufficient to perform patient assessment and daily care. The honors student probes more deeply by using information-seeking skills. For example, each member of a busy surgical team appreciates being provided with a copy of a timely, recent article from the literature summarizing new diagnostic approaches or management schemes.
- Nights on call provide another setting for the emergence of the honors student. The passing student responds to all requests for assistance from on-call house officers and enthusiastically assists in the emergency room and with new admissions. The honors student shadows the house officer during every waking hour, both to provide assistance and to learn techniques of intern survival on the ward and in the intensive care unit.
- The honors student recognizes the importance of the operating room in the overall scheme of clerkship learning. Textbooks and consultation services will be available throughout a nonsurgeon's practicing career, but there will never be a better opportunity to see surgery "on the inside." The honors student goes to the operating room on cases that are not assigned to him or her when there are opportunities to learn about rare or unfamiliar conditions. When a student shows interest in this type of learning, most faculty members take the time to point out interesting intraoperative findings to make the trip to the operating room worthwhile.
- The honors student looks for opportunities to work with faculty one on one. This experience makes it easier for faculty to provide useful end-rotation evaluation. The clinic may be the best such setting because in many centers, residents are not extensively involved in clinic practice. If these opportunities are available, an honors student arranges his or her daily schedule to allow for participation. In addition to these characteristics, the

honors student consistently demonstrates the five qualities addressed under Problem One.

- The true honors student works hard because he or she is intrinsically motivated to learn as much as he or she can so to become the best physician possible. The honors designation is not a means to an end, but a consequence of the student's effort.

SUMMARY

For the majority of medical students, the surgery clerkship may be their only opportunity to learn first-hand about surgical diseases and principles, as well as to experience the unique privilege of placing one's hands into one of the body's cavities. What percent of humanity ever gets this experience? There is much to be gained both from a knowledge and technical skill standpoint in the surgery clerkship, and we hope this chapter has offered some suggestions on how to set yourself up to succeed as a surgery clerk.

REFERENCES

1. Pauk W. *How to Study in College*. Boston, MA: Houghton Mifflin Company, 1990.
2. Kelman EG, Straker KC. *Study Without Stress*. Thousand Oaks, CA: Sage, 2000.
3. Johnson S. *One Minute for Myself*. New York, NY: Avon Books, 1987.
4. Calano J, Salzman J. *Managing Stress and Building Visibility. Success Shortcuts*. Chicago, IL: Nightingale-Conant, 1989.
5. Folse L, DaRosa DA, Folse JR. The relationship between stress and attitudes toward leisure among first-year medical students. *J Med Educ* 1985;60:610–617.

2

VIRGINIA A. EDDY, MD ■ RICHARD M. BELL, MD

Perioperative Management of Surgical Patients

OBJECTIVES

1 Describe the value of the preoperative history, physical examination, and selected diagnostic and screening tests.
2 Describe the important aspects of communication skills.
3 Discuss the role of outside consultation in evaluating a patient undergoing an elective surgical procedure.
4 Discuss the elements of a patient's history that are essential in the preoperative evaluation of surgical emergencies.
5 Discuss the appropriate preoperative screening tests.
6 Discuss the assessment of cardiac and pulmonary risk.
7 Discuss the effect of renal dysfunction, hepatic dysfunction, diabetes, adrenal insufficiency, pregnancy, and advanced age on preoperative preparation and postoperative management.
8 Describe the documentation required in the medical record of a surgical patient, including physician's orders and daily progress notes.
9 Describe the most commonly used surgical tubes and drains.
10 Discuss common postoperative complications and their treatment.

PREOPERATIVE EVALUATION

The ability to obtain an adequate history and perform a thorough physical examination is a critical skill for physicians. The importance of this skill lies in the diagnosis of surgical disease, the detection of comorbid factors, the determination of the severity of comorbidity, and an assessment of operative risk. The decision to proceed with an operative procedure is based on an analysis of the risk:benefit ratio. This analysis must begin with an accurate and complete database. Many surgical patients have coexisting medical problems or undiagnosed medical conditions that may affect risk assessment. Surgery and anesthesia profoundly alter the normal physiologic and metabolic states, and estimating the patient's ability to respond to these stresses in the postoperative period is the challenge of the preoperative evaluation. Perioperative complications are often the result of failure, in the preoperative period, to identify underlying medical conditions, maximize the patient's preoperative health, or accurately assess perioperative risk. Sophisticated laboratory studies and specialized testing are no substitute for a thoughtful and careful history and physical examination. Sophisticated technology has merit primarily in confirming clinical suspicion.

This chapter is not a review of how to perform a history and physical examination. Instead, this discussion is a review of the elements in the patient's history or findings on physical examination that may suggest the need to modify care in the perioperative period. Other chapters discuss the signs and symptoms of specific surgical diagnoses.

PHYSICIAN–PATIENT COMMUNICATION

Interviewing Techniques

The physician–patient relationship is an essential part of surgical care. The relationship between the surgeon and patient should be established, maintained, and valued. Good interviewing techniques are fundamental in establishing a good physician–patient relationship. Part of good interviewing comes from a genuine concern about people; another part relies on learned skills.

Effective interviewing can be challenging to the surgeon because of the variety of settings in which interviews occur. These settings include the operating room, the surgical intensive care unit, a private office, a hospital bedside, the emergency room, and an outpatient clinic. Each setting presents its own challenges to effective communication. To achieve good physician–patient relationships, surgeons adjust their styles to the environment and to each patient's personality and needs. Some basic rules are common to all professional interviews. The first rule is to make clear to the patient that during the history and examination, nothing short of a life-or-death emergency will assume greater importance than the interaction between the surgeon and the patient at that moment. This is the surgeon's first, and best, chance to connect with the patient. The patient must come to understand that a caring, knowledgeable, and dedicated surgeon will be the patient's partner on the journey through the treatment of surgical disease. The surgeon should observe certain other rules, including giving adequate attention to personal appearance to present a professional image that inspires confidence; establishing eye contact; communicating interest, warmth, and understanding; listening nonjudgmentally; accepting the patient as a person; listening to the patient's description of his or her problem; and helping the patient feel comfortable in communicating.

When the patient is seen in an ambulatory setting, the surgeon spends the first few minutes greeting the patient (using the patient's formal name); shaking hands with the patient; introducing himself or herself and explaining the surgeon's role; attending to patient privacy; adjusting his or her conversational style and level of vocabulary to meet the patient's needs; eliciting the patient's attitude about coming to the clinic; finding out the patient's occupation; and determining what the patient knows about the nature of his or her problem. Medical students should also acknowledge their own special role in the patient's care.

The next step involves exploring the problem. To focus the interview, the surgeon moves from open-ended to closed-ended questions. Important techniques include using transitions; asking specific, clear questions; and restating the problem for verification. At this point, it is important to determine whether the patient has any questions. Near the end of the interview, the surgeon explains what the next step will be and when he or she will examine the patient. Last, the surgeon should verify that the patient is comfortable.

Most of the techniques used in the ambulatory setting are also appropriate for inpatient encounters. Usually, more time is spent with the patient in the initial and subsequent interviews than in an outpatient setting. At the initial interview, patients are likely to be in pain, worried about financial problems, and concerned about lack of privacy or unpleasant diets. They may also have difficulty sleeping, be fearful about treatment, or feel helpless. It is important to gently and confidently communicate the purpose of the interview and state about how long it will take.

The patient is not only listening, but also is observing the physician's behavior and even attire. The setting also affects the interview. For example, a cramped, noisy, crowded environment can affect the quality of communication. Patients may have negative feelings because of insensitivities on the part of the physician or others. Examples include speaking to the patient from the doorway, giving or taking personal information in a crowded room, speaking about a patient in an elevator or another public space, or speaking to a patient without drawing the curtain in a ward.

Although the same interviewing principles apply in the emergency room as in the outpatient and inpatient settings, the emergency room encounter is tremendously condensed. The role of the student in the emergency room is to discover the patient's chief medical complaint, perform a physical examination, and present the findings to the resident or faculty member. Interviewing a patient in the emergency room requires communicating to the patient who you are and how you fit into the team. The following steps will help you conduct an effective patient interview:

1. Ask the patient or a family member to describe the problem briefly.
2. Focus on the primary medical problem.
3. Move from general to specific questions.
4. Provide a narrative for the patient.
5. Attend to the patient's privacy.
6. Be careful about expressing nonverbal attitudes about the patient or his or her behavior.
7. When the examination is finished, explain what will happen next and approximately how long the patient will have to wait.
8. After you interview and examine the patient, discuss the patient with the resident or faculty member in a location where the patient and family cannot hear or see you.
9. Finally, guard against any nonprofessional discussion or behavior in the emergency room.

Communication with patients is greatly influenced by both verbal and nonverbal behavior. Attention to these techniques can enhance the surgical student's communication skills and will have a profound influence on the quality of surgical care, particularly as patients perceive it.

Physician–Patient Compacts

The patient and the surgeon make a compact about the patient's care. The patient comes to the surgeon with a problem. The surgeon, in good faith, gathers information sufficient to identify the problem and its contributory factors. The surgeon then identifies a number of reasonable courses of action to pursue the evaluation or treatment of the patient's problem. The surgeon explains these strategies in layman's terms to the patient (and family where appropriate). Together, the patient and the surgeon select the course of action that seems best. This is what is meant by ***informed consent***. *Informed consent* is different from a *consent form*. A consent form is intended to serve as documentation of the compact between the physician and the patient. It is an unfortunate reality that consent forms must serve as a shield behind which care providers may take shelter should a tort claim be filed against them. The process of informed consent serves the more noble cause; consent forms serve the more mundane cause.

Sometimes, patients cannot speak for themselves. In these situations, the health care team will turn to those who might reasonably be thought to be able to speak on behalf of the patient. Usually, but not always, this is the next of kin. (The reader is strongly encouraged to familiarize himself or herself with pertinent state law on this matter.) These individuals are known as ***surrogate decision-makers***. Another concept that arises in this context is ***advance directives***. *Advance directives* are legal documents that inform care providers about the general wishes of the patient regarding level of care to be delivered should the patient not be able to speak for himself or herself. Most people wish to receive enough medical care to alleviate their suffering and to give them a reasonable chance of being able to enjoy the remainder of their life in a functional manner. The definitions of "reasonable" and "functional" will vary among individuals, but these are the causes that advance directive documents are intended to serve. Finally, it should be stated that there will be times when there is nobody present who can speak for the patient in a time frame that permits acceptable medical care. In these circumstances, the physician must remember that the first duty is to the patient, and that duty is to improve the patient's life. Improving life is not always the same thing as prolonging life. It is the duty of the physician to manage this aspect of the patient's care in a reverential and respectful manner. There will be times when physicians must make difficult judgments about matters of life and death. The responsible physician does so, expeditiously and thoughtfully, without attempting to evade the painful dilemmas that arise. The student is referred to any number of excellent sources for further information on the subject of medical ethics. An example is *The Hastings Center Report*, a journal devoted to ethical issues.

History

A careful history is fundamental to the preoperative evaluation of the surgical patient. It is here that the doctor learns about comorbidities that will influence the patient's ability to withstand and recover from the operation. This understanding begins with a careful review of systems intended to elicit problems that, although perhaps not the focus of the patient's surgical experience, are nonetheless important to their ability to recover from the operation. The following sections will consider the ways in which certain historical findings can be shown to impact a patient's perioperative risk, and what further evaluation should be prompted by the discovery of certain aspects of the patient's history.

Elective Surgical Procedures

Most clinical situations provide an adequate opportunity for a careful review of systems. Occasionally, patients cannot provide details of their illness, and the serious investigator must use every available resource, including family, friends, previous medical records, and emergency medical personnel. A specific review of systems, with special emphasis on estimating the patient's ability to respond to the stress of surgery, is imperative. Clinical suspicions are investigated with appropriate laboratory tests or special diagnostic studies. Specialty consultation may be required to determine the degree of medical illness. Consultants can provide important information about the risk:benefit ratio of a specific surgical procedure or suggest therapies to minimize perioperative risk. Medical consultants should not be asked to "clear" patients for a surgical procedure; their primary value is in helping to define the degree of perioperative risk and making recommendations about how best to prepare the patient to successfully undergo his or her operation and postoperative course. Once this risk is determined, the surgical team, in conjunction with the patient or the patient's family, may discuss the advisability of a planned surgical approach to the patient's illness. Postoperative consultation should be sought when the patient has unexpected complications or does not respond to initial maneuvers that are commonly employed to address a specific problem. For example, a nephrology consultation is in order for a patient who remains oliguric despite appropriate intravascular volume repletion, particularly if the creatinine level is rising. Likewise, consultation should be obtained from specialists who have expertise in areas that the treating physician does not. For example, a general surgeon would be well advised to obtain consultation from a cardiologist for a patient who had a postoperative myocardial infarction, no matter how benign the myocardial infarction appears.

Surgical Emergencies

The urgency of the surgical emergency should not preclude an attempt to acquire essential historical information about the patient. An emergency situation does force the physician to focus on the critical aspects of the patient's history. An AMPLE history (Allergies, Medications, Past medical history, Last meal, Events preceding the emergency) provides the important elements that will likely influence surgical care, as illustrated below.

Determining allergies and drug sensitivities is important and will influence selection of such critical interven-

Table 2-1 Perioperative Medication Management

Drug Type	Comment	Preoperative Management	Postoperative Management
Cardiac			
Beta blockers	Abrupt discontinuation can increase risk of MI	With sip of water a few hours before operation	Parenteral agent until taking p.o.
Atrial antiarrhythmics		With sip of water a few hours before operation	IV beta blockers, diltiazem or digoxin until p.o. intake resumed
Ventricular antiarrhythmics	Monitor Mg, K, and Ca levels perioperatively	With sip of water a few hours before operation	Parenteral amiodarone or procainamide
Nitrates	Transdermal (paste, patch) may be poorly absorbed intraoperatively	With sip of water a few hours before operation	Intravenous (most reliable) or transdermal until p.o. intake resumed
Antihypertensives	Abrupt discontinuation of clonidine can cause rebound hypertension	With sip of water a few hours before operation	Parenteral antihypertensives; if on clonidine, consider clonidine patch or alternative antihypertensive agents
Pulmonary			
Inhalers		No modification necessary	Can use nebulized or metered dose inhalers
Leukotriene inhibitors		With sip of water a few hours before operation	
Diabetes			
Insulin	5% dextrose solutions should be given intravenously intraoperatively and postoperatively in patients receiving insulin	1/2 dose usual long-acting agent at the usual time preoperatively	SSI until p.o. intake back to baseline
Oral agents (except metformin)		Hold a.m. of operation	SSI until p.o. intake back to baseline
Metformin	Can produce lactic acidosis, particularly in the setting of renal dysfunction or with administration of IV radiographic contrast agents	Hold for at least 1 day preoperatively	Monitor renal function closely. Resume metformin when renal function normalizes, usually 2–3 days postoperatively. SSI until then
Antiplatelet agents/ anticoagulants			
Aspirin, clopidogrel, ticlopidine		D/C 7 days preoperatively	Resume when diet resumed
Warfarin		Hold until INR normalizes, usually 3–5 days. If anticoagulation critical, maintain anticoagulation with heparin	Resume when diet resumed
Heparin		Discontinue 4 hr preoperatively	Resume 6–12 hr postoperatively, provided no increased risk of hemorrhage thought to exist
Osteoporosis agents			
SERMs	Associated with increased risk of DVT	Hold 1 week preoperatively for procedures with moderate to high risk DVT	
HIV agents		With sip of water a few hours before operation	Resume when taking p.o.

(continued)

Table 2-1 continued

Drug Type	Comment	Preoperative Management	Postoperative Management
Neurologic			
Antiparkinson agents Carbidopa/levodopa	Prolonged cessation of levodopa can lead to syndrome similar to neuroleptic malignant syndrome	With sip of water a few hours before operation	
Seligilene	Life-threatening syndrome similar to neuroleptic malignant syndrome reported when used with meperidine	Avoid use with meperidine	Avoid use with meperidine
Antiseizure medications		With sip of water a few hours before operation	Parenteral agents until p.o. intake resumed
Psychiatric			
Tricyclic antidepressants	Anticholinergic effects and conduction abnormalities can be seen		Monitor for anticholinergic side effects
MAOIs	Life-threatening hypertension reported when used with certain sympathomimetics; life-threatening syndrome similar to neuroleptic malignant syndrome reported when used with meperidine	Stop 2 weeks preoperatively	
SSRIs	"Serotonin syndrome" reported when used with tramadol; some agents have associated withdrawal syndrome	With sip of water a few hours before operation	Resume as soon as possible postoperatively
Antipsychotics	Can cause ECG abnormalities (prolonged QT interval)		Resume as soon as possible postoperatively
Lithium	Monitor levels perioperatively		Resume when p.o. intake resumes
Benzodiazepines	Abrupt cessation can cause withdrawal		Parenterally until diet resumed
Endocrine			
Levothyroxine		Can be held for a few days if needed without adverse effect	Parenterally until diet resumed
Propylthiouracil		Preoperative beta blockade for hyperthyroid patients; preoperative potassium iodide	Parenteral beta blockers; resume PTU when medications can be given via NG tube
Estrogen	Can increase risk of postoperative DVT	Consider stopping for 4 weeks prior to cases with high risk of DVT	
Rheumatologic			
Methotrexate	Does not interfere with wound healing or increase wound infection rate	Continue usual regimen	Resume when taking p.o.
COX-2 inhibitors	Can impair renal function	Hold 2–3 d preoperatively	Resume when taking p.o.

DVT, deep vein thrombosis; INR, international normalized ratio; MAOI, monoamine oxidase inhibitors; MI, myocardial infarction; NG, nasogastric; SSI, sliding scale insulin; SERM, selective estrogen receptor modulator; SSRI, selective serotonin reuptake inhibitor.
Reference: Mercado DL. Perioperative medication management. *Med Clin North Am* 2003;87(1):41–57.

tions as perioperative antibiotics and anesthetic technique. Many surgical emergencies occur in patients who have preexisting medical conditions. Many of these conditions (e.g., coronary artery disease, chronic obstructive pulmonary disease, diabetes) decrease the patient's ability to tolerate perioperative physiologic changes. Many patients with medical problems are being treated with drugs that may have important implications in perioperative patient management, for example, beta-blockers and anticoagulants (Table 2-1). Some drugs adversely interact with anesthetic agents or alter the normal physiologic response to illness, injury, or the stress of surgery. For example, patients who take beta-blocking agents cannot mount the usual chronotropic response to infection or blood loss. Anticoagulants may exert their effects on hepatic synthetic function (as with warfarin compounds) or platelet function (as with many agents given for atherosclerotic cardiovascular disease).

Information about the timing of the patient's last meal is important and will affect the timing of urgent (but not emergent) operations. A full stomach predisposes the patient to aspiration of gastric contents during the endotracheal intubation phase of the induction of anesthesia. Therefore, if the patient's disease process permits, it is generally best to allow gastric emptying to occur as much as possible prior to induction of anesthesia. This usually takes about 6 hours of strict *nil per os* status. If anesthesia must be induced emergently, the rapid sequence induction technique is used to optimize the chances for safe endotracheal intubation without aspiration.

A history of the events that preceded the accident or onset of illness may give important clues about the etiology of the problem or may help to uncover occult injury or disease. For example, the onset of severe substernal chest pain before the driver of a vehicle struck a bridge abutment may suggest that the hypotension that the driver exhibited in the emergency department may be related to acute cardiac decompensation from a myocardial infarction as well as from blood loss associated with a pelvic fracture. Such a situation might require modification of hemodynamic monitoring and volume restoration. Although such scenarios sound extreme, they are encountered in emergency departments on a daily basis. These historical elements add significantly to the physician's ability to provide optimal patient care.

Patients and/or families should be questioned about the patient's use of dietary supplements and over-the-counter medications. The popularity of complementary and alternative medicines and the use of herbal products (nutriceuticals) have dramatically increased worldwide. Estimates place the frequency of their use in North America at between 50% and 60% of the population. Patients do not volunteer information about the use of these products and should be asked specifically. Many of these nutriceuticals are thought to have the potential to adversely affect the administration of anesthetic agents, hypnotics, sedatives, and a variety of other medications. Some are thought to interfere with platelet function and coagulation, and oth-

Table 2-2 Nutriceuticals: Proposed Use and Adverse Effects[a]

Product	Use	Potential Side Effects
Echinacea *(Echinacea species)*	Prevent and treat upper respiratory infections	Immunosuppression (?)
Ephedra	Sympathomimetic	Vasoconstriction, MI, CVA, herb–drug interaction with MAOIs
Feverfew *(Tanacetum parthenium)*	Anti-inflammatory, arthritis, migraine headache	Oral ulcers, abdominal pain, bleeding
Garlic *(Allium sativum)*	Cholesterol reduction, anticoagulant, +/− antihypertensive, antimicrobial (?)	Irreversible antiplatelet activity (?) Excessive bleeding
Ginger *(Zingiber officinale)*	Digestive aide, diuretic, antiemetic, stimulant	Thromboxane synthetase inhibitor
Ginkgo *(Ginkgo biloba)*	Anticoagulant	Increased anticoagulant effects, bleeding
Ginseng *(Panax ginseng)*	Lowers blood sugar, inhibits platelet aggregation	Hypoglycemia, bleeding, potentiates warfarin
Glucosamine		Inhibits DNA synthesis (?)
Kava *(Piper methysticum)*	Sedation, anxiolytic	Addiction, withdrawal, increased sedative effects, extrapyramidal effects, (?) hepatitis, GI discomfort, false-negative PSA, hypertension, urinary retention
Saw Palmetto *(Serenoa repens)*	Prostatic health (BPH)	Contraindication in women
St. John's wort *(Hypericum perforatum)*	Cerebral failure	Inhibition of neurotransmitter uptake, multiple herb–drug interactions including cyclosporin, warfarin, steroids, calcium-channel blockers, and others
Valerian *(Valeriana officinalis,* vandal root)	Sedative	Withdrawal, enhanced sedative effects of hypnotics, sedatives, anxiolytics

[a] This table of commonly used supplements is neither all-inclusive nor comprehensive. Many of the potential adverse effects and herb–drug interactions are based on anecdotal reports or small uncontrolled case studies.
MI, myocardial infarction; CVA, cerebrovascular accident; MAOI, monoamine oxidase inhibitor; GI, gastrointestinal; PSA, prostate-specific antigen.

ers to potentiate or reduce the activity of anticoagulants and some immunosuppressants. These products have been classified as "supplements" and are not regulated by the Food and Drug Administration. As a consequence, robust scientific studies concerning their mechanism of action, herb–drug interactions, active-drug content, effectiveness, and potential side effects are difficult to identify. Further, reliable information regarding these products is difficult to obtain. The sheer number of preparations available, estimated to be over 20,000, makes it difficult, if not impossible, to compile detailed information on all of them.

Common nutriceuticals are listed in Table 2-2, along with their indications for use and potential adverse side effects. The American Society of Anesthesiologists recommends discontinuation of these supplements for 2 to 3 weeks prior to an operative procedure, but this recommendation is not based on sound scientific evidence.

Aspirin and nonsteroidal antiinflammatory medications are well known for their antiplatelet aggregation properties. Other over-the-counter, nonprescription pharmaceuticals should be noted and their actions and potential drug–drug interactions should be investigated. The hospital pharmacist or Doctor of Pharmacy is an excellent reference for questions in this area.

PREOPERATIVE SCREENING TESTS

Interpretation of Laboratory and Diagnostic Data

It is standard practice in most North American hospitals for doctors to order a battery of routine preoperative screening tests on otherwise asymptomatic patients under the mistaken belief that this practice improves patient safety, and outcome, by identifying unsuspected conditions that could contribute to perioperative morbidity and mortality. This indiscriminate practice is expensive and unwarranted. In fact, the potential harm caused by the routine screening of asymptomatic patients is greater than any benefit derived from uncovering occult abnormalities. The time and resources necessary to chase unanticipated results, the occasional performance of additional invasive (and risky) secondary procedures, and the fact that 60% of these abnormal results are ignored are arguments against unselected screening. If there is a legal liability issue surrounding preoperative screening, the latter is the most significant one. Obtaining data to establish a "baseline" is not recommended for the asymptomatic patient. Normal laboratory results obtained within 4 months of an elective operative procedure need not be repeated, since abnormalities could be predicted based on the patient's history. Preoperative screening tests are not a substitute for a comprehensive history and physical examination focused to identify comorbidities that may influence perioperative management. The need for emergency surgery, especially for patients who cannot provide historical data, obviously alters these recommendations.

Routine screening of hemoglobin concentration is performed only in individuals who are undergoing radical procedures that are associated with an extensive amount of blood loss. Patients with a history of anemia, malignant disease, renal insufficiency, cardiac disease, diabetes mellitus, or pregnancy should have baseline determinations of serum hemoglobin concentration. Individuals who cannot provide a history or who do not have physical findings that suggest anemia should have preoperative baseline hemoglobin determinations.

Evaluation of baseline serum electrolyte concentrations, including serum creatinine, is appropriate in individuals whose history or physical examination suggests chronic medical disease (e.g., diabetes; hypertension; cardiovascular, renal, or hepatic disease). Patients with the potential for loss of fluids and electrolytes, including those receiving long-term diuretic therapy, those with diabetes, and those with intractable vomiting, should also have preoperative determination of serum electrolytes. The elderly are at substantial risk for chronic dehydration, and testing is appropriate in these patients as well. Although there is no specific age that mandates automatic electrolyte screening, knowledge of the patient's medical history, medications, and systems review should guide decision making about testing.

Preoperative urinalysis is recommended only for patients who have urinary tract symptoms or a history of chronic urinary tract disease, or in those who are undergoing urologic procedures.

Screening chest radiography is rarely indicated. Despite the occasional incidental abnormality that is detected with a screening radiograph, these findings rarely receive further investigation and generally do not alter the surgical plans. Screening chest radiography in asymptomatic elderly patients is also controversial because the usefulness of this diagnostic study in this population is unclear. Chest radiography is recommended for patients who are undergoing intrathoracic procedures and for those who have signs and symptoms of active pulmonary disease.

Recommendations for screening electrocardiography are more firm, but likewise, definitive evidence about the utility of the procedure is lacking. Men who are older than 40 years of age and women who are older than 50 years of age should have a baseline recording. Patients with symptomatic cardiovascular disease, hypertension, or diabetes are candidates for preoperative electrocardiographic screening. Patients who are undergoing thoracic, intraperitoneal, aortic, or emergency surgery are also candidates for screening examinations. In summary, laboratory and other diagnostic screening tests should be performed only on those patients found to be at risk for specific comorbidities identified during the preoperative clinical evaluation. Students are encouraged to read the excellent review by Smetana and Macpherson (see Suggested Readings) for an in-depth discussion of preoperative testing. Table 2-3 is adapted from their review and should be used as a guide.

Cardiac Evaluation

Two primary alterations in physiology occurring in the postoperative period impose significant stress on the myo-

Table 2-3 Recommendations for Laboratory Testing before Elective Surgery

Test	Incidence of Abnormalities That Change Management	LR+	LR−	Indications
Hemoglobin	0.1%	3.3	0.90	Anticipated major blood loss or symptoms/history of anemia
White blood cell count	0.0%	0.0	1.0	Symptoms suggestive of infection, myeloproliferative disease, myelotoxic medications
Platelet count	0.0%	0.0	1.0	History of bleeding disorder/bruising, myeloproliferative disease, myelotoxic medications, splenomegaly
Prothrombin time	0.0%	0.0	1.0	History of bleeding disorder/bruising, chronic liver disease, malnutrition, recent or long-term antibiotic/warfarin use
Partial thromboplastin time	0.1%	1.7	0.86	History of bleeding diathesis, anticoagulant medication
Electrolytes	1.8%	4.3	0.80	Chronic renal insufficiency, CHF, diuretic use, other meds that affect electrolytes
Renal function tests	2.6%	3.3	0.81	Age 50, hypertension, cardiac disease, major surgery, medications that may alter renal function
Glucose	0.5%	1.6	0.85	Obesity, known diabetes or symptoms thereof
Liver function tests	0.1%			No indication, consider albumin measurement for major surgery or chronic illness
Urinalysis	1.4%	1.7	0.97	No indication
Electrocardiogram	2.6%	1.6	0.96	Men > 40, women > 50, known coronary artery disease, diabetes or hypertension
Chest radiograph	3.0%	2.5	0.72	Age > 50, known cardiac or pulmonary disease or symptoms or exam findings suggesting cardiac or pulmonary disease

CHF, congestive heart failure; LR+, likelihood ratio that a test will be abnormal in the absence of symptoms or signs; LR−, likelihood ratio that a test will be normal in the absence of symptoms or signs.
Adapted from Smetana GW, Macpherson DS. The case against routine preoperative laboratory testing. *Med Clin North Am* 2003; 87(1):7–40; used with permission.

cardium. The first is a catecholamine surge that may occur in response to the pain and anxiety associated with the operative procedure or the disease process itself. The result is an increase in the myocardial oxygen requirement secondary to an increase in heart rate and contractility. Concomitantly, myocardial blood flow is reduced by (1) the vasoconstrictive effect of the α_1-receptor stimulation and (2) the reduced time for blood flow through the myocardium as a result of a reduction in diastolic time (i.e., increased heart rate). The second alteration suppresses the fibrinolytic system, predisposing the patient to thrombosis. Myocardial ischemia can result in cardiac segments in which blood flow is reduced further by occlusive disease.

Evaluation of Patients Asymptomatic for Heart Disease

Special note is taken of the patient's overall status during the physical examination. Vital signs can give important clues about the status of the cardiovascular system (i.e., tachycardia, tachypnea, postural changes in blood pressure). Jugular venous distension at 30°, slow carotid pulse upstroke, bruits, edema, and a laterally displaced point of maximum cardiac impulse all suggest some type of cardiac disease. Auscultatory findings that suggest cardiac problems include rubs, third heart sounds, and systolic murmurs.

Determining which murmurs are clinically significant and which are innocent is perplexing for most medical students. Most innocent murmurs are apical. Innocent murmurs are never associated with a palpable thrill, and there are no innocent diastolic murmurs. Maneuvers that change blood flow (i.e., Valsalva) generally do not change the character or pitch of innocent murmurs. A patient who has hemodynamically significant aortic stenosis usually has a characteristically harsh holosystolic murmur, a slow carotid pulse upstroke, and a displaced primary myocardial impulse that is secondary to left ventricular hypertrophy. This latter finding, as well as poststenotic aortic dilation, may be seen on chest radiograph. Patients who have a history of mitral insufficiency also have an increased risk of postoperative congestive heart failure and arrhythmia.

Any abnormality seen on routine electrocardiography implies increased risk to the adult patient. Other than acute myocardial infarction or complete heart block, the abnormality rarely requires postponement of surgery, especially in asymptomatic patients.

Mild, chronic congestive heart failure is not associated with an increased occurrence of perioperative infarction. Patients with cardiomegaly on chest radiograph and even those whose clinical course is effectively managed medically do not represent high-risk groups. However, abnormal third heart sounds or signs of jugular venous distension indicate decompensation of cardiac function. These patients are in jeopardy of serious cardiac complications. Many patients with chronic congestive heart failure are treated with cardiac glycosides, and digitalis is a drug with a very narrow therapeutic:toxic ratio. Surgical patients frequently cannot take fluids orally and often have multiple tubes to remove fluids that are rich in electrolytes. These fluid shifts predispose the patient to electrolyte aberrations (specifically, hypokalemia) and further narrow the therapeutic:toxic ratio.

Evaluation of Patients With Heart Disease

The patient who is scheduled to undergo elective surgery should be questioned carefully about the nature, severity, and location of chest pain. Dates and details about infarctions, documented or suspected, should be noted, as should coronary artery bypass graft or revascularization procedures. Additional historical elements of significance include a history of dyspnea on exertion (which may signify underlying cardiac or pulmonary pathology). Other clues to the possibility of coexisting heart disease include syncope, palpitations, and arrhythmia. Patients with a history of rheumatic heart disease require prophylactic antibiotic therapy to prevent endocarditis, even for minor procedures.

In the patient with previous infarction, the risk of postoperative myocardial ischemia is between 5% and 10% overall, with an attendant mortality rate of 50%. This figure contrasts with a risk of less than 0.5% in patients with no history of infarct or clinically evident heart disease. If an elective operative procedure is performed immediately after a recent myocardial infarction, the risk of an additional acute cardiac event or death is approximately 30% within the first 3 months. The risk declines with time, and reaches a plateau of approximately 5% at 6 months. If possible, elective surgery should be postponed for 6 months after a myocardial infarction.

The patient who has unstable angina should avoid surgery, unless it is for coronary artery bypass grafting. Although the patient with stable angina is theoretically at increased risk, no clear answer about the extent of increased postoperative risk is available for this group. In contrast, patients who have undergone coronary artery bypass have a significantly reduced danger of postoperative infarct compared with those who have angina. The risk is estimated at slightly more than 1%, with a similar mortality rate. In a limited study, percutaneous angioplasty conferred myocardial protection in the postoperative period, but studies confirming the value of this procedure are not available. Patients with any cardiac history must be evaluated carefully, and the severity of their disease must be documented. If possible, maximum myocardial performance should be achieved before any operative procedure is undertaken.

A history of diabetes increases the index of suspicion for occult cardiac pathology. Of patients with a documented history of diabetes for 5 to 10 years, 60% have diffuse vascular pathology. After 20 years, nearly all patients with diabetes have some type of vascular abnormality. In addition, the risk of mortality after a cardiac ischemic event for the patient with diabetes is higher than that for people without diabetes. Silent infarctions, or ischemic events without symptoms, have also been reported in the diabetic population. Careful questioning, however, often discloses that these episodes involve some atypical symptoms (e.g., vague pain, breathlessness, syncope, mild congestive heart failure). Therefore, patients with diabetes, especially those with a long-standing history of the disease, should be viewed with suspicion and presumed to have some degree of cardiovascular abnormality.

The patient who has a history of rheumatic fever, a prosthetic heart valve, or other cardiac abnormalities requires preoperative antibiotic prophylaxis to prevent endocarditis before undergoing procedures that may cause transient bacteremia. Antibiotic recommendations for prophylaxis are listed in Table 2-4. These recommendations are derived by consensus of a panel of experts based on the stratification of the risk of endocarditis in the general population compared to the morbidity and mortality of the subset of patients at risk. High- and moderate-risk category patients generally receive prophylaxis, while low-risk category patients do not. These recommendations cannot be considered the "standard of care" or a substitute for sound clinical judgment, since they are not based on Class I data. Prophylaxis is individualized for patients who have other types of implanted devices or prosthetics. Evaluation of cardiac function is frequently accomplished with the insertion of a pulmonary artery catheter to monitor hemodynamics and maximize cardiac performance. The use of this tool has theoretical advantages; however, the clinical utility of pulmonary artery catheters, especially in terms of outcome, is difficult to substantiate in critically ill patients. A recent, prospective, multi-institutional trial failed to show any survival or therapeutic advantage in a group of critically ill patients who had pulmonary artery catheters placed for hemodynamic monitoring and guiding therapy.

Quantification of Surgical Risk

Based on the history, physical findings, and a few simple laboratory studies, efforts have been made to quantify surgical risk. The more commonly used system, the **Dripps-**

Table 2-4 Endocarditis Prophylaxis in Surgical Patients With a History of Rheumatic Fever, Cardiac Valvular Disease, or Prosthetic Heart Valve

	Dose for Adults	Dose for Children[a]
Dental and Upper Respiratory Procedures		
Oral[b]		
Amoxicillin[c]	3 g 1 hr before procedure and 1.5 g 6 hr later	50 mg/kg 1 hr before procedure and 25 mg/kg 6 hr later
Penicillin allergy:		
Erythromycin	1 g 2 hr before procedure and 500 mg 6 hr later	20 mg/kg 2 hr before procedure and 10 mg/kg 6 hr later
or clindamycin	300 mg 1 hr before procedure and 150 mg 6 hr later	10 mg/kg (300 mg maximum) 1 hr before procedure and 5 mg/kg 6 hr later
Parenteral[b]		
Ampicillin	2 g IM or IV 30 min before procedure	50 mg/kg IM or IV 30 min before procedure
plus gentamicin	1.5 mg/kg IM or IV 30 min before procedure	2 mg/kg IM or IV 30 min before procedure
Gastrointestinal and Genitourinary Procedures		
Oral[b]		
Amoxicillin[c]	3 g 1 hr before procedure and 1.5 g 6 hr later	50 mg/kg 1 hr before procedure and 25 mg/kg 6 hr later
Parenteral[b]		
Ampicillin plus gentamicin	2 g IM or IV 30 min before procedure 1.5 mg/kg IM or IV 30 min before procedure	50 mg/kg IM or IV 30 min before procedure 2 mg/kg IM or IV 30 min before procedure
Penicillin allergy:		
Vancomycin plus gentamicin	1 g IV infused slowly over 1 hr beginning 1 hr before procedure See dose above	20 mg/kg IV infused slowly over 1 hr beginning 1 hr before procedure See dose above

[a] Dose should not exceed the adult dose.
[b] Oral regimens are safer and more convenient. Parenteral regimens are more likely to be effective and are recommended for patients with prosthetic valves, those with a history of endocarditis previously, or those taking oral penicillin continuously.
[c] Amoxicillin is recommended because of its activity against streptococci and enterococci. *Viridans* streptococci are the most common cause of endocarditis after dental or upper respiratory procedures. Enterococci are the most common cause of endocarditis after gastrointestinal or genitourinary procedures.
IM, intramuscular; IV, intravenous.

American Surgical Association Classification, categorizes patients into five groups (Table 2-5). The system offers little guidance, however, for identifying patients who are at risk for postoperative myocardial ischemia.

In 1977, Goldman and associates published a prospective study that attempted to quantitate the perioperative hazards of myocardial infarction based on the history, physical findings, and simple laboratory data. Correlation and regression analysis of multiple recorded factors identified eight specific elements associated with an increased preoperative risk of infarction. Point values were assigned to each variable, and a quantitative estimate of the risk of postoperative myocardial infarction and death was determined (Tables 2-6 and 2-7).

Table 2-5 Dripps-American Surgical Association Classification

Class I	Healthy patient: limited procedure
Class II	Mild to moderate systemic disturbance
Class III	Severe systemic disturbance
Class IV	Life-threatening disturbance
Class V	Not expected to survive, with or without surgery

In this analysis, poor general health is assumed to reflect severe systemic disease, blood gas signs of respiratory insufficiency ($Pa_{O_2} < 60$ mm Hg or $Pa_{CO_2} > 50$ mm Hg), electrolyte abnormality ($K < 3.0$ mEq/dL) or metabolic acidosis ($HCO_3^- < 20$ mEq/dL), acute or chronic renal failure (creatinine > 3.0 mg/dL or blood urea nitrogen [BUN] > 50 mg/dL), or hepatic dysfunction (abnormal transaminase or stigmata of chronic liver disease). Patients who have a combination of risk factors (e.g., chronic renal failure and metabolic acidosis) could be assumed to have additive risk; however, Goldman's work does not address this issue. The danger of nonfatal or fatal postoperative cardiac ischemia is significantly greater if the risk factor is present.

A score of fewer than 25 total points implies minimal

Table 2-6 Assessment of Individual Risk Factors

Factor	Life-Threatening/Nonfatal Yes	Life-Threatening/Nonfatal No	Cardiac Death Yes	Cardiac Death No	Points	P
Third heart sound or JVD	14%	3.5%	20.0%	1.2%	11	< 0.001
MI in past 6 months	14%	3.7%	23.0%	1.4%	10	< 0.001
Rhythm other than sinus	10%	3.0%	9.0%	1.0%	7	< 0.001
> 5 PVCs/min	16%	3.3%	14.0%	1.4%	7	< 0.001
Age > 70 yr	6%	3.0%	5.0%	0.4%	5	< 0.001
Emergency procedure	8%	3.0%	5.0%	1.0%	4	< 0.001
Hemodynamically significant aortic stenosis	4%	4.0%	13.0%	1.6%	3	0.007
Aortic, intraabdominal, intrathoracic procedure	7%	1.2%	2.5%	1.4%	3	0.007
Poor general health	7%	2.0%	4.0%	1.0%	3	0.027
Total					53	

JVD, jugular venous distension; MI, myocardial infarction; PVC, premature ventricular depolarization.
Adapted with permission from Goldman L, Caldera DL, Nussbaum SR, et al. Multifactorial index of cardiac risk factor in noncardiac surgical procedures. *N Engl J Med* 1977;297:845–850.

risk; however, the threat of serious, but nonfatal, complications increases more than sevenfold between Class I and Class II and more than twice that between Class II and Class III on the Goldman scale. The risk of cardiac death for a patient with any score greater than 5 is increased by a factor of 10. In addition, a score of greater than 26 points suggests that the risk of a fatal coronary event is so great that elective surgery should not be considered. Patients who are categorized as Class II or Class III usually benefit from a period of medical management for several days before elective surgery, if possible, or from coronary angiography to determine the presence of a surgically correctable coronary lesion.

Qualification of Goldman's risk factors should be considered. Age in itself is not a straightforward risk factor. The difference between chronologic age and physiologic age may be substantial. For emergent intrathoracic and intraabdominal procedures, surgical risk is directly related to age. For nonemergent or minor procedures, the relation is less clear.

Table 2-7 Cardiac Risk Scale

Class	Points	Potentially Fatal Cardiac Complications	Cardiac Death
I	0–5	0.7%	0.2%
II	6–12	5.0%	2.0%
III	13–25	11.0%	2.0%
IV	> 26	22.0%	56.0%

Potentially fatal complications include postoperative myocardial infarction, pulmonary edema, and ventricular tachyarrhythmia.

A reliable indicator of hemodynamic reserve is made by quantitative estimate of the patient's cardiovascular functional class. A useful scale is outlined in Table 2-8. Activity is expressed in metabolic equivalents (METs). One MET represents an oxygen consumption of 3.5 mL/

Table 2-8 Energy Expenditure and Metabolic Equivalents

Class	Tasks Patient Can Perform to Completion
I	Activity requiring > 6 METs Carrying 24 lb up 8 steps Carrying objects that weigh 80 lb Performing outdoor work (shoveling snow, spading soil) Participating in recreation (skiing, basketball, squash, handball, jogging/walking at 5 mph)
II	Activities requiring > 4 but not > 6 METs Having sexual intercourse without stopping Walking at 4 mph on level ground Performing outdoor work (gardening, raking, weeding) Participating in recreation (rollerskating, dancing fox trot)
III	Activity requiring > 1 but not > 4 METs Showering, dressing without stopping, stripping, and making bed Walking at 2.5 mph on level ground Performing outdoor work (cleaning windows) Participating in recreation (golfing, bowling)
IV	No activity requiring > 1 MET Cannot carry out any of the above activities

MET, metabolic equivalent.
Adapted with permission from Paul SD, Eagle KA. A stepwise strategy for coronary risk assessment for noncardiac surgery. *Med Clin North Am* 1995;79:1241–1262.

kg/min, the average for a resting 70-kg man. Achieving a heart rate of more than 100 beats/min during cardiac stress is roughly equivalent to four METs.

The American College of Cardiology and the American Heart Association Task Forces have outlined a logical approach to the preoperative cardiac evaluation of patients who are undergoing noncardiac surgery. The general recommendation is that preoperative testing should be limited to the small subset of patients who are at very high risk, when results will affect patient treatment and, most important, outcome. The algorithm developed by the Task Force on Practice Guidelines (Fig. 2-1) shows an eight-step approach to preoperative cardiac assessment. Patients who need emergency noncardiac surgery require operative intervention without extensive preoperative testing. Postoperatively, these patients may require further cardiac evaluation. Step two concerns patients who need urgent or elective operative procedures. Patients who have undergone coronary revascularization within 5 years and who have had no recurring symptoms of myocardial ischemia may proceed to operative intervention without additional cardiac workup. Those who have recurrent signs or symptoms and have not undergone a recent coronary evaluation should be evaluated on the basis of clinical predictors. Patients with major clinical predictors (i.e., unstable coronary syndrome, decompensated congestive heart failure, significant arrhythmia, severe valvular disease) should be evaluated by noninvasive tests of myocardial perfusion. The objective of these noninvasive assessments is to identify patients who would benefit from coronary angiography and subsequent coronary artery bypass grafting before elective surgery. If the patient has only intermediate predictors or if no clinical predictors are present, then assessment for functional capacity can be estimated. Individuals who cannot meet a four-MET demand are at increased risk for perioperative cardiac ischemia and long-term complications. Those who exceed four METs are generally at low risk, and additional preoperative cardiac function testing may not be necessary. Individuals who are at high risk should undergo noninvasive testing and consideration for coronary angiography. Patients who show abnormalities by noninvasive testing and are considered candidates for coronary artery revascularization should undergo coronary angiography and subsequent intervention, as determined by the results of those studies.

Pulmonary Evaluation

Postoperative pulmonary complications are the most common cause of postoperative morbidity. For this reason, it is important to understand the factors that place a patient at risk for these problems. Unfortunately, there is no single predictor of increased risk. A careful history and physical examination will indicate which patients are most at risk; specialized testing is reserved for patients who have significant risk factors or who are expected to undergo an operation that carries a relatively high intrinsic risk of pulmonary complications.

Risk Factors

Surgical Factors

The first issue is the type of operation that the patient is to undergo. Obviously, a pneumonectomy carries a higher risk of pulmonary complications than does a hemorrhoidectomy. Elective lung resections carry specific risks and are considered later in this section. Even among nonpulmonary operations, the risk of pulmonary complications can be stratified by the type of operation. Abdominal operations that require an upper midline incision or involve dissection in the upper abdomen are associated with a much higher pulmonary complication rate than those that are restricted to the lower abdomen. Abdominal incisions are painful and are associated with diminished functional residual capacity. These problems contribute to the higher pulmonary complication rate. Any thoracotomy incision also predisposes the patient to pulmonary complications. Interestingly, the median sternotomy incision is associated with a low incidence of pulmonary complications, probably because it is associated with minimal discomfort during quiet breathing. Longer operations cause greater derangements in pulmonary function than do shorter ones.

Anesthesia Factors

Anesthesia predisposes the patient to pulmonary complications. Simply undergoing general anesthesia produces an 11% reduction in functional residual capacity (FRC). Patients do not cough under anesthesia, and postoperative sedation depresses respiratory drive and inhibits coughing. The lasting effects of neuromuscular blockade can also weaken the coughing effort. Mucociliary clearance is also depressed by anesthetic agents. Anticholinergic drugs commonly thicken the patient's mucus and make it more difficult to mobilize. Tracheal intubation promotes direct colonization of the upper airway by Gram-negative organisms and sets the stage for infection.

A significant portion of hospital-acquired infections are caused by iatrogenic introduction of nosocomial organisms into the tracheobronchial tree by suction catheters that are passed without attention to aseptic technique.

Figure 2-1 Stepwise approach to preoperative cardiac evaluation for noncardiac surgery. CHF, congestive heart failure; ECG, electrocardiogram; METs, metabolic equivalents. (Adapted with permission from Eagle KA, Brundage BW, Chaitman BR. Guidelines for perioperative cardiovascular evaluation for noncardiac surgery: report of the American College of Cardiology/American Heart Association Task Force on Practice Guidelines. *Circulation* 1996; 93:1278–1317.)

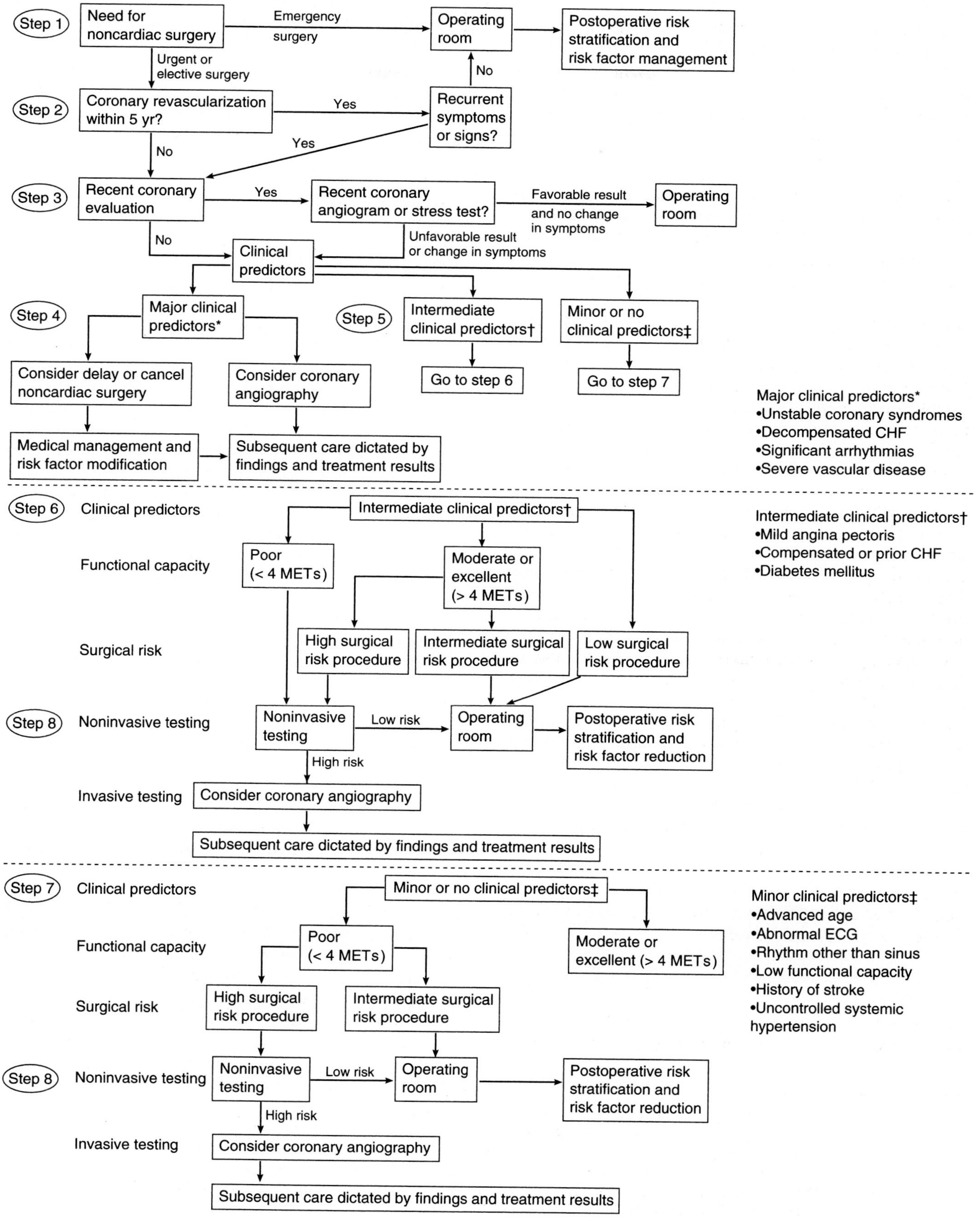
Step 1
Need for noncardiac surgery
Emergency surgery
Operating room
Postoperative risk stratification and risk factor management
Urgent or elective surgery
No
Step 2
Coronary revascularization within 5 yr?
Yes
Recurrent symptoms or signs?
Yes
No
Step 3
Recent coronary evaluation
Yes
Recent coronary angiogram or stress test?
Favorable result and no change in symptoms
Operating room
No
Clinical predictors
Unfavorable result or change in symptoms
Step 4
Major clinical predictors*
Step 5
Intermediate clinical predictors†
Minor or no clinical predictors‡
Consider delay or cancel noncardiac surgery
Consider coronary angiography
Go to step 6
Go to step 7
Medical management and risk factor modification
Subsequent care dictated by findings and treatment results
Major clinical predictors*
•Unstable coronary syndromes
•Decompensated CHF
•Significant arrhythmias
•Severe vascular disease
Step 6
Clinical predictors
Intermediate clinical predictors†
Functional capacity
Poor (< 4 METs)
Moderate or excellent (> 4 METs)
Intermediate clinical predictors†
•Mild angina pectoris
•Compensated or prior CHF
•Diabetes mellitus
Surgical risk
High surgical risk procedure
Intermediate surgical risk procedure
Low surgical risk procedure
Step 8
Noninvasive testing
Noninvasive testing
Low risk
Operating room
Postoperative risk stratification and risk factor reduction
High risk
Invasive testing
Consider coronary angiography
Subsequent care dictated by findings and treatment results
Step 7
Clinical predictors
Minor or no clinical predictors‡
Functional capacity
Poor (< 4 METs)
Moderate or excellent (> 4 METs)
Minor clinical predictors‡
•Advanced age
•Abnormal ECG
•Rhythm other than sinus
•Low functional capacity
•History of stroke
•Uncontrolled systemic hypertension
Surgical risk
High surgical risk procedure
Intermediate surgical risk procedure
Step 8
Noninvasive testing
Noninvasive testing
Low risk
Operating room
Postoperative risk stratification and risk factor reduction
High risk
Invasive testing
Consider coronary angiography
Subsequent care dictated by findings and treatment results

Gas exchange is directly affected by general anesthesia. Arterial saturation and a decline in PaO_2 occur because of changes in position and ventilation–perfusion (V/Q) mismatching. Even patients who have normal pulmonary function preoperatively may have a decrease in PaO_2 of as much as 33%. High levels of inspired oxygen also compound arterial hypoxemia because of the phenomenon of absorption atelectasis (which occurs when alveoli are filled with gas mixtures that contain high concentrations of oxygen and low concentrations of nitrogen). As oxygen is absorbed into the pulmonary capillaries, less gas is left in the alveoli to maintain FRC. As a result, atelectasis occurs.

It is tempting to assume that regional anesthesia would obviate these problems. In fact, this assumption may be true for procedures on extremities or procedures that can be done with a very specific regional blockade (e.g., axillary block). However, spinal anesthesia is also associated with postoperative pulmonary problems. As a rule, the important factor is not the type of anesthetic agent employed, but the circumstances to which the patient is exposed (e.g., abdominal procedures, loss of periodic hyperinflation by sighing). Positioning, pain, and sedation are not alleviated by spinal anesthesia alone.

Changes in ventilatory patterns also occur after general anesthesia. Within 24 hours, tidal volume is decreased by 20%, but the respiratory rate is increased by 25%. For the patient with normal pulmonary function, the net effect is essentially no change in minute ventilation. These alterations generally return to normal within 1 to 2 weeks. Significant changes in pulmonary compliance also occur; it may be reduced by as much as 33%. The average adult sighs nine or 10 times per hour. This effort normally hyperinflates the alveoli and prevents atelectasis. Observations in animals and humans indicate that FRC decreases by 10% when hyperinflation by deep breathing is discontinued.

Overall, the risk of pulmonary complications varies from approximately 10% to 70% (Table 2-9). Improvements in anesthetic technique and attention to improving pulmonary function preoperatively and postoperatively have reduced the incidence of respiratory problems, but as much as one-third of all postoperative mortality may still be related, directly or indirectly, to pulmonary insufficiency.

Patient Factors

In general, patients who have an obstruction to expiration flow for any reason are in greatest jeopardy. They may need specialized pulmonary function studies preoperatively and vigorous preoperative and postoperative pulmonary care for prophylaxis. The section on nonpulmonary operations in the discussion of evaluating a patient describes specific tests. Table 2-10 lists the categories of conditions that predispose patients to both infectious and noninfectious perioperative deterioration of respiratory function.

There is controversy about whether age itself is a risk factor for pulmonary complications. With increasing age, there is a progressive decline in static lung volume, maximum expiratory flow, and elastic recoil as well as a decrease in PaO_2 because of an increase in the alveolar–arterial oxygen gradient. The net effect is a loss of pulmonary reserve. The confounding factor is that many older persons also have independent risk factors for pulmonary complications. Age itself is not a contraindication to surgical intervention, but the normal changes that occur with the aging process should be kept in mind. However, pulmonary disease is a risk factor. In smokers, the relative risk of pulmonary complications is two to six times greater than that in nonsmokers. Smokers have abnormalities in mucociliary clearance, increased volume of secretions, increased carboxyhemoglobin levels, and a predisposition to atelectasis. Smokers should be asked to stop smoking at least 6 weeks before the procedure; however, compliance with this request is rare.

Chronic obstructive pulmonary disease increases perioperative risk for several reasons. Increased pulmonary secretions, small airway obstruction secondary to mucous plugging, inefficient clearing of secretions, and a general lack of pulmonary reserve predispose the patient to atelectasis and superimposed infection. Patients with asthma are also at higher risk. Perioperative stress and many medica-

Table 2-9 Risk of Postoperative Pulmonary Complications Associated With Specific Operative Proceduress

Procedure	Risk %
Elective thoracic/abdominal surgery	17.5
Elective cholecystectomy	14.8
Coronary artery bypass graft	18.7
Abdominal aortic aneurysm surgery (emergent)	60.0
Laparotomy	23.2
Abdominal aortic surgery (elective)	16.0

The definition of pulmonary complications varies widely in the literature and may account for some of the difference.

Table 2-10 General Factors That Predispose Patients to Pulmonary Complications

Cigarette smoking	Chronic bronchitis
Asthma	Occupational lung disease
Neuromuscular disease	Coma
Obesity	Tracheal intubation
Nutritional depletion	Hypotension
Acidosis	Hypoxemia
Chronic obstructive pulmonary disease	Azotemia
Prolonged operative time	Age > 60 years
Hypoalbuminemia	Thoracic/abdominal procedure
Extended stay in the hospital (preoperative)	

tions, including anesthetic agents, can provoke bronchospasm. Compliance with prescribed antiasthma medications and good pulmonary toilet are important in the preoperative phase.

Patients who have a history of occupational exposure to known irritants (e.g., silicone, asbestos, textile components) may have significant restrictive disease and a noticeable reduction in respiratory reserve. Also at high risk are patients who cannot cough or breathe deeply for any reason, such as those with an altered level of consciousness, neuromuscular disease, paraplegia, or weakness as a result of malnutrition.

Obesity contributes directly to the impairment of respiratory function. In simple obesity, FRC and expiratory reserve volume are decreased. As weight increases to 50% above ideal weight, a decrease in other parameters is noted as well. The work of breathing increases dramatically, producing an increase in oxygen consumption and carbon dioxide production. The effect of adipose tissue on the chest wall and the restriction of diaphragmatic excursion by the weight of abdominal contents when the obese patient is supine contribute to the reduction in tidal volume. This reduction results in atelectasis and hypoxemia and contributes to infection. Long-standing obesity may lead to pulmonary hypertension because of the increase in pulmonary blood volume and, later, because of hypoxic vasoconstriction. Eventually, the clinical picture is complicated by hypoxemia (because of a change in V/Q relations secondary to atelectasis and regional redistribution of blood flow and gas) and, ultimately, by hypercapnia (because of hypoventilation).

Pulmonary Evaluation for Nonpulmonary Operations

The pulmonary evaluation of the patient begins with an assessment of his or her functional status. Important historical factors were mentioned earlier, but it is crucial that a careful pulmonary history be obtained. One important question is whether the patient has a history of occupational exposure to known pulmonary irritants. Questions about activities in daily life should also be asked. For example, can the patient shovel snow (or rake the yard)? Is he or she out of breath after walking up a flight of stairs? The patient should be asked about his or her smoking history, sputum production, wheezing, and exertional dyspnea. Physical examination should begin with a general assessment of the patient's habitus. Are there signs of wasting or morbid obesity? Does the patient exhibit pursed-lip breathing? Does he or she have clubbing or cyanosis? What is the patient's respiratory pattern? Is there a prolonged expiratory phase, as in obstructive airways disease? What is the anteroposterior dimension of the chest? On auscultation, does the patient wheeze? A patient who cannot climb one flight of steps without dyspnea or blow out a match at 8 inches from the mouth without pursing the lips is a candidate for more sophisticated pulmonary function screening. Another useful bedside test is the loose cough test. A rattle heard through the stethoscope when the patient forcibly coughs is a reliable indicator of underlying pulmonary pathology and warrants investigation, beginning with a chest radiograph, with further studies ordered as appropriate to the patient's history, physical examination findings, and x-ray results.

Before the specific elements of pulmonary function tests are discussed, it is useful to review the physiologic definitions of standard lung volumes and capacities. Figure 2-2 shows a standard spirometry curve. Normal tidal ventilation is shown by **A.** At the end of passive tidal exhalation, the patient is said to be at FRC (shown by **B** in Figure 2-2). FRC is equal to the sum of expiratory reserve volume (the amount of air that can be expelled with a forced expiratory maneuver) and residual volume (the volume of air left in the lung after a forced expiration). This volume cannot be exhaled under normal circumstances. There is another volume that is worth considering: closing volume. Closing volume (CV) is the volume below which the alveoli become so structurally unstable that they cannot remain open, even with the benefit of surfactant. In Figure 2-2, normal CV is shown as being slightly lower than residual volume. In a smoker, however, CV requires a much higher volume of air. Consequently, patients with lung pathology tend to have spontaneous atelectasis at much higher volumes than they would otherwise. CV is actually greater than FRC in smokers and obese patients, whereas it is much lower than FRC in normal patients. Because FRC is the volume left in the lung after a passive tidal expiration, it is important to understand that certain lung diseases predispose the patient to atelectasis because CV is actually greater than FRC.

There is no evaluation strategy that precisely defines the pulmonary risk of a given patient. Although it is possible to indicate which patients are likely to fare extremely well or extremely poorly, the middle groups are difficult to stratify.

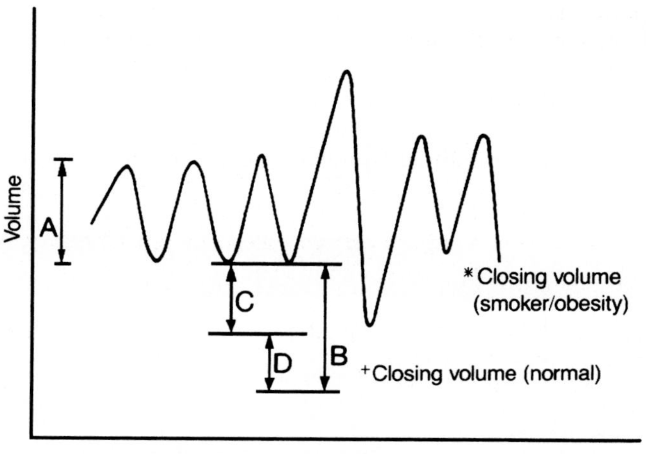

Figure 2-2 Spirometry. **A,** Tidal volume. **B,** Functional residual capacity. **C,** Expiratory reserve volume. **D,** Residual volume. *, Closing volume for smoker/obese patient. †, Closing volume for normal patient.

At a minimum, a patient with a preoperative FEV_1 (the amount of air that can be exhaled in 1 second during a forced expiration after the patient inhales to total lung capacity) of less than 1, a PaO_2 of less than 50 mm Hg, or a $PaCO_2$ of greater than 45 mm Hg should have the risks of operation explained in clear terms. These risks include not only death and pneumonia, but also the possibility of long-term ventilator dependence. Because of this possibility, some patients decide against proceeding with the operation.

Any patient who has significant abnormalities in respiratory function on routine history or physical examination may benefit from formal pulmonary function studies. In some patients, such information leads to a decision to postpone or modify the course of therapy. Pulmonary function studies that can potentially uncover or quantitate a condition that can be improved in the preoperative period (thereby lessening the risk of postoperative problems) are cost-effective and justifiable. Pulmonary function tests (PFTs) are often used in combination with arterial blood gas analysis to study the patient who is thought to be at high risk.

The most commonly used PFT is the FEV_1. During the forced vital capacity maneuver (part of obtaining the FEV_1), the patient is evaluated for intrinsic lung disease and also for problems with the ventilatory pump that moves air into and out of the lungs. The American College of Physicians outlined recommendations for preoperative specialized PFTs (Table 2-11).

Pulmonary Evaluation for Pulmonary Operations

Pulmonary resections present the special problem of removal of lung tissue in a patient who is already at risk for postoperative pulmonary complications. These patients are likely to have a significant smoking history. Patients who have a greater than eight-packs-a-year history are at particular risk for chronic bronchitis. In general, the goal is to leave the patient with an FEV_1 of at least 800 mL postoperatively. If the predicted postoperative FEV_1 is less than 800 mL, the chances are significant that the patient will never wean from the ventilator postoperatively. The predicted postoperative FEV_1 is estimated by a variety of methods, ranging from simple to complex. One of the easiest ways to estimate quickly whether the postoperative FEV_1 will be low is to multiply the preoperative FEV_1 by the percentage of lung tissue that will be left after resection. For example, consider a patient with an FEV_1 of 1.8 L who is scheduled to undergo a right upper lobectomy. The percentage of pulmonary tissue to be removed is one of five total lobes (20% of the total lung tissue). This patient's predicted postoperative FEV_1 is 1.8 L—80% lung remaining postoperatively equals 1.4 L.

In the very-high-risk patient who is to undergo pulmonary resection and whose predicted postoperative FEV_1 is less than 1 L, split perfusion radionuclide lung scanning is helpful in predicting the amount of functioning lung that will remain postoperatively. If, after careful study, the patient's predicted postoperative FEV_1 is less than 800 mL, the risk that the patient will not get off the ventilator is such that the patient is considered inoperable. Exercise testing is also useful in the evaluation of these patients and does not require a sophisticated pulmonary laboratory. The stair climb is a simple and reproducible method of assessing pulmonary function. The interested medical student can walk with the patient up stairs. A patient who can climb five flights of stairs can tolerate a pneumonectomy, and one who can climb three flights can usually tolerate a lobectomy. Patients with asthma and chronic obstructive pulmonary disease should be particularly careful to be compliant with their medication regimen preoperatively.

Evaluation of Patients With Abnormalities

The Patient With Renal Dysfunction

In the United States, more than 250,000 patients with end-stage renal disease are maintained on dialysis. An even greater number of patients have renal function that is significantly lower than normal. The metabolic and nutritional consequences of this disease frequently require special preparation of the patient for an elective surgical procedure. Most procedures can be performed with an acceptably low complication rate in patients who have chronic renal failure (CRF), provided that meticulous attention to perioperative care is given. Patients with CRF should not be denied a necessary or beneficial surgical procedure based on a history of renal disease alone.

Table 2-11 American College of Physicians Recommendations for Preoperative Pulmonary Function Testing

Type of Surgery	Spirometry	Blood Gas	Split Function Tests	Exercise Test
Pulmonary resection	All patients	All patients	Some patients	Some patients
Coronary artery bypass surgery	Smokers, history of dyspnea	Smokers, history of dyspnea	No	No
Upper abdominal	Smokers, history of dyspnea	Smokers, history of dyspnea	No	No
Lower abdominal	Suspected lung disease	No	No	No
Head and neck	No	No	No	No
Orthopedic	No	No	No	No

In CRF, the ability to excrete water and sodium and maintain homeostasis of the intravascular volume is impaired. Excessive preload usually does not appear, however, until renal function deteriorates to less than 10% of normal. Chronic volume depletion is encountered in these patients as frequently as volume overload. These patients often receive potent diuretic agents or have chronic volume contraction associated with hypertension. For this reason, fluid management is dictated by the patient's history and disease process, not by the fact that he or she has CRF. For example, a patient who has end-stage renal disease and is in septic shock because of a perforated sigmoid diverticulum requires crystalloid resuscitation to correct the relative volume deficit, even though he or she is dependent on dialysis. This patient should not be fluid-restricted. Invasive hemodynamic monitoring can be helpful in this patient group and allows precision in volume replacement. The ability to excrete potassium is also impaired, and patients with impaired renal function do not tolerate sudden changes in potassium level. The risk of malignant hyperkalemia is directly proportional to the serum potassium level before the last dialysis. Serum potassium levels should be less than 5 mEq/L before surgery. Achieving this level may require dialysis or the use of ion-exchange resins. Chronic renal failure is usually accompanied by chronic metabolic acidosis because excretion of fixed acids is reduced. These acids are the byproducts of metabolism and include sulfates, phosphates, and lactate. Respiratory compensation by hyperventilation can maintain the serum pH at an acceptable level that is slightly below normal. The serum bicarbonate level should be >18 mEq/L. Achieving this level may require exogenous bicarbonate administration or dialysis against a bicarbonate bath. Postoperatively, the acid load increases as hydrogen ions are released from damaged cells. Hyperventilation may provide temporary compensation for the metabolic acidosis. However, if $Pa{CO_2}$ increases even slightly, a profound exacerbation of acidosis may occur. This situation is seen in patients who cannot increase minute ventilation, who have increased **dead space,** or who are receiving an excessive carbohydrate caloric load. Aggressive pulmonary toilet to prevent hypoventilation, atelectasis, pneumonitis, and oversedation is prudent.

Another electrolyte abnormality that is often seen in patients with CRF is hypocalcemia secondary to hyperphosphatemia. Because hypermagnesemia is common, magnesium-containing antacids should be avoided in these patients. Oral phosphate binders and dietary restriction of phosphates may be required as well. Ionized calcium should be followed in these patients and supplemented as needed in the perioperative period.

Most patients with long-standing CRF are malnourished. Anorexia, which results from azotemia and the inability to handle the accumulation of nitrogenous end-products, promotes depletion of both skeletal muscle and visceral protein stores. Malabsorption syndromes are common, as are overt vitamin deficiencies. Patients who receive long-term peritoneal dialysis may lose as much as 6 to 8 g protein/day, and as a result, may have hypoalbuminemia. Anorexia and a history of weight loss suggest a catabolic state. Aggressive nutritional support should be provided. Patients should not be protein-restricted in the perioperative phase just because they have renal failure. Malnutrition significantly increases the risk of septic complications in the perioperative period.

The normochromic normocytic anemia that is often seen in patients with CRF is usually well tolerated. The added stress and oxygen requirements that follow a surgical procedure, however, may be poorly tolerated. Chronic dialysis is estimated to remove as much as 3 L blood/year, and the reduced production of erythropoietin hampers red blood cell replacement. The lifespan of red blood cells is also reduced in the uremic state. Immune responses are deficient, and as a result, the potential for infectious complications may be enhanced. Many patients with CRF are carriers of bloodborne pathogens because of multiple transfusions. Chronic coagulopathy secondary to heparinization during dialysis, or the coagulopathy associated with uremia, may exaggerate blood loss during surgery or in the perioperative period. D-desamino arginine vasopression promotes the release of **von Willebrand's** multimers from endothelial cells. These multimers may be useful in the preoperative preparation of patients with chronic renal disease.

Management of these patients requires careful attention to detail. Daily weighing and accurate intake and output records are essential. Baseline renal function studies should be obtained preoperatively and should include determinations of BUN and creatinine as well as an estimation of glomerular filtration rate. Exacerbation of renal failure is prevented if hypotension is avoided and medications are carefully administered. Most drugs can be nephrotoxic, and doses must be adjusted frequently based on an estimation of the degree of renal function. A coagulation profile may help to identify intrinsic deficiencies, and the anticoagulation effects of heparin may require reversal or time to clear. Patients with renal failure may require modifications in anesthetic techniques. For example, succinylcholine is generally avoided because it may promote or exacerbate hyperkalemia. Also, nondepolarizing neuromuscular blockage agents that are not renally metabolized and excreted should be selected. Cisatracurium undergoes Hoffman degradation and is often used in the anesthetic management of patients with renal failure. Many other examples of modifications are available in standard textbooks of anesthesiology. Aggressive pulmonary physiotherapy, attention to volume in electrolyte status, and nutritional support can substantially reduce many metabolic sequelae postoperatively. Modification of the timing and type of dialysis may be necessary, and close consultation with a nephrologist is advisable. Despite the formidable spectrum of potential problems faced by the surgical patient who has CRF, elective surgery can be performed safely with an acceptable level of risk. Precise fluid management may be assisted in these patients with the judicious use of invasive monitoring (e.g., pulmonary artery

Table 2-12 Common Problems in the Cirrhotic Patient

Hepatic Dysfunction	History and Physical Clues	Perioperative Effects or Complications
Drug metabolism	Nonspecific	Sensitivity to narcotics, oversedation, respiratory depression
Protein synthesis	Spider angioma	Abnormalities in coagulation or bleeding
	Petechiae	Reduced factors I, II, V, VII, VIII, IX, X, XI, XIII
	Bruises	Thrombocytopenia
	Changes in sensorium	Exacerbation of encephalopathy, delirium tremens (with alcohol withdrawal), seizures
	Ascites	Fluid retention/respiratory compromise
	Edema	Intraperitoneal sepsis, potential shifts in intravascular volume, potential electrolyte abnormalities
General nutrition	Weight loss (or weight gain with ascites), anemia, muscle wasting, fever, weakness	Vitamin deficiency (A, B, D, K): poor wound healing, poor handling of glucose, Wernicke's syndrome
	Nausea, anorexia, edema	Magnesium, phosphorus: multiple metabolic abnormalities, arrhythmias, reduced immunocompetence, infection

catheterization or esophageal doppler monitoring) as the situation dictates. Electrolytes, particularly potassium, magnesium, and phosphorous, must be followed carefully. The assistance of a clinical pharmacist is indispensable in providing advice regarding how to adjust the dosage and scheduled administration of medications to these patients. Renal function is monitored by accurate assessment of the fluid balance and periodic measurements of the markers of renal function (creatinine and BUN). Renal replacement therapy may be needed when the patient cannot manage his or her own fluid balance, or when the detoxification or excretory function of the kidney is not performing properly. Examples of this would include volume overload with overt congestive heart failure in an anuric patient, life-threatening hyperkalemia, and intractable acidosis.

The Patient With Hepatic Dysfunction

Although the liver has an extraordinary amount of reserve as well as the ability to regenerate, a significant number of patients (> 15 million) show evidence of hepatic dysfunction or overt cirrhosis. Usually, the etiology is nutritional and secondary to alcohol abuse, but it may also be secondary to an infectious event or idiopathic. General complications and the risk of impaired liver function are listed in Table 2-12. A careful search should be made for these conditions during the history and physical examination. Child's criteria have long been used to estimate the risk of nonhepatic surgery in the patient with cirrhosis (Table 2-13). These estimates of mortality are not absolute, and patients may have a significant reduction in risk if hepatic function is improved preoperatively.

Multiple metabolic aberrations exist in the patient with hepatic dysfunction or overt cirrhosis, even before the development of ascites. Perhaps the most important is a profound reduction in sodium excretion, frequently less than 5 mEq/24 hr, due to tubular reabsorption. The exact mechanism for this is unknown but is thought to be due to multiple hormonal factors. Challenging these patients with an oral sodium load further increases sodium and water retention. Many patients with hepatic dysfunction demonstrate, somewhat contrarily, intravascular volume depletion. The clinical implications of this derangement in sodium metabolism should be obvious, and extreme diligence must be paid to fluid and electrolyte issues in the perioperative period. There is nearly universal agreement that sodium and water restriction is the cornerstone of management of the patient with liver disease, with or without overt ascites.

The alcoholic patient is protected from withdrawal symptoms by the administration of proper sedatives. The onset of mild withdrawal symptoms can occur anywhere from 1 to 5 days after alcohol is discontinued. Major symptoms generally peak at approximately 3 days, but have occurred as long as 10 days after withdrawal. Benzodiaze-

Table 2-13 Child's Classification of Cirrhosis

Class	Albumin	Bilirubin	Ascites	Encephalopathy	Nutritional State	Mortality Rate (%)
A	> 3.5	< 2.0	Absent	Absent	Good	< 10
B	3.0–3.5	2.0–3.0	Minimal	Minimal	Fair	40
C	< 3.0	> 3.0	Severe	Severe	Poor	> 80

pines can prevent major withdrawal symptoms if they are instituted prophylactically. Untreated delirium tremens carries a postoperative mortality rate of as high as 50%. This rate is reduced to 10% with proper treatment. The use of intravenous ethanol has also been advocated, but it only postpones withdrawal.

Platelet abnormalities, both in number and function, are commonly found in patients with advanced liver disease. Further, the synthesis of vitamin K–dependent coagulation factors may be reduced, predisposing to excessive bleeding. Cirrhosis is frequently manifested by massive upper gastrointestinal hemorrhage from esophageal or gastric varices.

Vitamin and mineral deficiencies accompany the malnutrition associated with liver disease. Alcoholics should be given thiamine parenterally before intravenous glucose is administered. Ataxia, ophthalmoplegia, and the severe central nervous system disturbance **Wernicke-Korsakoff syndrome** (i.e., ataxia, ophthalmoplegia, and confusion) may follow if this therapy is not instituted. Magnesium and phosphate deficiencies are common, especially with refeeding, and these elements should be aggressively replaced to prevent abnormalities of glucose metabolism and cardiac arrhythmia.

For a more complete discussion of surgical diseases of the liver, see Chapter 19, Liver.

The Diabetic Patient

The task of the surgeon in managing the diabetic patient is to achieve euglycemia. It is well understood that if blood glucose levels are too low, death can quickly ensue due to starvation of glucose-dependent tissues (particularly, the brain) of their obligatory substrates. For decades, surgeons erred on the side of hyperglycemia, reasoning that modest hyperglycemia is better tolerated than hypoglycemia. Recently, information has become available that suggests that it is possible, at least in the critical care environment, to achieve euglycemia safely and with better outcomes using a continuous infusion of insulin. The safe application of this practice to the noncritical care environment has yet to be demonstrated, but is intriguing.

The patient who has diabetes is at increased risk in the perioperative period from a number of perspectives, particularly (1) metabolic (hyperglycemia or hypoglycemia), (2) cardiovascular, and (3) infectious. Those who require insulin to control their diabetes must have their dose adjusted to compensate for periods when food is not allowed or when the hyperglycemic response to the stress of illness, surgery, or trauma is clinically significant. Patients who have diabetes that was previously controlled by diet or oral agents may require insulin in the perioperative period for the reasons mentioned earlier. Infectious etiologies of surgical disease or postoperative infections may promote hyperglycemia and even ketoacidosis. On the other hand, overzealous administration of insulin may lead to hypoglycemia.

The perioperative management of patients with diabetes is approached as follows:

1. Patients who are instructed not to eat or drink after midnight in preparation for an operation the next morning should reduce their morning insulin dose to one-half the usual dose of intermediate- or regular-acting insulin to be taken the morning of the operation.
2. The patient should receive a continuous infusion of 5% dextrose to provide 10 g glucose/hr. Fingerstick glucose levels are monitored intraoperatively and followed postoperatively at least every 6 hours. The goal is to maintain a glucose level of between 150 and 200 mg/dL. It is generally considered preferable to have the patient at the higher end of this range because of the fearsome consequences of hypoglycemia. Alternatively, continuous intravenous infusion of insulin can be used. This approach is particularly helpful in the brittle diabetic. In the postoperative period, close attention should be paid not only to the patient's blood sugar, but also to the patient's carbohydrate intake. Diabetic ketoacidosis (DKA) can develop in patients with either type I or type II diabetes. DKA is deceptively easy to overlook, because it can mimic postoperative ileus. It may present as nausea, vomiting, and abdominal distension, or in association with polyuria (which is commonly mistaken for mobilization of intraoperative fluids). For this reason, patients with type I diabetes (and many with type II diabetes) should have their urinary ketone level monitored by dipstick. This method is faster and much less costly than following serum ketone levels, and it gives a fairly accurate picture of developing ketoacidosis. A glucose level that is less than 250 mg/dL does not mean that the patient is not at risk for DKA; DKA develops because of the metabolism of fuel in the absence of glucose. Hence, the development of DKA does not depend on a certain level of glucose, but on the absence of insulin. Patients with diabetes are best managed with a continuous infusion of intravenous insulin, usually 1 to 3 units/hr. If a sliding scale is needed, then the subcutaneous route is preferred, except when the subcutaneous tissue is not well perfused.

The cardiac effects of patients with diabetes were discussed previously. The incidence of vascular abnormalities found on physical examination increases with the age of the patient and the duration of the diabetes. Men with diabetes may have twice the risk of cardiovascular mortality as their nondiabetic counterparts. Women have approximately four times the risk. For unexplained reasons, tachycardia may be present in patients with diabetes. Tachycardia is believed to be secondary to autonomic cardiac neuropathy, which is often associated with orthostatic hypotension without an appropriate increase in pulse. These findings are associated with unexplained cardiopulmonary arrest postoperatively.

Gastroparesis, which is also believed to be caused by autonomic neuropathy, may delay gastric emptying and increase the likelihood of aspiration. Gastroparesis is suggested if the patient gives a history of prolonged fullness after eating, or of constipation. A splash of fluid heard with the stethoscope over the stomach at a time when the stomach should be empty may require the placement of a nasogastric tube for decompression.

The risk of infection is substantially greater for the patient with diabetes. Hyperglycemia has an adverse effect on immune function, especially phagocytic activity. The reduced blood flow in patients with vascular disease, especially to the extremities, retards wound healing. Because most peripheral vascular disease in the patient with diabetes is small vessel in nature, palpable pulses are common, even in the face of tissue ischemia. Often the extent of small vessel disease extends deep into the tissue, sparing the skin, much like a cone whose base is directed peripherally and whose apex extends in the central portion of the extremity proximally. For a patient with diabetes, ingrown toenails or minor injuries to the feet are potentially serious problems that can lead to amputation or mortality. Therefore, even minor procedures on the extremities of diabetic patients are approached with utmost caution. Patients with diabetes should always wear shoes.

The surgical patient who has diabetes should be carefully questioned about the duration of the disease, insulin requirements, diet, degree of glucose control, last insulin administration, and peripheral symptoms (i.e., numbness, extremity pain). During the physical examination, special attention is given to the feet, looking for minor injuries, evidence of poor hygiene, inadequate vascular supply, ulcers, or decreased vibratory sensation. Patients who have positive findings should give meticulous care to their feet (i.e., daily washing, careful drying, application of softening lotion, protection from minor trauma, avoidance of pressure sores).

The Adrenally Insufficient Patient

The role of steroids in the management of critically ill patients remains unresolved, despite recent multicenter, randomized, placebo-controlled studies. It is exceedingly difficult to conclusively demonstrate a beneficial effect of steroids in the critically ill, and the adverse effects of these agents are well described. Historically, any patient who had received even small doses of glucocorticoid within the 12-month period before surgery was given preoperative glucocorticoid coverage. This practice was based on reports of two patients from more than 40 years ago. These patients had complications that were believed to be caused by steroid-associated adrenal suppression. Recent advances in the understanding of the adverse effects of glucocorticoids, including increased susceptibility to infection, impaired tissue healing, abnormalities of glucose metabolism, and upper gastrointestinal hemorrhage, prompted a reconsideration of preoperative glucocorticoid coverage. New recommendations are based on the degree of surgical stress anticipated (i.e., minor, moderate, or major; see Table 2-14). For minor surgical stress, glucocorticoid replacement is the equivalent of 25-mg hydrocortisone over a 24-hour period. For moderate surgical stress (e.g., open cholecystectomy, colon resection, total joint replacement, hysterectomy), the glucocorticoid replacement is 50- to 75-mg hydrocortisone (or the equivalent) for 24 to 48 hours. For major surgical stress (e.g., cardiopulmonary bypass, esophagogastrectomy, pancreaticoduodenectomy), the glucocorticoid replacement is approximately 100- to 150-mg hydrocortisone (or the equivalent) for 48 to 72 hours. For comparison, patients with Cushing's syndrome produce the equivalent of 36-mg hydrocortisone/day.

Table 2-14 Stress Steroid Coverage

Level of Surgical Stress	Likelihood of HPA Axis Suppression: None (< 5 mg prednisone/day, or < 3 weeks duration steroid therapy	Likelihood of HPA Axis Suppression: Uncertain (prednisone 5–20 mg daily for 3 weeks in the year preceding operation), or Likely (> 20 mg prednisone for > 3 weeks)
Minor	Give usual dose a few hours preoperatively; continue usual dose postoperatively; no supplementation indicated	Give usual dose a few hours preoperatively; continue usual dose postoperatively; no supplementation indicated.
Moderate	Give usual dose a few hours preoperatively; continue usual dose postoperatively; no supplementation indicated	50 mg IV hydrocortisone prior to induction of anesthesia, 25 mg hydrocortisone every 8 hr, thereafter for 24–48 hr, then resume usual dose
Major	Give usual dose a few hours preoperatively; continue usual dose postoperatively; no supplementation indicated	100 mg IV hydrocortisone prior to induction of anesthesia, 50 mg hydrocortisone every 8 hr for 48–72 hr, then resume usual dose

The Pregnant Patient

Multiple anatomic and physiologic changes accompany a normal pregnancy, altering the presentation of many surgical diseases and mimicking others. The pregnant woman's response to these conditions can also be altered. The enlarging uterus displaces abdominal viscera and can alter the location of pain in some common intraabdominal conditions such as appendicitis. A gravid uterus can compress the inferior vena cava and reduce venous return when the woman assumes the supine position. Pelvic venous compression produces or exacerbates hemorrhoids in over one-third of pregnant women. Lower extremity venous insufficiency and the hypercoagulable state of pregnancy itself increase the risk of venous thromboembolic events, especially if the pregnant patient is placed at bed rest.

The surgeon caring for a pregnant woman is caring, in effect, for two patients, and the mother's physiology is often preserved at the expense of reduced uterine perfusion. Some of the most significant physiologic changes during pregnancy occur to the circulatory system. Heart rate, stroke volume, and plasma volume are increased. Erythrocyte volume is also increased but not to the same degree as plasma volume, resulting in a reduction of the hematocrit. This increase in blood volume can mask blood loss or delay the classic presentation of hypovolemia, especially after injury. The appearance of normal vital signs can be deceptive and obscure fetal distress. The leukocytosis associated with a normal pregnancy reduces the utility of this laboratory test.

Respiratory rate and tidal volume are increased. This increase in minute ventilation lowers the arterial partial pressure of carbon dioxide. This occurs despite a reduction in functional residual capacity and residual volume imposed by the restriction of diaphragmatic motion secondary to the enlarging uterus. Postoperatively, the potential for atelectasis and other pulmonary complications is increased.

Most pregnant women experience reflux symptoms to some degree. Gastric acid production is increased slightly, but the primary problem is the delay in gastric emptying, the result of the action of progesterone in reducing gastric smooth muscle contractility. Nausea and vomiting are common in the first trimester, and these symptoms can be confused with gastrointestinal conditions that are surgical in nature.

It is best when possible to avoid a surgical procedure during pregnancy, but surgical emergencies must be handled when they present. If surgery is necessary, it is best performed during the second trimester, when the risk of precipitating spontaneous abortion or early labor is lowest—approximately 5% in women undergoing general anesthesia and abdominal surgery. Precipitating labor, and perhaps fetal demise, appears to be related more to the underlying pathology than the anesthesia. Laparoscopy can be performed safely as well during the second trimester, albeit with changes in trocar positioning and reducing abdominal insufflation pressure.

Appendicitis and biliary tract disease are the most common reasons for gastrointestinal surgery in the pregnant woman. Pancreatitis occurring during pregnancy is usually related to biliary tract disease. Bulk laxatives, stool softeners, and suppositories are usually sufficient for hemorrhoids. Acute hemorrhoidal thrombosis can be drained with the use of local anesthesia. Rectal bleeding is also associated with colonic malignancy, and complaints of bleeding should not be blindly ascribed to hemorrhoids but investigated by endoscopy irrespective of gestational age.

Many women have delayed pregnancy until later in life, and historically women who were diagnosed with malignant conditions were advised to terminate the pregnancy. Fortunately, this is no longer the case. Women today share in the decision making regarding the pregnancy as well as therapeutic choices. Diagnostic delays, however, are still common in pregnant women with breast cancer. Mammography has an increased rate of false-negative results during pregnancy. Biopsy must not be delayed until after delivery but addressed promptly when the need becomes apparent. Breast cancer in pregnant women has the same prognosis when matched for age of the patient and stage of disease, despite being predominantly estrogen receptor negative. Breast conservation surgery can be performed when appropriate and chemotherapy administered after the first trimester. Radiation therapy is held until after delivery. Continuation of the pregnancy does not appear to adversely affect outcome in women with breast cancer. Rectal cancer is the most common colonic malignancy, and when discovered during the first half of the pregnancy should be resected. When discovered during the last half of the pregnancy, resection is generally postponed until after delivery. As in patients with breast cancer, chemotherapy is relatively safe after the first trimester, but radiation is withheld until after delivery.

One in every 14 pregnancies is complicated by injury. Every injured woman of childbearing age should be screened for pregnancy. As mentioned previously, the changes in a woman's physiology may mask severe fetal distress. Resuscitation of the fetus requires dutiful attention to preserving the mother's blood volume and oxygenation. The classic manifestations of hemorrhagic shock signify that the fetus has been in distress for some time. Early fetal monitoring is essential in the initial assessment and resuscitation of the pregnant trauma patient. Diagnostic studies should be obtained when needed and not withheld for fear of teratogenesis.

Fetal loss occurs in 15% of all women severely injured during pregnancy. Placental abruption can occur even after minor injury and is not consistently accompanied by vaginal bleeding. The presence of a hard uterus, larger than expected for gestational age, is suspicious for abruption. Disseminated intravascular coagulopathy is an ominous complication that can occur with hours of placenta abruption or amniotic fluid embolization. Because sensitization of Rh-negative women occurs with miniscule amounts of fetal Rh-positive blood, all injured Rh-negative women should be considered for Rh-immunoglobulin therapy, unless the injury is relatively minor and remote from the uterus.

The Geriatric Patient

The aging of the American population will continue for many decades to present some special challenges to surgeons. The elderly have less reserve than their younger counterparts. They are often on medications that can distort physiologic responses, for example, beta blockers. They are also often on medications that can impact the response to surgery, for example, warfarin or platelet aggregation–inhibiting agents. Their ability to negotiate everyday activities may be impaired at baseline, perhaps due to sensory impairment, difficulty in ambulation, or dementia. One of the conundrums that arises in the context of providing surgical care for an elderly patient is whether to proceed with an aggressive plan of intervention. It is critical to have repeated discussions with patients and their families about specific issues in their medical care. These discussions should begin preoperatively and continue in the postoperative phase. Generally, patients wish to feel that aggressive medical care will be rendered as long as there is a reasonable chance for meaningful survival. While these discussions are uncomfortable, they are as important to the patient's care as any component of the historical database. It is also important to remember that surgical care is rendered among individuals who take a personal interest in the overall well-being of the patient. Sometimes this means that medical care focuses more on alleviating pain than on prolonging life. These discussions are best held in a quiet, comfortable place, away from distractions. It is also important to note that discussions about end-of-life issues do not constitute some sort of legal activity. There are no forms to be signed. These discussions are just like any other conversation a doctor and patient might have about the patient's care, in which the strengths and weaknesses of different approaches are compared, until the physician and patient arrive at a plan of action. The special difference, of course, is that end-of-life discussions are the patient's best chance to determine his or her destiny. These discussions should be treated with the reverence that such subject matter would naturally evoke.

OPERATIVE MANAGEMENT

Documentation

The Medical Record

The medical record is a concise, explicit document that chronologically outlines the patient's course of treatment. There are three primary purposes of the medical record. The first purpose is to record in one common and accessible location the data and thought processes that form the basis for the treatment team's understanding of the patient's status and the rationale for the treatment plans proposed for the patient. This section of the chart contains progress notes from various disciplines (physicians; nurses; respiratory therapists; occupational, speech, and physical therapists; clinical pharmacists; clergy; nutrition support services; and so forth). It also contains data from laboratory and other diagnostic studies. The second purpose of the chart is to transmit instructions about the patient's care. This is the "orders" section. The final purpose of the chart is to provide a record of the events that occurred during the patient's care. Careful thought should be given to the information placed in the record; this information must be relevant to the course of treatment or diagnostic workup. Before notes are written, consideration should be given to the following six points:

1. Does the information pertain to patient care? Only information that pertains to the actual care of the patient should be entered into the medical record. The medical record should not be used to relay messages among consulting services. Extraneous information is inappropriate and may generate medicolegal liability. Examples include editorial comments about the appropriateness or inappropriateness of recommendations made by other physicians. If there is genuine disagreement about the appropriate plan of management, then the reasons supporting the plan of management chosen should be documented in the chart, without editorial comment about the competency of the physicians who have written dissenting opinions.
2. Is the information of value in documenting the treatment course? Little value is obtained in repeating what was previously documented. In teaching institutions, it is common to see history and physical examinations or progress notes recorded by students, house staff, and attending physicians. The delivery of care in an educational environment is by necessity repetitive. Students gain important experience in writing progress notes that reflect careful and thoughtful evaluation of the patient. Students often obtain important medical information, and their notes should be carefully written.
3. What details will be important for the future care of the patient? Operative notes are perhaps the best illustration of the importance of identifying potential needs for future care. For example, recording surgical findings is more important than noting the type of suture used to perform an anastomosis. A careful description of the abdominal organs as they are inspected and palpated may be of value if future review becomes necessary. Information about blood loss, blood and fluid replacement, and operative time is more relevant than many of the technical nuances of the operative procedure. The thought process used in diagnosing an illness or selecting a therapy is often more important than the technical details.
4. Is the information accurate? Extreme care should be taken to ensure the accuracy of information that is

entered into the medical record. Confusion may occur when verbal reports of diagnostic studies written into the progress notes do not agree with formal reports, once they are typed, signed, and filed. Erroneous information can lead to disastrous results, and may be more damaging than no information. Every effort should be made to maintain accuracy and consistency in the information that is recorded. In some circumstances, clinical decisions are made based on a verbal report. When this situation occurs, it is appropriate to note it (e.g., "Verbal report of positive blood culture received from the lab; plan removal of central line.").

5 Are suspicions and theories clearly defined as such? An inexperienced physician may not precisely differentiate suspicions, theories, and possibilities from reality. Incorrect documentation leads to distortion of the facts in the record and misconceptions on the part of others who are peripherally involved with the patient's care. Inaccuracy is a powerful deterrent to the quality of patient care at all levels.

6 Does the note serve the best interest of the patient, the physician, and the health care team? The medical record is kept on behalf of the patient to document the events, timing, and thinking relating to the care given during the period of hospitalization. The record is a confidential document and cannot be revealed to anyone who is not directly involved in the care of the patient, nor can it be revealed without the patient's or a responsible agent's written consent. An individual who discloses such information without this consent breaches the ethical contract between patient and physician.

Increasingly, health care providers are making the transition from a paper medical record to an electronic medical record (EMR). In 1991, the Institute of Medicine (IOM) released an influential report, "The Computer-Based Patient Record: An Essential Technology for Health Care." The IOM's vision for the electronic medical record is of a document that (1) has a standardized format and nomenclature, (2) is easily searchable, (3) is quickly accessible to those who need to participate in the care of the patient, and (4) can be linked with databases that could improve health care in an evidence-based manner and minimize errors in the delivery of health care. The rate of EMR use has remained relatively unchanged (5% to 10%) over the past decade. In 1996, a federal law known as the Health Insurance Portability and Accountability Act (HIPAA) was passed. Compliance is required of virtually all health care providers, and failure to comply can result in civil (monetary) or criminal (imprisonment) penalties. This law specifies the ways in which medical records may be accessed, and by whom. While it was not the intent of this law to hinder medical care, it is clear that there are many reasons why great care must be taken in being certain that the medical record accurately reflects the patient's care in a manner that respects each individual's privacy. In addition to the advantages surrounding data management, a computer order entry system is considered among the most important components of a hospital's overall program to promote and ensure patient safety.

The medical record can be the physician's and the patient's best ally or worst enemy. Documentation of all findings, results, and explanations to the patient, particularly in terms of risks, benefits, anticipated results, and therapeutic alternatives, can protect both the patient and the physician. The art in mastering the medical record is achieving a balance between brevity and completeness.

Physicians' Orders

The physician's order section of the medical record should be treated with care. Orders must be entered precisely, with the intent of being followed, not interpreted. Unfortunately, the latter is often the case because of the hasty scribblings of physicians that may be unclear, illegible, or inaccurate. Orders should be written with sufficient detail to eliminate possible misunderstanding. There is no excuse for illegible handwriting or imprecise orders. Every aspect of the patient's life, including diet, level of activity, access to the bathroom—even what the patient is to breathe—is the responsibility of the physician once the patient enters the hospital.

Orders include the elements listed in Table 2-15. Content and format may vary among institutions, but the principles are the same. Usually the first orders written concern general nursing care. Identification of the physician or team who is responsible for the patient is important so that the staff knows whom to contact if problems or questions arise. Listing the working diagnosis or reason for admission gives the staff a general idea of the problem and sets the tone for the delivery of services. The frequency of vital signs is next. Any special nursing evaluations (e.g., neuro-

Table 2-15 General Considerations for Writing Orders
Physician/team responsible
Diagnosis/condition
Immediate plans
Vital signs/special checks/notification parameters
Diet
Level of activity
Special nursing care instructions
Positioning
Wound care
Tubes/drains: management and care
Intake/Output: frequency
Intravenous fluids
Medications: drug, dose, route, frequency
Routine
Special
Laboratory orders
Special procedures/radiographs
Miscellaneous

logic function) are also indicated. If the physician wishes to be notified of any of these assessments (e.g., temperature > 38.5°C), the staff is informed.

Diet specifications or NPO (nothing by mouth) orders are also indicated. Special diets are required by some patients (e.g., those with diabetes, those undergoing special diagnostic procedures). Too frequently, hospitalization is prolonged or expensive procedures must be repeated because of lack of attention to the details of prescribing the appropriate diet. The level of patient activity is specified as well. Such orders are generally considered routine, and some hospitals may have standard protocols. Prudent physicians, however, specifically write their own routine in sufficient detail to ensure that their plans are carefully followed.

Some nursing care functions must also be identified. These include special positioning, turning, pulmonary exercises, and care of wounds or drainage tubes. Foley catheters are placed to gravity drainage, nasogastric tubes to some type of suction apparatus, and wound drains to either suction or dependent drainage. The staff is informed specifically about the management of these drains or tubes. Daily care of the incision site is clearly noted. Retrograde infection from incision sites, especially with urinary catheters and wound drains, is a major contributor to morbidity. Patient positioning is extremely important in preventing pulmonary problems and preventing aspiration of the gastric contents in patients who are receiving enteral tube feedings. Other nursing instructions include the recording of fluid intake or output from urinary catheters and drains; specific instructions for tube care, stripping, or irrigation; and notification of the physician in the event of a specific occurrence (e.g., urine output < 30 mL/hr, chest tube drainage > 100 mL/hr).

The type and rate of intravenous fluid administration are also specified. When multiple intravenous sites are used, it is helpful to specify which fluids are to be infused at which sites.

To prevent potentially fatal medication errors, meticulous attention to detail is mandatory when writing medication orders. The notation sequence is type of drug, dosage, route of administration, and frequency. These orders should be absolutely clear and legible. If a physician is uncertain of the spelling of a drug name, he or she should consult a reference. It is important to use only standard abbreviations. Writing medications on a separate section of the order sheet so that they are not mixed in with nonmedication orders may be advantageous; in this way, confusion and oversights are avoided. Orders for routine medications (e.g., analgesics, laxatives, sleeping pills) are written first, followed by medications for the patient's specific needs. Reviewing the medication lists daily is an excellent habit. Changes in drugs, dosage, or frequency are confusing for both the pharmacy and the nursing staff. If drugs are changed, writing an order to stop the original drug, then ordering the new one is the best approach. In most institutions, parenteral nutritional products are prepared in the pharmacy; therefore, total parenteral nutrition orders are placed with the medication orders.

Laboratory studies and special diagnostic procedures should be specified as well. Special procedures, such as radiographs, require additional thought. Request slips for these studies should specifically state the presumptive diagnosis and the reason for the test. Personal consultation with the radiologist or technician avoids confusion and prevents delays or unnecessary repetition of procedures. If those who perform the tests are aware of the reason for the testing, the results are nearly always more productive. Some procedures require special preparation of the patient; therefore, these instructions must be included in the orders. "Routine" or "daily" laboratory or radiology orders are wasteful, rarely contribute to care, and should be avoided. In the occasional situation in which serial studies are needed to follow some aspect of the patient's course, a stop time should be specified (e.g., "Please draw hematocrit q 6 hr × 24 hr."). Laboratory and diagnostic studies should be used to confirm clinical suspicions and not as a shotgun approach to reveal a diagnosis.

The miscellaneous category in Table 2-15 is intended for other orders that may be necessary, including requests for consultation, procurement of procedural permits or old records, or admission of a patient to a special study or protocol.

The orders are only as complete as you make them. Clarity and legibility allow for efficient and appropriate delivery of services. As previously noted, computerized order entry systems are increasingly common and are widely regarded as an essential component of any program to minimize medical error.

Progress Notes

A brief *preoperative note* to summarize the workup and the pertinent physical and diagnostic studies is usually written the day before surgery. These notes serve as a checklist to ensure that the important aspects of preoperative preparation are completed. An example is shown in Table 2-16. A *night of surgery note* should be recorded to document the condition of the patient after the operation. Important information to be included in this note would be the patient's comfort level and vital signs, fluid balance, pertinent examination findings, and any critical laboratory values caregivers would need to know within the next few hours.

Daily progress notes record the patient's clinical course throughout his or her hospital stay. Noting the hospital day number, the postoperative day, or the days after injury is helpful. The format for progress notes varies among hospitals and even among services within the hospital. All notes should be dated, timed, signed, and legible. A brief, handwritten operative note should list the important elements of the operation, with consideration given to recording information that might be important in the immediate perioperative period, before the official typed report is appended to the medical record. These important compo-

Table 2-16 Sample Preoperative Note

Diagnosis:	Cholelithiasis
Proposed surgery:	Cholecystectomy with operative cholangiogram
History and physical:	Completed (dictated)
	Grade II/VI systolic murmur at apex
	Hypertension (controlled)
Laboratory values:	CBC: 14.5/41.5% 7,500
	Electrolytes: 140 | 4.2 / 26 | 101
	BUN 10
	GLU 105
	CXR: NAD
	ECG: NSR-normal
	Present meds: HCTZ 50 mg qd
	Blood: type and hold (specimen in blood bank)
Operative permit:	Signed and on chart; risks, rationale, benefits, and alternatives have been explained in detail; patient understands and agrees to proceed with the surgical plans
Miscellaneous information:	
	Signature: ________

BUN, blood urea nitrogen; CBC, complete blood count; CXR, chest x-ray; ECG, electrocardiogram; GLU, glucose; HCTZ, hydrochlorothiazide; NAD, no appreciable disease; NSR, normal sinus rhythm.

nents are listed in Table 2-17. The important elements of the discharge note are listed in Table 2-18. *Event notes* should be recorded whenever there is an unexpected event in the patient's course. These should briefly summarize what the problem was and the reasons for the steps taken to address the problem. *Discharge notes* should be concise and list the patient's reason for hospitalization (also referred to as the "principal diagnosis"), a brief summary of the patient's hospital course, what medications the patient is to be discharged on, what medications the patient will take after discharge, where the patient is to go after discharge, what the patient's level of activity is, and what the plan for follow-up is. It is not necessary that the discharge summary recapitulate each detail of the patient's hospitalization.

Table 2-17 Operative Note

Procedure:	
Findings:	
Surgeons:	Attending surgeon:
Estimated blood loss:	
Crystalloid replaced:	Blood products:
Anesthesia:	
Complications:	
Tubes/drains:	
Disposition:	
	Signature: ________

Table 2-18 Discharge Note

Admission diagnosis:	Date:
Discharge diagnosis:	Date:
Operative procedure:	
Hospitalization course:	
Disposition:	
Home care instructions:	
Activity:	
Diet:	
Restrictions:	
Wound care:	
Other:	
Discharge medications:	
Follow-up instructions:	
Miscellaneous:	

In summary, the medical record is a legal document that contains important information about the patient's hospital course and his or her response to diagnostic and therapeutic interventions. It is also a place where information given to the patient by the health care providers can be documented. Despite the inconvenience involved, the time and effort devoted to thoughtful record keeping returns many dividends when future review is necessary.

Tubes and Drains

Gastrointestinal Tract Tubes

Nasogastric tubes are usually used to evacuate the gastric contents. They are most commonly used in patients who have ileus or obstruction. The modern nasogastric tube is a sump-type tube. The sump function is achieved by bonding a smaller diameter tube onto the larger-bore (usually 18 Fr) tube. When the main tube is placed to continuous suction, there is a small amount of air that will be drawn in by the sump tube, preventing the development of a suction lock between the main tube and the gastric wall. Therefore, sump tubes should be placed to continuous suction. You may occasionally see a nonsump tube; these should be to intermittent suction to break the seal that forms between the tube and the gastric wall. Nasogastric tubes may also be used to feed the patient in some cases. If feeding is the intended purpose of the tube, a soft, fine-bore tube is preferable to a stiff, large-bore tube.

Nasoenteric tubes are usually intended for feeding. These should be soft and fine bore. A word about safety is in order. Nothing should be instilled into a feeding tube of any kind (nasogastric or nasoenteric) unless the position of the tube is known. Auscultation of injected air over the epigastrium can be misleading; a tube can be intrabronchial and still transmit the sound of injected air to the epigastrium. The position of a feeding tube can only be definitively confirmed with a radiograph or by direct palpation at the time of operation. Instilling tube feeds, medications, or radiographic contrast material into an intrapulmonary (or intrapleural) tube can have lethal consequences.

Nasobiliary tubes are usually placed endoscopically, either to facilitate drainage of the biliary tree when there is an obstructing process (stone, tumor, stricture) or to facilitate drainage of bile via the biliary tract in cases of biliary fistula.

T-tubes are placed within the common bile duct for the purpose of drainage. They are kept to closed gravity drainage.

Gastrostomy tubes may be placed surgically. When placed endoscopically, they are referred to as percutaneous endoscopic gastrostomy (PEG) tubes. They may be used for drainage or for feeding.

Jejunostomy tubes can be placed surgically or endoscopically (via the stomach). When placed endoscopically, they may be placed in combination with a PEG tube. These are typically placed for long-term nutritional access.

Respiratory Tract Tubes

Chest tubes are placed into the pleural cavity to evacuate air (pneumothorax), blood (hemothorax), or fluid (effusion). They are connected to a special suction system that (1) permits a constant level of suction (usually 20 cm H_2O), (2) allows drainage of air and liquid from the pleural cavity, and (3) prevents air from entering the pleural space from the outside. This latter function is known as a "water seal." These three functions can be achieved with the use of a "three bottle system," or a proprietary manufactured chest drainage and collection system.

Endotracheal tubes for adults are cuffed to maintain a seal between the tracheal wall and the tube. These tubes are used when patients need short-term mechanical ventilation or when they cannot maintain a patent airway.

Tracheotomy tubes are placed directly into the trachea via the neck. They are used for patients who require long-term mechanical ventilation or who cannot maintain a patent airway over the long term.

Urinary Tract Tubes

Bladder catheters, commonly referred to as "Foley" catheters, are placed to straight drain.

Nephrostomy tubes are usually placed in the renal pelvis to drain urine above an area of obstruction or above a delicate ureteral anastomosis.

Tubes placed percutaneously to drain abscesses are often known as pigtail catheters. They are usually placed by interventional radiologists with the help of imaging technology.

Surgical Drains

Closed suction drains (Jackson-Pratt and Hemovac are two common types) are placed intraoperatively to evacuate actual or potential fluid collections. They are usually connected to a collapsible bulb or compressible box collection receptacle.

Sump suction drains, sometimes known as Davol drains, are very large. Although they are made of silicone, they tend to be stiff. They are placed to continuous suction and are used for situations when the drainage is expected to be thick or particulate.

Passive tubes (Penrose drains) simply maintain a pathway for fluid to follow, without suction to enhance flow. These are soft, cylindrical latex drains. Because suction is not applied to them, they are very much a two-way path for bacteria.

Wound Care

In general, surgical wounds heal either by primary intention or by secondary intention (see Chapter 8, Wounds and Wound Healing). To heal by primary intention means that the wound edges have been apposed, whether by sutures, wound clips, tapes, or dermal adhesives. To heal by secondary intention means that the wound edges have been left unapposed. Usually, there is a dressing of some sort used to collect wound fluids and help keep the wound from closing prematurely. A common situation in which healing by secondary intention would be encouraged would be in the management of an abscess. A saline-moistened cotton gauze dressing is used to gently fill the cavity. (The wound cavity should not be packed tightly, because this leads to tissue ischemia.) This helps to collect drainage and to prevent the abscess cavity from sealing over. A variety of substances are used to moisten the gauze for wounds managed in this way. Some examples include 0.25% acetic acid solution, Dakin's solution (sodium hypochlorite), and povidone-iodine solutions. Each of these can be shown to inhibit fibroblast proliferation in tissue culture, and neither has any special advantage over plain, sterile saline solution.

Pain Management

It is appropriate to consider the subject of pain management in surgical patients. Physicians are often justifiably criticized for neglecting to attend to the pain of their patients as closely as they might monitor, for example, their laboratory values. Asking the patient how their pain level is should be a routine part of the review of systems taken on daily rounds, in the clinic, or in the office. For patients who cannot report pain (e.g., those in the intensive care unit, who may be mechanically ventilated and unable to speak), attention to their facial expressions and vital signs will give clues as to their level of discomfort. The nature of the patient's disease process and his or her comorbidities will determine the type of pain management strategy he or she requires. For example, many patients with thoracic or abdominal incisions are well served with epidural analgesia administered by the Anesthesia Pain Service. Where possible, intravenous patient-controlled analgesia should be used for the intense pain that accompanies the early postoperative state. Once the patient is able to take medications orally, the transition to oral pain medication is simple. In the intensive care unit, where patients may not be able to manage the patient-controlled analgesia apparatus, continuous intravenous infusions of narcotics are appropriate, and should be titrated by the nurse to keep the patient comfortable without being overly sedated.

Deep Vein Thrombosis Prophylaxis

Venous thromboembolism will afflict 25% of postoperative patients if they are afforded no prophylaxis. Surgical patients are at particular risk for venous thromboembolism because they have each of Virchow's three risk factors for venous thrombosis: stasis, hypercoagulability, and endothelial injury. A variety of means have been examined in the effort to reduce the incidence of postoperative deep vein thrombosis (DVT).

Excellent evidence-based data show that surgical patients should routinely receive such prophylaxis. Low-dose unfractionated heparin is as effective in this population as low-molecular-weight heparin, and is usually less expensive. Use of any heparin compound carries a small but real risk of heparin-induced thrombocytopenia (HIT). The low-molecular-weight heparins have a lower risk of associated HIT. While this thrombocytopenia is usually transient, there is a form, known as "white-clot syndrome," that can result in stroke, loss of limbs, or death. Thus, patients on routine heparin prophylaxis should have their platelet counts monitored at least every other day. If heparin is chosen, it should be given preoperatively to obtain the greatest protection. Intermittent pneumatic compression (IPC) devices produce reductions in DVT rates similar to those of unfractionated heparin and may be viewed as adjunctive. Their main liability is poor patient tolerance. The data regarding the prevention of venous thromboembolism by IPCs are not strong. Presently, the mainstay of venous thromboembolism prophylaxis in surgical patients is some form of subcutaneous heparin. The routine general surgical patient is well protected by the unfractionated heparin. Low-molecular-weight heparin is recommended for the trauma patient. Close communication with the anesthesiologists is important if epidural analgesia is being considered in a patient who might receive low-molecular-weight heparin, because of the risk of spinal epidural hematoma formation.

POSTOPERATIVE COMPLICATIONS

Malignant Hyperthermia

This is a potentially fatal, hypermetabolic, autosomal dominant condition of skeletal muscle that is reported to occur in one in 14,000 children and one in 50,000 adults. Several genetic mutations are associated with malignant hyperthermia, but all result in a disruption of intracellular calcium metabolism. Problems with the ryanodine receptor (calcium-release channel) are found in over 50% of patients with this disorder, while problems with the dihydropyridine receptor are found in others. The result is a massive buildup of intracellular calcium released from the sarcoplasmic reticulum. This produces violent and sustained muscle contraction and rigidity, heat production, and acidosis. Muscle necrosis and rhabdomyolysis may occur. The clinical findings in heat stroke and neuroleptic malignant syndrome are similar, and individuals prone to malignant hyperthermia are thought to be more susceptible to these other conditions. Inhalational halogenated anesthetic agents and succinylcholine are known triggers of the syndrome as are extreme stress (heat) and vigorous exercise.

A family history of relatives who have had problems with anesthetic agents may be the only preoperative clue. Susceptible individuals may be confirmed with a muscle biopsy and stimulated contraction studies.

An abrupt rise in end-tidal carbon dioxide is the first sign. Masseter muscle rigidity is seen early in the syndrome in children, but not consistently in adults. Body temperature may climb by 1° to 2° every 5 minutes and reach extraordinary levels. Temperature elevation, on the other hand, may not present for up to 36 hours after exposure to the triggering agent. Tachycardia, cyanosis, and muscle rigidity are prominent features. Compartment syndromes may develop. Rhabdomyolysis may produce myoglobinuria. Cardiac rhythm disturbances appear to be associated with the hyperkalemia and hypercalcemia that accompany muscle necrosis. Mixed respiratory and metabolic acidosis is common, and a bleeding diathesis similar to disseminated intravascular coagulopathy has been reported.

Early recognition is the key to successful treatment. Thirty years ago mortality rates ranged as high as 70% but today have been reduced to less than 5%. The first step in management is to discontinue the triggering agent. Dantrolene, a muscle relaxant that blocks calcium release from the sarcoplasmic reticulum and disrupts excitation–contraction coupling, is the only agent available for treatment. It is given by rapid intravenous push in doses of 1 mg/kg (both adults and children) and continued until symptoms subside or a maximum dose of 10 mg/kg has been reached. Dantrolene is also available in oral form, and although the absorption is slow, it is consistent. Prophylactic oral dosing is 4 to 8 mg/kg in three to four divided doses 1 to 2 days prior to elective surgery and continued for 1 to 3 days following the procedure. Patients taking oral dantrolene may notice somnolence and muscular weakness. Hyperthermia is treated by cooling blankets, but not to the point where the patient is shivering. Renal support in the form of mannitol, bicarbonate (controversial), and volume infusion is provided in the case of myoglobinuria from rhabdomyolysis. A careful search for occult compartment syndrome is made and, if found, fasciotomy is performed. Respiratory support with mechanical ventilation is frequently required to correct the respiratory component of the acidosis. Dantrolene is usually effective in managing the metabolic component of the acidosis, and bicarbonate infusion is not generally recommended. Hyperkalemia is managed in the standard fashion with exchange resins and insulin therapy if necessary. Seizure activity is treated with benzodiazepines.

Atelectasis

Despite the frequent occurrence of atelectasis — in up to 90% of patients having a general anesthetic — there is no consensus regarding its etiology, its treatment, or even its clinical significance. The definition of atelectasis varies from that of a simple collapse of the adult alveolus to one that requires clinical features of collapse or consolidation, unexplained fever (temperature > 38°C), a positive chest radiograph, or evidence of infection on sputum microbiology. That alveolar unit collapse occurs with essentially all general anesthetics, regardless of the agents used, is evident.

General anesthesia results in a reduction of functional residual capacity by 400 to 500 mL in the adult. This reduction may fall below closing volume in many patients. The supine positioning loads the diaphragm, especially if mechanical ventilation and paralytic agents are used, compressing lung tissue in the basal segments by as much as 5%. Extrapolated to the entire lung, this represents up to 20% of all functioning alveolar units. It is easy to see that obesity multiplies this effect. Under anesthesia, patients do not sigh or cough, and mucociliary cleaning of the tracheobronchial tree is impaired. Mucous plugging of small airways may result. Absorption atelectasis, the uptake of gas from the alveoli in the face of proximal obstruction, further contributes to lung unit collapse. This is especially true if high concentrations of oxygen are used for induction or during the surgery. A loss or change in the physical properties of surfactant may further contribute to the process. The effect is an increase in shunt fraction, that is, low ventilation:perfusion ratio, resulting in hypoxia. The postoperative period is characterized by incisional pain, somnolence from analgesic use, suppressed cough, lack of mobility, and nasopharyngeal instrumentation. These factors all contribute to perpetuation of a situation in which tidal ventilation is reduced and periodic reexpansion of collapsed alveolar units by maximum inspiratory efforts is suppressed.

Debate continues over whether atelectasis is associated with fever or whether the condition predisposes (or is the prodrome) to more serious respiratory problems such as pneumonia or the adult respiratory distress syndrome. There is experimental evidence that atelectasis alters host defenses, but the clinical significance of these findings has yet to be elucidated.

Management of postoperative atelectasis should begin preoperatively, under ideal conditions, by encouraging cessation of smoking for 8 weeks preoperatively and the institution of inspiratory exercises. Chest physiotherapy may also begin, particularly for patients with productive cough or chronic bronchitis. Reexpansion techniques (incentive spirometry) are appropriate for all patients. Some may even benefit from chest physiotherapy. The most important strategies involve adequate postoperative pain management, frequently obtained with epidural analgesia, and early mobilization. One of the advantages of minimally invasive surgery is the significant reduction in atelectasis as well as other more serious pulmonary problems. Pharmacologic interventions and diaphragmatic pacing have not enjoyed much clinical success or enthusiasm, although these interventions are still practiced in some centers.

Surgical Wound Failure

Wound healing is a complex, but predictable and highly orchestrated, series of cellular, hormonal, and molecular actions that are initiated at the time of injury. The details of wound healing are discussed in detail in Chapter 8, Wounds and Wound Healing. Acute wound healing failure involves an alteration in this process as the result of mechanical forces, infections, or aberrations of the normal biologic response of injured tissue.

Dehiscence, or acute surgical wound failure resulting in disruption of the fascial closure, is acute mechanical failure of the surgical closure. The force exerted across the wound is greater than the strength of suture material or of the fascia itself. This latter failure is generally due to ischemia of the tissue from suture material placed too tightly or becoming too tight as edema develops at the site of wounding. Poor suturing technique is also to blame. Local infection can also lead to destruction of the fascia.

The spontaneous discharge of serous fluid from a wound is a sign heralding acute fascial dehiscence. These patients should be returned expeditiously to the operating room for examination and repair of the closure. Perhaps nothing is more dramatic, for both patient and doctor, than witnessing dehiscence of the abdominal closure and evisceration of the abdominal organs. In such a case, the exposed organs should be covered with sterile towels soaked in saline solution and the patient taken to the operating room immediately. Occasionally, a deep space infection — a subphrenic, pelvic, or interloop abscess — is associated with this problem. See Chapter 9, Surgical Infections, for further discussion of intraabdominal infections.

Surgical Site Infection

It is estimated that over 500,000 cases of surgical site infections occur in the more than 27 million operative procedures performed yearly, representing one-quarter of all nosocomial infections. The frequency varies from hospital to hospital, surgeon to surgeon, operation to operation, and patient to patient. There has been little change in the incidence or distribution of surgical site infections in the past 15 years, but emerging antibiotic-resistant organisms are becoming more of a problem. Surgical site infections increase the length of hospital stay and hospital costs. Furthermore, acute wound failure can have devastating consequences in the form of fascial dehiscence, pseudo-aneurysm formation, anastomotic leak, fistula formation, incisional hernia, deep space infection, and mortality.

Factors contributing to surgical site infections are discussed in Chapter 9, Surgical Infections. Signs of surgical site infections are those associated with inflammation: redness (rubor), swelling (tumor), localized heat and erythema (calor), and increased pain at the incision site (dolor). Tachycardia may be the first sign and fever may develop only later. Spontaneous drainage from the surgical wound indicates that there has been a delay in recognition of this postoperative problem. Delay in recognition leads to destruction of the fascia and contributes to dehiscence or incisional hernias. Prompt drainage minimizes these sequelae and antibiotics play a secondary role, unless there are extenuating circumstances. Failure of the patient's tachycardia, fever, or ileus to resolve should suggest a deeper site of infection, and additional diagnostic studies may be necessary. Occasionally the diagnosis is made by surgical exploration.

Guidelines have been developed by the Centers for Disease Control to minimize the incidence of surgical site infections and are shown in Table 2-19.

Table 2-19 Center for Disease Control Surgical Site Infections Prevention Guidelines, 1999

Recommendation	Strength of Recommendation
Do not remove hair unless it interferes with the operation	1A
If removed, remove immediately before operation with electric clippers	1A
Shower or bathe with antiseptic agent night before surgery	1B
Surgeon performs surgical scrub for 2–5 min with appropriate antiseptic	1B
After scrubbing, keep hands up and away from body; dry hands with sterile towel; don sterile gown and gloves	1B
Identify and treat all remote infections before surgery	1A
Keep hospital stay as short as possible	II
Administer antimicrobial agent only when indicated and select based on published recommendations for a specific operation and efficacy against most common pathogens	1A
Administer antimicrobial agents by IV timed to ensure bactericidal serum and tissue levels when incision made	1A
Maintain therapeutic levels during operation and, at most, a few hours after closure	1A
Before colorectal elective operations, in addition to IV antibiotics, mechanically prep the colon with cathartic agents and enemas; administer nonabsorbable oral antimicrobial agents in individual doses the day before surgery	1A
For cesarean sections in patients at high risk, administer IV antimicrobial agents immediately after cord is clamped	1A
Do not use vancomycin routinely for prophylaxis	1B

1A = Strongly recommended for implementation and supported by well-designed experimental, clinical, or epidemiologic studies.
1B = Strongly recommended for implementation and supported by some experimental, clinical, or epidemiologic studies and strong theoretical rationale.
II = Suggested for implementation and supported by suggestive clinical or epidemiologic studies or theoretical rationale.
Modified from Mangram AJ, Horan TC, Pearson MI, et al. The Hospital Infection Control Practices Advisory Committee. Guideline for prevention of surgical site infection 1999. *Infect Control Hosp Epidemiol* 1999;20:247–280; used with permission.

Fever

An elevation in a patient's core temperature postoperatively is so common that many mistakenly consider it a normal postoperative state. Next to requests for laxatives, analgesics, and sleep aids, calls from the nursing staff regarding temperature elevation are perhaps the most common. If asked to define fever, most will offer a simple thermal definition without the important corollaries as to time of day, anatomic site of temperature determination, or the apparatus used to take the measurement. The benchmark of 37°C as normal body temperature was established circa 1868 and has only recently been critically reviewed. To describe fever in purely thermal terms is a misleading oversimplification. The febrile response is a complex physiologic reaction to a stimulus that involves not only a cytokine-mediated rise in core temperature, but also the generation of acute phase proteins and activation of the endocrine and immune systems (Table 2-20). The pure thermal definition of fever is further flawed because it implies a single entity when in fact it represents a pasticcio of many different temperatures, each representing a different body region and state of activity. Additionally, fever should not be confused with hyperthermia, which is a rise in body temperature not associated with a pyrogen.

The causes of fever are multiple and include noninfectious (Table 2-21) as well as infectious etiologies (Table 2-22). The Society of Critical Care Medicine has adopted the guideline that a temperature elevation to 38.3°C is the trigger to initiate an investigation. The evaluation process begins with a review of the circumstances surrounding the patient: patient location (intensive care unit versus ward),

Table 2-20 Characteristics of the Febrile State

Endocrine and Metabolic
Increased production of glucocorticoids
Increased secretion of growth hormone
Increased secretion of aldosterone
Decreased secretion of vasopressin
Decreased levels of divalent cations (necessary for bacterial replication)
Secretion of acute phase proteins
Autonomic
Shift in blood flow from cutaneous to deep
Increased pulse and blood pressure
Decreased sweating
Behavioral
Shivering (rigors)
Search for warmth (chills)
Anorexia
Somnolence
Malaise

Adapted from Saper CB, Breder CD. The neurologic basis of fever. *New Engl J Med* 1994;330(26):1880–1886; used with permission.

Table 2-21 Noninfectious Causes of Fever

Alcohol/drug withdrawal
Atelectasis
Posttransfusion fever
Drug fever
Cerebral infarction/hemorrhage
Brain injury
Adrenal insufficiency
Myocardial infarction
Pancreatitis
Acalculous cholecystitis
Ischemic bowel
Aspiration pneumonitis
ARDS
Subarachnoid hemorrhage
Fat emboli
Transplant rejection
Deep vein thrombosis/phlebitis
Pulmonary emboli
Gout/pseudogout
IV contrast reaction
GI bleeding
Cirrhosis (without primary peritonitis)
Neoplasia
Decubitus ulcer

ARDS, adult respiratory distress syndrome; GI, gastrointestinal; IV, intravenous. Some conditions have been classified as both infectious and noninfectious, for example, acalculous cholecystitis, phlebitis. The classification, obviously, depends on whether the condition is associated with bacterial infection.
Adapted from Marik PE. Fever in the ICU. *Chest* 2000;117(3):855–869. Used with permission.

length of hospitalization, presence of mechanical ventilation and its duration, instrumentation (e.g., catheters, vascular lines, tubes in the nose or chest), duration of the instrumentation, medications, surgical sites and the reason for the surgical procedure (e.g., elective, emergent, trauma, gastrointestinal tract), current treatments, and diagnosis. This first step, if performed carefully and thoughtfully, will indicate the direction the doctor should take to investigate the cause of the fever. Secondly, a directed physical examination is performed to look for clues and/or confirmation of a suspected source. Table 2-22 can be used as a checklist to guide the evaluation process. Only after these two steps have been taken should consideration be given to ordering diagnostic studies. Undirected blanket ordering of laboratory tests, random cultures, and radiographs are appropriate only in very specific circumstances (for example, patients on prolonged mechanical ventilation, those who are immunosuppressed, or those with indwelling catheters or monitoring devices). For the majority of postoperative surgical patients, a selective approach to confirmatory testing is cost-efficient, effective, and high-quality medical practice.

The most common nosocomial infectious causes of fever in the intensive care units are ventilator-associated pneumonia, sinusitis, catheter-related sepsis (primarily Gram-negative), *Clostridium difficile* colitis, abdominal sepsis, and complicated wound infections. Notably absent from this list are urinary tract infections. Unless it is pyelonephritis, a urinary tract infection is rarely a cause of fever. The standard definition of a urinary tract infection (a colony count $> 10^5$ CFU/mL) does not apply to catheterized intensive care patients. Further, bacteriuria and urinary tract infection are not synonymous. Most patients with urinary catheters for more than 24 hours will have bacteria or white cells in the urine, and this should not trigger antimicrobial therapy.

Once the diagnosis is established, appropriate therapeutic steps can be taken. As mentioned previously, in a few select clinical circumstances it is appropriate to use broad-spectrum antibiotics. Generally speaking, these situations involve critically ill patients in whom withholding antibiotic therapy for 24 to 48 hours until definitive cultures or diagnostic studies are completed could lead to disastrous consequences. Most intensivists select broad-spectrum drugs, chosen on the basis of sensitivity profiles of their own units, and then switch to more focused therapy when the cultures return.

The question arises as to whether the fever itself should be treated with antipyretics. Much divergent opinion on this issue exists, and there is little prospective scientific evidence to support either position. Fever is an adaptive response that conferred a survival advantage on warm-blooded animals. Temperature elevation enhances immune function by increasing antibody production; increasing cytokine expression; enhancing neutrophil, lymphocyte, and macrophage function; and reducing bacterial replication. Temperature elevation also confers a resistance to bacterial invasion. Still, some health care pro-

Table 2-22 Physical Examination Checklist for Investigating Cause of a Fever

Anatomic Site	Clue
Head and Neck	
Sinusitis/Otitis	Nasal/oral instrumentation/facial fracture
Meningitis	Skull fracture/instrumentation/craniotomy/CSF leak
Parotitis	Elderly/periodontal disease/dehydration/oral instrumentation
Periodontal abscess	Periodontal disease
Peritonsillar/pharingeal abscess	Immunosuppression/facial fracture
Deep neck infection	Surgery/penetrating injury (especially digestive tract)/periodontal disease
Thorax	
Pneumonitis/lung abscess	Intubation/mechanical ventilation/contusion/penetrating injury/aspiration
Mediastinitis	Esophageal injury/sternotomy/neck exploration/penetrating thoracic injury
Empyema	Hemothorax/tube thoracostomy/duration of thoracic instrumentation
Endocarditis	Central vascular access/TPN/valvular disease (e.g., MVP)/periodontal disease
Pericarditis	Sternotomy/pericardial window/penetrating injury
Bronchitis/tracheitis (?)	Instrumentation
Esophagitis (?)	Immunosuppression/broad-spectrum antibiotics
Abdomen and retroperitoneum	
Intraabdominal abscess	Previous celiotomy/splenectomy/visceral organ repair/anastomosis/enteric contamination/bullet tract/possible missed injury
Acalculous cholecystitis	
Ischemic viscera	
Colitis	Age/hypotension/broad-spectrum antibiotics/diabetes
Pancreatitis (necrotizing)	Mesenteric injury/hypotension/pressors
Urinary tract	
Prostatitis	Broad-spectrum antibiotic use/diarrhea
Primary peritonitis	Hypotension/biliary stones/splenectomy/direct injury
Pylephlebitis	
Occult perirectal abscess	Bladder instrumentation/comorbid urinary tract disease/urinary tract injury/diabetes
Diverticular disease/appendicitis	Instrumentation/duration/age
TOA/endometritis	Hepatic failure/cirrhosis/ascites
	Intraabdominal process/abscess
	Hematogenous malignancy/diabetes/immunosuppression/perineal injury
	Preexisting condition/age/suspicion (?)
	Preexisting disease/direct injury
Extremities	
Occult compartment syndrome	Unconscious/extremity fracture/casts/hypotensive episodes/immobilization (gluteal compartments)/crush injury
Phlebitis/arteritis	Duration of hospitalization/instrumentation/injury
Wounds (surgical or traumatic)	
Superficial or deep abscess	Presence/contamination/time to definitive management/GI tract injury/diabetes/vascular disease
Necrotizing soft tissue infection	GI injury/diabetes/immunosuppression
Necrotizing myositis/ischemia	Occult compartment syndrome/unconsciousness
Decubitus ulceration/abscess	Immobilization

CSF, cerebrospinal fluid; GI, gastrointestinal; MVP, ; TOA, ; TPN, total parenteral nutrition.

viders feel that fever is harmful and noxious and should be suppressed. The conclusions that can be drawn from the literature are summarized as follows:

Short courses of antipyretics in approved doses carry a low risk of toxic side effects.

The benefits of antipyretic use to the patient are uncertain, other than perhaps the analgesic effect. The loss of the immunoprotective effects of fever is concerning and potentially harmful. There are no good comparative data on this issue.

The increase in metabolic demand (10% for each degree Celsius increase) associated with fever may be poorly tolerated in the elderly or debilitated, especially those with cardiac or pulmonary conditions.

Children should not be given aspirin.

Antipyretics do not prevent febrile seizures or raise the seizure threshold.

Cooling blankets should not be used to treat fever (although they are used to treat hyperthermia). The patient should not be cooled to the point of inducing shivering.

If antipyretics are used, they should be used on a scheduled basis and not as the occasion arises.

Indomethacin and nonsteroidal antiinflammatory drugs should not be used in patients with coronary artery disease.

Anything that increases the cerebral metabolic rate in patients with traumatic brain injuries (e.g., fever, seizures) increases cerebral oxygen demand and cerebral blood flow. This can increase intracranial pressure.

SUGGESTED READINGS

Ang-Lee MK, Moss J, Yuan CS. Herbal medicines and perioperative care. *JAMA* 2001;286(2):208–216.

Brooks-Brunn JA. Predictors of postoperative pulmonary complications following abdominal surgery. *Chest* 1997;111(3):564–571.

Dajani AS, Taubert KA, Wilson W, et al. Prevention of bacterial endocarditis: recommendations by the American Heart Association. *Circulation* 1997;96(1):358–366.

Denbrough M. Malignant hyperthermia. *Lancet* 1998;352(9134): 1131–1136.

Dubay DA, Franz MG. Acute wound healing: the biology of acute wound failure. *Surg Clin North Am* 2003;83(3):463–481.

Eagle KA, Berger PB, Calkins H, et al. ACC/AHA guideline update for perioperative cardiovascular evaluation for noncardiac surgery: a report of the American College of Cardiology/American Heart Association Task Force on Practice Guidelines (Committee to update the 1996 Guidelines on Perioperative Cardiovascular Evaluation for Non-cardiac Surgery). *J Am Coll Cardiol* 2002;39:542–553.

Geerts WH, Heit JA, Clagett GP, et al. Prevention of venous thromboembolism. *Chest* 2001;119(Suppl):132S–175S.

Hedenstierna G. Airway closure, atelectasis and gas exchange during anesthesia. *Minerva Anesth* 2002;68(5):332–336.

Hyers TM. Management of venous thromboembolism: Past, present and future. *Arch Intern Med* 2003;163:759–768.

Kearon C. Natural history of venous thromboembolism. *Circulation* 2003;107(23 Suppl 1):122–130.

Kroegel C, Reissig A. Principle mechanisms underlying venous thromboembolism: epidemiology, risk factors, pathophysiology and pathogenesis. *Respiration* 2003;70(1):7–30.

Marik PE. Fever in the ICU. *Chest* 2000;117(3):855–869.

Malangoni MA. Gastrointestinal surgery and pregnancy. *Gastroenterol Clin North Am* 2003;32(12):181–200.

Massard G, Wihlm JM. Postoperative atelectasis. *Chest Surg Clin North Am* 1998;8(3):503–528.

Nichols RL, Florman S. Clinical presentation of soft tissue infections and surgical site infections. *Clin Infect Dis* 2001;33(Suppl 2): S84–S93.

O'Grady NP, Barie PS, Bartlett J, et al. Practice parameters for evaluating new fever in critically ill adults. *Crit Care Med* 1998;26(2):392–408.

Platell C, Hall JC. Atelectasis after abdominal surgery. *J Am Coll Surg* 1997;185:584–592.

Roizen MF, Foss JF, Fisher SP. Preoperative evaluation. In: Miller RD, ed. *Anesthesia.* 5th Ed. Philadelphia, PA: Churchill Livingston, 2000:824–883.

Smetana GW, Macpherson DS. The case against routine preoperative laboratory testing. *Med Clin North Am* 2003;87(1):7–40.

3

SUSAN KAISER, MD ■ CLAUDIA CORWIN, MD
HILARY SANFEY, MD ■ DAVID ANTONENKO, MD

Fluids, Electrolytes, and Acid–Base Balance

OBJECTIVES

1 Know the range of normal values of Na^+, K^+, HCO_3^-, and Cl^- in serum, gastric aspirate, bile, and ileostomy aspirate.

2 Understand the contributions that extracellular, intracellular, and intravascular volumes make to body weight and how they vary with age and obesity.

3 List four hormones or substrates that affect renal absorption and excretion of sodium and water.

4 Compare the physical findings or symptoms of dehydration in the young and the elderly.

5 Understand the methods of determining fluid balance.

6 Describe the typical 24-hour fluid and electrolyte needs in the postoperative patient who has no complications.

7 Explain the composition of electrolytes in normal saline, lactated Ringer's solution, and 5% dextrose in water.

8 Given a patient with the condition in the left column, list the direction of change in values and pH for the serum electrolytes observed.

	Na K HCO_3 Cl pH
Excessive gastric losses	______
High-volume pancreatic fistula	______
Small intestinal fistula	______
Biliary fistula	______
Diarrhea	______
Closed head injury	______

9 Given a patient with the condition listed, determine an appropriate replacement fluid.

a. Pyloric outlet obstruction
b. Pancreatic fistula
c. Small bowel fistula
d. Biliary fistula
e. Diarrhea
f. Closed head injury
g. Massive blood loss

10 Indicate the direction of change in serum and urine values that might be obtained in patients with each condition listed in the left column.

Serum

	Na K HCO_3 Cl Osmolarity
Acute vasomotor nephropathy	______
Dehydration	______
Inappropriate ADH secretion	______
Diabetes insipidus	______
Congestive heart failure	______

Urine

	Na	K	HCO_3	Cl	Osmolarity
Acute vasomotor nephropathy	______				
Dehydration	______				
Inappropriate ADH secretion	______				
Diabetes insipidus	______				
Congestive heart failure	______				

11 List the differential diagnosis and treatment for each of the following conditions:

a. Hypernatremia
b. Hyponatremia
c. Hyperkalemia
d. Hypokalemia
e. Hyperchloremia
f. Hypochloremia
g. Hypercalcemia
h. Hypocalcemia
i. Hypermagnesemia
j. Hypomagnesemia
k. Hypophosphatemia

12 Indicate the directional change in values expected in patients with each condition listed in the left column:

Arterial Blood

	pH	Pao_2	$Paco_2$	HCO_3	Base Excess
Acute metabolic acidosis	______				
Acute respiratory acidosis	______				
Chronic respiratory acidosis	______				
Compensated metabolic acidosis	______				

Understanding and managing volume, electrolyte, and acid–base status is an integral part of the treatment of a surgical patient. Before discussing specific clinical problems, this chapter provides an overview of fluid, electrolyte, and acid–base balance. This chapter is intended to be an introduction to the subject material; for more complete and comprehensive information, see the many available texts and articles in the literature, some of which are listed at the end of this chapter. A table of **normal serum laboratory values** is provided in the glossary.

NORMAL PHYSIOLOGY

Total Body Water and Compartments

Total body water (TBW) in the adult is 45% to 70% of body weight. This value varies as a function of age, sex, and lean body mass. It is lowest in the aged and obese and highest in the very lean and young. TBW is estimated as 60% of body weight in the idealized 70-kg adult male and 50% to 55% in his female counterpart. In both, the TBW is directly proportional to muscle mass and inversely proportional to fat content, because muscle is about 70% water and fat is about 10% water. Consequently, TBW may be as little as 35% of weight in the morbidly obese or the very elderly, who lose muscle mass as they age.

TBW is partitioned into two main compartments. In the idealized lean male, the intracellular space represents about two-thirds of TBW (40% of body weight, or about 28 L in a 70-kg man), and the extracellular space one-third (20% of body weight, or about 14 L) in the average adult (Figure 3-1). This ratio changes as muscle mass decreases to a more common 60:40 ratio in most of today's population. The extracellular compartment is further divided into the interstitial space (16% TBW) and the intravascular fluid space (4% TBW).

There is little difference in the electrolyte composition of the two extracellular fluid subdivisions. In plasma (Table 3-1), sodium is the chief extracellular cation, with small amounts of potassium, calcium, and magnesium also

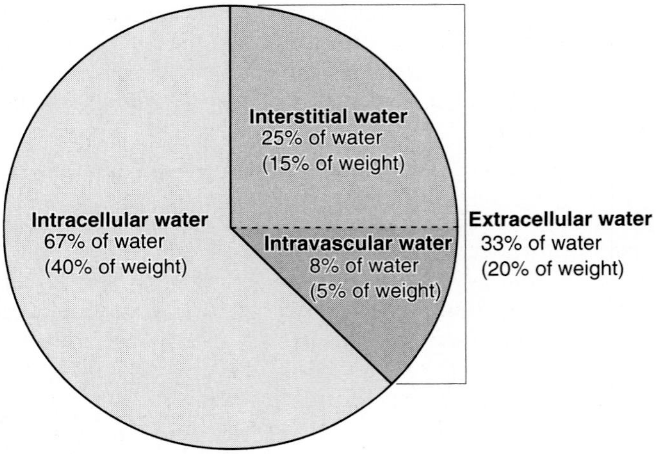

Figure 3-1 Total body water in the adult male, expressed as percentages of total body water and of body weight.

Table 3-1 Normal Plasma Values of Common Electrolytes

Electrolytes	Concentration	Units
Cations		
Sodium	135–145	mEq/L
Potassium	3.5–5.0	mEq/L
Calcium	8.0–10.5	mg/dL
Magnesium	1.5–2.5	mEq/L
Anions		
Chloride	95–105	mEq/L
Bicarbonate	24–30	mEq/L
Phosphate	2.5–4.5	mEq/L
Sulfate	1.0	mEq/L
Organic acids	2.0	mEq/L
Total protein	6.0–8.4	g/dL

present. The corresponding anions are chloride, bicarbonate, and smaller amounts of proteins, phosphates, sulfates, and organic acids. In the interstitial fluid space the ionic composition differs from plasma only with respect to its lower concentration of protein and the related minor changes in chloride and bicarbonate levels. In contrast to the extracellular compartment, the intracellular dominant cations are potassium and magnesium, and the dominant anions are phosphates, sulfates, and proteins. The striking differences in intracellular and extracellular electrolyte composition are maintained by the selective permeabilities of cellular membranes. Free diffusion of proteins, chloride, and multivalent ions is limited, and active metabolic "pumps" in the cell wall promote the movement of sodium out of the cell and the passage of potassium into it.

Movement of water from one compartment to another is passive and is determined by the action of physical forces exerted across the intervening membranes. The capillary membrane that separates the interstitial and intravascular spaces under most circumstances is freely permeable to water, electrolytes, and solutes, but not to proteins. Consequently, the net flow of water between these two spaces is a function of the balance between fluid pressures generated on either side of the membrane and the effective **colloid osmotic pressures** generated by the higher concentrations of nondiffusible protein in the plasma. On the other hand, the exchange of water between the intracellular and interstitial compartments is totally determined by osmotic gradients across the cell membranes. Normally, there is no gradient and no significant net water flow in either direction because the **osmolarity,** or number of osmotically active particles per liter of solution on either side of the membrane, is the same. When extracellular fluid becomes hypoosmolar relative to normal values, water flows into the cells in which the osmolarity is higher. A new equilibrium is reached, and the osmolarity of both compartments is less than the normal 285 mOsm/L. Similarly, hyperosmolarity develops in both compartments if extracellular osmolarity is increased. In this case, osmotic equilibrium is reached by an egress of water from the cell into the extracellular space. In contrast, isotonic fluid expansion or contraction of the extracellular space, which has no effect on osmolarity, does not include such movements of water between the cells and the interstitial fluid.

Sodium

Total body sodium is estimated as 40 mEq/kg. One-third is fixed in bone, and the other two-thirds, most of which is extracellular, is the exchangeable fraction. Sodium and its related anions represent 97% of the osmotically active particles that are normally present in the extracellular fluid compartments. Extracellular osmolarity is estimated by the formula:

$$\text{Osmolarity} = 2 \times [\text{Na}]_s + [\text{glucose (mg)/dL} \div 18] + [\text{blood urea nitrogen (BUN)} \div 2.8],$$

where $[\text{Na}]_s$ is serum sodium concentration. If the value approximates 290 ± 10 mOsm/L, it can be reasonably assumed that extracellular osmolarity is within normal limits.

The normal adult sodium requirement is 1 to 2 mEq/kg/day, although the usual intake far exceeds this amount. Fairly constant body sodium content is maintained by normal kidneys that excrete sodium when intake is high and conserve it when intake is low. Renal sodium resorption can be so efficient that nearly none is lost in the urine during maximum conservation. Assuming normal renal perfusion and membrane function, sodium and water are both filtered at the glomerulus. In the proximal tubules, large amounts of each are recovered. Ultimately, however, the determination of renal conservation or excretion of sodium or water depends on selective processes that occur at more distal tubular sites.

Sodium resorption in exchange for potassium and hydrogen ion secretion in the distal tubules is a direct effect of the adrenal cortical hormone **aldosterone.** This action helps to maintain both extracellular volume and osmolarity. Extracellular volume reduction, particularly in the intravascular space, is a potent stimulus for aldosterone release. This response is triggered by a decrease in renal perfusion, which causes the juxtaglomerular apparatus to secrete renin. Renin, in turn, cleaves angiotensinogen to produce angiotensin I, which is then converted by angiotensin-converting enzyme to angiotensin II, a potent stimulator of aldosterone secretion. Volume receptors in the right atrium, when activated, cause aldosterone secretion. The juxtaglomerular apparatus and its renin–angiotensin–mediated aldosterone secretion are also activated by low extracellular fluid sodium concentrations. Aldosterone secretion can also be stimulated by an increase in serum potassium levels and by the action of adrenocorticotropic hormone (ACTH). The secretion of aldosterone is suppressed by extracellular volume expansion, increased sodium concentration, and decreased potassium concentration.

Antidiuretic hormone (ADH), which is released from the posterior pituitary, has a potent direct effect on the kidney: it increases tubular resorption of water. This effect and its modulation are important in the regulation of fluid volume and osmolarity in the body. Intracranial osmoreceptors are the sensors that initiate the events that promote ADH secretion when plasma osmolarity increases. They also inhibit ADH secretion when plasma osmolarity decreases. The production and release of ADH also depend on the activity of volume receptors in the right and left atria. Decreased extracellular volume sensed in the right atrium leads to ADH secretion. Increased volume sensed in the left atrium leads to inhibition of ADH release. Volume-dependent responses usually override the effects of the osmoreceptor controlling system when the two are in conflict. ADH acts at the level of the collecting ducts, increasing the permeability of the apical membrane of the cell to water.

Potassium

In the normal adult, total body stores of potassium are approximately 50 to 55 mEq/kg, 98% of which is intracellular at a concentration of 150 mEq/L cell water. In the extracellular fluid compartment, a total of 70 mEq (including plasma) is present at a concentration of 3.5 to 5.0 mEq/L. Although the normal adult daily potassium requirement is 0.5 to 0.8 mEq/kg/day, the normal daily potassium intake averages 100 mEq, 95% of which is excreted in the urine and 5% of which is lost in feces and sweat. In the kidney, most of the filtered potassium is resorbed in the proximal tubular system. Nevertheless, selective secretion or absorption in the distal tubule determines net renal excretion or conservation. Unlike its ability to conserve sodium, the kidney can only decrease potassium excretion to approximately 10 mEq/L. Potassium excretion is directly related to circulating levels of aldosterone, cellular and extracellular potassium content, and tubular urine flow rates. Acid–base disturbances also exert significant influence.

Acid–Base Balance

Acid–base balance is in effect the management of large amounts of hydrogen ion that are produced endogenously each day. There is a 40- to 60-mmol load of fixed nonvolatile organic acids (i.e., sulfuric, phosphoric, and lactic acids), some of which are ingested and some of which are produced by metabolic activity. In addition, 13,000 to 20,000 mmol carbon dioxide constitutes the volatile acid load. Normally, the free hydrogen ion concentration of extracellular body fluids, measured as pH, is maintained at 7.40 ± 0.05 (40 nmol/L). Maintenance at this level is accomplished by the combined action of three mechanisms: (1) buffering systems that are present in body fluids and that immediately offset changes in hydrogen ion concentrations; (2) pulmonary ventilation changes that can promptly adjust the excretion of carbon dioxide; and (3) renal tubular function, which, over time, can contribute by modulating the urinary excretion or conservation of acid or base.

The bicarbonate–carbonic acid buffer system in extracellular fluid is one of the most important factors. Its relation to pH is described by the Henderson-Hasselbalch equation and its modifications:

$$
\begin{aligned}
pH &= pK^a + \log [HCO_3^-]/[H_2CO_3] \\
pH &= 6.1 + \log [HCO_3^-]/0.03 \times Pa_{CO_2} \\
7.4 &= 6.1 + \log 24\ mEq/L/1.20\ mEq/L
\end{aligned}
$$

A more useful variation of these equations is:

$$[H+] = 24 \times Pa_{CO_2}/[HCO_3^-].$$

The value for $[H_2CO_3]$ can be determined as the arithmetic product of a proportionality constant and the Pa_{CO_2}. In clinical practice, direct measurements of arterial pH and Pa_{CO_2} are readily available, and $[HCO_3^-]$ can be calculated or derived from a nomogram, assuming all measurements are reliable. The pH is determined by the ratio $[HCO_3^-]/[H_2CO_3]$, which normally is approximately 20:1. A change in either the numerator or the denominator can alter the ratio and the resulting pH value. In addition, a change of either $[H_2CO_3]$ or Pa_{CO_2} can be compensated for by a corresponding change in the same direction of the other, restoring the ratio to 20:1 and the pH to 7.40. Thus, pulmonary regulation of Pa_{CO_2} and renal tubular regulation of plasma HCO_3^- are important determinants of extracellular pH.

As effective as the $[HCO_3^-]/[H_2CO_3]$ buffer system is, and as available as its substrates are from metabolic sources, even in combination with all other extracellular buffers it cannot maintain arterial pH at normal levels in the face of all challenges. Intracellular buffer systems play a major role. As much as 50% of fixed acid loads and 95% of hydrogen ion changes that result from excessive retention or excretion of carbon dioxide are buffered in the cells. The movement of hydrogen into and out of the cell involves cationic exchanges that cause reciprocal shifts of potassium. Thus, **acidosis,** in which hydrogen ions move from an area of high concentration (extracellular) to an area of low concentration (intracellular), causes potassium to move out of the cell. As a result, the potassium concentration of extracellular fluid increases. On average, for every 0.1 change in pH, the K+ changes in an inverse manner by about 0.3 mEq/L. **Alkalosis,** in which hydrogen ions move from an area of high concentration (intracellular) to one of low concentration (extracellular), causes the opposite movement of potassium into the cell. As a result, the extracellular potassium concentration decreases. Thus, acidosis is associated with hyperkalemia, and alkalosis is associated with hypokalemia. The usual assumption of a direct relation between serum levels and total body stores of potassium is no longer valid. Changes in serum potassium concentration that are induced by acid–base alterations can have significant clinical implications, particularly with regard to myocardial irritability and function.

FLUIDS AND ELECTROLYTES IN THE PERIOPERATIVE PERIOD

The three components of fluid and electrolyte therapy for surgical patients are (1) maintenance, (2) resuscitation, and (3) replacement. The first component involves meeting the requirements for fluid and electrolyte intake that balance daily obligatory losses. The second component involves recognizing and repairing imbalances and deficits that are already present. The third component involves providing for ongoing and additional losses that occur during the course of therapy. Each component must be addressed in the three phases of surgical care (i.e., preoperative, intraoperative, and postoperative). With each component of therapy, comorbidities such as the presence of cardiac or renal disease and the pathophysiology of the clinical condition being treated must also be considered.

With no unusual stresses or losses and normal renal function, the fluid and electrolyte balance is maintained by the intake of adequate amounts of water, sodium, potassium, and chloride to balance daily obligatory losses. Intake is calculated to balance outputs of 12 to 15 mL/kg/day urine, 3 mL/kg stool water, 0 to 1.5 mL/kg sweat, 10 mL/kg combined insensible losses from lungs and skin, and an endogenous input of approximately 3 mL/kg water derived from the oxidation of carbohydrate and fat. These estimates apply to adults; more universal guidelines for calculating fluid and electrolyte requirements have also been devised. Probably the most accurate are based on surface area, but they are cumbersome, requiring measurements of height as well as weight and a nomogram for transposing the measurements into a value for surface. For this reason, the common practice is to determine water and electrolyte needs as a function of age and weight. Guidelines for using both methods are shown in Tables 3-2 and 3-3. If the entire intake is to be delivered intravenously, 5% dextrose in water is used to meet most of the fluid requirements because the kidney reabsorbs nearly all of the sodium and chloride that the body needs. The fluid used to replace ongoing losses or existing deficits should reflect the composition of the deficits or losses as much as possible. Usually, 0.45% or 0.9% saline can be given to provide the necessary sodium and chloride. Potassium is added in divided amounts to the various solutions. In this way, its delivery is spread out over time.

Table 3-3 Daily Electrolyte Requirements

Electrolyte	Per m^2	Example: 70 kg, 175 cm male
Sodium	50–75 mEq	92–140 mEq
Potassium	50 mEq	92 mEq
Chloride	50–75 mEq	92–140 mEq

Overall estimates of daily needs must be adjusted for fever and high ambient temperatures. Insensible skin and pulmonary losses increase with elevations of body temperature (10% to 15%/°C, 8%/°F), often requiring an additional 500 mL or more of salt-free water per day in febrile patients. Similar needs for more water because of increased pulmonary insensible losses occur in patients with tracheostomies who are inspiring unhumidified air or gas mixtures, especially with hyperventilation. In a slightly different way, requirements for both salt and water increase when ambient temperatures rise to more than 32°C (85°F). This increase is caused by hypotonic salt losses from sweating. Additional intravenous fluid replacement with 0.45% saline solution is appropriate in this case.

As with all aspects of good surgical care, the management of fluid and electrolyte balance starts with assessment. The surgeon uses the information obtained from a thorough history and physical examination to identify current or potential problems and determine what laboratory data are needed to confirm the problem. Preoperative risk assessment is essential before surgery. The initial workup could reveal underlying cardiac, pulmonary, renal, or hepatic disease. These findings may significantly influence the conduct of fluid therapy during and after the operation. In these cases, if stressful surgery is contemplated (e.g., abdominal aortic aneurysmectomy, pulmonary or pancreatic resection), the need for central venous or pulmonary arterial pressure monitoring in the perioperative period becomes apparent. A history of diuretic and digitalis therapy can call attention to the presence of hypokalemia or hyponatremia. Low preoperative serum potassium levels can fall even lower during surgery, particularly in patients who are under general anesthesia, are hyperventilated, and have hypocapnic respiratory alkalosis. If

Table 3-2 Daily Fluid Requirements

	Adult, Per Kilogram			Child > 5 kg, Per Kilogram		
Per m^2	25–55 YO	55–65 YO	> 65 YO	1st 10 kg	2nd 10 kg	> 20 kg
1200 mL	35	30	25	100	50	20

hyponatremia is present on admission, the margin of safety between asymptomatic and symptomatic low serum sodium concentrations is reduced, making even relatively small further decreases potentially hazardous. Depending on the extent of the planned surgery, a patient with chronic pulmonary obstructive disease may need an arterial blood gas evaluation as part of the preoperative workup. Similarly, BUN, serum creatinine, and electrolyte studies are indicated in a patient who has a history of chronic renal disease. With any of these disorders, any deficits and ongoing needs must be addressed in the preoperative period.

Fluid, electrolyte, and acid–base imbalances must be identified and treated promptly in patients who are acutely ill on admission. This requirement is even more important in patients who need urgent operation. The admitting history and physical examination should clarify the problem. Appropriate directed laboratory data should be obtained immediately. In patients who are vomiting or who have had prolonged gastric drainage, the presence of hypokalemic hypochloremic metabolic alkalosis should be anticipated, rapidly confirmed, and treated with replacement of volume, potassium, and chloride losses. In these circumstances, profound potassium depletion is present if the urine pH is acidic (this **paradoxical aciduria** is explained in more detail later). If emergency surgery is indicated, potassium replacement may need to be given in 10- to 20-mEq/hr boluses and the patient must be monitored electrocardiographically.

Isotonic volume depletion caused by **third-space fluid losses** (i.e., fluid sequestered into extracellular or interstitial space, not available in the intravascular space) is seen with peritonitis (bacterial or chemical), intestinal obstruction, extensive soft tissue inflammation, or trauma. This problem is common. Like hemorrhage, these extracellular fluid losses effectively reduce intravascular volumes, which must be replaced promptly. Balanced salt solutions (lactated Ringer's solution) are used to replace the isotonic losses. The indications of how much to give, however, are not always apparent. In this case, clinical observation of hemodynamic changes (i.e., tachycardia, narrowed pulse pressure, hypotension), decreasing urine output (i.e., $<$ 0.5 mL/kg/hr), and laboratory evidence of isotonic volume contraction (i.e., rising hematocrit, serum BUN:creatinine ratio $>$ 20:1, urine sodium concentrations $<$ 20 mEq/L) make it clear that the losses are significant. With continuous monitoring as intravenous fluid therapy is given, improvements in hemodynamic parameters and hourly urine output indicate when volumes have been restored to more normal levels. To avoid clinically significant dilutional hyponatremia, care must be taken to limit the intravenous administration of hypotonic fluid to patients who need large volumes.

During surgery, attention is focused largely on maintaining circulating volumes and adequate tissue perfusion, as monitored by urine flow rates and central venous or pulmonary arterial pressures. Crystalloid solutions are used initially to replace whole blood losses, but packed red blood cells and **colloid** solutions may also be used. At least 1 L lactated Ringer's or normal saline (NS) solution is used to replace third-space isotonic fluid losses in patients who undergo major abdominal or thoracic surgery. The use of hypotonic intravenous fluid should be limited to the replacement of evaporative water losses. Used freely to replace isotonic losses, these hypotonic fluids lead to dilutional hyponatremia. In patients who have compromised pulmonary function, arterial blood gas and pH studies are performed intraoperatively to monitor gas exchange and acid–base status.

In the immediate postoperative period, the fluid, electrolyte, and acid–base needs of the patient, for the most part, are related to monitoring and maintaining hemodynamic stability and the adequacy of ventilation. In many patients who have had relatively unstressful and uncomplicated elective surgical procedures (i.e., inguinal herniorrhaphy, cholecystectomy) and in whom oral intake will be resumed within 48 hours, this process is accomplished simply by physical examination and serial observations of pulse rate, arterial blood pressure, respiratory frequency, and urine output, and by the administration of intravenous fluids as described for maintenance in Table 3-2.

In patients who have had more surgically stressful procedures that involve extensive tissue dissection or resection, particularly those with known compromise of cardiac, renal, or pulmonary function, the needs are greater. Additional monitoring with central venous or pulmonary arterial pressure, hourly urine flow collected with an indwelling catheter in the bladder, and serial arterial blood gas and pH measurement may be necessary. Inadequate respiratory gas exchange may require the use of tracheal intubation and mechanical ventilation. Infusions are needed to replace third-space fluid losses that can continue for 48 to 72 hours, or even longer in the elderly. In addition to daily maintenance needs, gastric, intestinal, biliary, and pancreatic drainage should be replaced. If these losses are greater than 1000 mL in 24 hours, consideration should be given to replacing them milliliter for milliliter with an appropriate intravenous infusion. The electrolyte content of these infusions generally can be determined by knowing the electrolyte composition of the fluid that is lost, as described in Table 3-4. To determine more accurately what

Table 3-4 Composition of Normal Body Fluids[a]

Fluid	Na^+	K^+	Cl^-	HCO_3^-
Plasma	135–150	3.5–5.0	98–106	22–30
Stomach	10–150	4–12	120–160	0
Bile	120–170	3–12	80–120	30–40
Pancreas	135–150	3.5–5.0	60–100	35–110
Small intestine	80–150	2–8	70–130	20–40
Colon	50–100	10–30	80–120	25–30
Perspiration	30–50	5	30–50	0

[a] The composition of most gastrointestinal fluids varies according to the rate of secretion.

must be replaced, fluid samples are analyzed for their electrolyte composition. Daily weights are used to assess fluid volume depletion or retention, recognizing that gains or losses greater than 250 g (approximately 0.5 lb) represent changes in body fluid content. As valuable as it is to monitor extracellular fluid status, weight gains and losses relative to third-space fluid losses and their management must also be considered. During the replacement of third-space losses, weight gains do not represent hypervolemia. Rather, they are caused by the replacement of needed extracellular volume to compensate for the volume that was lost or sequestered. Similarly, diuresis and associated weight loss is expected 3 or more days postoperatively, when third-space fluid accumulations are mobilized (i.e., moved into intracellular or intravascular compartments). This fluid should be excreted, and not replaced. When this fluid is mobilizing, intravascular volumes are likely to be high, making additional intravenous volume loading undesirable. On the other hand, in patients who are receiving parenteral nutrition with hyperosmolar glucose solutions, increased urine output should not be interpreted simply as appropriate excretion of excess fluids. In fact, the high urine output in these patients is more likely to be caused by osmotic diuresis that is independent of the patient's volume status. This condition requires prompt recognition and correction with intravenous fluids to avoid severe hyperosmolar volume contraction.

The attention to fluid needs continues until the patient's renal and gastrointestinal function returns to normal and all fluid, electrolyte, and nutritional requirements are being met by oral intake. At this point, with the exception of chronically ill patients, who may have ongoing needs, concerns for this aspect of patient care end.

FLUID AND ELECTROLYTE DISORDERS IN THE SURGICAL PATIENT

Disorders of Volume

Volume disorders are common in surgical patients. Patients may lose volume through the loss of blood or gastrointestinal fluid (e.g., vomiting, diarrhea). Conversely, patients may gain excessive volume through volume replacement or physiologic disorders, such as renal failure or **syndrome of inappropriate secretion of antidiuretic hormone** (SIADH—discussed below).

Volume Depletion

Etiology

Blood lost at the time of surgery may be the most visible type of volume loss. However, gastrointestinal fluid losses, which are common in surgical patients, are related to vomiting, nasogastric suction, diarrhea, and external drainage from enteric, biliary, or pancreatic **fistulas.** For the most part, these losses are isotonic (Table 3-4) and result in extracellular fluid volume depletion. The intracellular compartment is affected only if osmolar concentrations change. Isotonic depletion of functional extracellular fluid volume also occurs with third-space losses. Particularly significant third-space losses occur in burns, crush injuries, long-bone fractures, peritonitis, severe pancreatitis, intestinal obstructions, pleural effusions, and large areas of soft tissue infection. Excessive urinary loss of water and electrolytes also can lead to volume depletion, as seen with diuretic therapy, high-output renal failure, and osmotic diuresis associated with nonelectrolyte hyperosmolar solute loading (e.g., glucose, mannitol, angiographic contrast media). Finally, some volume depletions involve losses of water in excess of solute. These losses include excessive renal free water excretion associated with primary deficiencies of ADH (i.e., central diabetes insipidus) or nephrogenic causes of diabetes insipidus, increased evaporative losses from burned surfaces, and increased sweating and evaporative losses from the skin and respiratory tract in febrile patients. These hypotonic losses create a hypernatremic hyperosmolar state in the extracellular compartment that draws water from the cell. This repletion of the extracellular space can blunt the clinical picture of volume depletion, which typically reflects extracellular deficits.

Presentation and Diagnosis

Extracellular volume depletion involves equivalent percentage reductions of interstitial and plasma fluid volumes. Signs of an interstitial fluid deficit include decreased tissue turgor, dry skin and mucous membranes, fissuring of the tongue, reduced tongue volume, and, if severe, sunken eyes. Signs of plasma volume deficits include reduced tissue perfusion similar to that seen with whole blood loss. The clinical signs and symptoms are directly related to the magnitude and rate at which the deficit occurs (Table 3-5). Further, as shown in Table 3-6, many of these findings are not reliable in elderly or chronically debilitated patients. Body weight can be a valuable measure of functional extracellular fluid deficits, but not if third-space sequestration occurs. Neurologic and cardiovascular signs are more prominent with acute losses, whereas tissue signs may not be evident for at least 24 hours. In such acute circumstances, the clinician is more dependent on hemodynamic parameters, elevated hematocrit, **oliguria,** and urinary concentration studies as guidelines. As renal perfusion becomes more restricted and levels of BUN and serum creatinine rise, it is important to verify that these signs are manifestations of prerenal azotemia and not acute renal failure. Urine sodium concentrations less than 20 mEq/L, BUN:creatinine ratio greater than 20:1, urine **osmolality** greater than 400 mOsm/L (in the absence of glucosuria or the excretion of other osmotically active particles), or a fractional excretion of sodium

$$[(U_{Na} \times P_{Cr}) / (P_{Na} \times U_{Cr}) \times 100]$$

less than 1% are characteristic of prerenal azotemia. With acute renal injury, however, urine sodium increases (usually > 40 mEq/L) as renal tubular resorption of sodium is impaired, BUN:creatinine ratio falls to 10:1 or less (be-

Table 3-5 Signs of Extracellular Fluid (ECF) Depletion

	10% Depletion	20% Depletion	30% Depletion
Clinical	2% weight loss Thirst Mildly reduced urine output	4% weight loss Apathy Drowsiness Decreased skin turgor Dry mucous membranes Longitudinal tongue furrowing Tachycardia Orthostatic hypotension Urine output < 30 mL/hr	6% weight loss Stupor or coma Skin cool, pale, cyanotic, with poor turgor Eyes sunken Tachycardia Pulse weak and thready Hypotension Urine output < 15 mL/hr
Laboratory	Slightly elevated hematocrit[a] Slightly elevated urine specific gravity	Elevated hematocrit[a] Elevated WBC count Modest elevation in BUN and creatinine Elevated BUN:creatinine ratio (> 10:1 up to 25:1) Urine specific gravity ≥ 1.020, urine osmolarity > 500 mOsm/L, urine sodium ≤ 10–15 mEq/L	Greatly elevated hematocrit[a] Elevated BUN:creatinine ratio (> 10:1 up to 25:1) Urine[b] specific gravity < 1.020, urine osmolarity < 500 mOsm/L, urine sodium > 20 mEq/L
Comments	Findings can be overlooked on evaluation	Findings are always evident	Findings are very obvious

[a] In the absence of bleeding, hematocrit falls about 1% for every 500 mL ECF deficit.
[b] These urine findings reflect acute tubular necrosis.
BUN, blood urea nitrogen; WBC, white blood cell.

Table 3-6 Responses to Extracellular Fluid Depletion in the Elderly

System	Signs or Symptoms in Younger Persons	In Persons > 65 Years Old
Intravascular	Orthostatic hypotension	Common in healthy elderly
	Hypotension	May be masked by preexisting hypertension
	Tachycardia	Maximal heart rate decreases with age
	Reduced pulse volume	Masked by rigid vessels
	Reduced CVP or PaOP	May not reflect heart function or volume status
	Oliguria	May be less marked if preexisting renal impairment is present
	No signs of fluid overload or heart failure	Preexisting hypoproteinemia and ankle edema may be present
Interstitial	Dry skin and mucous membranes	Common in the elderly
	Dry tongue	Unreliable at any age
	Reduced tongue volume	May be useful
	Sunken eyes	A late sign at any age
	Reduced skin turgor	Unreliable in the elderly
Miscellaneous	Reduced deep tendon reflexes	May be an age-related change
	Distal anesthesia	May be an age-related change
	Drowsiness	May be caused by infection, medication, hypothyroidism, or depression
	Apathy	May be caused by infection, medication, hypothyroidism, or depression
	Anorexia	May be caused by infection, medication, hypothyroidism, or depression
	Stupor or coma	A late, nonspecific sign
	Ileus	A late, nonspecific sign

CVP, central venous pressure; PaOP, pulmonary artery opening pressure.

cause creatinine starts to rise), and urine osmolality approaches plasma osmolality.

Treatment

Information gathered from the history and physical examination, knowledge of the volume and composition of body fluids lost (see Table 3-4), and appropriate laboratory tests are critical in determining proper fluid therapy. Correction of volume depletion also requires information about the composition of available intravenous fluids (Table 3-7). Treatment of isotonic extracellular volume deficits caused by intestinal, biliary, pancreatic, or third-space losses with intravenous infusion of lactated Ringer's solution or normal saline is usually appropriate. However, lactate-containing solutions should not be used to replace gastric losses that occur from vomiting or nasogastric suctioning. Inadequate chloride in lactated Ringer's solution plus in vivo conversion of a lactate to bicarbonate does not correct the hypochloremic hypokalemic metabolic alkalosis that occurs in this situation. A solution that more closely approximates the electrolyte composition of gastric fluid (e.g., 1/2 NS with 20 mEq KCl/L) is a better choice. Glucose solutions should not be used to correct volume deficits that result from an osmotic diuresis that is induced by hyperglycemia. Therapeutic needs are better served by infusion of isotonic crystalloid to restore vascular volume, followed by correction of osmolar and potassium abnormalities. As a rule, the rate of volume correction should be commensurate with the need and the ability of the patient to accept the fluid loads that are being delivered. When the deficits are moderate, complete replacement should be carried out over at least a 24-hour period. The longer the deficits have taken to occur, the more cautious the clinician should be in replacing them. If deficits are large and the consequences severe, the needs are more urgent. In these cases, the therapeutic priorities are first to correct hemodynamic and perfusion inadequacies as rapidly and safely as possible. Correcting these inadequacies may require rapid infusion of 1 L or more isotonic crystalloid solution to achieve hemodynamic stability. It is also wise to avoid using glucose-containing solutions during rapid correction of such a deficit, because these solutions can lead to an iatrogenic hyperglycemic-induced osmotic diuresis that may cause further fluid loss. The next priority is to correct potassium abnormalities that may be present, after adjusting for the pH effect (see the earlier section on normal physiology). Normalization of glucose and osmolality changes as well as volume correction of interstitial fluid and total body water can be carried out over the next 18 to 24 hours, or as symptoms dictate.

Measurements of weight change and cumulative fluid intake and output provide valuable information over an extended period. However, during vascular volume repletion, repeated physical examination to assess the physiologic response to fluid infusion, central venous or pulmonary artery monitoring (if necessary), and urine output measurements are the mainstay of monitoring the adequacy of replacement therapy. If there is no acute renal failure or significant chronically compromised renal function, osmotic diuresis, use of diuretics, septic-induced polyuria, or hypothermia, urine output at rates greater than 0.5/mL/kg/hr (1.0 mL/kg/hr in children) indicates adequate repletion of vascular volume. Similarly, in the absence of continuing blood loss, declining hemoglobin and hematocrit values signify extracellular volume correction. Reduction of BUN and creatinine toward normal levels is also consistent with restoration of adequate renal perfusion and extracellular volume expansion.

Prognosis

The prognosis for patients with volume depletion depends on the initial amount of depletion and the success of efforts toward volume resuscitation and cessation of ongoing losses. Some patients have such severe volume depletion or shock that, even with apparently adequate fluid resuscitation, the outcome is fatal. Most patients, however, have problems that permit correction and resuscitation (e.g., a patient with a massive gastrointestinal bleed who is given fluid and taken to the operating room, where a bleeding duodenal ulcer is oversewn).

Volume Excess

Etiology

Volume excess for any fluid compartment can be the result of excessive or inappropriate fluids for that compartment,

Table 3-7 Composition of Commonly Used Intravenous Solutions

	Glucose (g/L)	Na^+ (mEq/L)	K^+ (mEq/L)	Cl^- (mEq/L)	Lactate[a] (mEq/L)	Ca^{++} (mEq/L)
0.9% Sodium chloride ("normal" saline)		154		154		
Lactated Ringer's solution		130	4.0	109	28	3.0
5% dextrose water	50					
5% dextrose in 0.45% sodium chloride	50	77		77		
3% sodium chloride		513		513		

[a] Converted to bicarbonate.

abnormal fluid retention, or a combination of both factors. Excessive intravenous fluid therapy with balanced salt solutions is a common iatrogenic cause of isotonic fluid excess. This therapy causes extracellular expansion. This expansion, in the absence of attendant osmolar changes, is not shared intracellularly. This isotonic extracellular expansion causes both hypervolemia and excess interstitial fluid. These consequences are more likely to occur immediately after surgery or trauma, when maximal hormonal responses to stress (i.e., increases in both ADH and aldosterone) are operating to diminish sodium and water excretion by the kidney. The risk of fluid excess is even greater in the elderly and in patients in whom underlying cardiac, renal, or hepatic disorders contribute to fluid accumulation. Congestive heart failure, oliguric renal failure, and hypoalbuminemia secondary to hepatocellular dysfunction are other recognized causes of extracellular fluid volume expansion.

Hypotonic and hypertonic fluid excess can also occur. Inappropriate administration of salt-poor solutions to replace isotonic gastrointestinal or third-space fluid loss is a common cause of hyponatremic volume expansion. On the other hand, administration of sodium loads that are not balanced by appropriate water intake causes hypernatremic extracellular volume expansion. In this case, water moving out of the cells in response to increased extracellular osmolar concentrations may contribute to intravascular and interstitial fluid overload. The resulting hypervolemic state is even more pronounced when renal tubular excretion of salt or water is compromised. Hypertonic extracellular volume expansion can also be induced by the rapid infusion of nonelectrolyte osmotically active solutes (e.g., glucose, mannitol). This situation, however, is accompanied by hyponatremia, not hypernatremia. Plasma sodium concentration decreases as a result of dilution by the solution that is being infused and the sodium-free water drawn from the cells into the extracellular space in response to the osmolar gradient created by the infused nonelectrolyte solute load.

Syndrome of Inappropriate Secretion of ADH (SIADH). Hyponatremia results if vasopressin (antidiuretic hormone, or ADH) is excreted inappropriately. This may occur in the presence of surgical stress, endocrine disorders, pulmonary disorders (including chronic obstructive pulmonary disease [COPD], cystic fibrosis, pneumothorax, and infections), central nervous system (CNS) disorders (including head trauma, brain tumors, delirium tremens, and infections), certain drugs (including some diuretics, antidepressants, and nonsteroidal antiinflammatory drugs [NSAIDs]), and many malignancies (including lung, pancreas, prostate, and thymus). These clinically euvolemic patients display hyponatremia, urinary hyperosmolarity, and serum hypoosmolality, with normal adrenal, renal, and thyroid function. Treatment consists of fluid restriction to less than 1000 mL daily. If serum sodium is less than 110 mEq/L or neurologic symptoms of hyponatremia are present, hypertonic saline should be administered, but no attempt should be made to correct serum sodium rapidly (see central pontine myelinolysis, below). Treatment of SIADH requires severe fluid restriction to 1000 mL/day or less. For patients with chronic SIADH, long-term management options include butorphanol, lithium carbonate, and demeclocycline. Butorphanol inhibits ADH secretion. Lithium and demeclocycline block the effect of ADH on the collecting duct, and while both have side effects, demeclocycline 600 to 1200 mg daily is usually effective and well tolerated. Prognosis depends on the cause. Often, however, no etiology is ever established.

Presentation and Diagnosis

The clinical picture of extracellular volume excess can vary, depending on the cause, nature, and severity of the challenges. Thus, the signs can range widely. At the lower end of the severity scale are simple weight gain, small decreases of hemoglobin and hematocrit levels (signifying hemodilution), modest elevations of peripheral and **central venous pressure,** and dependent sacral or lower extremity edema. At the other end, there are extreme consequences of vascular and interstitial fluid overload, with frank congestive heart failure, as evidenced by pulmonary edema, pleural effusion, anasarca, and hepatomegaly.

Treatment

Treatment is adjusted according to the severity of fluid compartment changes and related clinical findings. Lesser problems are treated with fluid or sodium restriction. More severe problems require diuresis with loop diuretics as well as replacement of associated potassium losses. Cardiotonic drugs, oxygen therapy, artificial ventilation, or dialysis (if renal insufficiency is present) may also be needed to manage cardiac or respiratory failure. The therapeutic management of related hyponatremic and hypernatremic states is discussed in the next section.

Prognosis

After volume overload is corrected, most patients do well. The exceptions are patients whose volume overload leads to significant pulmonary edema or adult respiratory distress syndrome (ARDS) and those who have myocardial events associated with the hypervolemia.

Disorders of Electrolyte Concentrations

A good history is essential in determining the etiology and proper treatment of electrolyte imbalances. Electrolyte imbalances are rarely isolated, because the body must maintain electrical neutrality; complex homeostatic and metabolic mechanisms exist to maintain the neutral state. Attempts to correct a low serum level by simple oral or parenteral replacement of an ion may not improve the patient's condition because associated abnormalities are not treated. Although electrolyte abnormalities are often corrected easily, if untreated they may be fatal. Artifactual abnormalities of serum electrolytes may result from improper collection or handling of blood specimens. The range of normal values also varies somewhat from one laboratory to another.

Sodium

The sodium ion is the principal solute that determines extracellular fluid (ECF) osmolarity and volume balance in the body. An increase in extracellular sodium concentration creates an osmotic gradient that draws water out of cells. A decrease in extracellular sodium concentration does the reverse. These changes in cell volume produce the symptoms of abnormal serum sodium. Disorders of sodium balance are usually associated with disorders of fluid balance.

Hyponatremia

Hyponatremia results from the presence of excess body water relative to body sodium and the failure of the kidneys to excrete the excess water. The serum sodium concentration does not always reflect true total body sodium content, or even osmolarity. For example, total body sodium may be increased in patients with chronic cardiac, hepatic, or renal disease, but hyponatremia persists because of a proportionally greater increase in water.

Etiology. Hyponatremia may be associated with decreased, increased, or normal ECF volume. The causes of hyponatremia are shown in Table 3-8.

In surgical patients, dilutional hyponatremia occurs most commonly when hypotonic fluids are used to replace isotonic gastrointestinal or third-space losses. Catabolic breakdown of body tissues, which occurs with surgical stress and caloric deprivation, metabolically generates approximately 1 mL sodium-free water for each gram of fat or muscle that is catabolized. Further, the ability of the kidney to excrete excess water in response to decreased serum osmolarity is impaired after surgery or other trauma. Secretion of ADH is increased and uncontrolled by feedback inhibition.

Dilutional hyponatremia may occur with volume deficits, if isotonic fluid losses are replaced with hypotonic fluid. It also occurs in patients who have advanced cardiac, renal, or hepatic disease and increased total body sodium, because these patients accumulate proportionally more water.

Artifactually very low serum sodium values are seen in the presence of severe hyperglycemia and hypertriglyceridemia, or after intravenous infusion of lipids. In these cases, the water in the intravascular space is partially replaced, so the concentration of sodium in the total sample is low, even though the concentration of sodium in plasma may be normal, or even high.

Table 3-8 Causes of Hyponatremia

Excess water	Ingestion or infusion of excess free water (e.g., psychogenic polydipsia or replacement of isotonic gastrointestinal and third-space fluid losses with hypotonic fluid)
	Physiologic response to surgical stress, starvation, or hypovolemia (causing enhanced metabolic production of free water)
	SIADH (syndrome of inappropriate ADH secretion)
	Enhanced ADH activity
	Advanced cardiac, renal, or hepatic disease
Excess sodium loss	Thiazide diuretics
	Metabolic alkalosis
	Ketoacidosis
	Adrenal insufficiency
	Salt-wasting nephropathy
Artifactual	Hyperlipidemia
	Hyperproteinemia

ADH, antidiuretic hormone.

Presentation and Diagnosis. The primary clinical manifestations of hyponatremia are the signs and symptoms of central nervous system dysfunction. Osmotic forces draw water into the cells, and cerebrospinal fluid pressures increase because of cerebral and spinal cord swelling. Neurologic disturbances occur as a result. The severity of these disturbances is directly related to both the degree of the hyponatremia and the rapidity with which it develops. Serum sodium between 130 and 120 mEq/L may cause irritability, weakness, fatigue, increased deep-tendon reflexes, and muscle twitches if the hyponatremia developed rapidly (10 to 15 mEq/L in < 48 hours, or faster), but the patient may be completely asymptomatic if it developed slowly. Serum sodium levels of less than 120 mEq/L, if untreated, produce seizures, coma, areflexia, and death.

In diagnosing hyponatremia, serum and urine sodium, serum and urine osmolality, and pH are assessed. Blood tests can exclude associated electrolyte abnormalities (e.g., hyperglycemia, liver diseases, acid–base disorders). Volume status should also be assessed.

Treatment. Treatment of hyponatremia depends on the cause, severity, and nature of any associated volume abnormality. Psychogenic polydipsia is treated with water restriction. Most dilutional hyponatremia that is iatrogenically induced in the perioperative period, seen as an asymptomatic decrease in serum sodium along with modest extracellular volume expansion, is readily treated by simple fluid restriction. Thiazide diuretics cause hyponatremia by blocking the resorption of sodium and chloride in the cortical-diluting segment. However, because the resorption of salt in the ascending limb of the loop of Henle is not blocked, excretion of very concentrated urine is possible. This concentration permits the retention of water while sodium, potassium, and chloride are depleted. The best treatment for this condition is discontinuation of the diuretic. In patients who have chronic hyponatremia, even when serum sodium concentration is low, correction of serum sodium must be done slowly, 12 mEq/L/day or less. Disorders that involve body sodium excess in addition to disproportionate volume excess are treated by restriction of both sodium and water.

Hyponatremia associated with volume contraction is treated with combined sodium and volume repletion, usually with normal saline or lactated Ringer's solution. The rate of repletion is dictated by the degree of volume deficit. In most cases, rapid restoration of volume and sodium is not only unnecessary but also hazardous, because it can cause rapid shifts of intracellular water and undesirable neurologic consequences.

Hypertonic 3% saline solutions are indicated only when hyponatremia causes life-threatening neurologic disturbances. To estimate the amount of sodium needed to correct the serum deficit, multiply the decrease in serum sodium (in milliequivalents) by total body water (in liters) as a percentage of total body weight (TBW):

$$\text{mEq Na}^+ \text{ needed} = (140 - \text{measured serum Na}^+) \times \text{TBW},$$

where TBW $= 0.6 \times$ body weight (kg).

TBW is used because both intracellular and extracellular imbalances must be corrected. No more than one-half of the total calculated amount of sodium is given in the first 12 to 18 hours. The goal is to increase the serum sodium level sufficiently to eliminate the symptoms. Over the next 24 to 48 hours, the remainder of the deficit is corrected with normal saline. Any underlying conditions must also be treated. Responsible drugs should be discontinued, if possible. Rapid correction of chronic hyponatremia (e.g., $>$ 12 mEq/L/day) can cause osmotic demyelination syndrome. The patient usually improves for a day or so but then deteriorates, with a spectrum of neurologic findings that can include fluctuating levels of consciousness, seizures, pseudobulbar palsy, and paralysis. Some patients improve after several weeks, but others have significant permanent disability.

It is important to remember not to correct disturbances of sodium balance too quickly, as rapid extreme changes in body sodium levels may cause central pontine myelinolysis. In this entity, the myelin sheaths of nerve cells in the pons are destroyed. The resulting neurologic damage is usually permanent and may be debilitating.

Prognosis. Once treated, the prognosis of hyponatremia usually depends on the prognosis of the underlying condition. Severe neurologic symptoms may have irreversible sequelae.

Hypernatremia

Hypernatremia results from excess body sodium content relative to body water. Clinically significant hypernatremia, serum sodium greater than 150 mEq/L, is less common than hyponatremia, but it can be just as lethal if it is allowed to progress unchecked.

Etiology. Hypernatremia may result from the loss of water alone (e.g., hypothalamic abnormalities, unreplaced insensible losses); from the loss of water and salt together (e.g., gastrointestinal losses, osmotic diuresis, excessive diuretic use, central or nephrogenic diabetes insipidus, burns, excessive sweating); as a side effect of many drugs (e.g., alcohol, amphotericin B, colchicine, lithium, phenytoin); or from increased sodium without any water loss (e.g., Cushing's syndrome, hyperaldosteronism, ectopic production of ACTH, iatrogenic sodium administration, ingestion of seawater).

When body fluids become hypertonic, compensatory thirst is stimulated. Therefore, severe hypernatremia occurs only in situations in which a person cannot obtain water (e.g., infancy, disability, altered mental states).

Presentation and Diagnosis. The pathophysiologic consequences of hypernatremia reflect both extracellular volume losses and cellular dehydration that result from water shifts in response to osmotic pressure. As with hyponatremia, the severity of the clinical manifestations is directly related to both the degree of the hypernatremia and the rapidity with which it develops. Serum sodium concentrations greater than 160 mEq/L are cause for concern and may be symptomatic. Signs and symptoms include those of dehydration, including decreased salivation and lacrimation; dry mucous membranes; dry, flushed skin; decreased tissue turgor; oliguria (except when dehydrating renal water loss is the cause); fever; and tachycardia. Signs and symptoms also include those of neuromuscular and neurologic disorders, from twitching, restlessness, and weakness to delirium, coma, seizures, and death. Intracranial hemorrhage is a common postmortem finding in patients who die of hypernatremia; the hemorrhage is thought to result from cell shrinkage, with associated decreases in brain volume and decreased intracranial pressure, which disrupts the intracranial blood vessels.

In addition to the history and measurement of serum sodium, urine sodium and urine and plasma osmolality should be determined. Hematocrit may be high because of dehydration. The underlying cause should be diagnosed.

Treatment. Treatment of hypernatremia consists of correcting the water deficit, which can be estimated in several ways. The simplest accurate general rule is that for every liter of water deficit, serum sodium rises 3 mEq above the normal value of 140 mEq/L. If deficits are modest, they can be replaced orally or with intravenous 5% dextrose in water. If deficits are more severe, the TBW deficit is calculated as follows:

$$\text{mEq change in serum Na}^+ = (140 - \text{serum Na}^+) \times \text{TBW},$$

where TBW $= 0.6 \times$ body weight (kg).

The relative water deficit (in liters) is equal to the milliequivalent change in serum $Na^+/140$. The water must be replaced slowly, with no more than one-half given over the first 12 to 24 hours. For pure water loss, 5% dextrose is infused intravenously. Therefore, if a 70-kg patient has a serum sodium value of 150, the water deficit is calculated as follows:

$$\begin{aligned} \text{mEq change in serum Na+} &= (140 - 150) \times 0.6 \times 70 \\ &= 10 \times 42 \\ &= 420 \\ \text{Water deficit in liters} &= 420/140 = 3 \text{ L} \end{aligned}$$

In patients with associated sodium deficits, if symptoms of dehydration predominate, the volume deficit is initially replaced with normal saline. If neurologic symptoms are more prominent, half-normal saline is used. If the sodium loss is large (e.g., diabetic hyperosmolar coma), the volume is replaced initially with normal saline. The nature of the fluid required may change as different needs become apparent, and the process of reversing hypernatremia requires close monitoring. If water is replaced too rapidly, osmotic shifts can produce cellular edema. Brain cells accumulate intracellular solute slowly in response to slowly developing extracellular hypertonicity; a sudden decrease in extracellular osmolality leads to rapid swelling of brain cells, causing serious neurologic dysfunction.

As with other electrolyte disturbances, underlying problems must also be treated.

Prognosis. The prognosis depends on the severity of symptoms, the correct treatment, and the prognosis of the underlying disorder. Neurologic symptoms, once they develop, may be irreversible.

Potassium

As the principal intracellular cation, potassium is a major determinant of intracellular volume. It is a significant cofactor in cellular metabolism. Extracellular potassium plays an important role in neuromuscular function.

Hypokalemia

Hypokalemia is defined as a serum potassium level less than 3.5 mEq/L. When potassium is deficient, there may also be losses of magnesium and phosphorus. The exact relation between magnesium and potassium is unclear; however, many factors that cause renal potassium wasting also cause renal magnesium wasting (e.g., loop and thiazide diuretic use). The opposite is also true (e.g., potassium and magnesium sparing with amiloride). Hypophosphatemia and hypocalcemia often accompany hypokalemia. Potassium deprivation may impair calcium resorption by the kidney, resulting in a negative calcium balance. This change, in turn, alters phosphorous metabolism.

Etiology. Hypokalemia may reflect potassium deficiency that results from inadequate intake, gastrointestinal tract losses, or renal losses. Hypokalemia may also reflect shifts from the extracellular to the intracellular compartment (e.g., insulin administration or alkalosis).

Gastrointestinal losses (e.g., diarrhea, vomiting, biliary or pancreatic fistulae, villous adenoma, malabsorption) can be major factors in hypokalemia. The highest gastrointestinal concentrations of potassium are found in the colon and rectum. Prolonged vomiting or nasogastric aspiration causes hypokalemia through a combination of factors. In addition to the loss of potassium in the gastric fluid, the loss of hydrogen and chloride ions produces hypochloremic hypokalemic metabolic alkalosis. The increase in extracellular pH causes movement of potassium into the cells, which makes the hypokalemia worse. As a general rule, an increase in pH of 0.1 unit causes a decrease in serum potassium of 0.4 to 0.5 mEq. As the hypokalemia worsens, in the alkalotic state, the kidneys conserve hydrogen ions by excreting potassium. Further, high bicarbonate and low chloride concentrations in the renal tubules cause greater resorption of sodium in the distal tubule, causing additional urinary potassium loss. Finally, extracellular volume deficits stimulate aldosterone activity, which also increases renal potassium excretion. The interaction of these mechanisms, if uncorrected, produces noticeable intracellular and extracellular potassium depletion. At this point, because of the need to conserve potassium, renal tubular hydrogen ion excretion increases. Urinary potassium loss decreases, and paradoxical aciduria appears (i.e., acidic urine in the presence of severe alkalosis).

Renal potassium losses are caused by hyperglycemia, primary or secondary aldosteronism, renal tubular acidosis, elevated ACTH, licorice ingestion, acute leukemia, or corticoid excess. Hypokalemia is often iatrogenic, the result of treatment with thiazides, loop diuretics, or carbonic anhydrase inhibitors. By an unknown mechanism, magnesium deficiency decreases distal renal tubular potassium resorption. If the magnesium deficiency is not corrected, renal losses continue, and it is difficult to correct the hypokalemia.

Presentation and Diagnosis. Hypokalemia rarely becomes clinically significant until serum potassium decreases to less than 3.0 mEq/L. In general, the severity of symptoms is proportional to the degree of deficit and the rapidity with which it develops. Additionally, the consequences of hypokalemia are exacerbated by alkalosis, hypocalcemia, and digoxin therapy. Hypokalemia may cause neuromuscular symptoms that range from skeletal muscle weakness and fatigue to paresthesias, paralysis, and rhabdomyolysis. Deep-tendon reflexes may be diminished or absent. Hypokalemia causes increased production of ammonia in the renal tubules. This increase may worsen hepatic encephalopathy. Other symptoms include anorexia, polyuria, and nausea and vomiting associated with paralytic ileus. Total body potassium depletion produces cellular atrophy and negative nitrogen balance. Renal tubular function is impaired, which may result in polyuria and polydipsia because of decreased concentrating ability.

Cardiac abnormalities are the most important and worrisome consequences of hypokalemia, and intoxication may appear in the presence of digoxin, even with relatively mild deficits. Progressive electrocardiogram (ECG) abnormalities include low-voltage, flattened, or inverted T waves, with prominent U waves, depressed S-T segments, prolonged P-R intervals, and (at levels of $\leq$ 2.0 mEq/L) widened QRS complexes. A rapid decrease in serum potassium may lead to cardiac arrest.

If the deficiency is mild and the cause is clear from the history, serum potassium may be the only test required, with the digoxin level measured if the patient is being treated with this medication. If hypokalemia is more severe or refractory to treatment, other serum electrolytes, including calcium and magnesium, should be measured. An arterial blood gas determination may exclude acid–base disturbances, and urinary electrolytes can be used to exclude renal hyperexcretion. If the hypokalemic patient has normal blood pressure, serum bicarbonate and urine potassium should help distinguish among metabolic causes, gastrointestinal losses, dietary deficiency, and osmotic or drug-induced diuresis. If the patient is hypertensive, plasma renin and aldosterone levels may help identify the cause.

Treatment. Treatment of hypokalemia involves replacing lost potassium and correcting the underlying cause. Whenever possible, potassium is repleted orally, with pills or liquid. Most people find the taste of potassium solutions unpleasant. Enteric-coated tablets should not be used, because they can cause small bowel ulceration. In patients with normal kidneys, the oral dose should not exceed 40 mEq/4 hr. If the intravenous route is necessary, the rate should not exceed 10 mEq/hr, with the dose repeated as often as necessary to increase the serum level to within the normal range. Electrocardiographic monitoring is helpful during intravenous potassium repletion, and it is mandatory if a rate higher than 10 mEq/hr is used. Too rapid intravenous administration can cause hyperkalemia and fatal cardiac arrhythmias. Generally, dextrose-containing solutions are not used as the diluent; intravenous dextrose increases endogenous insulin, which induces the movement of potassium into cells and causes the serum level to decrease further, making repletion more difficult. A serum potassium level lower than 2.9 mEq/L may reflect depletions of the huge intracellular pool and thus require much more supplementation, with closer monitoring.

If hypokalemia is caused by hypomagnesemia, magnesium repletion will correct it. When hypokalemia and hypocalcemia occur together, they must both be treated; treatment of only one may cause the patient to become symptomatic from the other.

Prognosis. Most hypokalemia is moderate and relatively easy to correct. The prognosis depends on the severity of symptoms, correct treatment, and the prognosis of the underlying disorder.

Hyperkalemia

Hyperkalemia is a serum potassium level greater than 5.0 mEq/L.

Etiology. As in hypokalemia, the etiology of hyperkalemia is usually multifactorial. It can be caused by exogenous loading (e.g., from excessive dietary intake in a patient with renal failure or from parenteral sources, such as high-dose penicillin therapy), transfusions of many units of stored banked blood, or too vigorous correction of hypokalemia. Endogenous loading occurs whenever large amounts of intracellular potassium are released into the extracellular space (e.g., crush injuries, hemolysis, lysis and absorption of large hematomata, catabolism of fat and muscle tissue because of stress or starvation, rapid rewarming after severe hypothermia). Hyperkalemia can be caused by decreased renal excretion, which may result from adrenal insufficiency and impaired aldosterone activity, but most often it is caused by intrinsic renal disease. Shifts of potassium from the intracellular to the extracellular compartment also cause hyperkalemia (e.g., acute metabolic or respiratory acidosis, insulin deficiency, therapy with digitalis and related cardiotonic agents). In diabetic ketoacidosis, hyperkalemia may be seen, even with total body potassium deficit.

Numerous drugs cause hyperkalemia. Impaired renal excretion can be caused by diuretics (e.g., spironolactone, triamterene, amiloride) and by NSAIDs, β-adrenergic antagonists, and angiotensin-converting enzyme (ACE) inhibitors. Digitalis preparations, arginine, β-adrenergic antagonists, and some poisons, for example, can cause shifts of potassium out of the intracellular compartment.

Artifactually high serum potassium results from hemolysis of the blood specimen, from obtaining a blood specimen from a vein into which potassium is being infused, and occasionally from high platelet or leukocyte counts.

Presentation and Diagnosis. Although hyperkalemia causes peripheral muscle weakness that ultimately progresses to respiratory paralysis, the most important signs and symptoms are cardiac. The first ECG abnormality is peaked T waves, best seen in the precordial leads, at serum concentrations between 6.0 and 7.0 mEq/L. Further elevations produce multiple ECG abnormalities, including flattened P waves, increased P-R intervals, decreased Q-T intervals, widened QRS complexes, depressed S-T segments, and complete heart block with atrial asystole. At elevations of more than 8.0 mEq/L, more widened QRS complexes merge with T waves to produce a sine wave appearance. This change is followed by ventricular fibrillation and cardiac arrest.

Diagnosis is made by measuring serum potassium levels. It is usually relatively simple to determine the cause, but since significant hyperkalemia is uncommon if the kidneys are normal, serum BUN, creatinine, and urine output should be measured. Anuric patients accumulate potassium, but a source must be sought in hyperkalemic nonoliguric patients. Even in the presence of renal insufficiency, medication or excessive dietary intake is often responsible. A 12-lead cardiogram must be performed. If the patient is being treated with digoxin, a digoxin level should be obtained. If the patient had a crush injury, serum and urinary myoglobin should also be measured.

If spurious hyperkalemia is suspected (e.g., from a hemolyzed specimen, from blood drawn above an intravenous site), blood should be redrawn for a serum potassium level measurement or a plasma potassium level ordered. However, treatment of a very high serum potassium level should not be delayed while waiting for results.

Treatment. The primary goal of the treatment of hyperkalemia is to reduce serum potassium to levels that are not life threatening. In mild hyperkalemia (< 6 mEq/L), the simplest measures are to restrict potassium intake, eliminate causes such as potassium-sparing diuretics, and treat volume or acid–base disorders. Potassium-wasting diuretics may be administered, and hormone deficiencies may be replaced.

For potassium levels between 6.5 and 7.5 mEq/L, 10 units insulin is administered intravenously along with 25 g glucose intravenously over 5 minutes. This therapy shifts potassium from the extracellular to the intracellular compartment and may reduce serum potassium by as much as 1 mEq/L. A similar shift may be created by administering a bicarbonate infusion or by injecting 45 mEq sodium bicarbonate intravenously over 5 minutes to induce metabolic alkalosis. These compartment shifts last only a few hours. Sodium polystyrene sulfonate, a cation-exchange resin, administered orally or rectally actually removes potassium from the body. Each gram of the resin binds approximately 1 mEq potassium. The oral dose is 25 g resin suspended in 50 mL 20% sorbitol solution every 4 to 6 hours. The rectal dose is 50 g in 100 to 200 mL 35% sorbitol given as a retention enema every 4 hours. Patients with potassium levels greater than 6.5 mEq/L are monitored with continuous ECG.

Serum potassium levels greater than 7.5 mEq/L in a patient with evidence of cardiac toxicity should be treated with an intravenous infusion of 10 to 30 mL 10% calcium gluconate given slowly over 5 minutes to reduce cardiac muscle electrical excitability temporarily while other methods are used to rid the body of potassium. Rapid infusion of calcium is dangerous and is justified only when hyperkalemia is severe. Electrocardiographic monitoring is advisable during the treatment of hyperkalemia, and it is mandatory if calcium is being infused.

Hemodialysis and peritoneal dialysis also remove potassium from the body and may be necessary in patients with renal failure. They may be used along with more rapid methods to reduce serum potassium in moderate to severe hyperkalemia. In treating hyperkalemia with dehydration and acidosis in diabetic ketoacidosis, care must be taken not to allow serum potassium to decrease to subnormal levels.

Prognosis. Hyperkalemia itself does not affect recovery from illness or surgery, and it is usually correctable. However, cardiac events caused by hyperkalemia may be fatal if the hyperkalemia and its effects are not promptly treated. The prognosis of patients with hyperkalemia is often related to the underlying cause (e.g., renal failure).

Chloride

Chloride is the major extracellular anion. It is ubiquitous in the diet, absorbed in the small and large intestines, and excreted by the kidneys. Chloride balance usually parallels sodium balance, except when hypochloremia results from the loss of acidic gastric contents. The normal range of serum chloride is 98 to 108 mEq/L. Although no signs or symptoms are specific to abnormalities of chloride balance, changes in extracellular chloride content can significantly affect fluid, electrolyte, and acid–base balance and their management.

Hypochloremia

Hypochloremia is a serum chloride concentration of less than 95 mEq/L. In severe respiratory acidosis, metabolic compensation involves renal tubular resorption of bicarbonate to decrease the extracellular acidosis that is caused by carbon dioxide retention and chloride depletion. As respiratory acidosis resolves and carbon dioxide retention decreases, renal excretion of excess bicarbonate allows the pH to return to normal. Hypochloremia impairs renal bicarbonate excretion, however, and if serum bicarbonate remains high in the presence of decreased carbon dioxide tension, metabolic alkalosis results and persists until the chloride deficit is repleted.

Etiology. Hypochloremia classically results from the loss of acidic gastric contents, either by vomiting or by nasogastric suction. It can result from renal losses caused by diuretics, nonoliguric acute and chronic renal failure, or compensatory renal tubular resorption of bicarbonate in states of respiratory acidosis.

Presentation and Diagnosis. The signs and symptoms are those of the accompanying disorder. The diagnosis is made by measuring serum chloride.

Treatment. In general, hypochloremia is treated with solutions that contain sodium chloride and potassium chloride in a ratio determined by the underlying problem and by serum electrolyte concentrations. Ammonium chloride is not used in patients with advanced liver disease or hepatic failure because it may precipitate or increase encephalopathy. It is important to correct hypochloremia along with other deficits in the treatment of hypochloremic hypokalemic metabolic alkalosis. As noted earlier, hypochloremia must be corrected in the recovery phase after an episode of severe metabolic acidosis. Hydrochloric acid may rarely be used in severe refractory hypochloremic metabolic alkalosis.

Prognosis. Hypochloremia has no specific prognostic significance. The prognosis depends on the underlying disorder.

Hyperchloremia

Hyperchloremia is a serum chloride level greater than 115 mEq/L. It is uncommon in surgical patients.

Etiology. Hyperchloremia may occur in association with hypernatremia, in renal tubular acidosis, or after the administration of excess potassium chloride or ammonium chloride. It may be caused by surgical diversion of urine into segments of bowel (e.g., ileal urinary conduits, ureterosigmoidostomy). In these cases, the bowel mucosa absorbs excess chloride in exchange for bicarbonate, especially when evacuation of the urine is delayed.

Presentation and Diagnosis. The signs and symptoms are those of the accompanying disorder. Diagnosis is made by measurement of serum chloride.

Treatment. There is no specific treatment for hyperchloremia. Treatment is directed at the underlying disorder.

Prognosis. Hyperchloremia has no prognostic significance. The prognosis depends on the nature and treatment of the underlying disorder.

Calcium

Calcium is a common divalent cation, almost all of which is found in hydroxyapatite crystals in bone. On the surface of bone, calcium participates in exchange with calcium in the ECF. Of the small amount of calcium in the ECF, approximately 40% is bound to plasma protein and 10% is complexed with bicarbonate, citrate, and phosphate. Only the hormonally regulated ionized portion, the remaining 50%, is physiologically active. This small proportion is of vital importance, however, primarily because of its role in neuromuscular activity. The normal range of total serum calcium is 8.5 to 11.0 mg/dL, and that of ionized calcium is 4.75 to 5.30 mg/dL. Most bound calcium is bound to albumin, and total serum calcium is dependent on serum albumin. Total calcium values may appear artifactually subnormal in hypoalbuminemic patients unless a correction factor, such as the following, is used:

$$\text{Corrected total } Ca^{++} = [0.8 \times (4.0 - \text{patient's albumin})] + \text{patient's total serum } Ca^{++}$$

In this formula, 4.0 represents normal serum albumin. The proportion of calcium bound to proteins is dependent on pH; it is decreased by acidosis, with a concomitant increase in ionized calcium. The level of serum ionized calcium is a more accurate indicator of physiologic activity than total calcium, but it is a more expensive test and is not universally available.

The usual adult dietary intake of calcium is 1 g or more a day. Two-thirds of this calcium passes through the gut and is excreted in stool, and one-third is absorbed in the small intestine, regulated by vitamin D. In normal kidneys, approximately 10% of filtered calcium reaches the distal tubules, where resorption is increased by **parathyroid hormone** (PTH) and metabolic alkalosis, or is decreased by hypophosphatemia and metabolic acidosis. Overall calcium homeostasis, largely regulated by PTH, is the result of intestinal absorption, renal excretion, and calcium exchange between bone and the ECF. Although severe abnormalities of calcium metabolism are uncommon in surgical patients, symptomatic abnormalities are seen.

Hypocalcemia

Hypocalcemia is defined as total serum calcium less than 8 mg/dL. It is seen in many conditions common to surgical patients, several of which are acute problems.

Etiology. Hypocalcemia is often seen in surgical patients (Table 3-9). In acute pancreatitis, the etiology of hypocalcemia is unclear. It probably results from a combination of calcium binding in saponified tissue, PTH deficiency or dysfunction in the kidney and bone, and decreased protein-bound calcium as a result of hypoalbuminemia. Magnesium deficiency decreases PTH release and activity. Phosphate increases bone deposition of calcium, decreasing the available circulating pool. Inadequate intestinal absorption of calcium may result from inflammatory bowel disease, pancreatic exocrine dysfunction, or malabsorption syndromes. Excessive fluid losses from chronic diarrhea or pancreatic or intestinal fistulas may also seriously deplete extracellular calcium and cause other electrolyte abnormalities. Low serum calcium levels are seen with severe soft tissue infections, such as necrotizing fasciitis. Artifactual hypocalcemia is seen when serum albumin is low and total calcium, rather than ionized calcium, is measured. Vitamin D deficiency may result from synthetic failure in renal or hepatic disease, or from conversion to inactive metabolites caused by the anticonvulsants phenytoin and phenobarbital.

Another way to classify hypocalcemia is according to its relation to PTH, which may be (1) deficient or absent (e.g., hypomagnesemia, any type of true hypoparathy-

Table 3-9 Causes of Hypocalcemia in Surgical Patients

Artifactual as a result of hypoalbuminemia
Acute pancreatitis
Surgically induced hypoparathyroidism (transient or permanent)
Necrotizing fasciitis
Inadequate intestinal absorption
Inflammatory bowel disease
Pancreatic exocrine dysfunction
Mucosal malabsorptive syndromes
Excessive fluid losses from pancreatic or intestinal fistulae
Chronic diarrhea
Renal insufficiency with impaired calcium resorption
Hypomagnesemia
Hyperphosphatemia

roidism), (2) ineffective (e.g., vitamin D disorders, chronic renal failure, pseudohypoparathyroidism), or (3) overwhelmed (e.g., hyperphosphatemia).

Artifactual hypocalcemia occurs when the serum albumin is low and total calcium, rather than ionized calcium, is measured.

Presentation and Diagnosis. The clinical manifestations of hypocalcemia reflect the role of calcium in neuromuscular activity. Early symptoms of hypocalcemia include circumoral tingling, numbness and tingling of the fingertips, and muscle cramps. Hyperactive deep-tendon reflexes develop, with a Chvostek sign (unilateral facial spasm when the facial nerve on that side is lightly tapped), tetany, and Trousseau's sign (carpopedal spasm), eventually progressing to seizures. The patient may be confused or depressed. Prolonged Q-T intervals are seen on electrocardiogram.

In acidosis, the ionized fraction of serum calcium increases at the expense of the bound fraction. Because only the ionized fraction is active, symptoms may not appear, even with low total serum calcium. With severe alkalosis, the reverse occurs, and symptoms may appear even when the measured total serum calcium is normal.

Hypocalcemia can occur after blood transfusion, as a result of citrate binding and dilution. However, evidence suggests that at moderate rates of blood transfusion, endogenous release of calcium from bone is adequate to prevent hypocalcemia. Only with massive transfusion and volume replacement at rates of 100 mL/min or higher is there any need to give supplemental calcium.

Diagnosis is made by measuring serum calcium (the ionized portion if possible), along with serum potassium, magnesium, phosphate, and alkaline phosphatase. Other electrolyte abnormalities and acid–base disorders must be excluded. Serum albumin is measured, as well as BUN and creatinine. Measurement of urinary calcium can help assess calcium intake. It may ultimately prove necessary to measure vitamin D levels to help make the diagnosis. The response of urinary cyclic adenosine monophosphate to PTH infusion (increase) may help diagnose idiopathic hypoparathyroidism. During physical examination, a search should be made for a transverse surgical scar on the anterior neck, which would suggest previous thyroidectomy or parathyroidectomy.

Treatment. Treatment of symptomatic hypocalcemia is directed at correcting the calcium deficit, normalizing the relation between ionized and protein-bound calcium by correcting acid–base disorders, and treating the underlying causes. When the need for correction is urgent (e.g., severe, highly symptomatic hypocalcemia), calcium gluconate or calcium chloride is infused. Hypocalcemia associated with chronic disorders is treated over the long term with oral calcium lactate. Vitamin D supplements may be needed; the high doses required in hypoparathyroidism may be reduced if urinary calcium loss is decreased with thiazide diuretics.

Prognosis. Disorders of calcium balance can be treated with complete resolution of symptoms. Underlying disorders must also be identified and treated.

Hypercalcemia

Hypercalcemia is defined as an excessive amount of calcium in the blood, that is, total serum calcium greater than 11 mg/dL.

Etiology. The causes of hypercalcemia are classified in Table 3-10. In surgical patients, primary and secondary hyperparathyroidism and metastatic breast cancer are among the common causes. In fact, more than 90% of hypercalcemic patients who have no symptoms other than depression and fatigue have primary hyperparathyroidism. Malignancies cause hypercalcemia both by bony involvement and by the secretion of PTH-like substances that affect calcium metabolism. Malignancies that are sufficiently advanced to cause hypercalcemia are usually symptomatic. Mobilization of calcium from bone in bedridden patients can cause mild, asymptomatic hypercalcemia. The milk-alkali syndrome (i.e., hypercalcemia, alkalosis, and renal failure) results from excessive intake of calcium and absorbable antacids. Rare causes of hypercalcemia include Williams syndrome (a constellation of congenital defects and abnormal sensitivity to vitamin D) and vitamin A intoxication, possibly by increasing bone resorption.

Presentation and Diagnosis. The initial clinical manifestations of hypercalcemia are nonspecific: weakness, fatigue, anorexia, nausea, and vomiting. As serum calcium increases, severe headaches, diffuse musculoskeletal pain, polyuria, and polydipsia develop. The combination of decreased oral intake, vomiting, and polyuria leads to hypovolemia and dehydration, which may become pronounced. The ECG shows shortened Q-T intervals and

Table 3-10 Causes of Hypercalcemia

Hyperparathyroidism
Malignancy
Metastatic cancer
Lymphoma
Leukemia
Granulomatous disease
Sarcoidosis
Tuberculosis
Fungal infection
Excessive dietary intake
Milk-alkali syndrome
Vitamin A or D intoxication
Thiazide diuretics
Immobilization
Endocrine abnormalities
Thyrotoxicosis
Adrenal insufficiency

widened T waves. With normal or elevated phosphate, calcification may develop in the kidneys as well as in unusual locations (e.g., heart, skin). Pancreatitis and renal failure may develop as well. The renal failure has multiple causes, including volume depletion, nephrocalcinosis, and deposition of nephrotoxic myeloma proteins or light chains. When serum calcium increases to 15 mg/dL and above, confusion and depression progress to somnolence, stupor, and coma. This degree of hypercalcemia results in death unless it is corrected promptly.

Diagnosis is made primarily by a careful history, including all medications, and blood tests. PTH levels are assessed, and imaging procedures are used to locate a tumor. Squamous cell carcinoma of the bronchus and hypernephromas can produce PTH-related peptide. In a patient with a known malignancy, a search for bone metastasis is indicated. Hypercalcemia associated with bone metastases may be the initial presentation of some malignancies, such as those originating in the prostate or breast.

Treatment. Initially, calcium intake is restricted, hydration status improved, and urinary calcium excretion increased. If the patient is symptomatic or the calcium level is high, the patient should be hospitalized. Large volumes of intravenous normal or half-normal saline are infused. Loop diuretics enhance calcium excretion; however, their use is controversial except in patients with congestive heart failure, because they may increase resorption of calcium from bone and worsen hypercalcemia. Great care must be taken during this process of vigorous hydration and diuresis, with close monitoring of volume status to avoid overload. Meticulous assessment and replacement of electrolytes are necessary. Hypomagnesemia can develop as a result of forced diuresis. Bisphosphonates (e.g., pamidronate) are used in combination with calcitonin (which has a very rapid onset and short duration of action) to inhibit bone resorption. Gallium nitrate, which is nephrotoxic, is used in the treatment of cancer-related hypercalcemia unresponsive to hydration.

Corticosteroids are sometimes used as a longer-term treatment to suppress calcium release from bone in patients with granulomatous disease, vitamin D intoxication, or hematologic malignancies. The usual dose is hydrocortisone 3 mg/kg/day. This treatment may take 1 to 2 weeks to produce an appreciable reduction in serum calcium.

The antineoplastic agent plicamycin (formerly called mithramycin), a DNA-binding antibiotic and an RNA-synthesis inhibitor, acutely reduces serum calcium by an unknown mechanism. It is given in small intravenous doses, 25 μg/kg, for 3 to 4 days. Calcium levels decrease within 48 hours and remain low for several days to weeks. Contraindications include thrombocytopenia, coagulopathy or other bleeding diatheses, and bone marrow suppression from any cause. Plicamycin has significant renal and hepatic toxicity.

Oral or intravenous phosphate supplements are sometimes used to form complexes with ionized calcium. Given intravenously, these supplements may produce a precipitous decrease in serum calcium, resulting in tetany, hypotension, and renal failure. Therefore, phosphate supplementation is generally not recommended.

Prognosis. If the cause of hypercalcemia is treatable and the hypercalcemia itself is treated appropriately before neurologic symptoms become severe, the patient should recover completely. Many of the causes of hypercalcemia are life threatening (e.g., metastatic cancer), and this prognosis determines the outcome more than the hypercalcemia itself.

Magnesium

Magnesium plays an important role in metabolism because it is a cofactor for many enzymes. It also affects neuromuscular function. At least one-half the body's total magnesium is in bone. Most of the remainder is intracellular. Magnesium is the most common intracellular divalent cation, and most intracellular magnesium is bound to adenosine triphosphate. Less than 1% is extracellular. The average daily intake of magnesium is 25 to 30 mEq. Approximately 40% of the magnesium is absorbed, primarily in the jejunum and ileum, and it is excreted primarily by the kidneys. A higher percentage of intake is absorbed if body stores are deficient. The normal range of serum magnesium is 1.5 to 2.5 mg/dL. Normal kidneys conserve magnesium when intake is low, but hypomagnesemia develops if intake remains less than 0.3 mEq/kg/day.

Hypomagnesemia

Hypomagnesemia is common in surgical patients, who are often in a starvation state, experience gastrointestinal losses, or have absorption defects. When magnesium is deficient, losses of potassium and phosphorus, the other two major elements in cells, also occur. These elements are expelled from the cell, and the cells decrease in size to maintain normal intracellular composition. Severe hypomagnesemia also produces severe hypocalcemia by decreasing PTH secretion and by an apparent skeletal resistance and an impaired renal response.

Etiology. The most common cause of hypomagnesemia is dietary deficiency combined with gastrointestinal losses (e.g., diarrhea, nasogastric suction) and deficiencies in other elements. Other causes include chronic alcoholism (especially during withdrawal), malabsorption (especially steatorrhea), acute pancreatitis, improperly constituted hyperalimentation, and endocrine disorders. Hypomagnesemia also occurs as a side effect of many therapeutic drugs, particularly some diuretics, aminoglycosides, amphotericin, cyclosporine, cisplatinum, insulin, and pentamidine. Athletes and pregnant women may be mildly hypomagnesemic.

Presentation and Diagnosis. The effects of magnesium deficiency are not immediate. Like calcium, the body's other major divalent cation, magnesium affects neuromuscular function. Symptoms develop insidiously, first as nonspecific systemic symptoms that include nausea, vomiting, anorexia, weakness, and lethargy, then as neuromuscular symptoms that include muscle cramps, fasciculations, tetany, carpopedal spasm, paresthesias, irritability, inattention and confusion, and cardiac arrhythmias, along with other symptoms of associated hypokalemia and hypocalcemia.

Diagnosis is made by testing serum values. These values may be normal, even in the presence of a deficiency in body magnesium. Volume status should be assessed.

Treatment. Primary attention must be given to correcting the cause. If hypomagnesemia is mild and does not result from an absorptive defect, oral supplements are given. If it is moderate, then it is treated with intravenous magnesium sulfate at a rate of 50 to 100 mEq/day because the oral dose required can cause diarrhea. If symptoms are severe, an intravenous bolus of 8 to 16 mEq of magnesium sulfate is administered, followed by intravenous infusion at a rate of 1 to 2 mEq/kg/day. Concomitant or resultant deficiencies in other elements must also be corrected, and adequate hydration must be maintained. If the patient is in renal failure, extra care must be taken not to overcorrect hypomagnesemia.

Prognosis. Recovery from hypomagnesemia may be complete. The prognosis depends on the etiology, the severity of the deficiency and its symptoms, and the promptness of treatment.

Hypermagnesemia

Clinically significant hypermagnesemia is rare, especially if renal function is normal.

Etiology. Hypermagnesemia can result from renal failure; any injury that causes rhabdomyolysis (e.g., crush injuries, severe burns); dehydration; severe metabolic acidosis; adrenal insufficiency; familial benign hypocalciuric hypercalcemia; or overdosage with magnesium salts in cathartics. In addition, in either mother or newborn, it can occur after treatment for eclampsia. It also occurs in patients with renal failure who use magnesium-containing antacids. Renal excretion is decreased in metabolic alkalosis.

Presentation and Diagnosis. Symptomatic hypermagnesemia follows a progressive pattern, with increasing neuromuscular and central nervous system abnormalities as the serum level increases. Initial nausea is superseded by lethargy, weakness, hypoventilation, and decreased deep-tendon reflexes. The condition then progresses to hypotension and bradycardia, skeletal muscle paralysis, respiratory depression, coma, and death. Diagnosis is made by testing serum values.

Treatment. Mild hypermagnesemia is treated with oral hydration and by controlling magnesium intake (e.g., giving patients with renal failure non–magnesium-containing antacids). Severe symptoms are reversed temporarily by intravenous calcium, and the magnesium excess is treated with hydration and diuretics, or hemodialysis.

Prognosis. Recovery from hypermagnesemia may be complete. The prognosis depends on the etiology, the severity of the deficiency and its symptoms, and the promptness of treatment.

Phosphate

Phosphorus is a component of all body tissues, and it participates in virtually all metabolic processes. In a normal adult, approximately 85% of phosphorus is bound in bone and 15% is distributed in other tissues. Less than 1% is extracellular. The intestine, influenced by vitamin D, absorbs approximately 70% of ingested soluble phosphorus, and a higher proportion if dietary intake is low. The normal adult phosphorus requirement is 2 to 9 mg/kg/day. The amount of phosphorus excreted by normal kidneys is controlled by PTH and is proportional to the amount absorbed. The normal range of serum phosphate is 2.4 to 4.7 mg/dL. Circadian variation, mediated by the adrenal cortex, produces the highest serum levels during the afternoon and night and the lowest levels during the morning.

Hypophosphatemia

Hypophosphatemia is common in surgical patients. When phosphorus is deficient, there are also losses of potassium and magnesium, the other two major elements in cells. These elements are expelled from the cell, and the cells decrease in size to maintain normal intracellular composition.

Etiology. The causes of hypophosphatemia are categorized as (1) inadequate uptake as a result of inadequate dietary intake, malabsorption, gastrointestinal losses, prolonged antacid use, improperly constituted hyperalimentation, or vitamin D deficiency; (2) increased renal excretion as a result of diuretic use, hypervolemia, corticoid therapy, hyperaldosteronism, SIADH, or hyperparathyroidism; or (3) compartmental shifts as a result of hormones, nutrients that stimulate insulin release, treatment of diabetic ketoacidosis, recovery from hypometabolic states, rapidly growing malignancies, or respiratory alkalosis. It is also seen in chronic alcoholism, in burns, and after parathyroidectomy or renal transplantation. Occasionally, hypophosphatemia is the first clue to alcohol withdrawal in a hospitalized patient.

Presentation and Diagnosis. Severe phosphorus deficiency causes anorexia, dizziness, osteomalacia, severe congestive cardiomyopathy, proximal muscle weakness, visual defects, ascending paralysis, hemolytic anemia, and respiratory failure. Leukocyte and erythrocyte malfunction, rhabdomyolysis, hypercalciuria, and severe hypocalcemia are also seen. Central nervous system dysfunction occurs and can progress to seizures, coma, and death. If the hypophosphatemia is a result of vitamin D deficiency, metabolic acidosis may result from reduced renal hydrogen excretion.

Diagnosis is made by testing serum values, but total body phosphate deficiency may exist, even in the face of elevated serum values. Arterial blood gases, pH, and urine phosphate should be measured, along with serum potassium, calcium, and magnesium.

Treatment. Severe hypophosphatemia should prompt an aggressive search for and treatment of the cause. Phosphate salts may be given orally or intravenously. Other associated electrolyte abnormalities must also be treated. Diuretics may be withdrawn. VIPomas should be surgically removed.

Prognosis. Repletion of phosphorus corrects or decreases most abnormalities. Respiratory failure may not be reversed completely, and the ultimate outcome is likely to depend on the prognosis of the underlying condition.

Hyperphosphatemia

Hyperphosphatemia is relatively common in adults and is seen even in the presence of total body phosphate deficiency.

Etiology. The causes of hyperphosphatemia are categorized as (1) decreased renal excretion as a result of renal insufficiency or failure, hyperthyroidism, hypoparathyroidism or pseudohypoparathyroidism, or adrenal insufficiency; (2) increased intestinal absorption as a result of sarcoidosis or tuberculosis (both of which produce vitamin D), or excess phosphate or vitamin D ingestion; (3) iatrogenic, as a result of intravenous infusion of phosphate-containing fluids; or (4) shifts from the intracellular to the extracellular compartment as a result of acidotic states, tumor lysis, hemolytic anemia, thyrotoxicosis, or rhabdomyolysis.

Presentation and Diagnosis. Hyperphosphatemia has no symptoms, although in the presence of severe hypercalcemia, renal failure, or vitamin D intoxication, it may be accompanied by deposition of calcium phosphate in abnormal locations. It is diagnosed by testing serum values. Associated electrolyte abnormalities should also be identified and corrected.

Treatment. Aluminum-based antacids decrease absorption by binding phosphate, and diuretics increase the rate of urinary phosphate excretion. Dialysis is used in patients with renal failure. It is often unnecessary to treat hyperphosphatemia, except by correcting excess intake and addressing associated problems.

Prognosis. The prognosis of hyperphosphatemia depends on its cause.

Disorders of Acid–Base Balance

The management of acid–base disorders depends on prompt recognition and evaluation of the disturbances involved. A history and physical examination alert the physician to the nature and severity of disturbances that can occur in a particular clinical setting (see Table 3-11). Laboratory data pertinent to fluid and electrolyte status and renal function help to identify alterations that contribute to or result from the underlying disturbance. With the help of this information, the data provided by arterial blood gas and pH determinations are analyzed, an accurate diagnosis is made, and an appropriate course of treatment is defined. The measured arterial pH value (pHa) indicates whether alkalosis (pHa > 7.45) or acidosis (pHa < 7.35) is present. The arterial carbon dioxide tension [$Paco_2$] reflects whether any respiratory component is present. The bicarbonate concentration [HCO_3^-] derived from the Henderson-Hasselbalch equation (pHa = pK + log [HCO_3^-/H_2CO_3]) identifies a metabolic component, assuming that pHa and $Paco_2$ measurements are reliable. If an error in either measurement is suspected, the test is repeated or correlated with the [HCO_3^-] derived from the carbon dioxide content on the electrolyte measurements. Normally, the [HCO_3] is derived by subtracting 2–3 from the CO_2 content, to compensate for dissolved CO_2 and CO_2 bound to proteins. The measured Pao_2 and derived saturation values provide information about pulmonary gas exchange and its possible contribution to the acid–base status.

The need for accurate interpretation of blood gas data, especially when mixed disturbances are present, prompted

Table 3-11 Simple Disorders of Acid–Base Balance, With Examples

Respiratory alkalosis	**Metabolic alkalosis**
Congestive heart failure	Chronic diarrhea
Cirrhosis	Cushing's syndrome
Fever	Hyperaldosteronism
Hypermetabolic states	Loop or thiazide diuretics
Hyperventilation	Massive blood transfusion
Pregnancy	Milk-alkali syndrome
Pulmonary embolus	Vomiting
Sepsis	
Respiratory acidosis	**Metabolic acidosis**
Chest cage hypofunction	Anion gap
Central nervous system depression	Acid ingestion
Chronic obstructive pulmonary disease	Advanced renal failure
Drugs	Hypotension
Morbid obesity	Ketoacidosis
Pneumothorax	Renal failure
Sleep apnea	Sepsis
Status asthmaticus	Nonanion gap
	Acute diarrhea
	Moderate renal failure
	Renal tubular acidosis

the introduction of a variety of methods to facilitate their analysis. Some of these methods are too complex for use at the bedside on a busy surgical service. Others that use rules or guidelines for making simple, quick calculations seem more applicable in that setting. The information that they make available is equivalent to that provided when the Henderson-Hasselbalch equation and its modifications are used. Two rules that can be found in the text used to teach advanced cardiac life support (ACLS) are of particular value in practice. They provide simple means for quantitating the effects of changes of $Paco_2$ and $[HCO_3^-]$ on pHa. In turn, that information is used to assess the degree to which acidosis or alkalosis is caused by a respiratory or a metabolic disturbance and to quantitate the base excesses or deficits that contribute to the disturbance. Primary respiratory disturbances cause changes in the $Paco_2$ and produce corresponding effects on the blood hydrogen ion concentration. Metabolic disturbances primarily affect the plasma bicarbonate concentration. Because acute changes allow insufficient time for compensatory mechanisms to respond, the resulting pHa disturbances are often great and the abnormalities may be present in pure form. On the other hand, chronic disturbances allow the full range of compensatory mechanisms to come into play, so that blood pHa may remain near normal despite wide variations in plasma bicarbonate or blood $Paco_2$.

Rule 1. An increase or decrease in $Paco_2$ of 10 mm Hg is associated with a reciprocal decrease or increase, respectively, of 0.08 pH units (e.g., as $Paco_2$ goes up, pH goes down).

Rule 2. An increase or decrease in $[HCO_3^-]$ of 10 mEq/L is associated with a directly related increase or decrease, respectively, of 0.15 pH units (e.g., as $[HCO_3^-]$ goes up, pH goes up).

Acidosis

Whether acidosis has a respiratory or metabolic origin, the consequences of decreased pHa can be life threatening. At pHa levels less than 7.2, peripheral vascular and cardiac responsiveness to catecholamines is decreased. Cardiac dysfunction that occurs as a result of direct myocardial depression and arrhythmia can become significant, even lethal. Exchange of ions across cell membranes and changes in renal tubular transport of electrolytes induced by acidosis cause extracellular potassium concentrations to increase, at times to clinically symptomatic levels.

Respiratory Acidosis

Etiology. Respiratory acidosis is the result of carbon dioxide retention that occurs because of pulmonary alveolar hypoventilation. It can be acute or chronic. When acute, its causes can be numerous, including respiratory depression as a result of narcotics, sedatives, anesthetic agents, and muscle relaxants; limited ventilatory effort as a result of painful thoracic or upper abdominal incisions, or chest wall and pulmonary parenchymal trauma that interferes with the mechanics of breathing (e.g., fractured ribs, flail chest, hemopneumothorax); abdominal distension and impaired diaphragmatic function; and upper-airway obstruction as a result of tumor, foreign body, edema, laryngospasm, tracheobronchial injury, or improperly positioned endotracheal tubes. On the other hand, chronic respiratory acidosis is most often caused by advanced longstanding disorders of the lungs, especially COPD.

Presentation and Diagnosis. A primary respiratory acid–base disorder is present if the $Paco_2$ is abnormal and the $Paco_2$ and the pHa change in opposite directions. The clinical consequences of respiratory acidosis are caused by the effects of hypercapnia and the hypoxia that commonly occurs with it (assuming that the hypoxemia is not masked by increased inhaled oxygen concentrations). Acutely, mild hypertension and restlessness are evident. When $Paco_2$ levels continue to rise, somnolence, confusion, and ultimately coma (as a result of carbon dioxide narcosis) occur. In combination with hypoxemia, severe hypercapnia is also associated with significant cardiovascular dysfunction, including cardiac arrest. In patients with chronic respiratory acidosis, carbon dioxide narcosis is the major threat, although tolerance to hypercapnia is increased. In part, this increase is related to the compensatory increase in $[HCO_3^-]$ that is caused by the renal conservation of base, a phenomenon that is not apparent in the acute state because of the time needed for it to evolve.

Rules 1 and 2 can be used to determine whether respiratory changes are responsible for an acute acidotic state. According to rule 1, if the magnitude of the $Paco_2$ increase can account for the pH change, a pure respiratory acidosis exists. If the pH change is greater than can be accounted for, however, a metabolic component of acidosis must also exist. If the pH change is less than the increase in $Paco_2$ would predict, an element of metabolic alkalosis is present. The use of rule 2 in this case shows the contribution that an elevated $[HCO_3^-]$ makes to the mixed acid–base disturbance. In chronic respiratory acidosis, in contrast to the acute state, this finding is expected as a consequence of compensatory renal retention of bicarbonate.

Treatment. The treatment of respiratory acidosis is directed at removing the cause of the reduced alveolar ventilation while ensuring adequate oxygenation. Inadequate pain control is a common cause of respiratory acidosis. In the acute state, or with acute deterioration of a chronic situation, temporary use of mechanical ventilatory support and oxygen therapy may be necessary. In this case, acute hypercapnea should not be corrected too rapidly. Sudden decreases in $Paco_2$ cause sudden pH changes and ionic shifts between cellular and extracellular fluids, and this can produce severe cardiac dysrhythmias, including ventricular arrhythmias. Rapid decreases in $Paco_2$ may also decrease cerebral blood flow to critical levels in patients with head injury. The administration of bicarbonate to improve the buffering capacity of extracellular fluids in respiratory acidosis, without treating the cause, is not an appropriate treatment option.

Prognosis. In the acute state, once the underlying cause of decreased alveolar ventilation is treated, the hypercapnia will resolve. Chronic respiratory acidosis is generally well tolerated until severe pulmonary insufficiency leads to hypoxia. At this point, the long-term prognosis is poor.

Metabolic Acidosis

Metabolic acidosis (pH < 7.35) is a decrease in pHa related to a decreased arterial $[HCO_3^-]$ or increased hydrogen ion production. It can be acute or chronic.

Etiology. Metabolic acidosis occurs for two major reasons. The first is the loss of bicarbonate from the extracellular space. This loss occurs acutely with certain gastrointestinal disorders (e.g., diarrhea, external pancreatic fistula) and more chronically with increased urinary bicarbonate losses that occur with renal tubular disorders, ureterointestinal anastomoses, decreased mineralocorticoid activity, and diuresis induced with the carbonic anhydrase inhibitor acetazolamide. The second major cause of metabolic acidosis, most often as an acute process, is an increased metabolic acid load. This increase is seen with lactic **acidemia** secondary to cardiogenic, septic, and hypovolemic low-flow states or ischemia of major tissue beds (e.g., mesenteric infarction), ketoacidosis, and renal failure. Lactic acidosis is one of the most common causes of a high anion gap metabolic acidosis in critically ill patients. The differential diagnoses of lactic acidosis are historically classified in two groups: type A, due to hypoxia; and type B, not due to hypoxia. Causes of type A lactic acidosis include tissue hypoperfusion (such as that due to cardiac failure) and reduced arterial oxygen content due to pulmonary disease, severe anemia, or carbon monoxide poisoning. Causes of type B acidosis include liver failure, renal failure, cancer, strenuous exercise, seizure, ingestion of large amounts of alcohol by undernourished patients, toxicity due to biguanide therapy, and thiamine deficiency.

Presentation and Diagnosis. A primary metabolic acid–base disorder is present if the pHa is abnormal and the pHa and the $Paco_2$ change in the same direction. With both acute and chronic metabolic acidosis, respiratory compensation occurs. Ventilation is stimulated by the increased hydrogen ion concentration in arterial blood, and $Paco_2$ is reduced. The degree of compensation is determined by the extent of the hypocapnia that is induced and by estimates of its modifying influence on the pHa, as determined by application of rule 1. Similarly, the use of rule 2 to estimate whether measured decreases in $[HCO_3^-]$ can fully account for the measured changes in pHa identifies mixed acid–base disturbances.

Determination of the anion gap can help to distinguish metabolic acidosis caused by a loss of bicarbonate from that caused by an accumulation of a metabolic acid load. The anion gap is the difference between the serum sodium concentration and the sum of the serum bicarbonate and chloride concentrations:

$$Na - [Cl + HCO_3^-]$$

With losses of bicarbonate, decreases in the serum concentration of this anion are accompanied by reciprocal increases in chloride ion concentrations. The anion gap remains normal (~15 mEq/L). In contrast, with metabolic acid loads, chloride levels do not increase as the bicarbonate levels decrease, and the measured anion gap is greater than normal. Actually, the gap is more apparent than real, because unmeasured anions of metabolic acids are present in amounts that account for differences calculated solely on the basis of measured bicarbonate and chloride values.

Treatment. Treatment of metabolic acidosis depends on identifying the underlying disorder and correcting it. Often this is sufficient. In other conditions, particularly when there is an increased anion gap, intravenous replacement of bicarbonate is needed. The need to focus attention on the treatment of the underlying cause is critical in the management of metabolic acidosis caused by low-flow states. Hypovolemia must be corrected, sepsis must be controlled, and cardiovascular dynamics must be enhanced to improve tissue perfusion and satisfy cellular metabolic needs. Unless these goals are accomplished, no amount of infused bicarbonate by itself will succeed in returning the pHa to normal. Similarly, with diabetic ketoacidosis, treatment of the pHa with bicarbonate is of little value without concomitant administration of insulin and intravenous fluids.

If the patient is compensating fully for the metabolic acidosis by hyperventilating and the pHa is still less than 7.25, then bicarbonate may be used, assuming that the underlying disorder is being corrected. The amount needed to correct the pHa to normal is estimated as follows: (1) Using rule 1, the disparity between the pHa measured and the pHa calculated on the basis of the measured $Paco_2$ is determined. The difference defines the pHa decrease that is caused by a decrease in $[HCO_3^-]$. (2) Using rule 2, the pHa difference is translated into the decrease in $[HCO_3^-]$ that it represents. With that information and the assumption of a bicarbonate space that is approximately 50% TBW (25% to 30% body weight), the amount of bicarbonate needed to correct the total body base deficit is calculated as:

$$\text{mEq } HCO_3^- \text{ needed} = \text{mEq/L } [HCO_3^-] \text{ deficit} \times (\text{kg wt} \times 0.25)$$

In extreme circumstances (e.g., cardiac arrest), when a precipitous and life-threatening decrease in pHa will impair the effectiveness of efforts to resuscitate the patient, bolus administration of 1 mg/kg as an initial dose followed by one-half this dose every 10 minutes until the pHa is greater than 7.25 is justified. Otherwise, when the disturbance is less severe, it is better to proceed at a slower pace to avoid the consequences of overzealous and too rapid administration of intravenous bicarbonate. These consequences include cardiac irregularities, convulsions, metabolic alkalosis, hypokalemia, impairment of the delivery of red blood cell oxygen to tissues, and symptomatic hyperosmolarity as a result of the infusion of excessive amounts of sodium. Usually, it is advisable to replace no more than one-half of the calculated bicarbonate deficit in the first 3 to 4 hours and then, over the next 12 to 24 hours, to administer the remainder until serum bicarbonate and pHa values return to more normal levels. Again, it is imperative to treat the underlying cause of the metabolic acidosis.

Alkalosis

When the pHa rises to more than 7.45, regardless of the cause, alkalosis is present. The nature and importance of alkalosis with respect to fluid and electrolyte balance and oxygen carried by hemoglobin were discussed in the sections on hypokalemia, hypocalcemia, hypomagnesemia, and hypophosphatemia. Alkalosis also has clinical features that are specific to either respiratory or metabolic alkalosis.

Respiratory Alkalosis

When the increase in pHa is related to a decrease in Pa_{CO_2}, respiratory alkalosis is present. In the surgical patient, this problem is often caused by hyperventilation with short, shallow breaths because of pain in the young, but respiratory acidosis may occur instead in the elderly as pain decreases alveolar ventilation.

Etiology. Respiratory alkalosis is the consequence of pulmonary alveolar hyperventilation, which is commonly encountered in surgical patients. Apprehension, pain that does not limit respiratory effort, hypoxia, fever, CNS injuries, sepsis, and elevated serum ammonia levels in patients with chronic liver disease can stimulate respiration and cause hypocapnia and respiratory alkalosis. Hyperventilation, causing a decrease in Pa_{CO_2}, is common in patients who are mechanically ventilated during surgery or perioperatively.

Compensatory mechanisms for acute respiratory alkalosis are relatively ineffective in surgical patients. Renal compensatory efforts occur in the form of distal tubular excretion of bicarbonate. However, hyponatremia and increased aldosterone activity, which are common in surgically stressed patients, limit the effectiveness of this mechanism, which depends on renal excretion of sodium as the accompanying cation. Only with chronic respiratory alkalosis is any notable compensatory decrease in $[HCO_3^-]$ seen.

Presentation and Diagnosis. The clinical manifestations of acute respiratory alkalosis are paresthesias in the extremities, carpopedal spasm, and a positive Chvostek's sign. In addition to the consequences of disturbed potassium, calcium, magnesium, and phosphate metabolism that are seen in all alkalotic states, the low Pa_{CO_2} levels characteristic of respiratory alkalosis can, by themselves, exert significant pathophysiologic influences. Acute hypocapnia can cause cerebral vasoconstriction, which can reduce blood flow to the brain by as much as 50% (1% to 3% for each 1-mm Hg drop in Pa_{CO_2}). These effects can have particular significance in older patients whose cerebral arterial circulation might also be compromised by atherosclerotic disease.

Treatment. In the artificially ventilated patient, reduction of the amount of ventilation that is being provided can correct both the reasons for and the consequences of respiratory alkalosis. In the absence of mechanical hyperventilation as a cause, however, efforts are directed at treating the underlying conditions that are responsible for hypocapnia. Chronic respiratory alkalosis occurs in pulmonary and liver disease and generally does not require treatment.

Metabolic Alkalosis

When an elevated pHa is associated with an elevated $[HCO_3^-]$, metabolic alkalosis is present.

Etiology. Metabolic alkalosis is probably the most common acid–base disorder seen in general surgical patients. The ways in which gastrointestinal and renal losses of potassium and chloride ions can occur and can cause hypochloremic hypokalemic metabolic alkalosis were discussed in the sections dealing with disorders of those ions. The accumulation of exogenously infused excesses of base can also cause metabolic alkalosis in surgical patients. This situation can result from overzealous infusion of bicarbonate in the treatment of metabolic acidosis or the inadvertent administration of large amounts of citrate when multiple transfusions are given. Metabolic alkalosis can also occur through contraction of the extracellular volume from diuretic administration.

In metabolic alkalosis, the retention of carbon dioxide as a result of hypoventilation can help to compensate for the accumulation of base excess. In surgical patients, this mechanism may not be effective. On the other hand, renal tubular excretion of bicarbonate in an alkaline urine may be effective. However, as discussed with paradoxical aciduria that appears in the course of hypochloremic hypokalemic metabolic alkalosis, this mechanism for compensation cannot be sustained as the depletion of electrolytes grows more severe. The urine then becomes acidic as hydrogen ion is secreted and bicarbonate ion is reabsorbed. This situation enhances the severity of the existing metabolic alkalosis.

Presentation and Diagnosis. In general, the clinical problems seen with metabolic alkalosis are most often related to the hypokalemia, hypochloremia, and volume contraction caused by gastrointestinal or renal losses of fluid and electrolytes. Important clinical manifestations of potassium depletion, in particular, include paralytic ileus, digitalis toxicity, and cardiac arrhythmias.

Treatment. The successful treatment of metabolic alkalosis requires control of extrarenal losses of fluid and electrolytes and correction of fluid volume, potassium, and chloride deficits. With adequate volume repletion, the stimulus to tubular sodium reabsorption is diminished, and the kidneys can then excrete excess bicarbonate. Most patients will also require potassium supplementation. Only when all these issues are successfully addressed can appropriate renal tubular responses be restored and pHa returned to normal.

Chloride-responsive metabolic alkalosis, characterized by urinary chloride levels less than 10 mEq/L, as seen with significant uncorrected aspiration of gastric contents, generally responds to administration of chloride. Chloride-resistant metabolic alkalosis, characterized by urinary chloride levels greater than 20 mEq/L, as seen in primary hyperaldosteronism, generally responds to administration of glucocorticoids.

Mixed Acid–Base Disorders

As mentioned at the beginning of this section, the interpretation of mixed acid–base disorders can be complex. Such a disorder should be suspected when the changes in pH, $Paco_2$, and $[HCO_3^-]$ do not conform to the pattern expected for a simple acid–base disorder (see Table 3-12). Adequate understanding requires examination of serum electrolytes in addition to blood gas values. If $Paco_2$ and $[HCO_3^-]$ are markedly abnormal in the presence of normal or only slightly abnormal pH, a mixed disorder is extremely likely. If metabolic and respiratory components are abnormal in the same direction, extreme changes in pH may be seen. Discussion of mixed acid–base disorders is beyond the scope of this text.

Table 3-12 Mixed Acid–Base Disorders

Disorder	pH	$PaCO_2$	HCO_2
Metabolic acidosis + respiratory acidosis	↓↓	↑	↓
Metabolic acidosis + respiratory alkalosis	✓	↓	↓
Metabolic alkalosis + respiratory acidosis	✓	↑	↑
Metabolic alkalosis + respiratory alkalosis	↑↑	↓	↑

SUGGESTED READINGS

Gynn S. Kidney function and fluid balance in the elderly surgical patient. In: Gynn S, ed. *Medical Assessment of the Elderly Surgical Patient.* Rockford, IL: Aspen, 1986:189–223.

Halperin NL, Goldstein MB. *Fluid, Electrolyte and Acid–Base Physiology: A Problem-Based Approach.* 2nd Ed. Philadelphia, PA: WB Saunders, 1994.

Kokko JP, Tannen RL. *Fluids and Electrolytes.* 3rd Ed. Philadelphia, PA: WB Saunders, 1996.

Pestana C. *Fluids and Electrolytes in the Surgical Patient.* 5th Ed. Baltimore, MD: Williams & Wilkins, 1996.

Rose BD, Post TW. *Clinical Physiology of Acid–Base and Electrolyte Disorders.* 5th Ed. New York, NY: McGraw-Hill, 2001.

Sladen A. Acid–base balance. In: McIntyre KM, Lewis AJ, eds. *Textbook of Advanced Cardiac Life Support.* Dallas, TX: American Heart Association, 1994.

Valtin H. *Renal Function: Mechanisms Preserving Fluid and Solute Balance in Health.* 3rd Ed. Boston, MA: Little, Brown, 1995.

4

ANTHONY P. BORZOTTA, MD

Nutrition

OBJECTIVES

1. List at least four factors in a patient's medical history and physical examination that indicate malnutrition or risk for malnutrition.
2. Discuss the following objective assessments of nutritional status: anthropometric measurements, biochemical blood tests, immune function studies, and indirect calorimetry.
3. Determine a patient's protein and calorie requirements by estimation, with the Harris-Benedict equation or with specific laboratory tests.
4. List at least four water-soluble vitamins, three fat-soluble vitamins, and four trace elements that must be added to long-term parenteral nutrition.
5. Briefly describe the metabolic changes that occur in short-term and long-term starvation.
6. Discuss the effect of injury or infection on a patient's metabolism, and describe how nutritional support must be altered.
7. List at least five indications each for enteral and parenteral nutritional support.
8. Discuss the factors involved in choosing a route of nutritional support.
9. Describe the risks and benefits of enteral and parenteral nutritional support.
10. List at least four gastrointestinal, four mechanical, and four metabolic complications of enteral therapy, and describe appropriate prevention or treatment of each.
11. List four adverse sequelae of a total parenteral nutrition (TPN) catheter and four metabolic complications of TPN. Describe the appropriate treatment of each.

Nutrition is the study of the provision and use of foodstuffs in support of metabolic needs for immediate energy, protein synthesis, circulation and respiration, locomotion, energy storage, and waste product excretion. The surgeon often encounters patients who cannot eat normally, who are nutritionally depleted, or whose illness places them at risk for malnutrition. Consequently, surgeons care for patients needing a nutritional support program to maintain or restore normal body weight and composition. Many major advances in nutritional support were made by surgeons, including the first demonstration that intravenous nutrition alone could support normal growth, reported by Dudrick et al. in 1969.

This chapter describes and defines the current clinical and laboratory techniques for assessing nutritional status; the basic requirements for proteins, carbohydrates, lipids, and micronutrients; and the metabolic patterns found in normal, fasted, and stressed states. The indications for beginning (and the techniques for instituting, maintaining, and monitoring) enteral and parenteral nutritional therapy are outlined. New concepts will be introduced on the pharmacologic uses of some foods to manipulate the metabolic state or alter immune function. Finally, some areas of controversy and promise for the future are discussed.

ASSESSMENT OF NUTRITIONAL STATUS

History

Proper history taking and keen observation usually elicit clinical findings of malnutrition when present. Poverty, alcoholism, and the extremes of age are risk factors for malnutrition. Unplanned weight loss is identified by comparing current with earlier weights and determining whether the skin or clothing has become loose. A recent weight loss of 10% is considered significant, 15% is severe, and 20% may increase operative mortality 10-fold.

Malnutrition can develop in a number of ways that can be discovered by taking a careful nutritional history. Diminished intake may occur in people with severely restricted diets; anorexia of depression or illness; psychological diseases (e.g., bulimia, anorexia nervosa); and dysphagia as a result of esophageal cancer, bulbar palsy after stroke, or breathlessness while eating (e.g., severe obstructive pulmonary disease). Hospitalized patients who are maintained on 5% dextrose solutions are on enforced fasts that may unintentionally become prolonged. Increased losses may occur in malabsorption syndromes or inflammatory bowel disease and from gastrointestinal fistulas or chronically draining wounds. Subtle, chronic increases in metabolic workload may lead to malnutrition. Up to 60% of chronic obstructive pulmonary disease (COPD) patients are malnourished, and some cancers induce a catabolic state. Supranormal nutritional requirements unmet by usual feeding habits are seen in trauma, burns, fever, and sepsis. Catabolic medications (e.g., glucocorticoids, immunosuppressants, isoniazid) may alter nutrient requirements, whereas other therapeutic modalities (e.g., cancer chemotherapy, radiation therapy) often have side effects that reduce the appetite or ability to eat.

Many clinicians still rely on subjective global assessment, based on an individual surgeon's clinical experience. When history and physical examination alone were analyzed in comparison with other methods of nutritional assessment, they provided the best combination of sensitivity and specificity for detecting malnutrition. This finding indicates two things: (1) the value of close observation and personal clinical experience and (2) the lack of any independent, completely valid measure of nutritional status. The absence of a single standard is a major impediment to the analysis of the effect of nutritional therapy on acute disease.

The Joint Commission for Accreditation of Hospitals Organization requires that all hospitalized patients receive a nutritional assessment. However, patients are increasingly admitted on the same day that surgery is to take place, with little preoperative time for assessment by hospital personnel. Thus, the ability to screen for patients who might benefit from preoperative or perioperative nutritional support becomes more difficult. *This situation requires an increasingly greater awareness of nutritional assessment by the surgeon in the office setting.*

Many of the techniques described later should be used repeatedly to assess the effectiveness of nutritional therapy. The goals are positive nitrogen balance and repletion of diminished physical and chemical parameters, or their stabilization in the face of elevated metabolic demands.

Anthropometric Measurements

A variety of techniques are used to assess body fuel depots or body composition. The simplest are anthropometric measurements. Height and weight are universally attainable and are compared with standard tables of ideal values adjusted for age and sex and body frame. Obesity is defined as a body weight greater than ideal weight as follows: mild (15% to 30%), moderate (30% to 50%), severe (50% to 100%) and morbid (> 100%). Another method of defining obesity, used in bariatric surgery, is the body mass index (BMI). The BMI is the weight (kg) divided by the square of the height (meters). Normal BMI is 20 to 25. An index between 25 and 30 is borderline to moderate excessive body fat, and one greater than 30 reflects obesity.

Estimates of body composition can be made by other physical measurements. The triceps skinfold is the thickness of a pinch of skin and fat overlying the triceps of the nondominant arm, midway between the acromion and olecranon, measured with skinfold calipers. When compared with standard values, this measurement provides an estimate of subcutaneous fat stores. Skeletal muscle mass, the greatest body protein depot, is assessed with the arm-muscle circumference. This measurement is determined by taking the midarm circumference (in millimeters) minus 0.314 times the triceps skinfold (in millimeters). This measure of skeletal muscle mass, often referred to as *somatic protein status*, is compared with normal values specific for sex and age.

Measuring function rather than size is more germane to surgical concerns, if more difficult. Muscle strength is related to nutritional status and is measured by handgrip or forearm dynamometry. These techniques measure the amount of force that is generated by willed muscle contraction. Age- and sex-related norms in healthy volunteers were recently established. Patients who ranked below the 85% cutoff value had more postoperative complications.

Anthropometric measurements are more useful in population studies and less applicable to individual nutritional assessments, except over long periods of nutritional therapy. Deviation from normal does not reliably predict a malnourished state because the standards poorly account for individual variation in bone size, hydration, or skin compressibility. These measurements respond slowly to changes in nutritional status, and their interpretation may be complicated by simple fluid changes, especially in very ill hospitalized patients.

Biochemical Measurements

Although skeletal muscle mass reflects somatic protein status, concentrations of the plasma transport proteins reflect internal or visceral protein status. Albumin, transferrin, retinol-binding protein, and prealbumin (Table 4-1) are used to assess nutritional status and response to feeding. However, plasma concentration does not always reflect turnover rate or the production and destruction of a compound. Changes in the volume of distribution (e.g., expansion of the extracellular fluid space during a major resuscitation) can decrease the serum albumin level by dilution, regardless of nutritional status. Because of its short half-life, prealbumin is the most reliable choice for monitoring visceral protein response to therapy.

The creatinine–height index estimates somatic protein status because creatinine production from creatine is di-

Table 4-1 Visceral Proteins Used in Nutritional Assessment

Protein	Half-Life (days)	Normal Levels	Malnutrition		
			Mild	Moderate	Severe
Albumin	18	3.5–5.5 g/dL	3.0–3.5	2.1–3.0	< 2.1
Transferrin	8	200–400 mg/dL	150–190	100–150	< 100
Prealbumin	2–4	15.7–29.6 mg/dL	12–15	8–10	< 8

Normal ranges may vary according to laboratory.

rectly related to skeletal muscle mass. The 24-hour urine creatinine excretion divided by the value for a normal individual of the same sex, height, and ideal weight obtained from standardized tables equals the creatinine–height index. The normal creatinine excretion is 23 to 28 mg/kg ideal body weight/day in men and 18 to 21 mg/kg ideal weight/day in women. These values decrease with age. Creatinine–height indices of 60% to 80% of ideal weight indicate moderate depletion; indices of 40% to 50% indicate severe depletion of lean body mass.

Accurate measurement of nitrogen balance is key to nutritional support practices. Nitrogen balance is nitrogen intake minus nitrogen excretion. Nitrogen intake is determined from dietary history, calorie counts, or the known composition of enteral or parenteral formulations. The clinical standard for measuring nitrogen excretion is a 24-hour urine collection for urinary urea nitrogen (UUN) expressed in grams of nitrogen per 24 hours. To compensate for diurnal changes in nitrogen accretion and excretion related to cyclic eating, a 24-hour collection is necessary in the patient who is eating spontaneously. Shorter collection periods of as little as 6 hours are adequate in continuously fed patients. The UUN is 80% to 90% of total urinary nitrogen. The remainder consists of such compounds as ammonia, creatinine, and amino acids. Customarily, 3 or 4 g is added to the UUN value to account for unmeasured nitrogen losses. A highly stressed patient loses a greater proportion of nonurea nitrogen compounds than does a stable patient. In such conditions, the UUN is increasingly less accurate and should be replaced by total nitrogen measurements, if available. A positive nitrogen balance indicates that there is net protein synthesis; a negative balance indicates that more nitrogen is being lost than ingested. Zero, or balance point, varies with the premorbid customary intake, the metabolic state, and the quality of ingested protein. Protein quality is related to the proportions of essential and nonessential amino acids in a foodstuff.

Nitrogen losses are roughly proportional to the catabolic state, hence the following average losses in grams of nitrogen per day: starvation-adapted, 5; stable after elective surgery, 8 to 12; polytrauma, 15 to 20; and sepsis or burns, more than 20. Nitrogen balance measurements are taken before nutritional support is initiated and at least weekly thereafter to assess and ensure the adequacy of therapy.

For example, a 60-year-old man with esophageal cancer who has limited his food intake because of odynophagia may be in a starvation-adapted state on admission, excreting only 5 g N/day. After esophagectomy the next day, his nitrogen losses double to 10 g N/day, increasing further to 17 g N/day when pneumonia complicates his postoperative course a week later. Throughout this period, his nutritional support provided a steady 10 g N/day. Assuming unmeasured urine nitrogen losses of 3 g/day, his nitrogen balances would be as follows:

Admission: N_{in} (10 g) $-$ N_{out} (5 + 3 = 8 g) = $N_{balance}$ (2 g) per day
Postop: N_{in} (10 g) $-$ N_{out} (10 + 3 = 13 g) = $N_{balance}$ (-3 g) per day
With pneumonia: N_{in} (10 g) $-$ N_{out} (17 + 3 = 20 g) = $N_{balance}$ (-10 g) per day.

Immunologic Measurements

Nutrition and immunocompetence are closely linked. When entire populations are examined, for example, malnutrition correlates with an increased incidence of tuberculosis, epidemics of contagious diseases, and pneumonia. Malnourished individuals are prey to infectious complications of operations. Hence, immunologic functions are used to assess nutritional state. The absolute lymphocyte count reflects visceral protein status in the absence of nonnutritional variables, such as trauma, anesthesia, and chemotherapy, all of which depress the count. Low counts concurrent with hypoalbuminemia are correlated with an increased incidence of postoperative sepsis. The minimum normal level is 1500×10^6 cells/L.

Delayed hypersensitivity skin tests are anamnestic immune responses to a battery of antigens placed intradermally: mumps, purified protein derivative (PPD), streptokinase-streptodornase (SK-SD), *Candida*, and histoplasmin. A normal response is a 5-mm or greater area of induration in response to at least one antigen at 48 hours. Partial responses are smaller, and nonresponders are termed anergic. Response depends on previous exposure, an adequate dose of antigen, and proper technique of injection and measurement. Responses are depressed by malnutrition, infection, trauma, surgery, anesthesia, burns, corticosteroids, malignancy, and renal failure.

These tests are not specific measures of nutritional state. They may be applicable in stable patients, but are not of value for measuring nutritional state during acute illness.

Body Composition Analysis

The measurement of body composition by bioelectrical impedance analysis (BIA) is improving in accuracy and acceptance. This simple, rapid bedside technique uses a tetrapolar electrode array on a hand and foot. An electric current flows between the outer electrodes and the voltage drop is measured between the inner sensing electrodes. The measured resistance is combined with height, and sometimes weight, sex, or thigh circumference, into a computation that yields fat-free mass. Fat-free mass is composed of the body cell mass (all of the vital, oxygen-consuming tissues of the body), extracellular fluid, and extracellular solids. BIA-measured fat-free mass compares well with exchangeable Na/K measurements and with densitometry in well persons, those with AIDS, and those who are receiving nutritional support. It is used in both the outpatient and rehabilitation settings. Its precision in hospitalized patients who are experiencing rapid fluid shifts is under study.

BASIC NUTRITIONAL NEEDS

The supply and use of nutrients interact in a dynamic process. Metabolism varies with the amount of nutrient intake; the proportions of carbohydrate, lipid, and protein; the availability of micronutrients; and the homeostatic balance of the organism. This section describes essential substrate needs and how to estimate them.

Protein and Amino Acid Needs

The protein requirement is the amount needed to meet physiologic needs and is the lowest protein intake at which nitrogen balance can be achieved. *Proteins do not exist in storage form: they all have structural, enzymatic, immune, and transport functions.* Ingestion of amino acids in excess of needs results not in storage, but in deamination, nitrogen excretion as urea and ammonia, and reuse of the carbon skeletons. When intake is insufficient, functioning protein is mobilized, principally through skeletal muscle proteolysis. As a result, essential amino acids are added to endogenous, nonessential amino acids, and gluconeogenic substrates are provided to the liver. Although muscle wasting is the primary site of breakdown, the lungs, heart, kidneys, and white blood cells also contribute. If this self-consumption is unchecked beyond the point at which 50% of lean body mass is lost, death may ensue. The mechanisms of compensation during starvation are discussed later in the section on metabolic states.

Determining the patient's protein requirement is the first critical step in formulating a nutritional support program. The requirements for a normal, active person are 0.8 to 1.0 g protein/kg body weight daily (6.25 g protein = 1 g nitrogen). Requirements change with the clinical state, decreasing to < 1 g/kg/day early in refeeding after starvation and increasing to 2 to 2.5 g/kg/day in burned or severely septic patients. Total protein intake may need to be limited to 40 to 50 g/day in patients with hepatic failure. A 24-hour urine nitrogen loss measurement provides the most accurate and individualized estimate of nitrogen (protein) needs.

Protein balance cannot be achieved without protein intake, but the provision of nonprotein calories significantly enhances the efficiency of protein use. In the absence of nonprotein energy substrates, much exogenous protein intake is simply oxidized, not used to create new proteins. Protein sparing from oxidation is achieved with 150 to 200 g (700 kcal) glucose daily. This value is the basis for the common use of three liters per day of intravenous 5% glucose solutions. It also defines hypocaloric, 3% amino acid peripheral vein infusions (protein-sparing therapy) that are used by some clinicians in fasting clinical situations, such as repeated nothing by mouth (NPO) status during prolonged diagnostic evaluation, bowel obstruction, or adynamic ileus without previous weight loss. The remaining energy requirements are met by mobilization of fat stores.

Two further concepts concerning protein utilization should be kept in mind. First, at any fixed level of protein intake, nitrogen balance improves to a maximum as calorie intake increases from inadequate levels to levels that exceed energy requirements. That is, nonprotein calories supply energy to the body, allowing ingested protein to be used for synthetic purposes rather than being oxidized. Second, even when all energy needs are met by nonprotein calories, the nitrogen balance becomes increasingly negative at a fixed nitrogen intake as catabolism increases in disease states (e.g., burns, peritonitis, multiple trauma).

A practice to be faulted is the exogenous supply of albumin during nutritional support of hypoalbuminemic patients. In critically ill patients, the radioiodinated albumin half-life falls from 17 to 19 days to 5.5 to 12 days, with albumin catabolization per day similar to normal patients. This suggests a synthetic defect, perhaps associated with a shift to acute phase reactant production by the liver. Although an albumin infusion will increase serum concentration, morbidity or mortality is not improved.

Several amino acids are of special interest. The *branched-chain amino acids* (BCAAs; leucine, isoleucine, and valine) are essential amino acids that act as oxidative substrate in skeletal muscle; have protein synthesis–enhancing properties (particularly leucine); and inhibit protein breakdown. Several BCAA-enhanced solutions are available, but they have not been shown to improve clinical outcome. Further proof of their benefit is needed before they can be recommended as a routine supplement.

Glutamine, a nonessential amino acid, is the most abundant in the body, accounting for one-third of the amino acids released from muscle during stress. Glutamine is an ammonia donor in the kidney, aiding in acid–base balance; it is a primary fuel for rapidly proliferating tissues (enterocytes, colonocytes, fibroblasts, white blood cells); and it is a precursor of the antioxidant glutathione. It appears to be provisionally essential in catabolic states.

Arginine is considered a conditionally essential amino acid for T-cell growth and replication; it promotes nitrogen retention and wound healing; and supplemental levels promote immune function during metabolic stress. Two recent studies in trauma patients showed that L-arginine-enhanced enteral feeding (with several other potentially positive immunomodulators) significantly reduces septic complications compared with an isocaloric, isonitrogenous formula. To summarize, continuing research shows specific actions by individual amino acids beyond their simple contribution to nitrogen balance.

Energy Needs

Caloric requirements range from 25 to 80 kcal/kg/day, depending on age (greater in childhood) and stress. *Carbohydrate caloric value is 3.4 kcal/gram.* Glycogen, a carbohydrate storage form that is available for immediate energy needs, is in short supply. The approximately 75 g glycogen in the liver and the 200 to 400 g glycogen in adult muscle lasts only 1 to 2 days without replenishment. Muscle glycogen is glycolysed into lactate and pyruvate, which are then transported to the liver to be incorporated into glucose through the Cori cycle. Pyruvate is transaminated in muscle and released as alanine, a major substrate for hepatic gluconeogenesis. Lipolysis in adipose tissue releases triglycerides, which serve immediate energy needs for nonglycolytic tissues. Fat is the largest storehouse of energy and is the principal energy source during long fasts. Protein, especially from skeletal muscle, can be an energy source, but at the cost of destroying functional proteins. Conservation of protein occurs as a survival mechanism during long fasts.

The caloric values of major substrates are as follows:

Carbohydrates	3.4 kcal/g
Lipids	9.3 kcal/g
Proteins	4.0 kcal/g

The energy requirement can be *estimated* in several ways (Table 4-2). While each equation has its advocates, and special equations are available for subpopulations (e.g. obese, mechanically ventilated, geriatric), the Harris-Benedict equations (HBE) are among the most commonly used. The Harris-Benedict equations estimate the resting metabolic expenditure (RME), the energy needed to lie quietly in bed after an overnight fast. For each patient, the RME must be multiplied by both activity and stress factors to reach a total daily requirement. The factors are: fever, 1.13/1°C; bed rest, 1.15; ambulation, 1.2 to 1.3; major elective surgery, 1.2 to 1.4; trauma and fractures, 1.5 to 1.8; and severe sepsis and burns, 1.8 to 2.5. Obviously, a great deal of clinical experience is used to select a factor.

Table 4-2 Estimating Energy Needs

Harris-Benedict equations for resting metabolic rate (kcal/day):
Men: RME = 66.47 + 13.75 × weight (kg) + 5 × height (cm) − 6.76 × age (yr)
Women: RME = 665.1 + 9.56 × weight (kg) + 1.85 × height (cm) − 4.7 × age (yr)
World Health Organization, based on compilation of 11,000 measurements in people of all ages, both sexes, all ethnic groups, and all body mass indices (kj/24 hr). Convert kilojoules to kilocalories by dividing by 4.184:
Men: 18 to 30 yr: RME = 64.4 × weight (kg) − 113.0 × height (m) + 3000
30 to 60 yr: RME = 19.2 × weight (kg) + 66.9 × height (m) + 3769
Women: 18 to 30 yr: RME = 55.6 × weight (kg) + 1397.4 × height (m) + 146
30 to 60 yr: RME = 36.4 × weight (kg) − 104.6 × height (m) + 3619
General estimate based on weight alone:
25 to 30 kcal/kg/day in nonobese persons
Increase by 12% after major surgery, by 20% to 50% during sepsis, and up to 80% with major burns
For obese persons, use ideal body weight

RME, resting metabolic expenditure.

All of these equations are population-derived estimates and simply approximate individual needs. The HBE may significantly underestimate or overestimate individual needs in up to 40% of patients.

Individualized energy need can be assessed by *measuring* energy expenditure. A metabolic cart is a portable instrument that uses indirect calorimetry to quantify energy needs. A metabolic cart includes a paramagnetic oxygen analyzer and an infrared CO_2 analyzer to measure the volumes of oxygen consumed and carbon dioxide expired per unit time. The ratio $CO_2{:}O_2$ is the respiratory quotient (RQ) and reflects the proportions of different fuels that are being oxidized for energy needs. Carbohydrates produce equal volumes of CO_2 for O_2 consumed, with an RQ of 1.0. Lipids undergo β-oxidation, yielding both ketone bodies and CO_2. Therefore, they are associated with a lower RQ of 0.71, as found during fasting. When calories are supplied beyond the body's energy needs, the excess is converted to fat, and the RQ is greater than 1.0. A handheld device is now available, but it can only be used in spontaneously breathing patients and uses a fixed RQ of 0.85, a value that cannot be assumed to be accurate in sick or starved patients.

Indirect calorimeters compute the *measured resting energy expenditure* (MREE). Indirect calorimetry is more accurate than population-based estimates of energy needs. However, the equipment is moderately expensive, reliable results require that many technical features be rigorously observed, and the values measured over 5 to 30 minutes must still be extrapolated to 24 hours' worth of activity.

The MREE must be increased by 20% (or more) for such energy-consuming actions as movement (deliberate or agitated activity), digestion, or fever. The final value is called *total energy expenditure* (TEE). When available, a metabolic cart study should be ordered at the outset of nutritional support and at least weekly (more often if the patient's metabolic state is changing).

Another method of estimating energy needs uses nitrogen excretion and a clinical assessment of the patient's metabolic state. As patients become more catabolic, protein becomes a greater part of total energy expenditure. Certain ratios based on metabolic state can be multiplied by the nitrogen excretion to estimate nonprotein (carbohydrate plus lipid) calories. For example:

Stable (UUN + 3) × 150 = nonprotein calories
Moderately catabolic (UUN + 4) × 100 = nonprotein calories
Severely catabolic (UUN + 6) × 80 = nonprotein calories

The simplest method for estimating total energy expenditure is to multiply the patient's ideal weight by 25 kcal/kg/day. For example, a 75-kg man of normal habitus would have an estimated TEE of 1875 kcal per day.

Energy Needs in the Obese Patient

The obesity epidemic also weighs upon the question of accurate estimates of energy needs, particularly for the critically ill obese patient. Traditional nutritional management has been based on current bed weight. Using the obese patient's actual body weight will overestimate the calories needed during nutritional support, increasing the risk of hard to control hyperglycemia. One of the solutions coming into practice is hypocaloric feeding, whether enteral or parenteral. Using an adjusted body weight (equal to ideal body weight plus 50% of the difference between actual and ideal body weight) in the HBE and a stress factor of 1.25 appears to best fit indirect calorimetry values in hospitalized obese patients.

When hypocaloric feeding is delivered using enteral formulas, the reduced volumes used to lower the energy supply often result in incomplete provision of vitamins, minerals, and trace elements. Micronutrient supplementation or specially formulated hypocaloric feedings should be used.

Micronutrients: Vitamins

Vitamins are required in minute amounts for normal growth, maintenance, and reproduction. They are not endogenously synthesized. Essential vitamins in humans are the four fat-soluble and nine water-soluble vitamins (Table 4-3). The allowances for normal persons at varying ages are well defined by the National Academy of Sciences. The American Medical Association Nutrition Advisory Group published requirements during total parenteral nutrition (TPN) in 1979. These were revised in 2000 by the U.S. Food and Drug Administration (FDA). Needs during stress states are imprecise because of the variability of patient and disease.

The fat-soluble vitamins serve many functions. Vitamin A is an essential component of the visual photochemical mechanism and preserves the integrity of epithelial membranes by limiting keratinization. Vitamin D enhances gut absorption and resorption from bone of both calcium and phosphorus. Vitamin E is a family of seven tocopherols that have antioxidant properties and indefinite biologic roles. Vitamin K is a cofactor for the synthesis of coagulation factors II, VII, IX, and X. Vitamin K absorption in the jejunum requires the presence of bile salts, hence the abnormal coagulation times generally associated with bile duct obstruction. The destruction or alteration of colonic microflora by antibiotics also may induce vitamin K deficiency. Patients who are receiving TPN are usually given 10 mg vitamin K intramuscularly or in the solution once a week, to prevent coagulopathy. The FDA revised vitamin requirements for adult parenteral multivitamins in 2000, requiring daily vitamin K for the first time. In the future, patients treated with warfarin who begin TPN may require altered dosing with that anticoagulant.

The water-soluble vitamins include the B complex, which contains cofactors of enzymes that are vital to intermediary metabolism, energy supply, and nucleic acid synthesis. Folic acid deficiency is the most common hypovitaminosis in humans; it is often caused by poor nutritional intake, which is common with alcoholism. The B complex or multivitamin formulations must be added to TPN daily and probably should be included once daily in maintenance intravenous fluids. Increased amounts of B_1, B_6, C, and folic acid are in the new FDA requirements.

Micronutrients: Trace Elements

Trace elements are essential minerals: iron, iodine, cobalt, zinc, copper, selenium, and chromium (see Table 4-3). In addition, animal studies indicate important roles for manganese, vanadium, molybdenum, nickel, tin, silicon, fluorine, and arsenic. Zinc plays a key metabolic role in numerous metalloenzymes (e.g., carbonic anhydrase, alcohol dehydrogenase, alkaline phosphatase). Clinically, zinc is required for normal wound healing, normal immunologic function, taste and smell perception, and dark adaptation. In patients who are maintained on TPN without zinc supplements, serial zinc levels usually show progressive decreases. Approximately 60% of the total body zinc content is located within muscle. Therefore, conditions associated with muscle catabolism are associated with marked release of zinc and subsequent increased excretion in the urine. Zinc deficiency can also develop whenever there are protracted losses of gastrointestinal secretions. Acute zinc deficiency is manifested by diarrhea; central nervous system disturbances (including confusion and lethargy); eczematoid dermatitis of the nasolabial area, perineum, elbows, and digits; alopecia; and acute growth

Table 4-3 Micronutrients

Compound	Recommended Daily Amounts: Adults Usual to Stressed	Recommended Daily Amounts: NAG-AMA Guidelines	FDA Parenteral Dosage	Function	Deficiency States
Vitamins[a–c]					
Fat-soluble vitamins[b–c]					
A, retinol, IU	3300–5000	1 mg	1 mg	Retinal pigments; soft tissue and bone growth; functional integrity of epithelium	Xerophthalmia, night blindness, epithelial keratinization, delayed wound healing, anemia
D, cholecalciferol, IU	400	5 μg	5 μg	Mediates bone sensitivity to parathyroid hormones and gut absorption of calcium	Rickets (children); osteomalacia (adults)
E, tocopherol, IU	10–15	10 mg	10 mg	Placental implantation; sperm mobility; antioxidant of vitamin A and unsaturated fatty acids	Male and female infertility, vitamin A deficiency, serum deficiencies of phospholipids
K, mg	2–20	10 mg weekly	50 μg	Cofactor for synthesis of coagulant factors II, VII, IX, X	Bleeding disorders seen in hepatic disease, malabsorption states, certain antibiotic use
Water-soluble vitamins[a–c]					
B_1, thiamin, mg	1.5–10 (0.5 mg/1000 kcal)	3 mg	6 mg	Decarboxylation of pyruvate and ketoacids; coenzyme in carbohydrate metabolism	Beriberi; high-output cardiac failure; Wernicke's encephalopathy
B_2, riboflavin, mg	1.1–1.8	3.6 mg	3.6 mg	Cytochrome oxidase cofactors in cellular respiration	Cheilosis, seborrheic dermatitis, magenta tongue of pellagra, angular stomatitis
B_3, niacin, mg	12–20	40 mg	40 mg	Cofactor in redox reactions (NAD^+ and $NADP^+$) and energy metabolism	Pellagra; photosensitive dermatitis, diarrhea, gastrointestinal hemorrhage; dementia
B_5, pantothenic acid, mg	7–40	15 mg	15 mg	Synthesis of coenzyme A involved in amino acid; carbohydrate and fat metabolism	Malaise, headache, nausea, vomiting (only with a specific antagonist)
B_6, pyridoxine, mg	1.6–2.0	4 mg	6 mg	Coenzyme for amino acid deamination, transamination, decarboxylation, transulfuration, and glucose metabolism	CNS (irritation, depression somnolence); skin (seborrheic dermatitis, glossitis); microcytic, hypochromic anemia
Biotin, μg	150–300	60 μg	60 μg	Coenzyme in carboxylation reactions of CHO, lipids, and amino acids	Rare; seborrheic dermatitis
B_{12}, cyanocobalamin, mg	2–4	5 μg	5 μg	Coenzyme for purine and pyrimidine synthesis	Pernicious anemia; neural lesions
Folic acid, mg	100–300	400 μg	600 μg	Purine and thymine synthesis for DNA	Leukopenia; megaloblastic anemia; steatorrhea secondary to jejunal mucosal atrophy, sprue, glossitis

(continued)

Table 4-3 continued

Compound	Recommended Daily Amounts: Adults Usual to Stressed	Recommended Daily Amounts: NAG-AMA Guidelines	FDA Parenteral Dosage	Function	Deficiency States
C, ascorbic acid, mg	45	100 mg	200 mg	Anticorbutic; collagen cross-linking; hydroxylation of proline	Defective sulfonated copolysaccharides and chondroitin sulfate with retarded wound healing; scurvy; wound dehiscence; chronic skin ulcers
Trace elements[d]					
Zinc, mg	10–15		2.5–6.0	Metalloenzymes involved in lipid, CHO, protein, and nucleic acid metabolism	Hypogonadism; altered hepatic drug metabolism; diminished wound strength and healing rates; anorexia; diarrhea; abnormalities of taste and smell; mental depression; cerebellar dysfunction; alopecia; typical dermatitis of face
Copper, mg	1.2–3.0		0.5–1.5	Metalloenzymes; iron uptake in hemoglobin synthesis; normal CNS function	Anemia; skeletal defects, demyelination; reproductive failure (congenital deficiency); leukopenia
Chromium, μg	50–290		10–15	Insulin cofactor	Hyperglycemia; mental confusion; peripheral sensory neuropathy with ataxia
Iodine, mg	150		1–2 mg/kg	Thyroid hormone synthesis	Hypothyroidism; goiter
Iron, mg	10–18		Usefulness questionable	Constituent of hemoglobin, myoglobin, and cytochromes	Hypochromic anemia
Manganese, mg	2.0–5.0		0.15–0.8	Enzyme cofactor in protein and energy metabolism; fat synthesis	Sterility or diminished fertility; glucose intolerance, hypocholesterolemia, growth retardation

CHO, carbohydrate; CNS, central nervous system; IU, international unit; NAD^+, oxidized nicotinamide = adenine dinucleotide; $NADP^+$, oxidized nicotinamide = adenine dinucleotide phosphate; TPN, total parenteral nutrition.

[a] American Medical Association Department of Foods and Nutrition. Guidelines for multivitamin preparations for parenteral use. J Parenter Ent Nutr 1979;3:258–262.

[b] *Recommended Daily Amounts.* 9th Ed. Food and Nutrition Board of the National Research Council, National Academy of Science, 1980.

[c] Federal Register. Food and Drug Administration. *Parenteral Multivitamin Products* 2000;65(77):21200–21201.

[d] American Medical Association Department of Foods and Nutrition. Guidelines for essential trace element preparation for parenteral use: a statement by an expert panel. JAMA 1979;241:2051–2054.

arrest in children. Chronic deficiency is more subtle; inability to heal even superficial wounds should raise suspicion. In the stable adult who is receiving TPN, the daily intravenous zinc replacement is 2.5 to 4.0 mg/day. This amount is increased by an additional 2 mg/day in the acutely catabolic patient. In adults with intestinal losses, additional zinc is provided (12 mg/L small bowel fluid lost; 17 mg/kg stool or ileostomy output).

Copper is a component of several important enzyme systems, such as lysoxidase (involved in the maturation of collagen and elastin), ceruloplasmin (involved in iron metabolism), and tyrosinase (involved in melanin synthesis). Acquired copper deficiency is associated with anemia, leukopenia, and bone demineralization. Copper supplementation is usually 0.5 to 1.5 mg/day. Copper replacement is discontinued in the presence of biliary obstruction because copper is primarily excreted in bile.

Chromium is necessary in trace amounts because it acts as a cofactor for insulin. Chromium enhances the initial reaction of insulin with its receptor in insulin-sensitive tissues. Chromium deficiency in patients with prolonged parenteral nutrition without chromium supplementation leads to weight loss, glucose intolerance, and peripheral sensory neuropathy. Selenium is an essential trace element for many animal species and is now believed to be required for humans at doses of 50 to 70 μg/day. It is a component of the enzyme glutathione peroxidase in human red blood cells; this enzyme protects against damage from peroxidation of polyunsaturated fats. Occasional case reports of selenium deficiency have appeared. The manifestations include skeletal myopathy or cardiomyopathy. Selenium supplementation in patients who are receiving TPN is generally in the range of 30 to 100 μg/day. Selenium excess can cause central nervous system dysfunction, so serum selenium levels should be monitored when supplementation is given for an extended time.

Clinical trace element deficiency states are rare. In the United States, they appear among food faddists and severe alcoholics. They occur with prolonged TPN (i.e., months) when the trace elements are not routinely added, but are reversible and respond rapidly to supplementation. Parenteral administration bypasses the regulatory gut mucosa, a situation that is exacerbated by renal insufficiency. Monitoring of serum levels may be needed.

METABOLIC PATTERNS THAT AFFECT NUTRITION

An adequate energy supply is the critical need for living organisms. Metabolic adaptations serve this end; pathologic or iatrogenic maladaptations may subvert it. This section briefly describes energy flux in a variety of nutritional states. The reader is referred to more comprehensive resources for detailed information (Burzstein et al. 1989; Kinney et al. 1988).

Postprandial

The postprandial state exists after meals, serving immediate energy and synthesis needs as well as laying down stores for the future. Ingested carbohydrates provide glucose for the brain. The human brain consumes 20% of RME, a proportion that is remarkable among mammals. The blood-brain barrier blocks the entry of large free fatty acids (FFA) or chylomicrons, but allows the entry of small water-soluble compounds (e.g., glucose). In other words, the brain has discriminatory energy needs. Other glycolytic tissues are erythrocytes, bone marrow, renal medulla, and peripheral nerves. The remaining tissues oxidize lipids. There is net amino acid uptake into solid organs and muscle, and lipogenesis in adipose tissue (Fig. 4-1).

Postabsorptive

The postabsorptive state (Fig. 4-2) occurs after an overnight fast. Hepatic glycogenolysis is mildly supplemented by gluconeogenesis from amino acids derived from skeletal muscle. Lipolysis of fats stored in adipose tissue releases FFA to fuel liver and muscle, supplemented by products of hepatic ketogenesis that are also used by muscle.

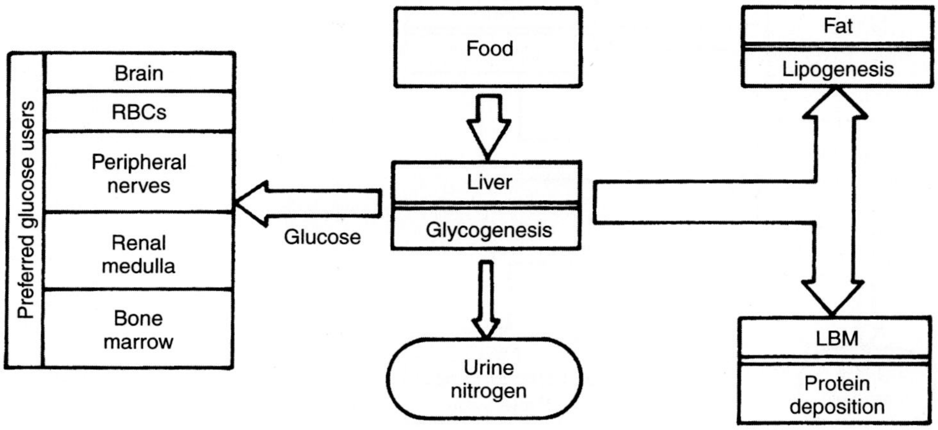

Figure 4-1 Postprandial state. LBM, lean body mass (principally skeletal muscle, but includes all viscera); RBCs, red blood cells.

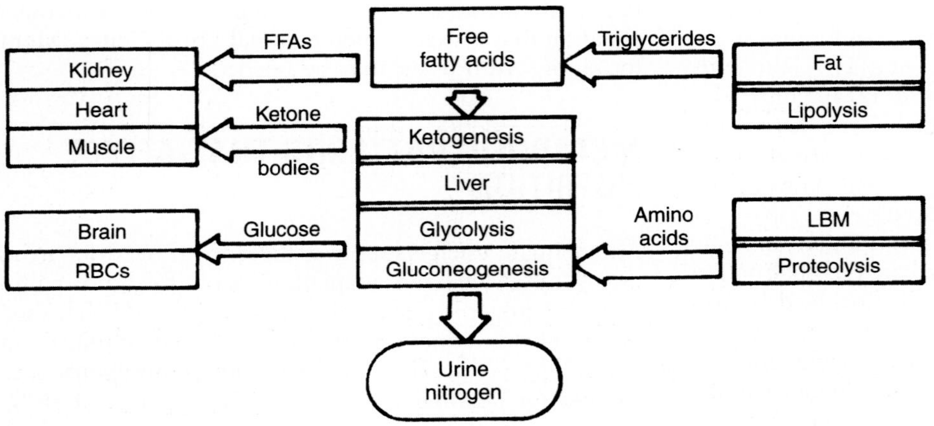

Figure 4-2 The postabsorptive, or early fasting, state. FFAs, free fatty acids; LBM, lean body mass; RBCs, red blood cells.

Early Starvation

In early starvation, glycogen stores are depleted in 12 to 24 hours. As blood glucose concentration decreases, insulin levels drop. An elevated glucagon:insulin ratio or an absolute glucagon increase plus chronic sympathetic nerve activity instigates catabolic changes. Glycogenolysis as the primary source of glucose is replaced by gluconeogenesis in the liver, supplied with substrate from enhanced protein breakdown, especially in skeletal muscle. Approximately 300 g wet muscle tissue/day is metabolized, and the excess nitrogen is excreted as urea. The UUN is 10 to 12 g/day. Lipolysis increases, and enhanced hepatic ketogenesis occurs. The partial oxidation of long-chain fatty acids in the liver produces ketone bodies (β-hydroxybutyrate and acetoacetate), which are then used as alternate fuels for extrahepatic tissues. Hepatic ketogenesis reaches a maximum after 2 to 3 days of starvation.

Starvation-Adapted

Prolonged starvation leads to the starvation-adapted state, a vital shift that minimizes protein breakdown (Fig. 4-3). Energy expenditure decreases 15% to 25% after 2 weeks of fasting. The peripheral (especially muscle) oxidation of ketone bodies decreases, allowing β-hydroxybutyrate and acetoacetate levels to reach maximal values in 8 to 10 days. Their rising concentrations form a transport gradient into erythrocytes and brain, allowing ketoacids to partially replace glucose as a primary metabolic fuel. After 2 weeks, more than two-thirds of brain oxygen consumption is for ketoacid oxidation. The remainder is for oxidation of glucose derived from glycerol and gluconeogenesis. Muscles burn more FFA as declining insulin levels permit enhanced lipolysis. Proteolysis decreases as the need for gluconeogenic substrate decreases, thus sparing protein. The UUN decreases to less than 5 g/day.

Catabolic

A different state of affairs exists in the stressed, hypercatabolic patient (Fig. 4-4). The difference begins with the presence of an injury or infection and the inflammation it evokes. A variety of mediators, including cytokines (e.g., interleukin-1, tumor necrosis factor), lipid mediators (prostaglandins and leukotrienes), bacterial products (e.g., en-

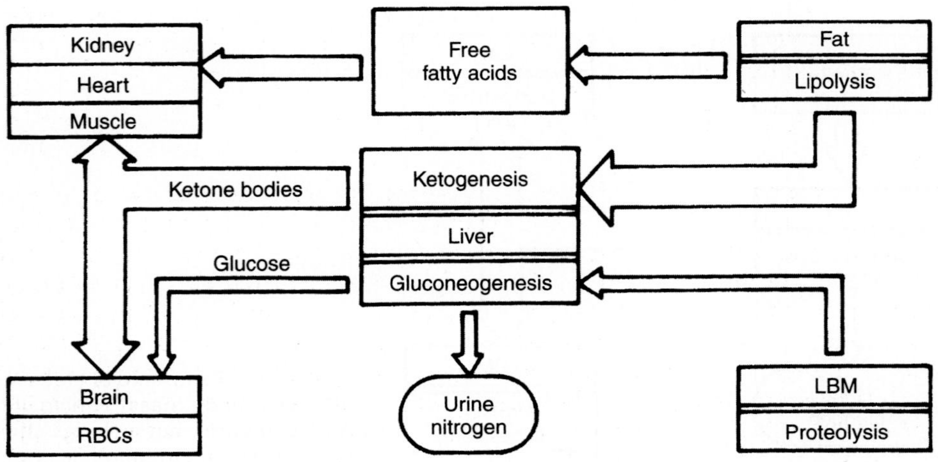

Figure 4-3 Starvation-adapted state. LBM, lean body mass; RBCs, red blood cells.

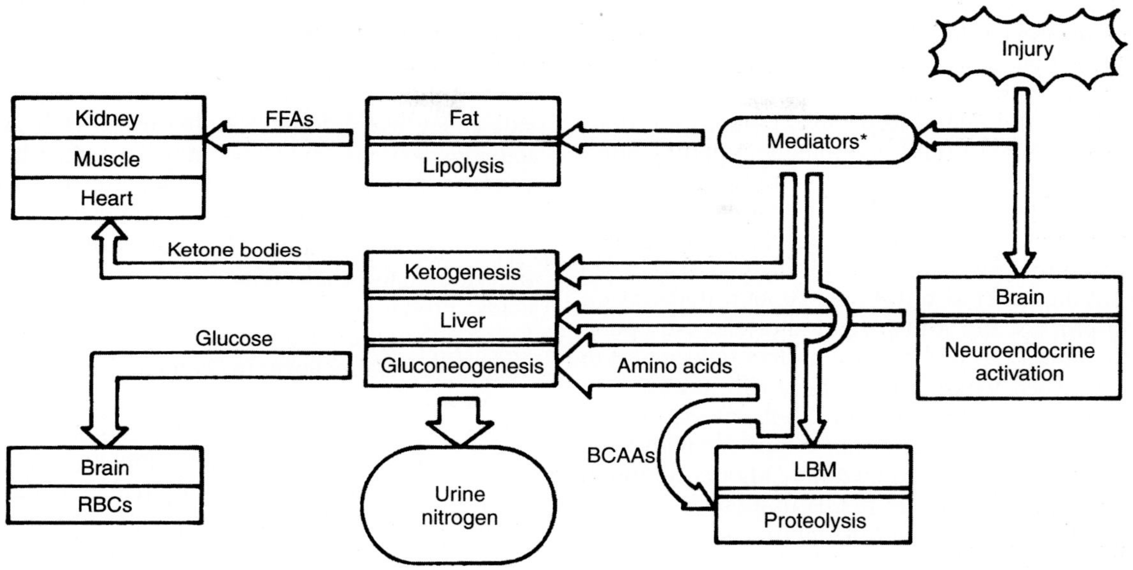

Figure 4-4 Hypercatabolic state. Interleukin-1, prostaglandins, kinins, superoxide radicals, leukotrienes, and pain. BCAAs, branched-chain amino acids; FFAs, free fatty acids; LBM, lean body mass; RBCs, red blood cells.

dotoxin), and pain, stimulate catabolic changes directly or through the neuroendocrine system. This mediator traffic, which is proportionate to the severity of injury, induces hemodynamic, thermal, hormonal, and metabolic alterations. The following changes occur: increased blood flow, hypermetabolism, increased energy expenditure, lean body mass wasting, and abnormal substrate use, lasting 1 to many weeks. Resting energy expenditure increases significantly after long bone fracture (10% to 30%), sepsis (20% to 45%), or burns (40% to 100%). Increased metabolic expenditure is needed for wound healing, synthesis of cellular and humoral immune components, and synthesis of acute-phase reactants until healing is complete. Central thermoregulation is adjusted upward (especially in burns), but increased metabolic expenditure is only slightly abated, even when ambient temperatures are elevated.

Increased catecholamine release is another major catabolic factor. Hypercortisolemia plays a permissive role with the catecholamines. Glucagon concentration rises, increasing proteolysis, gluconeogenesis, and ureagenesis. The anabolic hormone insulin increases, but to a smaller degree than glucagon. The production of glucose is accelerated, and is proportionate to the release of alanine and lactate from skeletal muscle. That is, muscle wasting provides alanine to meet increased energy needs. The efflux of amino acid from muscle also supplies the raw materials for acute-phase protein synthesis in the liver. The amino acid efflux profile, which contains disproportionate amounts of glutamine, reflects neither the protein composition of muscle nor the composition of newly synthesized protein. The fate of much of the effluxed amino acids is reflected by urine nitrogen losses of more than 20 g/day. Muscle oxidizes BCAA preferentially as an energy source. Ketogenesis is blocked in the liver. Increased lipolysis accelerates the release of FFA and triglyceride, but disposal is impaired, resulting in septic hyperlipidemia. This "autocannibalistic" situation continues until infection is controlled or wounds are stabilized by fixation (fractures) or coverage (burns). This hypercatabolic state cannot continue indefinitely. The late, uncontrolled hypermetabolic state is marked by hepatic failure of gluconeogenesis, hypoglycemia, severe amino acid profile abnormalities, and death.

Unique profiles of hormonal change, cytokine release, autonomic nervous system activation, and specific exogenous factors (microbes, kinetic energy, body part injured) modify details of the catabolic response. These variations are beyond the scope of this chapter. The interested reader is encouraged to conduct an independent review.

TECHNIQUES OF NUTRITIONAL SUPPORT

Either enteral or parenteral routes of nutritional support will meet a patient's needs. Although parenteral nutrition is well defined, is relatively easy to initiate, and has assured delivery systems, it is costly. Enteral nutrition is less expensive, but more difficult to maintain, and often is less well understood by physicians. During parenteral nutrition, the unused gut shows reduced villus height, enzyme content, and absorptive ability; immunoglobulin E production; and altered bacterial populations, both quantitatively and qualitatively. Gastrointestinal tract permeablility changes.

Combined, these changes may set the stage for transmigration of gut bacteria into the portal system, triggering a catabolic state that precedes multiple organ failure syndrome. (This is more apparent in rats than in mankind.) A meta-analysis from eight prospective, randomized trials that compared enteral and parenteral support found higher rates of infection and overall complications in patients who were assigned to TPN compared with those who were assigned to enteral feeding. Thus, the advice remains: when the gut is working, use it.

Timing of the onset of nutritional support depends on the disease process. For a fit patient after elective operation, consideration should begin on postoperative day 4 to decide the next day whether the patient will not eat for a more prolonged time. If the patient is not expected to eat, support is begun. Patients with major burns benefit from nasogastric tube feedings begun within 24 hours, although the human clinical results are not as impressive as those found in rats. Patients with multiple trauma must first have complete fluid resuscitation, especially before small intestinal feedings begin, because inadequate resuscitation impairs splanchnic perfusion, and food digestion and absorption increase the demands for splanchnic blood flow, potentially causing devastating bowel ischemia. In general, early feeding is considered to start within 6 to 48 hours after onset of lack of intake; late feeding, more than 5 days. The interim of 2 to 5 days is wholly a matter of study design, and collegial debate.

Rate of increase of feeding toward goal is another area of controversy. Studies from the 1970s and 1980s often required 5 to 7 days for feedings to reach target rates and concentrations. As delivery systems improved, target rates could be reached in as little as 48 hours. The result was the delivery of large amounts of nutrients while patients were still in the early catabolic phases of illness or injury. There are case reports of small bowel necrosis associated with too early, too much enteral nutrition after trauma laparotomy, probably due to marginal splanchnic perfusion. Exacerbation of hyperglycemia is associated with infusion of concentrated glucose solutions. Some authors now argue that deliberate hypocaloric but high-protein formulations are more appropriate early (first few days) in critical illness and injury.

Enteral Nutritional Support

A variety of enteral formulations are available to satisfy any patient's specialized needs along a whole continuum of disease stages. The products fall into three broad categories based on their composition: (1) polymeric, (2) chemically defined (or elemental), and (3) modular. The products differ in nutrient complexity, osmolarity, caloric density, and viscosity.

Polymeric foods contain intact macronutrients. Whole food that is blenderized naturally contains intact proteins, fats, polysaccharides, and fiber. For example, the willing family of a patient who has head and neck cancer may take a portion of the family meal, blenderize it, and administer it through a gastrostomy tube. Polymeric formulas contain combinations of intact macronutrients. These formulas are high in residue, viscosity, and osmolarity. They are nutritionally complete and cause few gastrointestinal side effects when delivered into the stomach. Because the feedings are viscous, they may be difficult to deliver through all but a large-bore tube. Energy is supplied as polysaccharides (either milk-based or lactose-free) and lipids, usually long-chain triglycerides, but may also include medium-chain triglycerides and even short-chain fatty acids. Protein is derived from whole milk, egg, or soy. Some polymeric formulas are nutritionally complete, but are low in residue, lower in osmolarity, and of only moderate viscosity. They contain vitamin and mineral supplements. Some flavored preparations are palatable and can be administered as oral dietary supplements.

Chemically defined diets are characterized by relative chemical simplicity. These products are intended for patients who have impaired digestive capacity or a metabolic state that requires substrate admixtures that are not found in natural foods. These products provide energy as lactose-free polysaccharides. They vary widely in carbohydrate: lipid ratio, and they may include medium-chain triglycerides. Protein is provided as single amino acids or dipeptides, tripeptides, and short polypeptides. Compared with the proportions of amino acids in "ideal" proteins (e.g., egg albumin), chemically defined formulas may provide enhanced proportions of BCAAs, glutamate, or arginine. They are also low in residue and nutritionally complete (include vitamins and minerals) but are hyperosmolar. They are often unpalatable, however, and must be administered through a feeding tube. For example, a trauma patient would benefit from a high-nitrogen, perhaps arginine-enhanced, polymeric formula administered by a continuous infusion pump through a jejunostomy tube.

Elemental diets are a subset of chemically defined diets that have substrates in forms requiring no digestive capacity, only absorption. For example, an elderly patient with short-bowel syndrome after resection of ischemic bowel caused by a mesenteric artery occlusion requires central parenteral nutrition but may also benefit from an elemental diet given by feeding tube, because of the remaining short length of absorptive surface area.

Modular products contain only single or a few macronutrients. Protein, fat, and carbohydrate modules are available. By definition, these components cannot provide complete nutrition. They selectively fulfill special nutritional needs in patients whose condition requires very specific proportions of substrates not available in routine formulations. For example, a diabetic patient fed a standard polymeric formulation experiences worsening hyperglycemia. Blood sugar control would benefit from a reduced amount of the original formula supplemented with a modular product of medium-chain triglycerides, maintaining the same total energy supply, but reducing the amount of carbohydrate.

Access for Enteral Nutrition

To a large extent, the route chosen for administration of nutritional support depends on a patient's particular circumstances. Patients with adequate appetite and a normally functioning gastrointestinal tract can usually be entirely supported with oral intake. Supplementation with snacks or high-calorie liquids may be appropriate in some patients. Such "sip feeding" is useful in elderly patients with hip fracture, stroke, or cardiac valve replacement. In other patients, the gastrointestinal tract is entirely normal, but little or no spontaneous oral intake takes place because of anorexia, depression, inability to swallow, or unconsciousness. Tube feedings permit the use of the functional gastrointestinal system.

The essential component of selecting the route for delivery of enteral feeding is choosing which portion of the patient's gastrointestinal tract to access. This decision is influenced by the anticipated duration of feeding, patient choice, and whether the patient is an operative candidate (Table 4-4). Either the stomach or the small bowel may be used. Delivery of enteral feeding into the stomach (prepyloric feeding) ensures exposure to the maximal gastrointestinal absorptive surface available, an important consideration in a patient who has a limited amount of small bowel remaining. In addition, because the stomach is a reservoir where diets are mixed and tonicity is adjusted, greater latitude in the selection of diet and the technique of administration results when intragastric delivery is chosen. The greater ease and flexibility with which intragastric feeding is performed must be weighed against the risks of gastroesophageal reflux, vomiting, and aspiration, especially in the patient who is already debilitated. Instillation of the diet into the small bowel (postpyloric feeding) virtually eliminates the problems of gastric retention, reflux, vomiting, and aspiration of feedings (if not aspiration of oral or gastric secretions). In addition, jejunal motility is usually not affected by most mechanical and inflammatory processes in the upper abdomen that may inhibit gastric emptying. The parenteral route is necessary when the gastrointestinal tract is nonfunctional or unavailable.

Several means of access to the gastrointestinal tract are available (Table 4-5). Transnasal intubation is the simplest and most widely used method. Nasal tubes are generally used for short-term programs because of their propensity to dislodge and to cause discomfort. Although individual differences exist in length and composition, most of the current feeding catheters are manufactured from silicone rubber or polyurethane. Weights incorporated into the

Table 4-4 Indications for Enteral Nutritional Support

Prolonged inadequate intake of nutrients
- Nothing by mouth for 5+ days
- Cancer: oral, esophageal, gastric, pancreatic
- Eating disorders: anorexia, bulimia, severe depression
- AIDS-related wasting
- Severe chronic obstructive pulmonary disease
- Dietary indiscretion: dietary fads, alcoholism, substance abuse

Sustained inability to eat
- Depressed level of consciousness: stroke, traumatic brain injury, metabolic disorders, encephalopathy
- Dysphagia: oropharyngeal cancer operations, advanced esophageal motility disorders, pseudobulbar palsy, mandibular fractures
- Pulmonary failure requiring prolonged mechanical ventilatory support
- Mechanical disability: quadriplegia, severe palsy, spinal cord neuropathy

Increased metabolic requirements
- Major burns
- Multiple torso and long bone trauma
- Severe brain injury
- Sepsis or systemic inflammatory response syndrome

Table 4-5 Enteral Routes for Nutritional Support, by Site of Nutrient Deposition

Oral: Supplements the usual diet or inadequate diet choices by increasing calorie or protein intake

PREPYLORIC DELIVERY

Gastric: Dependent on the emptying function of the stomach
- Nasogastric tube: Passed manually; position must be confirmed by chest radiograph (or by aspiration of 10+ mL gastric fluid) to be sure it is not in the lungs
- Gastrostomy tube (G-tube) placed during laparotomy (Stamm, Witzel), by laparoscopy, by percutaneous endoscopic gastrostomy (PEG), or by fluoroscopy
- Gastrocutaneous fistula (Janeway gastrostomy); often troubled by acid erosions at skin level, and largely abandoned

POSTPYLORIC DELIVERY

Duodenal: Dependent mainly on how well a tube can be kept in position without displacing back into the stomach
- Nasoduodenal tube: Passed manually or with fluor scopic control, often with the help of a dose of metoclopramide; position confirmed by abdominal radiograph or pH probe at the tip; often requires repeated repositioning
- Gastroduodenal tube: Placed during laparotomy to allow simultaneous gastric decompression and duodenal feeding

Jejunal: Feedings distal to the ligament of Treitz, with almost no chance of reflux of feedings into the stomach (can happen with severe ileus, as in peritonitis)
- Nasojejunal tube: Passed with fluoroscopic control
- Percutaneous endoscopic gastrojejunostomy (PEG/J or PEJ): A second, smaller-diameter tube passed within a PEG tube distally into the jejunum (allows simulteneous gastric decompression)
- Jejunostomy tube (J-tube): Placed at laparotomy or laparoscopy
- Needle catheter jejunostomy: Will accept only elemental diets due to its small bore

catheter tips facilitate neither introduction nor maintenance in the desired location. Most nasogastric feeding tubes are long enough to allow access to the duodenum. In approximately one-half of ambulatory patients, the feeding catheter spontaneously passes into the small bowel. The proximal small bowel may be successfully cannulated under fluoroscopic control, with the use of a rigid stylet to manipulate the tip of the catheter through the pylorus. Alternatively, the tip of the catheter may be guided into the small bowel with a fiberoptic gastroscope and its snare or biopsy forceps. All of the small, soft, nonreactive nasoenteral catheters are safe for extended use.

It is essential to confirm the intraabdominal location of the tip of the tube by radiography before feeding is instituted. The air insufflation test (blowing a syringe of air into the tube while listening over the left upper quadrant) does not protect the patient from inadvertent feeding into the airway as the result of a catheter misplaced into a bronchus.

Gastric or jejunal tubes are easily placed endoscopically (percutaneous endoscopic gastrostomy and percutaneous endoscopic jejunostomy) or under fluoroscopic control.

Operative access to the gastrointestinal tract for feeding can be achieved at a variety of levels. The proximal esophagus, stomach, and jejunum are all sites for operative feeding tube enterostomies. Although placement of a feeding tube may be the primary reason for an operation under general anesthetic, endoscopic procedures are becoming the norm. A feeding tube jejunostomy is strongly advised during major foregut, or hepatic operations; during a major trauma laparotomy; after pancreatic surgery; or in nutritionally bankrupt patients. Laparoscopic methods exist for the placement of gastric and jejunal tubes.

Implementation and Administration of an Enteral Feeding Program

Table 4-6 shows examples of enteral support programs by various routes. Bolus gastric feeding is advantageous because a pump is not needed, as in continuous feeding, but there may be little difference in nursing time. For intragastric feeding, enteral formulas are initiated at a caloric density of 1 kcal/mL (i.e., full strength). Initially, half-strength feedings may be better tolerated in elderly patients or those whose gut has been unused for a prolonged period. After the final rate is reached, feedings can be increased to full strength. Patients who are fed intragastrically should always be positioned with the head of the bed elevated 30°. These patients should be encouraged to ambulate frequently to minimize the risk of aspiration.

Intrajejunal feeding uses continuous administration by an infusion pump. Too rapid infusion of the diet or excessive caloric density can cause abdominal distension, weakness, sweating, hyperperistalsis, cramps, and diarrhea. Because the jejunum lacks the capacity of the intact stomach to serve as a reservoir while tonicity is adjusted, there is less flexibility with jejunal feeding than with intragastric feeding.

Table 4-6 Schedule for Enteral Nutritional Support

GASTRIC ROUTE

- **Adjunctive support** to oral diet
  - Daytime supplements: One can (250 mL), either orally or through a nasogastric tube, after each meal if <50% taken
  - Nighttime supplements: Continuous feeding from 10:00 p.m. until 6:00 a.m. of 30% to 60% of daily needs, based on daytime oral intake
- **Complete support**
  - Continuous: See the jejunal regimen, but advance rates every 24 hr
  - Bolus: Through a nasogastric or gastric tube
  - Full strength, 100 mL q 3 hr, for 24 hr (800 mL/day)
    - Check gastric residual before each feeding; hold for 1 hr if > 250 mL, and recheck. If residuals stay low, then:
    - Full strength, 200 mL q 3 hr, for 24 hr (1600 mL/day)
    - Check gastric residuals, as above
    - Full strength, 300 mL q 4 hr, for 24 hr (1800 mL/day)
    - Check gastric residuals, as above
    - Full strength, 400–500 mL q 4 to 6 hr (1600–3000) mL/day)
    - Check gastric residuals, as above

JEJUNAL ROUTE

- Continuous only (bolus feeding induces cramps, diarrhea, and gastric reflux)
  - Full strength, 25 mL/hr[a]
  - Advance rate by 25 mL/hr q 12 hr to final rate
  - Do not check jejunal residuals
  - Flush delivery system with 30 mL tap water at each tube feeding change, and after any medication is given through a tube
  - 24 hr after final rate is reached, add 300 mL tap water bolus twice a day to four times a day, depending on the patient's volume and electrolyte status

[a] Elderly patients or those whose gut has been unused for some time may not tolerate full-strength feedings. Start at half-strength, increasing to full strength after the final rate is reached.

All enteral feedings require some amount of free water to be coadministered to help renal excretion of metabolic byproducts and for insensible water losses. Typically, three or four boluses of 400 mL each day is sufficient.

Complications of Enteral Nutrition

The possible complications of enteral therapy are shown in Table 4-7. Gastrointestinal side effects occur in 10% to 20% of tube-fed patients. Patient interview and examination are the most critical tools for determining gastrointestinal tolerance of a defined-formula diet. Gastrointestinal overload may be signaled by symptoms of fullness, bloating, crampy abdominal pain, and nausea. Hyperactive bowel sounds and abdominal distension may also be noted. Vomiting may follow, particularly with intragastric feeding. Diarrhea may be caused by osmotic overload, rapid transit through the small bowel, incomplete absorption, bacterial contamination of feedings, coadministra-

Table 4-7 Complications of Enteral Therapy

Mechanical	
	Pulmonary aspiration
	Esophageal reflux
	Depressed cough
	Parotitis
	Otitis media
	Esophageal erosions
	Tube obstruction
	Inadvertent administration of feedings into airway or peritoneum
Gastrointestinal Function	
	Diarrhea
	Malabsorption
	Abdominal cramping
	Exacerbation of gastrointestinal disease
	Nausea and vomiting
	Distension
Metabolic	
	Prerenal azotemia
	Fluid and electrolyte abnormalities
	Hyperglycemia
	Hyperosmolar dehydration or nonketotic coma
	Inadvertent intravenous administration
	Essential fatty acid deficiency

tion of medications (especially sorbitol carriers used in liquid medicines), lactose solids in lactose-intolerant persons, and broad-spectrum antibiotics that alter normal gut flora. Voluminous diarrhea may affect fluid and electrolyte balance and worsen hypoalbuminemia.

To reduce the chances of reflux/regurgitation of feedings into the lungs, gastric residuals are measured. These are volumes measured 4 to 8 hours by nurses suctioning residual tube feedings from the stomach, and replacing them if below a threshold established by physicians to denote tolerance of feedings. Volumes above the threshold are an indication to hold feedings until the next scheduled time for a "residual check." It must be understood that establishing the threshold volumes is a matter of custom, not science. The best evidence suggests a threshold of 400 mL, which is three to four times the customary level. Aspiration events are often unpredictable, but seem to be reduced by head-up bed positioning, postpyloric deposition of feedings or jejunal feedings, and, in some patients, promotility drugs.

The signs and symptoms of gastrointestinal intolerance are managed by reducing both volume and caloric density until the patient becomes asymptomatic. Alternatively, feedings may be interrupted transiently if symptoms are severe or if the gastric residual is high. Antidiarrheal medications (e.g., paregoric, dilute tincture of opium) may be added directly to the feeding in refractory cases; however, obstipation and distension may occur with these agents. They should not be used if *Clostridium difficile* colitis is present or suspected. Critically ill patients with gastric emptying problems may benefit from administration of promotility drugs such as erythromycin or metaclopramide.

Mechanical problems include tube dislodgment, malposition (i.e., into the airway or esophagus), blockage, nasal sinus obstruction with consequent sinusitis, and tracheoesophageal fistula. It is essential to confirm the intra-abdominal location of the tip of the tube by radiography before feeding is instituted. The air insufflation test (blowing a syringe of air into the tube while listening over the left upper quadrant) does not protect the patient from inadvertent feeding into the airway as the result of a catheter misplaced into a bronchus. Small-bore tubes misplaced into the bronchus have pierced through the lung into the pleura, in debilitated patients.

Operations to place tubes may be complicated by bowel obstruction, wound infection, wound dehiscence, and peritonitis due to intraperitoneal instillation of feedings. Metabolic complications are similar to those seen with parenteral nutrition (Table 4-8).

Parenteral Nutritional Support

Formulations

When the gastrointestinal tract is not available for use in providing nutritional support, the parenteral route must be used. Common indications for parenteral nutritional support are shown in Table 4-9. Although the use of "bridging TPN" for a few days while initiating tube feedings is customary in some sites, there is no evidence of its value.

There are three categories of parenteral nutrition. Protein-sparing therapy uses a 3% amino acid solution in 5% dextrose with electrolytes and is administered through a peripheral vein. This hypocaloric protein source is used for the nutritionally fit patient who is undergoing fasting for a week or so. It probably serves no useful purpose. Peripheral parenteral nutrition uses a 3% amino acid solution in 10% dextrose with electrolytes, plus a lipid emulsion that supplies as much as 60% of estimated energy needs. It can be given by peripheral vein, but is relatively hyperosmolar. This solution is used to supply all estimated energy needs in nonstressed patients. TPN supplies all energy and nitrogen needs, even in hypercatabolic patients. Because of its hypertonicity, it must be delivered into a central vein (see Table 4-10 and Fig. 4-5).

Parenteral caloric requirements are most often met by the administration of 20% to 35% dextrose solution, with tonicity ranging from 1000 to 1500 mOsm/L. Parenteral nutritional programs require the administration of nitrogen in the form of pure L-amino acid solutions. Compared with naturally occurring proteins, synthetic amino acid solutions can be disproportionately essential amino acids for use in renal failure, or enhanced with BCAAs with restricted amounts of aromatic amino acids and methionine for use in hepatic failure. In addition, solutions with an enhanced BCAA content ($\leq$ 45% of protein as BCAA) are available for use in the management of hypercatabolic

Table 4-8 Metabolic Complications of Total Parenteral Nutrition and Their Treatment

Problem	Etiology	Prevention and Treatment
Glucose metabolism		
Hyperglycemia, glycosuria, osmotic diuresis, hyperosmolar nonketotic dehydration, and coma	Excessive total dose or rate of administration of glucose; inadequate insulin; glucocorticoids; sepsis with insulin resistance	Reduce or stop infusion rate; switch to lipid; add exogenous insulin; control infection (drainage, debridement, antibiotics); free-water resuscitation followed by electrolyte replacement; replace potassium
Ketoacidosis in diabetes mellitus	Inadequate endogenous insulin response; inadequate exogenous insulin therapy	Appropriately increase exogenous insulin; reduce glucose intake
Postinfusion (rebound) hypoglycemia	Persistently elevated islet cell production of insulin; decreased glycogen stores	Taper TPN slowly (over 24–48 hr); always infuse isotonic glucose for several hours after stopping hypertonic infusion
Respiratory failure; unable to wean from mechanical ventilatory support	Conversion of excessive glucose intake into CO_2, especially in patients with chronic obstructive pulmonary disease	Reduce total glucose load or switch to lipid system (40% of total calories as fat emulsion)
Amino acid metabolism		
Hyperchloremic metabolic acidosis	Excessive chloride and monohydrochloride content of crystalline amino acid solutions	Administer Na^+ and K^+ as lactate or acetate salts
Serum amino acid imbalance	Nonphysiologic amino acid pattern of the nutrient infusion; differential amino acid uptake in various disorders	Infuse essential amino acid–only formulations (renal failure); branched-chain amino acid–enhanced/aromatic amino acid–depleted formulations (sepsis, hepatic failure)
Hyperammonemia (rare)	Arginine-, ornithine-, aspartic acid–, or glutamic acid–deficient formulations; primary hepatic disorder	Infuse branched-chain amino acid–enhanced formulations in hepatic encephalopathy; reduce total amino acid intake
Prerenal azotemia	Excessive amino acid infusion; inadequate nonprotein calories	Reduce protein intake; evaluate other causes of prerenal azotemia; increase nonprotein calories:nitrogen ratio
Lipid metabolism		
Hyperlipemia	Decreased triglyceride clearance; sepsis	Reduce rate of infusion or discontinue; reassess after bloodstream is cleared of fat
Essential fatty acid deficiency (of phospholipid, linoleic, or arachidonic acids); eczematous, desquamative dermatitis of body folds	Inadequate essential fatty acid administration; inadequate vitamin E administration	Administer linoleic acid twice weekly as 500 mL 10% lipid emulsion; cure by daily lipid emulsion infusion
Calcium and phosphorus metabolism	Inadequate phosphorus administration	Monitor phosphorus levels, especially during repletion of malnourished patients; administer adequate phosphorus
Hypophosphatemia		
Neuromuscular: weakness, tremor, convulsions, coma, hyporeflexia, death	Decreased central nervous system ATP; inhibition of muscle glycolytic pathways	
Hematologic: hemolytic anemia, decreased oxygen release; decreased leukocyte function; decreased clot retraction and platelet survival	Decreased erythrocyte 2,3-diphosphoglycerate; decreased cellular ATP; abnormal membrane lipids	

(*continued*)

Table 4-8 continued

Problem	Etiology	Prevention and Treatment
Cardiac: impaired myocardial contractility, congestive cardiomyopathy	Decreased ATP	
Hypocalcemia	Inadequate calcium administration; reciprocal response to phosphorus repletion without calcium; hypoalbuminemia	Add calcium 3 to 4 mEq/kg/body weight to pediatric TPN; add to base solution as needed in adults
Hypercalcemia	Excessive calcium administration with or without high doses of albumin; excessive vitamin D administration	Withdraw calcium from future infusions; rehydrate; mithramycin, corticosteroids
Miscellaneous		
Hypokalemia	Inadequate potassium intake relative to increased requirements for protein anabolism	Add supplementary potassium to infusion at time of preparation
Hypomagnesemia	Inadequate magnesium intake for increased protein and carbohydrate metabolism	Add supplementary magnesium to infusions at the time of preparation

ATP, adenosine triphosphate; TPN, total parenteral nutrition.

Table 4-9 Indications for Parenteral Nutritional Support

GUT UNAVAILABLE
- Prolonged paralytic ileus
- Short-bowel syndrome*
- Enterocutaneous and enteroenteral fistulas*
- Necrotizing enterocolitis
- AIDS-related enteritis and malnutrition*
- Malabsorption syndromes
- Esophageal benign stricture or malignancy

INADEQUATE ORAL INTAKE or "BOWEL REST"
- Acute pancreatitis, hemorrhagic
- Symptomatic chronic pancreatitis*
- Catabolic states: burns, sepsis, polytrauma with ileus
- Extreme prematurity
- Tracheoesophageal fistula (infants; until gastrostomy performed)
- Hyperemesis gravidarum*
- Intractable diarrhea
- Wound dehiscence and evisceration

ADJUNCTIVE to OTHER THERAPY
- Cancer chemotherapy; continuous and high dose*
- Cancer radiation therapy–induced enteritis*
- Inflammatory bowel disease*
- Acute hepatitis and hepatic failure
- Perioperative nutritional repletion
- Bone marrow transplantation*

* Indications for home parenteral nutrition.

states. The efficacy of these preparations is limited to the period of hypercatabolism. After the hypercatabolism is resolved, standard amino acid preparations are more appropriate. A typical standard solution contains 25% dextrose and 4.25% amino acids, supplying 2700 nonnitrogen calories and 18.75 g nitrogen when 3 L/day is administered.

Electrolytes, vitamins, and trace elements are prescribed as well. Vitamin requirements are shown in Table 4-3. Electrolytes should be monitored frequently, particularly in the face of extraordinary losses. Hypokalemia commonly occurs after parenteral nutritional support is initiated. The use of glucose is associated with intracellular transport of potassium. The administration of carbohydrate and protein may profoundly decrease serum potassium levels if insufficient potassium is administered. Hypophosphatemia can also develop because of intracellular shifts of phosphorus, especially when initiating refeeding of the very depleted patient. The usual desired concentrations of electrolytes for TPN are: Na^+, 40 to 50 mEq/L; K^+, 40 mEq/L; Cl^-, 50 mEq/L; Mg^{2+}, 4 to 6 mEq/L; Ca^{2+}, 2.5 to 5.0 mEq/L; HPO^-, 20 to 25 mmol/L; and acetate, 40 to 60 mEq/L.

Access for Parenteral Nutrition

The most commonly used technique for central venous access is percutaneous cannulation of the subclavian or internal jugular vein. With either approach, the tip of the catheter must lie within the superior vena cava before any hypertonic solution is administered. Placement of the catheter under rigidly sterile conditions and a program of regular catheter care will prevent most infectious complications. When the catheter entry site is covered by a dry, sterile dressing, the dressing should be changed by trained personnel three times per week or immediately if wet or

Table 4-10 Examples of Parenteral Nutrition Solutions

Standard central formula (TPN)

A moderately malnourished patient underwent a major gastric resection 4 days ago and is not yet capable of eating. He is ordered a standard central formula at a rate of 100 mL/hr. Each day, he will receive in 2.4 L fluid:
120 g amino acids (19.2 g nitrogen)
422.4 g dextrose (1436 kcal)
67.2 g lipids (672 kcal)

Total calories = 2588 kcal (about one-third as lipids)
Nonprotein calories = 2108 kcal (109 : 1 nonprotein kcal/g N)

Standard peripheral formula (PPN)

A previously well-nourished patient has intractable nausea, but fluid and electrolyte abnormalities are corrected. Peripheral parenteral nutrition is ordered at a rate of 125 mL/hr. Each day, she will receive in 3.0 L fluid:
90 g amino acids (14.4 g nitrogen)
300 g dextrose (1020 kcal)
99 g lipids (990 kcal)

Total calories = 2370 kcal (about one-half as lipids)
Nonprotein calories = 2010 kcal (140 : 1 nonprotein kcal/g N)

Custom formula

A 70-kg man has adult respiratory distress syndrome complicating feculant peritonitis from a perforated colon. His nitrogen needs are measured (UUN = 28 g/24 hr + 4 g/day) as 32 g/day. Although he needs 200 g amino acids/day (32 × 6.25) for nitrogen balance (N_{output} [32] – N_{intake} [32] = N balance), the maximum amount that it is prudent to deliver, even to very catabolic patients, is 2.5 g protein/day, or (70 kg × 2.5 g/kg/day = 175 g amino acids, or 28 g N). His nonprotein energy needs are estimated by using an 80 : 1 NPC:N ratio, yielding 80 × 32 g N or 2560 kcal/day.
One-third lipids (853 kcal ÷ 10 kcal/g = 85 g)
Two-thirds dextrose (1706 kcal ÷ 3.4 kcal/g = 502 g).
ARDS suggests the need for fluid restriction, so the entire daily nutritional prescription is to be delivered in a 2-L volume.

Refer to Figure 4–5, which is an example of preprinted TPN orders. In each example, appropriate electrolytes, vitamins, and trace elements must also be ordered, based on the patient's laboratory tests or particular status each day.
ARDS, adult respiratory distress syndrome; PPN, peripheral parenteral nutrition; TPN, total parenteral nutrition; UUN, urinary urea nitrogen.

contaminated. The transparent occlusive dressings may be safely left in place for as long as 7 days. The catheter should be used only to deliver nutrient solutions. Blood should not be withdrawn from or administered through the catheter. Medications and supplemental intravenous infusions are not given through the catheter because they may serve as portals for microbes. When multiple-lumen catheters are used, one lumen is used exclusively for nutrition, whereas the other(s) can be used for such procedures as drug delivery and specimen withdrawal. The tubing that is used for parenteral nutrition should be changed daily. The ideal system consists of (1) a single-solution bottle that is connected to a drip chamber and (2) intravenous tubing that connects directly to the catheter. Infusion pumps keep the solutions running at a steady rate and prevent accidental rapid infusion of large amounts of hypertonic fluid. Volumetric infusion pumps with an occlusion alarm, an infusion-complete alarm, and an air-in-line detector are commonly used.

Once the catheter is properly positioned, the infusion is started slowly, usually at a rate of 40 to 50 mL/hr. Glucose tolerance is assessed by following the patient's urinary and blood sugar levels. If there is no evidence of glucose intolerance, the infusion is increased at the rate of an additional 1 L/day until the desired level is reached. Infusion rates are kept constant through the use of an infusion pump. The patient's weight is measured daily, and urine sugar and serum electrolyte levels, including calcium, phosphorus, and magnesium, are closely monitored. Liver function tests and lipid levels are tested weekly. Transferrin is measured weekly.

Parenteral Nutrition With Lipid Emulsion

An alternate regimen for TPN uses lipid as a supplementary, or occasionally a primary, calorie source. All of the lipid preparations are 10% or 20% emulsions of either safflower, soybean, or canola oil. These oils are mixtures of triglycerides, and they contain predominantly long-chain fatty acids, ranging from C:14 to C:24. The solutions are relatively isotonic and contain emulsified fat particles that approximate the size of a chylomicron (0.5 μm). Fat intake should not exceed 2.5 g/kg/day in adults and 4 g/kg/day in infants and children, assuming that clearance capacity is normal. The remaining calories are supplied by a 10% to 20% solution of dextrose, primarily to meet the requirements of the central nervous system. Typical ratios of carbohydrate:lipid vary from 95:5 to 60:40. Amino acids must be supplied to achieve positive nitrogen balance, usually as a 4.25% solution.

It had been common practice not to mix lipid emulsions with other substrates, administering them through a separate access site or with a Y connector near the point of entry. Increasingly, single bags containing 24 hours' worth of all three major substrates (three-in-one solutions), vitamins, and minerals are used when the nutritional prescription is stable. The use of fat emulsions has the potential advantage of permitting nutritional support through a peripheral vein. Fat emulsions may be helpful in patients who have glucose intolerance and in those who require volume restriction because of the greater caloric density of lipid emulsions. Fat metabolism is associated with a lower RQ than the carbohydrate metabolism, so the use of fat emulsions to provide calories may help to wean patients with CO_2 retention from ventilatory support.

Some fatty acids are essential nutrients. These include linoleic acid (C:18:2) (daily need is 1% of total energy) and linolenic acid (C:18:3) (0.5% of total energy). Fat emulsions prevent the development of essential fatty acid deficiency states. If not given daily as part of a three-in-one solution, then a minimum of 500 mL 10% lipid

LEGACY Health System

LPH - Adult Parenteral Nutrition
Formula Order Sheet
24 Hour TPN Orders

PRE-PRINTED ORDERS

USE BALL POINT PEN, PRESS FIRMLY

ALL LISTED ORDERS ARE IN EFFECT UNLESS CROSSED OUT. EXCEPTIONS: ORDERS PRECEDED BY A BOX (☐) REQUIRE A (✓) TO INITIATE. ORDERS WITH BLANKS INDICATE ADDITIONAL INFORMATION IS NEEDED.

DATE	TIME:	ORDERS: ANOTHER BRAND OF GENERICALLY EQUIVALENT OR APPROVED THERAPEUTICALLY EQUIVALENT PRODUCT MAY BE ADMINISTERED UNLESS CHECKED.	✓

ALL ORDERS MUST BE WRITTEN BY 1500 TO BE PREPARED AND ADMINISTERED BY 2100. ANY EXCEPTIONS TO THE 2100 START TIME MUST BE COORDINATED WITH THE PHARMACY.

____ **CONTINUOUS** ____ **CYCLIC** **Bag #** ____

For assistance with TPN orders contact Pharmacist at 34228 (EHHC), 37204 (GSH) or contact Dietitian at 34424 (EHHC), 37084 (GSH)

TPN SOLUTION CHOICES:

____ **Standard Central Formula**
Amino Acids 50g/L (Amino Acids 5%)
Dextrose 176g/L (Dextrose 17.6%)
Lipids 28g/L (Lipids 2.8%)

(= approximately 1 Kcal/ml)

NPC:N = 110:1
TC:N = 135:1

____ **Standard Peripheral Formula (PPN)**
Amino Acids 30g/L (Amino Acids 3%)
Dextrose 100g/L (Dextrose 10%)
Lipids 33g/L (Lipids 3.3%)

(= approximately 0.75 Kcal/ml)

____ **Custom Formula****
Protein ____ g/day x 4.0 = ________ Kcal
Dextrose ____ g/day x 3.4 = ________ Kcal
*Lipid 20% ____ g/day x 10.0 = ________ Kcal
TOTAL: ________ Kcal/24 hours

____ **Specialty Formula****
(Check one)
____ BCAA ____ Hepatic ____ Renal

NOTE:
* Lipids will be dispensed separately if not compatible.
** See reverse side for instructions and description of Custom & Specialty Formulas.
** BCAA and Hepatic Formula use must have prior approval of attending physician.

ADDITIVES / 24 HOURS:

____ Standard Formulation	____ Extra Additives	____ Other Additives	____ Custom Made Formulation
100 mEq NaCl	____ mEq NaCl	____ u Reg. Human Insulin	____ mEq NaCl
40 mEq K Acetate	____ mEq Na Acetate	____ mg Zinc	____ mEq Na Acetate
20 mEq K Phos	____ mEq Na Phos	____ mg Vit. C	____ mEq Na Phos
9 mEq Ca Gluconate	____ mEq KCl	____ mg Folic acid	____ mEq KCl
10 mEq $MgSO_4$	____ mEq K Acetate	____ Cimetidine	____ mEq K Acetate
1 vial 10 ml MVI	____ mEq K Phos	Other:	____ mEq K Phos
1 vial Trace Elements	____ mEq $MgSO_4$		____ mEq $MgSO_4$
*** 1000 u/L Heparin	____ mEq Ca Gluconate	________	____ mEq Ca Gluconate
VIT K 10mg q Monday	(✓)____ vial 10ml MVI	________	(✓)____ vial 10ml MVI
	(✓)____ vial TR Elements		(✓)____ vial TR Elements
		________	(✓)____ 1000 u/L Heparin

*** Unless otherwise ordered, 1000 units heparin will be added to each liter of TPN.

CONTINUOUS RATE

CPN: Day one infusion rate: Start Infusion at (i.e. 50% final rate) ________ ml/hr for ______ hr, then ________ ml/hr for ______ hours, then final infusion rate: ________.

Continuous Infusion Rate: ________ ml/hr.

NOTE: Substrate amounts must be adjusted proportionally (e.g. Kcal/24 hours) for rate changes.

PPN: Administration Rate: ________ ml/hr.

CYCLIC RATE:

Taper up ________ ml/hr for ______ hr, ________ ml/hr for ______ hr.
Taper down ________ ml/hr for ______ hr, ________ ml/hr for ______ hr.

INFUSE CYCLIC TPN from ______ hours to ______ hours.

OTHER INSTRUCTIONS:

I. Initiate "Inpatient Nutrition Support Orders" - Nutritional Assessment Orders, Parenteral Route Orders.
II. Hang TPN bags at 2100 unless otherwise specified and coordinated with the Pharmacy.

Physician's or Credentialed Provider's Signature________________________

All Pre-Printed Orders must have a Physician/Credentialed Provider's signature to initiate.

105133 (12/95) Original - Chart • Canary - Pharmacy • Pink - IV

Figure 4-5 Example of preprinted total parenteral nutrition (TPN) orders.

emulsion must be given twice weekly to prevent essential fatty acid deficiency. Essential fatty acid deficiency in humans is caused principally by a lack of linoleic acid. The clinical signs of deficiency are eczematous, desquamative dermatitis of body folds, anemia, thrombocytopenia, and hair loss. Growth retardation can also occur, especially in neonates. Lipid-free solutions can be given for as long as 3 weeks before risking lipid deficiency states.

Complications of Parenteral Nutrition

The complications of central venous catheterization are shown in Table 4-11. They may be categorized as technical mishaps, central venous thrombosis, and catheter sepsis. Infusion of a hyperosmolar solution is never started until chest radiographs confirm the correct positioning of the central venous catheter in the superior vena cava and exclude complications secondary to insertion. The overall complication rate of subclavian venous cannulation varies from 3% to 10%, with operator experience as the major variable. The internal jugular vein can be used as an alternate site for long-term central venous cannulation. Many believe that fewer technical complications occur with internal jugular venous cannulation; however, it is more difficult to stabilize and secure this catheter, and as a result, infectious morbidity is slightly increased.

Sepsis is one of the most serious complications of nutritional support with a central venous catheter. Solution contamination is rare. Catheter sepsis, defined as positive blood cultures and identical microbial growth from the cultured catheter, is a much more common problem. When a rigid aseptic protocol is followed for catheter insertion and maintenance, the incidence is 3% to 5%. The infusion line is used only for parenteral nutrition (or one port of a multilumen device is assigned the role), dressings are changed regularly, and skin care is provided at the entry site. The appearance of fever during TPN is an urgent problem because of the possibility of catheter sepsis. A thorough workup to identify the source of fever should be performed expeditiously. If no explanation for the fever is found, the catheter is considered suspect, removed, and cultured. Suspect catheters should be replaced at a new site. In some patients, venous access is difficult, and the TPN catheter may be salvaged by interrupting the flow of nutrients for a day and using an antibiotic solution instead of a heparin solution to "lock" the catheter. Catheter-related sepsis usually resolves within 24 to 48 hours after removal, and antibiotic therapy is often unnecessary.

The metabolic complications of TPN and their treatment are detailed in Table 4-8.

Table 4-11 Complications of Central Venous Catheterization

Upon Insertion	During Maintenance
Pneumothorax	Infection or sepsis
Tension pneumothorax	Central vein thrombosis
Subcutaneous emphysema	Thromboembolism
Subclavian or carotid artery injury	Hydrothorax
Subclavian hematoma	Hydromediastinum
Hemothorax	Cardiac tamponade
Caval or cardiac perforation	Endocarditis
Thoracic duct injury	Arteriovenous fistula
Brachial plexus injury	Air embolus
Horner's syndrome	
Phrenic nerve injury	
Improper position	

Home Parenteral Nutrition

Home parenteral nutrition (HPN) may be provided for patients whose gastrointestinal tract cannot meet their nutritional needs. There must be the potential to improve the quality of life, home placement must be appropriate for the clinical state, and family or other caregivers must be willing and capable of managing the complexities of home TPN if the patient cannot. Indications for home parenteral nutrition are highlighted in the list of general indications for TPN.

Patients are usually unstressed, so basal needs plus 25% for activity suffices. The solution composition is 1 g/kg/day protein, lipids 20% to 30% of total energy needs, and carbohydrates the remainder, with appropriate electrolytes, vitamins, and trace elements. These are mixed in a 2- to 3-L solution that is infused over a 10- to 12-hour period while the patient sleeps. Also called *cyclic parenteral nutrition*, this regimen is considered the least disruptive to the patient's lifestyle. These patients need central venous access with either peripherally inserted central catheter (PICC), nontunneled or tunneled and cuffed catheters (e.g., Hickman, Groshong), or completely implanted subcutaneous ports.

A team of people is necessary to deliver home parenteral nutrition safely and effectively. The team should include a physician familiar with HPN, a pharmacist, a nurse, a home care company, and a dietician.

NUTRITIONAL SUPPORT IN SELECTED SURGICAL SITUATIONS

For all of the reasons described in the section on nutritional assessment, it is difficult to definitively attribute particular elements of nutritional support to outcomes in specific disease states. As much as possible, the material below is drawn from class I and II data, but a great deal remains a matter of consensus opinion. Specific information on burns and pancreatitis are in the relevant chapters of this text.

Cancer

Protein-calorie malnutrition often occurs in patients with cancer, partly because of the presence of tumors that cause metabolic abnormalities. These abnormalities include inefficient energy metabolism, abnormal carbohydrate metabolism (including glucose intolerance), accelerated breakdown of body fat, abnormal protein metabolism causing host nitrogen depletion, decreased muscle protein synthesis, and increased muscle protein breakdown. Compounded by the associated stresses and side effects of surgery, chemotherapy, and radiation therapy, the patient's nutritional status is further compromised. Malnutrition and weight loss have long been known to predict increased morbidity. However, nutritional support in surgical oncology patients has not significantly reduced morbidity rates in objective clinical trials.

The Veterans Administration (VA) Total Parenteral Nutrition Cooperative Study showed that preoperative TPN benefited only cancer patients who were considered severely malnourished. Well-nourished or moderately malnourished patients did not experience a benefit, but had an increased risk of catheter-related infection. Patients who are not expected to have oral intake for more than 5 days may be helped by postoperative TPN. Patients who have postoperative complications need support. Although chemotherapy and radiation therapy place additional stresses on the patient, clinical trials showed no difference in response to therapy with the addition of nutritional support. There is a trend toward fewer side effects, and this trend alone may allow more patients to undergo or complete full courses of treatment.

The role of nutritional support in cancer therapy is controversial. Formulations with specific amino acid modifications may help to suppress tumor growth, but some research suggests that nutritional support accelerates tumor growth. Further study of the role of nutritional support in better defined subsets of cancer patients is needed.

Cardiac Disease

In cardiac surgery, two important points need to be noted. First, valve replacement patients who are malnourished will have a greater complication and mortality rate compared to a normally nourished cohort. It is not certain that immediate perioperative nutritional support will alter these associations.

Second, investigations have shown perioperative control of hyperglycemia to correlate closely with sternal wound infection rates. The original investigation simply held blood glucose levels to less than 180 mg/dL, beginning in the presurgical holding period and continuing intraoperatively and postoperatively. This effort contrasted with the typically postoperative effort at glucose control, which often accepted values as high as 200 to 250 mg/dL. Maintaining "tight" blood glucose control with exogenous insulin is now more widespread in general, vascular, and orthopedic surgery, and intervention at even lower threshold levels (as low as 100 mg/dL) is under investigation.

Inflammatory Bowel Disease (IBD)

Patients with Crohn's disease and ulcerative colitis are often malnourished and have weight and micronutrient depletion. Pubescent patients frequently exhibit growth failure because of deficient intake of nutrients or decreased absorption from diseased bowel. Acute exacerbations can lead to significant loss of body protein and physiologic impairment, but the increase in protein synthesis and breakdown rates is moderate, with an average combined fecal and urine nitrogen excretion of 15 g/day. Steroid therapy sharply increases nitrogen excretion. Specific attention should be paid to deficiencies in calcium, vitamin D, folate, vitamin B_{12}, and zinc.

The nutritional state of patients with inflammatory bowel disorders can be improved. Nutritional support has no primary therapeutic benefit in ulcerative colitis, but in Crohn's disease, individual diet counseling decreases disease activity, improves remission rates, and decreases the need for drug therapy, rehospitalization, and lost work days. Elemental diets have primary therapeutic efficacy in acute Crohn's disease, but randomized trials do not show them to be more effective than polymeric formulations. Several studies confirmed that an elemental diet is equal to or more effective than steroids in inducing remission in acute disease. The benefits of long-term diet supplementation are less clear. However, the long-term use of corticosteroids in IBD is a cause of concern. Enteral treatment failures are due to noncompliance because of feed palatability, inability to stay off a solid-free diet for weeks, social inconvenience, and occasional feed-related adverse reactions.

There is some promise that glutamine, arginine, glutamate, glutathione, short-chain fatty acids, antioxidants, zinc, and vitamin A may lead to a "Crohn's-disease-specific" formulation. The type of dietary fat may be a factor—high linoleate and low oleate diets had efficacy similar to that of prednisone for inducing remission in active disease. Efficacy is not altered by nitrogen source (amino acids or intact proteins). Glutamine enrichment was not found advantageous compared to a standard glutamine-containing diet.

TPN improves the general nutritional state, but is not useful as a primary therapy. Its main role is in managing fistula, intestinal obstruction, and short-bowel syndrome. A controlled, randomized trial of patients who were given postoperative TPN compared with standard intravenous fluids did not show a reduction in complication rate. HPN is effective in active Crohn's disease that is unresponsive to conventional medical management. HPN reduces hospital time and allows good quality of life at home.

Radiation Enteritis

Adjuvant radiation therapy may improve resectability, time to recurrence, or local control of several cancers. When directed to any portion of the gastrointestinal tract, radiation alters function, in turn affecting nutritional status. Symptoms of radiation enteritis are dependent upon dose, time, fractionation, and volume in the field. Acutely, mucosal brush border function is altered, and there may be bloody diarrhea. In a nonrandomized study of bladder cancer patients, jejunal delivery of an elemental diet during radiotherapy and postoperatively following radical cystectomy and ileal conduit prevented acute phase radiation injury.

Late complications of radiation enteritis include intestinal obstruction, short bowel, malabsorption, enterocutaneous and enteroenteral fistula, and dysmotility. HPN is a reasonable treatment option in such patients, with survival and complication rates similar to those of other HPN-treated patients. It may allow resumption of oral feedings in one-third of patients. TPN also enhances surgical options such as resection and stricturoplasty.

Short-Bowel Syndrome

Short-bowel syndrome is a serious consequence of massive bowel removal or dysfunction. When a large segment of the small bowel is removed, the ability of the intestine to absorb nutrients, fluids, and electrolytes is impeded. The result is known as short-bowel syndrome. Short-bowel syndrome causes a variety of complications, many of which are secondary to the lack of absorption of food and nutrients. These patients commonly experience protein-calorie malnutrition. They also have diarrhea, with or without steatorrhea, and often become dehydrated.

Therapy focuses on electrolyte and fluid replacement, early institution of enteral and parenteral nutrition, and symptomatic control of complications. Enteral feedings, even in the smallest amount, should begin as early as possible to prevent the remaining small bowel mucosa from degenerating. Once fluid and electrolyte balance is stabilized and nutrition is repleted, treatment consists of assisting the dietary intake and modifying it as needed. Patients need frequent nutritional assessments with the appropriate therapy. Weaning from TPN is attempted when the patient can tolerate oral feedings. If, after 1 year, the patient remains dependent on TPN, operative intervention may be considered. Restoration of continuity to lengths of bowel that are out of the enteral stream, construction of mucosal valves, reversed peristalsis of bowel segments to prolong bowel transit time, longitudinal splitting of lengths of remaining bowel or repeated Y-plasties to increase length, and small bowel transplantation have been described. These options, however, are controversial. Surgical intervention is experimental, and until recently, has not produced good results. Small bowel transplantation remains investigational.

FRONTIERS AND CONTROVERSIES

Clearly, the understanding of nutrition has moved from the simple provision of substrates into a better understanding of its influence upon numerous bodily functions. This is nowhere better seen than with the introduction of immune-enhancing nutrients. Arginine and glutamine have already been mentioned. Nucleotides, required for catalysis, energy transfer, and coordination of hormonal signals, can be synthesized endogenously. However, exogenous sources are preferred and enhance response to fungal infections in animal models. Omega-3 fatty acids do not stimulate the immune system, but compete with arachidonic acid for cyclooxygenase metabolism and thus reduce the inflammatory response. Numerous studies show benefits of immune-enhancing enteral formulations, particularly in surgical patients, but there is skepticism about their role in the critically ill. Much work remains to be done about each specific nutrient, dose ranges, interactions with other immunomodulating agents, and the effect of each in specific clinical states.

The role of anabolic steroid hormones as an adjunct to nutritional support is under investigation. Testosterone has both androgenic (virilizing) and anabolic (constructive) effects. Synthetic anabolic steroids attempt to minimize androgenic effects. Nandrolone decanoate reduces nitrogen loss, but increases total plasma amino acid levels; it also may enhance protein synthesis. Stanzolol improves nitrogen balance in postcolectomy patients who are given amino acids only, but provides no additional benefit to patients who are receiving amino acids, lipids, and carbohydrates. When coupled with nutrient supplements, oxandrolone has anabolic efficacy in HIV-associated wasting and cirrhosis. Oxymetholone has improved nitrogen retention in HIV-related wasting, and erythropoiesis in anemia.

Growth hormone (GH) has been studied as an adjunct to nutritional therapy since 1956. Recombinant human GH enhances nitrogen retention in patients who are receiving TPN and in those who have burns, chronic obstructive pulmonary disease, cancer, or other critical illnesses. Several investigations suggested that this effect occurs secondary to improved conservation of skeletal muscle protein mass and enhanced lipolysis. GH acts in a complex interrelation with insulin-like growth factor-1, and this factor may be a more effective anabolic agent in critical illness. Although GH accelerates protein gain and reduces fat and extracellular water gain during TPN, its influence on patient outcome is still in the early stages of definition. Two European trials reporting GH use early in critical illness found increased mortality in the recipients.

Internationally, diets vary in their content of polyunsaturated fatty acids, either omega-6 (vegetable oils) or omega-3 (fish oils). Their effect on cardiovascular disease is an area of intense epidemiologic study. Some investigators are using TPN to treat plaque regression in patients with premature atherosclerosis.

Alternative sources of energy are sought for use in clinical conditions that are marked by insulin resistance, hyperlipidemia, and carnitine deficiency. Long-chain fatty acids require carnitine to enter mitochondria for oxidation. Short- and medium-chain triglycerides (MCTs), however, do not. Consequently, much work is underway to define MCT absorption, uptake into organs, and interaction with long-chain triglycerides, as well as their role in nutritional therapy. Structured triglycerides are developed by mixtures of conventional fats and oils with MCTs on a single glycerol backbone. These unique structures are intended to modify the inflammatory state by reducing the number of prostaglandin precursors in long-chain fatty acids or to supply MCTs, which are carnitine-independent for their uptake into and metabolism by mitochondria.

Xylitol is metabolized through the pentose phosphate pathway. In combination with long-chain triglycerides, it is more effective than glucose in improving nitrogen retention in septic rats. Azelaic acid is a dicarboxylic acid that undergoes β-oxidation through carnitine-independent pathways. These acids are being studied in carnitine-deficient states of sepsis, cirrhosis, prematurity, and hemodialysis.

Functional food, *biotherapeutics*, and *nutraceuticals* are interchangeable terms coming into currency to describe foodstuffs used not so much to support metabolism as to manipulate specific functions of an organism. A *prebiotic* is defined as a nondigestible carbohydrate that stimulates the growth and/or activity of one or a limited number of bacterial species resident in the colon. Food fiber cannot be digested by human amylases, and is either insoluble (lignans, inulin, cellulose-bulking agents) or soluble (pectins, mucilages, gums). The latter are fermented by colonic anaerobes into short-chain fatty acids, which in turn stimulate colonocytes and beneficially alter glucose absorption. Synthetic fructooligosaccharides (oligofructoses or FOS) obtained by enzymatic synthesis of sucrose and lactose are used as mucosa reconditioners. *Probiotics* are live microbial food supplements that are beneficial to health. These include lactobacilli (yogurt), bifidobacteria, Gram-positive cocci (cheeses), and yeasts (*Saccharomyces* species). Health benefits of interest include prevention of antibiotic-associated diarrhea, treatment of *C. difficile* diarrhea, prevention of vaginal infections, enhancing gut-associated lymphoid tissue immunity, altering cholesterol levels, and improving calcium absorption. Most investigators are European or Japanese.

One last point should be made. Nutritional products from pharmacy and dietary services and their bedside delivery systems are heavily quality controlled, especially for bacterial contamination. Unhappily, there is growing evidence that some part of the emergence, spread, and human impact of bacterial antibiotic resistance is due to inappropriate antimicrobial use in animal and plant agriculture. Increased antibiotic exposure during food production leads to increased antibiotic resistance in food commensal microbes. Many such microbes are necessary for food production, and others are contaminants. These microbes enter the human system, and can (1) directly cause disease, (2) incite infections in the immunosuppressed, or (3) transfer resistance factors to human commensal bacteria. Investigation of the microbial life on and within us, their relationship to foods and to medical therapies, and the modifying actions of functional foods is an area of great importance.

SUGGESTED READINGS

ASPEN Board of Directors and Clinical Guidelines Task Force. Guidelines for the use of parenteral and enteral nutrition in adults and pediatric patients. *J Parenter Enter Nutr* 2001;26(Suppl).

Barza M, Gorbach SL, eds. The need to improve antimicrobial use in agriculture: ecological and human health consequences. *Clin Infect Dis* 2002;34(Suppl 3):S111–S125.

Burzstein S, Elwyn DH, Askanazi J, et al. *Energy Metabolism, Indirect Calorimetry, and Nutrition*. Baltimore, MD: Williams & Wilkins, 1989.

Elmer GW, Surawicz CM, McFarland LV. Biotherapeutic agents: a neglected modality for the treatment and prevention of selected intestinal and vaginal infections. *JAMA* 1996;275:870–876.

Heyland DK, Novak F, Drover JW, et al. Should immunonutrition become routine in critically ill patients? A systematic review of the evidence. *JAMA* 2001;286:944–953.

Kinney JM, Jeejeebhoy KN, Hill GL, et al., eds. *Nutrition and Metabolism in Patient Care*. Philadelphia, PA: WB Saunders, 1988.

Lipschitz DA. Approaches to the nutritional support of the older patient. *Clin Geriatr Med* 1995;11:715–724.

Patino JF, de Pimiento SE, Vergara A, et al. Hypocaloric support in the critically ill. *World J Surg* 1999;23:553–559.

Proceedings from Summit on Immune-Enhancing Enteral Therapy. *J Parenter Enter Nutr* 2001;25(2):1S–63S.

Rubin H, Carlson S, DeMeo M, et al. Randomized, double-blind study of intravenous human albumin in hypoalbuminemic patients receiving total parenteral nutrition. *Crit Care Med* 1997;25:249–252.

Sanders ME. Considerations for use of probiotic bacteria to modulate human health. *J Nutr* 2000;130:384S–390S.

Spiess A, Mikalunas V, Carlson S, et al. Albumin kinetics in hypoalbuminemic patients receiving total parenteral nutrition. *J Parenter Enter Nutr* 1996;20:424–428.

Tauxe RV. Emerging foodborne diseases: an evolving public health challenge. *Emerg Infect Dis* 1997;3(4):425.

5

HOLLIS W. MERRICK, III, MD ■ MARY R. SMITH, MD
BRUCE V. MACFADYEN, JR., MD

Surgical Bleeding and Blood Replacement

OBJECTIVES

1 Using a patient's physical examination and medical history, determine the likelihood and etiology of possible bleeding disorders.
2 Name five major etiologic factors that may lead to bleeding disorders.
3 Describe the common laboratory tests that are used to assess coagulation status, and explain how these tests apply to the diagnosis of the conditions discussed in Objective 2.
4 Identify the acute etiologic factors that might be responsible for extensive bleeding in a patient who has received massive transfusions.
5 Name the conditions that might lead to disseminated intravascular coagulation (DIC).
6 Describe the recommended component replacement therapy for the etiologic categories named in Objective 2, as well as the definitive treatment for the underlying cause of each.
7 Describe the process of obtaining and transfusing blood, the symptoms of a transfusion reaction, and the diagnosis and appropriate management of the different types of transfusion reactions.

Bleeding may occur during surgical procedures. Although the volume of blood lost is usually not large enough to create a major problem, certain operations are invariably associated with large blood losses that may impair the normal hemostatic process. Additionally, some patients with congenital or acquired clotting disorders require elective or emergency surgery. Therefore, surgeons must be prepared for significant blood losses that may have an adverse effect on patient recovery, and they must be able to manage blood loss in their patients. In addition, surgeons must be knowledgeable about common bleeding and clotting disorders, the components of blood replacement, and the problems associated with the transfusion of blood products.

THE HEMOSTATIC PROCESS

The hemostatic process involves an interaction among the blood vessel wall, the platelets, and the coagulation pathways. After injury, hemostasis begins with a brief period of **vasoconstriction** by the vessels that have muscular layers in their walls. This vasoconstriction in the region of injury only controls blood loss for a brief time and cannot offer significant control of bleeding.

The next step is mediated by **platelets,** which **adhere** to areas of vascular injury or to exposed subendothelial structures (Fig. 5-1). Platelets also adhere to structures other than platelets. After adhesion, the platelets extrude their contents, the most important of which is adenosine

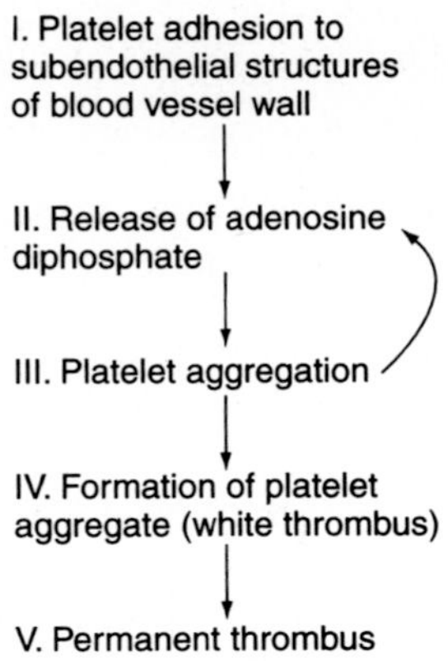

Figure 5-1 Platelets in the control of bleeding.

diphosphate. As a result, platelet **aggregation** occurs. This platelet-to-platelet sticking causes the initial **thrombus.** The process from initial injury to the white (platelet) thrombus occurs independently of the coagulation pathways; hemophiliacs, for example, can generate a normal white thrombus. However, a more permanent thrombus is required for control of bleeding and eventual healing. This thrombus is accomplished through the formation of **fibrin**.

The coagulation pathways use various **coagulation factors** to generate fibrin, which stabilizes the white thrombus (Fig. 5-2). The **extrinsic coagulation pathway** begins with tissue thromboplastin, which interacts with factor VII to convert factor X to factor Xa and initiates the common pathway. The **intrinsic coagulation pathway** requires factors XII, XI, IX, and VIII to interact and eventually convert factor X to factor Xa. The **common coagulation pathway** involves factors X, V, II (prothrombin), and I (**fibrinogen**). The end-product of coagulation is fibrin, which has a weak clot-stabilizing ability. Factor XIII (fibrin-stabilizing factor) is required to create fibrin of optimal strength (see Fig. 5-2).

Bleeding may occur in the presence of a deficiency of any of the factors of the coagulation pathways, except factor XII. Additionally, although normal hemostasis requires calcium, hypocalcemia does not cause bleeding.

EVALUATION OF THE PATIENT

Detecting and correcting bleeding disorders before surgery is the best way to avoid major bleeding problems during and after surgery. Therefore, a careful screening for bleed-

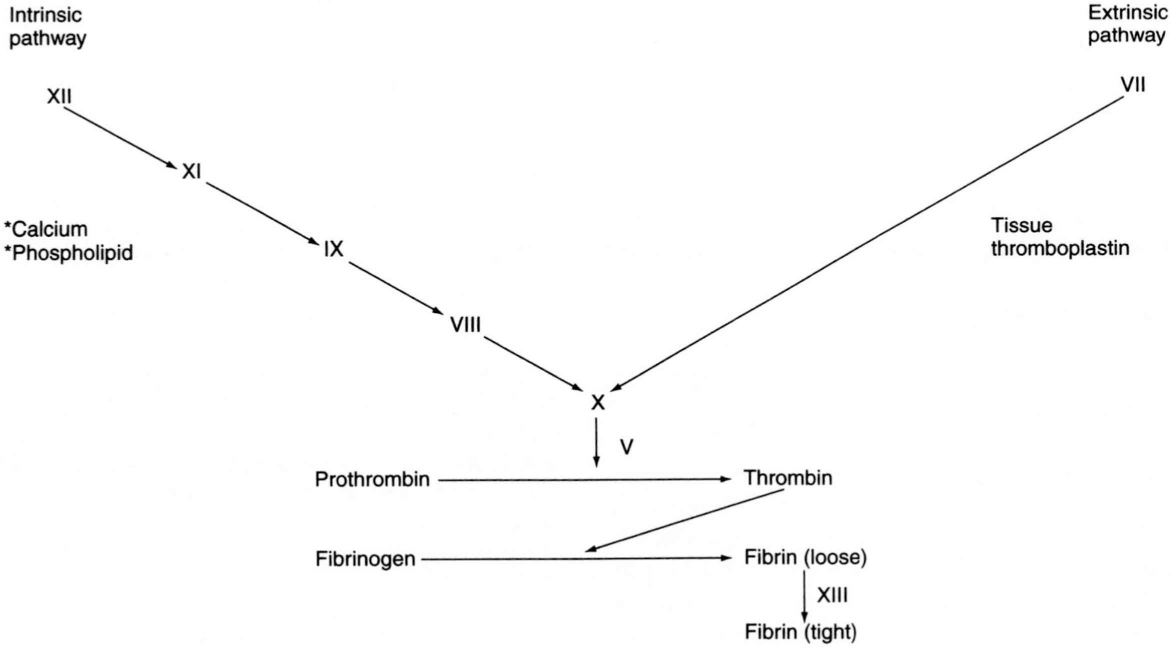

Figure 5-2 The coagulation pathways. *Calcium and phospholipid from platelets are needed to permit the coagulation pathways to proceed at optimum rates. Activated factor XI in turn activates factor IX to become factor IXa. Factor IXa, in the presence of factor VIII, platelet phospholipid, and calcium, activates factor X. The rate of this reaction is greatly increased by the presence of the platelet phospholipid.

Table 5-1 Preoperative Evaluation for Bleeding and Clotting Disorders

Study	When Performed
History	In all patients as part of routine preoperative evaluation
Physical examination	As part of routine preoperative evaluation
Laboratory studies: PT, APTT, platelet count, bleeding time, thrombin time	In patients with evidence of bleeding disorders or in whom excessive bleeding is anticipated because of the nature of the surgery

APTT, activated partial thromboplastin time; PT, prothrombin time.

ing risks is an essential part of the preoperative evaluation (Table 5-1).

History

Obtaining a detailed **bleeding history** is the most important step in evaluating patients for possible bleeding problems. Patients should be asked if they have had prolonged bleeding after dental extractions, minor cuts, or previous operations; if they have prolonged or frequent menses; if they have experienced bruising after minor injury; or if they experience nosebleeds. A history of "bleeders" in the family is also important to obtain. For the individual patient, a history of bleeding problems is the most important preoperative information that predicts unexpected bleeding complications. This information is even more reliable than laboratory tests.

Physical Examination

The physical examination is less helpful than the history in assessing bleeding risk, because most patients with mild to moderate bleeding disorders do not have physical signs. The examiner should seek signs of blood disorders, splenomegaly, hepatomegaly, hemarthroses, petechiae, or ecchymoses, which can be associated with bleeding disorders. Petechiae are typical of platelet disorders, whereas ecchymoses are more typical of abnormalities in the coagulation pathways.

Tests to Evaluate Hemostasis

Platelet count, prothrombin time (PT), and **activated partial thromboplastin time** (APTT) should be determined in patients who provide any history suggestive of a bleeding disorder as part of the routine preoperative evaluation to exclude thrombocytopenia, a coagulation factor deficiency, or an acquired coagulation factor inhibitor. Certain other screening tests, such as bleeding time, or **thrombin** time, are indicated when the history or physical examination suggests a bleeding or clotting disorder, or if major bleeding is expected because of the nature of the planned surgery. These studies should be carried out as a part of preoperative screening unless there has been a recent significant challenge to the patient's hemostatic competence. Acquired bleeding disorders (e.g., thrombocytopenia) or acquired inhibitors against clotting factors can lead to a bleeding disorder in a previously hemostatically healthy person. These tests are relatively inexpensive and may potentially avoid unexpected bleeding and the ensuing urgent need for transfusion of blood products.

Platelet Count

The platelet count verifies that an adequate number of platelets are available in the circulation. Platelet counts are done by automated methods in most institutions. However, automated counters may not be accurate at platelet counts of less than 40,000. Platelet counts may also be inaccurate if many red cell fragments are present or in cases of pseudothrombocytopenia due to ethylenediaminetetraacetic acid (EDTA)–sensitive platelets in a small number of patients. For this reason, very low platelet counts may need to be confirmed by manual methods. Review of the peripheral blood smear provides a reasonable estimate of platelet numbers and is recommended for patients before surgery if any past history of abnormal bleeding is known.

Platelets may be present in adequate numbers and yet may not function appropriately (e.g., von Willebrand's disease, qualitative platelet defects). In this case, bleeding time is prolonged and screening whole blood platelet aggregation is abnormal.

Prothrombin Time

The PT measures the ability of the blood to form stable thrombi. It evaluates the adequacy of factors VII, X, and V; prothrombin; and fibrinogen (Fig. 5-3), both extrinsic and common pathways. Its most common use is to monitor oral anticoagulation with warfarin (Coumadin). Today, PT is reported with the international normalized ratio (INR). The INR system overcomes the problem of variable sensitivity by standardizing the patient's PT ratio using the international sensitivity index (ISI) of the particular thromboplastin. The ISI compares the locally used thromboplastin to an international standard thromboplastin. Therefore, the INR is the PT ratio that would have been obtained if the international standard had been used. The formula is shown below:

$$\text{INR} = \left(\frac{\text{Patient}}{\text{Normal PT}}\right)^{ISI}$$

Mastery of the use of the INR as a tool for anticoagulation therapy is important for physicians. Although most patients are adequately anticoagulated when the INR is between

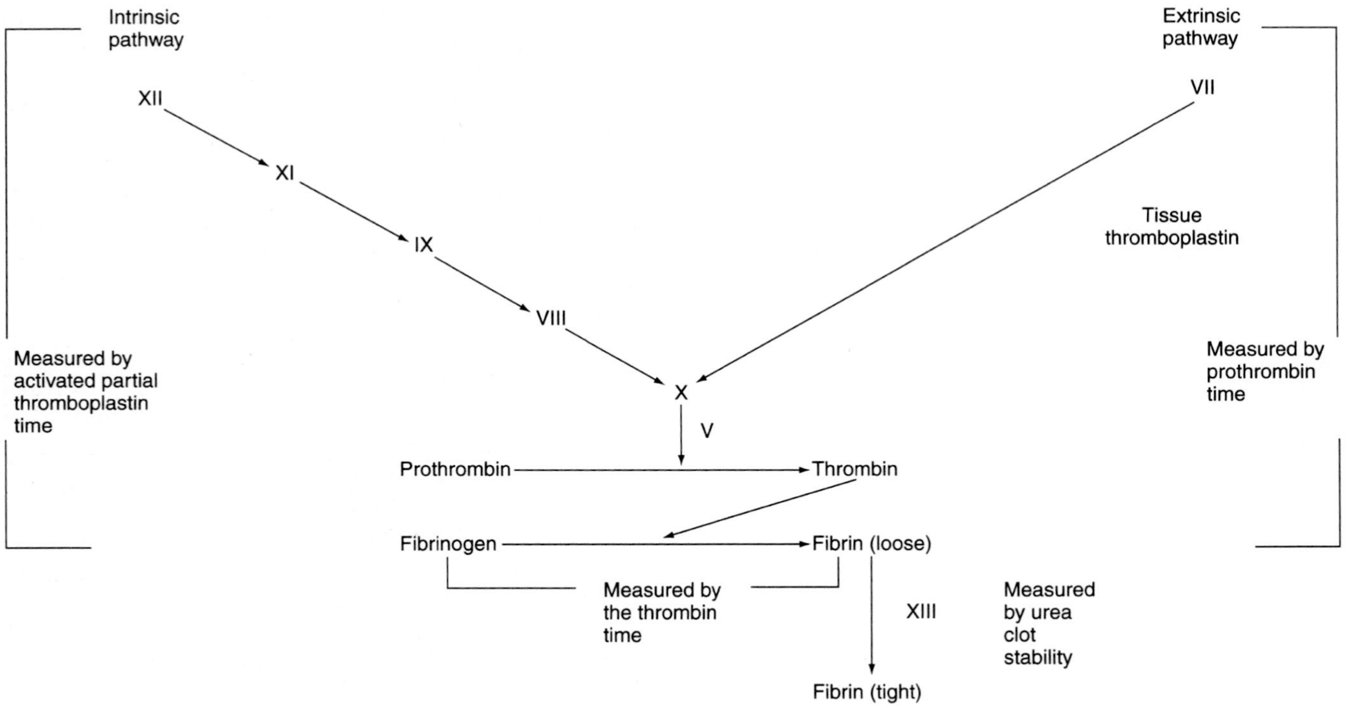

Figure 5-3 Tests of the coagulation pathways. Extrinsic pathway: measured by prothrombin time: monitor coumadin therapy. Intrinsic pathway: measured by activated partial thromboplastin time: monitor heparin therapy.

2.5 and 3.0, certain patients require more intensive therapy that results in an INR of up to 3.5.

Activated Partial Thromboplastin Time

The APTT evaluates the adequacy of fibrinogen, prothrombin, and factors V, VIII, IX, X, XI, and XII in the intrinsic and common pathways (see Fig. 5-3). It is the most commonly used test to monitor the effectiveness of unfractionated heparin therapy. The APTT is normal in patients with factor VII deficiency, but it is elevated during Coumadin therapy because of reductions in factors II, IX, and X. The APTT cannot be used to monitor most low–molecular-weight heparins.

Bleeding Time

The **bleeding time test** is conducted by making two standard wounds (6 mm long, 1 mm deep) in the forearm of the patient with a spring-loaded lancet. The time from injury until the cessation of bleeding from both wounds is measured. A normal bleeding time requires adequate numbers and function of platelets and normal blood vessel walls. A normal bleeding time range (in minutes) is established by each laboratory. The usual range is 5 to 10 minutes, but small variations are found from laboratory to laboratory. A mild prolongation of bleeding time may be caused by aging skin or long-term corticosteroid therapy. In both cases, senile ecchymoses may be seen, especially on the patient's forearms.

A prolonged bleeding time is often associated with significant bleeding at surgery. Bleeding time may be prolonged by certain drugs (e.g., aspirin, other nonsteroidal antiinflammatory drugs [NSAIDs], ticlopidine). An abnormal bleeding time in a patient without a history of associated drug use indicates a potential bleeding disorder. A newly found prolonged bleeding time may be caused by any of the following disorders:

1 Thrombocytopenia
2 Abnormal platelet function because of:
  a Medication (e.g., aspirin)
  b Dense granular disorders of platelets
3 Von Willebrand's disease (congenital or acquired)

Thrombin Time

The thrombin time evaluates fibrinogen-to-fibrin conversion with an external source of thrombin. Prolongation of thrombin time can be caused by: (1) low fibrinogen levels (hypofibrinogenemia), (2) abnormal fibrinogen (dysfibrinogenemia), (3) fibrin and fibrinogen split products, or (4) heparin (see Fig. 5-3). Thrombin time is used to evaluate disseminated intravascular coagulation (DIC) and chronic liver disease.

CAUSES OF EXCESSIVE SURGICAL BLEEDING

Most patients are hemostatically normal before they enter the operating room. However, in some patients with large blood losses, generalized oozing is noted after a certain period. In addition, some operations (e.g., cardiopulmonary bypass, liver transplant surgery, prostate surgery, construction of portacaval shunts) are frequently associated with large blood losses. These patients develop consumption of clotting factors and platelets, causing the syndrome of consumptive coagulopathy or disseminated intravascular coagulopathy.

Preexisting Hemostatic Defects

Preexisting hemostatic defects should be suspected when a prior history of bleeding exists or when abnormal bleeding begins within the first 30 minutes of the operative period.

Congenital Bleeding Disorders

Congenital bleeding disorders, such as hemophilia and **von Willebrand's disease,** are uncommon. Mildly affected patients may be asymptomatic. **Type A hemophilia** and von Willebrand's disease are both characterized by deficiencies of factor VIII clotting activity (VIII_c), but there are differences in the two disease processes. Hemophilia is seen almost exclusively in males, and platelet function is normal. Von Willebrand's disease affects people of both sexes. In addition to factor VIII_c deficiency, von Willebrand's disease is associated with platelet dysfunction, which is diagnosed by decreased aggregation in response to ristocetin and is corrected by normal **plasma.** Deficiency of von Willebrand activity is corrected with cryoprecipitate infusions or desmopressin (DDAVP) therapy. Cryoprecipitate is a fraction of plasma that contains von Willebrand's factor, factor VIII clotting activity, and fibrinogen. DDAVP is given as an intravenous infusion or as nasal "snuff." DDAVP is a hormone that, in addition to other properties, leads to the release of von Willebrand's factor from its endothelial cell storage sites.

Congenital platelet function disorders are uncommon and usually occur in patients who have a history of mucous membrane bleeding and easy bruising. Factor IX deficiency (e.g., Christmas disease, hemophilia B) is seen only in males and is less common than type A hemophilia. Type A hemophilia is treated with purified factor VIII concentrates. Factor XI deficiency is found almost exclusively in Jewish patients.

Acquired Bleeding Disorders

Acquired bleeding disorders are more common than congenital bleeding disorders and may have a variety of causes. Liver disease is a common cause of coagulation abnormalities. Inability of the liver to synthesize proteins leads to decreased levels of prothrombin and factors V, VII, and X (but not VIII), which may cause prolonged PT and APTT. Alcohol ingestion may result in acute thrombocytopenia. Hypersplenism may depress the platelet count moderately. Obstructive jaundice may lead to clotting factor deficiencies, which can usually be corrected with parenteral vitamin K. Cirrhosis may also cause clotting factor deficiencies. These respond less well to vitamin K. However, gastrointestinal bleeding in the patient who has cirrhosis is usually caused by varices or gastritis rather than by a coagulation defect.

Anticoagulant therapy with heparin or oral anticoagulants (e.g., Coumadin) leads to acquired bleeding disorders. Coumadin causes depression of the clotting activity of four coagulation factors (II, VII, IX, and X). Because both the intrinsic and extrinsic pathways are affected by Coumadin, both PT and APTT are prolonged. Heparin prolongs both APTT and thrombin time. Heparin (high–molecular-weight, or unfractionated, heparin) works by increasing the speed with which antithrombin III binds to and neutralizes factors IXa, Xa, XIa, XIIa, and thrombin. A number of different low–molecular-weight heparins are available for use. It is important to recognize the specifics of various low–molecular-weight heparin preparations when selecting an agent for clinical use in specific settings.

Acquired thrombocytopenia is caused by four mechanisms: (1) decreased platelet production in the bone marrow (e.g., aplastic anemia); (2) increased destruction of platelets in the peripheral blood (e.g., idiopathic thrombocytopenia purpura [ITP] or DIC); (3) splenic pooling in an enlarged spleen (e.g., cirrhosis); or (4) any combination of these disorders (e.g., alcoholic liver failure).

Platelet function disorders are usually associated with drugs (e.g., aspirin, other NSAIDs). Unlike other NSAIDs, however, aspirin induces a defect that does not reverse; thus, patients should be instructed to avoid aspirin for 1 week before elective surgery. Plavix, used commonly for platelet-inhibiting effects, also has an irreversible effect on platelets. As with aspirin, Plavix should be stopped 7 to 10 days before surgery.

A second important cause of acquired platelet dysfunction is uremia. Patients who are uremic and are bleeding require dialysis before surgery to correct their platelet dysfunction.

Intraoperative Complications

Several common conditions contribute to bleeding during a surgical procedure. Shock may cause or aggravate consumptive coagulopathy. Hypothermia is also associated with consumptive coagulopathy. Massive transfusion of stored packed red blood cells may lead to bleeding. This bleeding occurs after rapid transfusion of 10 units or more of stored blood over a 4- to 6-hour period. It is caused by low numbers of platelets and by dilution of the clotting factors as a result of the infusion of nonplasma fluids for volume support.

Acute hemolytic blood transfusion reactions may lead to DIC. When a patient is under general anesthesia, there may be no clues that incompatible blood has been infused until the onset of generalized bleeding as a result of DIC. The usual symptoms of an incompatible blood transfusion (e.g., agitation, back pain) do not occur under general anesthesia. Hemoglobinuria and oliguria provide additional clinical evidence of DIC.

Intraoperative bleeding from needle holes, vascular suture lines, or extensive tissue dissection can often be controlled through the use of local hemostatic agents. These include gelatin sponge (e.g., Gelfoam), oxidized cellulose (Surgicel), collagen sponge (Helistat), microfibrillar collagen (Avitene, Hemotene), topical thrombin (with or without topical cryoprecipitate), topical EACA, and topical aprotinin.

Postoperative Bleeding

Fifty percent of postoperative bleeding is caused by inadequate hemostasis during surgery. Other causes of postoperative bleeding include:

1. Circulating heparin that remains after bypass surgery.
2. Shock that results in consumptive coagulopathy.
3. Altered liver function after partial hepatectomy. If a large portion of the liver is removed, the remaining liver may need 3 to 5 days to increase its production of clotting factors sufficiently to support hemostasis.
4. Acquired deficiency of the vitamin K–dependent clotting factors (II, VII, IX, and X). This deficiency may develop in patients who are poorly nourished and are receiving antibiotics.
5. Factor XIII deficiency. In this case, bleeding occurs 3 to 5 days after surgery. The diagnosis of factor XIII deficiency is confirmed with a urea clot stability test, which evaluates the ability of a clot to remain intact. If the clot dissolves rapidly, it suggests a deficiency of factor XIII, which is an uncommon cause of postsurgical bleeding.
6. DIC and fibrinolysis.

COMMON BLEEDING DISORDERS IN THE SURGICAL PATIENT

Disseminated Intravascular Coagulation (Consumptive Coagulopathy)

As the name suggests, **disseminated intravascular coagulation,** or DIC, is characterized by intravascular coagulation and thrombosis that is diffuse rather than localized at the site of injury. This process results in the systemic deposition of platelet-fibrin microthrombi that cause diffuse tissue injury. Some clotting factors may be consumed in sufficient amounts to eventually lead to diffuse bleeding. DIC may be acute or clinically asymptomatic and chronic.

Etiology

The etiology of DIC may be any of the following: (1) the release of tissue debris into the bloodstream after trauma or an obstetric catastrophe; (2) the introduction of intravascular aggregations of platelets as a result of the activation of platelets by various materials, including adenosine diphosphate and thrombin (which may explain the occurrence of DIC in patients with severe septicemia or immune complex disease); (3) extensive endothelial damage, which denudes the vascular wall and stimulates coagulation and platelet adhesion (as seen in patients with widespread burns or vasculitis); (4) hypotension that leads to stasis and prevents the normal circulating inhibitors of coagulation from reaching the sites of the microthrombi; (5) blockage of the reticuloendothelial system; (6) some types of operations that involve the prostate, lung, or malignant tumors; and (7) severe liver disease.

Diagnostic Studies

The diagnosis of DIC is established by the detection of diminished levels of coagulation factors and platelets. The following laboratory results may be useful in diagnosing DIC: (1) prolonged APTT, (2) prolonged PT, (3) hypofibrinogenemia, (4) thrombocytopenia, and (5) the presence of fibrin and fibrinogen split (FDP) products. The euglobulin clot lysis is a simple and useful bedside test that can be performed while waiting for the laboratory results. The presence of fibrin and fibrinogen split products is caused by activation of the fibrinolytic pathway in response to activation of the clotting pathway. The D-dimer is a product of fibrin digestion by the fibrinolytic process.

Treatment

The most important aspect of the treatment of DIC is to remove the precipitating factors (e.g., treating septicemia). If DIC is severe, replacement of coagulation factors is required to correct the coagulation defect. Cryoprecipitate is the best method to replace a profound fibrinogen deficit. Platelet transfusions may also be required. **Fresh frozen plasma** is useful to replace other deficits that are identified, but it must be used judiciously if volume overload is a potential problem. In rare cases, the coagulation pathway must be inhibited with heparin or with drug therapy to prevent platelet aggregation.

The use of heparin to treat DIC is controversial. There is no conclusive evidence that using heparin alters the outcome of DIC. Because antithrombin III is consumed during DIC, the use of heparin as an anticoagulant may be severely compromised. Large trials are underway to evaluate the benefit of using antithrombin III concentrates and protein C concentrates as part of the treatment of DIC. Preliminary data from some trials are promising.

Bleeding Disorders Caused by Increased Fibrinolysis

Primary Fibrinolysis

Primary fibrinolysis is a disorder that occurs most commonly after fibrinolytic therapy with drugs such as tissue plasminogen activator (TPA) or urokinase, which are used to lyse coronary artery or peripheral artery thromboses. Primary fibrinolysis is also seen in conjunction with surgical procedures on the prostate gland, which is rich in urokinase. It also occurs in patients with severe liver failure. Very rare disorders of inhibitors of the fibrinolytic pathway (e.g., congenital deficiencies of α_2-antiplasmin) can also cause primary fibrinolysis. Treatment of these disorders is best accomplished by eliminating the precipitating cause.

If primary fibrinolysis becomes severe, ε-amino caproic acid can be used for therapy. This drug must be used cautiously because it blocks the fibrinolytic pathway and may predispose the patient to thrombotic events.

Secondary Fibrinolysis

Secondary fibrinolysis is most often seen in response to DIC. The coagulation pathway is activated, followed by the fibrinolytic pathway. Manifestations of this activation in laboratory tests include hypofibrinogenemia and the presence of fibrin split products. As the DIC is corrected, the secondary fibrinolysis resolves.

Hypercoagulable States in the Surgical Patient

Thromboembolism may occur for a number of reasons during the course of surgery and in the postoperative period. Both congenital and acquired disorders can put surgical patients at risk for thromboembolism.

Etiology

Congenital Disorders

The most common cause of congenital hypercoagulable states is activated protein C resistance (APCR). The most common cause of APCR is factor V Leiden. Activated protein C binds to and neutralizes factors VIII and V, thus acting to regulate the rate at which the intrinsic and common pathways proceed. Genetically abnormal factor V (factor V Leiden) lacks the binding site for activated protein C; thus, it cannot be neutralized. Patients with factor V Leiden abnormality are predisposed to thromboembolic events. Additional causes of congenital hypercoagulable states include deficiencies of antithrombin III and proteins C and S. Protein C is present in the plasma in an inactive form. When thrombin is attached to thrombomodulin on the endothelial cell surface, protein C is activated. Protein S functions as a catalyst to this activation. Activated protein C has two functions: (1) as an anticoagulant (as described earlier) and (2) as an inducer of fibrinolysis. Hyperhomocystinemia is also associated with an increased risk of thrombosis. Some patients with hyperhomocystinemia are found to have gene defects (e.g., MTHFR 677T). Prothrombin 20210 is an additional cause of a congenital hypercoagulable state.

A careful medical history and family history can often suggest the presence of a hypercoagulable state. Of particular note is the need to define the age of onset of thromboembolism. Events that occur in the 40s or younger should raise suspicion of an inherited hypercoagulable state.

Acquired Hypercoagulable States

Acquired hypercoagulable states may result from:

1 Decreased production of naturally occurring anticoagulants (e.g., liver failure).
2 Ineffective fibrinolysis secondary to reduced or defective plasminogen.
3 Very high levels of clotting factors, especially fibrinogen, which may occur in response to the stress of severe illness or trauma.
4 Platelet counts greater than $1000 \times 10^3/\text{mm}^3$ (1000×10^9/L).
5 The antiphospholipid syndromes (e.g., lupus anticoagulant).
6 Some cases of chronic DIC.
7 Hyperhomocystinemia (in patients with renal failure).

Diagnostic Laboratory Studies

The following laboratory studies should be considered when a patient is evaluated for a possible hypercoagulable state: (1) activated protein C resistance test; (2) antithrombin III activity assay; (3) proteins C and S activity assay; (4) assay for antiphospholipid antibody (especially if the patient had an arterial thromboembolism); (5) prothrombin activity as screening for prothrombin 20210; and (6) serum homocystine level.

Management of Hypercoagulable States

Therapy for hypercoagulable states is primarily directed at the following: (1) interfering with the coagulation pathways (with heparin, Coumadin, or both); (2) interfering with platelet function (with aspirin, ticlopidine, or other platelet-inhibiting drugs); and (3) treating hyperhomocystinemia (with folic acid, vitamin B_{12}, and other B vitamins). Therapy must be individualized both to the patient and to the site and severity of the thromboembolism. The duration of therapy requires careful consideration; the risks and benefits of protracted anticoagulation therapy must be weighed.

During the perioperative period, therapy for patients with a history of thromboembolism and a documented hypercoagulable state must be planned carefully by both the surgeon and the hematologist. Low-dose heparin (5000 internation units [IUs], subcutaneously administered) provides adequate protection from thromboembolism for short periods without compromising surgical hemostasis. For patients with a documented hematologic risk factor for thrombosis (e.g., activated protein C resistance) who have never had a thromboembolic event, prophylaxis with pneumatic compression boots or low-dose heparin is adequate.

BLOOD REPLACEMENT THERAPY

Collection and Storage of Blood and Blood Products

Whole blood is collected into plastic reservoir bags that contain an anticoagulant solution that binds to plasma calcium and prevents activation of the coagulation pathways. Whole blood is usually separated into four major components: (1) plasma, (2) platelets, (3) **white blood cells,** and (4) **red blood cells.** Administering only the specific components that are deficient in the patient is the preferred approach to therapy.

Packed red blood cells may be stored at 4°C for as long as 5 weeks. During storage at 4°C, platelets and leukocytes become nonfunctional within hours. A gradual reduction in red cell viability also occurs with prolonged storage. Red blood cells that are stored for 5 weeks have a mean recovery of approximately 70%. Survival of transfused red cells in patients depends upon the clinical setting; optimally, the survival is 5 to 6 weeks. Cellular metabolism during storage leads to progressive increases in plasma potassium and an increase in hydrogen ion concentration. The result is a lowered pH.

Platelet-rich plasma is obtained by gentle centrifugation of whole blood. The resulting suspension is rich in platelets and has a volume of 200 mL. Platelet concentrate is obtained by recentrifugation of platelet-rich plasma. Platelet concentrates contain approximately 6×10^{10} platelets and can be stored for 3 to 5 days in plastic containers at 22°C. They should not be refrigerated.

Platelet-poor plasma may be frozen and stored as fresh frozen plasma, or it may be fractionated into cryoprecipitate and other plasma fractions. A single 200-mL plastic bag of fresh frozen plasma contains all of the coagulation factors and can be stored for as long as 12 months at −30°C. A unit of cryoprecipitate measures 5 to 30 mL in a single plastic bag. It is rich in factor VIII, fibrinogen, and fibronectin, and can be stored for 12 months at −30°C. Stored plasma, which is available from some blood banking centers, contains coagulation factors other than factors V and VIII and can be stored for 5 weeks at 4°C or for 2 years at −30°C.

Blood Component Therapy

The major indication for the administration of fresh whole blood is the replacement of massive blood losses. The use of fresh whole blood for transfusion is limited to selected operations in small children. Otherwise, specific blood components are used. Blood components that carry oxygen include: (1) red cell concentrates, (2) leukocyte-poor blood, (3) frozen and thawed red blood cells, and (4) whole blood (no longer readily available in most centers). Platelet-containing components include: (1) platelet-rich plasma and (2) platelet concentrates.

The major blood groups are A, B, and O, and the major blood types are Rhesus (Rh)-positive and Rh-negative. There are also numerous minor groups that generally do not complicate transfusion. The universal donor red cells are O-negative red blood cells, but the plasma from type O donors is not universal donor plasma. Plasma from patients who are type O-negative contains varying levels of anti-A and anti-B antibodies. This plasma can cause some degree of hemolysis if it is given to individuals who are blood type A, B, or AB. In all but the most life-threatening emergency states, at least type-specific blood, or blood that has been crossmatched, must be given.

If transfusion of blood is expected during surgery or within 48 hours postoperatively, the patient is typed and crossmatched preoperatively. If the probability of transfusion is low, a "type and screen" is usually sufficient. In a type and screen, the patient's ABO group and Rh type are determined, and an antibody screen is carried out. Patients who have a positive antibody screen must have blood crossmatched to minimize the risk of hemolytic transfusion reactions.

Minor transfusion reactions occur frequently, and their management depends on their type and severity. Febrile transfusion reactions are the most common adverse reaction to the transfusion of blood products. They can be controlled with antipyretics and antihistamines. Repeated transfusion of blood products increases the possibility of a transfusion reaction. The removal of white cell debris from red cell, platelet, and plasma fraction transfusions may significantly reduce the risk of febrile transfusion reactions. If a patient has a febrile transfusion reaction, the use of antipyretics before future transfusions may prevent or reduce the severity of febrile transfusion reactions. If a major hemolytic transfusion reaction occurs, the administration of blood is stopped immediately, and the blood is returned to the laboratory for a repeated crossmatch. Hemolytic transfusion reactions require: (1) support of blood pressure, (2) maintenance of renal perfusion, and (3) management of DIC. Aggressive fluid support, diuretics, and renal dialysis may also be needed.

Many hospitals now allow appropriate patients to donate their own blood before elective surgery for possible use during the procedure (the safest blood transfusion practice). A healthy patient can bank two to three units of his or her own blood preoperatively.

Transfusion of Red Blood Cells

The transfusion of red blood cells is indicated when red cell mass is decreased, compromising oxygen transport and delivery to tissues. The decision to transfuse a patient with red blood cells must be individualized to the patient. The important considerations are as follows:

1 The patient's age
2 The presence of hemodynamic instability
3 Underlying medical conditions (e.g., cardiac, pulmonary, or cerebrovascular disease)
4 The etiology, degree, and time course of the patient's anemia.

Acute hemorrhage, with loss of 30% of blood volume, requires volume support and possibly red blood cell transfusion. Patients who have chronic anemia do not require red blood cell transfusions until the anemia causes systemic effects (as a result of the hypoxia that occurs secondary to the reduced oxygen-carrying capacity). Blood group and type must be considered when red cell transfusions are given.

Estimating Red Blood Cell Transfusion Needs

The formulas shown in Table 5-2 are used to calculate the number of units of red cell concentrate needed to raise the hematocrit to 40% (the normal value).

The total blood volume is calculated by multiplying the patient's weight by 7%, or 0.07. For example, in the case of a person who weighs 70 kg:

$$70 \times 0.07 = 4900 \text{ mL } (4.9 \text{ L})$$

One unit of red blood cell concentrate contains approximately 200 mL red blood cells. At transfusion, this concentrate is distributed throughout the total blood volume. Thus, administering one unit of red blood cell concentrate raises the hematocrit by 4%:

$$200 \text{ mL} \div 4900 \text{ mL} = 0.04, \text{ or } 4\%$$

This hypothetical patient had a hematocrit of 15%. Therefore, to raise the hematocrit from 15% to 40% (i.e., 25%), the patient must receive seven units of red blood cell concentrate:

$$25 \div 4 = 6.25, \text{ or 7 full units}$$

Table 5-2 Formula for Calculating Red Blood Cell (RBC) Transfusion Needs

1. Calculate total blood volume (TBV) (mL):	Patients weight (kg) × 7% × 1000 = TBV
2. Determine amount of increase (INC) in patient's hematocrit (Hct) from 1 unit of RBC concentrate:	200 mL/TBV = INC
3. Calculate number of units needed based on patient's current Hct:	40% (normal value) − Hct = Y%; Y%/INC = units needed

Plasma Component Therapy

Fresh frozen plasma can be used to correct all clotting factor deficiencies. Plasma products do not require crossmatch before use, but should be ABO-compatible with the patient.

Coagulation factor concentrates are also a part of plasma component therapy. Cryoprecipitate is used primarily to treat hemophilia A and von Willebrand's disease. There is a small risk of hepatitis and HIV transmission when cryoprecipitate is given. Monoclonal factor VIII concentrates have the advantage of being storable at 4°C. Factor VIII concentrates can be used in the treatment of hemophilia A, but not all are useful in the treatment of von Willebrand's disease. The level of von Willebrand's factor in factor VIII concentrates may not be adequate to support the patient's needs. A pasteurized intermediate-purity factor VIII concentrate (Humate-P) contains some high–molecular-weight von Willebrand's multimers and has been used successfully to treat some patients with von Willebrand's disease. Other intermediate-purity factor VIII concentrates contain only intermediate–and low–molecular-weight multimers. These preparations increase the factor VIII level, but may not correct the bleeding time abnormality. High-purity plasma factor VIII concentrates and recombinant factor VIII concentrates contain little or no von Willebrand's factor.

Estimating Factor VIII Transfusion Requirements

The formulas shown in Table 5-3 are used to calculate factor VIII transfusion requirements. Again, a 70-kg patient is used as an example.

The plasma volume in the body is equal to 4% of the total body weight. Therefore, in a 70-kg person, the plasma volume is 2.8 L:

$$70 \times 0.04 = 2.8 \text{ L, or } 2800 \text{ mL}$$

A clotting unit of a coagulation factor is the amount of that factor (arbitrarily called 100%) in 1 mL normal plasma. To calculate the number of clotting units needed to raise the patient's level to 50% (which controls most bleeding), the baseline level in the patient's blood is subtracted from

Table 5-3 Formula for Calculating Factor VIII Transfusion Needs

1. Calculate total plasma volume (TPV) (mL):	Patient's weight (kg) × 4% × 1000 = TPV
2. Determine number of units needed:	(0.50 − factor VIII level) × TPV = Y
3. Calculate number of bags of cryoprecipitate needed, based on 80 units per bag:	Y/80 = units needed

50%. The result is multiplied by the patient's plasma volume. For example, in a 70-kg patient who has a factor VIII level of 3% (as measured by an APTT-based testing method):

$$(0.50 - 0.03) \times 2800 \text{ mL} = 1316 \text{ units}$$

One bag of cryoprecipitate contains 80 clotting units of factor VIII. Therefore, the patient should receive 17 bags of cryoprecipitate:

$$1316 \div 80 = 16.45, \text{ or } 17 \text{ bags}$$

The amount of von Willebrand's factor in each bag of cryoprecipitate is similar to the amount of factor VIII clotting activity.

Management of Hemophilia

Hemophilia is an inherited bleeding disorder that affects males almost exclusively. It is caused by a reduction in factor VIII clotting activity. Recommended levels of factor VIII for the management of hemophilia type A have been established for minor and major trauma. After minor trauma or during the healing period after surgery, 15% to 20% activity of factor VIII should be maintained. After major trauma, major surgery, or bleeding at a dangerous site (e.g., intracranial bleed), 50% to 60% activity should be maintained. In the management of type A hemophilia, cryoprecipitate or monoclonal factor VIII is transfused every 12 hours to maintain the desired factor VIII level.

Management of von Willebrand's Disease

Von Willebrand's disease is a complex coagulopathy that is characterized by prolonged bleeding time and low levels of factor VIII_c. Factor VIII clotting activity increases slowly, reaching its maximum 6 to 12 hours after infusion. However, all transfused factor VIII is cleared from the patient's circulation within 48 hours after transfusion. The bleeding time is often shortened after transfusion with factor VIII–containing material, but the interval of this shortening is difficult to predict and may be only 2 to 3 hours. Therefore, transfusion support must be individualized for patients with von Willebrand's disease. Transfusion with cryoprecipitate may be required as often as every 2 to 3 hours or as infrequently as every 24 hours. NSAIDs should be avoided during therapy for von Willebrand's disease because they aggravate coagulopathy. To avoid the use of blood products, DDAVP therapy is used in many patients with von Willebrand's disease. If the use of DDAVP is being considered to protect a patient during surgery, a test dose of DDAVP is given 1 to 2 weeks before surgery to ensure that bleeding time and APTT are corrected. On the day of surgery, DDAVP is given 1 hour preoperatively as a 30-minute infusion. (The dose of DDAVP is 0.3 μg/kg.) A repeat dose of DDAVP is given 12 hours later if needed. Repeated doses, however, will not elicit desired responses. An interval of 2 to 3 days between doses usually permits good correction of bleeding time and APTT deficits in patients with von Willebrand's disease.

Other Indications for Plasma Component Use

Factor IX concentrates are used primarily to treat factor IX–deficient hemophilia or factor VIII–deficient hemophilia with severe factor VIII inhibitors. The major side effects of factor IX concentrates are hepatitis and HIV contamination. Some recipients may have DIC because of activated factors in the concentrate.

Albumin is prepared from whole plasma by ethanol fractionation. There is no risk of transmitting hepatitis with albumin transfusion. The primary role of albumin is as an oncotic agent.

Transfusion Safety

To ensure that blood transfusion products are as safe as possible, every effort must be made to avoid (1) immunologic transfusion reactions, (2) transmission of infections, (3) volume overload, and (4) massive transfusions.

Immunologic Transfusion Reactions

Immunologic transfusion reactions include hemolytic transfusion reactions, febrile transfusion reactions, posttransfusion thrombocytopenia, anaphylactic shock, urticaria, and graft-versus-host disease. Symptoms of immediate hemolytic transfusion reactions include fever, constrictive sensation in the chest, and pain in the lumbar region of the back. Signs include fever, hypotension, hemoglobinuria, bleeding as a result of DIC, and renal failure. Acute hemolytic reactions occur when A and B alloantibodies in the patient's plasma bind to antigens on the transfused donor red blood cells.

If a hemolytic transfusion reaction is suspected, the transfusion is stopped immediately, but the intravenous line is left in place. All of the documentation and other clerical information about the transfusion is checked to ensure that the blood that the patient is receiving is correctly crossmatched. Blood samples are taken from the patient to recheck the ABO blood group and Rh type and also to check for free-plasma hemoglobin. The crossmatch and Coombs' test are repeated. The investigator then retypes all donor units of blood for this patient, cultures the transfused blood to exclude bacterial infection, cultures the patient's blood, examines the patient for DIC caused by microaggregates and immune complexes, and initiates close monitoring of renal function.

Treatment of acute hemolytic transfusion reaction initially involves management of hypotension with volume expanders (e.g., lactated Ringer's solution) and vasoactive drugs. Good renal function is maintained with diuretic therapy (e.g., furosemide, mannitol). Bicarbonate is given to alkalinize the urine, and any depleted coagulation factor or platelets are replaced. Heparinization is rarely indicated, and dialysis is used only if acute renal failure develops.

Transmission of Infection

The transmission of infection through blood transfusion therapy is uncommon, but both patients and physicians have significant concerns about this possibility. There is a small possibility of transmitting a number of different types of infections. These include viral infections (e.g., viral hepatitis A, B, and C); HIV; cytomegalovirus; and human T-lymphotropic retrovirus (HTLV-I and HTLV-II). All blood is screened for hepatitis and HIV. Transmission of bacterial infections is rare. Parasitic infections, such as malaria and *Trypanosoma cruzi* (the cause of Chagas' disease), may also be transmitted through transfusion.

Careful screening of blood and blood donors has reduced transmission of infection to very low levels. Despite continuing improvement in the screening and handling of blood products, however, transfusion is not risk-free. The risk of acquiring a transfusion-transmitted disease ranges from one per 103,300 units for hepatitis C to one per 493,000 units for HIV. Thus, transfusion should be performed only after careful evaluation of the patient's clinical situation and specific blood component needs.

Volume Overload

Volume overload associated with blood transfusion usually occurs with plasma or plasma fraction therapy. These products contain proteins that hold or draw fluid into the vascular space and may cause volume overload. Transfusion with packed red blood cells is less often associated with volume overload. Careful planning of therapy and monitoring of the patient's cardiovascular status during transfusion therapy should identify volume overload (e.g., dyspnea, orthopnea, hypoxia) promptly and lead to therapy with diuretics to avoid harm to the patient.

Risks of Massive Transfusion

Massive transfusion is defined as "the transfusion of blood products greater in volume than a patient's normal blood volume in less than 24 hours." Massive transfusions may lead to complications that are not normally seen with lesser volumes or rates of transfusion. These include (1) coagulopathy, which may arise as a result of platelet and coagulation factor depletion; (2) hypothermia, which can cause cardiac dysrhythmias and coagulopathy; it may result from the use of chilled blood products but can be prevented by using blood warmers; (3) citrate toxicity, seen in patients with hepatic dysfunction; and (4) electrolyte abnormalities, including acidosis and hyperkalemia. Surgeons must be aware of the possibility of these complications and should consider hematology consultation whenever massive transfusions are required.

Blood Substitutes

Attempts to create blood substitutes date to the 17th century, with little success and an unacceptable rate of attendant mortality and morbidity. More recently, the HIV epidemic and predictions for increasing worldwide blood shortages have spurred renewed interest in the development of safe, abundant blood products and elements that can perform specific clinical functions. Examples of these products include oxygen carriers and plasma derivatives. Oxygen carriers, such as perfluorocarbons and hemoglobin-based oxygen carriers, could carry out the oxygen-transporting activity of red blood cells and provide volume expansion. Plasma derivatives, such as immune globulins, protease inhibitors, and coagulation products, have many clinical uses.

Clinical trials involving whole blood substitutes are ongoing. However, at the present time, no single blood substitute can duplicate the complex cellular composition of blood or its multiple long-term functions.

CONCLUSION

Surgeons should be able to perform preoperative screening evaluations for bleeding and clotting disorders, and they must be prepared to handle surgical hemostatic emergencies. However, a patient whose history or screening examination indicates a possible bleeding problem should also be evaluated preoperatively by a qualified hematologist. If a hemostatic disorder is found, the surgeon and hematologist should work in cooperation to manage the problem, thereby optimizing the patient's safety and well-being in the perioperative period.

SUGGESTED READINGS

Bauer KA, Rosendaal FR, Heit JA. Hypercoagulability: too many tests, too much conflicting data. *Hematology (Am Soc Hematol Educ Program)* 2002;353–368.

Beutler E, Coller BS, Lichtman MA, et al., eds. *Williams Hematology*. 6th Ed. New York, NY: McGraw-Hill, Medical Publishing Division, 2001.

George JN, Sadler JE, Lämmle B. Platelets: thrombotic thrombocytopenia purpura. *Hematology (Am Soc Hematol Educ Program)* 2002; 315–334.

Hambleton J, Leung LL, Levi M. Coagulation: consultative hemostasis. *Hematology (Am Soc Hematol Educ Program)* 2002;335–352.

Lumadue JA, Ness PM. Current approaches to red blood cell transfusion. *Semin Hematol* 1996;33(4):277–289.

Rosenberg RD. Biochemistry and pharmacology of low molecular weight heparin. *Semin Hematol* 1997;34(4):2–8.

Rosendaal FR. Risk factors for venous thrombosis: prevalence, risk, and interaction. *Semin Hematol* 1997;34(3):171–187.

Schuster HP. Epilogue: disseminated intravascular coagulation and antithrombin III in intensive care medicine: pathophysiological insights and therapeutic hopes. *Semin Thromb Hemost* 1998;24(1):81–83.

The Thrombosis Interest Group of Canada. Practical treatment guidelines. Guidelines for antithrombotic therapy. Available at: http://www.tigc.org/eguidelines/guidelines.htm

6

KENNETH W. BURCHARD, MD

Shock

OBJECTIVES

1 Define shock, and list the two primary mechanisms that may cause cellular malfunction consistent with shock.
2 List the etiologies of these primary mechanisms that are responsible for shock.
3 List the clinical information (i.e., history, physical examination, diagnostic tests, hemodynamic parameters) that helps to determine which of the two primary mechanisms is the predominant cause of shock in an individual patient.
4 Describe the interrelation between the two primary mechanisms of shock as a cause of cellular injury.
5 Describe the general principles of management that diminish cellular injury from the primary mechanisms of shock.

Traditional descriptions of **shock** often use systolic hypotension (< 90 mm Hg) as the defining variable. According to this criterion, classification schemes that use categories such as hypovolemic, septic, cardiogenic, and neurogenic shock are common and imply that evidence of an altered circulation is sufficient to make the diagnosis. However, certain etiologies of hypotension (i.e., neurogenic vasodilation after spinal cord injury) do not necessarily cause significant cellular or organ injury. In addition, cellular and organ injury may develop without hypotension reaching 90 mm Hg. Therefore, definitions of shock based on the circulatory measurement of systolic blood pressure are potentially misleading and narrow in scope.

A broader definition is that shock is a condition in which total body cellular metabolism malfunctions. This concept dates back to at least 1872 when S.D. Gross described shock as "a rude unhinging of the machinery of life." When treated aggressively, this cellular metabolic dysfunction, this "rude unhinging," is reversible. When allowed to continue, however, shock results in cellular death, organ damage, and eventual death.

During the 20th century, many theories were developed to explain this cellular injury and death (i.e., disorders of the circulation, disorders of the nervous system, toxemia). By 1950, two competing theories were predominant: (1) shock is secondary to inadequate oxygen delivery and (2) shock is secondary to a toxic cellular insult that can progress even when sufficient oxygen is delivered. Such conditions as severe hemorrhage and cardiac malfunction (i.e., **hypoperfusion**) were recognized throughout the century as etiologies of inadequate oxygen delivery. The recognition that the primary toxins of cellular injury are endogenous (the products of tissue injury or the consequent inflammatory response) rather than exogenous (endotoxin) emerged primarily over the last 3 decades. Tissue injury and the associated inflammatory response result in the production or activation of cellular molecules (i.e., cytokines, superoxide radicals, prostaglandins, adhesion molecules) that promote local cellular activation, tissue repair, and host defenses. However, sometimes this local response incites similar responses in cells that are distant from the primary insult. The result is systemic **inflammation** that can cause organ malfunction and shock.

Simultaneously, during the last 2 decades, experimental and clinical studies showed that these two mechanisms of cellular injury are not competitive or exclusive, but are most often additive during shock states. Simply stated, *hypoperfusion begets inflammation, and inflammation begets hypoperfusion.* The clinician must be alert to this association and must approach each patient who has the manifestations of total body cellular malfunction with the dual goals of carefully assessing the circulation for oxygen delivery and carefully assessing the state of inflammation for cell toxicity. Restoring excellent circulation and treating severe inflammation are the primary tenets for managing the patient with shock.

This chapter describes the pathophysiology that links hypoperfusion with inflammation and provides clinical guidelines for recognizing **hypoperfusion** and **severe inflammation** and managing these two mechanisms of cellular injury.

NORMAL PHYSIOLOGY OF THE CIRCULATION AND OF INFLAMMATION

The main function of the circulation is to deliver oxygen to the capillaries. The determinants of total body oxygen delivery are listed with other commonly measured or calculated hemodynamic variables in Table 6-1. As the formula for oxygen delivery shows, the pulmonary component is limited to providing adequate arterial oxygen saturation ($\geq$ 90% saturation is usually present when PaO_2 $\geq$ 60 mm Hg). This goal is usually readily achieved with modern respiratory therapy. Hemoglobin is frequently increased with transfusion. Usually, the most difficult component to treat is **cardiac output.** The determinants of cardiac output are organized by both the variables that affect **ventricular function** and the variables that affect **venous return.** Depending on clinical circumstances, sometimes it is more useful to use the logic associated with alterations in ventricular physiology to enhance the circulation, and sometimes it is more useful to use the logic associated with alterations in venous return physiology. This logical application of one circulatory physiology versus another ("physio-logic") is described in more detail in the hypoperfusion section.

Ventricular Physiology

The major determinants of ventricular performance are listed in Table 6-2. **Preload** is the magnitude of myocardial stretch, the stimulus to muscle contraction that is described by the Frank-Starling mechanism (Fig. 6-1), whereby increased stretch leads to increased contraction until the muscle is overstretched (commonly recognized

Table 6-1 Hemodynamic and Oxygen Delivery Variables

Item	Definition	Normal
CVP	Central venous pressure; CVP = RAP; in the absence of tricuspid valve disease, CVP = RVEDP	5–15 mm Hg
LAP	Left atrial pressure; in the absence of mitral valve disease, LAP = LVEDP	5–15 mm Hg
PCWP	Pulmonary capillary wedge pressure; PCWP = LAP, except sometimes with high PEEP levels	5–15 mm Hg
MAP	Mean arterial pressure, mm Hg; MAP = DP + 1/3 (SP − DP)	80–90 mm Hg
CI	Cardiac index; CI = CO/m^2 BSA	2.5–3.5 L/min/m^2 BSA
SI	Stroke index; SI = SV/m^2 BSA	35–40 mL/beat/m^2
SVR	Systemic vascular resistance; SVR = (MAP − CVP) × 80/CO	1000–1500 dyne-sec/cm^5
PVR	Pulmonary vascular resistance; PVR = (MAP − PAOP) × 80/CO	100–400 dyne-sec/cm^5
Cao_2	Arterial oxygen content (vol %); Cao_2 = 1.39 × Hgb Sao_2 + (Pao_2 × 0.0031)	20 vol %
$C\bar{v}o_2$	Mixed venous oxygen content (vol %); $C\bar{v}o_2$ = 1.39 × Hgb × $S\bar{v}o_2$ + ($P\bar{v}o_2$ × 0.0031)	15 vol %
$C(a - v)o_2$	Arterial venous O_2 content difference; $C(a - v)o_2$ = Cao_2 − $C\bar{v}o_2$ (vol %)	3.5–4.5 vol %
O_2D	O_2 delivery; O_2D = CO × Cao_2 × 10; 10 = factor to convert mL O_2/100 mL blood to mL O_2/L blood	900–1200 mL/min
O_2C	O_2 consumption; O_2C = (Cao_2 − $C\bar{v}o_2$) × CO × 10	250 mL/min 130–160 mL/min/m^2

BSA, body surface area (m^2); CO, cardiac output; DP, diastolic pressure; LVEDP, left ventricular end-diastolic pressure; Pao_2, partial pressure of oxygen, arterial; PAOP, pulmonary artery occlusion pressure; PEEP, positive end-expiratory pressure; $P\bar{v}o_2$, partial pressure of oxygen, mixed venous; RAP, right atrial pressure; RVEDP, right ventricular end-diastolic pressure; Sao_2, arterial oxygen saturation; $S\bar{v}o_2$, mixed venous oxygen saturation; SP, systolic pressure; SV, stroke volume.

Table 6-2	Determinants of Ventricular Function
Preload	
Afterload	
Contractility	
Heart rate	

clinically as congestive heart failure; see the hypoperfusion section). Preload is most appropriately measured as end-diastolic volume. Because volume is not easily measured clinically, the direct proportion between ventricular volume and ventricular end-diastolic pressure allows the measurement of pressure to estimate volume. This pressure is measured as central venous pressure (CVP) for the right side of the heart and pulmonary capillary wedge or pulmonary artery occlusion pressure (PAOP) for the left side of the heart.

Ventricular **afterload** is determined primarily by the resistance to ventricular ejection that is present in either the pulmonary (pulmonary vascular resistance) or systemic arterial tree (systemic vascular resistance). With constant preload, increased afterload diminishes ventricular ejection, and decreased afterload augments ejection (see Fig. 6-1).

Contractility is the force of contraction under conditions of a predetermined preload or afterload. Factors that increase and decrease contractility are listed in Table 6-3. A change in contractility, like a change in afterload, results in a different cardiac function curve (see Fig. 6-1).

The combined influence of increasing contractility and decreasing afterload to improve ventricular function is also shown in Fig. 6-1.

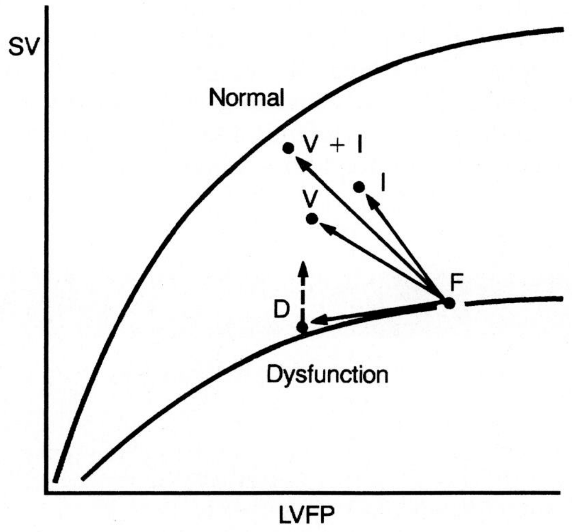

Figure 6-1 Expected hemodynamic response in severe left ventricular dysfunction to administration of diuretics (D), inotropic drugs (I), vasodilators (V), and a combination of vasodilators and inotropics (V + I). F, failure; LVFP, left ventricular filling pressure; SV, stroke volume.

Table 6-3 Factors That Affect Myocardial Contractility

Increased	Decreased
Catecholamines	Catecholamine depletion and receptor malfunction
Inotropic drugs	Alpha and beta blockers Calcium channel blockers
Increased preload	Decreased preload
Decreased afterload	Overstretching of myocardium Severe inflammation and ischemia

Heart rate is directly proportional to cardiac output (not to cardiac muscle mechanics) until rapid rates diminish ventricular filling during diastole.

Venous Return

Venous return is described by the following formula:

$$VR = (MSP - CVP)/(RV + RA/19),$$

where MSP = mean systemic pressure, CVP = central venous pressure (right atrial pressure), RV = venous resistance, and RA = arterial resistance.

This equation (including the constant, 19) was formulated by Guyton in 1973 using both calculations and empirical observation. As might be expected, alterations in arterial resistance have much less effect on venous return than alterations in venous resistance, as indicated in the formula.

Mean systemic pressure (MSP) is not the same as mean arterial pressure. MSP is the pressure in small veins and venules. This pressure must be higher than CVP in the periphery so that blood can flow from the periphery to the thorax. Venous resistance occurs primarily in the large veins in the abdomen and thorax. Arterial resistance occurs mostly in the arterioles.

Factors that alter venous return variables are listed in Table 6-4. Surgical patients frequently have diseases or therapeutic interventions that may inhibit venous return.

Physiology of Inflammation

The normal response to tissue injury is essential for eliminating infectious organisms, wound healing, and restoring normal tissue function. The initial response to tissue damage by trauma is bleeding and coagulation. This response is less likely, but not impossible, with tissue damage from ischemia or infection. Platelet activation results in the release of important chemoattractants (i.e., platelet-derived growth factor [PDGF], transforming growth factor-β [TGF-β]).

Table 6-4 Factors That Alter Venous Return Variables

Increased venous return
Increased MSP
Increased vascular volume
Increased vascular tone
External compression
Trendelenburg position (increased MSP in lower extremities and abdomen)
Decreased CVP
Hypovolemia
Negative pressure respiration
Decreased venous resistance
Decreased venous constriction
Negative pressure respiration
Diminished venous return
Decreased MSP
Hypovolemia
Vasodilation
Increased CVP
Intracardiac
Congestive heart failure
Cardiogenic shock
Tricuspid regurgitation
Right heart failure
Extracardiac
Positive pressure respiration
PEEP
Tension pneumothorax
Cardiac tamponade
Increased abdominal pressure
Increased venous resistance
Increased thoracic pressure
Positive pressure respiration
PEEP
Increased abdominal pressure
Tension pneumothorax
Increased abdominal pressure
Ascites
Bowel distension
Massive edema in the abdominal cavity
Intraabdominal hemorrhage
Retroperitoneal hemorrhage
Tension pneumoperitoneum

CVP, central venous pressure; MSP, mean systemic pressure; PEEP, positive end-expiratory pressure.

Damaged blood vessels initially vasoconstrict, but this constriction is soon followed by vasodilation and increased capillary permeability secondary to the action of agents such as prostaglandin E_2, prostacyclin, histamine, serotonin, and kinins. When blood flow is present, this vascular response results in the accumulation of protein-rich edema fluid (exudate).

Attracted by chemoattractants (e.g., PDGF), polymorphonuclear cells (PMNs) are the first white cells to migrate to the inflammatory site (within minutes if the circulation is good). White cells adhere to damaged, leaky vessels as a result of an increase in adhesion molecules, first P-selectin, then E-selectin, as well as intracellular adhesion molecules (ICAM-1). The adhesion molecules enhance the migration of PMNs into the interstitium. PMNs move to the site of tissue injury down a concentration gradient of another type of molecule called a chemokine.

PMNs then phagocytize dead tissue and foreign objects, sometimes assisted by opsonins and preformed antibodies in the removal of bacteria. PMNs produce proteases and intracellular oxygen radicals that are critical for beneficial PMN activity. Besides proteases and oxygen radicals, PMNs can also release interleukin-1 (IL-1). IL-1 mediates temperature elevation through the thermoregulatory center and also stimulates other inflammatory activity (e.g., migration of macrophages). Another cytokine, interleukin-8 (IL-8), is a potent PMN attractant that is produced by many cell types after exposure to IL-1 and the cytokine tumor necrosis factor (TNF). The PMNs last only for a period of hours.

Within hours, tissue macrophages and circulating monocytes are attracted by such substances as PDGF, TGF-β, and IL-1; they migrate into the injured area, and last for days to weeks. The continuing inflammatory process is largely regulated by macrophages through such mediators as IL-1, TNF, PDGF, TGF-β, TGF-α, and fibroblast growth factor.

For instance, fibroblast migration and angiogenesis begin next. Fibroblasts are influenced by IL-1, TNF, PDGF, TGF-β, TGF-α, insulin-like growth factor, and epidermal growth factor (EGF). Angiogenesis is influenced by TNF, TGF-β, TGF-α, and EGF. The combined process of fibroblast proliferation and capillary budding produces granulation tissue that is friable and bleeds easily.

Fibroblasts produce collagen. This process usually accelerates 5 days after tissue damage occurs. Collagen synthesis is influenced by IL-1, TNF, PDGF, TGF-β, and EGF.

A summary of cellular activity in inflammation is shown in Tables 6-5 and 6-6. As emphasized below, much of the local effect of inflammation (increased vascular permeability, nearby cellular activation, and injury) can result in the production of cytokines and other molecules that gain access to the circulation. These molecules that are

Table 6-5 Normal Inflammation

Event	Cells Responsible
Coagulation	Platelets
Early inflammation	Polymorphonuclear leukocytes (first few hours)
Later inflammation	Monocytes (days) macrophages
Collagen and mucopolysaccharide	Fibroblasts (maximum deposition 7–10 days)
Capillary budding	Endothelial cells (maximum 7–10 days)

Table 6-6 Functions of Inflammatory Cells

Cells	Function
Platelets	Coagulation, release PDGF, IL-1
Polymorphonuclear leukocytes	Phagocytosis, especially microbes, release IL-1, IL-8
Macrophage	Phagocytosis; stimulate fibroblast migration and growth; stimulate endothelial cell migration and growth; release FGF, PDGF, IL-1, TNF, TFG-β, TGF-α
Fibroblast	Collagen deposition
Endothelial cells	Release of adhesion molecules Capillary budding

FGF, fibroblast growth factor; IL, interleukin; PDGF, platelet-derived growth factor; TGF, transforming growth factor; TNF, tumor necrosis factor.

Table 6-7 Neurohumoral Response to Hypoperfusion

Increased	Decreased
Epinephrine	Insulin
Norepinephrine	Thyroxine
Dopamine	Triiodothyronine
Glucagon	Luteinizing hormone
Renin	Testosterone
Angiotensin	Estrogen
Arginine vasopressin	Follicle-stimulating hormone
Adrenocorticotropic hormone	
Cortisol	
Aldosterone	
Growth hormone	

necessary for effective **local** inflammatory activity can cause distant or **systemic** tissue injury by the endocrine effect of these proinflammatory substances. This is particularly important as it relates to PMN and endothelial cell activation.

Effective inflammation controls infection, heals wounds, and then abates. Therefore, in addition to the proinflammatory physiology described above, there are antiinflammatory responses that develop simultaneously to limit the action of inflammatory cells. Such cytokines as IL-6 (another pyrogen), IL-10, IL-13, and the adrenal secretion of cortisol are some of the agents that serve this function.

A perfect inflammatory response, then, represents a precise balance between the proinflammatory and antiinflammatory physiology that results in the resolution of infection and/or the healing of wounds without any deficit in either of these positive outcomes and no distant organ malfunction or failure.

HYPOPERFUSION STATES

Hypoperfusion is a decrease in total body or regional blood flow that is sufficient to result in cellular malfunction or death. Hypoperfusion is the primary mechanism that is responsible for inadequate oxygen delivery; the immediate effects of hypoperfusion on cell viability are secondary to the interruption of oxidative metabolism.

The Neurohumoral Response to Hypoperfusion

Total body hypoperfusion usually manifests as a reduction in cardiac output. The most frequently studied models of total body hypoperfusion cause a reduction in cardiac output from loss of volume (hypovolemic hypoperfusion, i.e., hemorrhage) or loss of cardiac function (cardiogenic hypoperfusion). Either of these etiologies may result in the neurohumoral response shown in Table 6-7.

The clinically apparent effects of this neurohumoral response are tachycardia (epinephrine, norepinephrine, dopamine), vasoconstriction (norepinephrine, arginine vasopressin, angiotensin), diaphoresis (norepinephrine), oliguria with sodium and water conservation (adrenocorticotropic hormone [ACTH], cortisol, aldosterone, arginine vasopressin), and hyperglycemia (epinephrine, glucagon, cortisol, insufficient insulin). This activation of the neuroendocrine system attempts to preserve blood flow to vital organs (heart, lungs, brain) while diminishing flow to less vital organs (kidneys, gastrointestinal tract). In this way, it maintains or increases intravascular volume by limiting urine output. This response is more homeostatic under conditions of hypovolemic hypoperfusion compared with cardiogenic hypoperfusion. In the latter, tachycardia, vasoconstriction, and sodium and water retention may aggravate rather than diminish hypoperfusion by decreasing ventricular filling time, increasing afterload, and increasing myocardial stretch, respectively.

The Effects of Hypoperfusion on Inflammation

The most clearly documented association of hypoperfusion with inflammation is the effect of ischemia followed by reperfusion (**reperfusion injury**). Clinically, this effect is most obvious in patients with isolated limb ischemia (compartment syndrome) and in some patients with localized intestinal ischemia. However, severe systemic hypoperfusion may cause a similar response in many tissues, particularly the gastrointestinal tract.

The mechanism that is responsible for ischemia reperfusion injury appears to require both local and systemic factors. A complex interaction of oxygen free radicals, thromboxane, leukotrienes, phospholipase A_2, and leukocytes participates in both regional and total body alterations in capillary permeability and organ function. Anatomic and physiologic damage to the intestine, limb, kidney, liver, and lung may occur after reperfusion, even when a specific organ (i.e., lung) was not initially hypoperfused. Because PMNs are potent producers of oxygen free radicals, these cells are central to this pathophysiology.

In the last decade more evidence has demonstrated that hypoperfusion itself can stimulate inflammatory cell (PMN) and mediator (complement) activity, even before reperfusion.

In clinical hypoperfusion, particularly with trauma, it is difficult to separate tissue injury that is secondary only to hypoperfusion from damage from other mechanisms (e.g., a direct blow). Whatever the cause, hypoperfusion and inflammation commonly occur together.

The Effects of Hypoperfusion on Cellular Metabolism

The classic effect of hypoperfusion on cellular metabolism is anaerobic metabolism caused by an oxygen deficit. The reduction in adenosine triphosphate (ATP) production that occurs secondary to the loss of mitochondrial function can result in inadequate energy to meet cellular needs, with cell death as a consequence. Elevated levels of lactic acid, with low pyruvate levels, characterize anaerobic glycolysis as the primary means of ATP production in anaerobic states.

Besides an elevation in lactic acid, cell membrane function may be impaired by decreased intracellular ATP production and from a circulating protein that can depolarize cell membranes. As a result of such cell membrane alterations, sodium and calcium can move into cells, with water following the sodium. Sequestration of water in cells can cause a deficit in extracellular fluid, which may accentuate the fluid requirements during resuscitation.

ETIOLOGIES, DIAGNOSIS, AND MANAGEMENT OF HYPOPERFUSION STATES

The primary etiologies of hypoperfusion states in surgical patients are decreased venous return and decreased myocardial function (Table 6-8).

Table 6-8	Etiologies of Hypoperfusion
Decreased venous return	
Hypovolemia	
Pericardial tamponade	
Tension pneumothorax	
Increased abdominal pressure	
Bowel obstruction	
Tension pneumoperitoneum	
Massive bleeding	
Diagnostic laparoscopy	
Pneumatic antishock garment	
Ascites	
Positive end-expiratory pressure	
Decreased myocardial function	
Congestive heart failure	
Cardiogenic shock	

Decreased Venous Return: Hypovolemia

Hypovolemia (especially from hemorrhage) is the most common etiology of decreased venous return secondary to decreased MSP. Common etiologies of hypovolemia are listed in Table 6-9. Hypovolemia is the most common cause of hypotension.

Severe hypoperfusion secondary to hypovolemia (i.e., hypovolemic shock) has been studied most frequently in experimental and clinical hemorrhage. Hemorrhagic shock not only diminishes venous return, but also may cause cardiovascular alterations (Table 6-10). Cellular effects (other than lactic acidosis from anaerobic glycolysis) are listed in Table 6-11. As mentioned earlier, ischemia-induced activation of local and systemic inflammation has also been described.

The metabolic and toxic phenomena associated with hypovolemic shock, even without severe inflammation, result in loss of plasma and interstitial volume beyond what is accounted for by the primary disease process (i.e., hemorrhage, vomiting). Migration of interstitial fluid into cells and increased capillary permeability are implicated as mechanisms.

Physical Examination in Hypovolemic Hypoperfusion

In the patient who has hypovolemia, vital signs and physical findings show evidence of hypoperfusion roughly in proportion to the degree of hypovolemia. A 10% loss of blood volume (560 mL, approximately the amount donated for transfusion) produces little, if any, disturbance. A 20% loss may cause tachycardia and orthostatic hypotension. A 30% loss may produce hypotension while the patient is supine. However, a patient may be normotensive when supine, even with greater loss of blood volume (Table 6-12).

Agitation, tachypnea, and peripheral vasoconstriction

Table 6-9	Common Etiologies of Hypovolemia
Hemorrhage	
Severe inflammation or infection	
Trauma	
Pancreatitis or other causes of peritonitis	
Burns	
Vomiting or other intestinal losses	
Excess diuresis	
Inadequate oral intake	

Table 6-10	Cardiovascular Effects of Hemorrhagic Shock
Decreased venous return	
Increased systemic vascular resistance	
Decreased ventricular contractility	
Decreased ventricular compliance	
Increased atrial contractility	
Transcapillary refill of water to restore plasma volume	
Intravascular protein replenishment from preformed extravascular protein	

are common with any etiology of hypoperfusion. Hypotension, however, most commonly develops secondary to hypovolemia. Hypotension as a result of disruption of intrinsic cardiac function (cardiogenic shock) is much less common (discussed later). Congestive heart failure, a distinct clinical entity from cardiogenic shock, frequently causes increased blood pressure.

The neck veins are not distended unless hypovolemia is accompanied by an extracardiac increase in central venous pressure (tension pneumothorax, pericardial tamponade, severe effort during expiration, increased abdominal pressure). An S_3 gallop is not usually present. An etiology of hypovolemia may also be apparent (open wound with hemorrhage, distended abdomen, femur and pelvic fractures).

Common Laboratory Aids

Hypovolemic hypoperfusion that is severe enough to cause hypotension is associated with metabolic acidosis that is recognized either from serum electrolytes or, more precisely, arterial blood gases. Elevated serum blood urea nitrogen (BUN) and creatinine levels that are indicative of renal malfunction are common. CVP and PAOP are low, as are cardiac index and oxygen delivery.

Other tests (e.g., hemoglobin level, other serum chemistries, radiographic studies) are usually used to determine the etiology of hypovolemic hypoperfusion rather than to document the severity of the perfusion deficits.

Treatment of Hypovolemia

In the patient who has severe hypovolemic hypoperfusion, the circulation must be restored simultaneously with diagnostic and therapeutic interventions to correct the underlying cause of the hypovolemic state. The circulatory, metabolic, and toxic effects of hypovolemic hypoperfusion are best treated by rapid (within minutes) restoration of intravascular volume, thereby increasing MSP, venous return, and oxygen delivery. In general, two types of fluid, **crystalloid** and **colloid**, are used for volume replacement (Table 6-13).

Table 6-11	Cellular Effects of Hemorrhagic Shock
Diminished transmembrane potential difference	
Increased intracellular sodium	
Decreased intracellular adenosine triphosphate	

Red blood cells are effective when needed. After hemorrhage is arrested (the premier method of treating hemorrhagic shock), the administration of red cells causes increased cardiac output, increased oxygen-carrying capacity, and little, if any, leakage of red cells into the interstitium, even in the face of increased capillary permeability. The primary disadvantage of red cell transfusion is the increasing evidence that these exogenous cells increase the risk of subsequent nosocomial infection. There is less risk of infection with a transmissible disease (e.g., hepatitis C, HIV). Incompatible red cell hemolytic transfusion reactions are very rare. Febrile episodes that do not represent true transfusion incompatibility are more common, and are most often secondary to antibodies to the small numbers of white cells that remain in the packed red cell unit.

Potential advantages and disadvantages of various resuscitation fluids other than red cells are shown in Tables 6-14 and 6-15.

Fresh frozen plasma (FFP) should not be used primarily as a colloid. Only when hypovolemia is accompanied by bleeding and a deficiency in intrinsic or extrinsic coagulation (partial thromboplastin time $> 1.5 \times$ control, prothrombin time $< 50\%$) should FFP be used. In general, red blood cells are used to replace lost red cells and are administered until the serum hemoglobin approaches 8 g/100 mL. Little advantage is documented for increasing the hemoglobin to greater than 10 g/100 mL, except possibly for patients with significant underlying cardiovascular disease. Although hemoglobin concentrations of as low as 7 g/100 mL are now considered acceptable for some acute illnesses, cautious assessment of oxygen delivery and consumption variables is recommended if a plan to avoid red cell transfusion for such concentrations is considered advantageous (see section on endpoints of resuscitation of the circulation).

Much more controversial than the appropriate use of FFP and red blood cells are the advantages and disadvantages of the various crystalloid and colloid solutions previously listed. Most investigators agree that colloid administration results in less sodium and water administration compared with crystalloid solutions. In addition, plasma oncotic pressure is higher after the administration of colloids. Still debated is whether increased total body sodium and water gain are detrimental to organ function after resuscitation of the circulation. Curiously, recent evidence has suggested that lactated Ringer's solution may actually augment the inflammatory response, especially when ischemia/reperfusion is the mechanism.

When a patient who has hypovolemia is receiving large volumes of crystalloid or colloid and is not responding well to therapy (most often seen in severe systemic inflammation, e.g., septic shock), dopamine administration is a logi-

Table 6-12 Hemodynamic Effects of Intravascular Volume Loss in Supine Subjects

Amount	Rate	Blood Pressure	Pulse	Mentation	Skin Vasoconstriction	Urine Output
≤ 10%	5 min	NL	NL	NL	NL	NL
≤ 10%	1 hr	NL	NL	NL	NL	NL
20%	5 min	↓	↑	NL	↑	↓
20%	1 hr	NL	↑	NL	NL	↓
30%	5 min	↓↓	↑↑	↓	↑↑	↓↓
30%	1 hr	↓	↑	↓	↑	↓
50%	5 min	↓↓↓	↑↑	↓↓	↑↑↑	↓↓↓
50%	1 hr	↓↓	↑↑	↓↓	↑↑	↓↓

NL, normal.

cal adjunct. Dopamine increases left ventricular filling pressures as it increases cardiac output, probably as a result of constriction of the veins and decreased venous capacitance. This increase may occur at the expense of increasing myocardial oxygen demands. After adequate vascular volume is attained, the dopamine can usually be discontinued. Therefore, dopamine can serve as a pharmacologic surrogate for fluid administration. Since left ventricular end diastolic pressure increases with dopamine administration, left atrial pressure will increase, and the clinician should not presume that dopamine will lessen any deleterious effect that elevated left atrial pressure might exert on the lungs.

Decreased Venous Return: Pericardial Tamponade

The primary mechanism for decreased venous return during pericardial tamponade is an extracavitary increase in CVP. The etiologies of tamponade are most commonly chest trauma (penetrating and blunt) and bleeding after cardiac surgery. Physical examination usually shows evidence of hypoperfusion, along with distended neck veins, muffled heart sounds, and an increased paradoxical pulse (> 15 mm Hg). The electrocardiogram may show low voltage, the CVP is often elevated, and a chest radiograph may show an enlarging heart. With severe hypovolemia, the CVP may be normal despite tamponade and may become elevated only after fluid resuscitation. An echocardiogram shows fluid surrounding the heart, with diminished ventricular volumes.

It is important to distinguish this etiology of hypoperfusion from congestive heart failure (CHF) or cardiogenic shock because reducing fluid intake and administering a diuretic would reduce venous return further in tamponade. As stated, CHF usually results in normal or elevated blood pressure. Severe tamponade results in hypotension. Therefore, tamponade simulates cardiogenic shock more closely than CHF. Because cardiogenic shock requires a major insult to myocardial function (see later), hypotension with elevated CVP should increase suspicion of tamponade or a tension pneumothorax unless obvious evidence of severe myocardial malfunction is found.

The incidence of cardiac tamponade in surgical patients is low, and it is most often seen in patients with chest trauma or in those undergoing cardiac surgery. Removal of the fluid surrounding the heart (pericardiocentesis/peri-

Table 6-13 Fluids for Hypovolemia Resuscitation

- Crystalloid
  - Isotonic
  - Ringer's lactate
  - 0.9% saline
  - Hypertonic saline
- Colloid
  - Red blood cells
  - Fresh frozen plasma
  - Albumin
  - Processed human protein
  - Low–molecular-weight dextran
  - Hydroxyethyl starch

Table 6-14 Crystalloid Solutions

- Isotonic solution advantages
  - Inexpensive
  - Readily available
  - Replenishes epidermal growth factor
  - Freely mobile across capillaries
  - No increase in lung water
- Isotonic solution disadvantages
  - Rapid equilibration with interstitial fluid
  - Lowers serum oncotic pressure
  - No oxygen-carrying capacity
  - Increase in systemically perfused interstitial fluid
  - ? if some formulations (i.e., Ringer's lactate) augment the inflammatory response

Table 6-15	Colloid Solutions (Other Than Red Cells)

Advantages
- Less water administered (more resuscitation per milliliter)
- Less sodium administered
- Less decrease in oncotic pressure
- Acid buffer (fresh frozen plasma)

Disadvantages
- Expensive (albumin, fresh frozen plasma)
- Transmissible disease (fresh frozen plasma)
- Increased interstitial oncotic pressure
- Depressed myocardial function (albumin: 50% reduction in left ventricular stroke work index at a pulmonary capillary occlusion pressure of 15 mm Hg)
- Depressed immunologic function (albumin: decreased immunoglobulins, decreased response to tetanus toxoid)
- Delayed resolution of interstitial edema
- Coagulopathy: infrequent in low doses (low–molecular weight dextran: platelet malfunction; hydroxyethyl starch: decreased factor VIII:c concentrations; albumin: decreased fibrinogen, decreased prothrombin, decreased factor VIII)

cardial window/repair of a cardiac wound) is the most effective therapy, and it can result in a dramatic improvement in cardiac output. However, venous return also improves as a result of increasing MSP with intravenous fluid. Therefore, vigorous fluid administration should be provided despite an elevated CVP.

Decreased Venous Return: Tension Pneumothorax

Tension pneumothorax reduces venous return by producing an extracavitary increase in CVP and by increasing venous resistance in the chest. Tension pneumothorax may occur spontaneously from rupture of a bleb or, more commonly, after penetrating or blunt trauma. Physical examination shows evidence of decreased perfusion, along with decreased breath sounds and tympany over the affected thorax, tracheal deviation away from the affected thorax, and distended neck veins. A chest radiograph may be the first clue to a tension pneumothorax, but most often, the diagnosis is made at the bedside without radiologic assistance.

Treatment consists of emergently releasing the tension (e.g., placing a 14-gauge needle into the chest, placing a finger in a large penetrating injury), followed by closed thoracostomy. Administration of intravenous fluid to increase MSP is also beneficial, and neck vein distension may not be evident with severe hypovolemia.

Decreased Venous Return: Increased Abdominal Pressure

Increased abdominal pressure ($\geq$ 25 mm Hg) diminishes venous return by increasing intrathoracic pressure, producing an extracavitary increase in CVP, and increasing venous resistance in abdominal veins. Increased abdominal pressure may be particularly detrimental to renal blood flow, but it can cause marked total body hypoperfusion despite a well-maintained mean arterial blood pressure from increased systemic vascular resistance.

Abdominal pressure is increased by a variety of mechanisms (see Table 6-4). It is most easily measured with a bladder catheter. Through the fluid sampling port on a Foley catheter, 50 to 100 mL of fluid is inserted into the bladder. The catheter is then clamped distal to the sampling port. Pressure is measured by connecting the needle in the sampling port to standard hemodynamic monitoring tubing, using the pubis as the zero pressure level.

Physical examination often shows evidence of hypoperfusion along with a tensely distended abdomen and possibly distended neck veins. The most effective treatment is to relieve the pressure. However, aggressive fluid management to increase MSP may be the only option in some cases where, for instance, exploration of the abdomen is considered prohibitively risky. When hemodynamics and respiratory function are severely impaired by increased abdominal pressure, then opening the abdomen and closing it with a prosthesis or leaving it packed open may be the best alternative.

While intraabdominal pressure in the 25 mm Hg range is well understood to cause marked alterations in circulatory physiology, any increase above 0 is potentially detrimental to venous return, especially in patients who have a compromised circulation for other reasons in addition to the abdominal process. Therefore, some patients with an abdominal pressure less than 25 mm Hg will benefit from interventions to reduce this impairment to venous return.

Cardiogenic Hypoperfusion and Cardiogenic Shock

To cause cardiogenic shock, or hypotension, on a cardiac basis, cardiac function must be severely disrupted (cardiac index < 2.2 L/min/m^2) from etiologies such as those listed in Table 6-16. Hypoperfusion of this magnitude, especially when it is secondary to myocardial infarction, is associated with a high mortality rate. Cardiogenic shock is a clinical entity distinct from CHF. In CHF, arterial blood pressure is characteristically well maintained or increases. This characteristic distinguishes cardiogenic shock (the term applied to significant reductions in systolic pressure) from CHF.

In general, the diseases listed in Table 6-16 are not subtle and do not cause gradual alterations in cardiac function. Hypotension is more often a disease of hypovolemia than a disease of severe impairment of cardiac function. When a clinician decides not to administer fluid to a hypotensive patient, he or she is actually making a diagnosis of cardiogenic shock. Cardiogenic shock is the only major circulatory deficit that can be worsened by the administration of fluid. Because cardiogenic shock is secondary to

Table 6-16 Etiologies of Cardiogenic Shock

Acute ischemia	
	Ventricular wall infarct
	Papillary muscle infarct
	Ventricular septal defect
Acute valvular disease; mitral, tricuspid, or aortic regurgitation	
Arrhythmias	
	Rapid supraventricular
	Bradycardia
	Ventricular tachycardia
Miscellaneous	
End-stage cardiomyopathy	
	Severe myocardial contusion
	Severe myocarditis
	Severe left ventricular outflow obstruction
	Severe left ventricular inflow obstruction

severe, usually obvious, cardiac disease, the clinician should be able to document the occurrence of a marked insult to cardiac function. Without such documentation and the associated recognition of a disease that requires aggressive monitoring and management in a critical care setting, the clinician should consider the hypotensive patient to be hypovolemic and not in cardiogenic shock.

Physical Examination

Physical examination shows hypotension, tachycardia, tachypnea, peripheral vasoconstriction, distended neck veins, agitation, and confusion. An S_3 gallop may be apparent, and when valvular dysfunction is present, associated murmurs may be auscultated.

Laboratory Aids

Cardiogenic shock is associated with chest x-ray evidence of hydrostatic pulmonary edema, metabolic acidosis (lactic acidosis), increased CVP and PAOP, and increased BUN and creatinine. A cardiogram often shows evidence of acute ischemia, infarct, or arrhythmias. An echocardiogram can provide information about ventricular wall motion and valve function. The cardiac index is low (< 2.2 L/min/m^2), and both systemic and pulmonary vascular resistance are high.

Treatment

As always, treatment is based on the etiology. Arrhythmias are usually the most readily treated etiology of severe cardiac impairment. Arrhythmias are diagnosed and treated as described in textbooks that cover advanced cardiac life support. When the etiology is not an arrhythmia, the same sequence of interventions used to increase cardiac output

Table 6-17 Treatment of Cardiogenic Shock

Reversal of underlying disease	
	Coronary artery bypass
	Valve replacement
	Rx myopathy
	Repair ventricular septal defect
Reduce preload	
	Decrease water intake
	Diuretics
	Venous dilation
	Nitroglycerin
	Calcium channel blockers
	Narcotics
Reduce afterload	
	Nitroprusside
	Antihypertensives
	Diuretics
	Narcotics
Increase contractility	
	Intravenous inotropes
Increase arterial oxygen	
	Supplemental O_2
	Mechanical ventilation

in CHF may be used for cardiogenic shock (Tables 6-17 and 6-18). However, hypotension (often < 90 mm Hg systolic) makes the use of vasodilators alone less attractive. Therefore, a combination of **inotropic drug support** and vasodilation is frequently used. Mechanical support of the heart with an intraaortic balloon pump (IABP) increases cardiac output while reducing preload and afterload. IABP may be more successful than high-dose dobutamine in supporting patients during severe cardiac impairment. IABP may be adequate to support a patient until cardiac function improves, or may be required until surgery (e.g., replacement of the aortic valve, coronary revascularization) is performed. Complications of IABP are listed in Table 6-19.

Table 6-18 Hemodynamic Effects of Inotropic Drugs and Vasodilators

	Hemodynamic Parameters			
	Heart Rate	Contractility	Preload	Afterload
Dopamine	↑↑	↑	↑	↑ or NC
Dobutamine	↑	↑↑	↓	NC or ↓
Isoproterenol	↑↑	↑↑	↓	↓
Nitroprusside	±	NC	↓	↓↓
Nitroglycerin	±	NC	↓↓	↓

NC, no change.

Table 6-19	Complications of the Intraaortic Balloon Pump
Injury to femoral vessels	
Ischemic extremity	
Hemolysis or thrombocytopenia	
Infection	

Endpoints for Resuscitation of the Circulation

Endpoints for resuscitation of the circulation depend on such variables as the primary etiology of the circulatory deficit, the underlying state of the patient's circulation, and the magnitude of cellular and organ malfunction recognized during the hypoperfusion insult. However, for most clinical conditions, bedside recognition of normal circulation is adequate for assessing the outcome of resuscitation. Such variables as normal (the designation of normal depends on knowledge of the patient's premorbid blood pressure) or increasing blood pressure, pulse rate of less than 80/min, normal or improved mental status, urine output greater than 0.5 mL/kg/hr, warm extremities, and resolution of metabolic acidosis usually suffice.

However, patients who have had a severe cellular insult may require more complicated hemodynamic monitoring and adjustment of the circulation. Certainly, patients who are in cardiogenic shock require precise hemodynamic monitoring (i.e., pulmonary artery catheterization, echocardiogram, cardiac catheterization) to make the proper diagnosis and adjust therapy. In such cases, return of the cardiac index from low (< 2.2 L/min/m^2) to normal (2.5 to 3.5 L/min/m^2), along with normal amounts of oxygen delivery (400 mL/min/m^2) and consumption (130 mL/min/m^2), may allow cellular and organ function to recover. A normal cardiac index may also be adequate in patients with underlying heart disease who have a further reduction in cardiac function from noncardiac causes and then undergo resuscitation of their circulation close to baseline. Unfortunately, despite the achievement of **normal** cardiac index and oxygen parameters, patients with or without severe acute or chronic heart disease may continue to have cellular malfunction that progresses to organ failure and death after a severe hypoperfusion insult.

The recognition that normal circulation, oxygen delivery, and oxygen consumption may be inadequate for cellular and organ recovery after severe hypoperfusion was inferred from epidemiologic data that associated an increase in these parameters (cardiac index > 4.5 L/min/m^2; oxygen delivery > 600 mL/min/m^2; oxygen consumption > 170 mL/min/m^2) with eventual survival. In patients who achieve these endpoints, metabolic acidosis usually resolves. This situation also portends a favorable outcome. Therefore, several investigators champion the use of fluids, inotropic drugs, and sometimes vasodilators to push for these hemodynamic endpoints in every critically ill patient. The results of such management remain controversial, with some studies supporting these endeavors and others finding an increase in mortality rates.

What can be used in the individual patient to determine if sufficient oxygen is being provided to the tissues? The pulmonary artery catheter allows the measurement of mixed venous oxygen saturation ($S\bar{v}O_2$), measured by taking a sample from the pulmonary artery port. Healthy adults deliver hemoglobin that is close to 100% saturated with oxygen and consume about 25%. This results in a [$S\bar{v}O_2$] of 75%. When the [$S\bar{v}O_2$] measures in the 50s, most would argue that cells are demanding more oxygen than the circulation is delivering. When this value is in the 70s, oxygen delivery would appear sufficient for the demand. Values in the 60s could be interpreted either way.

As with any clinical measurement, [$S\bar{v}O_2$] is subject to inaccuracies, and any value obtained should be juxtaposed with the other clinical variables described above before deciding that more therapy for the circulation must be provided.

In summary, clinical evaluation is usually sufficient to recognize the "end points of resuscitation"—normal blood pressure for that individual, a slow pulse, warm extremities, good urine output, normal mental status, and resolution of metabolic acidosis (e.g., resolution of elevated lactic acid). However, many patients will continue to exhibit abnormalities in these clinical parameters even after aggressive efforts. Such patients can be more precisely evaluated with the pulmonary artery catheter and echocardiographic data, recognizing that the information so obtained must not be used in isolation. Once the clinical and cellular evidence of shock has resolved (see below), then such monitoring techniques are no longer necessary.

SEVERE INFLAMMATORY STATES

As described above, inflammation is a normal response to tissue injury. However, although localized inflammation in response to an insult is usually beneficial, severe tissue injury from a variety of causes (Table 6-20) can result in inflammation distant from the original disease (systemic inflammation). This inflammation may cause cellular malfunction and death in remote organs. As catalogued

Table 6-20	Etiologies of Systemic Inflammation (Partial List)
Infection (meets definition of sepsis)	
Trauma	
Burns	
Ischemia or reperfusion: regional or total body	
Pancreatitis	
Drug reactions	
Hemolytic transfusion reactions	

in the concept of the **systemic inflammatory response syndrome (SIRS),** many disease states can cause systemic inflammation, probably as a result of the activation of cellular mediators of inflammation at remote sites.

To meet the definition of SIRS, a patient must have two or more of the following conditions: (1) temperature greater than 38.5°C or less than 36°C; (2) heart rate greater than 90 beats/min; (3) respiratory rate greater than 20 breaths/min or $Pa{CO_2}$ less than 32 torr; and (4) total leukocyte count greater than 12,000 cells/mm, less than 4000 cells/mm^3, or greater than 10% immature forms. Many patients with systemic inflammation but without evidence of significant cellular and organ malfunction (i.e., not in shock) may meet the definition of SIRS. The SIRS variables of hypothermia ($<$ 36°C) and leukopenia ($<$ 4000 cells/mm^3) are associated with more severe inflammation, as are systolic hypotension and evidence of organ malfunction (e.g., elevated BUN and creatinine, oliguria, altered mental status, decreased arterial oxygenation, increased bilirubin, decreased platelets). These patients are in shock, even if infection is not present and the term sepsis cannot strictly be applied. Therefore, the traditional concept of septic shock is too narrow. Patients with severe systemic inflammation who exhibit these alterations are in shock. When infection is the cause of severe systemic inflammation, then septic shock can be considered the diagnosis.

Effects of Severe Inflammation on the Circulation

Severe systemic inflammation is associated with alterations in both total body and regional perfusion. Mechanisms that reduce cardiac output during systemic inflammation are listed in Table 6-21.

The most common etiology of inadequate cardiac output during inflammation is decreased venous return, which results from both loss of intravascular fluid and vasodilation. Intravascular volume decreases as plasma exudes into the primary focus of inflammation (area of injury or infection). When systemic inflammation develops in response to the primary focus of inflammation, plasma may also exude into some or all of the other tissues. Such exudation causes an increase in interstitial fluid, which becomes protein-rich compared with normal. In general, interstitial fluid is maintained in the extracellular space by active cellular processes that maintain cell membrane integrity and perform such functions as sodium-potassium exchange, which keeps potassium in the cell and sodium out of the cell. Severe inflammation may interfere with active cell membrane function, decrease ion-exchange capabilities, and allow more interstitial water and solutes to enter cells. Depletion of interstitial fluid is another mechanism that aggravates plasma volume loss.

Ileus is common during severe inflammation, regardless of the location of the primary focus. Ileus can cause fluid to accumulate in the lumen of the gastrointestinal tract that can be as voluminous as that sequestered during bowel obstruction.

Collectively, the exudation of plasma volume into inflammatory foci, the accumulation of fluid in the gastrointestinal tract, and the migration of fluid into cells is known as the third space, to distinguish it from normal plasma and interstitial fluid spaces. The magnitude of the third-space effect is roughly proportional to the magnitude of tissue injury or infection that is present. The primary effect of **third-space fluid accumulation** is to deplete intravascular volume and impair venous return.

Vasodilation of the systemic veins and arterioles is characteristic of severe inflammation, and several inflammatory mediators are implicated as causative (e.g., histamine, kinins, prostacyclin, nitric oxide). Increasing the capacitance of veins decreases MSP and may decrease venous return, especially if CVP (discussed previously and in the section on venous return) does not decrease proportionally because of increased pulmonary vascular resistance.

Severe inflammation may directly depress the function of previously normal myocardial cells. Less severe inflammation may result in augmented malfunction of previously abnormal cardiac tissue. Therefore, cardiac output may be impaired and result in a physiology that is consistent with an excess, rather than a deficit, of intravascular volume (i.e., CHF, cardiogenic shock physiology). Recognition of such **cardiogenic states** of hypoperfusion during inflammation is important for proper therapeutic intervention (see later).

Severe inflammation is associated with increased pulmonary vascular resistance. This increase in right ventricular afterload may cause dilation of the right ventricle, decreased right ventricular ejection, and impaired filling of the left ventricle. Right atrial pressure may increase and impair venous return.

In addition to the recognized effects on cardiac function and cardiac output, which can reduce total body perfusion, severe inflammation may cause deficits in the microcirculation that in turn can result in regional ischemia to organs or within organs. This ischemia will accentuate cell

Table 6-21	Circulatory Disorders in Severe Inflammation: Reduced Cardiac Output
Hypovolemia	
Peripheral vasodilation	
Increased capillary permeability, local or total body	
Intracellular migration of fluid	
Sequestration in gastrointestinal tract lumen	
Myocardial depression	
Increased pulmonary vascular resistance	
Hypoxia	
Platelet emboli	
Thromboxane release	
Serotonin release	
White blood cell aggregation	
Deficits in the microcirculation	
Gastrointestinal tract	
Renal	

and organ injury. The gastrointestinal tract and kidneys appear to be particularly prone to such alterations.

Effects of Severe Inflammation on Cellular Function

Severe inflammation can result in alterations of cellular metabolism that are independent of inflammation-induced reductions in oxygen delivery, but similar to abnormalities recognized with hypoperfusion, a condition called "cytopathic hypoxia." In cytopathic hypoxia the cells behave as if there is too little oxygen because of an inflammation-induced alteration in cellular function, not because there is too little oxygen for cellular function. For instance, the elevation in lactic acid level that is associated with severe inflammation is not characteristically secondary to cellular anaerobic metabolism. Increased lactic acid production can also develop secondary to alterations in glucose metabolism that are associated with increased pyruvate production or decreased pyruvate metabolism without mitochondrial malfunction (i.e., aerobic glycolysis). Therefore, in inflammatory states an elevated lactic acid level does not necessarily support the conclusion that a patient has inadequate oxygen delivery.

There are other physiologic disturbances that demonstrate how cells have difficulty distinguishing the insults from too little oxygen and too much inflammation. For example, the same cell-depolarizing molecule that appears in the circulation after hypovolemic hypoperfusion is present after inflammatory insults. Such cell depolarization can result in sodium and water accumulation in the cells. Further, a decrease in serum ionized calcium is common in both hypoperfusion and inflammatory states. This decrease, shown experimentally to be associated with increased intracellular calcium, is also likely a marker for cell membrane malfunction.

Therefore, several cell function alterations—production of lactic acid, decreased cell membrane function, increased intracellular sodium and calcium—can all result from either true cellular hypoxia or as a result of inflammatory toxins, namely, cytopathic hypoxia.

DIAGNOSIS AND MANAGEMENT OF SEVERE INFLAMMATION

The clinical manifestations of severe systemic inflammation (Table 6-22) are as potentially varied as the many organs that may manifest malfunction. Most patients have hemodynamic alterations, but sometimes abnormal lung, central nervous system, hematologic, or other organ function is the primary evidence of inflammation, rather than hemodynamic changes. Therefore, a high index of suspicion of the patient at risk, augmented by evidence gathered during physical examination and with selected laboratory tests, supports the diagnosis of significant inflammation.

Table 6-22 Common Clinical Manifestations of Severe Inflammation

Vital signs
Temperature elevation, hypothermia
Tachycardia
Tachypnea
Hypotension with warm or cold extremities
Change in mental status
Respiratory insufficiency
Ileus
Oliguria, increased urine protein
Elevated hemoglobin, thrombocytopenia, leukocytosis, leukopenia
Increased serum glucose, decreased ionized calcium

The Patient at Risk

The first category of risk is a patient who recently acquired a disease (e.g., severe pancreatitis) or had an injury (e.g., unstable pelvic fracture with ruptured spleen) that is characterized by severe inflammation. The second category of risk is a patient who has an underlying condition (e.g., immunosuppression after liver transplantation) or who recently underwent a procedure (e.g., elective colon resection for carcinoma) that makes systemic inflammation, particularly from infection, more likely. Any patient who has had a significant episode of hypoperfusion (e.g., cardiogenic shock after an acute myocardial infarction, upper gastrointestinal hemorrhage sufficient to result in hypotension) is also at risk for systemic inflammation, either at the time of the hypoperfusion or days later.

Physical Examination

Outward Manifestations

The patient is usually restless and may have alterations in mental status ranging from delirium to coma. In fact, mental status changes may precede obvious hemodynamic or respiratory findings. These alterations sometimes lead the clinician to a misdirected evaluation (i.e., computed tomography of the brain). Such alterations in central nervous system function are rarely focal and are most consistent with a metabolic encephalopathy.

If intravascular volume is decreased, the skin is cool and possibly mottled, with vasoconstriction most often evident in both the upper and lower extremities. Capillary refill time is also decreased.

Vital Signs

Usually, severe systemic inflammation is seen as a decrease in blood pressure, an increase in heart rate, an increase in respiratory rate, and elevated temperature. Patients who have underlying cardiac disease may have hemodynamics that are more consistent with congestive heart failure (i.e., elevated blood pressure, tachycardia). Hypothermia may be present in the most severe cases.

Lung Examination

At lung examination, the lungs may be clear, even when acute respiratory distress syndrome (ARDS) is present. However, rales, rhonchi, and bronchospasm may be found. Examination findings consistent with consolidation (e.g., tubular or tubulovesicular breath sounds, egophony) may assist in locating an inflammatory process, but they are clearly not specific to systemic inflammation. The lung examination is not sufficiently specific to permit a diagnosis of systemic inflammation or other etiology of diffuse pulmonary malfunction.

Cardiovascular Examination

Hypotension and tachycardia are usually present, along with crisp heart tones. After intravascular volume is restored, the extremities are usually warm, demonstrating good capillary refill. Hypotension with warm hands and feet most often represents the response to inflammation, although anaphylaxis and a high spinal cord injury can produce similar findings. Jugular venous pressure is low by clinical examination.

As a result of plasma exudation and the other causes of plasma volume loss, the patient usually is sequestering fluid. This sequestration can be sudden or, if the patient has been monitored in a hospital setting, the positive fluid balance and an increase in weight may have been documented for several days before acute deterioration is noted.

Myocardial depression from inflammation might cause elevated jugular venous pressure, hypertension, and an S_3 gallop. Myocardial depression that is severe enough to result in hypotension and a clinical picture identical to cardiogenic shock is possible. However, such myocardial malfunction is much less common than are circulatory deficiencies secondary to hypovolemia. The clinician must be careful to distinguish the fluid sequestration and positive fluid balance associated with severe inflammation (which is universal) from the same phenomena seen with cardiogenic states. Treating hypovolemia with fluid restriction and diuretics causes further circulatory embarrassment.

Fluid administration is directed at restoring and maintaining the plasma and blood volume that is threatened by the fluid sequestration associated with severe inflammation. Thus, the primary reason for fluid administration is to support the circulation. Often the circulation is assessed with urine output. Decreased urine output secondary to severe inflammation is most often caused by inadequate cardiac output. Therefore, it is a marker of inadequate circulation.

Laboratory Studies

Hematologic Studies

An increase in total white blood cell count, particularly young PMNs, is most common. Leukopenia denotes more severe disease and consists mostly of immature PMNs. The platelet count usually falls, and evidence of consumption of coagulation proteins, with breakdown of fibrinogen (increased prothrombin time, increased partial thromboplastin time, and increased fibrin split products or D-dimer), denotes more severe disease. Hemoglobin may increase as plasma exudes into inflammatory sites. This increase indicates hemoconcentration, and may be a useful tool in assessing intravascular volume resuscitation because plasma volume is likely to be inadequate until the hemoglobin returns to the patient's baseline value.

Lung Studies

A decrease in arterial P_{O_2} and P_{CO_2} is characteristic of severe systemic inflammation as well as many other lung disease states. The increase in physiologic shunt, which results in a decrease in arterial P_{O_2}, is associated with stimuli that increase minute ventilation and decrease arterial P_{CO_2}. A chest radiograph may be clear or may demonstrate loss of lung volume as well as evidence of pulmonary fluid accumulation, most often from a noncardiogenic pathophysiology (i.e., ARDS). The clinician should recognize that respiratory signs and symptoms and laboratory data during severe inflammation (shortness of breath, tachypnea, crackles, wheezing, decreased arterial P_{O_2}, chest radiograph showing increased lung water) may be indistinguishable from those seen with CHF. In addition, the clinician should recognize the dangers of misdiagnosing the effects of severe lung inflammation as CHF.

Urine Studies

Oliguria is common during severe inflammation and is most often secondary to low intravascular volume and inadequate circulation. It causes laboratory test results that are consistent with a prerenal state (e.g., elevated urine specific gravity, low urine sodium, increased urine osmolality, elevated BUN:creatinine ratio).

Serum Chemistries

An elevated blood glucose level is common during inflammation from such alterations as increased gluconeogenesis, glycogen lysis, and relative insulin resistance.

For many years, decreased total serum calcium has been recognized as associated with one particular severe inflammatory disease, pancreatitis. The amount of decrease correlates with the severity of disease. Ionized calcium is the calcium that is not bound to albumin. Therefore, it is not affected by albumin concentrations, which can change significantly during critical illness. Ionized calcium is also better correlated with parathyroid hormone release compared with total calcium.

Ionized calcium decreases with any disease that causes either severe hypoperfusion or inflammation. This decrease is not secondary to inadequate parathormone secretion. Several recent studies showed an increase in intracellular calcium during or after hypoperfusion or inflammatory states. In addition, the magnitude of the decrease correlates with the severity of disease. Although it is not specific for inflammation, ongoing severe inflammation must be considered in any patient who has decreased ionized calcium. In contrast, a normal ionized calcium level is unusual during severe inflammation or hypoperfusion. Therefore, a normal value suggests that a severe acute systemic insult is not present.

The combination of electrolyte or arterial blood gas levels that are consistent with metabolic acidosis and an elevated lactic acid level is often seen in severe inflammation. An elevated lactic acid level may develop secondary to anaerobic metabolism, suggesting hypoperfusion as the cause. However, an elevated lactic acid level can also result from metabolic alterations associated with inflammation in the presence of normal oxygen concentrations. Therefore, like ionized calcium, these abnormalities do not distinguish severe inflammation from a decrease in either regional or global perfusion. Persistent metabolic acidosis could mean that either disease is present and should prompt further diagnostic and, possibly, therapeutic efforts.

Treatment

Treating the Underlying Cause

Once severe inflammation is recognized, the first principle of treatment is to determine the underlying cause and initiate appropriate therapy (Table 6-23). Infection and infection-like processes (i.e., endotoxin) are the most commonly considered etiologies of severe inflammation. However, reactions to drugs or transfusions and tissue injury without infection (i.e., early severe pancreatitis) can also cause severe systemic inflammation that is indistinguishable from that seen with the invasion of microorganisms.

While the search for the primary disease is underway and therapy is initiated, vital organ function must be supported until the primary process is under control. Unfortunately, systemic inflammation may continue despite adequate resolution of the initiating insult. In some patients, inflammation appears to become self-sustaining, as though a positive feedback system developed in one or more of the organs with systemic inflammation. For instance, ARDS initiated by an inflammatory process in the abdomen causes inflammatory cells to accumulate in the lungs. The inflammation caused by these pulmonary cells usually, but not always, subsides when the underlying illness is effectively treated. Sometimes the lung inflammation becomes subacute despite resolution of the first inflammatory focus.

Table 6-23 Treatment of Severe Inflammation

Control etiology
Drug or transfusion reaction
Tissue injury
Infection
Support organ function
Antagonize inflammatory and metabolic mediators

As discussed later, novel therapies that focus on interrupting various steps in the inflammatory process are being studied to determine whether they can ameliorate the adverse effects of severe inflammation and improve clinical outcome. In addition, therapies designed to enhance immunologic function may prevent subsequent inflammatory insults from infection or microbiologic byproducts.

Supporting Organ Function: Cardiovascular and Pulmonary

Rapid restoration of the circulation during severe inflammation has been shown to reduce mortality. Support of the circulation usually starts with treatment of hypovolemia. The result is usually an increase in cardiac output such that hypotension is alleviated, if not completely reversed. The temperature of the extremities also changes from cool to warm. For most patients, the combination of restoration of intravascular volume, peripheral vasodilation, and the neurohumoral response to inflammation produces a hyperdynamic (cardiac index $>$ normal) circulatory state. Urine output and mental status usually improve. Unfortunately, pulmonary function does not characteristically improve dramatically with treatment of hypovolemia alone. Ionized calcium alterations and metabolic acidosis may or may not improve as a result of simple improvement in the circulation.

Red blood cell transfusion is reserved for patients who have ongoing hemorrhage or hemoglobin levels of less than 9 g/100 mL and who have abnormalities that are consistent with inadequate oxygen delivery. For patients with hemoglobin levels of more than 10 g/100 mL, simply increasing hemoglobin does not appear to significantly improve oxygen consumption.

Dopamine, usually in low concentrations, is commonly administered during severe inflammation. Because dopamine, even at these low doses, tends to increase left ventricular end-diastolic pressure as cardiac output increases, this drug has a physiologic effect that is similar to fluid infusion, and is most useful when hypovolemia is the primary abnormality.

The diagnosis and treatment of a cardiogenic state usually requires more complicated monitoring than simply recording blood pressure, pulse, skin color, mental status, urine output, and electrolyte concentrations. Insertion of a pulmonary artery catheter (PAC) allows more precise measurement of cardiac filling pressures and the response to inotropic and vasodilator manipulations.

The primary advantage of PAC insertion is the ability to acquire hemodynamic data to assist in hemodynamic diagnostic and therapeutic decision making. Given the evidence that achieving excellent circulation is associated with improved outcome in patients who have severe hypoperfusion or inflammation, using technologic devices (which might include echocardiography) to evaluate the circulation and possibly avoid continuing hypoperfusion clearly appears beneficial. This argument is not supported by data accrued during routine use of PACs, however, because critical assessment of the circulation is not likely to be crucial for any common illness or surgical intervention (e.g., major vascular surgery). Likewise, it may be difficult to discern a survival advantage to using such equipment in large groups of patients in the intensive care unit. However, an individual patient may achieve a distinct advantage, especially when a therapeutic intervention that reverses hypoperfusion is documented.

The disadvantages of PAC insertion include complications related to central venous access (e.g., pneumothorax, central venous thrombosis) as well as those associated with the cardiac location (e.g., ventricular arrhythmias, damage to the tricuspid or pulmonic valves, rupture of the pulmonary artery). Ventricular arrhythmias are usually not sustained, and anatomic injuries are rare. Despite the relatively low risk, PAC insertion should be used when the potential advantage, as described earlier, is considered worth the risk.

During severe inflammation, myocardial depression may be a manifestation of decreased function of the myocardial catecholamine receptors. Phosphodiesterase inhibitor drugs (e.g., amrinone), which do not require this receptor function for action, may be particularly useful inotropic agents during severe inflammation.

In a patient who is hyperdynamic, has elevated cardiac output, and has low systemic resistance states, the use of a vasoconstrictor (e.g., norepinephrine, neosynephrine, vasopressin) may be indicated, especially when certain vessels with fixed stenoses (e.g., atherosclerotic plaques in renal, carotid, or coronary arteries) are likely to require higher mean arterial pressure for adequate perfusion. Under these circumstances, the use of such vasoconstrictors (with simultaneous documentation of no significant reduction in cardiac output) may increase mean arterial pressure and provide evidence of better organ perfusion (e.g., increased urine output).

Endpoints for resuscitation of the circulation during severe inflammation are as controversial as those described in the hypoperfusion section. Because severe inflammation commonly increases cardiac index, one indicator that inflammation is resolving may be a decrease in cardiac index (e.g., from 5.0 to 3.5 L/min/m^2) and an increase in systemic resistance (e.g., from 350 to 900 dynes-sec/cm^5).

Support of pulmonary function often requires mechanical ventilation and various associated techniques of ventilator management. Such management is sufficient when arterial oxygen saturation is greater than 90%.

Achieving a Balance in the Effects of Inflammation

Much experimental and clinical research has evaluated the antagonism of inflammatory and metabolic mediators in severe inflammatory states (Table 6-24). Many studies show promise, but few are emerging as "standard" therapy.

As previously stated, inflammation has beneficial effects (e.g., wound healing, defense against invasive organisms) that are important for survival during critical illness. Therefore, a successful outcome depends significantly on a balance between the beneficial and the detrimental effects of inflammation. Therapy that aggressively suppresses inflammation (i.e., pharmacologic doses of antiinflammatory steroids) may provide short-term benefits (e.g., improvement in hemodynamic and pulmonary function), but the loss of the beneficial effects of inflammation may result in death secondary to recurrent infection or wound breakdown.

For all of the therapies listed in Table 6-24, this balance must be considered. The benefits of inflammation are primarily local (i.e., at the focus of tissue injury or infection). The detrimental effects are primarily systemic (e.g., alterations in circulation or pulmonary function). Therapies that allow local inflammation to continue while the systemic inflammation is suppressed may allow the proper inflammatory balance.

Table 6-24 Antagonism of Inflammatory and Metabolic Mediators

- Interference with effects of endotoxin
  - Clear endotoxin from the circulation
    - Antiendotoxin antibody
    - Bind toxin to membrane
    - Filter toxin out
  - Interfere with binding of endotoxin to effector cells (i.e., bactericidal or permeability-increasing protein)
- Interference with the activation of proinflammatory cytokines
  - Steroids
  - Nonsteroidal antiinflammatory agents
  - Inhibition of IL-1-converting enzyme
- Interference with the activity of increased proinflammatory cytokines
  - Anti-TNF, anti-IL-1 antibodies
  - Binding of TNF and IL-1 with excess receptors
  - Blocking of effector cell receptors (i.e., administration of IL-1 receptor antagonist)
  - Continuous blood filtration
- Administration of antiinflammatory cytokines
- Interference with superoxide activity
  - Decrease production
  - Increase scavenging
- Interference with secondary mediators
  - Cyclooxygenase system
  - Nitric oxide system
  - Complement
  - Histamine, serotonin, kinin system
  - Coagulation system
- Interference with inflammatory cell activation by blocking activation receptors (i.e., inhibition of leukocyte integrin and selectin)

IL, interleukin; TNF, tumor necrosis factor.

In general, these therapies are most helpful in patients who appear to have severe systemic inflammation despite usually adequate therapy for the underlying illness. For instance, consider a 65-year-old previously healthy woman who has perforated diverticulitis and undergoes a sigmoid resection with end-sigmoid colostomy. Ordinarily, fluid resuscitation, surgery, and antibiotics are sufficient to reverse the detrimental effects of this severe inflammatory illness and support the proper balance between the beneficial and detrimental effects of inflammation. However, if organ malfunction (e.g., ARDS, hyperdynamic circulation, impaired renal function) consistent with ongoing severe inflammation is still present 3 to 4 days later, then one possible explanation is that the inflammation stimulated in other organs by the perforated diverticulitis is responsible for the lack of resolution, despite therapy that is often sufficient. In other words, the detrimental and beneficial effects of severe inflammation are out of balance. Under such circumstances, therapy directed at the systemic inflammation may be warranted.

Recently, two such therapies have shown limited benefit: (1) the use of recombinant human activated protein C and (2) the use of physiologic (rather than pharmacologic) doses of hydrocortisone.

A PRACTICAL GUIDE TO THE PATIENT IN SHOCK

Once a patient is recognized to be in shock, the guiding principles are to (1) provide an excellent circulation and (2) treat severe inflammation.

Recognize the Patient in Shock

Clearly, the first step in the evaluation and management of the patient who is in shock is to recognize that a deficit in total body cellular function is present, that is, that there is a "rude unhinging." The history is the first clue to the patient who is at risk (Table 6-25). Next, bedside examination can provide clues, but severe hypotension and marked tachycardia may not always accompany other evidence of shock (Table 6-26). Next come common laboratory data, which are frequently abnormal during shock (Table 6-27) and may provide the first clue of threatened cellular function.

Table 6-25	Characteristics of the Patient Who Is at Risk for Shock
Trauma or burn	
Vascular catastrophe	
Acute cardiac disease	
Acute abdominal disease	
Severe extraabdominal infection	
Drug exposure	

Table 6-26	Bedside Examination Indicators of Shock
Hypotension	
Tachycardia	
Tachypnea	
Hyperthermia or hypothermia	
Peripheral vasoconstriction and cool extremities	
Hypotension with warm extremities	
Agitation and altered mental status	
Oliguria	

Provide an Excellent Circulation

An accurate diagnosis of the state of the circulation is critical (see the section on hypoperfusion states).

The patient who is in cardiogenic shock requires aggressive hemodynamic monitoring as well as pharmacologic and possibly mechanical assistance of the circulation (see earlier sections). This level of care clearly requires a critical care environment and physician expertise. The decision may be made to perform emergency cardiac catheterization or cardiac surgery.

The hypotensive supine adult who does not have a cardiogenic process most often has lost at least 30% of intravascular volume (approximately 1500 mL in a 70-kg person). Replacement with isotonic crystalloid solution requires a 3:1 ratio as the crystalloid distributes throughout the extracellular space. Therefore, 4500 mL crystalloid solution is required to begin plasma volume restitution in this patient. Because there is no organ in the body that is improved by hypoperfusion, and because prolonged hypoperfusion induces or aggravates tissue inflammation, restitution of an adequate circulation should be accomplished rapidly (within minutes, if possible, with two large-bore intravenous lines wide open).

When decreased venous return (most often as a result of hypovolemia) is the cause of hypoperfusion, a diagnostic evaluation of the etiology of impaired venous return must occur simultaneously with restoration of the circulation. Venous return can improve with fluid infusion, regardless of the underlying etiology of the decrease (e.g., hypovolemia vs. pericardial tamponade).

As described in previous sections, the circulatory param-

Table 6-27	Common Laboratory Abnormalities With Shock
Metabolic acidosis	
Elevated blood urea nitrogen and creatinine	
Leukocytosis or leukopenia	
Elevated blood glucose	
Decreased platelet count	
Decreased ionized calcium	

Table 6-28 Bedside Indicators of an Excellent Circulation

Normal blood pressure and pulse for the individual
Normal mental status
Warm extremities
Urine output ≥ 0.5 mL/kg/hr
Resolution of metabolic acidosis

eters that indicate an excellent circulation may vary from patient to patient, but general bedside guidelines are listed in Table 6-28. More sophisticated indicators of an excellent circulation have been proposed and may be of particular value when evidence of organ malfunction is present, despite bedside indicators that the circulation is adequate (i.e., BUN and creatinine levels are increasing when the blood pressure and pulse are normal) (Table 6-29).

Treat Severe Inflammation

Treating severe inflammation requires recognition that an inflammatory state is present (see discussion of severe inflammatory states). Next, the focus of severe inflammation must be localized and treated (e.g., antibiotics for pneumonia, colon resection for perforated diverticulitis). Usually, these interventions suffice. Occasionally, the other methods described in the section on severe inflammatory states are used to diminish the effects of severe inflammation.

Table 6-29 Monitors of Circulation Status

Cardiac index	> 4.5 L/min/m^2
Mixed venous O_2 saturation	≥ 70%
Oxygen delivery	> 600 mL/min/m^2
Oxygen consumption	> 170 mL/min/m^2
Gastric mucosal pH (tonometer measurement)	> 7.35
Right ventricular end-diastolic volume index	> 100 mL/m^2

Ideal values indicate a good prognosis.

Hypoperfusion can cause inflammation or aggravate established inflammation. Therefore, providing an excellent circulation is as much a treatment of inflammation as is the use of antibiotics or surgery. As a corollary, because inflammation can induce both total body and regional hypoperfusion, treating inflammation improves the circulation.

CONCLUSION

Total body cellular malfunction (i.e., shock) can result from various insults that may be broadly categorized as severe hypoperfusion or severe inflammatory disturbances. Almost invariably, hypoperfusion and inflammation coexist in patients who have shock. Restoring an excellent circulation and treating severe inflammation are the keys to preserving cellular and organ function and preventing death from shock.

SUGGESTED READINGS

Baue AE. MOF/MODS, SIRS: an update. *Shock* 1996;6:S1–S5.

Bernard GR, Vincent JL, et al. Efficacy and safety of recombinant human activated protein C for severe sepsis. *N Engl J Med* 2001; 344(10):699–709.

Burchard, K. A review of the adrenal cortex and severe inflammation: quest of the "eucorticoid" state. *J Trauma* 2001;51(4):800–814.

Califf RM, Bengtson JR. Cardiogenic shock [review]. *N Engl J Med* 1994;330:1724–1730.

Eastridge BJ, Darlington DN, Evans JA, et al. A circulating shock protein depolarizes cells in hemorrhage and sepsis. *Ann Surg* 1994;219: 298–305.

Fink MP. Bench-to-bedside review: cytopathic hypoxia. *Crit Care* 2002; 6(6):491–499.

Livingston DH, Mosenthal AC, Deitch EA. Sepsis and multiple organ dysfunction syndrome: a clinical-mechanistic overview. *N Horizons* 1995;3:257–266.

Rivers E, Nguyen B et al. Early goal-directed therapy in the treatment of severe sepsis and septic shock. *N Engl J Med* 2001;345(19): 1368–1377.

Szebeni J, Baranyi L, et al. Complement activation during hemorrhagic shock and resuscitation in swine. *Shock* 2003;20(4):347–355.

Society of Critical Care Medicine. Practice parameters for hemodynamic support of sepsis in adult patients in sepsis. Task Force of the American College of Critical Care Medicine, Society of Critical Care Medicine. *Crit Care Med* 1999;27(3):639–660.

7

WILLIAM MILES, MD ■ GAMAL MOSTAFA, MD

Surgical Critical Care

OBJECTIVES

1 Understand the multidisciplinary needs of the critically ill surgical patient and the coordination of care required of health care providers practicing in the intensive care unit (ICU).
2 Describe the hazards of transporting ICU patients for procedures, diagnostic tests, and transfer of care.
3 Understand the potential benefits and complications of total parenteral nutrition.
4 Describe the method and importance of performing the Allen test prior to placing a radial arterial catheter.
5 List the potential benefits of central venous catheterization and its complications.
6 Review the differences between sedation and analgesia and the effects these medications have on patients.
7 Describe the differences in the diagnosis and management of ICU delirium and alcohol withdrawal.
8 Understand the pathophysiology and management of abdominal compartment syndrome.
9 Understand the difference between systemic inflammatory response syndrome and severe sepsis; review the guidelines in the prevention and management of sepsis.
10 Describe the arterial blood gas findings that typically correlate with respiratory failure and the need for mechanical ventilation.
11 Understand the effects of multisystem organ failure on morbidity and mortality in the surgical patient.
12 Understand the importance of ICU monitoring techniques of the major organ systems in the prevention of multisystem organ failure.
13 Understand the definition of brain death and procedures to assist in determining brain death.
14 Understand the importance of using low tidal volume ventilation in the mechanical
15 Describe the effects of oxygen toxicity.
16 Outline the differences between the basic modes of mechanical ventilation and the advantages and disadvantages of each mode.

The intensive care unit (ICU) of a hospital is where all medical disciplines provide highly organized and technologically advanced care to patients. It is the most challenging of the hospital wards and can be an intimidating rotation for a medical student. The ICU is where the developing clinician must learn to use all skills and senses to care for critically ill surgical patients. Although challenging, the ICU rotation can also be among the most rewarding; over 96% of critically ill patients admitted are discharged alive.

The surgical ICU is truly the place where the analogy of "team sports" comes into play, and medical students should be a part of the team. "Multidisciplinary" refers not only to other physician consultants, but also to other health care providers such as nurses, respiratory therapists, nutritionists, pharmacists, and physical therapists. Getting to know these practitioners and their responsibilities will help fortify a student's experience in the ICU.

This chapter describes basic management and support techniques for patients requiring critical care as well as some of the diseases and conditions likely to be encountered in the ICU. Some of these diseases and conditions are discussed in other chapters of this textbook. To understand the needs of the ICU patient, it is necessary to understand all of the potential pathophysiologic processes a patient may develop.

UNIQUE NEEDS OF THE ICU PATIENT

Transport

The surgical patient comes to the ICU from the emergency department, the recovery room, or, most commonly, the operating room. This transfer of care is actually a continuation of critical care from the patient's point of origin to the intensive care unit. Surgical patients, whether in the operating room or the ICU, usually require invasive monitoring, mechanical ventilation, and resuscitation maneuvers during the perioperative period. This "intensive care" is best performed in an area of the hospital having the expertise and resources needed to accommodate a patient's needs. There are several types of ICUs, depending on the hospital. Some institutions have combined general medical–surgical ICUs, whereas some have separate specialty ICUs, such as cardiac, neurosurgical, and trauma.

The transport of the ICU patient is potentially a hazardous undertaking. The rate of complications related to transport is reported to be as high as 37%. These complications include changes in vital signs, unplanned tube removal, cardiac dysrhythmias, and even cardiac arrest. Whether being transported to radiology or to surgery, most ICU patients are unable to support themselves and often have lines, tubes, or ventilators that must accompany them. To make the transport safe, a team of health care workers should accompany the patient. If the patient is critically ill, this team should include a nurse, a respiratory therapist, and a physician, all carrying the equipment necessary to sustain the patient during transport. A cardiac defibrillator may be required for the transport itself.

Complications of transportation may be avoided by observing certain guidelines. Unless transport is required for lifesaving intervention, it should be avoided in an unstable patient. Maintaining airway patency is crucial. If there is concern about the ability of the patient to maintain airway patency or spontaneous breathing, endotracheal intubation should be performed before transportation. In the intubated patient, sedation and neuromuscular blocking agents can be administered to control agitation and prevent accidental extubation during transport. The physician should acknowledge the potential for respiratory decompensation in ventilated patients during transport. Significant changes in gas exchange may occur in the transition from mechanical to manual ventilation. The patient should have adequate oxygenation with a manual ventilation system (mask–bag-valve) before leaving the unit. Patients dependent on positive end-expiratory pressure (PEEP) may need a special manual ventilation system with a PEEP valve to maintain oxygenation during transportation. Adequate oxygen supply and vasoactive and cardiac medications should be readily available during transportation, along with essential monitoring equipment and personnel.

Due to the potential risks of transport, many surgical ICUs have developed guidelines and protocols for "bedside" surgery. Many of these procedures (e.g., tracheostomy, wound debridements, vena caval filters) were once routinely performed in the operating room. This "bedside" surgery should be considered only if the patient's risk of transport is too great and if the procedure can be performed safely.

The Stress Response

Most ICU patients undergo a systemic stress response. This response is characterized by endocrine, metabolic, and immunologic alterations. The inciting injury may be surgical, traumatic, or infectious; its severity is the main determinant of the magnitude of the stress response. The stress response to injury, surgery, infection, or critical illness is mediated through several cascades involving hormones and cytokines, with extensive degree of overlap and interaction between these important mediators.

The hormones released in response to injury may be regulated by the hypothalamic–pituitary axis or the autonomic nervous system. Most injuries are characterized by an elevation in corticotropin-releasing hormone from the hypothalamus and adrenocorticotropic hormone (ACTH) from the anterior pituitary. The release of ACTH leads to the release of cortisol from the adrenal cortex. Cortisol is essential for survival after significant physiologic stress. Adequate cortisol levels after bleeding are a prerequisite for restoration of blood volume after hemorrhage. Cortisol has a significant role in the metabolic stress response. It potentiates the actions of glucagon and epinephrine, while decreasing insulin binding to insulin receptors in adipose tissue. In the liver, cortisol stimulates hepatic gluconeogenesis. Overall, the metabolic effects of cortisol will result in a hyperglycemic response associated with trauma or critical illness. ACTH is also a potent stimulus for aldosterone release in the injured patient. The main action of aldosterone is maintenance of intravascular volume by conserving sodium in the distal renal tubules.

Elevation of arginine vasopressin (AVP) secretion is another characteristic of the stress response. The major stimulus for AVP release is elevated plasma osmolality, which is detected by special hypothalamic receptors. Depletion of the effective circulating intravascular volume is also a potent stimulus to AVP release. AVP induces water absorption from the distal renal tubules and collecting ducts and stimulates peripheral vasoconstriction.

Catecholamines (e.g., endogenous epinephrine) exert

significant influence on the stress response to surgery, trauma, or critical illness. They modulate the hypermetabolic state observed after the acute stress response. Catecholamines stimulate glucagon secretion, decrease insulin release, and inhibit insulin-dependent glucose uptake by skeletal muscles. In the liver, catecholamines stimulate glycogenolysis, gluconeogenesis, and ketogenesis. These actions are responsible for the stress-induced hyperglycemia.

In the critically ill patient, insulin release has a biphasic pattern. In the early phase, occurring a few hours after surgery or injury, insulin production is suppressed as a consequence of increased levels of catecholamines. In the later phase, insulin production is normal or even excessive. However, persistent hyperglycemia is noted mainly due to peripheral resistance to insulin actions.

Cytokines are protein mediators that are secreted by one cell to influence another cell and are, therefore, important in the biologic process of cell signaling. Cytokines play an important role in regulating the immune response to injury and wound repair (see Chapter 8, Wounds and Wound Healing). Important cytokines in the mediation of stress response include tumor necrosis factor-α (TNF-α), interleukin-1 (IL-1), and interleukin-6 (IL-6). The overall effect of TNF is to favor thrombosis, and this effect may be important in the pathogenesis of the hypercoagulable state associated with inflammation. IL-1 shares many properties with TNF. It induces fever in acute illness through its interaction with the endothelial cells of the hypothalamus. The most important function of IL-6 appears to be the regulation of the hepatic acute phase response. Changes in the circulating level of the so-called acute phase proteins during or after injury or infection are mostly related to the hepatic effect of IL-6. IL-6 induces the production of C-reactive protein, fibrinogen, α_1-antitrypsin, and haptoglobin. It inhibits the production of albumin and transferrin.

Nutrition and Metabolism

The ICU patient undergoes metabolic alterations that result in unique nutritional requirements. Hypercatabolism is a prominent feature of the stress response. Energy requirements are increased by 30% to 50% during critical illness, and endogenous substrates are mobilized to meet this increased demand. After depletion of glucose stores, hepatic gluconeogenesis provides glucose to obligatory cell-type (brain, heart, and inflammatory cells). Protein catabolism is increased and amino acids become an important substrate for acute phase protein synthesis and gluconeogenesis. Skeletal muscle proteolysis is the initial source of amino acids, which leads to reduction in the total body mass. As catabolism continues, visceral and structural proteins are also depleted.

To determine the amount of nutrients needed, a weight-based goal (25 to 30 kcal/kg) is often used. An alternative method is the Harris-Benedict equation, where basal energy expenditure is calculated based on age, sex, height, and weight (see Chapter 4, Nutrition). The assessment of protein needs is important. The goal is to place patients in a positive nitrogen balance. Nitrogen intake is determined from the dietary protein intake knowing that 1 g of nitrogen = 6.26 g of protein. Daily nitrogen output is determined by measuring urine urea nitrogen (UUN) in a 24-hour urine collection and adding 4 g of nitrogen (i.e., daily nitrogen output = UUN + 4).

The route of nutrition in the ICU can be enteral or parenteral. Recent research provides compelling evidence in support of enteral nutrition, even in the postoperative patient. The benefits of the enteral route include better delivery of substrates, prevention of mucosal atrophy, and preservation of gut flora. Enteral nutrition is therefore associated with fewer septic complications than parenteral nutrition. In the critically ill patient, enteral nutrition is better tolerated if it is begun early in the course of illness.

Complications of Total Parenteral Nutrition

A multitude of complications is associated with total parenteral nutrition (TPN). Problems may arise in the placement and maintenance of venous access or in the formulation and delivery of parenteral solutions. One of the more common and serious complications associated with long-term parenteral feeding is sepsis secondary to contamination of the central venous catheter. Usually it is a result of failure to observe strict aseptic precautions during preparation and administration of the solutions. One of the earliest signs of systemic sepsis may be the sudden development of glucose intolerance (with or without temperature increase) in a patient who previously has been maintained on parenteral alimentation without difficulty. When this occurs or if fever develops without obvious cause, a diligent search for a potential septic focus is indicated. Other causes of fever also should be investigated. If fever persists, the infusion catheter should be removed and cultured. It may be advisable to wait a short period before reinserting the catheter, especially if bacteremia or hemodynamic instability is present (see section on infectious diseases below). Other complications related to catheter placement include the development of pneumothorax, hemothorax, or hydrothorax; subclavian artery injury; cardiac arrhythmia if the catheter is placed into the atrium or the ventricle; air embolism or catheter embolism; and, rarely, cardiac perforation with tamponade.

Hyperosmolar nonketotic hyperglycemia may develop with normal rates of infusion in patients with impaired glucose tolerance or in any patient if the hypertonic solutions are administered too rapidly. This is a particularly common complication in latent diabetics and in patients who have had severe surgical stress or trauma. Treatment of the condition consists of volume replacement with correction of electrolyte abnormalities and the administration of insulin. This serious complication can be avoided with careful attention to daily fluid balance and frequent determinations of serum glucose and electrolyte levels.

It is important not to "overfeed" the parenterally nourished patient. This is particularly true of the depleted patient in whom excess calorie infusion may result in carbon dioxide retention and respiratory insufficiency. Excess feeding also has been related to the development of hepatic steatosis or marked glycogen deposition in certain patients. Mild abnormalities of serum transaminase, alkaline phosphatase, and bilirubin levels may occur in many parenterally nourished patients. Failure of the tests to plateau or return to normal over 7 to 14 days should suggest another cause.

Two indirect complications of TPN are related to the absence of bulk nutrients in the bowel: mucosal atrophy and acalculous cholecystitis. The absence of bulk nutrients in the bowel produces atrophy and disruption of the bowel mucosa. These changes may predispose to translocation of enteric pathogens across the bowel mucosa and subsequent septicemia. Because TPN is usually accompanied by bowel rest, one indirect complication of TPN is bacterial translocation and sepsis of bowel origin. The absence of lipids in the proximal small bowel prevents cholecystokinin-mediated contraction of the gallbladder. The bile stasis that results may promote acalculous cholecystitis.

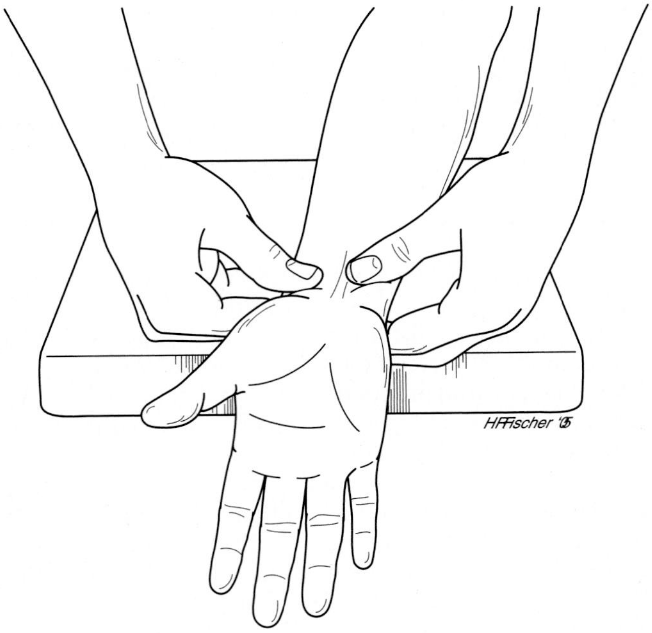

Figure 7-1 Allen test.

MONITORING IN THE ICU

The surgeon's role in bedside critical care is to recognize and correct pathophysiologic problems. These problems may develop in all organs of the body due to the defects in perfusion related to shock, stress responses, disease processes, or trauma. To monitor effectively, the surgeon must understand the requirements, benefits, and limitations of physiologic monitoring.

Hemodynamic Monitoring

Clinical evaluation is often unreliable in critically ill patients, since there can be major changes in cardiovascular function that do not produce obvious clinical findings. Invasive hemodynamic monitoring at the bedside provides information about cardiorespiratory performance and guides treatment on a rational physiologic basis.

Arterial Catheterization

Arterial catheterization is used whenever there is a need for continuous monitoring of blood pressure and/or frequent sampling of arterial blood. Conditions during which precise and continuous blood pressure data are needed include shock of any etiology, acute hypertensive crisis, use of potent vasoactive or inotropic drugs, and high levels of respiratory support. Information on sequential blood gas tensions and pH values is needed in acute illness involving cardiovascular or respiratory dysfunction. With an indwelling arterial catheter and monitoring system, the systolic blood pressure (SBP), diastolic blood pressure (DBP), and mean arterial pressure (MAP) are displayed continuously. Many anatomic sites have been used to access the arterial circulation for continuous monitoring. The dual blood supply to the hand and the superficial location of the vessel make the radial artery the most common site for arterial catheterization. Cannulation is technically easy, and there are few complications.

Most authors recommend assessing the adequacy of collateral circulation before cannulation of the radial artery. The test most often used for this is the modified Allen test (Fig. 7-1). The patient elevates one hand, makes a fist, and clenches it firmly, squeezing the blood from the vessels of the hand. After the examiner simultaneously compresses both the radial and ulnar arteries, the patient lowers and opens his relaxed hand. The examiner then releases the pressure over the ulnar artery and measures the time for return of color. It is considered normal if the capillary blush of the hand is complete within 6 seconds. Failure to perform the Allen test may cause permanent tissue ischemia and necrosis of the hand, resulting in a "claw hand." Table 7-1 lists some of the common problems associated with arterial catheterization.

Table 7-1	Complications Associated With Arterial Catheters
Bleeding	
Pain	
Tissue ischemia	
Embolization	
Paresthesia	
Arterial occlusion	
Claw hand	

Central Venous Catheterization

Central venous catheterization secures access for fluids, drug infusions, parenteral nutrition, and central venous pressure (CVP) monitoring. The CVP measurement can differentiate between pericardial tamponade and hypovolemia in a hypotensive trauma patient. A CVP measurement can also assist in trending the volume status in a critically ill patient. The most commonly chosen sites include the subclavian and the internal jugular veins, which can be fairly easily cannulated, although the external jugular, femoral, and brachiocephalic veins can also be used.

The subclavian vein should be used in patients with profound volume depletion. Disadvantages of using the subclavian vein include a higher risk of pneumothorax and the inability to compress the vessel if bleeding occurs.

The major advantages of internal jugular vein catheterization are the lower risk of pneumothorax and the ability to compress the insertion site if bleeding occurs. The internal jugular vein, however, can be more difficult to cannulate in patients with volume depletion or shock. Technical or mechanical complications occur during catheter placement, and long-term complications are related to the length of time that the catheter remains in place. Technical and mechanical complications include catheter malposition, dysrhythmia, embolization (air or catheter fragments), vascular injury, pleural injury (pneumothorax, hemothorax, or hydrothorax), mediastinal injury, and neurologic injury (phrenic nerve, brachial plexus, or recurrent laryngeal nerve). Arterial puncture is the most common immediate complication of internal jugular vein cannulation. Long-term complications are due to infection or thrombosis.

Pulmonary Artery Catheterization

Pulmonary artery catheterization provides information about CVP, pulmonary artery diastolic pressure (PADP), pulmonary artery systolic pressure (PASP), mean pulmonary artery pressure (MPAP), pulmonary artery occlusion ("wedge") pressure (PAOP), cardiac output (CO) by thermodilution, and mixed venous oximetry. When the pulmonary artery catheter balloon is inflated (1.5 mL), the blood flow in a distal segment of the pulmonary artery is occluded, creating a conduit through which the pulmonary capillary wedge pressure (PCWP) can be measured. Barring other influences (such as ventilator pressures or valve disorders), the left atrial pressure (LAP), the left ventricular pressure (LVP), and the left ventricular volume (LVV) are felt to be similar to the PCWP. In addition to the complications attributed to central venous cannulation, complications can occur during passage of the pulmonary artery catheter or after the catheter is in place. The most common complication during passage of the catheter is the development of dysrhythmias. Coiling, looping, or knotting of the catheter in the right ventricle can occur during catheter insertion. Complications that can occur after the catheter is in place include infections, thromboembolism, and rupture of the pulmonary artery. Infections from pulmonary artery catheters are directly related to the length and severity of illness. In addition to the complications associated with catheter insertion, complications can result from delays in treatment due to time-consuming insertion problems and from inappropriate treatment based on erroneous information or erroneous data interpretation.

Respiratory Monitoring

Monitoring ventilation and gas exchange in critically ill surgical patients is important in determining problems with mechanical ventilation. A disposable, noninvasive, and inexpensive calorimetric device permits detection of the expired CO_2. This device, attached between an endotracheal tube and a manual ventilation system, is one of the most reliable means of determining proper endotracheal tube placement. Esophageal intubation can produce one or a few breaths containing CO_2 during expiration, but because there is no CO_2 in the stomach, expired CO_2 rapidly becomes nondetectable by the CO_2 calorimeter. The detection of expired CO_2 correlates with cardiac output and coronary perfusion pressure during cardiopulmonary resuscitation (CPR) and with successful resuscitation from and survival after cardiac arrest. Because circulatory arrest creates total dead space, if mechanical ventilation is continued, then expired CO_2 disappears. Any detection of expired CO_2 provides an immediate bedside validation of the efficacy of CPR, and if the presence of CO_2 is detected abruptly, it provides the earliest evidence of successful resuscitation.

Pulse oximetry provides a reliable, real-time estimation of arterial hemoglobin oxygen saturation (SaO_2). Pulse oximeters estimate arterial hemoglobin saturation by passing an infrared light through the skin to detect and indirectly measure oxygen bound to the hemoglobin in well-perfused tissue, such as the finger or ear. Various physiologic and environmental factors interfere with the accuracy of pulse oximetry. These include hypovolemia, hypotension, hypothermia, vasoconstrictor infusions, motion artifact, electrosurgical interference, backscatter from ambient light, and dyshemoglobinemias. The pulse oximeter can only distinguish oxyhemoglobin and deoxyhemoglobin. If other hemoglobin species are present, an error can occur.

The oxygen saturation of mixed venous hemoglobin ($S\bar{v}O_2$) is the amount of oxygen-saturated venous blood returning to the heart. It is usually measured at the pulmonary artery, with a newer-model pulmonary artery catheter, where all of the blood is "mixed" as it returns to the heart. Measurement of $S\bar{v}O_2$ is helpful in the assessment of the oxygen supply–oxygen demand relationship in critically ill patients. The use of improved fiberoptic oximetry systems in conventional pulmonary artery catheters has permitted continuous monitoring of $S\bar{v}O_2$ and has made bedside monitoring of this relationship practical. The normal range for $S\bar{v}O_2$ in healthy subjects is 0.65 to 0.75, with an average value of 0.70. An $S\bar{v}O_2$ of less than 0.65 implies that the amount of oxygen being delivered to the body is low or the amount being used is too high. An $S\bar{v}O_2$ of more than 0.80 is usually associated with a hyperdynamic physiologic state consistent with sepsis or massive systemic inflammation. In this situation, the body is delivering the oxygen to the end organs. However, due to capillary endothelial inflammation, the oxygen is not being used effectively. This process is called "peripheral shunting" of oxygen.

Renal Monitoring

In most situations, the kidney serves as an excellent monitor of the adequacy of perfusion, and monitoring kidney function can help prevent acute organ failure. Blood urea nitrogen (BUN) often has been used to estimate renal function. BUN is affected by the glomerular filtration rate (GFR) and urea production. Production can be increased if large amounts of nitrogen are administered during parenteral nutritional support, or as a result of gastrointestinal bleeding. Because these factors are often interrelated in an unpredictable manner in critically ill patients, BUN is not a reliable monitor of renal function. The value of plasma creatinine as a measure of renal function far exceeds the value of BUN. In contrast to BUN concentration, plasma creatinine levels are not influenced by protein metabolism. When creatinine production is constant, the serum creatinine level reflects GFR. The plasma creatinine level will double with a 50% reduction in GFR. Acute reductions in the GFR are not immediately reflected, however, because it takes 24 to 72 hours for equilibration to occur. Serial determination of creatinine clearance is currently the most reliable method for clinically assessing GFR and the most sensitive test for predicting the beginning of perioperative renal dysfunction. Although measurements are usually made using a 24-hour urine collection, a 2-hour collection is reasonably accurate and easier to perform.

Measuring the concentrating ability of the renal tubules helps distinguish oliguria due to prerenal causes from that caused by intrinsic renal failure due to tubular dysfunction (see Chapter 3, Fluids and Electrolytes). With prerenal azotemia, the tubules can appropriately reabsorb sodium and water. In intrinsic renal failure, tubular function is markedly compromised, and the ability to reabsorb sodium and water is impaired. Tubular function tests are useful in oliguric patients (urine output < 500 mL/day), because nonoliguric individuals typically have less severe tubular damage. The fractional excretion of sodium (FE_{Na}) is the most reliable laboratory test for distinguishing prerenal azotemia from acute tubular necrosis. This test requires only simultaneously collected "spot" urine and blood samples. The FE_{Na} value is normally less than 1% to 2%. In an oliguric patient, a value of less than 1% is usually due to a prerenal cause. A value of more than 2% to 3% suggests compromised tubular function.

Intracranial Pressure Monitoring

The most significant cause of death and secondary injury in patients with traumatic brain injury is severe intracranial hypertension. Therefore, measurement of intracranial pressure (ICP) is vital to improving outcomes in this patient population. The most common indication for ICP monitoring is severe head injury. Patients with a **Glasgow Coma Scale** score (Table 7-2; discussed under neurologic dysfunction below) of 8 or less (in the absence of neurodepressive agents) probably need ICP monitoring. Intracranial pressure may be monitored using a subarachnoid bolt, an intraparenchymal fiberoptic pressure monitor, or an intraventricular catheter (Fig. 7-2). An intraventricular catheter offers excellent waveform characteristics and permits drainage of cerebrospinal fluid (CSF), offering a ther-

Table 7-2 Glasgow Coma Scale

	Response	Points
Opens eyes	Spontaneously	4
	To verbal commands	3
	To pain	2
	No response	1
Best motor response (Verbal/painful stimuli)	Obeys	6
	Localizes pain	5
	Flexion withdrawal	4
	Flexion (decorticate)	3
	Extension (decerebrate)	2
	No response	1
Best verbal response	Oriented and converses	5
	Disoriented and converses	4
	Inappropriate words	3
	Incomprehensible sounds	2
	No response	1

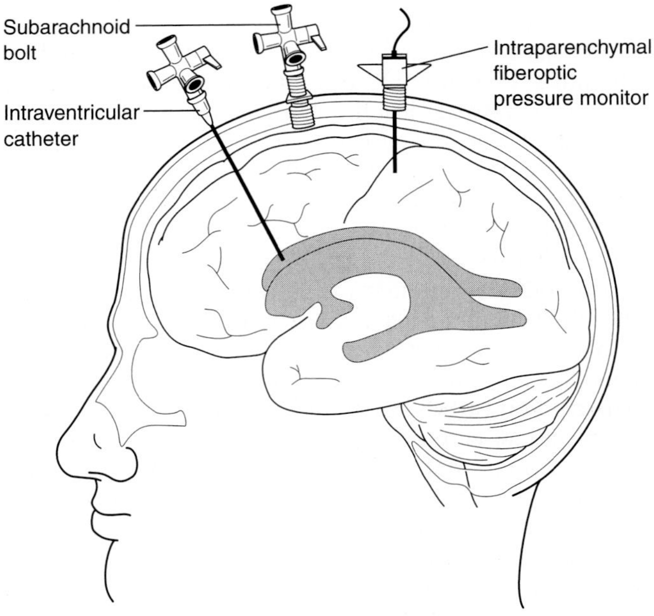

Figure 7-2 Intracranial pressure monitoring.

apeutic maneuver. A subarachnoid bolt is easily inserted, although it can give erroneous readings, depending on its placement relative to the site of injury. Compared with ventricular catheters, the waveforms obtained are not as good, and CSF drainage is usually not possible. Complications of ICP devices include infection, hemorrhage, malfunction, obstruction, and malposition. Bacterial colonization of ICP devices increases after 5 days of implantation.

Measuring ICP permits calculation of cerebral perfusion pressure (CPP), which is the difference between the MAP and ICP (CPP = MAP − ICP). Thus, isolated increases in ICP or decreases in MAP will cause a reduction in CPP. The CPP can be insufficient if ICP increases to more than 20 mm Hg. In brain-injured patients, a higher CPP level is required to maintain cerebral blood flow. This level is at least 60 mm Hg. Controlling ICP is the best way to maintain adequate CPP and appears to be one of the most important factors in reducing secondary brain injury. Maintaining adequate intravascular volume as well as administering vasopressor agents as needed may improve CPP when lower than normal MAPs are encountered.

PREVENTING COMPLICATIONS IN THE ICU

Stress ulceration of the gastric mucosa and deep vein thrombosis (DVT) of the lower extremities with its associated threat of fatal pulmonary embolism (PE) are two well-recognized complications of critical illness, multiple trauma, or major surgery. The term *prophylaxis* is often used by ICU physicians to refer to the specific measures taken to prevent these complications.

Stress Ulcers

Stress ulcers are superficial erosions that are confined to the gastric mucosa. These lesions can develop within hours of admission to the ICU. The major threat associated with stress ulcers is the development of clinically significant upper gastrointestinal bleeding. Although bleeding related to stress ulcers occurs in up to 20% of critically ill patients, only 5% of cases are clinically evident. The basic mechanism believed to result in stress ulcers is inadequate blood flow to the gastric mucosa, which results in disruption of the gastric mucosal barrier to the intraluminal hyperacidity. The incidence of stress ulceration has decreased over the last 2 decades due to better prophylactic measures and earlier recognition and treatment of inflammatory processes.

Several measures are used for the prevention of stress ulcers. Prophylaxis is specifically indicated in high-risk patients, including those needing prolonged mechanical ventilation and those with coagulopathy, shock, burns, and head injuries. Preventive measures involve: (1) gastric acid reduction using histamine 2 (H_2) receptor antagonists or, more recently, proton pump inhibitors (PPIs); (2) gastric acid neutralization with antacids; or (3) protection of the gastric mucosal integrity with the use of sucralfate, which does not influence the gastric acid output. Gastric feeding will, however, be as effective as the above-mentioned agents in preventing stress gastric ulceration. It also has the major additional benefit of meeting the nutritional requirements while avoiding the complications of parenteral nutrition. Therefore, whenever possible, early use of enteral feeding should be encouraged as long as it can be tolerated.

Deep Vein Thrombosis

Patients in the ICU are often at risk for the development of DVT of the lower extremities. Propagation of the clot to proximal veins carries the threat of fatal PE. High-risk patients include those who have undergone hip/knee surgery, those who have undergone extensive pelvic/abdominal operations, those with cancer or hypercoagulable states, and those with spinal cord injury or major pelvic fractures. Prophylactic measures for DVT include the use of graded compression stockings or pneumatic compression devices, and the administration of low-dose heparin. Color duplex ultrasonography of the lower extremities may be used for surveillance of DVT at regular intervals. Though not 100% sensitive, this noninvasive procedure can be safely performed at the bedside. Surgical prophylaxis for the prevention of PE entails the percutaneous placement of an inferior vena caval filter (IVCF). This measure is primarily indicated in patients in whom anticoagulants are contraindicated (e.g., patients with intracranial hemorrhage), or in patients who develop pulmonary embolism while on anticoagulation therapy.

Heparin-Induced Thrombocytopenia

An important complication of the frequent use of heparin in ICU patients is the development of thrombocytopenia. Up to 15% of patients who receive heparin experience acute thrombocytopenia, which spontaneously reverses and has no clinical sequelae. It is caused by transient sequestration of platelets and is termed heparin-induced thrombocytopenia-I (HIT-I). This is in contrast to heparin-associated antiplatelet antibodies (HAAbs), which develop in 2% to 4% of patients and lead to platelet activation and aggregation. This causes another type of heparin-induced thrombocytopenia (HIT-II), which occurs an average of 8 days after the beginning of heparin administration (5 days if a patient was previously sensitized). Because HIT cannot be predicted, patients receiving heparin should be monitored with serial platelet counts. The diagnosis should be suspected if a patient develops resistance to anticoagulation, thromboembolic events, a fall in the platelet count greater than 30%, or a platelet count less than 100,000/mm^3. If HIT is suspected, heparin should be stopped and the patient tested for HAAbs. If there are no antibodies, heparin can be resumed. If the patient has HAAbs, options for anticoagulation include nonreactive heparins and heparinoids, direct thrombin inhibitors (lepirudin, argatroban), defibrinogenating agents (ancrod), and platelet function inhibitors (glycoprotein IIb/IIIa inhibitors). The direct thrombin inhibitors should be considered the preferred agents. HAAbs typically disappear in a few weeks to months, but patients should be retested for antibodies before subsequent heparin administration.

CONDITIONS AND DISEASES TREATED IN THE ICU

The Agitated Patient: Sedation and Analgesia

The first goal in evaluating the patient with agitation is to determine and treat the etiology. The causes of agitation in the ICU may include hypoxia, pain, sepsis, hypercapnia, and substance withdrawal. Therefore, careful history, physical examination, and use of appropriate laboratory tests are essential in the evaluation of the agitated patient. It is crucial to identify and treat the potentially life-threatening causes of agitation prior to controlling the agitated patient with the liberal use of pharmaceutical agents (Fig. 7-3).

Common pharmacologic agents used for sedation include benzodiazepines, haloperiodol (Haldol), and propofol (Diprivan). Benzodiazepines are either short-acting (midazolam or Versed) or long-acting (lorazepam). The use of these sedating agents may be associated with certain side effects. The prolonged use of the short-acting benzodiazepines can lead to a buildup of metabolites with prolonged duration of action, and the use of haloperiodol may result in extrapyramidal manifestation. Propofol has a short half-life, and its effects are reversed within 10 minutes of stopping infusion. The main drawback of propofol use is the possibility of profound hypotension. Propofol is best used in the intubated patient when quick reversal of sedation is necessary, such as in the case of a head injury, when the patient must undergo serial neurologic examination.

Most patients in the surgical ICU require pain control. It is important to remember that most sedatives do not have analgesic properties and that additional medications are required for this purpose. Intravenous narcotics are

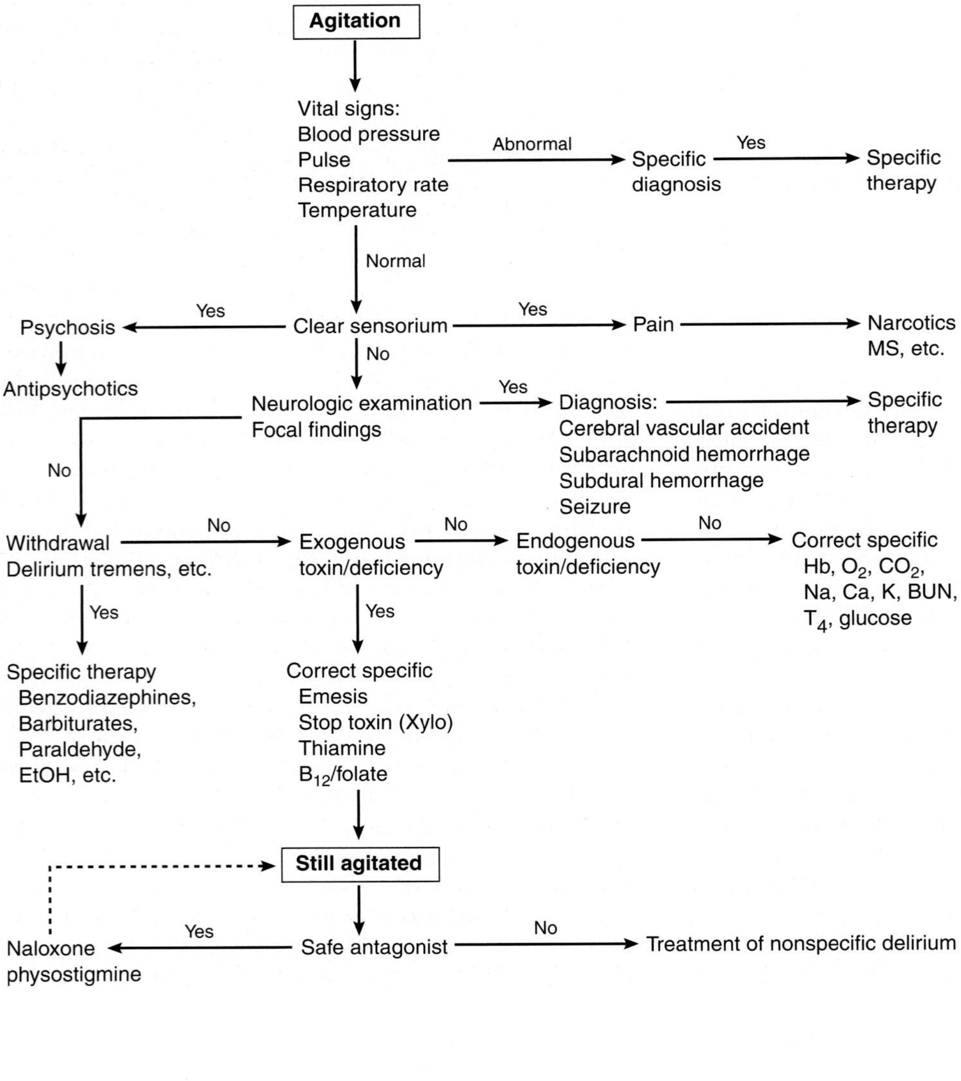

Figure 7-3 Algorithm for the diagnosis and treatment of agitation and specific abnormalities. BUN, blood urea nitrogen; Hb, hemoglobin; MS, ; T_4, thyroxine. (From Cased NH. Psychiatric problems. In Parillo JE, ed. *Current Therapy in Critical Care Medicine.* Toronto, Ontario: BC Decker, 1987. Used with permission.)

the most commonly administered analgesics. The onset of action of morphine sulphate (MSO_4) is 15 minutes after intravenous administration. It has a half-life of 2 hours. Some patients release a large amount of histamine with MSO_4 injection, leading to hypotension from peripheral vasodilation. Fentanyl acts more rapidly, and potent analgesia occurs within 60 to 120 seconds after intravenous injection. It does not result in histamine release and is, therefore, ideal for hemodynamically unstable patients.

Neuromuscular blocking agents are commonly used in the ICU. Common indications include bedside procedures, maximum mechanical ventilatory support for critical hypoxemia or hypercarbia, and refractory intracranial hypertension. Again, it is important for the physician and the nursing staff to understand that neuromuscular blocking agents do not have any analgesic or sedating properties. Additional coverage with appropriate medication should therefore be provided along with neuromuscular paralysis. It is equally important to realize that the use of neuromuscular blocking agents has certain adverse consequences. Complications of paralysis in the ICU include immobility with pressure ulceration and a variety of cardiovascular effects based on the specific agent used. Prolonged paralysis has been described after the discontinuation of neuromuscular blockades. This could be due to excessive dosing and decreased clearance due to hepatic or renal impairment. Administration of the lowest effective dose as monitored by peripheral nerve stimulation is recommended to avoid complications.

A major initiative in ICU care is the daily cessation of sedatives in patients that are improving. Allowing patients to awaken from their sedation daily and, importantly, in a controlled manner has been shown to reduce their ventilation requirements, sedation needs, and their length of stay in the ICU.

ICU Psychosis

Acute delirium is a very common problem in critical care and has many causes: older patients devoid of common surroundings; constant daylight and disruption of sleep patterns; withdrawal from drugs; and side effects of medications. Pain itself, or the effects of the pain medicine, may cause agitation in a delirious patient. As an example, morphine used as an analgesic may cause confusion. Whatever the source, psychosocial measures are not effective in treating delirium of unknown cause. Management in these cases includes medications, restraints, and trying to identify the source.

Because agitated critical care patients may harm themselves by pulling out necessary tubes and drains, reduction in agitation is the goal in management. Benzodiazepines should be given first since they are effective in mild agitation. Higher doses of benzodiazepines may cause severe confusion or respiratory compromise in older patients. Delirium is often treated with antipsychotic medications in combination with benzodiazepine.

Haloperidol is a very useful and commonly used medication to treat agitation and delirium in the ICU. It is very useful in patients who are older or who may have impaired cardiac or pulmonary function. The usual dose of haloperidol may vary depending on the patient and his or her needs. Initially, 2 mg is used for mild agitation, 5 mg is used for moderate agitation, and 10 mg is used for severe agitation. Doses of haloperidol may be given over 30-minute intervals until the desired calm state is achieved.

Though given enterally or parenterally in this setting, haloperidol has not been approved by the U.S. Food and Drug Administration (FDA) for intravenous administration. Intravenous haloperidol is generally safe for most patients, though some institutions have reported that IV haloperidol may be infrequently associated with torsade de pointes (a form of ventricular tachycardia) and prolonged QT widening. Haloperidol should not be administered in patients with low levels of potassium or magnesium or in patients with liver failure or prolonged QT on their cardiac monitors.

Delirium Tremens

Delirium tremens, the most alarming manifestation of the ethanol withdrawal syndrome, occurs in about 5% of alcoholics. It consists of agitated arousal, global confusion and disorientation, insomnia, and vivid, often threatening hallucinations and delusions. Signs of sympathetic hyperactivity include tremor, mydriasis, tachycardia, fever, and intense diaphoresis. Delirium tremens begins abruptly within 2 to 4 days of abstinence, sometimes as a surprising development in an unrecognized alcoholic admitted to the hospital for other reasons. Episodes of delirium tremens last from 1 to 3 days and end as abruptly as they begin. However, relapses occur, and the disorder may continue for days to weeks with intervening periods of lucidity.

Alcoholics stop drinking for many reasons, including serious alcohol-related medical, surgical, or psychiatric conditions. Hence, symptoms or signs of trauma, infection, liver disease, gastritis, pancreatitis, arrhythmia, or electrolyte disturbance should be sought. One hundred milligrams of thiamine should be given intravenously to all patients undergoing ethanol withdrawal to prevent or treat Wernicke's encephalopathy. This treatment should be followed by daily multivitamins. The alarming symptoms of ethanol withdrawal are best managed by substituting another central nervous system depressant. However, alcoholics undergoing withdrawal are very resistant to sedatives (cross-tolerance), so large doses are often required to calm their agitation.

Benzodiazepines are widely used to manage tremulousness and disordered perceptions during ethanol withdrawal. The goal is to suppress symptoms and produce mild sedation, and the drug dosage is adjusted to the severity of the withdrawal reaction. Treatment includes managing delirium and autonomic stability, and preventing seizures. A sedative-hypnotic agent, typically a benzodiazepine, is prescribed as a substitute for alcohol, and the dose is tapered over several days. Beta-blockers are useful ancillary therapy; they attenuate the symptoms of autonomic hypersensitivity. The first several days of severe alcohol withdrawal may require intravenous administration of total daily diazepam doses exceeding 400 mg (or the equivalent of other benzodiazepines) to achieve mild sedation. Multivitamin and thiamine supplementation should be continued, as should meticulous attention to electrolyte status. The benzodiazepine dosage can then be tapered by approximately 20% to 25% on successive days, with an increase in dosage if withdrawal symptoms recur. Once the symptoms of ethanol withdrawal are suppressed, it is necessary to avoid oversedation and the danger of respiratory depression by carefully titrating the dose of diazepam to just keep the patient calm. Volume depletion accompanying delirium tremens may cause circulatory collapse, so maintaining adequate intravascular volume is essential.

Abdominal Compartment Syndrome

Intraabdominal hypertension (IAH), resulting in abdominal compartment syndrome (ACS), is a clinically serious condition in the critically ill surgical or trauma patient. The syndrome results from an increase in the volume of any retroperitoneal or intraperitoneal contents. Causes of ACS may include capillary-leak edema, intraabdominal hemorrhage, and complicated intraabdominal operations such as liver transplantation, abdominal trauma, and retroperitoneal hematoma. The resulting intraabdominal hypertension can be measured at the ICU bedside via a urinary catheter connected to a pressure transducer (Fig. 7-4).

Increased intraabdominal pressure (IAP) adversely affects cardiac output, pulmonary mechanics, and renal function. It also results in decreased perfusion of intraabdominal viscera due to impaired splanchnic blood flow. Clinically, these consequences are manifested as increased inspiratory pressures or decreased tidal volumes, decreased cardiac output, and oliguria. These manifestations are observed with an IAP above 25 mm Hg.

Clinically significant IAH should be managed by abdominal decompression. Following decompression, the abdominal skin and fascia are left open. The abdominal viscera are covered with one of several temporary closure methods, including towel suction closure, bogata bag, or absorbable mesh. These techniques permit a moist environment to protect the viscera while maintaining abdominal compartment decompression. Complications may occur, causing significant problems for the management of the patient. The anticipation and prevention of the development of ACS is crucial. To avoid ACS, forceful closure of the abdomen in patients with significant abdominal trauma or massive intraabdominal hematoma should be avoided.

Fever Resulting From Noninfectious Causes

The appearance of fever in a patient in the ICU is not always a sign of impending disaster. However, it is a sign that requires attention. The operational definition of fever proposed by a consensus conference on sepsis and inflammation is a body temperature above 38°C (100.4°F). It is important to remember that this definition has several shortcomings (i.e., it does not take into account the measurement site, time of day, or age of the patient). Fever is an adaptive process where the normal body temperature is set at a higher level in response to circulating pyrogens,

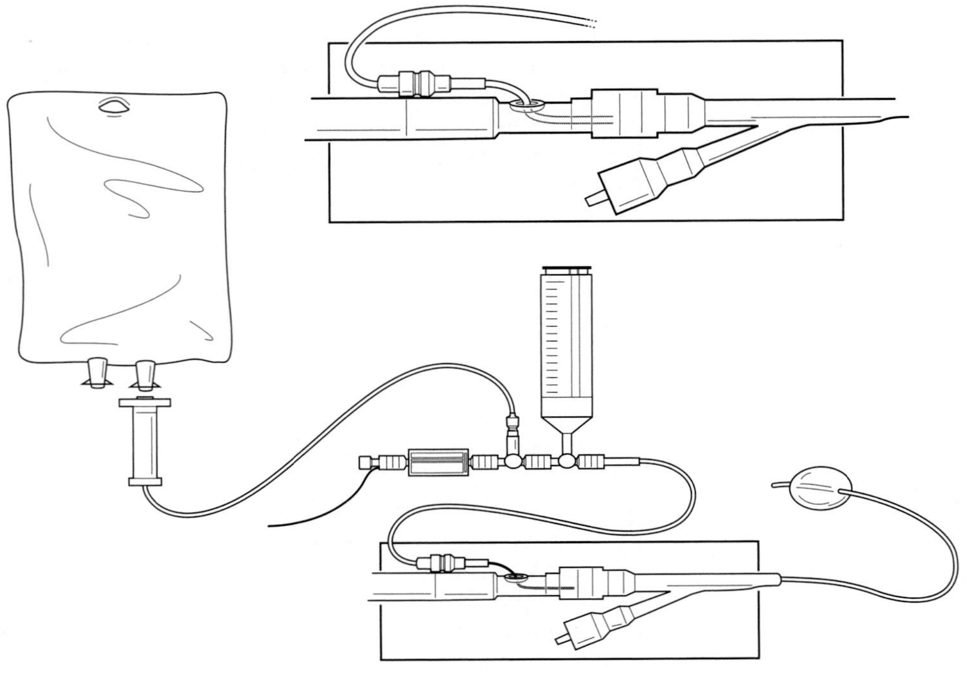

Figure 7-4 Bladder pressure measurement. With the patient in a supine position and using the patient's symphysis pubis as a reference point, a bladder catheter is inserted and the bladder is filled with 100 mL of saline solution. The catheter is connected to a pressure transducer and the pressure is read. A neurogenic, contracted bladder or a pelvic hematoma may alter the reading.

or chemicals released by the body that increase body temperature. This process is distinct from hyperthermia (also called hyperpyrexia), which is not an adaptive response but a condition in which the body is unable to control the core body temperature. The following aspects of the febrile response deserve attention. Fever is a sign of inflammation, not infection (see Chapter 2, Perioperative Management of Surgical Patients). The febrile response is initiated by inflammatory cytokines (e.g., TNF and IL-1B). Therefore, fever is not a specific response to infection, but a response to whatever incites the production of inflammatory cytokines. In many instances, the inciting event is tissue injury, not infection. In fact, approximately 50% of fevers in patients in the ICU are not the direct result of infection. The distinction between inflammation and infection is an important one, not only for the evaluation of fever, but also for the popular practice of using antimicrobial agents to treat a fever. The severity of the febrile response is not an indication of the presence or severity of infection. High fevers and rigors can be associated with noninfectious processes, and minor temperature elevations can accompany life-threatening infections. Noninfectious causes of fever that may be encountered in the ICU are drug fever, neuroleptic malignant syndrome, and systemic inflammatory response syndrome, which are discussed below. Additional causes include thromboembolism, pancreatitis, and adrenal insufficiency.

Drug Fever

Drug fever can be caused by a variety of pharmacologic agents. The diagnosis of drug fever usually is suggested by excluding all other potential causes of fever. When drug fever is suspected, as many drugs as possible should be discontinued and replaced with suitable alternative agents. The fever should disappear in 2 to 3 days if a drug is responsible. The diagnosis can be confirmed by reintroducing the suspected drug, which should produce a fever within hours.

Neuroleptic Malignant Syndrome

A variant of malignant hyperthermia that is triggered by neuroleptic agents (e.g., haloperidol) is known as neuroleptic malignant syndrome. The clinical presentation and management are the same as described for malignant hyperthermia. Haloperidol is a popular sedative in many ICUs, so awareness of this syndrome is important in selected patients (see the discussion of malignant hyperthermia in Chapter 2, Perioperative Management of the Surgical Patient).

Systemic Inflammatory Response Syndrome

Evidence of systemic inflammation (i.e., fever and leukocytosis) in the absence of documented infection or other noninfectious source of fever may represent a clinical entity known as the systemic inflammatory response syndrome (SIRS) (Table 7-3). This syndrome can be triggered by traumatic tissue injury or translocation of endotoxin across the bowel mucosa. Evidence of multiorgan dysfunction may be present. This syndrome can lead to progressive multiorgan failure and death. If perfusion of the intestinal mesentery is reduced, mesenteric ischemia and even infarction can occur. These are often accompanied by abdominal pain and tenderness, but these symptoms may be masked in patients with an altered mental status. Unfortunately, the diagnosis is often difficult because physical findings and laboratory tests are neither sensitive nor specific. Plain radiographs of the abdomen rarely reveal gas in the bowel wall or portal venous gas. Usually, radiographic findings are nonspecific and the diagnosis often requires laparotomy.

Infectious Diseases

Sepsis

Sepsis is a major problem in ICUs throughout the world. It is a leading cause of morbidity, mortality, and health

Table 7-3 Definitions of Systemic Inflammatory Response Syndrome and Sepsis

Systemic inflammatory response syndrome (SIRS): systemic inflammatory response to a wide variety of severe clinical insults. Present if patient has a response greater than or equal to two of these signs or symptoms:
- Temperature > 38°C or < 36°C
- Heart rate > 90 beats per minute
- Respiratory rate > 20 breaths per minute
- Partial pressure of CO_2 < 32 mm Hg
- White blood cell count > 12,000 or < 4000 or an increase in abnormal cells > 10% bands

Sepsis: characterized by generalized inflammatory response that can include abnormal bleeding or clotting in the presence of infection

Septicemia: sepsis that begins with a blood-borne infection

Severe sepsis: sepsis with associated acute organ dysfunction

Septic shock: severe sepsis with cardiovascular system dysfunction. Perfusion of vital organs falls and the organs are deprived of an adequate blood supply care expense. It is estimated to strike 750,000 people every year, with one-third succumbing to death. In addition, the incidence is expected to rise to over 1 million people by 2010 due to the aging population. Severe sepsis has a higher mortality than breast, pancreatic, colorectal, and prostate cancers combined. It is also very expensive to treat, with annual costs recently estimated to be $17 billion in the United States. The clinical manifestation of sepsis ranges from mild to severe and can include shock (see Table 7-3).

Sepsis is caused by an infection, either bacterial, fungal, or viral, which itself may be a complication of trauma, burns, cancer, or other severe illness. While the events that cause an infection to evolve into sepsis are as yet unknown, it is linked to widespread inflammation, coagulation, and suppression of a patient's fibrinolytic response (ability to break down blood clots). It seems that immune modulators (cytokines), usually released by the body to fight an infection, increase to a level that affects the lining of all blood vessels, causing an uncontrolled activation of the coagulation system. The body usually is able to control this increase in cytokine levels with an endogenous substance known as activated protein C. At the endothelial level, activated protein C increases fibrinolysis, prevents adhesion of macrophages and neutrophils to cell membranes, and reverses the activation of the clotting system. Unfortunately, with widespread sepsis, levels of endogenous activated protein C are depleted. The inflammatory process and clot formation causes organ function to deteriorate due to poor perfusion at the end-organ level.

The diagnosis of sepsis should begin by recognizing the signs and symptoms of widespread inflammation (see Table 7-3). When these signs are present, an attempt should be made to obtain appropriate cultures and diagnostic studies. At least two blood cultures should be obtained from two different sites before antimicrobial therapy is initiated. Other diagnostic studies may include specific cultures of body sites suspected to be the source of the infection, quantitative bronchoalveolar lavage for pneumonia, and computed axial tomography for cavitary abscesses.

Treatment usually begins with identifying and eliminating the offending infection with antibiotics. When an abscess is diagnosed, source control may be achieved with surgical or procedural drainage. Supportive care with adequate physiologic monitoring along with vasopressor and volume support should be initiated. New treatment modalities include early goal-directed therapy and recombinant activated protein C. Early therapy directed at achieving normal physiologic goals of resuscitation is necessary to improve survival in sepsis. This early therapy should begin at the first suspicion of sepsis, even before a patient arrives in the ICU. Recombinant activated protein C may be useful in the management of severe sepsis. In a phase 3 trial of 1690 patients, recombinant activated protein C was shown to reduce the mortality in sepsis compared to placebo. The drug had a low incidence of a potentially severe complication of bleeding compared to placebo (2.4% versus 1%).

A campaign called "Surviving Sepsis," supported by all major critical care societies and many health care organizations, has begun an attempt to reduce the high mortality and morbidity of sepsis. A panel of international experts has developed evidence-based guidelines for the systematic and rational approach to the diagnosis and management of sepsis. Though the specific details are beyond the scope of this chapter, it is important to note that this systematic approach for the prevention, diagnosis, and management of such a life-threatening disease is important. The adoption of a "daily goals" sheet addressing all aspects of a patient's ICU management has been shown to assist in consistent management of patients. These daily goals may include such items as head-of-bed elevation (to prevent aspiration), strict glucose control (between 80 mg/dL and 120 mg/dL), appropriate antimicrobial management, mechanical ventilator management guidelines, and deep venous thrombosis prophylaxis. The use of such an organized approach has been shown to reduce the incidence of nosocomial infections and mortality by as much as 35% in a surgical ICU.

Catheter-Related Sepsis

Catheter-related sepsis, usually a preventable, iatrogenic problem, is defined as clinical sepsis that resolves with central venous catheter (CVC) removal. It is diagnosed when there are positive cultures for the same pathogen on the catheter tip and simultaneous positive cultures with alternate-site venous sampling, and no other source of infection. It usually develops from contamination of the catheter at the skin insertion site or contamination of the hub of the catheter. Preventive measures include decontaminating the skin adequately (chlorhexidine is preferred), using barrier precautions, using gauze instead of transparent dressing, and changing the dressing or tubing every 48 hours. Antibiotic- and silver-ion–impregnated catheters have been shown to reduce catheter-related sepsis. In the past, periodic CVC removal and guide-wire exchange were strategies to reduce catheter-related sepsis; however, removing the CVC only when there are clinical signs of sepsis is just as effective.

Ventilator-Associated Pneumonia

Pneumonia is the most common hospital-acquired infection in the ICU, occurring in up to 40% of patients on mechanical ventilation. The clinical criteria used to diagnose pneumonia include fever, leukocytosis, purulent sputum, and a new or progressive radiographic infiltrate, combined with a pathogen on sputum cultures. In mechanically ventilated ICU patients, however, the presence of a potential pathogenic microorganism in sputum samples is unreliable, usually reflecting colonization of the upper airways. For this reason, bronchoscopic sampling techniques using a protected specimen brush or bronchoalveolar lavage are used to bypass upper airway contamination. These techniques are relatively invasive and expensive and should be used only when the diagnosis is not clear.

Pneumonia can be prevented by limiting risk factors such as prolonged intubation and by initiating aggressive respiratory therapy (i.e., early mobilization, incentive spirometry, and selective use of intermittent positive-pressure breathing). Sufficient pain control to allow normal ventilation is critical. Bronchoscopic suctioning and lavage for lobar collapse may be needed when pneumonia fails to resolve despite conventional therapy. The best outcome is achieved when therapy is started in the early stages of pneumonia and when the initial empirical antibiotics are correct. Early pneumonia occurs within 3 days of admission to the surgical ICU. Predominant organisms include oral flora, *Haemophilus influenzae*, and *Staphylococcus aureus*. Late pneumonia (after 3 days) is associated with prolonged mechanical ventilation. Predominant organisms are drug-resistant Gram-negative aerobes; however, resistant Gram-positive aerobes are becoming more common isolates in nosocomial pneumonia.

Urinary Tract Infection

Urinary tract infections (UTIs) are responsible for 35% to 45% of nosocomial infections. In many cases, the predisposing factor is an indwelling bladder catheter. The association between urethral catheters and UTIs may be related to retrograde migration of skin microbes up the urethra along the catheter. Most of the isolates in cases of UTI are Gram-negative enteric pathogens. *Escherichia coli* accounts for one-third of the cases. The second most common organism is *Enterococcus*. *Candida* is also becoming an important pathogen in the etiology of UTI.

Like other cases of nosocomial infection and sepsis related to indwelling catheters, the diagnosis of UTI in the ICU may be difficult. The definition of UTI based on the presence of urine cultures showing 100,000 colony-forming units (CFU) per mL may simply represent contamination in the chronically catheterized patient. On the other hand, significant urosepsis may be present with a bacterial count of less than 100,000 CFU/mL. This difficulty may be overcome by repeated urine cultures showing progressively increasing bacteriuria and estimation of urine leukocyte count. A leukocyte count above 10 cells/mm^3 indicates infection as opposed to contamination.

Most cases of candiduria represent simple colonization, since *Candida* grow readily in the urine of patients maintained on antibiotic therapy, a therapy commonly used in the ICU. It is therefore important to distinguish simple contamination from cases of disseminated candidiasis that require aggressive therapy. The presence of endophthalmitis is pathognomonic of systemic candidiasis. Other findings that suggest systemic candidiasis include the growth of *Candida* from three or more body sites and the sudden deterioration of renal function.

Paranasal Sinusitis

Nasogastric and nasotracheal tubes can block the ostia that drain the paranasal sinuses; this can lead to the accumulation of infected secretions in the paranasal sinuses. The maxillary sinuses are almost always involved, and the resulting acute sinusitis can be an occult source of fever. This complication is reported in 15% to 20% of patients with nasal tubes. Surprisingly, paranasal sinusitis is also found in patients who are intubated orally and have free nares. Purulent drainage from the nares may be absent, and the diagnosis is suggested by radiographic features of sinusitis (i.e., opacification or air-fluid levels in the involved sinuses). Radiographic detection of sinusitis can be accomplished by conventional radiography. The maxillary sinuses can be viewed with a single occipito-mental radiograph, called a Water's view, obtained at the bedside. Computed tomography is also commonly used, especially when a source of sepsis is being sought. It is important to emphasize that 30% to 40% of patients with radiographic evidence of sinusitis do not have an infection documented by culture of aspirated material from the involved sinus. Therefore, radiographic evidence of sinusitis is not sufficient for the diagnosis of purulent sinusitis. The diagnosis must be confirmed by sinus puncture and isolation of one or more pathogens by quantitative culture. Responsible pathogens include streptococci, staphylococci (including *Staphylococcus epidermidis*), enteric pathogens, and yeasts (mostly *Candida albicans*). Polymicrobial infections are common. A brief course of systemic antibiotics is indicated, because septicemia is a complication of purulent sinusitis in critically ill patients. Nasal tubes should also be removed when possible.

Acalculous Cholecystitis

Acalculous cholecystitis is an uncommon but serious disorder reported in up to 1.5% of critically ill patients. It is most common in postoperative patients, trauma victims, and patients receiving parenteral nutrition. The inciting event is edema of the cystic duct, which blocks drainage of the gallbladder. The resulting clinical syndrome includes fever (70% to 95% of cases) and right upper quadrant tenderness (60% to 100% of cases). Diagnosis is often possible with right upper quadrant ultrasound. Perforation of the gallbladder can occur within 48 hours after onset. The treatment of choice is cholecystectomy, or percutaneous cholecystostomy in patients who are too ill to undergo surgery.

Clostridium difficile Colitis

Clostridium difficile colitis is associated with broad-spectrum antibiotic therapy and is the most common cause of infectious diarrhea in hospitalized patients. Pathogenic strains of *C. difficile* produce two exotoxins (toxins A and B), which cause colonic mucosal injury and inflammation. Infection can cause mild diarrhea, self-limited colitis, fulminant pseudomembranous colitis, or life-threatening toxic megacolon. Patients present with fever, abdominal distension, and diarrhea. The diagnosis is made by identification of *C. difficile* toxin in the stool, or by endoscopy in some cases. Treatment includes withholding antibiotics or changing to an antibiotic less likely to cause *C. difficile* colitis. Narcotic antidiarrheal agents should be avoided, so that continued bowel activity can evacuate the toxins. Intravenous fluids and oral metronidazole should be given. Intravenous metronidazole, which is less effective, can be used if the patient cannot take medications orally. Oral vancomycin is also effective. Rarely, fulminant colitis or toxic megacolon can require colectomy.

Neurologic Dysfunction

Daily examination of the critically ill patient is required to detect newly developing neurologic problems. The Glasgow Coma Scale (GCS) is a scoring system that includes individual scores of eye opening, best motor, and best verbal responses (see Table 7-2). It is a simple way of monitoring a patient's global neurologic function. A computed tomography scan of the head is often needed to establish a specific diagnosis in patients with focal neurologic deficits, risk of stroke, or history of head trauma. Lumbar puncture is performed in cases of suspected meningitis.

Brain dysfunction presents as an alteration in mental status ranging from delirium to coma. The most common manifestation of neurologic dysfunction in the ICU is disorientation and agitation. The pathophysiology of this phenomenon is poorly understood, and diagnosis is often difficult to make. Potential causes of neurologic dysfunction in the ICU include organ failure (renal or hepatic), septic encephalopathy, drug withdrawal, cerebrovascular events, and meningitis.

Metabolic encephalopathy is a global neurologic derangement associated with critical illness. Specific etiologies include hypoglycemia, hypercalcemia, acidemia, hyperosmolarity, hypoxia, and uremia. In most surgical ICUs, encephalopathy is a side effect of sedative medications, such as benzodiazepines. In such a case, all other potential etiologies in the differential diagnosis must be excluded. Daily interruption of sedatives in the improving patient can prevent oversedation and reduce a patient's ICU requirements. It should be noted that most acute encephalopathy is often due to severe systemic inflammation; this type of encephalopathy tends to persist and resolves with overall improvement of the patient.

Endocrine Dysfunction

Adrenal Insufficiency

The hypothalamic–pituitary–adrenal axis is stimulated by stress, resulting in proportional increases in corticotropin-releasing hormone (CRH), ACTH, and cortisol. An impairment in this stress response may result in adrenal insufficiency, with potentially catastrophic consequences. It may be difficult to recognize adrenal insufficiency in the ICU. An acute adrenal crisis may present as unexplained hypotension, fever, abdominal pain, or weakness. If adrenal crisis is suspected, 200 mg of hydrocortisone should be administered, along with glucose and saline, while awaiting confirmatory laboratory values (hyponatremia, hyperkalemia, hypoglycemia, azotemia, cortisol < 20 μg/dL). If adrenal insufficiency is present, hydrocortisone should be continued at 100 mg every 8 hours for 2 days, and then the dosage should be tapered. If there is a concern about adrenal insufficiency, the serum cortisol level should be measured. This may be a random level, because there is loss of diurnal variation of cortisol secretion in critical illness. A level greater than 34 μg/dL suggests normal adrenal function, and no further testing is required. On the other hand, less than 15 μg/dL is consistent with hypoadrenalism and corticosteroids should be administered (hydrocortisone, 50 mg, every 6 hours). For cortisol levels between 15 and 34 μg/dL, a cosyntropin stimulation test should be performed. Cosyntropin, 250 μg, is administered, with plasma cortisol measured at 0, 30, and 60 minutes. An increase of less than 9 μg/dL is consistent with hypoadrenalism and should prompt corticosteroid therapy.

Glucose Disorders

Diabetic ketoacidosis (DKA) is typically seen in patients with type I diabetes mellitus, owing to noncompliance with insulin therapy, an illness, or injury. Patients may present with symptoms such as nausea, abdominal pain, excessive thirst, or fatigue. They may be hemodynamically unstable, with an altered level of consciousness. Laboratory findings include hyperglycemia (400 to 800 mg/dL), a high anion gap, metabolic acidosis, and the presence of serum and urine ketones. Hyperkalemia is common despite total body potassium deficit. Mortality from DKA can approach 10% to 15%, so aggressive treatment is critical. Normal saline is infused to replace intravascular volume, along with regular insulin (0.1 to 0.2 U/kg bolus followed by 0.1 U/kg/hr). Glucose should be monitored frequently. Once it is below 250 mg/dL, the intravenous fluid should be changed to 5% dextrose in hypotonic saline. The insulin infusion should be titrated but continued until ketoacidosis abates. Hypokalemia and hypophosphatemia commonly develop during therapy and should be corrected.

Hyperglycemia (defined as blood glucose level > 200 mg/dL) in the absence of a diagnosis of diabetes mellitus is quite common in critically ill patients. The phenomenon of stress-related hyperglycemia appears to be related to insulin resistance resulting from the release of counterregulatory hormones (e.g., glucagon, epinephrine, norepinephrine, glucocorticoids, growth hormone) and cytokines (e.g., TNF, IL-1, IL-6). It is typically seen shortly after admission to an ICU and resolves as the catabolic illness subsides. However, ongoing metabolic dysregulation and protracted hyperglycemia may persist in some patients, particularly those with untreated infection or ongoing injury. The consequences of protracted hyperglycemia include increased postoperative infectious complications and worse outcomes following myocardial infarction, stroke, and head injury. Increasing attention has been directed toward insulin as a therapeutic drug in critical illness. It has potent anabolic as well as immunomodulatory effects that may favorably impact the course of critical illness. In fact, maintaining serum glucose levels strictly between 80 and 120 mg/dL with insulin drips has been shown to reduce the infection rates in ICUs.

Thyroid Storm

Thyroid storm occurs in patients with existing thyrotoxicosis that is unrecognized or uncontrolled. The abrupt administration of iodides without the protection of antithyroid drugs may also precipitate a thyroid storm. Any traumatic event, such as surgery, or infection may complicate thyrotoxicosis and provoke thyroid storm. Tachycardia, high fever, and mental status changes are the most prominent early symptoms. Patients are intensely irritable and manifest confusion, delirium, or perhaps coma. Tachycardia is initially sinus, but if thyroid storm persists, high-output cardiac congestive failure may result. Irreversible cardiac failure usually is the mode of death. Treatment of thyroid storm, which has a mortality of 10% to 20%, involves control of the catecholamine-induced cardiac symptoms. Propranolol or other beta-blockers are given 1 mg/min intravenously to a maximum of 10 mg to control the tachycardia and stabilize the cardiovascular system. Propylthiouracil, 200 mg, and potassium iodide, 5 to 10 drops, are given to decrease triiodothyronine (T_3) and thyroxine (T_4) release. Hydrocortisone, 200 mg intravenously as an initial dose and 100 mg every 8 hours thereafter, diminishes thyroid hormone release.

Cardiac Dysfunction

Abnormalities in cardiac function in the ICU may be related to abnormal cardiac rhythm, impaired ventricular contractility, or the occurrence of cardiac tamponade. Abnormal cardiac rhythm, such as sinus tachycardia, may be a normal physiologic response to the underlying stress or a response to other problems commonly encountered in the ICU, such as fever or hypovolemia. The prime concern with any cardiac arrhythmia is to determine if the arrhythmia is symptomatic. Symptomatic arrhythmias will be associated with hemodynamic instability and should be treated aggressively. All cardiac arrhythmias should be evaluated with a 12-lead electrocardiogram (ECG). Serum electrolytes and arterial blood gas should be measured and any abnormality corrected (abnormal potassium or magnesium levels, and hypoxia or hypercapnia).

In cases of left ventricular failure, signs of hypoperfusion, or sepsis with hypotension, the use of a pulmonary artery catheter may be essential for directing therapy. Prior to using inotropic agents for impaired cardiac contractility, it is essential to determine the adequacy of preload or ventricular filling. The ischemic myocardium loses compliance and higher filling pressure may be needed to achieve effective diastolic distension and improve contractility (Fig. 7-5). Once this has been achieved, inotropic agents can be used. Dobutamine infusion (starting at 5 μg/kg/min) is the inotropic agent of choice. It increases myocardial contractility and has a beneficial mild vasodilatory effect that reduces afterload and augments ventricular stroke volume (Table 7-4).

Respiratory Failure

Respiratory failure is caused by a variety of disease processes (Table 7-5). It occurs when the pulmonary system is unable to adequately provide gas exchange, that is, the absorption of oxygen and the excretion of carbon dioxide. The inability to absorb oxygen (hypoxemia) and the inability to excrete carbon dioxide (hypercapnia) are difficult to diagnose on physical exam. As mentioned earlier, pulse oximetry is a noninvasive and reliable means to assess hypoxemia. Noninvasive detection of hypercapnia is not as reliable as the measurement of hypoxemia. The end tidal carbon dioxide monitor can give an estimate of the carbon dioxide level, a measurement that can be trended. However, the best way to accurately diagnose acute respiratory failure is to measure arterial blood gases.

It is generally accepted that a partial pressure of arterial oxygen (PaO_2) less than 50 mm Hg, a partial pressure of arterial carbon dioxide ($PaCO_2$) greater than 50 mm Hg, or a blood pH less than 7.30 are signs of respiratory failure. These correlate with a failure of oxygenation or ventilation, which means the failure of oxygen and/or carbon dioxide to diffuse across the alveolar membrane. Hypoxemia or hypercapnia or both can be present in a single patient. If they are present, the patient requires urgent treatment.

Hypoxemia requires raising the arterial PaO_2 to greater than 50 mm Hg. This can be done by providing supplemental oxygen to the cooperative patient. Nasal cannulas usually cannot exceed a fractional inspiratory concentration of oxygen (FIO_2) greater than 30%. Various facemasks can supply oxygen, but at best these supply an FIO_2 of only up to 60%. Only oxygenation via an endotracheal tube can supply inspired oxygen up to 100%.

The treatment for hypercapnia or failure of ventilation almost always requires endotracheal tube intubation and mechanical ventilation (MV). This is usually evident when a patient manifests an increase in the work of breathing, evident by tachypnea, agitation, and fatigue of respiratory muscles, while trying to maintain arterial blood gases. Overall, the decision to artificially ventilate a patient is based on the patient developing signs of respiratory failure; however, in isolated circumstances, MV is used to assist in managing other conditions, such as reduction of intracranial pressure in patients with closed head injuries. A fuller description of MV appears at the end of the chapter.

Liver Failure

The most common cause of liver failure is preexisting liver disease. Patients with cirrhosis, alcoholic hepatitis, or fatty infiltration caused by alcoholism requiring surgical inter-

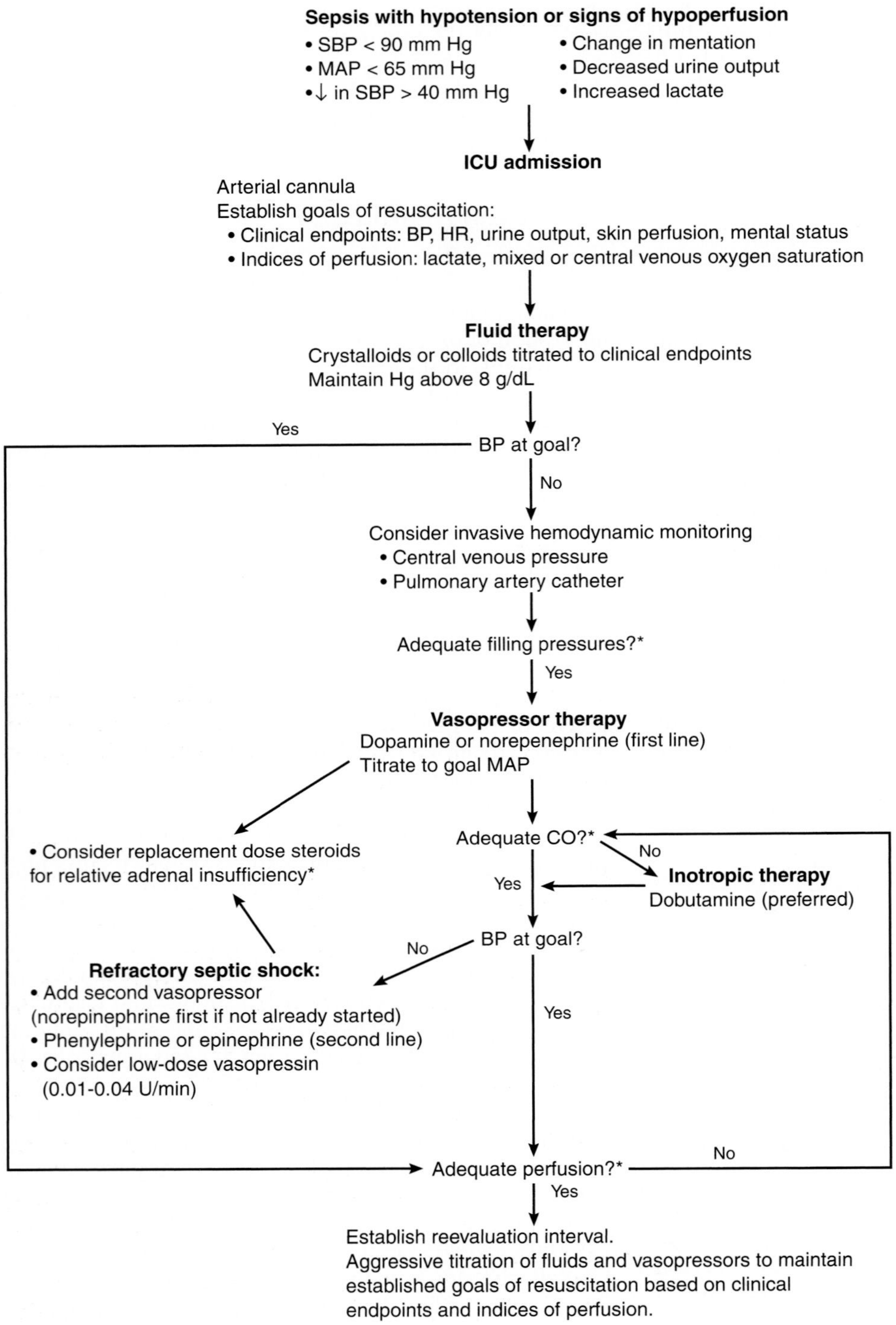

Figure 7-5 Suggested algorithm for hemodynamic support of adult patients with severe sepsis and septic shock. BP, blood pressure; CO, cardiac output; Hg, hemoglobin; HR, heart rate; ICU, intensive care unit; MAP, mean arterial pressure; SBP, systolic blood pressure. *Adequate cardiac filling pressures can be assessed by response of cardiac output (CO) to increases of pulmonary artery occlusion pressure. Maximal benefit is usually achieved at pulmonary artery occlusion pressure, 12–15 mm Hg.

vention are prone to liver failure postoperatively. In patients with established liver disease such as cirrhosis, general anesthesia should be avoided if possible. In cirrhosis, the portal vein's contribution to hepatic perfusion of the liver is diminished, and the hepatic artery supplies at least 50% of hepatic blood flow. Since the hepatic artery is a splanchnic artery, general anesthesia, hypotension, shock, blood loss, and hypovolemia cause splanchnic vasoconstriction and hepatic ischemia. Thus, both portal flow and hepatic artery flow are markedly decreased. A regional or epidural anesthetic is preferred in patients with liver disease.

Any stress, even without infection, can cause liver failure beginning on the third to fifth postoperative day. Som-

Table 7-4 Vasoactive Drugs and Receptor Activities for the Treatment of Shock

Class and Drug	Blood Pressure	Systemic Vascular Resistance	Cardiac Output	Heart Rate
Alpha only				
Phenylephrine	↑↑↑	↑↑↑↑	↓↓↓	↓↓↓
Alpha and beta				
Norepinephrine	↑↑	↑↑↑	↓↓	↓↓±
Epinephrine	↑±	↑±	↑↑	↑↑↑
Dopamine	↑↑	↑↑	↑↑	↑
Beta only				
Isoproterenol	↑±	↓↓	↑↑↑↑	↑↑↑↑
Dobutamine	↓↓	↓↓↓	↑↑↑	↑↑
Beta-blocker				
Propanolol	+↓	±	↓↓↓	↓↓↓↓
Metoprolol	↓↓↓	↓	↓↓	↓↓↓
Other				
Nitroglycerine	±↓	↓↓	↑↑	±
Hydralazine	↓↓↓	↓↓↓	↑↑	↑↑
Prazosin	↓↓↓	↓↓	↑↑	±
Nitroprusside	↓↓	↓↓↓	↑↑↑	±↑

Source: Pettit TW, Cobb JP. Critical care. In: Doherty GM, Bauma DS, Creswell LL, et al., eds. *The Washington Manual of Surgery.* Philadelphia, PA.: Lippincott Williams & Wilkins, 1996:166.

nolence, jaundice, diminished urine output, and ascites are signs of incipient hepatic failure. Other signs include an elevated bilirubin level, usually of the indirect fraction, minor elevation of transaminase level, a decreased albumin level, and a lengthening of prothrombin time. Reversible causes include hypovolemia, hypokalemia, hypomagnesemia, gastrointestinal bleeding, constipation, and remote infection. Treatment of postoperative liver failure includes the correction of electrolyte abnormalities (especially hypokalemic alkalosis); the administration of neomycin, cathartics, or lactulose orally or by enema; and nutritional support. Enteral nutrition is best if the patient tolerates tube feedings.

Table 7-5 Common Causes of Respiratory Failure

Inadequate Ventilation
Airway obstruction
Atelectasis
Reactive airway disease (e.g., asthma)
Drug overdose
Nerve injury (e.g., spinal cord, phrenic nerve)
Respiratory muscle weakness
Inadequate Perfusion
Pulmonary embolism
Right-to-left shunt
Inadequate Ventilation and Perfusion
Chronic obstructive pulmonary disease (COPD)
Acute respiratory distress syndrome (ARDS)
Pneumonia
Pulmonary venous hypertension (e.g., congestive heart failure)
Tension pneumothorax

Adapted from Norton J, et al. *Essential Practice of Surgery: Basic Science and Clinical Evidence.* New York, NY: Springer Verlag, 2003.

Acute Renal Failure

In the presence of hypotension, catecholamine release and norepinephrine stimulation by the sympathetic nervous system decreases renal blood flow. When caring for an emergency patient, it is important to normalize urine output before surgery and, if time permits, resuscitate the patient. In the elderly, it is not *rapid* rehydration or transfusion, but *over*hydration and *over*transfusion that cause congestive failure. If the patient's volume status is in question before surgery, a pulmonary artery catheter should be placed, the patient's fluid and volume status corrected, and the operation delayed, if feasible, until urine output is adequate. In transfusion reaction, sepsis, myocardial dysfunction, or crush injury, diuresis should be established using mannitol and furosemide given only when volume status is restored.

Prerenal dysfunction is identified by a BUN:creatinine ratio of 20:1 or greater. This occurs often with dehydration or underresuscitation of patients before or after a surgical procedure. If a patient with prerenal azotemia undergoes surgery without adequate resuscitation, acute renal failure likely ensues. The diagnosis is fairly clear when the patient is hypotensive, is overtly hypovolemic with decreased skin turgor, and has sunken eyes and flaccid skin.

Intrinsic damage that can occur following surgery includes a series of merged forms of tubular damage, known as acute tubular necrosis. The most common cause is diminished renal perfusion. Prolonged and sustained hypotension in the presence of sepsis, blood loss, hypovolemia, dehydration, or myocardial infarction results in prolonged ischemia of the renal parenchyma. In addition to acute tubular necrosis, pigment nephropathy and drug nephrotoxicity are prominent.

Preventing Acute Renal Failure

Certain measures can be taken to prevent acute renal failure. A patient with inadequate urine output should not be subjected to general anesthesia, because acute tubular necrosis can result. Radiographic contrast agents cause renal failure in 1% to 10% of ICU patients. Injury is due to direct nephrotoxic effect and hypovolemia from osmotic diuresis. Prestudy hydration is partially protective. If possible, antibiotics that are not nephrotoxic should be used. In low-flow states, mannitol, bicarbonate, and diuresis induced by furosemide should be used. Mannitol increases renal cortical blood flow and produces an osmotic diuresis. It can protect the tubules by preventing tubular precipitation of metabolite. Renal perfusion may be increased by a low dose of dopamine, 2 to 5 μg/kg/min, which increases systolic function. If the volume status is in question, central venous pressure monitoring or, preferably, monitoring of left-sided filling pressure with a pulmonary artery catheter is advisable.

In a patient with renal failure, there are a number of goals: (1) avoid overhydration, which results in congestive heart failure and the need for hemofiltration or dialysis; (2) avoid dialysis, if possible; (3) avoid toxic ionic damage, such as hyperkalemia; and (4) provide nutrition. The most immediate threat in many patients with acute renal failure is hyperkalemia. Serum electrolyte levels should be monitored closely. When the serum potassium level reaches 5.5 mEq/dL, a sudden rise in potassium can occur, causing ECG changes. ECG changes include peaked T-waves with progression to a sinus bradycardia and a sine-wave rhythm with hypotension and death. Deaths from hyperkalemia are avoidable. The emergency treatment of hyperkalemia includes the infusion of calcium, hypertonic dextrose solution, and insulin. Thereafter, sodium polystyrene sulfonate (Kayexalate), 5 g given by enema or by mouth, should be administered. Dialysis is undertaken in patients with acute renal failure for critical ionic excesses, volume overload, or a BUN concentration of greater than 80 to 100 mg/dL.

Renal Replacement Therapy

Renal replacement therapy is indicated in the treatment of complications of renal failure that failed medical treatment. These include hypervolemia, acidemia, refractory hyperkalemia, uremic pericarditis, and platelet dysfunction. A large catheter inserted in a central vein is required for dialysis. Renal replacement therapy can be intermittent or continuous. Hemodynamic instability often ensues during intermittent renal replacement therapy as a result of rapid fluid shifts from the intravascular compartment through the filter. This is usually well tolerated. Continuous venovenous hemodialysis (CVVHD) is used in patients with hemodynamic instability, usually in the setting of shock. It decreases the rate of fluid shifts and improves hemodynamic stability. The main disadvantage of CVVHD is the need for continuous heparinization.

Multiple Organ Dysfunction Syndrome

Multiple organ dysfunction syndrome (MODS) is characterized by progressive but potentially reversible physiologic failure of two or more organ systems that begins after resuscitation from a life-threatening event. The syndrome involves variable degrees of dysfunction affecting several organ systems. With each successive organ dysfunction, the mortality increases significantly (Fig. 7-6). Though the mortality from MODS has improved over the last decade due to earlier monitoring and successful resuscitation, it still is quite high. Progression of organ dysfunction can lead to complete organ failure. Patients with two-organ dysfunction approach 60% mortality.

Acute respiratory distress syndrome (ARDS) is the prototypical expression of respiratory dysfunction in MODS. In its mildest form, this type of respiratory dysfunction is characterized by tachypnea, hypocapnia, and hypoxemia. As lung injury evolves, increases in both hypoxemia and the effort of breathing makes mechanical ventilation necessary. Increased capillary permeability and neutrophil influx are the earliest pathologic events in ARDS. Further lung injury is caused by the process of repair, which involves fibrosis and the deposition of hyaline material, and by further lung trauma, resulting from positive-pressure mechanical ventilation. Lung involvement in ARDS is heterogeneous, with areas of functional and aerated alveoli interspersed with areas of nonfunctional alveoli. Impaired lung function is reflected in a reduced alveolar PAO_2. To ensure adequate oxygen delivery to the tissues, mechanical ventilation must be instituted and FIO_2 increased. The ratio of PAO_2 to FIO_2 is a sensitive and objective measurement of oxygenation impairment and is a reliable measure of physiologic respiratory dysfunction. By consensus, ARDS is defined as a PAO_2:FIO_2 ratio less than 200 mm Hg

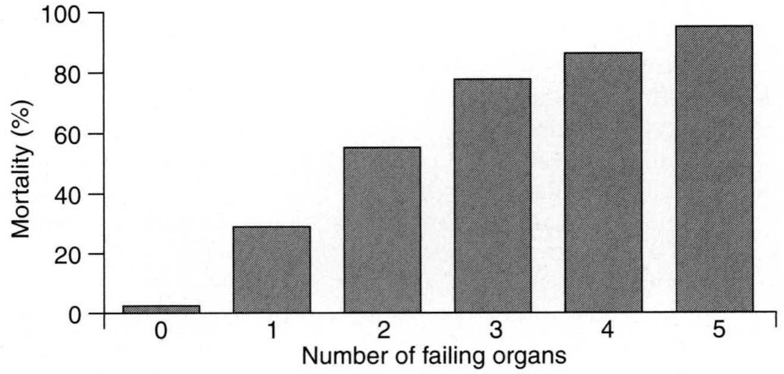

Figure 7-6 Increase in mortality as a function of number of failing organs. (From Awad S. State of the art therapy for severe sepsis and multiorgan system dysfunction. *Am J Surg* 2003;186:5[A]. Used with permission.)

associated with bilateral fluffy pulmonary infiltrates and a pulmonary capillary wedge pressure less than 18 mm Hg.

Endotracheal intubation and positive-pressure ventilation are the mainstay of support for critically ill patients with respiratory failure. In unstable patients, it is best to use a controlled ventilatory mode (e.g., pressure-control ventilation) rather than a spontaneous breathing mode (e.g., pressure-support ventilation). Oxygenation can be optimized through the use of PEEP, which can also decrease the accumulation of interstitial fluid and minimize ventilator-associated lung injury. Ventilation with large tidal volumes and high peak inspiratory pressures contributes to lung injury, and it has been shown that the survival of ARDS patients can be improved by using low tidal volumes (6 mL/kg). Pressure-controlled ventilatory techniques limit peak airway pressures to a maximum predetermined level, optimizing gas exchange by inverting the inspiration:expiration ratio (I:E) from its normal value of 1:2 to 1:1 or higher. They also change the shape of the inspiratory flow curve (normally square) to one in which flow initially is rapid, then decelerates. Although oxygenation can be maintained with low tidal volumes, ventilation is jeopardized and CO_2 levels rise (called permissive hypercapnia). Hypercapnia per se does not appear to be deleterious; animal studies suggest that increased levels of CO_2 can be independently beneficial to critically ill patients. For patients with refractory hypoxemia, high-frequency oscillation appears to be a promising ventilatory mode.

Clinical or subclinical renal dysfunction is common in MODS. Early-onset renal dysfunction is usually caused by hypotension and decreased renal blood flow. The etiology of late-onset renal failure is multifactorial and includes prerenal factors (e.g., decreased cardiac output and hypovolemia) and the cumulative renal effects of nephrotoxic agents (e.g., medications and radiocontrast material). Physiologic signs of renal dysfunction in MODS are decreased urine output and a rising serum creatinine level. Preventing renal ischemia and hypoperfusion through the maintenance of cardiac output and treatment of cardiac dysfunction is essential. The use of nephrotoxic medications should be avoided.

Hepatic dysfunction in multiple organ failure involves two clinical syndromes. The first, ischemic hepatitis or shock liver, usually follows profound hypotension with splanchnic hypoperfusion. Early elevations of aminotransferase levels are striking and can be associated with an increased international normalized ratio and hypoglycemia; centrilobular necrosis is evident histologically. Successful resuscitation of the shock state results in rapid normalization of these biochemical abnormalities. The second syndrome, ICU jaundice, is more common than ischemic hepatitis and usually evolves many days after the physiologic insult. Conjugated hyperbilirubinemia and aminotransferase levels are elevated along with alterations of hepatic synthetic function. This leads to hyperbilirubinemia and cholestatic jaundice. Histologic features include intrahepatic cholestasis, steatosis, and Kupffer cell hyperplasia. The pathogenesis is multifactorial and includes ongoing hepatic ischemia, cholestasis induced by total parenteral nutrition, and drug toxicity. Elevated serum bilirubin is the most common sign of hepatic dysfunction of MODS. The hepatic dysfunction of critical illness is not considered to be life threatening in itself, and no hepatic-specific supportive therapy is indicated.

Both peripheral vascular and myocardial function are altered in MODS. Characteristic changes in the peripheral vasculature include a reduction in vascular resistance and an increase in microvascular permeability, causing a hyperdynamic circulatory profile and peripheral edema. Both alterations jeopardize tissue oxygenation. Reduced vascular resistance causes shunting in the microvasculature. Edema increases the distance across which blood oxygen must diffuse to reach the cell. Shunting is signaled by reduced arteriovenous oxygen extraction and increased mixed venous oxygen saturation ($S\bar{v}O_2$). Biventricular dilation with a reduction in the right and left ventricular ejection fractions may occur. Right ventricular dysfunction is particularly prominent, perhaps because of increased pulmonary vascular resistance caused by concomitant lung injury. Cardiovascular dysfunction of MODS appears clinically as increased peripheral edema with hypotension that is refractory to volume challenge and therapeutically in the use of vasoactive agents to support the circulation. Nitric oxide is being considered as an associated factor in both the peripheral vasodilatation and the myocardial depression associated with critical illness.

Abnormalities of central and peripheral nervous system function are common in critical illness. Central nervous system (CNS) dysfunction occurs in up to 70% of critically ill patients, usually presenting as reduced consciousness without localizing signs. Its pathophysiology is incompletely understood. Proposed mechanisms include the direct effects of proinflammatory mediators on cerebral function, vasogenic cerebral edema, areas of cerebral infarction related to hypotension, and alterations in the blood-brain barrier causing changes in the composition of the interstitial fluid. Peripheral nervous system dysfunction, known as critical illness polyneuropathy, is also common in MODS, though its clinical presentation is more subtle than CNS dysfunction. Peripheral nervous system dysfunction can present as failure of weaning from mechanical ventilation or as limb weakness with relative sparing of the cranial nerves.

The most common hematologic abnormality of critical illness is thrombocytopenia, occurring in approximately 20% of all ICU patients. Causes include increased consumption of platelets, intravascular sequestration, and impaired thrombopoiesis caused by suppression of bone marrow function. In addition, heparin-induced thrombocytopenia, resulting from antibodies to complexes of heparin and platelet factors, develops in as many as 10% of patients receiving heparin (see heparin-induced thrombocytopenia section above). The most fulminant expression of hematologic dysfunction in MODS is disseminated intravascular coagulation (DIC), which is characterized by

Table 7-6 Features Evaluated in Brain Death

Feature	Evaluation	Response Confirming Brain Death
Coma or unresponsiveness	Assess patient's motor response to painful stimuli (e.g., supraorbital pressure or nail-bed pressure)	Absent
Absence of brainstem reflexes	Assess patient's corneal, pharyngeal, and tracheal reflexes	Absent
Apnea	Assess patient's spontaneous respiration	Sustained apnea when disconnected from respirator

derangements in platelet numbers, clotting times, and fibrin degradation products in plasma.

Gastrointestinal dysfunction in the context of MODS most commonly involves stress gastric ulceration leading to upper gastrointestinal bleeding. This was once a relatively common complication, but improved techniques of resuscitation and hemodynamic support, earlier diagnosis of infection, and the widespread use of stress ulcer prophylaxis have reduced its incidence to fewer than 4% of ICU patients. Other manifestations of gastrointestinal dysfunction in MODS include ileus and intolerance of enteral feeding, pancreatitis, and acalculous cholecystitis.

Determining Brain Death

Brain death refers to the irreversible cessation of activity in the cerebrum and brainstem. A qualified physician should determine brain death. The surgeon must recognize conditions that can mimic brain death, know the procedure for the apnea test, know indications for confirmatory tests, and know how to manage physiologic changes associated with brain death. Early identification of potential organ donor candidates is important, but selection of these candidates can proceed only after the clinical diagnosis of brain death has been established and family members have given their consent (see Chapter 24, Transplantation).

The guidelines for determining brain death in adults and children have been published. The clinical diagnosis of brain death requires the following: (1) the presence of a cause compatible with brain death; (2) the absence of complicating medical conditions that can confound clinical assessment; (3) the absence of drug intoxication or poisoning; (4) a core temperature of at least 32°C, because brainstem reflexes may be absent at lower temperatures.

In most patients, a computed tomography (CT) scan will show an abnormality that is compatible with brain death. In patients with normal CT scans, the diagnosis should be reconsidered, unless there is certainty about the mechanism that has led to brain death (e.g., ischemic–anoxic brain death caused by cardiac arrest or asphyxia). Severe electrolyte, acid–base, and endocrine disturbances should be excluded, and a drug screen may be helpful to detect a specific drug or poison. Table 7-6 shows the cardinal features of brain death that are evaluated during clinical testing, and Table 7-7 lists the precautions taken to minimize such confounding factors as marked hypotension, severe cardiac dysrhythmias, and desaturations.

Tests can be repeated after 6 hours to confirm the clinical diagnosis. When the specific components of clinical testing cannot be evaluated reliably (e.g., because of drug intoxication, altered metabolic status, shock, or hypothermia), other confirmatory tests are needed. These tests include electroencephalogram, cerebral angiography, single-photon emission CT, and transcranial Doppler ultrasonography. Angiography is the most reliable and rapid way of establishing brain death. In children younger than 5 years, caution is needed in applying the neurologic criteria for brain death. Compared with adult brains, the brains of infants and young children are more resistant to cerebral damage, and children are more likely to recover substantial functions, even after exhibiting prolonged unresponsiveness.

MECHANICAL VENTILATION

MV is an important tool in supporting patients, not only through surgery, but also during the postoperative period,

Table 7-7 Precautions Taken to Minimize Confounding Factors When Evaluating Brain Death

Core temperature must be 32°C or more (rewarm the patient if temperature is less)
Systolic blood pressure (BP) must be 90 mm Hg or more (use dopamine if BP is lower)
Fluid balance must be positive for 6 hours or more (use vasopressors if this cannot be accomplished)
Arterial P_{CO_2} must be 40 mm Hg or more (decrease minute ventilation if P_{CO_2} is lower)
Arterial P_{O_2} must be 200 mm Hg or more (inspired oxygen fraction = 1.0 for 10 minutes)

should respiratory failure persist. MV is the use of machines or devices to provide oxygenation and/or ventilation from the atmosphere to a patient's alveolar capillary interchange. Its purpose is to provide appropriate levels of gas exchange and to allow a patient's physiologic processes to function normally. A student entering the critical care rotation or following a postoperative patient must understand the basic mechanics and interactions of machine-produced ventilation. The mechanisms of flow, pressure, and the patient's own effort all intertwine to challenge the practitioner in the management of MV. This section discusses only the most basic modes of mechanical ventilation and leaves the newer modes to more advanced texts.

Early devices attempting artificial ventilation, known as iron lungs, applied negative pressure, which is the physiologic basis of human ventilation. In humans the synaptic firing of the diaphragm and the mechanics of the extraaccessory muscles expanding the chest wall cause atmospheric air to move into the lungs, expanding the alveoli and allowing gas exchange to take place.

Today, positive-pressure ventilation is the most common mode of providing air exchange and pulmonary support in patients. This mode of ventilation was developed during the Danish polio epidemic of the mid-1900s. The need for pulmonary support was so enormous and the lack of iron lungs so prevalent that techniques for supporting patients in the operating room were used to support patients stricken by polio. Using cuffed endotracheal tubes, artificial breaths were applied by forcing positive-pressure air into the patient's lungs. Machines using these techniques were soon developed and evolved into the basic ones used today. The development of modern-day mechanical ventilators corresponds with the development of ICUs.

The basic goal of mechanical ventilation is to provide oxygen and remove carbon dioxide in a safe, efficient manner. Lung inflation occurs during mechanical ventilation when positive pressure is applied at the airway. Positive-pressure ventilation occurs when air is blown into the lungs by way of a mask or endotracheal tube. This inflation occurs due to the buildup of positive pressure from the mouth and is transformed down into the alveoli. The alveoli expand from the pressure that builds up and becomes more positive. This positive pressure is transmitted across the pleura. At the end of inspiration, the ventilator stops insufflation, and positive pressure stops being delivered. Mouth pressure returns to ambient pressure (zero), and alveoli air, still being more positive, flows out of the lungs due to the pressure gradient.

Although ventilators are an essential part of patient support and are credited with saving countless lives, lung injury related to ventilators occurs and can be due to many causes. These causes are referred to as ventilator-induced lung injury (VILI) and include barotrauma, volutrauma, biotrauma, atelectatic trauma, and oxygen toxicity. When alveoli are stretched excessively by positive pressure, they can tear and cause significant damage. This is often recognized by extraalveolar air in the mediastinum, pericardium, subcutaneous tissues, pleura, and vasculature. This risk increases with greater alveoli distension over time. However, this alveolar distension and injury can be minimized by using low tidal volume ventilation.

Using high concentrations of oxygen has been shown to cause significant scarring of alveolar membranes similar to that seen in ARDS. Amounts greater than 0.80 are more hazardous, but some animal studies show that amounts above room air (0.21) can, over time, cause histologic changes similar to ARDS. The goal is to minimize problems and maintain the lowest possible fraction of inspired oxygen needed to keep alveolar SAO_2 at greater than 91%.

Atelectasis occurs when alveolar air is reabsorbed, and the pressure difference causes the alveoli to collapse. The alveoli then require a significant amount of inflation to reopen. This inspiratory force can cause significant damage if performed by too much positive pressure or tidal volume.

Though a detailed discussion is beyond the scope of this chapter, biotrauma is fast becoming a better understood part of mechanical ventilation. As discussed in the stress response section above, cytokines released by inflamed or damaged tissues circulate throughout the body. These chemicals cause reactions at the endothelial level of all end organs. If the lung is involved, these reactions can further inflame the lung, decreasing alveolar gas exchange. The harmful effects of MV have now been shown to facilitate cytokine release, thus increasing pulmonary inflammation in a potentially vicious cycle. Consequently, to minimize ventilator-induced lung damage, the lowest possible settings necessary for adequate ventilation and oxygenation should be used.

Basic Ventilator Modes

Lung protective strategies have been developed to minimize the effects of ventilator-induced lung injury. To provide appropriate pulmonary support, the critical care practitioner must balance the need for pressure, volume, and inspired oxygen to the benefit of gas exchange. Ventilator settings should provide basic levels of gas exchange while preventing overdistension of alveoli at end inspiration.

Of the many types and modes of mechanical ventilators, the basic modes of ventilation are assist-control, pressure-control, pressure-support, synchronized intermittent mandatory, and controlled mechanical. These modes are discussed below and detailed in graphic form in Figure 7-7. The advantages and disadvantages among the common modes of mechanical ventilation are found in Table 7-8. Many newer modes of ventilation are frequently being developed and used in critical care areas, but they need further evaluation and clinical study before they are widely accepted.

When the patient is placed on mechanical ventilation, the mode is chosen based on patient comfort and requirements. The rate and volumes are adjusted to allow improved exchange of carbon dioxide to appropriate levels. In all the modes of ventilation, whether time-cycled, volume-

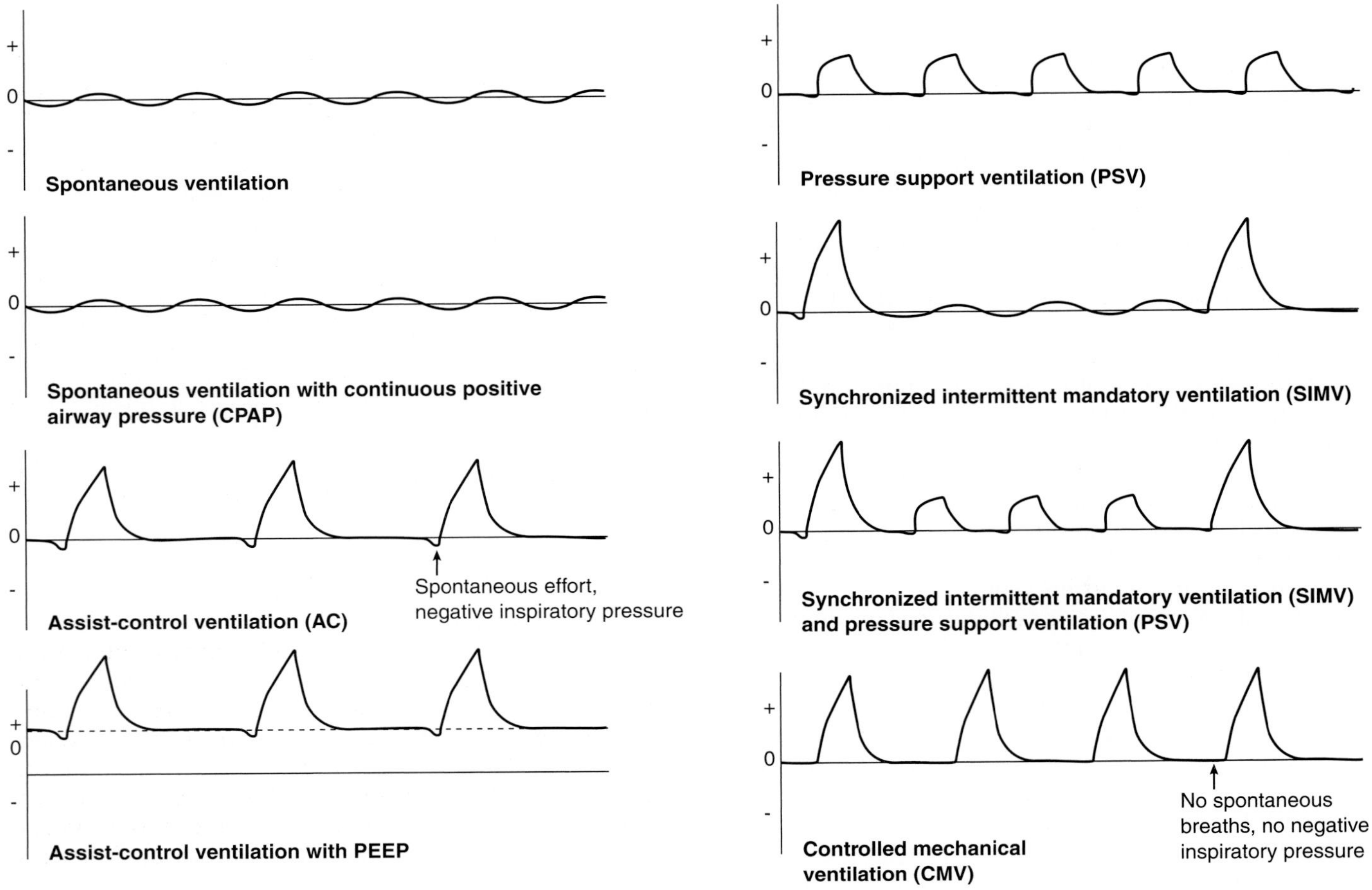

Figure 7-7 Airway pressure and flow tracings for spontaneous breathing, for continuous positive airway pressure, and for commonly used modes of mechanical ventilation. Time is represented on the horizontal axis and pressure on the vertical axis. The zero line reflects atmospheric pressure. PEEP, positive end-expiratory pressure. (From *Fundamentals of Critical Care Support Manual*. DesPlaines, IL: Society of Critical Care Medicine, 2001:5-4. Used with permission.)

Table 7-8 Potential Advantages and Disadvantages of Selected Modes of Mechanical Ventilation

Mode	Advantages	Disadvantages
Assist-control ventilation (AC)	Patient can increase ventilatory support; reduced work of breathing compared to spontaneous breathing	Potential adverse hemodynamic effects; may lead to inappropriate hyperventilation
Pressure support ventilation (PSV)	Patient comfort; improved patient–ventilator interaction; decreased work of breathing	Apnea alarm is only backup; variable patient tolerance
Synchronized intermittent mandatory ventilation (SIMV)	Less interference with normal cardiovascular performance	Increased work of breathing compared to AC
Controlled mechanical ventilation (CMV)	Rests muscles of respiration	Requires use of sedation/neuromuscular blockade; potential adverse hemodynamic effects

Source: *Fundamentals of Critical Care Support Course Manual*. DesPlaines, IL: Society of Critical Care Medicine, 2001:5–5.

cycled, or pressure-cycled breaths, the fraction of inspired oxygen and PEEP are adjusted independently. To improve a patient's oxygenation, these are increased to allow improved oxygen gas exchange. By increasing the percentage of oxygen into the alveoli, more is allowed to diffuse across the alveolar membrane. Increasing PEEP allows alveoli to open over time, thus increasing the number of alveoli participating in gas exchange (Table 7-9). Likewise, to improve a patient's ventilation, carbon dioxide needs to be eliminated. This is done with increasing minute ventilation, either by increasing the respiratory rate or inspired tidal volume.

The three types of ventilator breaths can best be explained by what is called the cycling mechanism of the ventilator. The "cycle" mechanism is the variable that terminates inspiration and is usually either the volume, the time, or the flow. A *volume-cycled breath* allows delivery of a preset tidal volume. With volume breaths, if there is significant resistance or poor lung compliance, there will be increases in the peak pressure of inspiration with the continued delivery of the set tidal volume. In a *time-cycled breath*, also called a pressure-control breath, the total amount of positive pressure is delivered over a preset time. With this type of breath, any change of airway resistance or compliance will alter the tidal volume delivered. A *flow-cycled breath* is one with a constant pressure applied throughout the inspired breath; the breath is terminated when the flow rate decreases to around 25% of the initial flow rate. In this breath, the patient's own decrease in inspiratory flow will end inspiration.

In general, a ventilator can be set to deliver volume or pressure over a set period of time. In a volume-control mode, the ventilator delivers volume and the pressure generated is dependent on the compliance of the lung and the resistance of the airway system. In a pressure-control mode, pressure is delivered and the tidal volume is then dependent on the resistance and compliance of the respiratory system. In pressure-support mode, a patient's inspiratory flow triggers the ventilator; the ventilator augments a patient's breath by providing supporting pressure only throughout the patient's own inspiratory flow.

Table 7-9 Oxygenation Versus Ventilation

Improving oxygenation
Increase FIO_2
Reopen alveoli with PEEP
Increase mean airway pressure
Increase PEEP
Increase I:E ratio
Improving ventilation
Increase minute ventilation
Increase respiratory rate
Increase tidal volume

I:E, inspiration:expiration; PEEP, positive end-expiratory pressure.

Assist-Control Ventilation

An assist-control mode guarantees that the patient will receive a preset minimum number of breaths and a preset tidal volume with every breath. The added benefit with assist-control is that it allows the patient to trigger a mechanical breath with spontaneous breathing. This is made possible by a pressure or flow transducer built into the system that delivers a machine breath when it senses a patient providing a specific negative inspiratory force. Patients are therefore able to have mechanical breaths delivered that are synchronized to their own spontaneous breathing efforts in addition to the mandatory mechanical breaths (Fig. 7-7). Assist-control breaths are delivered with either volume-cycled breaths or time-cycled breaths. This mode works well with a patient in respiratory failure, but if the patient is agitated or not synchronous with the ventilator, a significant increase in the work of breathing can result.

Pressure-Control Ventilation

Pressure-control ventilation is similar to assist-control ventilation in that a preset pressure and time of breath are delivered at a preset minimum rate. It is used when there is a need to limit the high-peak inspiratory pressures caused by volume ventilation and noncompliant lungs. Inspiratory flow can vary with patient effort and may be more comfortable. Inversing the ratio of inspiration to expiration may improve oxygenation but is a more uncomfortable mode of ventilation and the patient usually requires heavy sedation.

Pressure Support Ventilation

Pressure support is a patient-friendly mode of ventilation in that it augments a patient's own breath to help overcome the work of breathing caused by the resistance of the circuit, the mechanics of the ventilator, and the endotracheal tube. The amount of pressure support is set and applied only when the patient has a spontaneous breath. The patient controls the inspiratory flow and respiratory rate (Fig. 7-7). The breath delivered is directly influenced by the elasticity of the lungs and the resistance to the system (compliance). Pressure support is often used with other modes of ventilation, such as synchronized intermittent mandatory ventilation, to augment spontaneous breaths. It is important to remember that if a patient is being ventilated with pressure support ventilation alone, to increase their minute ventilation, they only are able to do so by increasing their spontaneous respiratory rate. The patient's spontaneous tidal volume is elevated by increasing the pressure support on the ventilator, thus adjusting to their pulmonary compliance.

Synchronized Intermittent Mandatory Ventilation

Volume-cycled breaths are more commonly used with synchronized intermittent mandatory ventilation (SIMV). With this mode, the physician sets the desired number of delivered breaths, which can be either volume-cycled or time-cycled. It is synchronized so that the ventilator can deliver the machine breaths at times separate from the patient's breaths. This synchronization is to prevent stacking the two volumes, the patient's and the ventilator's, causing overdistension of the alveoli. If the ventilator does not sense a patient breath, it delivers the preset volume at a preset rate. In this mode, the breaths can be from the patient and from the ventilator (Fig. 7-7). In addition, pressure support is often used along with SIMV to augment the patient's spontaneous breaths. This support aids the patient in two ways: It prevents excessive breathing work on the part of the patient, and it improves cardiac function as the negative pressure produced by the patient increases venous return to the heart. When pressure support is added to SIMV, minute ventilation improves, due to the increase in the patient's augmented, spontaneous volumes (Fig. 7-7).

Controlled Mechanical Ventilation

In controlled mechanical ventilation (CMV) mode, only machine breaths are delivered. They can be either time-cycled or volume-cycled, and the rate is preset. This mode does not allow for any patient breaths (Fig. 7-7). Though there are no CMV settings on most ventilators, this is the most commonly used mode. It is the default mode when patients are on assist-control or synchronized intermittent mandatory ventilation and do not take a spontaneous breath. This is usually due to the patient being chemically paralyzed, heavily sedated, or unable to take spontaneous breaths for any reason.

Ventilation Concepts

Inspiratory Time

Inspiratory time is the specific time over which the tidal volume, or the pressure, is delivered, depending on the mode of ventilation. This includes the time it takes to inspire as well as the pause time just prior to expiration. In time-cycled modes, the inspiratory time is set. In volume-cycled modes, the flow is set and inspiration ends when the set tidal volume is delivered. In pressure-support mode, the patient determines the inspiratory time.

The inspiration:expiration ratio (I:E) is the time it takes to inspire plus the time to expire. It is usually set at 1:2, more expiration time, to mimic a more physiologic breathing pattern. The inspiratory times can be increased by reversing the I:E ratio. Longer inspiratory times may improve oxygenation by increasing mean airway pressure and allowing redistribution of air from less compliant alveoli to more compliant ones. This alveolar recruitment allows more alveoli to participate in gas exchange. By this maneuver, oxygenation is usually improved, since it diffuses more slowly than carbon dioxide. This reversal of I:E is usually performed in pressure-control ventilation. It is a very uncomfortable mode of ventilation and the patient usually requires sedation and occasionally neuromuscular blockade.

Positive End-Expiratory Pressure

PEEP is a baseline positive pressure maintained at end of expiration. It was first introduced in the 1960s for the treatment of ARDS. PEEP provides continuous pressure at end expiration that is greater than atmospheric pressure. This improves oxygenation by increasing functional residual capacity of the lung, opening up alveoli previously collapsed due to edema. The positive pressure that PEEP provides is measured in the upper airways and not at the alveoli level. PEEP is dissipated depending on lung compliance and airway resistance. Using greater than 10 cm H_2O, PEEP may be associated with increased complications, depending on how a patient is managed. These complications can include either alveolar rupture from the increased pressure or a decrease in cardiac output due to decrease in venous return of blood to the heart. It should be remembered that these complications can also occur from alveolar overdistension secondary to high tidal volume ventilation.

Ventilator Weaning

To prevent complications of mechanical ventilation, a patient should be weaned from the ventilator as soon as possible. Complications include nosocomial pneumonia, hoarseness, tracheal stenosis, pneumothorax, and cardiovascular collapse. Weaning from mechanical ventilation may seem like an arduous task, but if it is broken down into a few simple steps, the process becomes manageable. First, the patient's overall physiologic condition must be stable. Second, the patient must be assessed for the ability to maintain adequate oxygenation and ventilation comfortably, without the mechanical ventilator. This assessment may be done with the use of weaning parameters as well as with spontaneous breathing trials. Specific physiologic parameters (Table 7-10) may be used to assess a patient's ability to be removed from the ventilator. However, these parameters should be used as only a guide. None has been validated as always predicting successful extubation from mechanical ventilation.

Spontaneous Breathing Trial

The use of spontaneous breathing trials (SBTs) has been more successful. This test allows a more physiologic assess-

Table 7-10 Weaning Parameters for Patients on Mechanical Ventilation

$F_{IO_2} < 0.50$
Positive end-expiratory pressure < 10 mL H_2O
$P_{AO_2}/F_{IO_2} > 200$
Forced vital capacity ≥ 10 mL/kg/body weight
Negative inspiratory force ≤−30
Minute ventilation < 10 L/min
Rapid shallow breathing index (Rate/V_T).

ment of a patient's ability to oxygenate and ventilate, because the evaluation is conducted while the patient is breathing spontaneously. By assessing a patient's tolerance during an SBT, the patient's respiratory pattern, hemodynamic stability, adequacy of gas exchange, and comfort are tested. A patient able to tolerate a spontaneous breathing trial for 30 to 120 minutes should be considered for permanent discontinuation of the mechanical ventilator.

Inspiratory Force

Inspiratory force is measured as the maximal pressure below atmospheric that a patient can exert against an occluded airway. A maximal inspiratory pressure (PI_{max}) or negative inspiratory force (NIF) value less than -20 to -25 cm H_2O is one of the clinical parameters to confirm recovery from neuromuscular block after general anesthesia. Negative inspiratory force values less than -30 cm H_2O have been used to assist in predicting successful weaning from mechanical ventilation. Compliance, a measure of the elastic properties, or stiffness, of the lung and chest wall, is expressed as a change in volume divided by a change in pressure (V/P). Decreased values are observed with disorders of the thoracic cage or a reduction in the number of functioning lung units (resection, bronchial intubation, pneumothorax, pneumonia, atelectasis, or pulmonary edema).

Rapid Shallow Breathing Index

The rapid shallow breathing index (RSBI) has been used as a predictor for weaning success. It is calculated by dividing the patient's respiratory rate by the tidal volume in liters (RWSBI = Rate/V_T). An index of less than 100 is a predictor of success, but an index of greater than 100 is not necessarily a predictor of failure. Some institutions have shown that serial measurements of the rapid shallow breathing index during spontaneous breathing may be a better predictor of successful weaning from mechanical ventilation.

No single method of assessing ventilator weaning is 100% predictive. The physician should be vigilant, observing a patient's breathing pattern and comfort after removing the endotracheal tube. If the patient develops significant hypoxemia or hypercapnia that is refractory to initial conservative treatment, the patient should have the endotracheal tube replaced and be reconnected to mechanical ventilation immediately. The patient should then be reassessed to explain the unsuccessful extubation. Reasons usually include muscle weakness, oversedation, or occult infection.

CONCLUSION

Treating a patient in the surgical critical care unit can be a demanding but worthwhile experience, if it is approached with a basic understanding of disease processes and management. Understanding the basics of mechanical ventilation will allow a heightened learning experience when managing a patient in the ICU. With this basic knowledge and clinical experience, the student can optimize support while minimizing damage. Though most disease processes encountered in the ICU are complex, a systematic approach to the overall patient management has been shown to improve survival. A multidisciplinary team approach with consistent collaboration is essential in the successful management of these patients.

SUGGESTED READINGS

Bernard GR, Vincent JL, Laterre PF, et al. Efficacy and safety of recombinant human activated protein C for severe sepsis. *N Engl J Med* 2001;344(10):694–709.

Caples SM, Hubmays RD. Respiratory monitoring tools in the intensive care unit. *Curr Opin Crit Care* 2003;9(3):230–235.

Centers for Disease Control and Prevention. Guidelines for the prevention of intravascular catheter-related infections. *MMWR* 2002;1–29.

Dellinger RP, Carlet JM, Masur H, et al. Surviving sepsis: campaign guidelines for management of severe sepsis and septic shock. *Crit Care Med* 2004;32(3):858–873.

Egol AB, Fromm RE, Kalpalatha KG, et al. Guidelines for ICU admission, discharge, and triage. *Crit Care Med* 1999;27(3):633–638.

Fisher JE, Fegelman E, Johannigman J. Surgical complications. In Schwartz SI, ed. *Principles of Surgery*. 7th Ed. New York, NY: McGraw-Hill, 1999:441–484.

Hogarth DK, Hall J. Management of sedation in mechanically ventilated patients. *Curr Opin Crit Care* 2004;10(1):40–46.

Hollenburg S, Ahrens T, Annane D, et al. Practice parameters for hemodynamic support of sepsis in adult patients. *Crit Care Med* 2004; 32(9):1928–1948.

MacIntyre NR, et al. Evidence-based guidelines for weaning and discontinuing ventilatory support. *Chest* 2001;120(6):375–395.

Malbrain ML. Is it wise not to think about intra-abdominal hypertension in the ICU? *Curr Opin Crit Care* 2004;10(2):132–145.

Marvin RG, Cocanour CS, Moore FA. Critical care. In Townsend CM, ed. *The Biological Basis of Modern Surgical Practice*. 16th Ed. Philadelphia, PA.: WB Saunders, 2001:375–393.

Patel GP, Gurka DP, Balk RA. New treatment strategies for severe sepsis and septic shock. *Curr Opin Crit Care* 2003;9(5):390–396.

Pronovost P, Berenholtz S, Dorman T, et al. Improving communication in the ICU using daily goals. *J Crit Care* 2003;18:71–75.

Rivers E, Nguyen B, Havstad S, et al. Early goal-directed therapy in the treatment of severe sepsis and septic shock. *N Engl J Med* 2001; 345(19):1368–1377.

Schein M, Ivatury R. Intra-abdominal hypertension and the abdominal compartment syndrome. *Br J Surg* 1998;85:1027–1028.

Szem JW, Hydo LJ, Fischer E, et al. High-risk intrahospital transport of critically ill patients: safety and outcome of the necessary "road-trip." *Crit Care Med* 1995;23(10):1660–1666.

Varon AJ, Kirton OC, Civetta JM. Physiologic monitoring. In Schwartz SI, ed. *Principles of Surgery*. 7th Ed. New York, NY: McGraw-Hill, 1999:485–510.

Warren J, Fromm RE, Orr RA, et al. Guidelines for the inter- and intrahospital transport of critically ill patients. *Crit Care Med* 2004;32(1): 256–262.

8

GLENN E. TALBOY, JR., MD ■ IAN GORDON, MD, PHD

Wounds and Wound Healing

OBJECTIVES

1. Define a wound, and describe the sequence and approximate time frame of the phases of wound healing.
2. Describe the three types of wound healing and the elements of each. Describe the three phases of wound healing that are distinct to each type of wound.
3. Describe the essential elements and significance of granulation tissue.
4. Describe the growth factors and cytokines involved in wound healing, their cells of origin, and their target cells.
5. Describe the clinical factors that decrease collagen synthesis and retard wound healing.
6. Describe the rationale for the uses of absorbable and nonabsorbable sutures.
7. Describe the appropriate use and toxic doses of local anesthetics.
8. Discuss the functions of a dressing.
9. Define clean, contaminated, infected, and chronic wounds, and describe the management of each type.
10. Develop a basic understanding of methods to assist in wound healing, when their use is indicated, and when it is contraindicated.

A wound, in the broadest sense, is a disruption of normal anatomic relations as a result of an injury. The injury may be intentional (e.g., elective surgical incision) or unintentional (e.g., trauma). Regardless of the cause of injury, the biochemical and physiologic processes of healing are identical, although their time course and intensity may vary. The process of wound closure is classified into three distinct types: (1) primary, (2) secondary, and (3) tertiary, based on the timing of replacement of the epithelium over the wound. Wound healing is also divided by physiologic process into three stages, or phases: (1) inflammatory or substrate, (2) proliferative, and (3) maturation or remodeling. These biochemical and physiologic events are correlated with gross morphologic changes in the wound. Knowledge of these events and changes allows the physician to maximize the chances of successful healing and minimize scarring.

PHYSIOLOGY OF WOUND HEALING

Inflammation is the basic physiologic process that is common to all wounds. Clinically, inflammation is identified by the cardinal signs of redness (rubor), heat (calor), swelling (tumor), pain (dolor), and loss of function. These signs of inflammation are also seen in wound infections, which ultimately may cause wound disruption. All wounds, whether acute, chronic, or infected, have varying time courses after the primary events that lead to normal wound healing. The physiology underlying these clinical signs is a complex interaction of biochemical and cellular events.

Biochemical Aspects

Trauma activates a cascade of chemoattractants and mitogens that recruit phagocytes, fibroblasts, and endothelial cells. These chemoattractants, which include platelet-derived growth factors (PDGF) and complement peptide (C5A), are produced during the clotting of blood by degradation of the surrounding tissue and by cells entering the wound. The initial event of clotting blood and recruitment of cells occurs in the first 1 to 2 hours after injury. The first cells that enter the wound are platelets, which come into contact with the damaged **collagen** at the time of injury. The platelets degranulate and release alpha granules that contain multiple growth factors, including PDGF and transforming growth factor-β (TGF-β).

Inflammatory cells are attracted and release a variety of cytokines and growth factors. Cytokines are soluble proteins that are secreted by a cell and influence activities of other cells. Growth factors are proteins that bind to cell receptors and initiate cellular proliferation and differentiation. Macrophages release TGF-β, macrophage-derived growth factor (MDGF), TGF-α, heparin-binding epidermal growth factor (HB-EGF), and basic fibroblast growth factor (bFGF). Keratinocytes also enter the wound and release TGF-β, TGF-α, and keratinocyte-derived autocrine factor (KAF). All of these cytokines and growth factors are involved in synthesis of extracellular matrix and new capillary formation. Many also act as attractants for fibroblasts and neutrophils. Table 8-1 lists growth factors and cytokines by cell of origin and their target tissues.

In addition to cytokines and growth factors, arachidonic acid is contained in the walls of cells. It is released when the cells are injured. The degradation of arachidonic acid into prostanoid derivatives of prostaglandins and thromboxanes causes a number of responses associated with the inflammatory response, including vasodilation, swelling, and pain.

Physiologic Aspects

At the same time that these biochemical events are developing, leukocytes are marginating, attaching to vessel walls, and migrating through the walls toward the site of injury (Fig. 8-1). In addition, venules are dilating, and lymphatics are being blocked. This inflammatory response in the wound occurs for a variable period, depending on

Table 8-1 Cytokines and Growth Factors

Name	Cell of Origin	Target Cells/Tissue	Effect
TGF-α	Macrophages	Fibroblasts, epithelial cells, and endothelial cells	Migration of target cells
	Keratinocytes		Extracellular matrix proteins, proliferation, and capillary formation
TGF-β	Platelet alpha-granules	Inflammatory cells	Chemotactic for target cells
	Macrophages	Fibroblasts, epithelial cells, and endothelial cells	Migration of target cells
	Fibroblasts and keratinocytes		Extracellular matrix proteins, proliferation, and capillary formation
EGF	Platelet alpha-granules	Inflammatory cells	Chemotactic for target cells
PDGF	Platelet alpha-granules	Inflammatory cells	Chemotactic for target cells
	Fibroblasts and endothelial cells		Extracellular matrix proteins, proliferation, and capillary formation
IL-1	Macrophages, monocytes, and keratinocytes		Increase collagen synthesis, activate neutrophils, increase keratinocytes migration
IL-2	T lymphocytes	Fibroblasts, inflammatory cells, and T cells	Attract fibroblasts and inflammatory cells, activates T cells
IL-6	Fibroblasts and inflammatory cells	Fibroblasts	Fibroblast proliferation
		Inflammatory cells	Chemotactic for inflammatory cells
IL-8		Leukocytes	Recruitment and activation
IFN-γ	T lymphocytes	Monocytes and macrophages	Activation of target cells
TNF-α	Macrophages, monocytes, fibroblasts, mast cells, and keratinocytes	Macrophages, monocytes, endothelial cells, and neutrophils	Mediates tissue repair, endothelial cell activation, and tissue remodeling

EGF, epidermal growth factor; IL, interleukin; PDGF, platelet-derived growth factor; TGF, transforming growth factor; TNF, tumor necrosis factor.

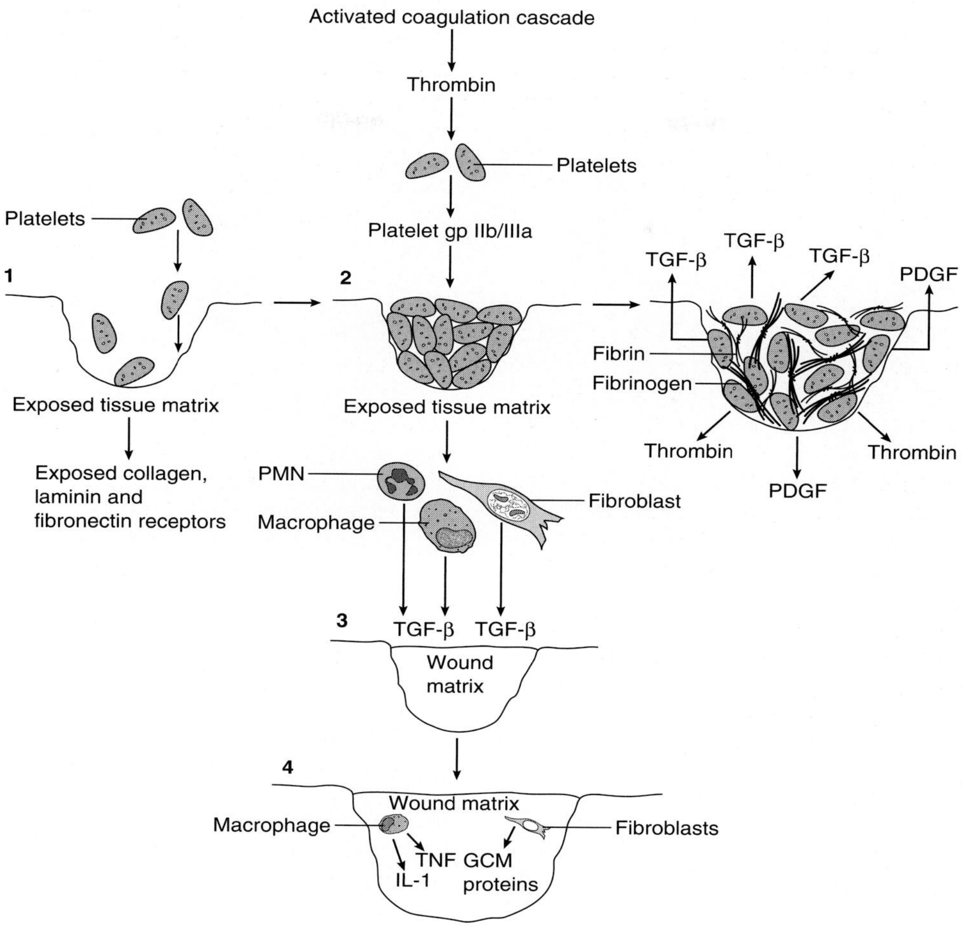

Figure 8-1 At tissue injury a provisional wound matrix is established. (1) Platelets bind to exposed wound matrix receptors. (2) After wounding, the coagulation cascade is activated, generating thrombin, which activates platelet glycoprotein (Gp) IIb/IIIa and increases platelet aggregation. A provisional wound matrix is formed and is made up of platelets, fibrin, fibrinogen, and fibronectin. The activated platelets in the wound generate transforming growth factor-β (TGF-β), platelet-derived growth factor (PDGF), and thrombin. (3) TGF-β is strongly chemotactic for neutrophils, macrophages, and fibroblasts, recruiting these cells into the provisional wound matrix, where they are also subsequently activated by TGF-β. (4) Increasing concentrations of TGF-β result in macrophage activation, producing increased amounts of tumor necrosis factor-α (TGF-α) and interleukin-1 (IL-1). TGF-β also stimulates fibroblast production of extracellular matrix proteins. These reactions further enhance migration of macrophages and fibroblasts into the wound, facilitating tissue repair. Based on Greenfield LJ. *Surgery: scientific principles and practice.* Baltimore, MD: Lippincott Williams & Wilkins, 2001:Fig. 5.15.

local tissue and host factors. Some of these factors are responsive to manipulation by the physician.

PHASES OF WOUND HEALING

Understanding the phases of wound healing is important in treating conditions and diseases that affect various stages of the healing cascade (e.g., diabetes mellitus, malnutrition, and chronic illnesses). The three phases of wound healing are (1) inflammatory or substrate, (2) proliferative, and (3) maturation or remodeling. The second and third phases are relatively constant, regardless of the type of wound healing. These phases begin only when the wound is covered by epithelium. Figure 8-2 shows the phases of healing, comparing cells and collagen concentrations with wound strength over time.

Substrate Phase (Inflammatory)

The substrate phase is also known as the inflammatory phase, lag phase, or exudative phase. The main cells in-

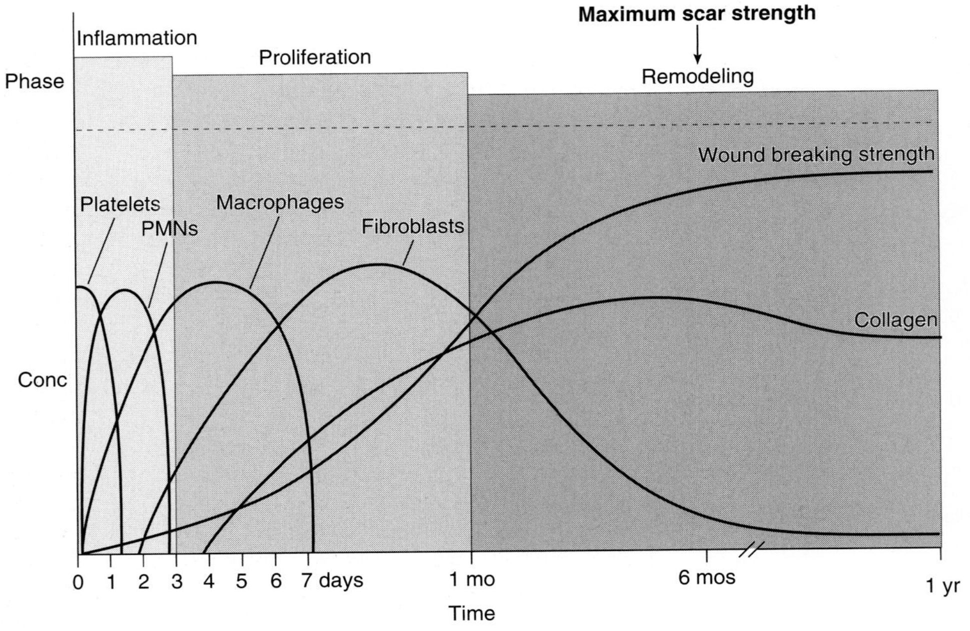

Figure 8-2 Phases of wound healing comparing cells and collagen concentrations with wound strength over time.

volved in this process are polymorphonuclear leukocytes (PMNs), platelets, and macrophages. Shortly after a wound occurs, PMNs appear and remain the predominant cell for approximately 48 hours. These leukocytes may be the origin of many inflammatory mediators, including complement and kallikrein. Small numbers of bacteria are handled by the macrophages that are present in the wound. However, if a large number of bacteria are present, especially in the neutropenic patient, clinical infection will occur. The neutrophil is not crucial for normal wound healing, but the macrophage is. Monocytes enter the wound after the PMNs, reaching maximum numbers approximately 24 hours later. They evolve into macrophages, which are the main cells involved in wound debridement. Another biochemical event associated with debridement is activation of tissue matrix metalloproteinases (TMMPs). In the absence of injury or inflammation, these degradative, proteolytic enzymes normally are quiescent, in part due to TMMP inhibitors, which also reside in normal tissue. After injury, TMMP inhibitor activity dramatically falls and TMMP activity is stimulated. Activated TMMP enzymes, working in conjunction with leukocyte enzymes, degrade surrounding matrix proteins such as collagen and necrotic cellular macromolecules. These enzymes break down devitalized tissue structures, which is required for subsequent events in wound healing. Experimental wounds that are depleted of macrophages and monocytes show marked inhibition of fibroblast migration, proliferation, and loss of collagen production. Macrophages, which can secrete more than 100 different molecules, are an important producer of growth factors. Some of these factors are TGF-β, which stimulates the proliferation of fibroblasts, and interleukin-1 (IL-1), which is partially responsible for regulating the repair of damaged tissue. IL-1 is an important growth factor in the regulation of many processes in the inflammatory response; it may induce fever, promote hemostasis by interacting with endothelial cells, enhance fibroblast proliferation, and activate T cells.

As clot, debris, and bacteria are being removed from the wound, substrates for collagen synthesis are being arranged. In primary wound healing (discussed later), the substrate phase occurs over approximately a 4-day period. The wound is edematous and erythematous. This normal process may be difficult to distinguish from early signs of wound infection. In healing by secondary or tertiary intention (discussed later), this phase continues indefinitely until the wound surface is closed by ectodermal elements (i.e., epithelium for skin, mucosa in the gut).

Proliferative Phase

The second and third phases of wound healing are relatively constant, regardless of the type of wound healing. These phases begin only when the wound is covered by epithelium. The proliferative phase is the second stage of healing. It is characterized by the production of collagen in the wound. The wound appears less edematous and inflamed than before, but the wound scar may be raised, red, and hard. The primary cell in this phase is the fibroblast, which produces collagen.

Collagen is the principal structural protein of the body. It has a complex, three-dimensional structure. Collagen synthesis begins with the production of amino acid chains in the cytoplasm of the fibroblast. These α-chains are unique in that each third amino acid is glycine. Two amino acids, hydroxyproline and hydroxylysine, are found only in collagen. These amino acids are required for hydroxylation during collagen synthesis by specific enzymes. Important cofactors involved in the hydroxylation process are ferrous ion, α-ketoglutarate, and ascorbic acid. Insufficient consumption of one of the cofactors can lead to an interruption of the proliferative phase. The absence of ascorbic acid leads to the production of defective, unhydroxylated collagen, which leads to wound breakdown. Most physicians are familiar with scurvy, which is caused by vitamin C deficiency.

Maturation Phase (Remodeling)

The third, and final, phase of wound healing is the remodeling, or maturation, phase. It is characterized by the maturation of collagen by intermolecular cross-linking. The wound scar gradually flattens and becomes less prominent and more pale and supple. This phase is a time of great metabolic activity. Collagen is deposited in the wound and existing collagen is remodeled and removed, thus there is no net collagen gain in the wound. The maturation process clinically corresponds to the flattening of the scar. Wound maturation in an adult takes from 9 to 12 months.

CLASSIFICATION OF HEALING WOUNDS

Wounds are often classified as acute, chronic, clean, or contaminated. Acute wounds tend to progress through the phases of wound healing in an orderly fashion and without delays. Chronic wounds will progress through the phases of wound healing at a much slower rate. Chronic wounds become arrested in the inflammation phase and fail to advance. Many factors influence the development of chronic wounds, including nutritional status, chronic disease states (diabetes mellitus), oxygen delivery (peripheral vascular disease or smoking), and chronic edema (coronary heart disease). Clean wounds are any wounds that have minimal bacterial or particulate loads and are opened less than 12 hours. Contaminated wounds can have high bacterial counts ($> 10^5$organisms/gram of tissue) or a large amount of particulate matter. Classification of the wound type and determination of the potential for successful closure is determined by the physician.

The depth of skin injury also distinguishes wounds. Partial thickness wounds result from injuries that do not completely penetrate the top epithelial layer of the skin. Although the top layer of the epithelium is devitalized in superficial wounds such as blisters or mild burns (first- and second-degree thermal burns, sunburns), the basal stem cells that reside in the deepest portion of the skin epithelium remain active and will proliferate sufficiently to replenish the damaged superficial layer. Full-thickness (third-degree) wounds entail damage to the entire layer of keratinocyte epithelium including sweat glands and hair follicles that contain stem cells. Such wounds cannot regenerate simply by proliferation of stem cells resident in the base. Although most of the physiologic events of wound healing occur in full-thickness wounds, spontaneous reepithelialization depends upon migration of keratinocytes from the edge of the wound. Large full-thickness wounds may require skin grafting or other surgical interventions to achieve closure.

Primary Healing

In **primary healing** (healing by first intention), the wound is closed by direct approximation of the epithelial wound edges. Primary healing of a wound can be performed in clean and contaminated wounds. All wounds should be cleaned and debrided, if necessary, prior to closure. In contaminated wounds it is essential to thoroughly clean the wound. The use of normal saline under pressure and with a pulsatile action (syringe and 18-gauge needle) can be used to clean the wound. Simple irrigation with normal saline can be beneficial but is less effective than pressure irrigation. The physician needs to determine whether or not a contaminated wound can be closed after irrigation. The volume and character of the contamination needs to be considered. Delayed closure can be performed when the wound is clean (see tertiary healing below). In a large defect that has lost skin and/or subcutaneous structures, pedicle flaps or skin grafts are used to close the wound primarily. This process is still considered primary wound healing because the healing occurs by immediate coverage with epithelial elements in some form. Epithelialization of the primarily closed wound occurs in 12 to 24 hours, allowing removal of dressings and cleansing of the surrounding skin. Figure 8-3 shows the strength of a primarily closed wound as a function of time.

Secondary Healing

In **secondary healing** (spontaneous wound closure), the wound is left open and allowed to heal spontaneously from the edges of the wound. The wound closes by contraction and epithelialization (Fig. 8-4). Contraction occurs from the wound edges in a centripetal fashion. Epithelialization is the other component of healing by secondary intention. Under optimal circumstances, the epithelium proliferates from the wound margins to the center of the wound at the rate of 1 mm/day. This proliferation occurs only in a wound that is not infected. The inflammatory phase of wound healing continues and creates granulation tissue. Granulation tissue is the result of proliferation of capillaries and other tissue components. Normal progression of wound healing is for the epithelium to migrate over the granulation tissue and result in a closed wound. If the wound fails to epithelialize the granulation tissue will continue and result in an unclosed wound with friable tissue outgrowing the epithelial edges. To avoid this, wounds that have formed granulation tissue beds can be skin grafted to prevent excessive growth of the granulation tissue and achieve wound closure in a more timely fashion.

Tertiary Healing

In tertiary healing (healing by third intention), the wound is closed by active means after a delay of days to weeks. Delayed closure should be performed only in wounds that have a quantitative bacterial count of less than 10^5 organisms/gram of tissue. Currently, this is estimated by clinical ap-

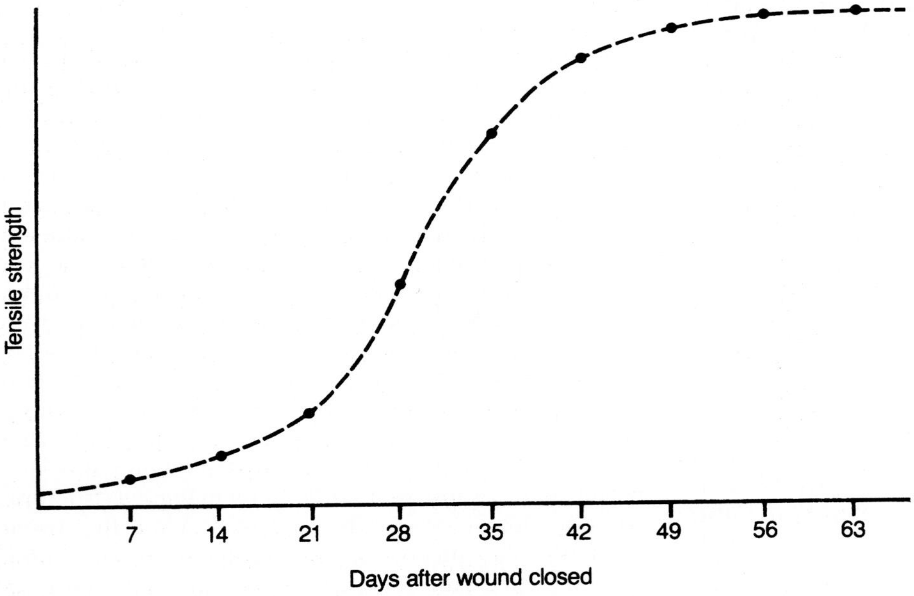

Figure 8-3 Strength of primarily closed wound as a function of time.

pearance, although quantitative bacterial counts can be measured. Delayed primary closure can be accomplished when there is an adequate decrease in the contamination (bacterial load) and formation of granulation tissue. Repeated irrigation, debridement, and dressing changes are used to accomplish this goal. The use of such items as negative pressure devices, hyperbaric oxygen, and growth factors can accelerate granulation tissue formation (see methods for promoting wound healing). When it is determined that the wound is at the proper stage (usually 5 to 7 days), the epithelial portion of the wound can be closed primarily.

FACTORS THAT AFFECT WOUND HEALING

There are many local and systemic factors that affect wound healing. The physician should be actively working to correct any abnormality that can prevent or slow wound healing.

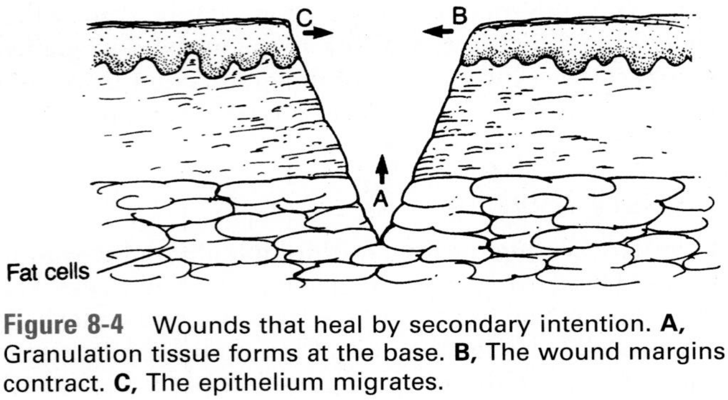

Figure 8-4 Wounds that heal by secondary intention. **A,** Granulation tissue forms at the base. **B,** The wound margins contract. **C,** The epithelium migrates.

Local Factors

A health care provider can improve wound healing by controlling local factors. He or she must clean the wound, debride it, and close it appropriately. Avulsion or crush wounds (defined below under general management of wounds) need to be debrided until all nonviable tissue is removed. Grossly contaminated wounds should be cleaned as completely as possible to remove particulate matter (foreign bodies) and should be irrigated copiously.

Bleeding must be controlled to prevent hematoma formation, which is an excellent medium for bacterial growth. Hematoma also separates wound edges, preventing the proper contact of tissues that is necessary for healing.

Radiation affects local wound healing by causing vasculitis, which leads to local hypoxia and ischemia. Hypoxia and ischemia impede healing by reducing the amount of nutrients and oxygen that are available at the wound site.

Infection decreases the rate of wound healing and detrimentally affects proper granulation tissue formation, decreases oxygen delivery, and depletes the wound of needed nutrients. Care must be taken to clean the wound adequately. All wounds have some degree of contamination; if the body is able to control bacterial proliferation in a wound, that wound will heal. The use of cleansing agents (the simplest is soap and water) can help reduce contamination. A wound that contains the highly virulent *streptococci* species should not be closed. Physicians should keep in mind the potential for *Clostridium tetani* in wounds with devitalized tissue and use the proper prophylaxis.

Systemic Factors

In addition to controlling local factors, the physician must address systemic issues that can affect wound healing. Nutrition is an extremely important factor in wound healing. Patients need adequate nutrition to support protein synthesis, collagen formation, and metabolic energy for wound healing. Patients need adequate vitamins and nutrients to facilitate healing; folic acid is critical to the proper formation of collagen. Adequate fat intake is required for the absorption of vitamins D, A, K, and E. Vitamin K is essential for the carboxylation of glutamate in the synthesis of clotting factors II, VII, IX, and X. Decreasing clotting factors can lead to hematoma formation and altered wound healing. Vitamin A increases the inflammatory response, increases collagen synthesis, and increases the influx of macrophages into a wound. Magnesium is required for protein synthesis, and zinc is a cofactor for RNA and DNA polymerase. Lack of any one of these vitamins or trace elements will adversely affect wound healing.

Uncontrolled diabetes mellitus results in uncontrolled hyperglycemia, impairs wound healing, and alters collagen formation. Hyperglycemia also inhibits fibroblast and endothelial cell proliferation within the wound.

Medications will also affect wound healing. For example, steroids blunt the inflammatory response, decrease the available vitamin A in the wound, and alter the deposition and remodeling of collagen.

Chronic illness (immune deficiency, cancer, uremia, liver disease, and jaundice) will predispose to infection, protein deficiency, and malnutrition, which, as noted previously, can affect wound healing.

Smoking has a systemic effect by decreasing the oxygen-carrying capacity of hemoglobin. Smoking may also decrease collagen formation within a wound. Every physician should encourage patients to stop smoking for general health reasons.

Hypoxia results in a decrease in oxygen delivery to a wound and retards healing.

GENERAL MANAGEMENT OF WOUNDS

Local Anesthetics

To reduce patient discomfort when debriding or suturing wounds, local anesthesia may be required. Of the two pharmacologic classes of local anesthetics, the amide group is most commonly used and includes xylocaine, bupivacaine, mepivacaine, and prilocaine. The second pharmacologic class is the esters and includes procaine, chlorprocaine, tetracaine, and cocaine. If a patient has a known sensitivity to one family of local anesthetics, the physician may select the other. However, the ester anesthetics may not be used in individuals with sensitivity to p-aminobenzoic acid (PABA).

All local anesthetics reversibly inhibit the conduction of nerve impulses by decreasing the membrane permeability to sodium, which decreases the rate of depolarization and leads to an increase in the excitability threshold of the nerve and inhibition of the nerve impulse. Clinically, the order of loss in nerve function is pain, temperature, touch, proprioception, and skeletal muscle tone.

Solubility, protein binding, and the pH and the vascularity of the tissues determine duration of action of the local anesthetics. Another important factor is the inclusion of a vasoconstrictor, which is most commonly epinephrine. Amides are protein-bound and are metabolized in the liver by ring hydroxylation, oxidative N-dealkylation, ring hydroxylation, cleavage of the amide linkage, and conjugation. Esters are metabolized by pseudocholinesterase to PABA and diethylaminoethanol. Individuals with sensitivity to PABA therefore should not receive an ester local anesthetic.

The physician needs to evaluate carefully the wound size and consider whether excessive amounts of local anesthetic will be required to treat a wound. If the maximum dose will be exceeded, general anesthesia will need to be employed. For example, the toxic limit of xylocaine, a frequently used local anesthetic, is 7 mg/kg given in 1 hour. The clinician should remember that 1 mL of xylocaine 1% contains 10 mg of drug. Another way to consider this is that 50 mL of xylocaine 1% is the toxic level for a 70-kg person. Major side effects of local anesthetics include central nervous system (tinnitus, blurred vision, tremors, and depression) and cardiovascular effects (myocardial depression, atrioventricular [AV] block, and decreased cardiac output). Table 8-2 gives the name, maximum dose, onset of action, and duration of action of the more commonly used local anesthetics.

Local anesthetics containing vasoconstrictors (i.e., epinephrine) should not be used in tissues supplied by end arteries, such as the nose, digits, penis, and ear. Necrosis of this tissue can result from vasoconstriction

Table 8-2 Local Anesthetics

Type/Name	Maximum Dose	Maximum Dose With Epinephrine	Onset of Action	Duration of Action
Amides				
Xylocaine	4.5 mg/kg–350 mg	7 mg/kg–500 mg	1–5 min	60/90 min
Bupivacaine	2.5 mg/kg–175 mg	3.5 mg/kg–225 mg	5–10 min	12/18 hr
Esters				
Procaine			2–5 min	60 min
Chlorprocaine	11 mg/kg–800 mg	14 mg/kg–1000 mg	6–12 min	60/90 min

Classification of Wounds

A **clean wound** is one that is relatively new (< 12 hours) and has minimal contamination. Clean wounds are classified according to presentation and method of injury. The clean wound needs to be debrided, if necessary, and closed using the proper suture material (see below). Wound edges should be approximated without tension. Skin edges should not be overlapped, since this would result in undergrowth of the epithelial layer. Table 8-3 lists the steps in wound care.

An **avulsion** injury occurs when the skin has been violated by shearing forces and underlying tissue has been undermined and elevated, creating a flap or total loss of skin. The flap or avulsed tissue is composed of skin with or without the underlying fat and muscle. This type of wound needs thorough cleaning, debridement of necrotic tissue, and closure if appropriate. Efforts should be made to suture the "flap" of tissue down with absorbable suture and then close the wound edges. It is also helpful to place a pressure dressing over this wound to decrease fluid collection. If an open wound has been created, a full-thickness flap containing the appropriate layers of tissue or a skin graft may be required to cover the defect.

An **abrasion** is a superficial loss of epithelial elements, with portions of the dermis and deeper structures remaining intact. Usually, only cleansing of the wound is required, because the remaining epithelial cells regenerate and migrate to close the wound. Careful cleansing is critical to prevent traumatic tattoos, which can result from debris in the wound. Desiccation of an abrasion should be avoided by applying a layer of petroleum jelly or antibiotic ointment.

Puncture wounds generally do not require closure. Management consists of assessment of the damage to underlying vital structures and examination for a foreign body. Radiographs are often helpful in assessing the presence of a foreign body. This wound must be carefully followed clinically to detect any developing infection at an early stage.

Crush injuries are often accompanied by the loss of significant amounts of tissue that may initially appear viable. Nonviable tissue must eventually be debrided, and the wound closed with either a skin graft or a myocutaneous flap.

Table 8-3	Steps in Wound Care
1. Sterile preparation and draping	
2. Administration of local anesthetic	
3. Hemostasis	
4. Irrigation and debridement	
5. Closure in layers	
6. Dressing and bandage	

Suture Material

Suture material, size, and type should be chosen based on the type of tissue that is being sutured (Table 8-4). Suture size is graded by a number or by a zero (0). The more zeros, the smaller the suture. Suture size number 1 is larger than 0, which in turn is larger than 2-0 (00). Suture can be as small as 9-0 or 10-0. A 3-0 or 4-0 suture is used for skin on the torso and extremities, whereas a 5-0 or 6-0 suture is appropriate for the more delicate tissues of the face and neck. A 2-0 to 4-0 suture is appropriate for closure of deeper tissues.

Wound Closure

It is important that the wound be prepared properly prior to closure by thorough cleaning and debridement (Fig. 8-5), as discussed above. When suturing, the physician should remember several important details:

1. There should be no tension on the wound edges, because tension can lead to necrosis of the skin. If the wound will not close without excessive tension, another management plan (e.g., rotational flaps, skin graft) should be considered.
2. Sutures in the skin of the torso and extremities should be left in place for 7 to 10 days.
3. Sutures on the face and neck should be left in place for only 4 days.
4. Knots should be secure but not so tight as to strangulate the tissue.
5. Monofilament nonabsorbable suture should be used on the skin because it is less reactive.
6. Deep suture should be absorbable and placed in the tissues that have the greatest strength. For closure of muscle, it is the fascia that provides the greatest strength. For closure of the skin, the dermis provides the strength (Fig. 8-6).

Dressings

A dressing is usually placed over the closed wound to protect the wound, immobilize the area, compress the area evenly, absorb any secretions, and be aesthetically acceptable. Proper wound dressing should fulfill all of these criteria without compromising adequate coverage of a wound. The dressing should provide sufficient bulk to protect the wound from trauma. The bulk provided by fluffed gauze and gauze pads allows for adequate absorption of wound secretions and helps to immobilize the area. A plaster splint or cast may provide further immobilization. An outer layer of firmly wrapped rolled gauze and a loosely but evenly applied elastic roll can provide even compression and an aesthetically acceptable appearance.

Suture Removal

Sutures used for skin closure are removed when they have done the job for which they were placed. Sterile forceps

Table 8-4 Suture Material

Suture	Trade Names	Raw Material	Stranding	Type	Retention of Tensile Strength	Where Used
Nylon	Neurolon	Synthetic	Mono/polyfilament	Nonabsorbable		Skin
Polyester	Dacron, Tevdek, Ethibond	Synthetic	Polyfilament			Below skin
Silk		Natural	Polyfilament	Permanent*	2 yr	Below skin
Catgut		Natural	Monofilament	Absorbable	7 days	Below skin
Chromic Catgut	Chromic	Natural	Monofilament	Absorbable	14 days	Below skin
Polyglycolic acid	Vycril, Dexon	Synthetic	Polyfilament	Absorbable	14–30 days	Below skin
Polypropylene	Prolene	Synthetic	Monofilament	Permanent		Skin, fascia, vasculature, and tendon/bone
Polyglyconate	Maxon	Synthetic	Monofilament	Absorbable	30–60 days	Below skin, fascia, bowel, ducts
Polydioxanone	PDS	Synthetic	Monofilament	Absorbable	60 days	Below skin, fascia, bowel, ducts
Poliglecaprone	Monocryl	Synthetic	Monofilament	Absorbable	30–50 days	Subcuticular skin closure
Poly (L-lactide/glycolide)	Panacryl	Synthetic	Polyfilament	Absorbable	90 days	Bone, tendon, and fascia
Stainless steel			Mono/polyfilament	Nonabsorbable		Bone, fascia, and skin

* Absorbs over 2 years but is considered permanent.

and fine scissors are the basic instruments that are used to remove sutures. The use of sterilized supplies is important for infection control. The suture is grasped with forceps and cut, then gently removed.

Figure 8-7 shows the stages of wound healing, from debridement of necrotic skin and soft tissue, to formation of a granulation bed and placement of a skin graft, to a healed wound with a combination of skin graft and advancement flap.

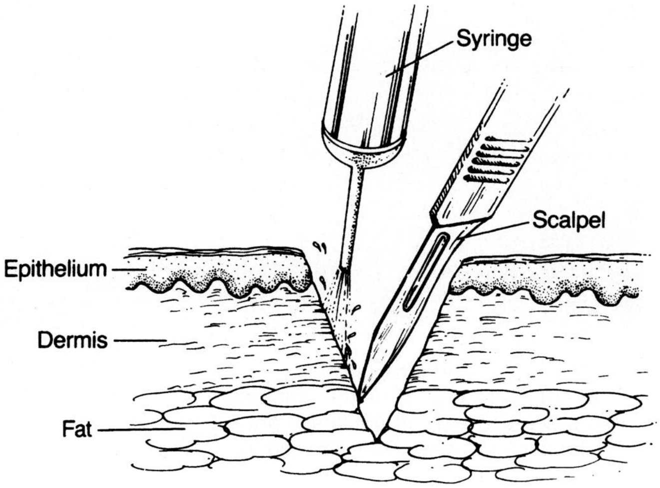

Figure 8-5 Sharp debridement and saline lavage to prepare the wound for closure.

MANAGEMENT OF THE CONTAMINATED, INFECTED, AND CHRONIC WOUND

The Contaminated Wound

All wounds are contaminated to a greater or lesser extent. Even the wounds that are considered clean have a bacterial

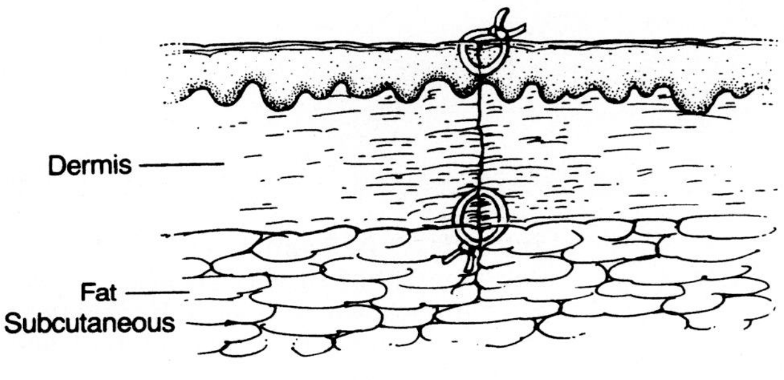

Figure 8-6 The dermis is approximated for strength, and the epidermis is closed to seal the wound and align the surface cells.

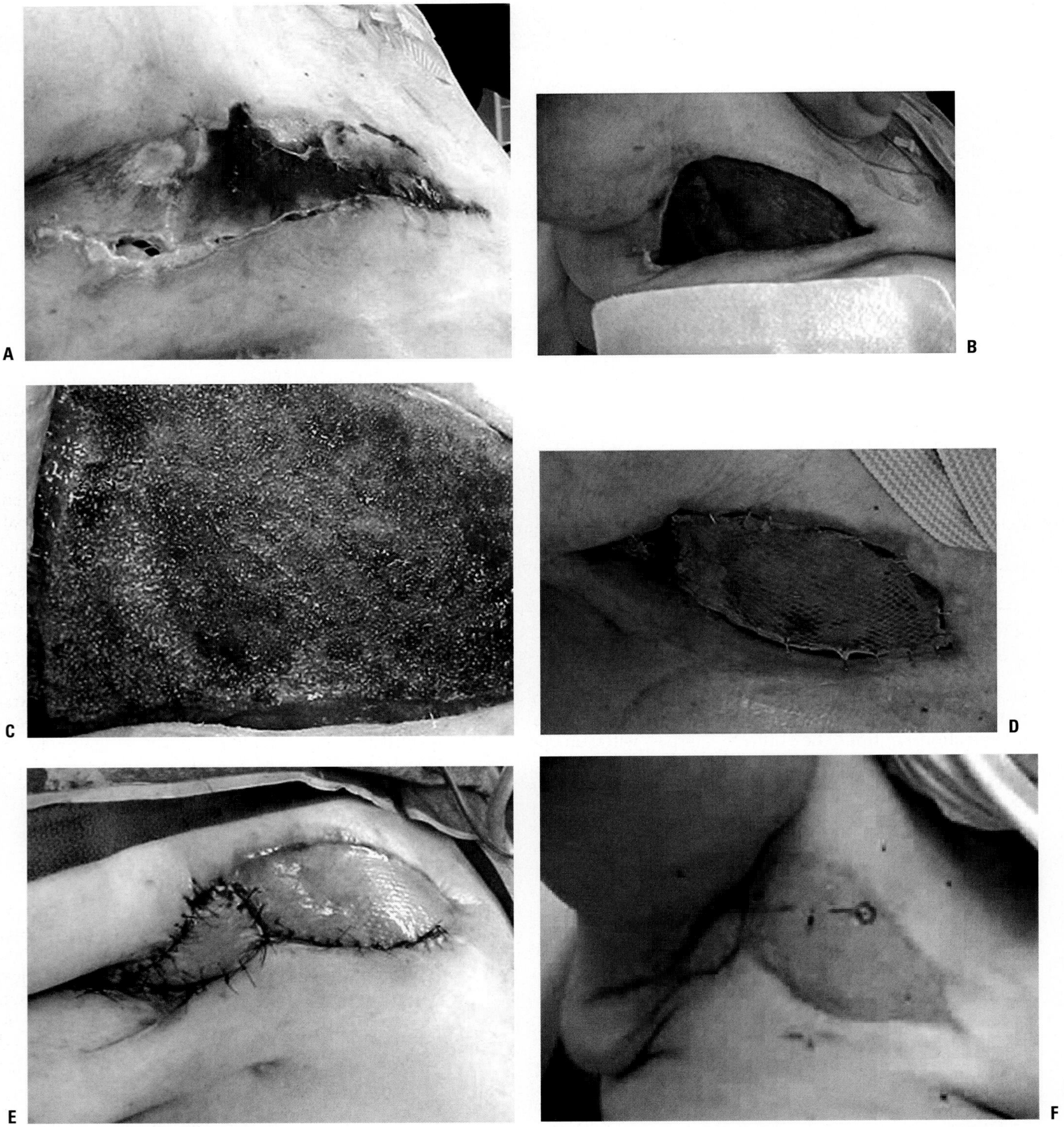

Figure 8-7 **A,** Example of necrotic skin and soft tissue. **B,** Wound after proper debridement of all necrotic skin and soft tissue. **C,** Granulation bed. **D,** Initial placement of split-thickness skin graft. **E,** Skin graft with lateral advancement full-thickness graft. **F,** Healed wound with combination of skin graft and advancement flap. Note the radiation tattoo markings.

Table 8-5 Wound Classification

Wound Classification	Average Infection Rate	Examples
Clean	3%	Atraumatic, no GI, GU, or R tract involvement
Clean-Contaminated	8%	Minor sterile breaks, entrance into GI, GU, or R tract without significant contamination
Contaminated	15%	Entrance into GI, GU, or R tract with spillage of contents, traumatic wounds with soil and particulate matter
Dirty	35%	Infection within tissue (i.e., abscess)

GI, gastrointestinal; GU, genitourinary; R, respiratory.

inoculum (see Table 8-5 for classification of wounds). Proper wound care, with debridement and adequate lavage, can markedly diminish the inoculum and result in successful primary wound healing. Exceptions to primary closure of these contaminated wounds include a very high bacterial inoculum (e.g., human bite, farm injury), a long time lapse since the initial injury, the suspected or known presence of species, and a severe crush injury. In these instances, delayed closure is the preferred management.

Keeping buried sutures to a minimum is important when closing any wound. Excessive use of buried suture provides foreign body for bacterial contamination. Monofilament skin sutures are used to reduce the possibility of wound infection. If the surgeon has doubts about the extent of contamination or the safety of the closure, delay is the judicious approach to wound management. Delay allows time for further debridement and reduction of the bacterial count to less than 10^5 bacteria/gram of tissue. Follow-up within 48 hours detects early signs of clinical infection.

The Infected Wound

Infected wounds are sometimes difficult to detect. Proper management begins with identifying the truly infected wound. Any layperson can observe **pus** exuding from a severely inflamed wound and tell that the wound is infected. On the other hand, the most experienced surgeon will have no better chance than the flip of a coin in identifying the level of bacterial contamination in a chronically granulating wound.

The number of bacteria that can be tolerated and still allow successful wound closure is the most precise definition of an infected wound. A wound is considered infected when the level of contamination is greater than 10^5 organisms/gram tissue. The proper management of the infected wound is to decrease the bacterial count to 10^5 or less organisms/gram of tissue so that the wound may be closed. Debridement is the most important technique to decrease the bacterial count. Frequent cleaning of a wound can also decrease the bacterial count. Dressing changes should be limited to twice per day to prevent adversely affecting the progression of healing within an open wound. Systemic antibiotics are of little use in local bacterial control because they do not penetrate the granulating wound bed. However, topical antibacterials (e.g., mafenide acetate, silver sulfadiazine) are effective and may be used. Because of possible corneal irritation, mafenide acetate or silver sulfadiazine should not be used on the face. Biologic dressings (e.g., allograft, amniotic membrane) also decrease the bacterial level. Successful adherence of a biologic dressing indicates a reduced bacterial count and accurately predicts success with either wound closure or autograft. Successful wound management requires diligent preoperative, intraoperative, and postoperative care as well as meticulous surgical technique. Proper handling of tissues, adequate debridement, careful placement of sutures, and bacteriologic knowledge of the wound are critical aspects in wound closure.

Chronic Wounds

Wounds that are slow to heal are classified as chronic. They include diabetic foot ulcers, venous stasis ulcers, and open wounds that have failed to close. These wounds are stalled in the inflammatory phase of healing. They have poor granulation tissue formation, altered cell cycles, and biochemical imbalances. Studies have shown that chronic wounds have elevated levels of inflammatory cytokines and tissue matrix metalloproteinases (TMMPs). The presence of both inhibits or slows the natural progression of healing. The increased concentration of TMMPs is enhanced by the associated decrease in protease inhibitors. In addition, there is an increase in degradation of fibronectin and other important matrix components. Chronic wounds are difficult to deal with and take time and patience. Debridement of the wound, careful cleaning, and dressing changes have been the only hope in advancing healing in a chronic wound. Negative pressure devices, recombinant growth factors, hyperbaric oxygen, and enzymatic debridement ointments are some of the methods that have been used to assist in wound healing.

Chronic wounds develop when normal healing mechanisms are not capable of repairing the tissue injury. They are a consequence of the equilibrium between the systemic and local factors favoring healing and those that oppose it being tilted towards chronicity. Malnutrition, uremia, and the hyperglycemia of diabetes are examples of systemic factors that retard healing. Edema, infection, arterial insufficiency (ischemia), fecal soiling, and pressure on the wound are examples of local factors that can impair healing. Appreciation of the role of these factors and judicious intervention to counter them often are key to successful management.

Four types of chronic wounds are generally encountered in clinical practice: pressure ulcers, venous stasis ulcers, arterial insufficiency ulcers, and diabetic neuropathic ulcers. All are more common in the elderly. Each type of ulcer reflects local factors that promote repeated bouts of trauma or injury in the wound bed, leading to prolonged or repetitive inflammatory stimulation of the wound, including promotion of leukocyte activity, TMMP degradation, and, in some, repeated infection. Successful management starts with the correct diagnosis of the type of ulcer. It continues with specific steps to alleviate the continuing pathologic influences, which usually include local factors specific to the type of chronic wound, but may include systemic factors that need to be addressed.

Pressure Ulcers

Pressure ulcers develop in neurologically impaired patients or those with critical illness who are bedridden and cannot protect their skin with appropriate reflexes and spontaneous movement to relieve pressure. As many as 10% of acutely hospitalized patients develop bed sores, which progress from partial- to full-thickness injuries if not well managed. Patients with chronic spinal cord injury are at particular risk for pressure ulceration due to a loss of both sensation and motor function below the level of spinal injury. The common sites for pressure ulceration are the heel, sacrum, and ischial tuberosities (bony prominences that bear increased pressure in the bedridden or wheelchair-bound patient). Pressure ulcers can be classified and graded using the information in Table 8-6.

Pressure ulcer prevention starts with frequent turning and repositioning of the patient at risk. Particular attention to the heel is necessary, and protective devices such as foam heel pads are not as effective as floating the foot off the bed with a pillow under the calf. Rotating the patient from side to side with pillows helps to prevent pelvic ulceration. Once a pressure sore has developed, it may be necessary to use specialized pressure relief mattresses, including elaborate air-fluidized supports, to minimize pressure. Pelvic pressure ulcers often have small skin defects overlying large cavities and become severely infected from fecal soiling. Aggressive surgical debridement and drainage to control infection may be required, and ultimately rotational skin or myocutaneous flaps are necessary to close the defect and achieve primary healing. The most common local care applied to pelvic pressure ulcers is probably saline-moistened gauze with twice daily changing. A particularly useful new modality is the negative pressure wound vacuum device (Wound VAC—Vacuum Assisted Closure system, Kinetic Concepts, Inc., San Antonio, TX), which is a porous sponge packed into the wound connected to negative pressure. The negative pressure applied by the VAC stimulates more rapid closure of the wound, while simultaneously promoting drainage and creating a moist wound environment favorable for the ingrowth of granulation tissue.

Table 8-6 Pressure Sore Classification/Grade

Grade	Description
Grade 1	This is a nonblanching erythematous area on intact skin
Grade 2	Partial thickness skin loss with the involvement of the epidermis and/or the dermis. This is usually superficial and can appear as a blister or abrasion.
Grade 3	Full thickness skin loss with necrosis of subcutaneous tissue that can extend to the fascia.
Grade 4	Full thickness skin loss with necrosis. Destruction can involve muscle, bone, and tendons.

Venous Stasis Ulcers

Venous stasis ulcers are the most common chronic wounds developing in adults. Venous insufficiency from venous valvular incompetence affects approximately 15% of adults, with typical symptoms of leg discomfort, heaviness, and edema. Ulceration in patients with chronic venous insufficiency is relatively uncommon, with an overall incidence of one per 1000 per year. Venous ulcers generally are superficial wounds in the anteromedial aspect of the leg ("gaiter zone"), not involving the foot. The underlying pathophysiology is a consequence of venous hypertension transmitted to the microcirculation of the skin. Incompetent valves in the deep and superficial veins draining the lower extremity lead to the transmission of elevated pressure to the venous side of the capillaries in the skin. This effect is exacerbated when the leg is dependent and alleviated when the leg is elevated. The consequences include anatomic changes in the capillaries that slowly enlarge and become tortuous. Additionally, the increased filtration and subsequent deposition of plasma proteins and red cells alter the interstitium around the capillaries. The red cells break down in the tissue, causing deposition of hemosiderin pigment. The chronic consequence is hyperpigmentation and edema (termed *dermatofibrosis*) of the leg above the ankle. Patients with chronic venous insufficiency who develop a wound have impaired healing both because of (1) decreased skin perfusion as a consequence of elevated venous pressures in the capillaries and (2) decreased delivery of oxygen and glucose to tissues as a consequence of edema and protein deposition in the interstitium. An additional factor is the tendency of the wounds to weep fluid copiously, with maceration of the surrounding normal tissues and further skin damage.

Management of venous ulcers starts with compression, either with paste bandages (Unna boots) or with multiple-layer dry bandages (Charing Cross or dry boots). Multiple-layer dry dressings are generally more effective, because they provide more pressure and allow variation in the medications and topical devices applied directly to the wound bed. Routine management of venous ulcers starts with establishing a clean wound bed with sharp debridement of necrotic tissue, using systemic antibiotics when infection is present, as well as teaching the patient to elevate the limb as much as practical. Local care requires weekly or biweekly application of compression bandages, often with topical application of medications or devices directly to the wound, which promotes healing. Most venous wounds will heal in several months with continued compression therapy. Refractory wounds may require surgery to ablate the abnormal veins transmitting pressure to the involved skin or skin grafting.

Arterial Insufficiency Ulcers

Arterial insufficiency ulcers result from atherosclerotic obstruction of the main conduit arteries supplying the lower extremity, although other causes of occlusion such as thromboembolism may apply. Chronic arterial ulcers may resemble venous ulcers or any chronic wound, with variable appearances and degree of granulation. They tend to excite little inflammation, and may extend into deeper structures to expose bone or tendon. Typically, arterial ulcers involve the toes, which can be mummified and black (dry gangrene) or have suppuration with oozing (wet gangrene), but any part of the foot, ankle, or leg may develop ulceration or nonhealing wounds. The presence of black, infarcted skin or multiple wounds should strongly raise the suspicion for arterial disease. Pedal pulses are usually absent, but in doubtful cases diagnostic vascular ultrasound to assess the arterial circulation is very reliable. Arterial wounds are the harbinger of limb loss from infection, and the presence of an arterial wound should prompt timely and aggressive intervention to salvage the limb and prevent major amputation.

Management of arterial wounds usually entails mechanical arterial interventions to improve tissue perfusion. Focal obstructions and occlusions are occasionally present and can be treated with endovascular balloon angioplasty or stenting, but most often long segments of arterial occlusion mandate bypass surgery with synthetic conduits or autologous saphenous veins. Without arterial reconstruction, approximately 25% of wounds can be healed with local care alone. It is hard to predict which wounds will respond to local care; therefore, the impetus to perform arterial surgery is high. Local care before revascularization is generally conservative: wet-to-dry gauze or antibiotic ointments are widely employed modalities. After arterial reconstruction, management options include excision of the wound and primary closure (e.g., toe amputation), or skin grafting. These interventions are occasionally successful without revascularization, but the chance for success with these minor surgical procedures depends greatly on the adequacy of arterial perfusion, and generally should be deferred until after successful arterial reconstruction.

Diabetic Neuropathic Ulcers

Diabetic neuropathic ulcers result from a combination of factors. Diabetic patients tend to develop polyneuropathy of the long neurons supplying the foot and lower extremity. Motor neuropathy leads to atrophy of the intrinsic muscles of the foot, leading to derangements in bony architecture that depends on intrinsic muscle tone for proper alignment. The resulting deformities include Charcot's foot, which is a collapse of the midfoot with plantar subluxation of the ruined bones, and clawing of the toes with plantar subluxation of the metatarsal heads. In both cases the change in bony architecture leads to excessive weight-bearing on surfaces at risk for pressure ulceration. In addition, diabetic polyneuropathy often causes sensory deficits, and a lack of proper protective reflexes contributes to promoting the chronic wound. Elevated glucose in poorly controlled diabetes independently retards wound healing and inhibits the leukocyte response to infection; often all measures to promote healing will fail without tight control of glucose. Arterial disease is frequently present in diabetics. Approximately 40% of diabetic neuropathic ulcers have an element of contributing arterial ischemia, which adds to the difficulty of treating these wounds. Typically, diabetic neuropathic ulcers are found at a site of increased weight bearing, such as a subluxed plantar surface of a metatarsal head, the heel, or on the dorsal surface of a toe that is rubbing against a shoe. Wounds typically have a fibrotic granulated bed surrounded by hypertrophic skin (callus), which identifies the exposure to excess pressure. Proper care for the diabetic wound starts with an appreciation of the burden imposed by the nonhealing wound. For each year a diabetic wound remains open, a 25% risk of limb loss is present. As a conseqeunce, aggressive and timely intervention is mandated.

Management starts with control of infection. Wounds that penetrate into bone or joint usually require surgical debridement followed by secondary healing or, when possible, primary closure after limited amputation. Specialized shoe gear to alleviate pressure is generally indicated. The most effective means to reduce pressure on a foot wound is a wheelchair, which will remove all pressure on the foot until the wound is healed. Another option, which is often successful, is to immobilize the foot in a cast to redistribute pressure and eliminate shear. Many different types of specialized shoes with cushioned soles and pressure relief features are available, and custom-made shoes with deep toe boxes and accommodative insoles are appropriate for management of the healed foot. Minor surgical procedures to treat bony deformity such as extensor tendon tenotomy to correct clawing or Achilles tendon lengthening to correct equinus deformity may be very helpful interventions and should be considered when local care measures are not successful. Arterial surgery may be required when ischemia is a prominent factor. Local wound care to keep the granulating wound clean and free of infection can be supplemented with topical medication in lieu of moist gauze. Frequent debridement of the wound and regular shaving of surrounding calluses are important steps, as well as aggressive treatment of nail diseases.

Advanced Care for Chronic Wounds

Management of chronic wounds requires a significant investment of resources, and many novel and technically sophisticated methods for stimulating healing of wounds have been devised in recent decades. Compared to medical interventions for other diseases, wound care therapy has not been as rigorously subjected to randomized prospective trials, and there is not much clear evidence that any one of these modalities has better efficacy compared to conventional care or other advanced modalities. Nonetheless, all of these newer treatments have developed proponents and seem to have a place in the management of chronic wounds. These newer modalities include:

1. Intermittent negative pressure devices
2. Topical foams and occlusive bandages to promote a moist wound environment
3. Topical application of growth factors and collagen preparations to promote healing
4. Topical use of broad-spectrum antimicrobial compounds to decrease the bacterial burden of the wound
5. Topical enzyme preparations
6. Use of engineered living skin substitutes
7. Hyperbaric oxygen therapy

Negative pressure applied to the wound using the Wound VAC (described earlier) is a method of wound healing that promotes new tissue growth, removes edema fluid, reduces TMMPs, and assists in contraction of the wound. This device is used in wounds that are not infected and have undergone adequate debridement. It is contraindicated in wounds that have cancer growth, untreated osteomyelitis, or necrotic tissue.

Topical foams and occlusive bandages are devices that, when placed over an open wound, prevent loss of moisture and desiccation. The typical moist-to-dry gauze dressing change regimen that is normally adequate for acute wounds may be suboptimal for chronic wounds. With gauze-packing methods, the wound tends to become overly dry, leading to damage to the wound tissue. With topical occlusive covers, however, desiccation is prevented, and the resident proteolysis enzymes (TMMPs) can better promote autolytic debridement. Foams typically are porous and allow absorption of exudates from a wound, but do not have an adhesive backing. Other devices are impermeable or permeable membranes made of polyurethane or other synthetic polymers that allow variable flux of water vapor. Occlusive dressings that allow sufficient flux of water to prevent excessive fluid in the wound often are optimal. One risk with occlusive dressing methods is that without regular changes, bacterial overgrowth may be promoted.

Growth factor therapy with topically applied platelet derived growth factor (PDGF) can stimulate chronic wounds to heal. It seems to be particularly useful in diabetic ulcers, where prospective, randomized, multicenter clinical trials showed complete wound healing to be almost twice as likely to occur with PDGF therapy compared to wounds treated otherwise. Venous ulcers appear to respond well to PDGF therapy. A new growth factor, keratinocyte growth factor II (KGFII), is in clinical trials with promising early results. KGFII has the unique ability to stimulate keratinocyte migration. Topical application of devitalized tissue (thin sheets of animal skin or intestinal submucosa) and purified collagen preparations are widely used to promote healing. These biologics may work to counteract excessive TMMP activity in the wound. Some evidence indicates that TMMPs are bound and inactivated by topical collagens. An alternative hypothesis for how collagen and tissue products stimulate healing is that they mimic the architecture found in healing acute wounds, and thus stimulate chronic wound cells by providing growth factors or other cues that promote normal wound healing.

Topical broad-spectrum antimicrobial preparations include 1% silver nitrate solution, which has been used for over a century to inhibit bacterial growth in burns and other chronic wounds. Other silver preparations such as silvadene cream and films that slowly release silver into wounds are widely used. Topical iodine solutions have good antimicrobial activity, but are too cytotoxic for recurrent use. A better preparation is cadexomeric iodine, a formulation of starch granules with elemental iodine, which both absorbs exudate from the wound and promotes a sterile environment. This is one of the few topical antimicrobials supported by randomized clinical trials. Specific topical antibiotics such as gentamicin and metronidazole ointment also can be useful in promoting wound healing, especially when wound cultures indicate that sensitive organisms are present. Dilute acetic acid (e.g., 0.25%) suppresses pseudomonas colonization and infection and is widely used in lieu of saline to moisten gauze when wet-to-dry gauze-packing regimens are employed.

Debriding wounds of necrotic tissue or fibrinous exudates is an important adjunct to wound management. An alternative to sharp surgical debridement is the use of ointments containing degradative enzymes such as collagenase or papain. These products can significantly expedite healing. Cross-hatching the crust or necrotic tissue covering the wound with a scalpel prior to starting topical enzyme therapy increases the efficacy. One product, a combination of papain with copper and chlorophyll (Panafil), appears to be a particularly useful adjunct for many chronic wounds, but to date supporting randomized clinical trial data is absent.

Recent advances in tissue engineering have led to the commercial production of synthetic living skin substitutes. These are bilayers of fetal fibroblasts growing over collagen layers mimicking the dermal layer of skin. These products are increasingly employed to promote healing of burns and chronic wounds. They appear to have some ability to promote healing by providing keratinocytes to cover the wound and possibly through the elaboration of growth factors.

Hyperbaric oxygen therapy is another of the newer modalities used to stimulate wound healing. Treatment entails placing a patient in a chamber of pure oxygen at three atmospheres of pressure, with daily exposures of up to 8 weeks. Exposure to high-pressure oxygen increases tissue oxygen levels, which seems to promote healing in some refractory wounds, although other effects of high oxygen levels may be important. Osteoradionecrosis of the mandible and anaerobic soft tissue infections are particularly sensitive to hyperbaric therapy, but randomized clinical trials have shown disappointing efficacy with this therapy for chronic diabetic and arterial ulcers.

SUGGESTED READINGS

Armstrong DG. Improvement in healing with aggressive edema reduction after debridement of foot infection in persons with diabetes. *Arch Surg* 2000;135(12):1405–1409.

Bennett NT. Properties of growth factors and their receptors. *Amer J Surg* 1993:165(6):728–737.

Bennett NT. Growth factors and wound healing. Part 2: role in normal and chronic wound healing. *Amer J Surg* 1993:166(1):74–81.

Black E. Decrease of collagen deposition in wound repair in type 1 diabetes independent of glycemic control. *Arch Surg* 2003;138(1): 34–40.

Cross KJ. Growth factors in wound healing. *Surg Clin North Am* 2003; 83(3):531–545.

Enoch S. Wound bed preparation: the science behind the removal of barriers to healing. *Wounds* 2003;15(7):213–229.

Ginard H. Inflammatory mediators in wound healing. *Surg Clin North Am* 2003;83(3):484–507.

Greenfield, LJ, Mulholland MW, Oldham KT, et al. Cytokines. In *Surgery: Scientific Principles and Practice*. 3rd Ed. Philadelphia, PA: Lippincott Williams & Wilkins, 2001:111–133.

Greenfield, LJ, Mulholland MW, Oldham KT, et al. Wound healing. In *Surgery: Scientific Principles and Practice*. 3rd Ed. Philadelphia, PA: Lippincott Williams & Wilkins, 2001:69–86.

Hackman DJ. Cellular, biochemical and clinical aspects of wound healing. *Surg Infect* 2002;3:S23–S35.

Jeschke MG. Nutritional intervention high in vitamins, protein, amino acids and [omega]3 fatty acids improves protein metabolism during the hypermetabolic state after thermal injury. *Arch Surg* 2001; 136(11):1301–1306.

Mani R. Science of measurements in wound healing. *Wound Care Regener* 1999;7:330–334.

O'Leary PJ. Wound healing biology and its application to wound management. In *The Physiologic Basis of Surgery*. 3rd Ed. Philadelphia, PA: Lippincott Williams and Wilkins, 2002:107–132.

Saap LJ. Debridement performance index and its correlation with complete closure of diabetic foot ulcers. *Wound Repair Regener* 2002; 10:354–359.

Stamm J. Growth hormone does not attenuate the inhibitory effects of sepsis on wound healing. *Wound Repair Regener* 2000;8:103–109.

Williams JZ. Nutrition and wound healing. *Surg Clin North Am* 2003; 83(3):571–596.

Wysocki AB. Evaluating and managing open skin wounds: colonization versus infection *AANC Clin Issues* 2002:13(3):382–397.

9

RICHARD N. GARRISON, MD ■ DONALD E. FRY, MD
DAVID A. SPAIN, MD

Surgical Infections

OBJECTIVES

1 List the factors that contribute to infection after a surgical procedure.
2 List the four classes of surgical wounds and the frequency with which each type becomes infected.
3 Describe the principles of prophylactic antibiotic use.
4 List the clinical variables that affect antibiotic sensitivity when compared with in vitro tests.
5 Describe the events that lead to antibiotic resistance in a surgical patient who has an infection.
6 Discuss four common hand infections, and describe the treatment of each.
7 List the clinical variables that contribute to foot infections in patients with diabetes.
8 Identify the most likely bacterial species encountered initially with infection from a dog bite, from acute cholecystitis, and from acute perforated appendicitis, and infection found 2 hours after a perforated duodenal ulcer.
9 List three viruses that pose an occupational hazard for surgeons, and discuss methods to protect against infection.
10 List the causes of postoperative fever, and discuss the diagnostic steps for evaluation.

Treatment of the diverse surgical infections that a surgeon encounters requires an understanding of the etiology of the invading organism, the physiologic response of the host, and mechanisms of the treatment. Currently, a limiting factor in advanced surgical care is the inability to control infectious processes that are ubiquitous. The wholesale use of antibiotics has caused the emergence of virulent bacteria, fungi, and viruses that are resistant to standard methods of treatment. In addition, patients have become more vulnerable as such factors as aging, transplantations, tumor therapies, foreign body implants, and prolonged intensive care have weakened both the immune system and the ability of the host to respond. Thus, the surgeon must be familiar with both the simple and the complex challenges of modern care of surgical patients with infections. This chapter describes the diagnostic methods and the therapy indicated for common infections that are encountered by the surgeon and introduces some of the complex issues of **sepsis** that are prominent within surgical intensive care units.

PATHOGENESIS OF INFECTION

Surgical procedures, traumatic injuries, and nontraumatic local invasion can lead to severe bacterial insult. Regardless of the anatomic site, bacterial soilage of host tissues initiates well-defined processes of host defense. Potent mediators of the inflammatory response (e.g., kinins, histamine) are released from mast cells, platelets, and fixed granulocytes, altering capillary permeability in the area of injury and contamination. Plasma proteins, such as **complement,** fibrinogen, and specific or nonspecific **opsonins,** are delivered into the area of the bacterial invaders. Circulating neutrophils then "marginate" as a result of upregulation of adhesion molecules at the site of increased vascular permeability in the capillary. Through the process of diapedesis, these molecules move out of the intravascular compartment and into the interstitium. Neutrophils are directed toward the site of infection by chemoattractants from tissue macrophages, platelets, and vascular endothelial cells. Chemoattractants include complement cleavage products, leukotrienes, kinins, and proinflammation cytokines. Neutrophils subsequently make contact with the foreign particles or bacteria. Opsonins bind to the foreign particle and facilitate adherence to the neutrophil plasma membrane, where phagocytosis is initiated. The engulfed organism or foreign particle is then surrounded within the phagosome, and intracellular killing and digestion are initiated by the release of lysosomal enzymes, hydrolases, reactive intermediators, and other enzymes into the surrounding vacuole. Ingestion of microorganisms in excess of the ability of the neutrophil to achieve intracellular killing results in death and dissolution of the phagocytic cell with the subsequent release of activated digestive enzymes and reactive oxygen intermediates that further local inflammation. Dead phagocytic cells, fibrin, opsonic proteins, dead and viable microorganisms, and bacterial products are the essential components of **pus.** The inflammatory microenvironment that develops is relatively hypoxic and acidic. As a result, cellular and enzyme function is inhibited. The primary determinant of establishing a local infection for a given level of contamination is the density of bacteria present versus the efficiency and effectiveness of the host in disposing of the organisms.

Numerous local and systemic factors affect bacterial virulence and cellular host response and thus may alter the host–pathogen interaction in favor of the bacteria (Table 9-1). Hemoglobin potentiates bacterial virulence because ferric iron may enhance bacterial growth, and hemoglobin diminishes the efficiency of the neutrophil in eradicating the microorganism. Therefore, it is advisable to rid the wound of blood before closure. Likewise, dead tissue and foreign bodies are potent adjuvants. Dead tissue is not readily penetrated by host defense mechanisms, and it provides a haven for bacterial proliferation. Thus, wound debridement and cleansing are essential for healing. Foreign bodies, regardless of whether they are suture material or drains in the surgical wound, Foley catheters in the urinary bladder, or intravenous cannulae, protect bacteria against the host response.

Systemic factors (e.g., shock, hypovolemia, hypoxia) cause acidosis and weaken host defenses. Hemorrhagic shock causes tissue hypoperfusion and increases septic complications in patients who have traumatic injury or who have undergone surgical procedures. Oxygen is an essential metabolic component of phagocytosis and intracellular killing. Inadequate oxygenation results in acidosis at the site of contamination and significantly enhances the likelihood of subsequent infection.

Other coexisting systemic variables also diminish host response. Patients with diabetes have impaired neutrophil mobility, probably as a result of hyperglycemia. Obesity facilitates local wound infection because the blood supply to adipose tissue is poor. Starvation with protein-calorie malnutrition increases the vulnerability of the host to infection, and acute or chronic alcoholism impairs host response. Systemic drug therapy with corticosteroids, cancer chemotherapeutic agents, and immunosuppression during transplantation also increases vulnerability to invasive infection.

The systemic response to the initial injury and changes in the microenvironment is mediated by several factors. Tissue macrophages are stimulated to produce cytokines that have profound stimulatory effects on other systemic cellular and humoral cascades. The best characterized of these cytokines is tumor necrosis factor (TNF). When produced in excess, this factor is associated with tissue destruction and a hypermetabolic state. Similarly, the endothelial cell, whether injured or stimulated, causes local changes in blood flow, coagulation, and (through the release of vasoactive substances) a systemic vascular response.

In summary, the interaction between the pathogen and the host determines whether contamination has no sequelae or clinical infection occurs. Numerous local and systemic variables swing the biologic balance of power in favor of the bacterial invaders and determine whether the infection remains local or causes a systemic inflammatory state. The objective of surgical therapy is to reduce the bacterial concentration and alter the tissue environment so that supremacy of the host defense is established.

Table 9-1 Surgical Infection

Local	Systemic
High bacteria concentrations	Advanced age
Wound hematoma	Shock (hypoxia, acidosis)
Necrotic tissue	Diabetes mellitus
Foreign body	Protein-calorie malnutrition
Obesity	Acute and chronic alcoholism
	Corticosteroid drug therapy
	Cancer chemotherapy
	Transplant immunosuppression

PREVENTION OF SURGICAL INFECTION

Preventing infection in patients who are injured or undergo elective surgical procedures is essential for quality surgical care. Numerous soft tissue local adjuvant factors must be managed mechanically to avoid infection. Steps include debridement of nonviable tissue, irrigation to remove bacteria-laden clot and fibrin, control of bleeding, and meticulous removal of dirt and other foreign bodies. The wound can then be closed with a reasonable prospect for uncomplicated healing. Preservation of systemic oxygenation and tissue perfusion is also important in the prevention of infection.

Surgical wounds have different degrees of risk of infection. Infection in surgical wounds is primarily a consequence of contamination and adjuvant factors that are present in the wound at the time of closure. These different degrees of risk are organized into several classification

Table 9-2 Classification of Surgical Wounds

Wound	Bacterial Contaminants	Source of Contamination	Infection Frequency	Examples
Clean	Gram-positive	Operating room environment, surgical team, patient's skin	3%	Inguinal hernia, thyroidectomy, mastectomy, aortic graft
Clean-contaminated	Polymicrobial	Endogenous colonization of the patient	5%–15%	Common duct exploration, elective colon resection, gastrectomy
Contaminated	Polymicrobial	Gross contamination	15%–40%	"Spill" during elective gastrointestinal surgery, perforated gastric ulcer
Dirty	Polymicrobial	Established infection	40%	Drainage of intraabdominal abscess, resection of infarcted intestine

schemes to allow stratification of similar operations. Only when operative wounds at similar risk are examined can the effect of different preventive measures be assessed. The classification system that is most commonly used for surgical wounds is shown in Table 9-2.

Universal Precautions

Universal precautions and isolation are applied to bacterial (e.g., staphylococcal) infections and selected viral infections (e.g., hepatitis A) to prevent the organisms from being carried out of the room or treatment area. Gowns and gloves should be worn and then removed upon leaving the patient's room, and traffic into the patient's room is restricted. The objective is to prevent nurses, hospital personnel, and physicians from serving as vectors in transmission of the organism to others. Isolation is contrasted with reverse isolation, where the objective is to prevent pathogens from being introduced into contact with severely immunosuppressed patients. In this situation, nurses, physicians, and others who attend these patients wear masks to prevent airborne organisms from being introduced into the controlled environment.

Surgical Asepsis

In clean procedures, surgical asepsis is of paramount importance in the prevention of operative site infection. The frequency of **clean wound** infection is the most sensitive indicator of quality surgical care and is a surveillance tool that is used to judge overall sterile technique in the operating room. Certain techniques are used to obtain a low rate of infection in this category of wounds. Preoperative hospitalization should be limited to avoid colonization of the patient with antibiotic-resistant, hospital-acquired bacteria. Preoperative showers with specific cleansing of the proposed operative site are useful. Hair removal should be performed immediately before the procedure in the operating room to avoid colonization of small razor nicks and cuts. Adhesive plastic skin drapes actually increase clean wound rates of infection. Shorter operative times are associated with lower wound infection rats. Operations that last more than 2 hours have a 40% greater infection rate than those that last less than 1 hour. A careful preoperative examination of all patients who are about to undergo an elective procedure should include a search for areas of coexisting infection (e.g., boil, furuncle, urinary tract). These sources of infection should be treated before the surgeon performs the procedure to avoid endogenous wound contamination.

Intraoperative efforts should minimize the introduction of bacteria and reduce adjuvant factors. Hemostasis is important, but excessive use of suture material and the indiscriminate use of electrocautery, which may leave large areas of devitalized tissue, should be avoided. Wound drains are seldom indicated, but when needed, they should be closed-suction drains that have a separate stab wound to exit the subcutaneous space. The purpose of drains is to remove adjuvant material (e.g., blood), and they should be used only when they are actively removing debris or fluid. At the time of wound closure, the patient's fate is sealed with respect to wound infection. A postoperative dressing is generally applied, but it does not prevent wound infection after the first few hours when the wound coagulum has formed.

Although most surgical infections originate from the patient's endogenous microflora and the degree of contamination present at the time of the procedure, the operating room environment also contributes to wound infection. Personnel (i.e., surgeons, anesthetists, nurses, students) are a common source of bacterial contamination in this setting. Respiration and mouth secretions, along with the bacteria shed from exposed skin and hair, are measurable threats to clean incisions. Operating room attire is designed to minimize this source of contamination. Scrubbing of the hands and arms with an antiseptic solution and donning of sterile gowns and gloves are the last barriers against contamination. When infections occur after clean operative procedures, a break in this routine should be suspected. Appropriate scrubbing and the maintenance of a sterile environment are necessary for all procedures performed within the operating room. Other prevention techniques (e.g., ultraviolet irradiation, laminar flow air-handling systems, space suit attire for operating room personnel) are expensive and are most often used when the patient requires implantation of a permanent foreign body, such as an orthopedic joint or a vascular graft. However, the efficacy of such techniques is not proven.

Perioperative Antibiotics

Since their introduction in the 1940s, antibiotics have been used in an effort to prevent infection in patients who are undergoing elective operations. Studies show that **prophylactic antibiotics** must be present in the tissue at the time of bacterial contamination to be effective. Antibiotics that are given after contamination occurs are not effective. Clinical studies show the effectiveness of preoperative systemic antibiotics in reducing the incidence of tissue infection, especially in **clean-contaminated** and **contaminated** wounds. Few studies support the use of antibiotic prophylaxis for clean operative procedures. The risk from the antibiotic complication (e.g., allergic reaction) is greater than the minimal benefit that could be obtained. For clean procedures in which a foreign body is implanted (e.g., aortic graft, total hip replacement), prophylaxis is used because a septic complication, although infrequent, is a very morbid or lethal event. The important issues in surgical prophylaxis with antibiotics, regardless of the clinical setting, are to give the drug preoperatively and to select a drug that is active against the anticipated pathogens. Antibiotics that have a long half-life are preferable to those that have a short half-life, which require frequent re-dosing to maintain tissue concentrations; they should be given within 60 minutes of the time of incision, and again 4 to 6 hours later. Antibiotics used in a perioperative prophylactic manner should not be continued past two postoperative doses to avoid the emergence of resistant bacteria.

Prophylactic systemic antibiotics are of little value when the period of bacterial contamination is longer than a short defined period of exposure. When used over a prolonged time, the growth of multiple generations of microbes favors the development of resistance to the antibiotic utilized. Antibiotics alone or in combination will not prevent infection in open wounds, passive wound drains, burns, Foley catheters, ischemic tissue, endotracheal tubes, intravenous catheters, or percutaneous monitor devices. In such settings, the risk of colonization and subsequent invasive infection with aggressive resistant bacteria actually is enhanced when systemic therapy is used.

Because elective colon surgery, which is classified as a clean-contaminated wound, is associated with high rates of infection, it is considered a special area for antibiotic prophylaxis. Orally administered, poorly absorbed antibiotics reduce the numbers of aerobic and anaerobic species that reside in the bowel and can ultimately contaminate the surgical wound during colon resection. Oral antibiotics are effective in reducing wound infection rates to less than 10% for elective colon resections. Oral neomycin–erythromycin base antibiotics are most commonly used, along with a mechanical bowel preparation. Whether prophylactic systemic antibiotics and preoperative oral neomycin–erythromycin base antibiotics used together are superior to either type used individually is unproven, but this practice is commonly used in colon surgery.

For grossly contaminated wounds or dirty procedures, the risk of a wound infection exceeds 15% to 20%. Therefore, many surgeons close only the fascial layers, with the skin and subcutaneous tissues left open. The open wound can then be managed with wet-to-dry saline dressings, and may be closed by delayed primary closure on postoperative day 4 or 5. Small open wounds rarely become infected when the underlying tissue is viable, although the wound surface may become colonized. Prolonged postoperative systemic antibiotics do not facilitate the process of delayed primary closure.

MANAGEMENT OF ESTABLISHED INFECTION

Established surgical infections are organized into community-acquired infections and hospital-acquired, postoperative (**nosocomial**) infections. Community-acquired infections are active processes that were initiated before the patient presented for treatment. Hospital-acquired infections include all infections that occur after surgical procedures. Thus, **peritonitis** is usually a community-acquired infection, but intraperitoneal abscess is most commonly a postoperative problem. Potential choices for antibiotic selection for each type of infection are shown in Table 9-3.

Several caveats must be considered in choosing a **therapeutic antibiotic.** Antibiotic sensitivity to an identified organism should always be determined for serious invasive infections and, if necessary, the antibiotic should be switched according to the sensitivity profile. However, because of the arbitrary testing environment of the laboratory, in vitro sensitivity does not always indicate clinical responsiveness. Factors that must be considered in choosing an appropriate agent include bacterial counts, tissue environment (e.g., pH, tissue hypoxia), antibiotic concentration (as a function of drug metabolism), function of organs that either metabolize or excrete the drug, and inherent toxicity of the agent. Regardless of the drug used, an ongoing daily assessment of the response of the host to the therapy is an essential component of care for surgical infections. If therapy is effective, that course of action should be sustained; however, if there is little or no sign of effectiveness, both the drugs used and the infection source that is being treated should be reevaluated.

Antibiotic resistance is a prominent concern in the treatment of surgical infection. Resistance means that a structural or functional change within the microorganism enables formerly sensitive bacteria to resist the antimicrobial effects of specific antibiotics. The bacterial changes may be mediated primarily by acquired genetic material

Table 9-3 Antibiotic Selections for Common Infections

Infection Site	Anticipated Organism	Antibiotic Choice
Soft tissue cellulitis	Group A *Streptococcus, Staphylococcus*	Nafcillin/oxacillin
Breast abscess	Usually *Staphylococcus*	Nafcillin/oxacillin
Synthetic vascular graft		Nafcillin/oxacillin
Hip prosthesis		
Heart/valve prosthesis	*Staphylococcus, Streptococcus viridans, Enterococcus,* etc.	Specific sensitivity needed
Biliary tract infection	*Escherichia coli, Klebsiella, Enterococcus*[a]	Aztreonam, cefazolin
Peritonitis; intraabdominal abscess	*E. coli,* other *Enterobacteriaceae, Bacteroides fragilis,* other obligate aerobes	Clindamycin/aminoglycoside, metronidazole/aminoglycoside, third-generation cephalosporin[b]
Antibiotic-associated colitis	*Clostridium difficile*	Oral metronidazole, vancomycin
Hospital-acquired pneumonia	*Pseudomonas, Serratia,* resistant Enterobacteriaceae, *Staphylococcus*	Ciprofloxacin, amikacin (or expanded-spectrum penicillin) quinolones, vancomycin (Gram+)
Catheter-associated bacteremia	*Staphylococcus,* Enterobacteriaceae	Specific sensitivities (beware methicillin-resistant *Staphylococcus epidermidis*)
Urinary tract (postcatheterization)	*E. coli, Pseudomonas, Klebsiella* spp., Enterobacteriaceae	Specific sensitivity
Candidiasis	*Candida albicans*	Amphotericin, fluconazole
Pneumocystis	*Pneumocystis carinii*	Trimethoprim/sulfamethoxazole

[a] *Enterococcus* is not specifically covered primarily—either in the biliary tract or in intraabdominal infection. Consideration for treatment should be given when *Enterococcus* emerges as a secondary pathogen or when it is isolated in blood culture.
[b] Includes cefotaxime, cefoperazone, moxalactam, ceftizoxime, and ceftriaxone.

(through plasmid transfer from other organisms) or by spontaneous chromosomal mutation. Once genetic changes are established within a given bacterial population, sustained use of the antibiotic preferentially promotes the resistant organisms by effectively eliminating the sensitive microbial population. Although this resistance is an evolutionary process and new techniques and drugs with different mechanisms of action have outpaced the surge of resistance, clinical practice concerning antibiotic selection and use is of utmost importance. Antibiotic therapy should be initiated only when there is clear evidence that an infection that is amenable to that form of therapy is present. Most surgical infections require drainage or debridement, and antibiotics should be used as an adjuvant to mechanical treatment. Finally, with the exception of only a few narrow indications, antibiotic therapy should not be used to prevent infection over an extended period. Application of these principles will at least forestall the development of resistant strains of microorganisms within both the individual patient and the surgical unit.

Community-Acquired Infections

Skin and Soft Tissue Infections

Soft tissue infection, which is usually due to a break in the skin barrier, usually after a minor cut or puncture, ordinarily presents with spreading cellulitis. The blanching erythema of cellulitis is usually caused by group A streptococci and responds to penicillin therapy. Staphylococci may also be the cause of cellulitis, particularly if gross suppuration (pus) is present at the injury site. Common soft tissue infections are listed in Table 9-4.

Necrotizing streptococcal gangrene is rarely seen in surgical patients. These infections are characterized by nonblanching erythema, with blisters and frank necrosis of the skin. Nonblanching erythema indicates subdermal thrombosis of the nutrient blood supply of the skin. Extensive surgical debridement of the affected area, in combination with high-dose penicillin and clindamycin, is the appropriate treatment. A Gram stain of blister fluid is useful in differentiating this infection from other necrotizing infections of the skin and subcutaneous tissue.

Severe staphylococcal soft tissue infections are usually identified by Gram stain of the pus. Nafcillin and oxacillin are first-line antibiotics that are used in addition to surgical drainage and debridement of the primary focus of infection. Because staphylococci are readily passed to other patients by health care personnel or by objects passed between patients, sterile isolation techniques must be used for any patient contact or treatment. Sensitivity data are important to confirm that methicillin-resistant staphylococci (MRSA) are not present. MRSA will require antibiotic therapy with vancomycin or linezolid.

Breast Abscess

Breast abscess is a common staphylococcal soft tissue infection. Postpartum women with galactoceles are particularly at risk for this infection. These abscesses are characterized

Table 9-4 Common Soft Tissue Infections

	Etiology	Usual Organism	Physical Findings	Treatment
Cellulitis	Break in skin barrier	Group A *Streptococcus*	Diffuse blanching erythema, tenderness	Systemic penicillins, cephalosporins, local wound cleansing
Furuncle, carbuncle	Bacterial growth within skin glands and crypts	*Staphylococcus aureus*	Localized induration, erythema, tenderness, swelling, creamy pus formation	I & D of abscess, systemic antibiotics against staph for surrounding cellulitis
Hidradenitis suppurativa	Bacterial growth within apocrine sweat glands	*Staphylococcus aureus*	Multiple abscesses, drainage, thick pus from axilla and groin regions	I & D of small lesions, wide debridement, excision and grafting of large areas
Lymphangitis	Infection within lymphatics	*Staphylococcus aureus*	Swelling and erythema of distal extremity, inflamed streaks along involved lymphatic channels	Local wound cleansing, removal of any foreign body, systemic penicillins or cephalosporins
Gangrene, necrotizing fasciitis	Destruction of healthy tissue by virulent microbial enzymes	Synergistic *Streptococcus/Staphylococcus,* mixed aerobic–anaerobic organisms, *Clostridium*	Necrotic skin/fascia, extremity swelling, grayish liquid discharge, crepitation/gas formation within tissue planes	Radical debridement of necrotic tissues, parenteral broad-spectrum antibiotics
Diabetic fetid foot	Ischemia, neuropathy, injury, pressure, ulceration, bone involvement	Mixed aerobic–anaerobic organisms	Foot erythema, swelling, malodorous discharge	Radical debridement including soft and bony tissues, broad-spectrum antibiotics

I & D, incision and drainage.

by localized severe tenderness, swelling, and redness associated with a mass that may or may not be fluctuant. Aspiration with a needle is helpful to confirm the presence of purulent material; however, the treatment requires urgent incision and drainage. Antibiotics for staphylococci are directed at the cellulitis but alone will not suffice, and a delay in surgical drainage may result in necrosis of large amounts of breast tissue. MRSA is currently very uncommon in breast abscess.

Perirectal Abscess

These abscesses result from infection within the crypts of the anorectal canal that subsequently suppurates; they are identified as tender masses in the perianal area. Perirectal abscess can extend into the pelvis above the rectal sphincter and, in diabetic or immunocompromised patients, can be fatal. Because both perirectal and breast abscesses are exquisitely tender, they usually must be examined and adequate drainage established under general anesthesia. Antibiotics for the patient with a perirectal abscess are usually broad-spectrum for both anaerobes and aerobes, but are probably necessary only to protect the patient from the **bacteremia** that is associated with drainage, which is the appropriate treatment. Perianal infection and resultant subcutaneous tissue necrosis can be extensive if drainage is not adequate. In this instance, fecal diversion should be considered to avoid further soilage to the area.

Gas Gangrene

Clostridial soft tissue infections include both cellulitis and myonecrosis. This combination is referred to as gas gangrene. These infections occur when contaminated objects (e.g., nail in the foot) penetrate the skin. These infections commonly cause a brown, watery drainage from the wound site and are associated with marked tenderness. Palpable crepitance is commonly present, but may be subtle when the myonecrosis extends along a subfascial plane. Roentgenograms may show soft tissue gas.

Tetanus toxoid immunization, along with adequate surgical debridement without primary wound closure, prevents clostridial myonecrosis or cellulitis in most patients

Table 9-5 Wound Classification

	Tetanus Prone	Nontetanus Prone
Age	> 6 hr	< 6 hr
Type	Crush Avulsion Extensive abrasion Burns or frostbite	Sharp/clean
Contaminants (soil, saliva)	Present	Absent

who are at risk. Tetanus antitoxin is administered to patients with high-risk wounds who have an uncertain history of immunization. When clostridial gas gangrene is diagnosed, immediate radical surgical debridement is necessary. Massive doses of penicillin are necessary to kill the organism *Clostridium perfringens,* but penicillin is not useful in the absence of aggressive debridement of the affected tissue. Metronidazole and clindamycin are alternative antibiotic choices when penicillin cannot be used because of an allergic history. Hyperbaric oxygen is an unproved but often employed treatment in these patients.

Tetanus

Tetanus (lockjaw) is caused by the exotoxin produced by the organism *Clostridium tetani.* After an incubation period of 2 days to several weeks, a prodromal symptom complex of restlessness, headache, stiffness of the jaw muscles, and muscular contractions in the area of the wound evolves. Violent generalized tonic muscle spasms usually follow within 24 hours, and respiratory arrest occurs. The keystone of management is the prevention of exotoxin production by debridement and cleansing of all wounds in which devitalized, contaminated tissue is present, along with a program of immunization. All patients who have traumatic wounds should receive tetanus prophylaxis in accordance with the recommendations of the Committee on Trauma of the American College of Surgeons (Tables 9-5 and 9-6). Patients with tetanus-prone wounds should be given tetanus toxoid. The only contraindication to the use of tetanus toxoid is a history of a neurologic or hypersensitivity reaction to a previous dose. Patients who have not been immunized within 10 years should receive additional therapy with tetanus immune globulin (human). The use of systemic antibiotics specific for clostridia (e.g., penicillin) should be considered for all tetanus-prone wounds to eliminate residual tetanus bacilli.

Hand Infections

Hand infections are common. They are described in Table 9-7. Although they are not life threatening, hand infections can lead to severe morbidity because of the loss of hand function. **Paronychia** is usually a staphylococcal infection of the proximal fingernail that ordinarily points in the sulcus at the nail border. Simple drainage and hot soaks are usually adequate therapy for these infections. **Felons** are deep infections of the pulp space of the terminal phalanx. These infections usually occur after penetrating injuries of the distal phalanx and are treated by drainage. A subungual abscess is the extension of a deep paronychia. It is identified by fluctuance beneath the nail. Removal of the nail is usually necessary to permit adequate drainage. Neglected infections of the fingers may result in **tenosynovitis,** an infection that extends along the tendon sheath of the finger. Drainage requires opening the sheath along its entire length to prevent necrosis of the tendon, with its functional implications.

Penetrating trauma or spread from a contiguous fascial compartment can result in an infection in one of three **deep-space compartments** in the hand. A thenar space infection causes swelling and pain directly over the thenar prominence. The thumb is held in abduction. Loss of normal concavity as a result of tense, painful swelling of the palm is characteristic of a midpalmar space abscess. Rarely, the hypothenar space presents in a similar fashion,

Table 9-6 Immunization Recommendations

	Tetanus Prone		Nontetanus Prone	
History of Immunization	Tetanus Toxoid	Tetanus Immune Globulin	Tetanus Toxoid	Tetanus Immune Globulin
Unknown or incomplete	0.5 mL[a]	250 units	0.5 mL[a]	No
Complete, last booster > 5 yr ago	0.5 mL	No	No[b]	No
Complete, last booster < 5 yr ago	No	No	No	No

[a] In unimmunized children, DT (diphtheria, tetanus) or DPT (diphtheria, pertussis, tetanus) is used. Completion of immunizations is necessary.
[b] Yes, if booster > 10 yr ago.

Table 9-7 Common Hand Infections

	Location	Signs	Treatment
Felon	Pulp space of digits	Swollen, indurated, tense, throbbing distal finger; point tenderness	I & D over length of phalanx along side of finger
Paronychia	Skin over mantle of nail and lateral nail folds	Swelling/induration of nail folds, point tenderness, purulent drainage	I & D at base of nail; removal of nail if infection beneath nail
Tenosynovitis	Tendon sheath	Throbbing, pain with movement, entire finger swollen, tenderness over sheath, finger held semi-flexed	I & D over length of sheath and bursa; systemic antibiotics usually indicated
Fascial space	Spaces of hand/thenar regions	Tenderness of involved space, swelling over region involved, limited motion	I & D along surface lines of projection; systemic antibiotics indicated
Human bites	Point of skin penetration and underlying regions	Injury site wound, induration and swelling, purulent drainage, limited motion	Wide debridement and irrigation; systemic antibiotics and tetanus immunization indicated

I & D, incision and drainage.

with swelling and painful movement. In all cases, incision and drainage are urgently required, and antibiotics are empirically initiated and then continued, based on culture and sensitivity reports, for at least 10 days.

Human bites of the hand are common, but their potential infectious nature should not be underestimated. These infections are caused by contamination with **polymicrobial** aerobic and anaerobic mouth flora. Deep-space infections, including tenosynovitis, may be consequences of these bites. Copious irrigation, debridement, hand elevation, and systemic antibiotics are required initially to prevent infection. Human bites are the only penetrating injury of the hand in which primary closure is not employed. The hand is often injured by animal bites as well. Debridement and irrigation are required (as for human bites), but the pathogens involved are more likely to be aerobic *Pasteurella* species.

Foot Infections

Foot infections result from direct trauma or, more commonly, from mechanical and metabolic derangements that occur in patients with diabetes. Trauma-related infections are best prevented by adequate wound cleansing at the time of injury. Established infections raise concern that a foreign body or osteomyelitis is present. Radiographs and bone scans, along with aggressive debridement and cultures, should establish the extent of the infection and identify the organisms involved.

Foot infections in patients with diabetes are a common problem because of neuropathy, the resultant bone deformities, and the vascular compromise that occurs in this population, which results in ischemic pressure ulceration. Ulcers on the plantar aspect of the forefoot underneath a metatarsal head are termed "mal perforant" ulcers. A thorough examination of the infected foot should determine the extent of vascular and neurologic impairment. Osteomyelitis is a frequent component, and any persistent or extensive infection should be evaluated for bone involvement. Cultures should always be obtained, followed by broad-spectrum antibiotic therapy, debridement, and drainage. In addition, mechanical external support devices can be fitted to relieve pressure points and provide protection. All efforts should focus on limb salvage in these patients, because amputation is a frequent morbid consequence of these complex infections.

Biliary Tract Infections

Biliary tract infections are usually a consequence of obstruction within the biliary tree, involving either the cystic or the common bile duct. The bacteria that are likely to be involved include *Escherichia coli, Klebsiella* species, and the enterococci. Anaerobes are not commonly encountered. Antibiotics to cover these organisms are usually used, but surgical intervention in the biliary tract is often necessary for effective drainage and resolution.

Acute cholecystitis is the most common inflammatory process in the biliary tract. It begins as a nonspecific inflammatory process secondary to obstruction of the cystic duct. Entrapped bacteria convert inflammation to an invasive infectious process. Empyema of the gallbladder occurs when infection in the gallbladder is undrained, leading to purulent distension and, often, severe systemic sepsis. Increased intraluminal pressure combined with invasive bacterial infection into the wall may impede the blood supply of the gallbladder, resulting in gangrene and perforation. Prevention of these complications can best be achieved by early operation.

Infection proximal to a common duct obstruction causes ascending cholangitis. Patients have fulminant fever, leukocytosis, and jaundice. These patients are usually toxic and often have hemodynamic instability. Prompt surgical intervention is imperative. The common duct must be drained by open operation or by percutaneous radiologic methods. Endoscopic drainage of the common duct through the ampulla of Vater provides adequate drainage in selected patients.

Acute Peritonitis

Acute peritonitis occurs when bacteria are present within the peritoneal cavity after mechanical perforation of a hollow viscus. Primary peritonitis may occur without a perforation, but it is uncommon and is usually seen in alcoholics with ascites or in immunocompromised patients. Secondary peritoneal infection can occur as a result of cathetic contamination in patients undergoing peritoneal dialysis for chronic renal failure. Peritonitis causes acute abdominal pain, usually accompanied by fever and leukocytosis. Palpation of the abdomen usually shows marked tenderness with rebound and also may show a boardlike rigidity. An upright chest roentgenogram commonly shows free air beneath the diaphragm from the perforated viscus.

Peritonitis is variable in severity. Different segments of the intestine that may perforate have different bacterial and chemical compositions and microorganism densities; therefore, it is probably inappropriate to consider all of the illnesses that are classified as peritonitis as a single disease entity.

Perforated gastroduodenal ulcers usually occur as precipitous events with acute abdominal pain. Approximately 80% of patients have free air on an upright chest film (Fig. 9-1). Patients may or may not have antecedent symptoms of ulcer disease. The peritonitis may be entirely chemical, with no bacteria culturable from the peritoneal cavity in the first 12 hours. If the perforation persists for longer than 12 hours, however, bacterial infection becomes increasingly severe. Operative repair of the perforation, usually with a definitive ulcer operation (e.g., vagotomy and pyloroplasty), is the treatment of choice. Antibiotics for common Gram-negative bacteria are usually used but provide minimal benefit, except in patients with delayed operation.

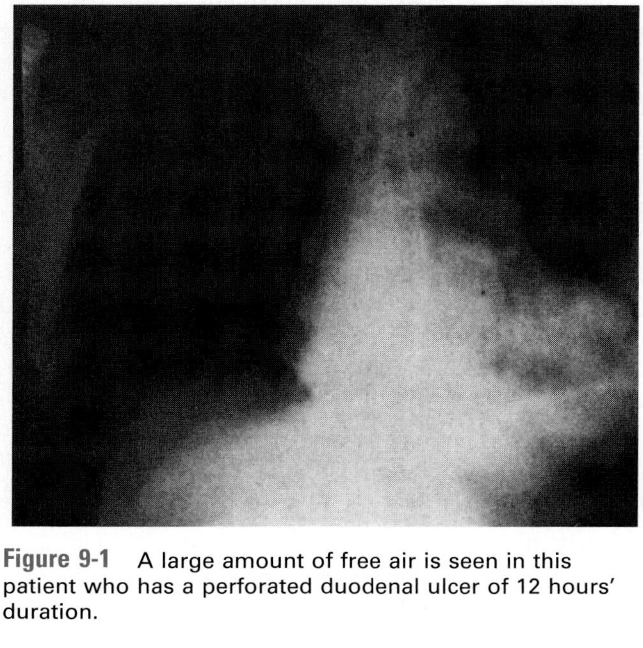

Figure 9-1 A large amount of free air is seen in this patient who has a perforated duodenal ulcer of 12 hours' duration.

A perforated appendix is another common cause of peritonitis that starts as acute appendicitis. In the absence of an appropriate operation, perforation may occur after 24 hours of symptoms. Patients usually have diffuse tenderness and generalized rebound tenderness. Antibiotic therapy is directed against both aerobic (*E. coli*) and anaerobic (*Bacteroides fragilis*) enteric organisms. Treatment requires appendectomy and drainage of any right lower quadrant abscesses. When a localized abscess is identified, external drainage is indicated. External drainage is unnecessary and ineffective for diffuse peritoneal spillage in the absence of a localized abscess.

Colonic perforation from either carcinoma or diverticular disease is the most virulent cause of peritonitis. Colonic microflora have high densities of both aerobic and anaerobic bacteria. Patients usually have marked peritoneal signs and are systemically toxic. After volume resuscitation and the initiation of broad-spectrum systemic antibiotics, operation is mandatory to manage the perforation, drainage (of pus), and debridement of nonviable tissue within the peritoneal cavity. Left colon perforations usually require diversion of the fecal stream as part of their management.

Peritonitis can occur from other sources as well. If sufficient physical findings are present (e.g., diffuse rebound tenderness), a celiotomy (laparotomy) is justified. It is important to diagnose peritonitis and not to delay operative intervention while radiologic studies are performed to define the offending organ system. Exploration and direct visualization will define the specific diagnosis and etiology.

Viral Infections

The diagnosis and treatment of viral infections is not usually the province of the surgeon, except in cases of severely immunosuppressed patients, in whom invasive infection may mimic a bacterial etiology. However, occupational exposure of health care workers to patients who are infected with hepatitis or HIV requires an understanding of the route of transmission so that preventive measures can be taken.

The DNA virus hepatitis B is the pathogen of greatest concern for surgeons because blood or body fluid exposure is the primary route of transmission. In 5% to 10% of infected patients, a chronic carrier state develops and the individual becomes a lifetime risk to infect others. It is estimated that over 1 million people in the United States have chronic hepatitis B. Many of these chronic carriers progress to cirrhosis, end-stage liver disease, or hepatocellular carcinoma. An acute infection may result in hepatic failure and death. Once an infection is established, effective therapy is limited; however, a highly effective hepatitis B vaccine is available. All health care workers who are at risk should undergo vaccination, with follow-up antibody titers determined to ensure protection.

Hepatitis C, an RNA virus, poses a similar risk because it is also transmitted by blood and body fluids. Although acute infection from hepatitis C virus is usually mild or occult, the chronic carrier state occurs in approximately 60% of patients. In these patients, chronic active hepatitis and cirrhosis eventually develop. There appears to be an increased risk of hepatocellular carcinoma in cirrhotics who have hepatitis C. Because there is no vaccine and because over 4 million people in the United States have chronic hepatitis C, it is important that health care workers exercise universal precautions in all patient contacts.

Infections secondary to the retrovirus HIV have been a focus of public concern. Although our understanding of this viral disease and its treatment continues to evolve, it is clear that blood and body fluid exposure is the primary mode of transmission. Therefore, the disease presents a potential risk to surgical care providers. With few exceptions, HIV infection appears to progress to clinical AIDS, a fatal illness. The best strategy to combat HIV is prevention, although a large array of antiretroviral chemotherapy has significantly prolonged life for patients with HIV infection. Modification of professional behavior, with universal precautions and strict limits on contact exposure by workers (e.g., physicians, nurses, students), is mandatory.

Hospital-Acquired Infections

The discussion of hospital-acquired infections in surgical patients is by definition a discussion of postoperative fever. The onset of fever usually heralds an evolving infectious problem. The student of surgery should understand the pathogenesis of fever and its many causes.

Fever is a consequence of the synthesis and release of the endogenous pyrogens, of which interleukin-1 is the most notable. Macrophages come into contact with foreign particles (usually bacteria) and stimulate the synthesis of interleukin-1. Interleukin-1 is released into the inflammatory environment and transported by the circulation to the hypothalamus, which then acts to increase body temperature. This temperature increase is accompanied by neutrophilia, hypoferremia, hypozincemia, hypercupremia, and the synthesis of acute-phase proteins by the liver (e.g., C-reactive protein). All acute responses that are mediated by interleukin-1 are adaptive responses mediated by the host, presumably to bolster defenses against evolving infections.

To manage fever in surgical patients, the source of the pathogen–macrophage interaction must be identified. The causes of postoperative fever are multiple, and it is helpful to think about the etiology utilizing the five "W" mnemonic: *Wind* (atelectasis, pneumonia, pulmonary embolus); *Wound* (incision, devitalized tissue, abscess); *Water* (urinary tract, IV fluids); *Walk* (deep venous thrombosis, IV site phlebitis); and *Wonder* drugs (blood product transfusion, drug infusions). Based on the timing of onset relative to the operation and a careful physical and radiologic exam focused on the common causes, an etiology can usually be identified. The practice of bacterial culture of all possible sites for infection is not usually indicated with an initial febrile episode unless the patient is unstable. Empiric use of antibiotics as an initial response to fever should not be a customary practice without first identification of the source unless the patient is severely septic, hypotensive, hypermetabolic, or hypoxic; when meningitis is a possible cause; and in immunocompromised patients. The primary focus of surgical infection must be identified and then disrupted, usually by mechanical means (e.g., drainage of infected sites), before or during the administration of systemic antibiotics.

Pulmonary Infection

Pulmonary infection in the postoperative patient may have three pathologically distinct causes. First, non–respirator-associated **pneumonia** results from atelectasis. Poor postoperative tidal volumes as a result of anesthesia, analgesia, and painful abdominal or thoracic incisions can cause small airways to collapse. Entrapped organisms plus alveolar macrophages cause fever, usually within the first 48 hours after operation. Early ambulation, coughing, deep breathing, and even nasotracheal suctioning (in refractory cases) of postoperative patients can prevent and manage atelectasis. Various incentive spirometers are helpful when used correctly in the prevention and management of atelectasis. When a new fever and suspected atelectasis are present in the first 48 hours after surgery, laboratory and radiographic studies are usually unnecessary. If fever persists despite aggressive pulmonary chest physical therapy, a chest roentgenogram is often informative. When infiltrates are identified on chest roentgenograms and leukocytosis evolves, then invasive infection has occurred and systemic antibiotics are warranted. Drug selection requires culture and sensitivity data. Organisms in this setting may be either Gram-positive or Gram-negative.

Second, postoperative pneumonitis may be respirator-associated. Critically ill patients are very vulnerable to infection while they are receiving ventilatory support. In these patients, the lung has usually been assaulted by large volumes of intravenously administered fluids. The endotracheal tube is a foreign body that prevents bacterial and secretion clearance, injures tracheal mucosa, and permits bacterial proliferation. The ventilator then serves as a reservoir to "shower" the vulnerable pulmonary tissues with multiresistant hospital-acquired microflora. Weaning the patient from the ventilator promptly is the most important preventive measure. When infection occurs in this setting, opportunistic Gram-negative species endogenous to the hospital unit (e.g., *Pseudomonas, Serratia*) predominate, although Gram-positive staphylococci (including MRSA) are being seen with increasing frequency. Endotracheal aspiration and culture remains a common method for identification of the pathogen. Pulmonary cultures may be obtained by bronchoscopy with bronchoalveolar lavage or protected-brush sampling. In addition, frequent suction through the endotracheal tube removes purulent material and retained secretions.

Third, aspiration is an ever-present risk in the postoperative patient. The patient who is at risk for aspiration usually has gastric distension and altered mental status. Patients who have a head injury or are elderly are particularly at risk. Gastric decompression does not totally obviate the risks of aspiration, but certainly reduces the probabilities. After aspiration occurs, bronchoscopy is diagnostic and may also permit evacuation of particulate matter from the tracheobronchial tree. If hypoxemia is present after aspiration, bronchoscopy must be approached cautiously to avoid causing cardiopulmonary arrest. Management of aspiration requires support of systemic oxygenation. Antibiotics are withheld until clinical and culture evidence identifies an organism for specific therapy. Systemic corticosteroid therapy has no role in aspiration.

Urinary Tract Infection

Postoperative **urinary tract infections** are usually consequences of an antecedent indwelling Foley catheter. These catheters traumatize the bladder and urethral tissues and provide ready access for pathogens. To-and-fro movements of the catheter provide a "sump" effect to dislocate catheter and urethral microorganisms into the bladder. Prevention requires aseptic placement of the catheter, firm fixation after placement, maintenance of the closed drainage system, daily periurethral catheter care, and removal of the catheter as soon as it serves its purpose. Although systemic antibiotics do not prevent postoperative urinary tract infection, they modify the microflora that are potential pathogens.

The diagnosis of postoperative urinary tract infection has traditionally been made with a quantitative bacterial culture. When more than 100,000 organisms/mL urine are identified, surgeons should not assume that the source of postoperative fever has been located. Bacteriuria does not indicate invasive urinary tract sepsis, and it does not cause fever. In most cases, cultures that are positive after Foley catheterization clear with removal of the catheter and an adequate "flush" by volume-induced diuresis. Systemic bacteremia from the urinary tract is uncommon in surgical patients who do not have functional or anatomic obstruction to urine flow. Significant postoperative fever from the urinary tract is always a presumption, even with positive cultures. Constant surveillance for other sources of fever must be pursued.

Urinary infections that develop after catheterization are not caused by the usual urinary tract pathogens (e.g., *E. coli*). They are usually caused by *Pseudomonas*, *Serratia*, and other resistant Gram-negative organisms. Treatment almost always requires culture and sensitivity data. *Candida* and enterococci are being cultured from the urinary tract in more and more patients. Systemic treatment for these presumed urinary tract pathogens should be deferred in the absence of positive blood cultures.

Wound Infections

Postoperative fever should alert the clinician to look where "the hands of man" have been. The wound is always a prime suspect, especially when tenderness, redness, heat, or a mass effect is noted when inspecting the wound. The discharge of pus from the wound is definitive. The absence of a "healing ridge" in one portion of the incision is also a useful clinical sign of wound infection.

A wound infection requires the wound to be opened. Pus is evacuated, fibrin is debrided, and subcutaneous suture material is removed. Systemic antibiotics are not an alternative to drainage. Antibiotics are necessary only for patients who have severe or progressive cellulitis or necrotizing infection. In the latter case, frequent wound debridement is an essential component of management.

Intraabdominal Infection

Postoperative intraabdominal infection generally occurs in two settings. First, complications of elective gastrointestinal or biliary surgery may result in postoperative peritonitis or abscess. Major dehiscence of anastomoses is usually associated with florid sepsis, and reoperation for management of this complication is usually based on clinical criteria. Abdominal tenderness and pain, fever, leukocytosis, and the toxic septic state (rather than roentgenograms, contrast studies, or other sophisticated diagnostic methods) are the most important indicators of the need for reoperation. Patients who underwent an initial laparotomy for infection or penetrating trauma often have a degree of bacterial contamination that makes a subsequent abdominal abscess a common event. Most postoperative intraabdominal infectious complications are abscesses in contrast to diffuse inflammation of peritonitis.

Intraabdominal abscess is difficult to diagnose. Physical examination is significantly compromised by the painful abdominal incision of a previous procedure. Localized tenderness is a useful indicator in only approximately one-third of patients, and palpable masses are helpful in fewer than 10% of patients with abscess. Rectal examination is a particularly valuable method of diagnosis when pelvic abscess is a concern.

Roentgenograms of the abdomen are helpful in the few cases in which positive findings are identified. An abdominal series is occasionally ordered, but is useful in fewer than 20% of patients (Figs. 9-2 and 9-3).

Upper or lower gastrointestinal studies with Gastrografin may show filling defects or intestinal leaks but may not be useful in patients who underwent recent construction of anastomoses. Under fluoroscopic guidance, installation of water-soluble contrast agents through drain sites

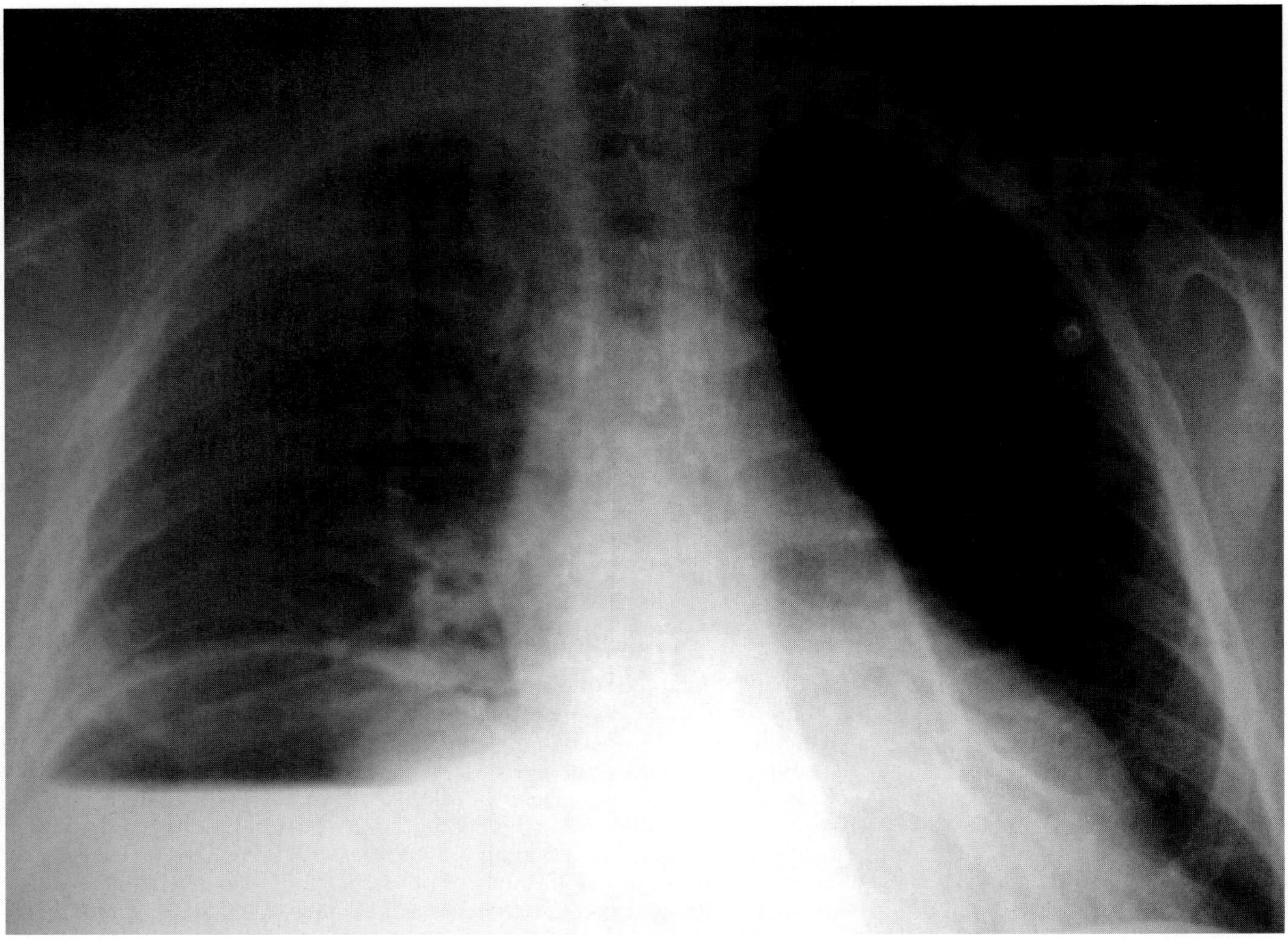

Figure 9-2 An upright chest radiograph showing an air-fluid level below the right hemidiaphragm and a reactive pleural effusion in a patient with a subphrenic abscess.

may also help to identify undrained collections within the abdomen.

Ultrasound is also used to identify intraabdominal abscesses. It is inexpensive, it allows for immediate interpretation, and the equipment can be taken to the bedside (which eliminates the need to transport critically ill patients to another area of the hospital for evaluation). However, the receiver surface must make direct contact with the skin of the abdomen. For this reason, ultrasound may not provide a complete examination in patients with dressings, open wounds, or stomas. Ultrasound provides poor anatomic detail, and intestinal gas, which is commonly encountered in septic postoperative patients, leads to limited anatomic detail and outline of abscesses.

With an accuracy rate of more than 90%, computed tomography (CT) is the fastest and most useful diagnostic study for suspected intraabdominal abscess (Fig. 9-4). CT routinely demonstrates retroperitoneal collections (Fig. 9-5). A water-soluble contrast agent can be given orally and intravenously to help distinguish abscesses and fluid collections from gastrointestinal, vascular, and urinary structures. However, when adynamic ileus prevents filling of the gastrointestinal tract, the oral contrast agent is contraindicated. In addition, when the patient has ascites (making identification of specific fluid collections difficult), CT results are frequently equivocal. In these cases, diagnosis can be made by radionuclide scanning after the injection of indium-111–labeled autologous leukocytes. Total body scanning can be done within 1 day after injection, and all sites of infection can be shown. If indium-111 leukocyte scanning is added to CT in equivocal cases, abdominal abscess can be diagnosed accurately in nearly all instances.

Drainage is the primary treatment of an intraabdominal abscess. Drainage allows removal of the bacteria, fibrin, and debris that fuel the septic process. After the abscess is precisely located in a patient who is tolerating the septic process, localized drainage with CT or other radiologically guided percutaneous methods or a limited operative pro-

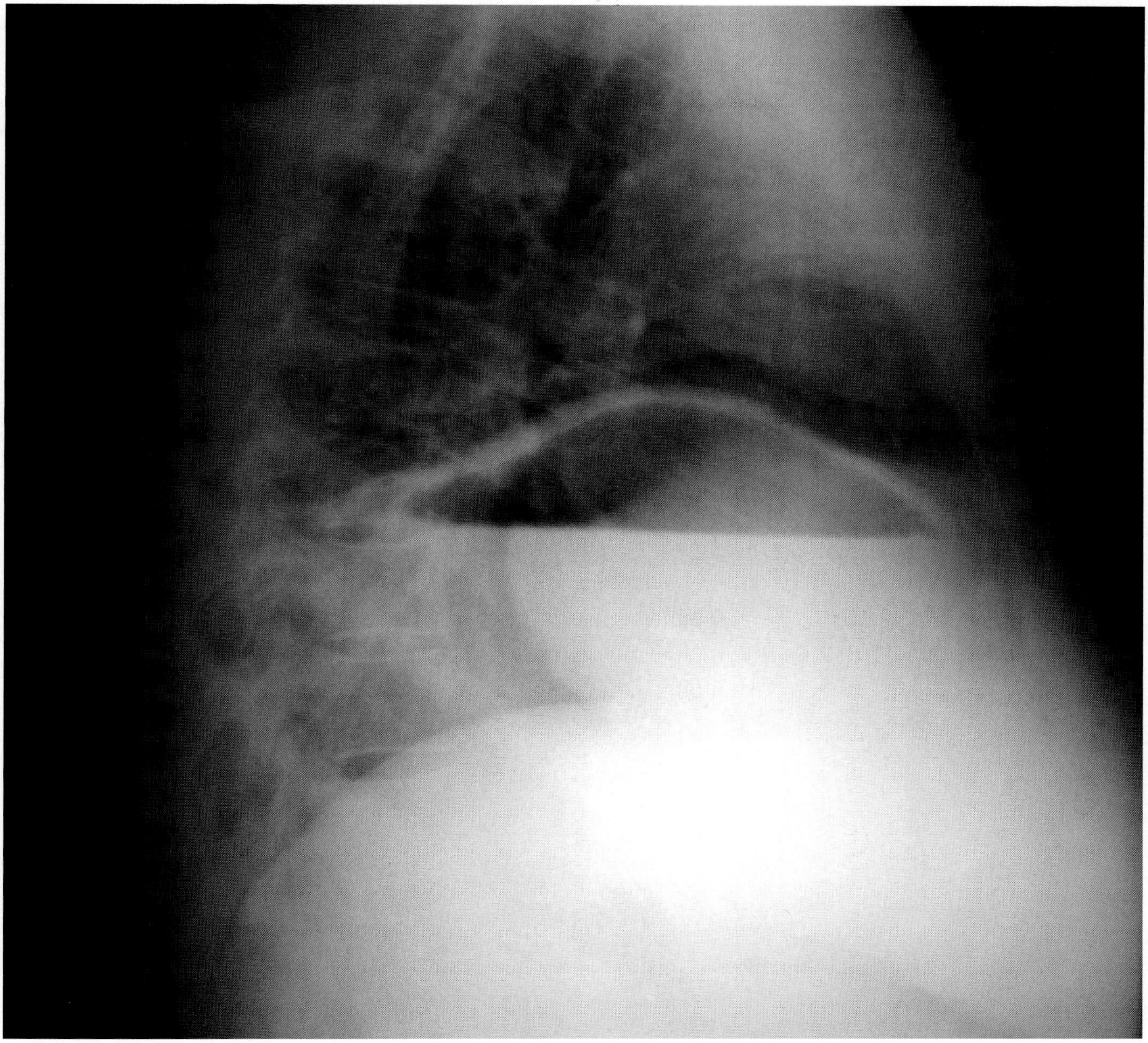

Figure 9-3 A lateral upright chest radiograph of the patient shown in Figure 9-2.

cedure is justified. However, patients who have severe metabolic and physiologic decompensation as a result of the septic process, particularly those with associated organ failure, must undergo comprehensive reexploration to ensure complete surgical drainage and debridement.

Infection in the peritoneal cavity is usually polymicrobial. These infections usually have lipopolysaccharide-laden organisms (e.g., *E. coli*) and obligate anaerobes (e.g., *B. fragilis*). These organisms appear to have a complex synergistic relation. Conventional antibiotic coverage for patients with peritonitis or intraabdominal abscess requires coverage of both halves of the synergistic pair. Regardless of the antibiotic used, treatment of intraabdominal infection is destined to failure without adequate surgical drainage, intestinal diversion or exteriorization when enteral perforation is present, and debridement of the infected soft tissues that surround the focus of infection.

Pleural Empyema

Empyema may be a complication in the postoperative period after thoracotomy or chest tube placement. Occasionally, it occurs spontaneously in association with a bacterial

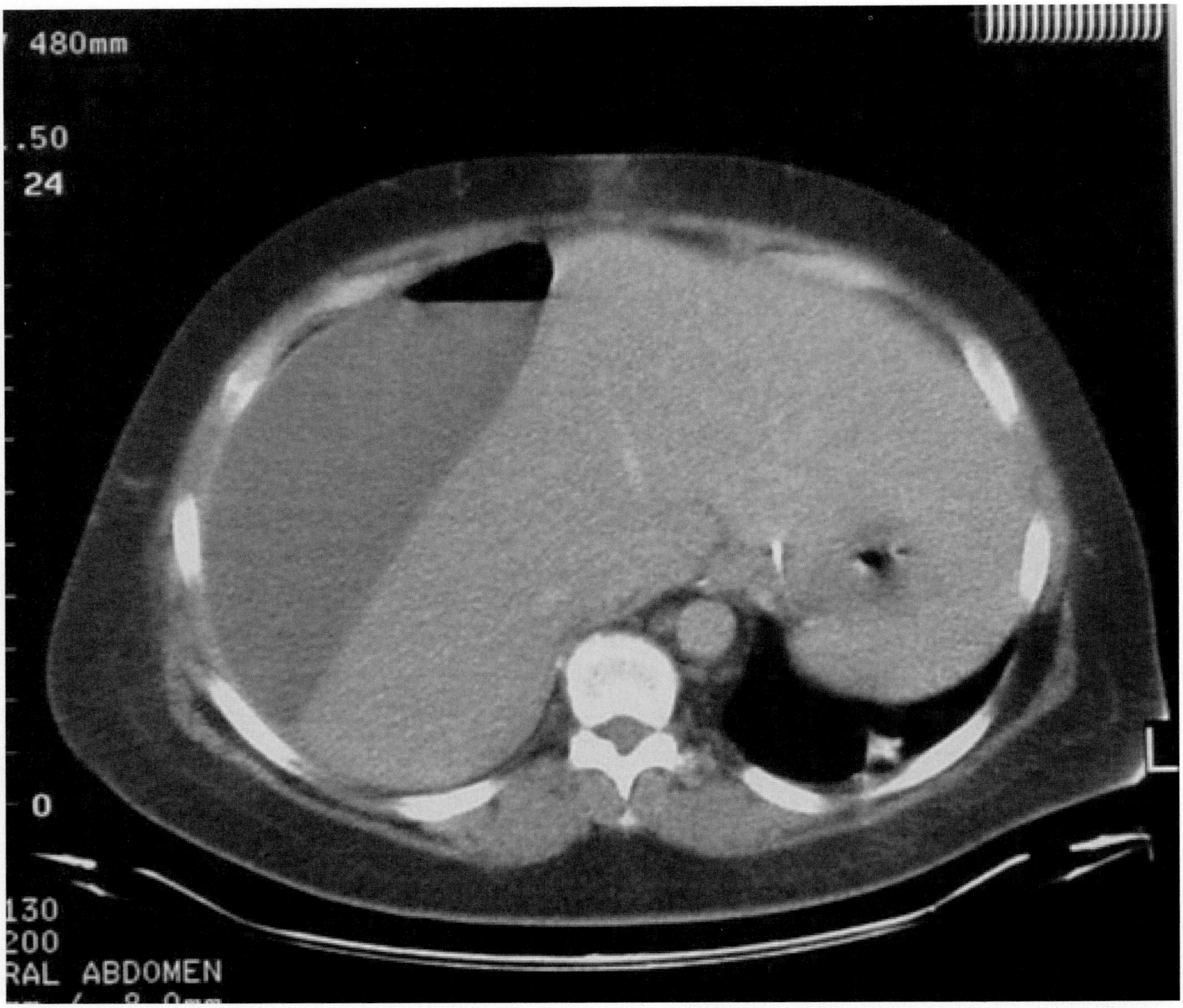

Figure 9-4 An abdominal computed tomography (CT) scan showing the large subphrenic and perihepatic abscess with air fluid level in the patient shown in Figure 9-2.

pneumonic process or tuberculosis. Endogenous flora from pulmonary or esophageal resection or from technical failures of these resections may cause empyema. Inadequate drainage of blood and tissue fluid following blunt or penetrating thoracic trauma is a common etiologic factor. Chest tubes are "two-way" streets that may allow blood and fluid to exit the pleural space, but may also allow exogenous bacteria to enter this space. Roentgenograms show an effusion, usually in the dependent portion of the pleural space. Because patients may be lying down most of the time, a loculated empyema cavity may be posterior. Thus, a lateral chest film, CT, or ultrasound is often helpful in the diagnosis. CT is particularly useful for distinguishing among loculated empyema, lung abscess, and combinations thereof. The diagnosis of empyema is confirmed by aspiration of pus by needle thoracentesis. Ultrasound guidance during needle placement is helpful. CT guidance is invaluable to depict the anatomy when multiple loculations require tube drainage. Treatment of empyema is drainage of the infection.

Pathogens in an empyema are highly variable, and Gram stain of the pus is useful for selecting antibiotics. In patients with empyema after previous placement of a chest tube, Gram-positive staphylococcal organisms predominate. Antibiotic failure in patients with appropriate coverage usually reflects inadequate drainage. In this case,

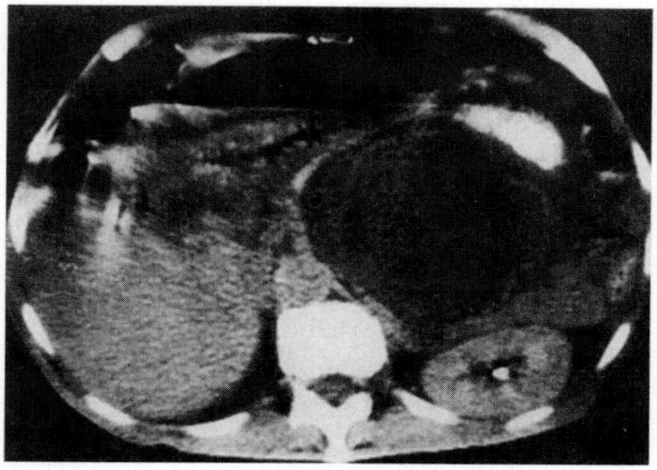

Figure 9-5 A large lesser sac abscess is noted on the abdominal computed tomography (CT) scan of a patient who has severe pancreatitis.

rib resection to marsupialize the empyema cavity may be necessary.

Foreign Body–Associated Infection

Surgical patients are inundated with invasive intravascular catheters and devices. Peripheral intravenous cannulae, Swan-Ganz catheters, percutaneous pacemakers, and arterial lines are only a few of the devices that are used in patients in the intensive care unit. These portals of entry into the intravascular compartment are being recognized with increasing frequency as sources of postoperative nosocomial bacteremia. Indwelling lines permit organisms to migrate from the skin level into the intravascular compartment of the device. Bacteremia then occurs from the catheter. Intimal injury, with localized clot formation, may provide an additional growth medium for bacteria. Newly designed subcutaneous implanted infusion ports decrease the chance of contamination through the skin entrance site, but are still a potential source of infection because of the need for percutaneous access and pericatheter clot formation. To prevent this complication, all percutaneous peripheral intravenous cannulae, central venous catheters, and monitor devices (e.g., Swan-Ganz catheters, arterial lines) must be placed with sterile technique and removed or replaced within 72 hours. Only parenteral nutrition catheters should be maintained for longer periods, and they must be handled with meticulous sterile technique. Asepsis must be exercised in the care of all intravascular devices. Silver-impregnated catheters may be a newer method that will reduce catheter-associated infection.

The diagnosis of intravascular device bacteremia is suspected in any postoperative patient who has positive blood cultures, particularly when either *Staphylococcus aureus* or *Staphylococcus epidermidis* is recovered. A semiquantitative culture of the suspected catheter tip may help to confirm the diagnosis. The essential component of treatment of intravascular device–associated bacteremia is removal of the foreign body. In a bacteremic patient the clinical response to removal of the catheter usually confirms the diagnosis. Persistent fever, leukocytosis, and bacteremia suggest suppurative thrombophlebitis; therefore, the sites of previous intravascular devices must be examined carefully. Local incision and drainage to identify pus within the vein dictate excision of the entire length of involved vein. Antibiotics specific to the bacteremic organisms are used until clinical resolution occurs. Longer courses of antibiotics (e.g., 14 days) are recommended for patients with *S. aureus* bacteremia to prevent the complications of bacterial endocarditis.

Fortunately, infection of implanted vascular grafts, orthopedic joints, or other permanent devices occurs infrequently. Infection of implanted prosthesis usually is initiated during the operative procedure. The diagnosis is considered either because of purulent drainage or a part of a fever evaluation in a patient at risk. A fluid collection around the prosthesis, identified by ultrasonography or CT scan, is strong evidence of infection. When infection of these implants does occur, the device must be surgically removed for therapy to be effective. In most cases, removal of these devices requires alternate prosthetic implants (e.g., extra-anatomic vascular bypass for an infected aortofemoral graft). Management of these complex clinical problems dictates the prolonged use of culture-specific systemic antibiotics. The organisms frequently encountered are *S. aureus* or *S. epidermidis*. Recently, antibiotic-impregnated beads have been used adjacent to the infected site to permit the delivery of higher doses of antibiotic to the area. This technique had dramatic effects in selected anecdotal cases.

Postsplenectomy Sepsis

Young patients who have not developed specific bacterial immunity or older immunocompromised patients are at risk to develop fulminant systemic sepsis following splenectomy. The efficient clearance of transient encapsulated bacteria (e.g., pneumococcus, meningococcus, or *Haemophilus influenzae*) requires splenic function. Prevention of this entity with efforts to avoid splenectomy is the first order of management. Whenever splenectomy is necessary, vaccination is directed at the most common serotypes of encapsulated bacteria. This technique does not cover all possible serotypes and thus does not completely remove the risk. This diagnosis requires an awareness of the postsplenectomy condition and a prompt response with systemic antibiotic directed at the most likely bacteria promptly initiated to any significant febrile illness. Blood cultures should be drawn to document the infection.

Clostridium Difficile Enterocolitis

Systemic antibiotic administration can result in diarrhea as a result of a change in the normal gut bacteria population. Most commonly there results an overgrowth of the pathogenic bacteria C. *difficile,* which produces specific enterotoxins. The diagnosis is suspected in any patient who develops diarrhea while receiving antibiotics. Detection of the toxin in a stool specimen confirms the diagnosis. Oral metronidazole or vancomycin is the treatment of choice, and resumption of enteral feeding is helpful in reestablishing the normal gut flora.

Fungal Infections

Fungal infections are being identified with increasing frequency in surgical patients. The use of antibiotics with an expanded scope of coverage has caused the ubiquitous fungi to become opportunistic pathogens. Patients who are immunosuppressed, are undergoing advanced cancer chemotherapy, or are older and have chronic debility have provided an abundance of susceptible hosts for these fungi. Most of these fungi can be isolated from the patient or environment routinely because they are part of the natural microbial milieu. It is only under selected environmental conditions that fungi cause clinical invasive infection. The most common of these microbes seen in the clinical setting is the *Candida* species. Because of the ubiquitous and, at times, subtle nature of most fungi, systemic or invasive infection must be documented by blood or tissue culture to confirm the diagnosis. Therapy consists of debridement of infected tissue when applicable, along with prolonged systemic antifungal chemotherapy. Amphotericin B is the mainstay of therapy for most invasive infections, but careful dosing is needed because of the toxicity of the drug. Fluconazole is another widely used antifungal, but it is unclear whether this less toxic drug is clinically comparable to amphotericin B.

Sepsis, Septic Shock, and Multiple Organ Failure

Infection results in the local activation of the human inflammatory response due to the proliferation of bacteria. When microbes are disseminated (e.g., bacteremia), when microbial cell products are disseminated (e.g., endotoxemia), or when proinflammatory mediators are released systemically, then inflammation becomes a systemic event. Systemic activation of inflammation secondary to infection is sepsis.

The clinical diagnosis of sepsis is made when patients have tachycardia, tachypnea, fever, and leukocytosis. The septic response is characterized by increased cardiac output, reduced systemic vascular resistance, and altered systemic utilization of oxygen. Thus, patients will commonly have a metabolic acidosis. Sepsis is a clinical diagnosis and does not require positive blood cultures, because circulating bacteria are not a requirement for this illness.

When sepsis rapidly develops, patients may have septic shock. Septic shock has both vasoactive and cardiogenic components. The vasoactive component exists when the loss of vascular resistance from vasodilation cannot be compensated by increased cardiac output. The cardiogenic component exists when cardiac output is inadequate due to intrinsic cardiac disease or due to the systemic toxicity of the septic state. Treatment of septic shock requires intravascular volume support, inotropic support to maintain cardiac output, and effective systemic oxygenation. Control of the primary source of the septic condition is essential for recovery of the patient.

Sustained systemic activation of inflammation results in multiple organ dysfunction syndrome (MODS). MODS represents the failure of the lungs, liver, kidneys, and heart as a consequence of the microcirculatory consequences of systemic inflammation. Even with control of the primary source of infection, MODS may continue because the syndrome becomes a dysregulated systemic inflammatory response. It is treated with oxygenation, cardiac support, and antibiotics. Many systemic therapies to reduce the effects of inflammation have been tried. Recently, the use of activated recombinant protein C appears to have benefit in the treatment of these patients.

THE FUTURE OF SURGICAL INFECTION

The evolution of pathogens in the surgical patient continues to change the face of infection. The influence of systemic antibiotics upon microbial resistance and the increasingly immunosuppressed surgical host means that older pathogens will continue to be problems and that newer pathogens will emerge.

Newer treatments will continue to evolve. Newer antibiotics will be necessary to combat resistance. Strategies to rotate antibiotic use in the critical care unit have been advocated as a means to reduce resistance problems. Clearly, the reduction in the unnecessary use of antibiotics for prevention and for prolonged therapy needs to occur.

Enhancement of host responsiveness has been a goal that has not yet been achieved. However, recent evidence that demonstrates better control of blood glucose, supplemental oxygen delivery, and intraoperative temperature control would indicate that optimization of the host at the time of operation may achieve a more responsive host.

Finally, the arena of sepsis and its sequelae require a better understanding of the human septic response. To date, mediator blockade or modification has largely failed in the treatment of the septic surgical patient. It can be anticipated that as our understanding of the host response to sepsis improves, newer and more innovative therapies will evolve to combat the consequences of severe infection in the surgical patient.

SUGGESTED READINGS

American College of Chest Physicians/Society of Critical Care Medicine Consensus Conference. Definition of sepsis and organ failure and guidelines for the use of innovative therapies in sepsis. *Crit Care Med* 1992;20:864.

Bohnen JMA, Solomkin JS, Dellinger EP, et al. Guidelines for clinical care: anti-infective agents for intra-abdominal infection. *Arch Surg* 1992;127:83.

Cruise PJE, Ford R. The epidemiology of wound infection: a 10-year prospective study of 62,939 wounds. *Surg Clin North Am* 1980;60:27.

Gozal D, Ziser A, Shupak A, et al. Necrotizing fasciitis. *Arch Surg* 1986;121:233.

Hausman MR, Lisser SP. Hand infections. *Orthop Clin North Am* 1992;23:171.

Luster AD. Chemokines—chemotactic cytokines that mediate inflammation. *N Engl J Med* 1998;338:436–445.

Rodriguez JR, Gibbons KJ, Bitzer LG, et al. Pneumonia: incidence, risk factors, and outcome in injured patients. *J Trauma* 1991;31:907

Stamm WE, Hooton TM: Management of urinary tract infection in adults. *N Engl J Med* 1993;329:1328.

Vincent JL, Anaissie E, Bruining H, et al. Epidemiology, diagnosis and treatment of systemic Candida infection in surgical patients under intensive care. *Intensive Care Med* 1998;24:206

10

MATTHEW O. DOLICH, MD ■ JEFFREY G. CHIPMAN, MD

Trauma

OBJECTIVES

1 Outline the steps that must be followed to assess the patient who has multiple injuries.

2 Describe the principles and methods that are used in the initial assessment, resuscitation, and definitive care phases of trauma management.

3 Define shock, discuss the pathophysiology related to shock, and outline the management of hemorrhagic shock.

4 Describe the pathophysiology and initial treatment of both immediately life-threatening and potentially life-threatening thoracic injuries.

5 Describe the diagnostic and therapeutic procedures that pertain to abdominal trauma, including the indications, contraindications, and limitations of ultrasound, computed tomography, and peritoneal lavage.

6 Outline the initial management of the unconscious trauma patient and discuss the complications that can develop after head injury.

7 Define the Glasgow Coma Scale, and describe its point scale and its prediction of neurologic recovery.

8 Describe the therapeutic interventions that reverse or delay the consequences of increased intracranial pressure.

9 Outline the management of a patient with a suspected spine or spinal cord injury, including proper immobilization techniques.

10 List the types of extremity injuries, and prioritize their assessment and management.

11 Describe the issues involved in the transportation or transfer of injured patients.

OVERVIEW AND EPIDEMIOLOGY

Trauma is the number one cause of death in the first 4 decades of life (ages 1 to 44 years) and is the fourth leading cause of death in all age groups. In 2002, a total of 152,467 people died in the United States of accidents, suicides, and homicides. Approximately one-half of these deaths are related to motor vehicle or firearm use. As impressive as these numbers are, they do not tell the entire story. For each trauma-related death in the United States, three trauma victims will suffer permanent disability. Trauma-related costs are estimated at more than $400 billion annually. This monumental figure is approximately 40% of the health care dollar. The real cost of trauma, however, is not measured in dollars, but in lives lost. It is estimated that trauma causes the loss of approximately 4.7 million years of potential life before age 75 in the United States. Trauma robs society of some of its youngest and potentially most productive members. For the most part, trauma is a preventable problem that involves multiple (and controversial) social issues. Until our society increases injury prevention efforts, management of the traumatized patient will remain a critically important skill for physicians.

The time of death from trauma has a trimodal distribution. The first peak includes immediate deaths that occur within seconds to minutes of injury; these patients die of lacerations to the brain, brainstem, spinal cord, heart, or major blood vessels. Most of these patients die before they reach the hospital. The second peak includes early deaths that occur within minutes to hours of injury; these patients die of major hemorrhage of the head, chest, or abdomen, or of multiple injuries that cause significant blood loss. Most of these injuries can be treated if the patient is rapidly assessed and resuscitated according to the Advanced Trauma Life Support (ATLS) program within the first hour after injury. The third peak includes deaths caused by sepsis and multiple organ dysfunction syndrome (MODS) that occur several days to weeks after injury. The outcome of this third group of patients is related to their initial care.

If proper care is delivered during the initial "golden hour" after injury, the number of early and late trauma deaths will be decreased.

This chapter describes the principles of the ATLS program and describes the care of the patient with multiple injuries. The ATLS program was developed by the American College of Surgeons to save the lives of patients who would otherwise die an early death, defined as one occurring in the minutes to hours after injury.

INITIAL ASSESSMENT

The initial assessment of an injured patient is based on a logical sequence of steps. Conceptually, the process is organized into four phases: (1) **primary survey,** (2) **resuscitation,** (3) **secondary survey,** and (4) **definitive care.** The ongoing care of the injured patient requires frequent repetition of the primary and secondary surveys to confirm the patient's response to therapy. In practice, these activities often occur simultaneously. For example, the resuscitation phase typically begins during the primary survey when circulation is assessed. This algorithm provides the physician with a method to mentally check and recheck the management of the injured patient.

Primary Survey

The primary survey involves the diagnosis and treatment of all immediately life-threatening injuries. This process is organized into an ABCDE algorithm. In a sequential fashion, the physician protects the cervical spine while assessing the *A*irway, *B*reathing, *C*irculation, and neurologic *D*isability of the injured patient. *E*xposure of the patient, by removing all clothing, and the prevention of hypothermia, by keeping the patient warm with blankets, are the last steps of this phase. The physician treats all immediately life-threatening injuries in sequence before proceeding to the next phase.

Airway Maintenance With Cervical Spine Protection

The physician's first priority in managing an injured patient is the assessment of the airway. For this discussion, the term airway is used interchangeably with airway management, which refers to maintaining patency of the upper airway, specifically the mouth, oropharynx, larynx, and trachea. Because patients die rapidly if they are deprived of oxygenated blood, every injured patient should be given supplemental oxygen. One common cause of preventable death is failure to recognize the need for an adequate airway. Other causes are esophageal intubation, aspiration of gastric contents, and failure to provide adequate ventilation. Patients at particular risk are those who are unconscious or who have sustained injures to the head, face, neck, or chest. Those who are intoxicated with alcohol or other drugs are also at risk for **airway compromise.**

Initial Airway Maneuvers

The physician who arrives at the side of the trauma patient must rapidly determine whether the patient is unconscious. The physician should listen and feel for air movement from the victim's mouth. The physician should touch the patient and say, "Are you OK?" When the patient's response is appropriate and his or her voice is normal, the *talking patient* informs the astute physician that the airway is patent, the brain is perfused, and ventilation is adequate. However, when there is airway compromise, the physician may hear abnormal sounds coming from the mouth. The presence of stridor, snoring, or gurgling suggests a supraglottic problem. Dysphonia, hoarseness, or pain when speaking suggests a laryngeal problem. Other signs to look for are tachypnea, agitation, cyanosis, and the use of the accessory muscles of ventilation. Agitation suggests hypoxia, and obtundation suggests hypercarbia. The agitated, abusive, or belligerent patient is considered hypoxic until proven otherwise, regardless of whether the patient is intoxicated with alcohol or other drugs. In the worst case, there is no air movement from the mouth and the patient is unconscious. In this situation, an adequate airway must be provided immediately.

It is important to assume that any patient with a head injury, altered level of consciousness, or multisystem blunt trauma has an unstable cervical spine injury until proven otherwise. Movement of the unstable cervical spine can cause spinal cord injury and resultant quadriplegia. Therefore, it is imperative to stabilize the cervical spine while opening the airway. The physician or another health care provider who is positioned at the head of the stretcher holds the head and neck in the neutral position. This maneuver is called *in-line immobilization of the cervical spine*.

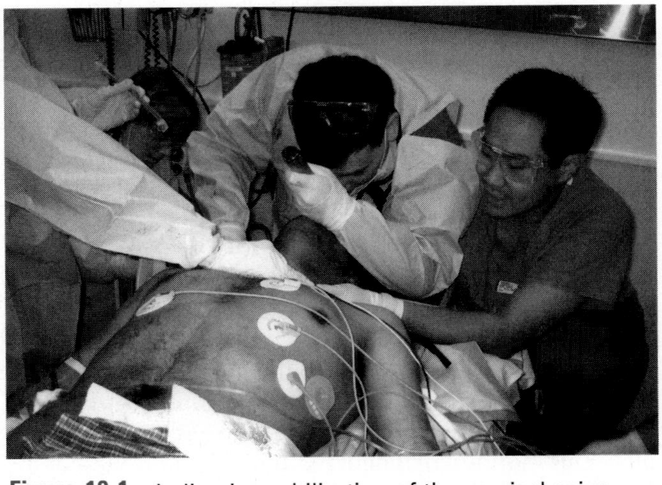

Figure 10-1 In-line immobilization of the cervical spine. The assistant kneels at the head of the bed and places his or her hands on the patient's shoulders with the wrists alongside the patient's head. The assistant's wrists and forearms prevent the patient's head from moving, while the physician inserts the laryngoscope and orotracheally intubates the patient.

It cannot be accomplished with a soft or rigid cervical collar alone because these types of collars do not ensure complete stabilization of the cervical spine. A cervical collar can also hide the trachea and hinder frequent visual inspection and palpation. Patients are often brought to a trauma center immobilized on a backboard, with a cervical collar in place. Adequate immobilization of the spine for transport requires immobilization of the entire patient. An adequately immobilized patient has a cervical collar in place and is secured to a rigid backboard with straps and tape. The patient's head, neck, and shoulders are bolstered to prevent movement of the cervical spine.

If the patient is lying supine on a stretcher, immobilization of the neck while the airway is assessed is best accomplished by designating an individual to kneel at the head of the stretcher and grasp the patient's shoulders with both hands while immobilizing the neck and head with both forearms (Fig. 10-1). Next, the mouth is opened with a **jaw-thrust** or **chin-lift maneuver.** In the unconscious supine patient, the relaxed muscles cause the jaw to fall posteriorly. The tongue can then fall back against the hypopharynx and obstruct the airway. The **jaw-thrust** is accomplished by standing behind the patient's head, placing one's fingers behind the angle of the jaw, grasping it on both sides, and lifting the jaw forward. The thumbs are used to open the mouth by drawing the mouth and chin downward, revealing the oral cavity for inspection. The disadvantage of this maneuver is that it requires the use of both hands; therefore, an assistant is needed to suction or remove any foreign objects. The **chin-lift** is accomplished by placing the fingers under the chin while placing the thumb anteriorly below the lips. The chin is grasped and lifted forward and downward, opening the mouth for inspection. A more secure grip on the jaw can be accomplished by placing the thumb inside the mouth and behind the lower incisors. The disadvantage of this maneuver is that in the semiconscious patient, the thumb can be bitten. The jaw-thrust and chin-lift maneuvers must be done carefully to avoid extending the neck and moving the cervical spine. The chin-lift and jaw-thrust maneuvers are illustrated in Figure 10-2.

Next, the oral cavity is illuminated, inspected, and suctioned. Any foreign objects are removed. A rigid (Yankauer) suction device (Fig. 10-3*F*) is preferred because it can be better controlled than a soft, flexible suction catheter. After excess secretions are removed, the airway can be maintained with an **oropharyngeal (oral) airway** (Fig. 10-3*B*) or a **nasopharyngeal (nasal) airway.** The oropharyngeal airway is made of plastic. It is inserted into the mouth over and behind the tongue. A tongue blade is used to depress the tongue to allow airway insertion. An alternate method of insertion involves putting the airway in upside down so that the concave side is up. When the soft palate is reached, the oral airway is rotated 180° into the proper position. The oropharyngeal airway, if inserted improperly, can push the tongue backward and block the entrance to

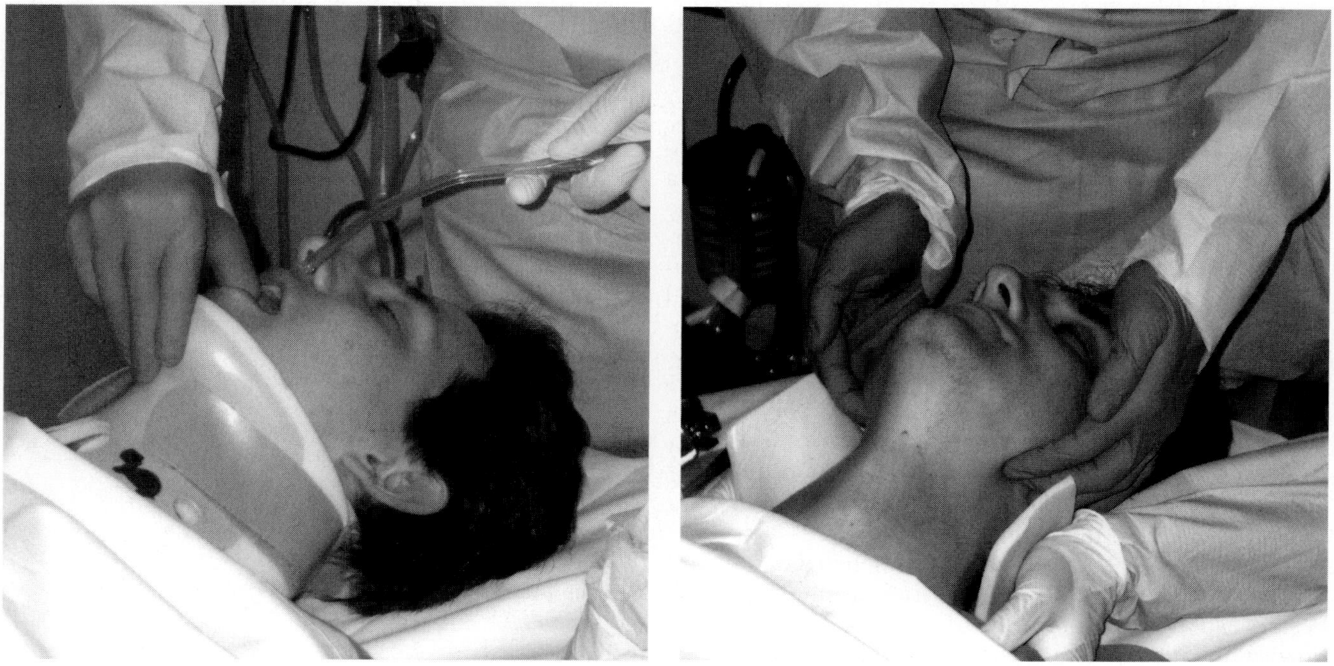

A B

Figure 10-2 Chin-lift maneuver (**A**) and jaw-thrust maneuver (**B**). In the chin-lift maneuver, the physician's thumb is placed behind the patient's lower incisors to securely lift the jaw and open the mouth for suctioning with a rigid (Yankauer) sucker. During the jaw-thrust maneuver, the physician's fingers are positioned behind the angle of the mandible to move the jaw anteriorly, opening the airway.

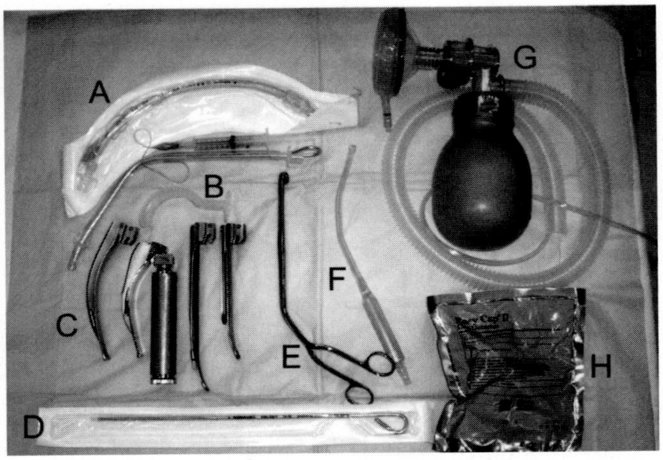

Figure 10-3 Airway equipment. **A,** Endotracheal tube. **B,** Oropharyngeal airway. **C,** Laryngoscope and blades. **D,** Stylet for endotracheal tube. **E,** McGill forceps (for removal of foreign body obstructing airway). **F,** Rigid (Yankauer) sucker. **G,** Bag-valve–mask (BVM) device. **H,** Colorimetric CO_2 detector.

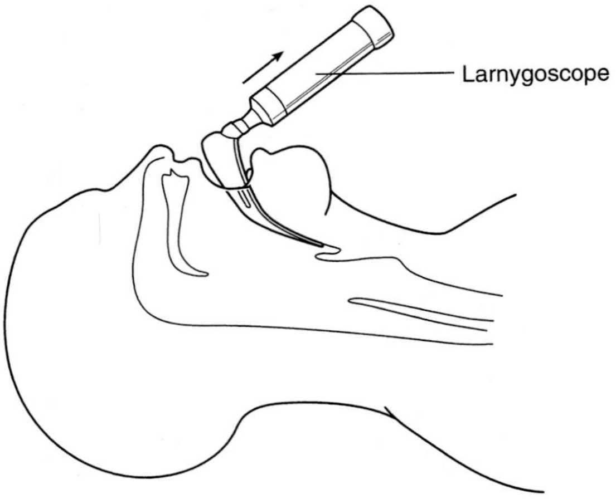

Figure 10-4 Visualization of the vocal cords for oral tracheal intubation with a laryngoscope that is fitted with a curved blade. The epiglottis is displaced anteriorly by upward traction on the laryngoscope while the tip of the blade is placed in the epiglottic vallecula. In the trauma patient, the neck is not extended during this procedure.

the larynx. This airway should not be used in the conscious patient who has an intact gag reflex because it can cause gagging, vomiting, and possible aspiration. The nasopharyngeal airway is a soft, flexible tube that has a trumpet-like flange on one end. It is commonly made of rubber. The nasopharyngeal airway is well lubricated and passed gently through one of the nostrils into the hypopharynx. This airway is generally well tolerated in awake patients who have an intact gag reflex.

Tracheal Intubation: The Definitive Airway

If the patient's airway cannot be secured by an oropharyngeal or nasopharyngeal airway, then he or she needs a definitive airway provided by a cuffed tube placed in the trachea. There are several ways to provide definitive airways: orotracheal intubation, nasotracheal intubation, surgical **cricothyroidotomy,** needle cricothyroidotomy, and tracheostomy. Emergency surgical airways include the surgical cricothyroidotomy and needle cricothyroidotomy. Because tracheostomy is a more complex, time-consuming procedure than cricothyroidotomy, it is not considered an emergency surgical airway. A tracheostomy is normally performed in the operating room because of the anatomic position of the thyroid gland, its generous blood supply, and its relation to the trachea.

Indications for a definitive airway are based on the physician's knowledge of the mechanism of injury and concern that the patient will need mechanical ventilation, may aspirate blood or gastric contents, or may obstruct the airway because of edema or expanding hematoma. Mechanical ventilation is needed in cases of apnea, hypoxia despite supplemental oxygen by face mask, hypercarbia, and head injury that requires controlled ventilation. Before a definitive airway is inserted, supplemental oxygen must be provided by face mask or bag-valve–mask device (Fig. 10-3G), and the physician must inspect and palpate the neck to determine whether the trachea is in the midline, the larynx or the trachea is fractured, or the neck veins are distended. The significance of these conditions is discussed later.

Orotracheal intubation is performed under direct visualization of the vocal cords (Figs. 10-4 and 10-5). In-line cervical immobilization is maintained throughout the procedure. The laryngoscope (Fig. 10-3C) is inserted, the vocal cords are visualized, and an endotracheal tube (Fig. 10-3A) is inserted through the cords, approximately 1 to 2.5 cm beyond the cuff. The cuff is inflated, and the endotracheal tube is attached to a bag-valve device, which al-

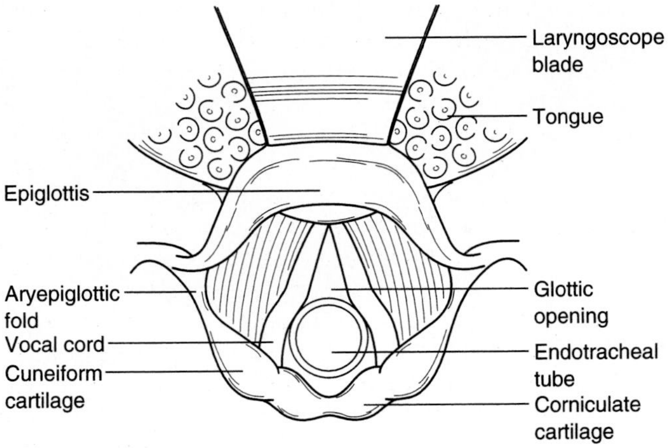

Figure 10-5 Laryngoscopic view of the vocal cords with the endotracheal tube in place.

lows the patient to be ventilated with oxygen. As the bag is squeezed, the patient's chest is inspected for movement. Auscultation is performed over the lateral aspect of the right and left sides of the chest, in the midaxillary line, and over the epigastrium. The presence of breath sounds bilaterally confirms proper intubation. A colorimetric CO_2 detector (Fig. 10-3*H*) is placed to confirm proper ventilation and tube placement, or continuous end-tidal CO_2 monitoring may be used. The presence of gurgling in the epigastrium confirms an esophageal intubation; in this case, the tube should be removed immediately. Before another attempt at intubation is made, the patient should be ventilated and oxygenated with a bag-valve–mask device. Absent or decreased breath sounds on the left side of the chest may indicate a right mainstem bronchus intubation, in which case the tube should be pulled back a few centimeters. However, absent or decreased breath sounds on either side of the chest can suggest **pneumothorax** or **hemothorax.**

Nasotracheal intubation is an option for airway control in the breathing adult patient. It is contraindicated in apneic patients, in patients with basilar skull fractures, and in children under 12 years of age. In the conscious patient, the nasal canal is sprayed with a topical anesthetic and a vasoconstrictor (to shrink the nasal mucous membranes). An endotracheal tube is well lubricated with anesthetic jelly and passed gently through a nostril without a stylet. It is then guided into the pharynx. At this point, airflow can be heard coming from the end of the tube. The tube is then advanced slowly until the sound of airflow is maximal. At the point of inhalation, the tube is quickly advanced into the trachea. Successful intubation is confirmed with a rush of air, water vapor condensing within the endotracheal tube, or expulsion of respiratory secretions from the end of the tube. Finally, the cuff is inflated, and the patient is ventilated with supplemental oxygen.

When it is impossible to insert an orotracheal or a nasotracheal tube, an emergency surgical airway is required. This type of airway is usually necessary in patients with massive facial trauma with no recognizable normal anatomy or when the vocal cords cannot be visualized because of bleeding, glottic edema, or laryngeal fracture. In this situation, there are two options: surgical cricothyroidotomy or needle cricothyroidotomy. Surgical cricothyroidotomy is performed by first locating the cricothyroid membrane. The index finger is placed in the sternal notch and moved up the trachea. As the finger moves cephalad, the tracheal rings are palpated. The cricoid cartilage is more prominent than the first tracheal ring, and as the finger passes over this distinctive cartilage, it falls into a depression, the cricothyroid membrane. This membrane is located just below the thyroid cartilage. Next, the cricoid cartilage is stabilized between the thumb and index finger. The skin is held taut to occlude any subcutaneous veins. A 2-cm transverse incision is made through the skin and cricothyroid membrane. The knife handle is then inserted through the incision and rotated 90° to allow insertion of a size 6 cuffed endotracheal tube or tracheostomy tube (Figs. 10-6 and 10-7). The cuff on the tube is inflated. The patient is allowed to ventilate spontaneously or, if necessary, is manually or mechanically ventilated. This procedure is not recommended for children younger than 12 years of age

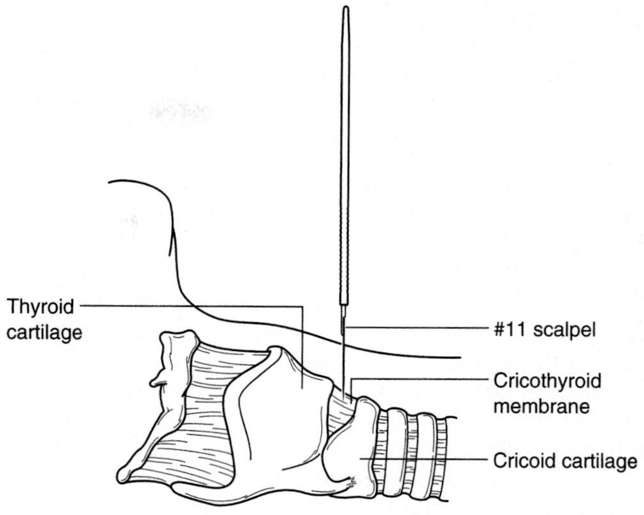

Figure 10-6 Surgical cricothyroidotomy. With the patient in the supine position, a 2-cm transverse incision is made through the skin and cricothyroid membrane. The incision is made in a single motion with a scalpel blade. The scalpel blade is kept perpendicular to the skin. The cutting edge of the blade is swept upward as it is removed, making the transverse incision.

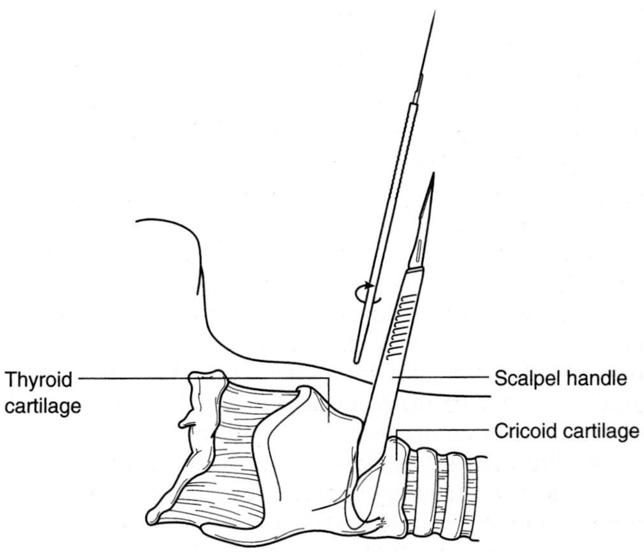

Figure 10-7 Surgical cricothyroidotomy. After the cricothyroid membrane is cut, the handle of the scalpel is inserted through the incision and rotated 90° to allow insertion of a size 6 cuffed endotracheal tube.

because of potential damage to the cricoid cartilage and the small size of the trachea.

Needle cricothyroidotomy is performed similarly to surgical cricothyroidotomy, except that the cricothyroid membrane is pierced with a standard intravenous catheter. In adults, a 12- to 14-gauge (16 to 18 gauge in children), 5-cm-long, over-the-needle catheter attached to a 3- to 10-mL syringe is used to pierce the cricothyroid membrane. The catheter is inserted at 45° caudally while aspirating on the syringe. Aspiration of air confirms entry into the trachea. The needle is removed while the catheter is advanced. The catheter is then attached to wall oxygen at 15 L/min (40 to 50 psi) through tubing with a side hole cut into it. Intermittent insufflation is accomplished by placing the thumb over the side hole for 1 second and releasing it for 4 seconds. An alternate method is placing a Y-connector between the oxygen source and the catheter. Adequate oxygenation can be maintained for approximately 30 to 45 minutes. However, because exhalation is inadequate, hypercarbia will gradually occur. Needle cricothyroidotomy is the emergency surgical airway of choice in children under 12 years of age. In adults and children, this method provides a rapid, temporary airway that allows time to place another type of definitive airway, including a tracheostomy.

Breathing

Breathing is the "B" component of the trauma ABCDE algorithm. Once the airway is deemed patent, the physician must quickly ascertain whether respiration is adequate. The central question is whether air is moving in and out of both lungs equally. The chest is inspected for symmetrical rise and fall and auscultated for presence or absence of breath sounds. Percussion of the chest may reveal areas of dullness suggestive of hemothorax, or hyperresonance associated with pneumothorax. These maneuvers must be repeated often during the evaluation of the injured patient. Specifically, they should be repeated after any therapeutic maneuver that can affect pulmonary function. These maneuvers include, but are not limited to, the placement of a definitive airway, tube thoracostomy, and central venous catheter placement.

Circulation

After ventilation is confirmed by the presence of bilateral breath sounds, the next step is assessment and management of the patient's circulation. Initial maneuvers include auscultation of heart sounds and palpation of peripheral pulses. Initial management of the circulation involves controlling obvious external hemorrhage with direct pressure, assessing tissue perfusion, and administering intravenous fluids. External hemorrhage is best managed by placing a dressing on the wound and applying direct pressure. Application of a tourniquet is not recommended because it crushes underlying tissue and causes distal ischemia. Tissue perfusion is assessed by the patient's pulse, skin color, and level of consciousness. Pulse quality, rate, and rhythm provide an estimate of stroke volume and cardiac output. A weak, rapid pulse denotes a narrow pulse pressure and low cardiac output; a palpable radial pulse indicates a systolic blood pressure that is usually at least 80 mm Hg; inability to palpate a carotid or femoral pulse generally indicates a systolic blood pressure that is less than 60 mm Hg. The patient who is ashen gray with pale nailbeds is severely hypovolemic. As blood volume decreases, so does cerebral perfusion, resulting in a progressive change in mental status. First the patient displays anxiety, then confusion, then lethargy, and finally unconsciousness.

Hemorrhagic Shock

The management of trauma requires a thorough knowledge of **shock,** which is defined as inadequate organ perfusion. The first step in managing shock is to recognize its presence. The second step is to identify its cause. In trauma, shock is directly related to the mechanism of injury. The most common cause is hypovolemia secondary to hemorrhage. In hemorrhagic shock, treatment is directed at stopping the bleeding and restoring intravascular volume. Therapy should not be directed at merely restoring the patient's blood pressure. It is not appropriate to use vasoconstrictors in patients with hemorrhagic shock because these drugs increase afterload, which in turn increases myocardial oxygen consumption. Vasoconstrictors also promote ongoing ischemia to the kidneys and splanchnic viscera, which can contribute to the progression of the shock state until it becomes irreversible.

Pathophysiology of Blood Loss. The pathophysiology of blood loss is a compensatory progressive vasoconstriction to preserve oxygen delivery to the brain and heart. A generalized adrenergic response to hemorrhage causes elevated plasma catecholamine levels. The skin becomes cool and moist as a result of vasoconstriction and stimulation of the sweat glands by a generalized sympathetic discharge. The degree of vasoconstriction or perfusion of the extremities can be measured by capillary refill time. The patient's fingernail is depressed and released; the interval until the normal color returns is timed. Normal capillary refill time is approximately 2 seconds, or the time it takes to say "capillary refill." It should be noted that this test may be unreliable in the hypothermic patient. In addition to peripheral vasoconstriction, the catecholamine response to hemorrhage results in tachycardia.

Cells that are inadequately perfused switch to an anaerobic metabolism and the formation of lactic acid. Intracellular adenosine triphosphate (ATP) stores become depleted, the sodium potassium adenosine triphosphatase (ATPase) pump is inhibited, and membrane potentials approach neutrality. Cell membrane dysfunction occurs, leading to an influx of fluid into the cell and concomitant cellular swelling. The administration of intravenous lactated Ringer's solution fights this process by restoring intravascular volume and increasing tissue perfusion. Resuscitation is often accompanied by interstitial edema, which is the result of vascular endothelial injury that allows electrolytes, water, and protein to leak out of the capillaries. This capillary leak usually causes larger volumes of resuscitation fluid to be used than initially predicted.

Classification of Blood Loss. The human response to hemorrhage is directly related to the volume of blood loss (Table 10-1). In the 70-kg adult, blood volume is approximately 7% of body weight, or approximately 5000 mL. Class I hemorrhage is defined as blood loss of less than 15%, or 750 mL in a 70-kg person. When a person donates blood, the donation is usually approximately 10% of blood volume, or approximately 450 to 500 mL. If a blood donation is roughly equal to a class I hemorrhage, then it is easy to understand the hemodynamics of this category of hemorrhage. Heart rate is less than 100 beats/min, and there is no measurable change in blood pressure, pulse pressure, or respiratory rate. Urine output is normal at greater than 30 mL/hr. Slight anxiety may be present. Capillary refill time is normal. Treatment is administration of crystalloid solution (lactated Ringer's solution is preferred). Class II hemorrhage is defined as blood loss of 15% to 30% of circulating blood volume, or 750 to 1500 mL in a 70-kg person. Tachycardia is present, with a heart rate greater than 100 beats/min. Blood pressure remains normal. Pulse pressure (systolic minus diastolic pressure) is decreased because systolic pressure is unchanged, but diastolic pressure is elevated as a result of catecholamine-induced vasoconstriction. Tachypnea is present, with a respiratory rate of 20 to 30 breaths/min. Urine output is 20 to 30 mL/hr. The patient has mild anxiety that may be expressed as fear or hostility. Capillary refill time is greater than 2 seconds. Treatment is also administration of crystalloid solution. Class III hemorrhage is defined as blood loss of 30% to 40% of circulating blood volume, or 1500 to 2000 mL in a 70-kg person. Heart rate is greater than 120 beats/min, and blood pressure is measurably decreased. Pulse pressure is also decreased, and tachypnea is present, with a respiratory rate of 30 to 40 breaths/min. Urine output is low at 5 to 15 mL/hr. The patient is very anxious and confused. Capillary refill time is greater than 2 seconds. Treatment is administration of lactated Ringer's solution; blood transfusions are typically required as well. Class IV hemorrhage is defined as a blood loss of more than 40% of circulating blood volume, or greater than 2000 mL in a 70-kg person. This magnitude of exsanguination is immediately life threatening. Heart rate is greater than 140 beats/min, and blood pressure is markedly decreased. Often, it cannot be obtained with a standard sphygmomanometer. Pulse pressure is very narrow if it is measurable at all. Respiratory rate is greater than 35 breaths/min, and urine output is almost nonexistent. The patient is confused and lethargic. Capillary refill time is greater than 2 seconds. Treatment is administration of lactated Ringer's solution and blood transfusions.

Resuscitation Phase: Treatment of Hemorrhagic Shock. During the circulation step of the primary survey, resuscitation is commenced when circulation is deemed inadequate. The initial management of hemorrhagic shock involves rapid diagnosis, replacement of intravascular volume, and control of obvious external hemorrhage. Two large-bore (minimum 16-gauge) peripheral intravenous catheters should be inserted and intravenous infusion begun with lactated Ringer's solution. These lines should be placed in uninjured extremities using percutaneous techniques. However, in patients with class IV hemorrhage, the peripheral veins are often collapsed and difficult to cannulate percutaneously. Alternatively, the saphenous vein at the ankle may be cannulated by performing a surgical cutdown procedure to isolate and access the vein. Central venous access using a large-bore catheter (e.g., introducer sheath) may be obtained at the femoral, subclavian, or internal jugular veins when peripheral access is unobtainable. In children under 6 years of age, vascular access may be obtained by intraosseous infusion into the marrow cavity of a long bone (usually the tibia) in an uninjured extremity.

Lactated Ringer's solution is the initial resuscitation fluid of choice. Normal saline is the second choice be-

Table 10-1 Classification of Hemorrhage

	Class I	Class II	Class III	Class IV
Blood loss (mL) 70-kg person	< 750	750–1500	1500–2000	> 2000
Blood volume loss (%)	< 15	15–30	30–40	> 40
Heart rate	< 100	> 100	> 120	> 140
Blood pressure	Normal	Normal	Decreased	Decreased
Pulse pressure	Normal	Decreased	Decreased	Decreased
Respiratory rate	14–20	20–30	30–40	> 35
Urine output (mL/hr)	> 30	20–30	5–15	Negligible
Capillary refill (sec)	Normal	> 2	> 2	> 2
Mental status	Slight anxiety	Mild anxiety	Anxious/confused	Confused/lethargic
Fluid management	Crystalloid	Crystalloid	Crystalloid and blood	Crystalloid and blood

cause massive amounts may cause hyperchloremic metabolic acidosis. This potential is increased if the patient has impaired renal function. Normal saline, 0.9%, has an electrolyte content as follows: $Na^+ = 154$ mEq/L, $Cl^- = 154$ mEq/L. Lactated Ringer's solution has an electrolyte content as follows: $Na^+ = 130$ mEq/L, $K^+ = 4$ mEq/L, $Ca^{++} = 3$ mEq/L, $Cl^- = 109$ mEq/L, lactate = 28 mEq/L. When large volumes of resuscitative fluid are required, fewer electrolyte and metabolic abnormalities result from use of lactated Ringer's solution.

The amount of fluid and blood needed to resuscitate a given trauma patient is difficult to predict. However, a rough estimate can be made based on the patient's clinical presentation. A general rule of thumb is that it takes 3 mL of crystalloid fluid to replace 1 mL of blood loss. This 3:1 ratio allows for the redistribution of crystalloid into the interstitial and intracellular spaces. For example, if a 70-kg patient loses 30% of blood volume, or 1500 mL, it will take 4500 mL of crystalloid to replace it. It is not unusual to give this amount of crystalloid in the first hour of resuscitation.

The patient's initial response to fluid is the best guide to subsequent fluid therapy. When a hypotensive trauma patient comes to the emergency room, two large-bore intravenous lines are started and a 1-L bag of lactated Ringer's solution is attached to each line. The fluid is allowed to run in as rapidly as possible (≤ 10 minutes if the fluid is pumped in manually). This method of rapid intravenous fluid infusion is called a fluid bolus, or fluid challenge. The initial fluid bolus in adults is usually 1000 to 2000 mL; in children, it is 20 mL/kg body weight. After the initial bolus, the patient's vital signs and urine output are reassessed. If the patient does not respond to a bolus of intravenous fluid, type-specific or O-negative blood is transfused, along with more crystalloid. The response to this initial fluid challenge identifies patients who have greater blood loss than expected or those who continue to bleed, and patients generally fall into one of three categories. The "rapid responder" becomes hemodynamically normal after the initial fluid bolus, and fluid rates can be set to maintenance levels. The "transient responder" responds to the initial intravenous fluid bolus, but experiences subsequent deterioration of vital signs or requires additional resuscitation to maintain hemodynamic stability. The "minimal responder" or the "nonresponder" does not achieve normal blood pressure despite the administration of large volumes of crystalloid and blood. These patients usually have exsanguinating blood loss and frequently require emergent surgical intervention to control hemorrhage.

Nonhemorrhagic Shock

Nonhemorrhagic causes of shock include cardiogenic shock, **tension pneumothorax,** neurogenic shock, septic shock, and hypoadrenal shock. The patient's initial response to therapy usually allows recognition and management of all forms of shock.

Cardiogenic shock in the trauma patient is myocardial dysfunction that usually occurs as a result of blunt cardiac injury ("myocardial contusion"), **cardiac tamponade,** air embolus, or, rarely, myocardial infarction. Tension pneumothorax and cardiac tamponade produce shock by impeding venous return and direct compression of the heart, respectively. These entities are generally caused by blunt or penetrating thoracic trauma and are discussed in more detail later in this chapter.

Neurogenic shock results from injury to the descending sympathetic pathways in the spinal cord. It is caused by high thoracic and cervical spinal cord injuries. Patients who are in neurogenic shock are hypotensive without tachycardia. Loss of sympathetic vasomotor tone causes hypotension secondary to vasodilation and intravascular pooling of blood. Loss of sympathetic innervation to the heart produces bradycardia. Primary treatment involves the administration of intravenous fluids to restore intravascular volume. Vasopressors (e.g., phenylephrine) can be used as an adjunct to fluid therapy. Atropine can be used to counteract bradycardia in these patients. Management can be challenging when neurogenic shock is combined with hemorrhagic shock in the patient with multiple injuries. Neurogenic shock is not caused by isolated closed head injuries.

Septic shock results from the body's systemic inflammatory response to an infection. Cytokine and inflammatory mediator release result in peripheral vasodilation and hypotension. Septic shock is not common immediately after injury. It occurs in patients for whom definitive care is delayed (e.g., a patient with a bowel injury who presents in delayed fashion with fever and peritonitis). Septic patients who are hypovolemic resemble patients who are in hypovolemic shock. Normovolemic septic patients have warm extremities, wide pulse pressures, and elevated cardiac output. Treatment consists of intravenous fluid, antibiotics, and eradication of the source of infection.

Hypoadrenal shock is caused by adrenal insufficiency. Patients who are taking exogenous corticosteroids are at particular risk because the exogenous steroids cause adrenal suppression, although the syndrome may occur in patients who have no history of exogenous corticosteroid use. Circulatory collapse can be triggered by the stress of injury. The diagnosis is suggested by the presence of shock that does not respond to resuscitation with fluids and inotropic agents. Confirmation of the diagnosis can be made by performing a cosyntropin stimulation test, with lack of appropriate response suggesting hypoadrenalism. Therapy requires replacement with intravenous hydrocortisone (100 mg every 6 to 8 hours).

Disability

The neurologic disability assessment establishes the patient's level of consciousness, pupillary size and reaction, and motor response to stimuli. The level of consciousness is assessed quickly with the mnemonic **AVPU.** Is the patient Alert, responsive to *V*ocal stimuli, responsive to *P*ainful stimuli, or *U*nresponsive? A more detailed quantitative neurologic evaluation is performed with the **Glasgow Coma Scale** (GCS), which is explained later.

Exposure and Environment

This portion of the initial assessment refers to completely disrobing the patient so that a complete physical examination can be performed. Many injuries have been missed because of failure to perform this simple maneuver. Frequently, clothing must be cut off to facilitate this process and avoid compromising spinal precautions or causing further injury. It is important to remember that once undressed, a trauma victim may rapidly become hypothermic, especially if hemorrhage is present. The patient should be covered with warm blankets and the temperature of the room raised to prevent hypothermia. During this phase of initial assessment, other environmental factors are controlled as well (e.g., removal of burned or gasoline-saturated clothing).

Secondary Survey

The secondary survey follows the initiation of resuscitation and a reassessment of the primary survey. A detailed head-to-toe evaluation, including an **AMPLE history** and a complete physical examination, is undertaken to identify all injuries: *A*llergies, *M*edications, *P*ast illnesses, *L*ast meal, and the *E*vents surrounding the injury are noted. ATLS guidelines refer to the concept of "tubes and fingers in every orifice." Urinary and gastric catheterization should be performed in any seriously injured patient, and urinary output is assessed as an indicator of organ perfusion. Continuous electrocardiogram (ECG) and pulse oximetry measurements are monitored. Baseline laboratory studies are drawn at this time if they were not drawn when the intravenous lines were started. Portable radiographs are taken at this time, but should not interrupt resuscitation efforts. Three essential x-ray views are the lateral cervical spine, anteroposterior (AP) chest, and AP pelvis. Other diagnostic procedures (e.g., ultrasound, peritoneal lavage, radiography) are also performed during this phase.

Gastric and Bladder Catheters

Nasogastric (NG) and bladder intubations are integral to the management of the injured patient. The placement of an NG tube is both diagnostic and therapeutic. When placed with low continuous suction, it removes air and gastric contents. The presence of blood in the NG aspirate may represent oropharyngeal injury (swallowed blood), traumatic insertion of the tube, or distinct injury to the esophagus, stomach, or duodenum. An NG tube reduces the risk of vomiting and aspiration. It also prevents acute gastric dilation that is associated with aerophagia and assisted ventilation with a bag-valve–mask device. Air can be forced down the esophagus almost as easily as it can be forced down the trachea with a bag-valve–mask device. Acute gastric dilation may cause a vasovagal reaction that can lead to hypotension and bradycardia. The outcome of a vasovagal reaction in a hypotensive trauma patient can be cardiac arrest. Caution must be exercised in patients with severe facial fractures because these injuries are associated with fractures of the cribriform plate. In these cases, the NG tube should be inserted orally to avoid inadvertent insertion of the tube through the cribriform plate fracture and into the brain.

Bladder (Foley) catheter insertion serves several purposes: (1) it decompresses the bladder, and (2) it provides a means to monitor urine output, both in color and in volume. Hematuria (red urine) implies genitourinary trauma. Myoglobinuria (red-brown urine) is associated with severe crush injury and muscle damage. Concentrated (dark yellow) urine means hypovolemia. Urine output provides an index of tissue perfusion and is one of the best initial ways to ensure that resuscitation is adequate. Appropriate resuscitation should produce urine output of at least 30 mL/hr in adults, 1 mL/kg/hr in children, or 2 mL/kg/hr in infants younger than 1 year old. Before a transurethral bladder catheter is inserted, the perineum and rectum must be examined. The presence of blood at the urethral meatus, a perineal hematoma, or an abnormal finding on prostate examination requires that a retrograde urethrogram be performed to ensure continuity of the urethra. A suprapubic bladder catheter is normally required if the urethra is injured. Urethral injuries are commonly associated with pelvic fractures in men. In women, urethral injury is rare because the urethra is short.

Definitive Care

The definitive care phase follows the secondary survey. The patient is reevaluated, and all injuries are prioritized. The care plan is based on the mechanism of injury, the patient's physiologic status, anatomic injuries, and concomitant disease conditions that may affect the patient's survival. During this phase, further diagnostic and therapeutic procedures may occur, such as computed tomography (CT) scanning, angiography, and surgical procedures.

This algorithm—primary survey, resuscitation (begun simultaneously with the primary survey), secondary survey, and definitive care—forms the basis for the early care of the injured patient. Later care, which involves management of specific injuries that are common to the trauma patient, is discussed below.

THORACIC TRAUMA

Thoracic trauma accounts for one-fourth of trauma deaths and is second only to head trauma as the most common type of fatal injury. Although some of these injuries are immediately or rapidly fatal, others can be treated with simple interventions if they are recognized. Knowing the signs and symptoms of these injuries and having a high index of suspicion are critical for early recognition. Of thoracic injuries, approximately 85% can be treated with simple maneuvers that are taught in medical school. The

Table 10-2 Categories of Thoracic Trauma

Immediately Lethal Injuries	Potentially Lethal Injuries	Nonlethal Injuries
Airway obstruction	Pulmonary contusion	Simple pneumothorax
Tension pneumothorax	Blunt cardiac injury	Simple hemothorax
Open pneumothorax	Traumatic aortic rupture	Scapula and rib fractures
Massive hemothorax	Traumatic diaphragmatic rupture	
Flail chest	Tracheobronchial tree disruption	
Cardiac tamponade	Esophageal injury	

other 15% usually require operative intervention. It is convenient to divide these injuries into groups according to their severity (Table 10-2).

Immediately Lethal Thoracic Injuries

Airway obstruction, the first entity in this category, was previously discussed. Tension pneumothorax, the second type, occurs when there is a continuous buildup of air in the pleural space, with no means of escape. This can occur after blunt or penetrating chest injury. As the intrapleural pressure rises, the ipsilateral lung collapses, the mediastinum is displaced to the opposite side, and the contralateral lung is compressed. As a result, compression, distortion, and kinking of the superior and inferior vena cavae occur. Venous return to the heart is significantly decreased, thereby compromising oxygen delivery. Unless this condition is rapidly treated, death ensues. Tension pneumothorax should never be diagnosed by chest radiography; it is a clinical diagnosis that is made by physical examination. Waiting for x-ray confirmation may have disastrous consequences. Physical signs include respiratory distress, tachycardia, hypotension, jugular venous distension, and tracheal deviation toward the noninjured side of the thorax. On the injured side, breath sounds are absent or markedly decreased, with hyperresonance (tympany) to percussion (Table 10-3). If tension pneumothorax is suspected, rapid decompression with a needle is indicated. A 14-gauge (or larger), 5-cm-long, over-the-needle catheter is inserted into the pleural cavity through the second intercostal space (just over the top of the third rib) in the midclavicular line. A rush of air from the needle signifies decompression of the tension. The needle is removed, but the catheter is left in place to prevent recurrence. Needle decompression is a rapid, temporary treatment that converts a tension pneumothorax into a simple pneumothorax.

Definitive treatment requires a chest tube placement, usually through the fifth intercostal space in the midaxillary line. The tube is connected to an underwater seal device to remove air, fluid, and blood from the pleural space, thus allowing the lung to expand. Suction is commonly applied to this device to ensure adequate evacuation of the pleural cavity and expansion of the lung.

Open pneumothorax, or a sucking chest wound, occurs when a large chest wall defect permits equilibration of intrapleural and atmospheric pressures. This situation leads to lung collapse. As the patient breathes, air is heard or seen bubbling from the wound. If the size of the opening in the chest wall is two-thirds the diameter of the trachea or larger, resistance to flow is lower through the injury than through the trachea. Air then moves preferentially in and out of the pleural space instead of into the trachea, thus preventing effective ventilation. Therefore, this wound is immediately life threatening. The fastest and easiest way to stop this abnormal air movement is to cover the wound with an impermeable dressing (e.g., Vaseline gauze, plastic wrap), taped on three sides, to create a one-way flap valve. During exhalation, as pressure in the pleural space increases, air can escape under the open side of the dressing. During inspiration, as pressure in the pleural space decreases, the dressing is sucked down, occluding the wound and preventing air from entering the pleural space. It is crucial not to tape the dressing on all four sides because doing so might convert an open pneumothorax to a tension pneumothorax. Definitive care in-

Table 10-3 Signs of Tension Pneumothorax and Cardiac Tamponade

Tension Pneumothorax	Cardiac Tamponade
Respiratory distress	Respiratory distress
Tachycardia	Tachycardia
Hypotension	Hypotension
Jugular venous distension (elevated CVP)[a]	Jugular venous distension (elevated CVP)[a]
Ipsilateral absent or markedly decreased breath sounds	Muffled or distant heart sounds
Ipsilateral hyperresonance to percussion (tympany)	Pulsus paradoxus >10 mm Hg
Contralateral tracheal deviation	

[a] In the hypovolemic patient, this sign may not be present.
CVP, central venous pressure.

volves placement of a chest tube and surgical closure of the chest wall defect.

Massive hemothorax is the rapid loss of more than 1500 mL blood into the thoracic cavity. It is a class III or greater hemorrhage into the chest. Diagnosis is made when a hypotensive patient has decreased or absent breath sounds and dullness to percussion on one side of the chest. Initial management is the same as that of any patient who is in hemorrhagic shock. A portable supine chest radiograph usually shows complete opacification on the injured side. Treatment typically begins with the insertion of a large (#36 to 40 Fr) chest tube. An autotransfusion device should be set up, if available. Initial evacuation of greater than or equal to 1500 mL of blood or ongoing blood loss of greater than or equal to 200 mL/hour requires thoracotomy for control of hemorrhage. Sometimes, there is no further significant blood loss from the chest tube, and thoracotomy is avoided. A post–chest tube chest radiograph should be obtained to verify complete drainage of the hemothorax.

Flail chest occurs when consecutive ribs are fractured in multiple places (i.e., each rib is fractured in at least two places). This results in a free-floating, or flail, segment of the chest wall that moves paradoxically with inspiration and expiration. Paradoxical motion occurs because the flail segment is not in bony continuity with the rest of the thoracic cage. As the patient inhales, the ribs rise and the diaphragm descends, creating negative pressure in the pleural space. The uninjured chest wall expands, but the flail segment, responding to the negative intrapleural pressure, moves inward. Similarly, as the patient exhales, the normal ribs retract, but the flail segment moves outward. Seeing or palpating this paradoxical motion makes the diagnosis. The ventilatory insufficiency that is commonly seen in patients with flail chest is not simply caused by the abnormal chest wall motion. Instead, the underlying lung injury in combination with hypoventilation produces respiratory failure. A significant amount of force is required to break multiple ribs in multiple places. Some of this energy is transmitted through the chest wall into the underlying lung, causing a **pulmonary contusion,** which involves extensive intraparenchymal hemorrhage and alveolar collapse. As a result, ventilation–perfusion mismatch occurs and results in hypoxemia. The pain associated with multiple rib fractures causes the patient to splint the injured chest wall by inhibiting its movement during ventilation. Hypoventilation is the consequence. Patients with significant ventilatory impairment need intubation and mechanical ventilation to prevent hypoxia and hypercarbia. Positive end-expiratory pressure (PEEP) may also be required to maintain adequate oxygenation. Optimization of intravascular volume and myocardial performance often requires placement of a central venous or pulmonary artery catheter. Definitive treatment requires reexpansion of the lung, adequate oxygenation, judicious use of fluids, and adequate analgesia to improve ventilation.

Cardiac tamponade as a result of trauma occurs when blood accumulates within the pericardial sac and compresses the heart. It is associated with blunt and penetrating injuries to the heart (e.g., a motor vehicle crash that thrusts the driver's sternum into the steering wheel). Even isolated injuries to the small pericardial and coronary vessels can cause tamponade. When blood leaks into the fibrous, nondistensible pericardium, it compresses the cardiac chambers and restricts ventricular filling during diastole. As a result, stroke volume and cardiac output decrease. The increased pressure within the pericardial sac is transmitted to each cardiac chamber, resulting in equalization of the right atrial, right ventricular diastolic, pulmonary artery diastolic, pulmonary capillary wedge, left atrial, left ventricular diastolic, and intrapericardial pressures. Three classic clinical signs, known as **Beck's triad,** are related to these hemodynamics: (1) muffled (distant) heart sounds; (2) elevated central venous pressure (jugular venous distension); and (3) hypotension. Other signs include **pulsus paradoxus** (a decrease of $>$ 10 mm Hg in systolic blood pressure during inspiration) and **Kussmaul's sign** (an increase in central venous pressure [CVP] with inspiration). However, one or more of these findings may be absent in a significant number of patients with hemopericardium. Muffled heart sounds and pulsus paradoxus may be difficult to elicit in a noisy emergency department. Distended neck veins associated with elevated CVP may not be present in the hypovolemic patient. Cardiac tamponade and tension pneumothorax are included in the differential diagnosis in patients who manifest pulseless electrical activity (PEA). Bedside ultrasonography is the diagnostic modality of choice, although measurement of elevated CVP in the appropriate clinical setting may be helpful as well.

The initial treatment of a patient who is suspected of having cardiac tamponade is administration of large volumes of intravenous fluid. Raising CVP higher than the intrapericardial pressure temporarily increases cardiac output, allowing time to prepare for definitive therapy. Emergent thoracotomy is usually required to release the pericardial tamponade and repair the underlying cardiac injury. **Pericardiocentesis** may be diagnostic and therapeutic when an experienced surgeon is not immediately available. A 16- to 18-gauge, 15-cm-long, over-the-needle catheter attached to a 30- to 60-mL syringe is used for the procedure. The needle is inserted 1 to 2 cm to the left and inferior to the xiphochondral junction at a 45° angle to the skin. The needle is directed toward the left shoulder and slowly advanced while the syringe is aspirated. Return of blood into the syringe signifies entry into the pericardium. The procedure should be performed under ultrasound or ECG guidance. The patient's ECG reading is monitored with standard leads or a precordial lead that can be attached to the needle with a sterile alligator clip. Removal of as little as 10 mL blood can significantly improve cardiac function. The catheter (not the needle) is advanced into the pericardial sac, the needle is withdrawn, and the catheter is anchored in place and capped with a three-way stopcock to allow for repeat aspirations, if necessary. Pericardiocentesis may be unsuccessful if the pericardial blood is clotted. If the needle enters the heart, the

ECG reading will show an injury pattern (i.e., ST-T wave changes, QRS widens and enlarges). If a precordial ECG lead is attached to the needle, the tracing inverts when the epicardium is entered. It should be emphasized that pericardiocentesis is a temporizing maneuver. Definitive therapy requires opening the pericardium, finding the source of bleeding, and repairing it. This repair requires a qualified surgeon. If one is available, then it becomes a clinical decision as to whether to first perform the pericardiocentesis followed by operative exposure of the heart or to proceed directly to the operating room without pericardiocentesis. In extreme cases, there may not be time to go to the operating room, and a left anterior thoracotomy must be done in the emergency room.

Potentially Lethal Thoracic Injuries

Pulmonary contusion is an injury to the lung parenchyma that causes interstitial hemorrhage, alveolar collapse, and extravasation of blood and plasma into alveoli. It causes a ventilation–perfusion mismatch that results in hypoxemia. Physical examination may show a blunt or penetrating injury to the chest. Blunt injuries are associated with chest wall contusions, rib fractures, sternal fractures, and flail chest. The radiographic appearance is that of a poorly defined opacification that develops over time. These findings on chest radiography are usually present within 1 hour of injury, but may take as long as 6 hours to become visible. Treatment includes observation, supplemental oxygen, and analgesics. Mechanical ventilation and PEEP may be required in patients with worsening pulmonary insufficiency.

Blunt cardiac injury is a difficult diagnosis to make. The diagnosis of blunt cardiac injury requires a high index of suspicion, especially in patients who have had deceleration or crush injuries to the anterior chest. These injuries are associated with motor vehicle collisions that involve the driver's sternum being propelled into the steering wheel or dashboard. Fractures of the sternum or ribs may be present. The anterior myocardium (right ventricle) is primarily involved, and when severely injured may lead to right-sided heart failure, hypotension, arrhythmia, and rarely, myocardial rupture. Initial diagnostic methods include blood pressure monitoring, continuous ECG monitoring, and 12-lead ECG. Significant blunt cardiac injury may be safely excluded in normotensive patients without cardiac dysrhythmia. Prolonged monitoring and cardiac enzyme measurement are not indicated for asymptomatic patients with a normal ECG. The diagnosis should be considered in trauma patients with blunt thoracic injury and unexplained hypotension, or in those with significant dysrhythmia. Such patients may require further diagnostic maneuvers, such as echocardiography or pulmonary artery catheterization. Antiarrhythmics or inotropic support may be indicated depending on patient presentation.

Traumatic aortic rupture, or blunt aortic injury, is a common cause of immediate death in abrupt deceleration injuries associated with motor vehicle collisions or falls from great heights. For survivors, salvage is possible with early diagnosis and treatment. Shear forces cause injury of the aorta at sites of anatomic fixation. Common sites are just distal to the origin of the left subclavian artery at the ligamentum arteriosum, at the root of the aorta near the aortic valve, and at the diaphragmatic hiatus. In a horizontal deceleration, seen in high-speed motor vehicle collisions, the heart and aortic arch continue to move forward, while motion of the descending aorta is limited because of its posterior attachments. In a vertical deceleration, seen in falls from great heights, the heart, weighted with blood, moves rapidly downward, stretching the aortic arch and causing injury in this location. Anterior–posterior compression of the chest and abdomen can also result in fracture or dislocation of the lower thoracic spine, which can injure the aorta at the diaphragmatic hiatus. The forces involved in these types of injury are complex and interrelated. For example, in motor vehicle collisions, the body moves forward, the heart and aortic arch decelerate at a different rate than the descending aorta, the chest hits the steering wheel (causing anterior–posterior compression), and the heart is displaced caudally and to the left. As a result, the aorta is exposed to shearing, bending, and torsion stresses that are beyond its ability to maintain structural integrity. If the initial tear involves the intima and media, the aortic blood is contained by the aortic adventitia and a pseudoaneurysm forms. If the initial tear involves all three layers of the aortic wall, the patient exsanguinates into the chest. Ruptures at the aortic root carry a high mortality rate; those at the diaphragmatic hiatus are rare. Of the survivors, most have contained injuries at the ligamentum arteriosum. Specific symptoms include severe chest or back pain. Radiographic signs that suggest blunt aortic injury are listed in Table 10-4. Often, however, there are no specific symptoms or signs, and chest radiography has a false-negative rate of up to 15% for aortic injury. Having a high index of suspicion in patients with deceleration trauma may be the only indication for further evaluation. Arteriography is considered the "gold standard" for diagnosing blunt aortic injury, but it is invasive, time consuming, and labor intensive. Because of its accuracy and ease, contrast-enhanced CT has become the screening test of choice at most trauma centers in the United States. Radiologists equipped with modern spiral or multidetector

Table 10-4 Radiographic Signs Suggestive of Blunt Aortic Injury

Widened mediastinum (> 8 cm)
Indistinct aortic knob
Opacification of the aortopulmonary window
First or second rib fracture
Deviation of the esophagus or nasogastric tube to the right
Presence of pleural apical cap
Depression of the left mainstem bronchus
Widened paratracheal or paraspinous stripe

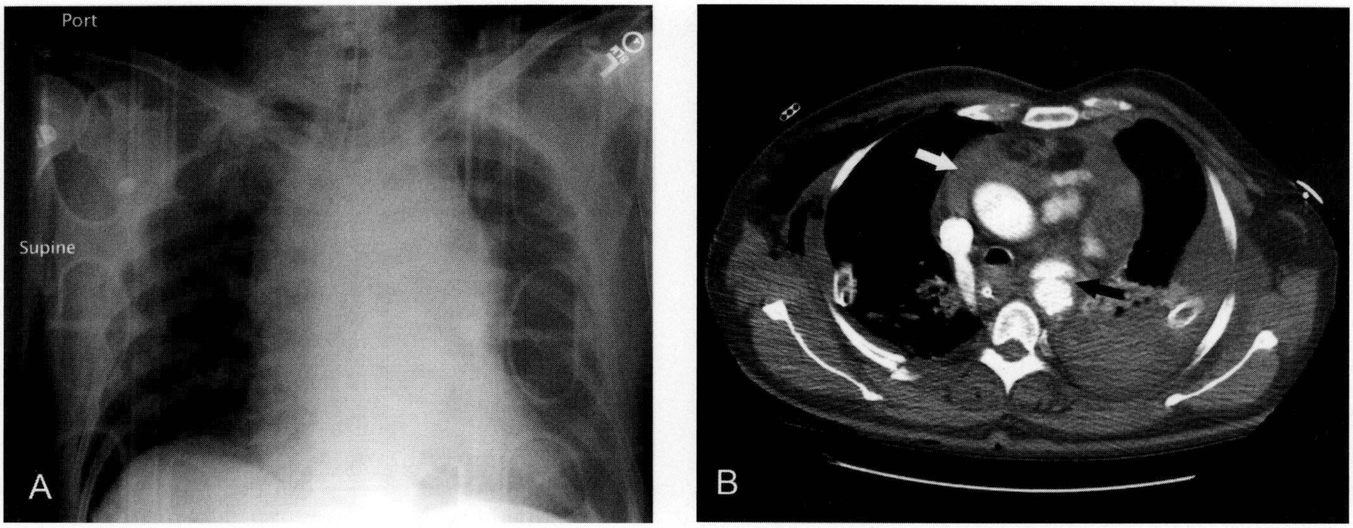

Figure 10-8 Blunt aortic injury. **A**, Chest radiograph reveals significantly widened mediastinum, right second rib fracture, left apical cap and pleural effusion, deviation of the endotracheal tube to the right, and obliteration of the aortic knob and aortopulmonary window. **B**, Subsequent contrast-enhanced spiral computed tomography of the chest reveals blood in the mediastinum (white arrow) and blunt injury of the descending aorta with pseudoaneurysm (black arrow).

CT scanners can diagnose or rule out this potentially lethal injury in fewer than 10 minutes (Fig. 10-8). Transesophageal echocardiography (TEE) is an alternate diagnostic test that is quite accurate in the hands of a skilled operator. Rapid operative repair, usually with partial cardiopulmonary bypass, is necessary if these patients are to survive. Preoperative preparation includes control of blood pressure, as well as definitive treatment of other immediately life-threatening injuries (e.g., splenectomy for splenic rupture). Hypotension is treated with intravenous fluids or blood, whereas hypertension must be controlled pharmacologically to avoid free rupture before surgical repair. The risk of postoperative paraplegia secondary to spinal cord ischemia is best minimized by using cardiopulmonary bypass techniques during surgical repair.

Traumatic diaphragmatic rupture is associated with blunt trauma to the lower chest and abdomen. The rupture can occur at any site on the diaphragm, but 90% of cases involve the left hemidiaphragm. The pressure gradient between the pleural and peritoneal cavities of 5 to 10 cm of water favors the movement of abdominal viscera into the chest. Blunt trauma produces large radial tears that can permit the stomach, spleen, colon, or small bowel to herniate into the thorax. Physical examination may reveal bowel sounds in the chest. Chest radiography may be misinterpreted as showing elevated left hemidiaphragm, gastric dilation, loculated pneumothorax, pleural effusion, or subpulmonic hematoma. If diaphragmatic rupture is suspected, an NG tube should be inserted to decompress the stomach. In such cases, chest radiography may show the NG tube curling up into the chest. This finding is diagnostic of diaphragmatic rupture, and no further diagnostic studies are needed (Fig. 10-9). If the diagnosis is still in question after an NG tube is inserted, then an upper gastrointestinal contrast study can be performed. On the right side, the liver usually prevents the abdominal contents from entering the thorax. Thus, making the diagnosis of a right diaphragmatic laceration may be difficult. Penetrating trauma may produce

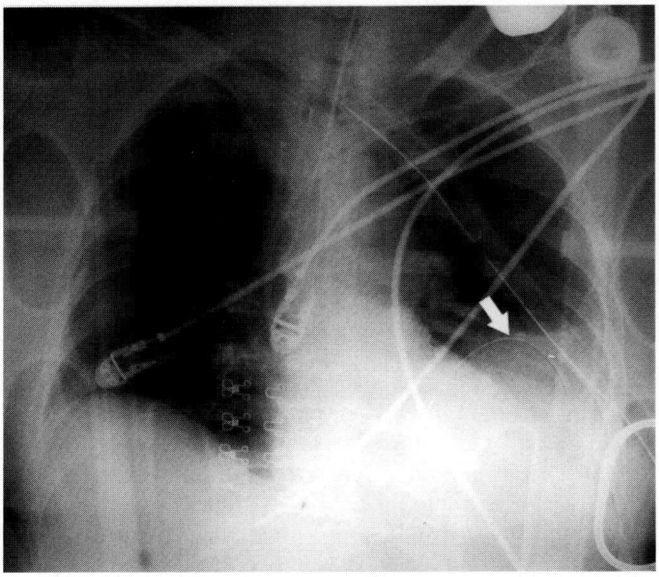

Figure 10-9 Chest radiograph of a patient with a traumatic diaphragmatic rupture. The nasogastric tube is curling up into the chest (arrow). This finding is diagnostic of diaphragmatic rupture.

small holes in the diaphragm that may take years to develop into a diaphragmatic hernia. Treatment of acute diaphragmatic rupture is direct repair from an abdominal approach. The high incidence of associated intraabdominal injuries makes exploratory laparotomy mandatory.

Disruption of the tracheobronchial tree is an uncommon injury. However, because of the high mortality rate associated with airway obstruction, subtle signs must be investigated thoroughly. Laryngeal and tracheal injuries may cause hoarseness, subcutaneous emphysema, palpable fracture, **crepitus,** hemoptysis, and respiratory distress. Severe anteroposterior crush injuries to the chest cause lateral deformation to the thorax, which can result in a traction injury to the trachea and mainstem bronchi. Such injuries to the mainstem bronchi usually occur within 2 cm of the carina. These patients may have hemoptysis, subcutaneous emphysema, pneumothorax, or pneumomediastinum. The diagnosis is confirmed by bronchoscopy. Treatment may require only airway maintenance with an endotracheal tube. Major disruptions require operative repair.

Esophageal injury is usually caused by penetrating trauma. If the potential path of a penetrating object is near the esophagus, this injury should be suspected. Blunt injury to the esophagus is rare but can result from a severe blow to the lower sternum or upper abdomen, which causes a forceful eruption of gastric contents into the esophagus. A linear tear may occur through the left posterior wall of the esophagus. Symptoms associated with esophageal trauma are severe epigastric or left-sided chest pain, dysphagia, hematemesis, left pleural effusion, subcutaneous emphysema, pneumothorax, and pneumomediastinum. A chest tube thoracostomy may show food particles in the chest. The diagnosis can be confirmed with an esophagogram or esophagoscopy. Acute perforations are treated with operative repair and drainage. Patients with missed esophageal injuries typically develop sepsis; treatment usually requires wide drainage and esophageal exclusion, including proximal diversion with a cervical esophagostomy, gastrostomy, and feeding jejunostomy. Mediastinitis is often fatal.

Nonlethal Thoracic Injuries

Simple pneumothorax is caused by a lung laceration or a chest wound that extends into the pleural space. Breath sounds may be decreased or normal. Diagnosis is made by chest radiography. An expiratory chest radiograph can make a small pneumothorax more visible. A simple pneumothorax may become a tension pneumothorax and therefore should be treated with a chest tube.

Simple hemothorax is the presence of less than 1500 mL blood in the pleural cavity. It is caused by laceration of the lung or intercostal blood vessels. Blood in the pleural cavity can lead to restrictive lung disease if it is not evacuated. Placement of a chest tube is not only a means to evacuate the chest but also a means to monitor blood loss from the chest. The bleeding is often self-limited, and no further therapy is needed.

Rib fractures are the most common injury in patients with blunt thoracic trauma. Pain with movement causes the patient to splint the chest wall. As a result, ventilation is reduced, and the clearance of respiratory secretions is impeded. Fractured ribs are characteristically diagnosed by physical examination with findings of localized pain, tenderness, and crepitus. A chest radiograph is appropriate to exclude associated pneumothorax or other thoracic injuries. The upper ribs and scapula are protected by the shoulder girdle and clavicle. Fractures of the scapula and upper ribs 1 to 3 require significant force. As a result, these fractures are associated with major injuries to the head, neck, cervical spine, lung, and aorta and its major branches. Fractures of ribs 9 through 12 may be associated with injuries to the spleen and liver. Treatment of isolated rib fractures is supportive and consists of pain control. Intercostal nerve blocks may be necessary if oral or parenteral analgesics do not control pain adequately. Analgesics allow the patient to cough and breathe deeply, thus preventing atelectasis by clearing respiratory secretions. Binders or rib belts should not be used to treat rib fractures because they promote atelectasis.

ABDOMINAL TRAUMA

Physical Examination of the Abdomen

Abdominal evaluation occurs during the secondary survey. In trauma patients, unrecognized intraabdominal hemorrhage is one of the leading causes of preventable death. Patients with significant abdominal trauma often have no significant physical findings to indicate intraabdominal injury. The classic signs of abdominal pain, tenderness, and rebound tenderness are often camouflaged by other extra-abdominal injuries or masked by an altered level of consciousness as a result of head trauma, drugs, or alcohol. In trauma patients with hypotension, normal breath sounds, and no external signs of blood loss, the abdomen is a likely source of occult hemorrhage. As many as 20% of patients with acute intraperitoneal hemorrhage have a normal abdominal examination. For this reason, the astute physician must have a high index of suspicion when managing patients who have blunt or penetrating trauma to the torso. In evaluating abdominal trauma, the initial goal is to determine whether a significant intraabdominal injury exists, not to determine which organ is injured.

The abdominal cavity extends from the diaphragm to the pelvic floor. It is divided into four zones: (1) upper abdomen, (2) lower abdomen, (3) pelvis, and (4) retroperitoneum. The upper, or intrathoracic, abdomen is confined by the rib cage. During expiration, the diaphragm is elevated to as high as the fourth intercostal space anteriorly (the male nipple line) and the seventh intercostal space, or the tip of the scapula, posteriorly. Thus, trauma to the mid- and lower thorax may injure the abdominal viscera.

Organs located in the upper abdomen include the liver, spleen, stomach, transverse colon, and diaphragm. The lower abdomen contains the small bowel and the ascending and descending colon. Pelvic organs include the bladder, rectum, and iliac vessels; in females they also include the uterus and ovaries. The retroperitoneum contains the kidneys, ureters, duodenum, pancreas, aorta, vena cava, and parts of the colon. Figure 10-10 shows the surface landmarks that define the abdominal cavity.

Physical examination of the abdomen begins with inspection, auscultation, percussion, and palpation. Inspection of the abdomen begins with the patient fully undressed. A careful inspection of the anterior, lateral, and posterior surfaces of the torso is made, looking specifically for abrasions, contusions, lacerations, and penetrating wounds. When the possibility of a spine injury exists, the patient is cautiously log-rolled to reveal the dorsum. Other clues to injury come from noting whether the abdomen is scaphoid, flat, or distended. Auscultation of the abdomen in a noisy emergency department is often difficult. The absence of bowel sounds implies ileus. A search should be made for vascular bruits. If any are found, a specific note should be made about their relation to the cardiac cycle. A continuous bruit implies a left-to-right shunt or, more precisely, an arteriovenous fistula. For example, a loud supraumbilical continuous bruit can be caused by an **aortocaval fistula.** Percussion can elicit subtle signs of peritoneal irritation, and it is another way to test for rebound tenderness. It can also detect gastric distension when there is tympany in the left upper quadrant. Normally, there is dullness to percussion over the liver; however, the absence of this sign or the presence of tympany in the right upper quadrant may indicate free air in the abdomen. Palpation of the abdomen is crucial to the evaluation of the trauma patient. Gentle palpation may show tenderness, guarding, or the presence of an abnormal mass. Voluntary muscle guarding usually indicates a fear of pain, whereas involuntary muscle guarding means significant peritoneal inflammation. Rebound tenderness signifies peritoneal irritation and may occur after hollow viscus injury. Evaluation of the abdomen also includes palpation of the iliac crests and symphysis pubis. Manual compression of the iliac wings, inward and outward, may show abnormal movement that indicates pelvic fracture.

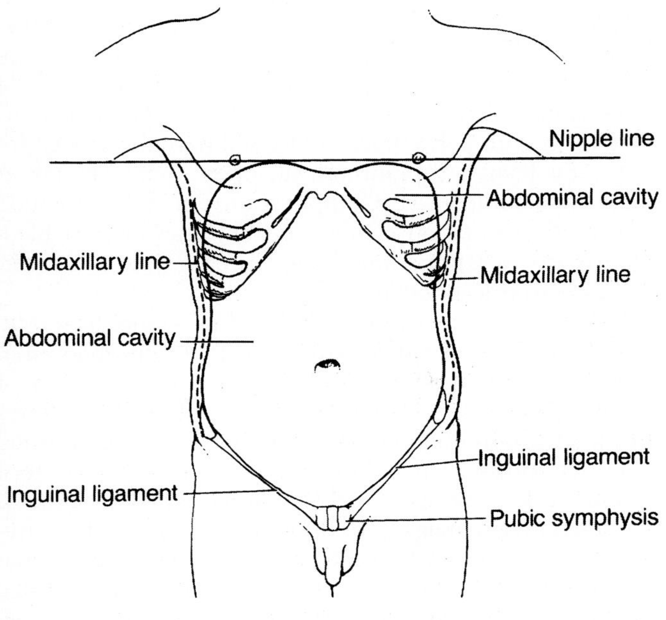

Figure 10-10 Surface landmarks of the abdominal cavity.

Perineal and rectal examinations are essential to the complete abdominal evaluation. Inspection of the perineum begins with gentle separation of the thighs and buttocks. The presence of blood at the urethral meatus or a scrotal hematoma suggests significant lower genitourinary tract injury. Digital rectal examination is mandatory in all trauma patients. Abnormal sphincter tone implies a neurologic injury. A boggy, spongy, or soft prostate may indicate periurethral bleeding, and a nonpalpable or high-riding prostate may indicate a urethral transection. Blood in the rectum indicates a rectal injury until proven otherwise. In female trauma patients, a bimanual pelvic examination should be performed. Vaginal lacerations are easily overlooked in patients with pelvic fracture or penetrating injuries. Speculum examination of the vagina is often required to identify these injuries.

Diagnostic Evaluation

Physical examination of the abdomen is unreliable in patients who are unconscious, intoxicated, or insensate below the nipple line from spinal cord injury. Lower rib fractures may imitate abdominal pain when the bony ends move with palpation of the upper abdomen. In these situations, a more accurate method to evaluate the abdomen is required. Abdominal ultrasonography, CT scan, and diagnostic peritoneal lavage (DPL) are the primary diagnostic modalities in abdominal trauma. Each test has certain advantages and disadvantages, which will be outlined below.

Bedside abdominal ultrasound in the emergency department can be used to search for the presence of intraabdominal fluid, which is assumed to be blood in the trauma patient. In the trauma setting, a limited abdominal ultrasound, termed FAST (Focused Assessment with Sonography for Trauma) is utilized (Fig. 10-11). This study, which may be performed by surgeons, emergency physicians, radiologists, or ultrasound technologists, involves the examination of two quadrants for the presence of fluid (blood) in four areas: right upper quadrant, for fluid in Morison's pouch; left upper quadrant, for fluid in the splenorenal recess, the pelvis, and the pericardium. An advantage of ultrasound is that it can be easily repeated in the event of a change in the patient's status. Ultrasound does have certain limitations, however. It is a poor examination for hollow viscus injury, and may be difficult in obese patients or in patients with subcutaneous emphysema (crepitus)

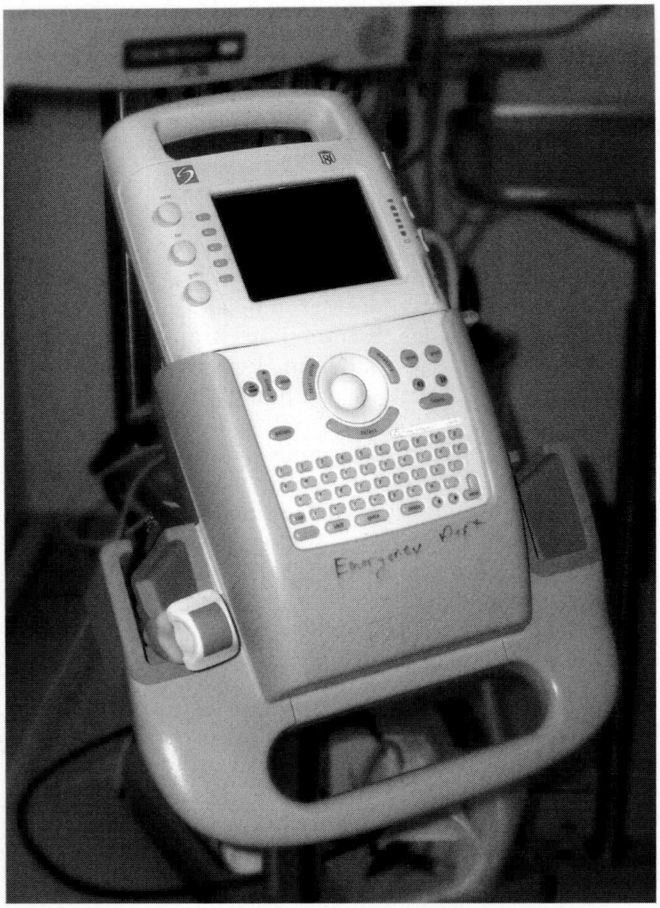

Figure 10-11 Portable ultrasound unit. These ultrasound machines may be used to perform FAST (*F*ocused *A*ssessment with *S*onography in *T*rauma) in the emergency department.

from chest injuries, since ultrasound waves do not penetrate well through air or fat. Use of ultrasound in penetrating abdominal trauma is controversial, largely because of its insensitivity for bowel injury (which is common after penetrating injury). However, ultrasound may reveal hemopericardium, hemoperitoneum, or hemothorax, facilitating definitive operative treatment in unstable patients with penetrating wounds that violate more than one body cavity. Despite certain limitations, FAST is a rapid, noninvasive, and highly accurate method for determining the presence of hemoperitoneum in traumatized patients and is the initial diagnostic modality of choice in blunt abdominal trauma.

Diagnostic peritoneal lavage (DPL) is an effective method of evaluating the abdomen of a critically injured patient. It is 98% sensitive for intraperitoneal hemorrhage and takes approximately 5 to 10 minutes to perform. DPL is a surgical procedure that is performed to determine whether an intraperitoneal injury exists. The procedure begins after the stomach and bladder are decompressed, a critical step to avoid injury to these organs. Therefore, the patient must have a gastric tube and a bladder catheter in place before the procedure begins. After the abdomen is cleansed with antiseptic solution, the DPL typically is performed through a midline incision just below the umbilicus (except in cases of suspected pelvic fracture, as explained later). The area is infiltrated with a local anesthetic (e.g., 1% lidocaine with epinephrine 1:100,000). Epinephrine is needed to maintain hemostasis and prevent contamination of the peritoneal cavity by blood from the incision. A small (2 to 5 cm) vertical midline incision is made and carried down through the skin and subcutaneous tissue to the linea alba. The linea alba is incised, and the peritoneum is identified and grasped with forceps. A small hole is made in the peritoneum, and through it, a peritoneal catheter is advanced into the peritoneal cavity and into the pelvis. In addition to the aforementioned open technique, DPL may be performed percutaneously using a commercially available prepackaged kit. Once the catheter is satisfactorily positioned, a syringe is attached and the catheter aspirated. If 10 mL gross blood is aspirated, the procedure is terminated and the patient is taken to the operating room for laparotomy. Otherwise, 10 mL/kg (1 L in adults) of warm lactated Ringer's solution or normal saline is infused through the catheter. The lavage fluid is retrieved after 5 to 10 minutes by gravity siphon technique, with the empty fluid bag placed on the floor. A 50-mL sample of the lavage fluid is sent to the laboratory for microscopic analysis, cell count, bile, and amylase analysis. Positive findings for blunt trauma are 100,000 red blood cells/mm^3 or more; greater than 500 white blood cells/mm^3; the presence of bacteria, bile, or food particles; or amylase greater than serum amylase. A negative finding does not exclude retroperitoneal injury to the duodenum, pancreas, kidneys, diaphragm, aorta, vena cava, or retroperitoneal portions of the colon. An absolute contraindication to DPL is an existing indication for laparotomy. Relative contraindications include previous abdominal operations (because of adhesions), morbid obesity, pediatric trauma, advanced cirrhosis (because of portal hypertension and the risk of bleeding), and preexisting coagulopathy. Pregnant patients and those with pelvic fractures should have the procedure performed via a supraumbilical, open approach, rather than percutaneously. Complications of DPL include bleeding; perforation of the stomach, intestines, or bladder; injury to retroperitoneal organs or vessels; and insertion-site wound infections.

Abdominal CT scan is considered to be the diagnostic standard for most *stable* patients with blunt abdominal trauma. CT scanning provides excellent delineation of solid organs, blood vessels, and retroperitoneal structures (Fig. 10-12). In the trauma setting, it is usually performed with administration of oral and intravenous contrast agents. CT scanning of stable trauma patients facilitates nonoperative management of less severe solid organ injuries. The major disadvantage of abdominal CT scan is that the patient must be moved from the resuscitation area. Therefore, CT scan is reserved for hemodynamically stable patients. CT scanning has a lower diagnostic accuracy

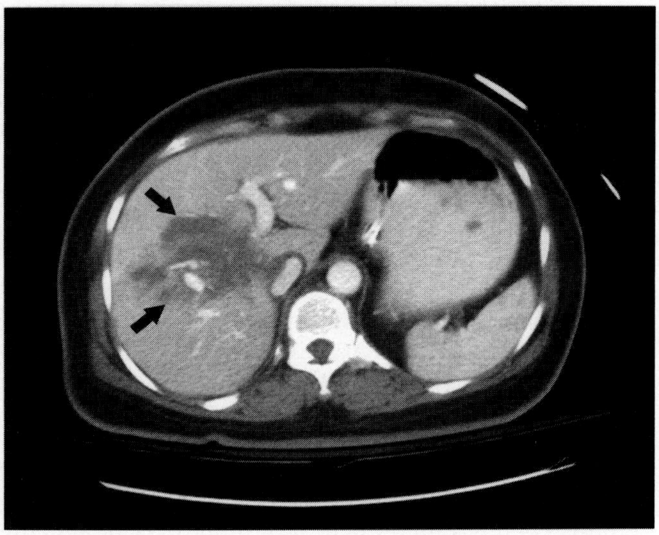

Figure 10-12 Computed tomography scan of the abdomen. A large intraparenchymal liver laceration is demonstrated (arrows).

Table 10-5	Splenic Injury Scale
Grade[a]	**Injury Description**
I Hematoma	Subcapsular, nonexpanding, < 10% surface area
Laceration	Capsular tear, nonbleeding, < 1 cm depth
II Hematoma	Subcapsular, nonexpanding, 10%–50% surface area Intraparenchymal, nonexpanding, < 5 cm diameter
Laceration	Capsular tear, active bleeding; 1–3 cm parenchymal depth that does not involve a trabecular vessel
III Hematoma	Subcapsular, > 50% surface area or expanding; ruptured subcapsular hematoma with active bleeding Intraparenchymal hematoma > 5 cm or expanding
Laceration	> 3 cm parenchymal depth or involving trabecular vessels
IV Hematoma	Ruptured intraparenchymal hematoma with active bleeding
Laceration	Laceration involving segmental or hilar vessels producing major devascularization (> 25% of spleen)
V Laceration	Completely shattered spleen
Vascular	Hilar vascular injury that devascularizes spleen

[a] Advance one grade for multiple injuries up to grade III.

for hollow viscus injury, although certain indirect CT findings (e.g., free intraperitoneal fluid without solid organ injury, bowel wall thickening) are highly suggestive of bowel injury. Other disadvantages of CT include high cost and the relatively long time it takes to obtain the study (as compared with FAST and DPL). Despite these disadvantages, CT scan plays a critical role in the evaluation of retroperitoneal and solid organs and has greater specificity than DPL.

Treatment of Abdominal Injury

Blunt Abdominal Trauma

Patients with blunt abdominal trauma and hemodynamic instability or peritonitis generally require exploratory laparotomy for definitive diagnosis and repair of intraabdominal injuries. Hemodynamically unstable patients with positive FAST ultrasound or DPL should be taken expeditiously to the operating room. Blunt trauma patients who are stable should undergo CT scanning to better delineate their injuries. Patients with solid organ injuries who remain hemodynamically stable may be managed nonoperatively. Deterioration of vital signs, falling hematocrit, or worsening abdominal exam are usual indications for laparotomy.

Specific Organ Injuries in Blunt Abdominal Trauma

The spleen is the most commonly injured organ in the setting of blunt abdominal trauma. Splenic injuries range in severity from small capsular tears to complete devascularization (Table 10-5). Bleeding from low-grade splenic injuries is frequently self-limited and can be managed expectantly in hemodynamically stable patients without signs of peritonitis. Such patients are closely observed with frequent vital signs, serial abdominal examinations, urinary output monitoring, and hemoglobin levels. Stable patients with radiographic signs of active splenic hemorrhage (e.g., extravasation of intravenous contrast) may be successfully treated by selective transcatheter embolization of the bleeding vessel. Interventional radiographic techniques have increased the rate of splenic salvage at many trauma centers. However, patients with persistent hemodynamic instability should be transported to the operating room for surgical exploration. Surgical options include repair (splenorrhaphy) when the patient's condition permits, or splenectomy. Overwhelming postsplenectomy infection (OPSI) is a rare (< 1% incidence) but frequently fatal complication of splenectomy. Accordingly, splenectomized patients should receive 23-valent pneumococcal vaccine, meningococcal vaccine, and *Haemophilus influenzae* type b (Hib) vaccine prior to discharge from the hospital.

Injury to the liver may occur with blunt trauma to the abdomen or lower thorax. Classification of liver injuries is detailed in Table 10-6. Low-grade liver injuries almost never require operative management unless injury to another intraabdominal organ is present. Grade III to V injuries may also be managed nonoperatively, provided the patient remains hemodynamically stable. Liver injury pa-

Table 10-6 Liver Injury Scale

Grade[a]	Injury Description
I Hematoma	Subcapsular, nonexpanding, < 10% surface area
Laceration	Capsular tear, nonbleeding, < 1 cm depth
II Hematoma	Subcapsular, nonexpanding, 10%–50% surface area
	Intraparenchymal, nonexpanding, < 10 cm diameter
Laceration	Capsular tear, active bleeding; 1–3 cm parenchymal depth, < 10 cm in length
III Hematoma	Subcapsular, > 50% surface area or expanding; ruptured subcapsular hematoma with active bleeding
	Intraparenchymal hematoma > 10 cm or expanding
Laceration	> 3 cm parenchymal depth
IV Hematoma	Ruptured intraparenchymal hematoma with active bleeding
Laceration	Parenchymal disruption involving 25%–75% of hepatic lobe or 1–3 segments within a single lobe
V Laceration	Parenchymal disruption involving > 75% of hepatic lobe or > 3 segments within a single lobe.
Vascular	Juxtahepatic venous injuries (i.e., retrohepatic vena cava/central major hepatic veins
VI Vascular	Hepatic avulsion

[a] Advance one grade for multiple injuries up to grade III.

tients selected for conservative management should be closely monitored in an intensive care unit, because major hemorrhage may be rapidly lethal if not detected early. As in splenic injury, angiographic transcatheter embolization is a useful adjunct when hepatic arterial bleeding is noted on CT scan. Patients with liver injury and signs of shock who fail to respond to initial resuscitation should undergo emergent exploratory laparotomy. Operative management is directed at cessation of hemorrhage and control of bile leakage. Techniques include parenchymal suturing, electrocautery, and topical hemostatic agents. Temporary occlusion of the portal triad (Pringle maneuver) may be useful during hepatic repair. Operative techniques for higher-grade liver injuries include perihepatic packing and temporary abdominal closure ("damage control" laparotomy), and atrio-caval shunting during retrohepatic vena cava repair.

Hollow viscus injury after blunt trauma most frequently involves the small bowel and duodenum. Types of injury include serosal tearing, full-thickness perforation, devascularization, and mesenteric injury. The presence of a "seatbelt sign" or ecchymosis on the anterior abdomen is associated with an increased risk of these injuries. Early diagnosis may be challenging. Abdominal CT scan with free intraperitoneal fluid in the absence of solid organ injury should raise concern for hollow viscus or mesenteric injury. DPL is a useful adjunct and typically reveals a white blood cell count of greater than $500/mm^3$ in the lavage fluid. Operative treatment includes repair or resection of the injured bowel segment.

Penetrating Abdominal Trauma

Gunshot Injuries

Gunshot wounds of the abdomen that involve peritoneal violation almost always result in visceral injury. Thus, if physical or radiographic examination of the abdomen reveals a missile trajectory that clearly involves peritoneal traverse, laparotomy is indicated, regardless of the patient's hemodynamic status. However, in stable patients with apparently tangential abdominal gunshot wounds, further evaluation may result in avoidance of nontherapeutic laparotomy. High-resolution helical or multidetector abdominal CT has been shown to reliably predict peritoneal violation in gunshot injuries. DPL and diagnostic laparoscopy may also be used to determine the presence of peritoneal violation.

Stab Wounds

Hemodynamically unstable patients with abdominal stab wounds should be transported emergently to the operating room for laparotomy. Peritonitis is an additional indication for operative management. However, stable patients with abdominal stab wounds may undergo further diagnostic evaluation to ascertain whether visceral injury exists. Exact location of stab wounds determines the type of evaluation. Anterior abdominal stab wounds (those located between the anterior axillary lines) are initially evaluated by wound exploration under local anesthesia. If no fascial penetration is noted, the wound may be treated as a simple laceration. If fascial penetration is noted, a DPL may be performed to assess for visceral injury. Stable patients with stab wounds of the flank and back (i.e., wounds posterior to the anterior axillary lines) are best evaluated with triple contrast CT scan (CT with intravenous, oral, and rectal contrast). Thoracoabdominal stab wounds, especially those on the left side, warrant a high level of suspicion for diaphragmatic injury. Imaging studies have notoriously poor sensitivity for diaphragmatic injury; therefore, patients with suspected diaphragmatic lacerations should undergo laparoscopy or laparotomy.

Pelvic Fractures

Pelvic fractures are associated with high energy forces (e.g., motor vehicle accidents, falls from great heights). The large bones of the pelvis have an abundant blood supply, and when fractured, the ends of the bones bleed. Forces that injure the pelvis can also rip the sacral venous plexus and cause lacerations to branches of the internal iliac artery. Ongoing bleeding causes the blood to dissect in the retroperitoneal and preperitoneal spaces, forming a pelvic hematoma. As expected, hemorrhage can be massive.

Management of a hypotensive patient with pelvic fracture is challenging. After initial fluid resuscitation is begun, a search for unrecognized blood loss must be made, despite obvious identification of a pelvic fracture. If a force is great enough to fracture the pelvis, it can also injure the intraabdominal viscera. If there are significant associated intraabdominal injuries, a laparotomy is required.

As mentioned, DPL is useful in assessing the peritoneal cavity for associated injuries. In patients with pelvic fractures, DPL is performed through a supraumbilical open incision rather than through the usual infraumbilical incision to avoid entering a pelvic hematoma. From a surgical standpoint, it is important to avoid entering a pelvic hematoma because attempting to control a bleeding pelvic fracture surgically is extremely difficult. Therefore, management centers around stabilizing the pelvis and permitting the closed retroperitoneum to tamponade. Most of the time, the bleeding is low-pressure hemorrhage from the fracture sites, venous plexus, and contiguous tissues. However, in major crush injuries to the pelvis in which the iliac wings, sacrum, and pubic rami are fractured, the patient can lose several liters of blood into the retroperitoneum. Bleeding can be temporarily controlled by wrapping a sheet around the pelvis and tying it tightly. The best method is to stabilize the pelvic fracture with external pelvic fixation (a metal C-clamp or vise-type mechanical device that is applied externally to the pelvis). If external fixation does not control the bleeding, arteriography should be performed to identify any arterial bleeding that can be treated with embolization.

Genitourinary tract injuries are associated with both pelvic fracture and abdominal trauma. Hematuria, whether gross or microscopic, is a sensitive clinical indicator of genitourinary trauma. Patients with blunt trauma to the genitourinary tract and microscopic hematuria usually have renal contusion. Those with penetrating trauma to the genitourinary tract usually have hematuria, but may not. Urethral injuries, suspected when blood is found at the urethral meatus, are diagnosed with a urethrogram; bladder injuries are diagnosed with a cystogram; kidney and ureteral injuries are usually diagnosed by a CT scan.

HEAD INJURY

Head injury is the most common cause of trauma-related mortality, accounting for approximately one-half of all deaths and more than 60% of motor vehicular deaths. Head injury is also the leading cause of disability in trauma patients. Primary injury to the brain can be caused by either penetrating or blunt trauma. Blunt trauma may injure the brain by direct transmission of energy at the point of impact, or at a point distant from impact because the brain rebounds against the inner surface of the skull (i.e., contrecoup injury). Regardless of the mechanism, primary injuries to the brain include lacerations, contusions, and shear injuries. Although primary brain injury is difficult to treat, secondary brain injury is preventable or treatable and thus is the focus of head trauma management. Secondary brain injury occurs when local processes within the skull or systemic processes worsen the initial brain injury and cause further damage. Local processes include intracranial hematomas and local or diffuse brain swelling, which can increase intracranial pressure and decrease cerebral perfusion. Systemic processes that can worsen the primary injury include hypoxia, hypotension, and anemia. Hypotension in a patient with a head injury should prompt a search for hemorrhage. Isolated closed head injuries do not cause hypotension.

Cerebral Anatomy and Physiology

A review of the anatomy and physiology of the cranium is essential to understanding the issues involved in the management of head trauma. The mnemonic **SCALP** is useful in recalling the five layers of the scalp: Skin, subCutaneous tissue, galea Aponeurotica, Loose areolar tissue, and Periosteum (pericranium). Dense connective tissue within the subcutaneous tissue accounts for the firm attachment of the first three layers, allowing them to move together in wrinkling the scalp. Blood vessels are held securely by the dense subcutaneous connective tissue and are prevented from retracting when severed. For this reason, scalp laceration can cause major hemorrhage, especially in children. This problem occurs with superficial lacerations into the subcutaneous tissue as well as with deep lacerations through the galea. The galea is attached anteriorly to the frontalis muscle and posteriorly to the occipitalis muscle. When the galea is lacerated, these muscles pull the galea in opposite directions. Consequently, the wound is held open, which causes prolonged bleeding from scalp wounds. The irregular surface of the base of the skull can cause damage to the brain if the brain moves inside the cranium during acceleration or deceleration. The dura mater is a thick, dense fibrous layer that encloses the brain and spinal cord. It forms the dural venous sinuses, diaphragm sellae, falx cerebri, falx cerebelli, and tentorium cerebelli. Cerebral venous blood flows into the dural sinuses through bridging veins, such as the superior cerebral veins that terminate in the superior sagittal sinus. These bridging veins can be torn and are, along with cerebral lacerations, a cause of subdural hemorrhage. The meningeal artery lies between the skull and the dura. Nondisplaced linear fractures in the temporoparietal region that cross the middle meningeal artery can lacerate this artery and cause an epidural hematoma. Beneath the dura is the arachnoid, and cerebrospinal fluid circulates in the subarachnoid space. The vascular pia mater is the final covering of the brain. Injuries to the blood vessels of the pia as well as the underlying brain can cause subarachnoid hemorrhage.

The brain and spinal cord are housed within a rigid bony case, the skull and vertebral column. Changes of pressure within this bony case are transmitted to its contents and affect blood flow into the case. The skull and vertebral column can be compared with a funnel with a long tube attached. The cerebrum is in the mouth of the funnel, the brainstem is in the neck of the funnel, and the spinal cord is in the tube. The brainstem enters the neck of the funnel through the incisura of the unyielding tentorium cerebelli. Within this opening, the oculomotor nerve exits the midbrain and enters the superior orbital fissure. An increase in supratentorial pressure, from hemorrhage or brain edema, pushes, or herniates, the brain through the neck of funnel. The temporal lobe uncus is easily herniated through the tentorial incisura. This herniation compresses the oculomotor nerve and causes the ipsilateral pupil to become fixed and dilated. As herniation progresses, the corticospinal (pyramidal) tract in the cerebral peduncle can be compressed on either side, but the side ipsilateral to the injury is usually jeopardized, causing contralateral spastic weakness and a positive Babinski sign. Further compression can cause dysfunction of the cardiorespiratory centers that reside in the medulla. The hypotension and bradycardia that follow usually signal impending death. The reticular activating system is essential for the alert state of wakefulness, and is located in the midbrain and upper pons. Altered consciousness can result from decreased cerebral perfusion, increased intracranial pressure, injury to the cerebral cortex, or injury to the reticular activating system.

Cerebral blood flow (CBF) is affected by many factors, including cerebral vascular resistance (CVR) and intracranial pressure (ICP). CBF is **cerebral perfusion pressure** (CPP) divided by CVR:

$$CBF = CPP/CVR$$

Under normal circumstances, CBF is constant over a wide range of CPP (approximately 50 to 150 mm Hg), and is autoregulated by CVR. After a brain injury, autoregulation is usually disrupted; in such cases, a clinically acceptable CPP is approximately 70 mm Hg in adults. CPP is the difference between mean arterial pressure (MAP) and ICP:

$$CPP = MAP - ICP$$

Normal ICP is usually less than 10 mm Hg. Generally, an ICP of greater than 20 mm Hg requires treatment to prevent herniation or cerebral ischemia. When ICP rises, the body attempts to maintain CPP by increasing the systemic blood pressure. This early response to increased ICP is known as the **Cushing reflex.** In addition to hypertension, this reflex is associated with bradycardia and a decreased respiratory rate. Brain death occurs as ICP approaches MAP and CPP decreases to less than 50 mm Hg.

Carbon dioxide is a potent cerebral vasodilator that decreases CVR and increases CBF. Conversely, low CO_2 levels increase CVR and decrease CBF. The effect of CO_2 on CBF is linear in the $PaCO_2$ range of 20 to 80 mm Hg. These changes in CBF are mediated primarily by changes in interstitial cerebral pH associated with rapid diffusion of CO_2 across the blood-brain barrier. Changes in CBF produced by changes in $PaCO_2$ are relatively short-lived because of the brain's ability to restore the interstitial pH toward normal. In patients with head injury, hyperventilation can transiently decrease ICP, but it carries the risk of cerebral ischemia. Thus, the role of hyperventilation in head injury is largely as a bridge to definitive therapy (e.g., surgical evacuation of subdural hematoma). CBF is also influenced by sympathetic tone.

Neurologic Evaluation

Important information that is obtained from an AMPLE history includes the patient's neurologic status at the scene. Was the patient initially alert, with a later loss of consciousness? Was the patient moving all four extremities? Did the patient have any seizures? In the primary survey, the state of consciousness is assessed with the AVPU mnemonic. In the secondary survey, a complete neurologic examination is performed that focuses on the level of consciousness, pupillary function, sensation, and the presence of lateralizing extremity weakness. The neurologic evaluation is repeated periodically to detect deterioration. Hypotension in a patient with a head injury indicates blood loss until proven otherwise. Hypertension, bradycardia, and a slow respiratory rate signify increased ICP. Hypertension, either alone or with hyperthermia, can indicate central autonomic dysfunction. Abnormal respiration (e.g., periods of apnea separated by equal periods of hyperventilation [Cheyne-Stokes respiration] and periods of rapid, deep breathing [central neurogenic hyperventilation]) may be associated with herniation.

The Glasgow Coma Scale (GCS) is a widely accepted and reproducible method that is used to quantitatively assess the patient's level of consciousness. This rapidly performed assessment assigns scores for eye opening (E), verbal response (V), and best motor response (M). The sum total of the E, V, and M scores is the GCS score (Table 10-7). A neurologically normal person has a GCS score of 15; a comatose person has a score of less than 9; and a dead person has a score of 3. It is important to memorize the GCS so that the evaluation can be performed quickly. The GCS score is a prognostic indicator that is closely correlated with outcome, especially in the early stages of coma. It is a useful indicator of the severity of head injury. A score of 3 to 4 is associated with a probability of mortality or a vegetative state of approximately 97%. A score of 5 to 6 corresponds with a probability of death of approximately 65%, and a score of 7 or 8 has a mortality rate of approximately 28%. It is important to note that multiple factors may contribute to an altered level of consciousness. Traumatic brain injury, shock, alcohol consumption, and recreational drug use all depress consciousness and may result in a low GCS score. A common pitfall is the assumption that combativeness or somnolence in a trauma patient is due to alcohol or drug use. Although this may be the case, it is more prudent to assume that a multiple trauma victim has a head injury or inadequate perfusion. Once those etiologies are ruled out as a source of altered mental status,

Table 10-7 Glasgow Coma Scale (GCS)[a]

Test	Response	Points
Eye opening (E score range 1–4)	Spontaneous	4
	To verbal command	3
	To painful stimuli	2
	No response	1
Best verbal response (V score range 1–5)	Oriented conversation to person, place, and time	5
	Disoriented, confused conversation	4
	Inappropriate words without sustained conversation	3
	Incomprehensible sounds, moans, and groans	2
	No response	1
	Intubated	1T
Best motor response (M score range 1–6)	Follows verbal commands (moves extremity as directed)	6
	Localizes pain (reaches for the painful site)	5
	Withdraws from pain (moves away from painful stimulus)	4
	Abnormal flexor posturing to pain (exhibits decorticate posturing)	3
	Abnormal extensor posturing to pain (exhibits decerebrate posturing)	2
	No response	1
GCS score range	Extubated	3–15
	Intubated	3–11T

[a] GCS score = E score + V score + M score. Head injury severity = severe GCS < 9, moderate GCS 9–12, minor GCS > 12.

further evaluation of an alcohol- or drug-related coma is warranted.

The patient's pupils are assessed for equality, size, and briskness of response to light. Differences of greater than 1 mm are abnormal. Extremity weakness is identified by observing spontaneous movements and response to painful stimuli. Neurologic deterioration is recognized on repeat examination by a decrease in the GCS score of two points or more, increased severity of headache, change in pupillary response, or the development of unilateral weakness.

In the secondary survey, the patient's scalp is inspected for lacerations and the skull is palpated. Wearing sterile gloves, the examiner palpates for step-offs that indicate depressed skull fractures. Bleeding is controlled first with direct pressure. Periorbital ecchymoses (raccoon eyes), perimastoid ecchymoses (Battle's sign), hemotympanum, and leakage of cerebrospinal fluid (CSF) from the nose or ear are signs of a basilar skull fracture. In basilar skull fractures, blood from the fracture site tracks along the base of the skull, becoming visible as ecchymoses. Cribriform plate fractures are associated with raccoon eyes; their presence alerts the astute physician to the dangers of inserting an NG tube into the cranium. CSF otorrhea and rhinorrhea are difficult to detect when there is bleeding. Placing a drop of the bloody fluid on filter paper and looking for the **ring sign,** or **target sign,** helps to make the diagnosis. Standard laboratory filter paper works best, but if it is not readily available, then a paper towel or bedsheet may be used. CSF diffuses more quickly than blood, and as a result, the blood remains in the center, and one or more concentric rings of clearer (pink) fluid forms around the central red spot.

Noncontrast brain CT is enormously useful and should be obtained in any patient who is suspected of having a head injury. The CT scan can show intracranial hematomas, areas of swelling in the brain, midline shift, and skull fractures. Plain radiography of the skull adds little to the evaluation in view of the information provided by CT scan and is usually not necessary. Although recognizing a skull fracture is important, diagnosing the underlying brain injury is more important. Brain injuries can occur with or without skull fractures, and vice versa. Occult cervical spine injuries are found in as many as 15% of patients with head injury. For this reason, cervical spine radiographs should be obtained for all patients with head injuries. Table 10-8 summarizes the clinical findings associated with common types of brain injuries.

Management of Head Injuries

The management of head injury begins with the ABCDE algorithm of the primary survey. The rates of morbidity and mortality for head trauma are profoundly affected by resuscitation. In a recent large multicenter study of head-injured patients, the presence of hypoxia, hypotension, or both at the time of arrival at the emergency room was associated with a mortality rate of, respectively, 33.3%, 60.2%, and 75%. Therefore, it is imperative for the trauma surgeon to establish respiratory and hemodynamic stability rapidly in patients with head injuries.

Patients with significant nonoperative head injuries are admitted to the intensive care unit and usually require tracheal intubation, mechanical ventilation, and ICP monitoring. There are several methods of ICP monitoring. The ventricular catheter method consists of placing a catheter into the lateral ventricle of the brain through a hole drilled into the skull. The catheter is connected to a transducer that allows continuous ICP monitoring as well as withdrawal of CSF as indicated to reduce ICP. Many neurosurgeons consider the ventricular catheter the "gold standard" of ICP monitoring. A second method is placement of a subarachnoid bolt. With this technique, a bolt is screwed into a hole drilled into the skull and positioned in the subarachnoid space. The bolt is connected to a transducer for ICP monitoring. This method is used when there is no need for ventricular drainage or when the ventricles cannot be cannulated. A third technique involves placement of a fiberoptic transducer into the epidural space, subdural space, or lateral ventricle. The appropriate method for a specific patient should be left to the judgment and experience of the neurosurgeon.

Table 10-8 Types of Brain Injury

Injury	Clinical Findings
Diffuse brain injuries	
Concussion	A diffuse brain injury associated with brief loss of neurologic function with little or no apparent cerebral tissue damage. This injury is exceedingly common. Unconsciousness is usually short (minutes) and usually disappears before the patient gets to the hospital. There is usually some degree of posttraumatic amnesia. It represents approximately 59% of head injuries.
Diffuse axonal injury (DAI)	Brain injury caused by rotational or deceleration forces, resulting in tissue injury greatest at the gray-white matter junction. Coma may be present for weeks. As many as 90% of patients may remain in a persistent vegetative state. CT scan shows no mass lesion. Treatment is mainly nonsurgical, with control of intracranial pressure. It represents approximately 44% of severe (GCS < 9) head injuries.
Focal brain injuries	
Contusion	A focal injury that is directly related to the site of impact (coup contusion) or an area remotely related to the point of impact (contrecoup contusion). The tips of the frontal and temporal lobes are frequently involved. Focal deficits, confusion, obtundation, and coma can be seen. It represents approximately 15% of head injuries.
Acute hemorrhage	
Epidural hemorrhage	Usually results from a tear in the middle meningeal artery. Classical signs are loss of consciousness (concussion) followed by a lucid interval, then depressed consciousness and contralateral hemiparesis. The prognosis is usually excellent with prompt treatment because there is minimal underlying brain injury. Treatment is evacuation of the hematoma. It represents 0.5% of head injuries.
Subdural hemorrhage	Caused by ruptured bridging veins, tears in cortical arteries, or cerebral laceration. Clinical problems are caused by severe underlying brain injury as well as mass effect. It accounts for approximately 30% of head injuries.
Subarachnoid hemorrhage	The most common intracranial hemorrhage. It is caused by injury to vessels in the pia that bleed into the cerebrospinal fluid, producing meningeal irritation (headache, stiff neck). It has little surgical significance by itself because the blood distributes throughout the subarachnoid space and no mass effect is produced.
Intracerebral hemorrhage	Severe brain injury. It is commonly associated with DAI, cerebral lacerations, and gunshot wounds.

CT, computed tomography; GCS, Glasgow Coma Scale.

Care of the patient with head trauma focuses on supporting CPP and preventing elevation of ICP. Reverse Trendelenburg position, or elevation of the head of the patient's bed to 30° in the neutral position, facilitates venous drainage and helps to decrease ICP. Other methods that lower ICP include sedation, moderate hyperventilation, prudent fluid administration, and diuretics. Sedation with narcotics or chemical paralysis with appropriate nondepolarizing neuromuscular-blocking agents (e.g., vecuronium) reduces posturing and combative behavior, both of which increase ICP. Moderate hyperventilation to a $PaCO_2$ of 30 to 35 mm Hg lowers ICP in most cases without causing cerebral ischemia. Intravenous fluids are administered judiciously to ensure filling pressures that preserve adequate cardiac output. This goal can be accomplished by monitoring CVP, pulmonary capillary wedge pressure, and urine output. Mannitol is a free-radical scavenger and osmotic diuretic that effectively reduces brain swelling and lowers ICP. Caution must be used when administering mannitol to patients with multiple injuries, because the diuretic effect of the drug may cause hypotension in patients with occult hemorrhage. Sometimes loop diuretics are given in an attempt to reduce brain edema, but they must be used with caution. Hypovolemia is best avoided in patients with multiple injuries, who may already have volume deficits, because hypotension increases both secondary brain injury and mortality. Patients with head injuries should be closely observed for seizures and treated appropriately when they occur. Diazepam is a common first-line therapy; when it is unsuccessful, longer-acting phenytoin may be used. Early enteral nutrition is an important adjunct once the initial resuscitation of a brain-injured patient has concluded and should be commenced within the first 24 to 48 hours of injury.

OTHER INJURIES

Penetrating Neck Injuries

Penetrating injuries to the neck are associated with injuries to the trachea, esophagus, great vessels, and spinal cord.

Spinal cord injuries are discussed in the next section. To evaluate penetrating neck injuries, the anterior neck is divided into three zones, illustrated in Figure 10-13. Zone I is the base of the neck. It extends from the sternal notch to the inferior border of the cricoid cartilage. Injuries in this area carry a high mortality rate because of major vascular and tracheal injuries. Zone II is the central portion of the neck. It extends from the inferior border of the cricoid cartilage to the angle of the mandible. Injuries in zone II carry a lower mortality rate because they are relatively easy to diagnose and treat. Zone III is the distal portion of the neck. It extends from the angle of the mandible to the base of the skull. Operative exposure in this region can be difficult. Any injury that involves violation of the platysma muscle carries risk of underlying severe injury and requires further evaluation.

Unstable patients with vascular or aerodigestive injuries in any zone of the neck require urgent surgical exploration and treatment. Stable patients with penetrating injuries in zone II may be managed by selective or mandatory surgical exploration. Routine surgical exploration of zone II injuries is not technically difficult due to easy proximal and distal exposure of the carotid and jugular vessels. An alternative to routine surgical exploration of zone II involves diagnostic evaluation with angiography, esophagography, and endoscopy. More recently, CT angiography has been used with good results, and duplex ultrasonography has been shown to be accurate for diagnosing carotid injuries in zone II. Stable patients with injuries in zones I and III usually require further evaluation. Diagnostic evaluation of zone I penetrating injuries is advisable because proximal vascular control of vessels in this area frequently requires surgical entry into the chest via sternotomy or thoracotomy. Zone III penetrating injuries need further study because gaining control of the distal internal carotid at the base of the skull can be extremely challenging. Preoperative diagnostic studies include arteriography, esophagography, and endoscopy. Endoscopic evaluation often involves laryngoscopy, bronchoscopy, and esophagoscopy.

Spine and Spinal Cord Injury

Any patient who has significant multiple injuries should be assumed to have a potential spine injury. In these patients, the entire spine is immobilized with a rigid cervical collar and a long spine board. Spinal injury precautions continue until the spine is radiographically and clinically evaluated and fractures, dislocations, and ligamentous injuries are excluded. Patients with injury above the clavicles should be considered to have a cervical spine injury until proven otherwise. As many as 10% of patients who are unconscious on presentation have an associated cervical spine injury.

Physical examination begins with assessment of the vital signs. Hypotension associated with bradycardia suggests

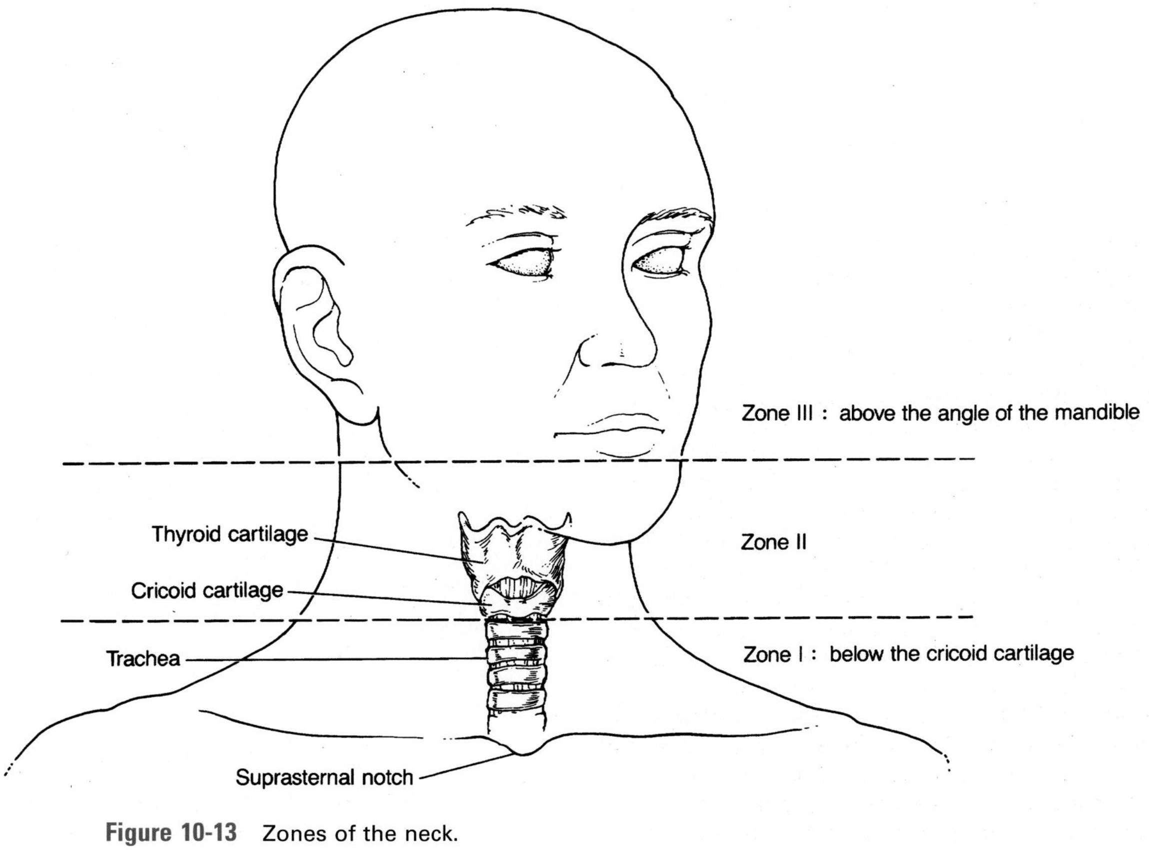

Figure 10-13 Zones of the neck.

neurogenic shock, especially in high thoracic and cervical cord injuries (usually above the T-5 level). Other findings that suggest cervical spine injury include flaccid areflexia; diaphragmatic breathing; the ability to flex, but not extend the elbow (in which case the injury involves the C-7 nerve root, which supplies the triceps); grimaces to pain above, but not below, the clavicles; and priapism. Spinal injury is commonly associated with local pain and tenderness. Patients with these symptoms require careful evaluation. Less frequently, an anatomic deformity or step-off is palpated. Examination requires the patient to be carefully log-rolled: while in-line vertebral immobilization is maintained, the back is inspected and the spine is palpated from the base of the skull to the tip of the coccyx. The unconscious patient should be considered to have an occult spine injury until proven otherwise. A patient who is mentally alert, sober, and normal neurologically; has no neck pain; and can actively move his or her neck through a complete range of motion usually does not have a clinically significant cervical spine injury.

Motor and sensory function is assessed, and based on this assessment, the diagnosis of complete or incomplete cord lesion is made. In a complete spinal cord transection, there is no motor or sensory function below the injury. This situation has a dismal prognosis, with minimal recovery, if any. Patients with incomplete cord injury have some sensory or motor function and are more likely to have significant recovery. The corticospinal tract is located in the posterolateral portion of the cord and is involved in motor function on the same side of the body. Pain and temperature are transmitted by the lateral spinothalamic tract, which is located in the anterolateral portion of the cord. Proprioception, deep touch, two-point discrimination, and vibration are carried in the posterior columns. Light touch is often preserved in incomplete cord injuries because it is conveyed by both the lateral spinothalamic tract and the posterior columns. Sparing of the sacral dermatomes is also seen in incomplete spinal lesions. Preservation of rectal tone and the bulbocavernosus reflex are signs of sacral sparing.

Spinal shock is a neurologic condition that occurs after spinal cord injury. It is caused by acute loss of stimulation from higher levels. This shock, or stun, to the injured cord makes the cord appear functionless. There is complete flaccidity and areflexia instead of the predicted spasticity, hyperreflexia, and positive Babinski sign that are seen in the classic upper motor neuron lesion. Spinal shock may last days to weeks after injury. As it abates, motor tone becomes spastic, reflexes are accentuated, and the Babinski sign becomes positive. Spinal shock is not synonymous with neurogenic shock.

Radiologic assessment of vertebral injury usually begins during resuscitation. In most cases, lateral cervical spine, AP chest, and AP pelvis radiographs are taken first. An acceptable lateral cervical spine radiograph is required to show the base of the skull, seven cervical vertebrae, and the superior aspect of the first thoracic vertebra (T-1). If the top of T-1 is not visualized, then a "swimmer's view" is taken (i.e., radiograph through the axilla of the lower cervical and upper thoracic spine). During the secondary survey, other spine radiographs, including an open-mouth odontoid view, an AP cervical view, and thoracolumbar AP and lateral radiographs, are obtained as indicated by the patient's condition. More recently, CT scanning of the cervical spine has gained popularity as a replacement for plain radiography, especially in head-injured patients.

Initial management focuses on the ABCDE algorithm and on spine immobilization. Hypotension is initially managed with intravenous fluids (described earlier). In clinical trials, patients who received high-dose methylprednisolone sodium succinate within 8 hours of spinal cord injury had improved neurologic recovery. Based on this evidence, many neurosurgeons treat blunt spinal cord injuries with 30 mg/kg methylprednisolone, followed by an infusion of 5.4 mg/kg/hr for 23 hours. For this therapy to be effective, it must be started within the first 8 hours after injury. Definitive care involves spinal stabilization followed by rehabilitation, which is an important part of long-term management.

Pediatric Trauma

Trauma is the leading cause of death in children over 1 year of age. Although the resuscitation priorities (ABCDE algorithm) are the same for children as for adults, anatomic differences require modifications to the approach. Because of their greater surface area to body mass ratio, children lose heat more quickly. For this reason, particular care must be taken to keep an injured child warm. Airway management also differs because the child's larynx is more cranial and anterior, and the trachea is shorter. Orotracheal intubation is the preferred route. Nasotracheal intubation is contraindicated because of anatomic factors that increase the risk of injury to the nasopharynx as well as the risk of penetration into the calvarium. Uncuffed endotracheal tubes are used in young children because, in a child, the cricoid is the narrowest part of the airway, and it forms a natural seal around the tube. Tube size can be estimated by the diameter of the child's fifth finger or external nares. In a child, as in an adult, the first response to hypovolemia is tachycardia. However, because tachycardia can also be caused by fear or pain, it is important to monitor other signs of organ perfusion (e.g., urine output). Children have an enormous physiologic reserve and usually do not become hypotensive until they lose more than 45% of their blood volume. At this point, tachycardia can quickly convert to bradycardia, and unless the child is resuscitated rapidly, circulatory arrest occurs. Normal systolic blood pressure for a child is approximately 80 mm Hg plus twice the child's age in years, and diastolic pressure is two-thirds (67%) of the systolic blood pressure. Therefore, a 10-year-old child's systolic blood pressure should be $80 + 2\,(10) = 100$ mm Hg, and the diastolic blood pressure should be $100\,(0.67) = 67$ mm Hg.

Management priorities are the same for children as for adults. Volume resuscitation begins with the placement of two peripheral intravenous lines. If percutaneous access fails after at least two attempts in a child who is younger than 6 years of age, an intraosseous infusion needle can be inserted into the tibia for bone marrow infusion of crystalloid solution. In children who are 6 years of age or older, a venous cutdown may be necessary if percutaneous access is not possible. Common femoral lines should be avoided in infants and children because of the high incidence of venous thrombosis and limb ischemia from iatrogenic arterial injury. Warm, lactated Ringer's solution is used for resuscitation, beginning with an initial bolus of 20 mL/kg. If there is no improvement, a second bolus is given. If, after two boluses, the child shows minimal or no improvement, a third bolus is given. If the patient remains hemodynamically unstable, a transfusion of 10 mL/kg of packed red blood cells is promptly instituted. It is important to remember that a child's blood volume is approximately 8% of body weight, or 80 mL/kg.

Because a child's skeleton is softer and more pliable than an adult's, a child's bones can take a great deal of force without breaking. Therefore, in a child, a broken bone is evidence of injury from significant force. However, the absence of broken bones does not exclude serious injury. Diagnostic workup is largely the same as in adults; however, abdominal evaluation is generally limited to ultrasound and CT scanning. DPL is generally not used in children because hemoperitoneum infrequently requires surgical intervention in the pediatric population. Child abuse should be suspected when a child has repeated episodes of injury, when there is a delay in seeking medical attention, when parental response is inappropriate, or when there are discrepancies between the history and the degree of injury. Certain types of injuries suggest abuse: multiple old scars or fractures, scars that resemble cigarette or rope burns, long bone fractures in children younger than 3 years of age, genital or perineal injuries, perioral trauma, internal injuries without a history of trauma, multiple subdural hematomas, and retinal hemorrhage. Health care personnel are required by law to report suspected child abuse to local authorities.

Trauma in the Elderly

Trauma is the eighth leading cause of death in persons over 65 years of age. More than half of these deaths are due to falls, motor vehicle collisions, and pedestrians being struck by vehicles. Elderly persons are significantly more likely to experience complications and death after trauma. Lack of physiologic reserve, changes in cardiopulmonary function, osteoporosis, malnutrition, and altered immune function may exist in elderly individuals and may result in significant morbidity after relatively minor trauma. Medications commonly taken by elderly patients may mask physical findings (e.g., prevention of tachycardia by chronic usage of a β-adrenergic antagonist) or lead to complications (e.g., intracranial hemorrhage in a traumatized patient taking warfarin or aspirin).

Resuscitation priorities are similar in the elderly as compared with younger persons. Certain caveats exist, however. Obtaining a careful history is of critical importance, since an underlying medical problem may have precipitated the trauma (e.g., a driver's myocardial infarction results in an automobile crash). Because hypertension is quite prevalent in the elderly, relative hypotension from hypovolemia may go unnoticed if the treating physician is not astute. Fluid resuscitation must be done in a judicious manner, since volume overload and heart failure may ensue after overenthusiastic intravenous fluid boluses. Urinary output may poorly reflect intravascular volume status in patients with renal disease or in those who take diuretics. Frequently, invasive hemodynamic monitoring in an intensive care unit setting is required for adequate resuscitation of elderly patients with preexisting cardiac disease.

Specific types of injury are common in elderly patients. Head injuries are a major cause of mortality in geriatric trauma patients. An admission GCS of less than or equal to 8 is associated with a mortality rate of 80% in patients over 65 years of age. Underlying medical illnesses frequently worsen secondary brain injury after trauma, and functional outcomes tend to be poor. Chest injuries are associated with increased morbidity as well. A brittle rib cage and decreased vital capacity make rib fractures quite serious in elderly patients. Multiple rib fractures are commonly associated with respiratory failure, pneumonia, and prolonged hospitalization. Abdominal injuries have a fourfold higher mortality rate in elderly patients. A high level of suspicion for abdominal injury is warranted, and diagnostic imaging modalities such as FAST and CT should be used for a thorough evaluation. Hip fractures after falls are extremely common, and may present with subtle signs or with gross deformity. Hip fractures in the elderly are associated with a 13% to 30% 1-year mortality rate.

Trauma in Women

Domestic violence is the leading cause of death in women 15 to 44 years old. Trauma is now the leading cause of death in pregnant women. The most important principle in managing the pregnant trauma victim is that resuscitating the mother will resuscitate the fetus. Once obvious shock develops in the mother, the chances of saving the fetus are approximately 20%. The uterine vascular bed is a passive, low-resistance system, without autoregulation. Thus, uterine blood flow is dependent on uterine perfusion pressure. Significant maternal hemorrhage causes uterine artery vasoconstriction, which reduces uterine blood flow. Uterine perfusion can decrease by as much as 20% before changes in the mother's vital signs are seen. If low uterine perfusion is uncorrected, the fetus becomes hypoxic and ultimately bradycardic. Maternal hypotension is best managed with vigorous resuscitation with lactated Ringer's solution. The use of vasopressors to support blood pressure is contraindicated because these drugs further decrease uterine perfusion and increase fetal distress.

Several important physiologic changes occur during pregnancy. Plasma volume expands by 40% to 50% and is proportionately greater than the expanded red blood cell mass. This expansion causes a decrease in hematocrit and accounts for the physiologic anemia that is seen in pregnancy. Systolic and diastolic blood pressure decrease by 5 to 15 mm Hg because of decreased systemic vascular resistance (SVR). Auscultation of the heart may show grade I to II systolic flow murmurs and S3 heart sounds. ECG may show left axis deviation. Cardiac output is increased by 1 to 1.5 L/min. Compression of the vena cava by the gravid uterus can significantly decrease cardiac output by 30% to 40%, especially in the last trimester. Therefore, all visibly pregnant trauma victims should be placed in the left lateral tilt position, while maintaining spinal precautions. Initially, this may be accomplished by placing a wedge or pillow under the left side of the patient's backboard. Once spine injury has been ruled out, the patient may be moved to the left lateral decubitus position.

The respiratory system is affected by the size of the uterus. Upward displacement of the diaphragm causes a decrease in residual volume and increases the patient's susceptibility to atelectasis. Progesterone stimulates hyperventilation, with an increase in minute ventilation and tidal volume. Hypocapnia is common with $Pa{CO_2}$ of approximately 30 mm Hg. Impaired function of the lower esophageal sphincter, delayed gastric emptying, and decreased intestinal motility predispose these patients to aspiration. Early NG tube placement is therefore indicated. The white blood cell count is commonly 10,000 to 12,000 cells/mm^3 and may increase to 20,000 cells/mm^3 in late pregnancy.

Management priorities remain largely unchanged in pregnancy. The major difference is that two or more lives are at risk. Because of their physiologically expanded blood volume, pregnant women can lose 30% to 35% of their blood volume before becoming hypotensive. In addition, some effort should be made to limit unnecessary exposure to radiography and anesthesia to minimize the teratogenic risk to the fetus. Evaluation of the pregnant trauma patient includes an obstetric history and physical examination. Important information includes the date of the last menses, the expected due date, the number and outcome of past pregnancies, and the most recent fetal movement. Abruptio placentae is associated with uterine tenderness and contraction, with or without vaginal bleeding. Ruptured chorioamniotic membranes are associated with excess vaginal fluid with a pH of 7 to 7.5. Uterine rupture may occur with blunt abdominal trauma and is suspected when fetal extremities are palpable on abdominal examination.

Fetal evaluation consists of assessing the uterus and fundal height and documenting fetal heart tones, heart rate, and movement. The normal fetal heart rate is 120 to 160 beats/min. A heart rate of less than 100 beats/min indicates bradycardia. A Doppler ultrasonic cardioscope is the best method of monitoring fetal heart rate and rhythm. Early decelerations of heart rate associated with uterine contractions are not considered significant; however, late decelerations that occur after uterine contractions imply fetal hypoxia. Continuous fetal monitoring is usually indicated in pregnant trauma victims who are past 24 weeks gestation. In Rh-negative women, the Kleihauer-Betke test can detect fetomaternal hemorrhage, and the administration of Rh immunoglobulin can prevent Rh alloimmunization of the mother and subsequent erythroblastosis fetalis.

Medically indicated radiographic studies should not be avoided simply to spare the fetus possible exposure to ionizing radiation. The greatest period of risk for radiation-induced anomalies is during the first 16 weeks of gestational life. This risk also appears to be directly proportional to the amount of exposure. In general, a fetal dose of less than 10 rad is believed to be reasonably safe. Low-dose exposure is defined as less than 1 rad, or 1000 mrad. A standard chest radiograph delivers approximately 10 mrad to the chest, and with proper shielding, it delivers negligible amounts of radiation to the fetus (< 1 mrad). An AP view of the abdomen delivers approximately 220 mrad to the skin and 70 mrad to the fetus.

When there is a concern about intraabdominal injury, ultrasound is the initial diagnostic modality of choice, because, in addition to providing information about the presence of intraperitoneal fluid or blood, it can provide information about the fetus, placenta, and uterus. Indications for DPL in a pregnant woman are the same as those in a nonpregnant patient. However, when performed during pregnancy, DPL should be performed using open surgical technique with a supraumbilical incision. Percutaneous DPL should not be performed in pregnancy.

Extremity Trauma

Extremity injuries are usually not immediately life-threatening, except in the case of uncontrolled hemorrhage. Potentially life-threatening injuries are major crush injuries, severe open fractures, proximal amputations, and multiple fractures. Limb-threatening injuries are vascular injuries, **compartment syndromes**, open fractures, crush injuries, and major dislocations. In the primary survey, proper management includes controlling obvious hemorrhage with direct pressure. A tourniquet is applied only as a last resort because it crushes the tissue beneath it and makes the distal extremity ischemic by occluding collaterals. In the secondary survey, the limbs are thoroughly examined and appropriate radiographs are taken. Early care involves alignment and splinting of the extremity, restoration of perfusion, wound care, and tetanus prophylaxis.

The physical examination begins with complete exposure of the extremities. Inspection of the limbs involves noting the color and looking for wounds, deformities, and swelling. Palpation begins with an assessment of temperature, tenderness, crepitation, capillary fill, and quality of the pulses. Every long bone is palpated, and range of motion assessed. Sensory and motor function is tested. An injury to a major blood vessel is likely if there are hard signs of vascular injury (e.g., history of significant blood loss at the scene, brisk arterial bleeding from the wound, expanding hematoma, bruits, thrills, abnormal pulses). A vascular injury is possible if the injury is near a major blood vessel, especially in the case of gunshot and stab wounds. In these cases, the circulation to the extremity is assessed with a continuous-wave Doppler flow probe. Doppler pressures are taken by placing an appropriately sized blood pressure cuff around the extremity distal to the suspected injury. The recorded blood pressure of an artery is based on the location of the blood pressure cuff, not the location of the Doppler. It is useful to compare the pressures in all four extremities. When the Doppler ankle pressure is compared with the Doppler brachial pressure, it is called an ankle–brachial index (ABI). Pressures in the legs are normally higher than in the arms, so the ABI is greater than 1. Normally, pressures are equal between segments in the same extremity. Any deviation from the norm implies a traumatic, flow-restricting lesion until proven otherwise. For example, arterial injuries that cause vessel transection, thrombosis, intimal flap, or vasospasm are flow-restricting lesions. Other injuries that cause a pseudoaneurysm (hole in the arterial wall) or an arteriovenous fistula may not be flow restricting. As a result, pulses and Doppler pressures may be normal.

Vascular injuries can be obvious or occult. Transmural arterial wall injuries rarely heal spontaneously, and if they are not treated appropriately, may cause ischemia or hemorrhage. Because missed arterial injuries can produce serious complications hours to years after injury, early diagnosis and treatment are essential. Diagnostic vascular imaging is often necessary to completely evaluate the structural integrity of the vascular system. These studies are used to augment the physical and Doppler examination, to exclude the presence of an injury, to locate an injury exactly, and to identify anatomic features that may affect operative management. Arteriography is considered the gold standard when extremity arterial injury is suspected. However, other less invasive modalities (e.g., duplex scan, spiral CT angiography, magnetic resonance angiography) are also useful.

The management of blunt and penetrating injuries to the extremities requires a thorough knowledge of vascular anatomy. Supracondylar fractures of the humerus, severely displaced fractures of the knee, and knee dislocations are frequently associated with significant injuries to the brachial and popliteal arteries, respectively. Diagnostic evaluation is usually indicated in these injuries, despite the lack of any clinical signs of vascular injury. Gunshot and stab wounds that are in close proximity to major blood vessels require careful physical examination for subtle signs of vascular injury. Determination of the need for operative exploration, angiography, or duplex ultrasound generally requires the expertise of a surgeon skilled in vascular anatomy and procedures. Additional information regarding extremity vascular injury can be found in Chapter 23, Diseases of the Vascular System.

Traumatic amputations, especially of the proximal limb, are severe open wounds that carry significant risk to life and limb. These amputations can be complete or incomplete. When the amputated part has been crushed and there is severe soft tissue damage, there is frequently little hope for replantation. However, when the ends have been sharply severed, with minimal distal soft tissue injury, there is potential for replantation. The more distal the amputation, the better is the prognosis for replantation. The amputated part should be cleansed of gross dirt, wrapped in a saline-moistened sterile towel, placed in a sterile plastic bag, sealed, and transported in an insulated container filled with crushed ice and water. Keeping the part cold, but not allowing it to freeze, is essential for successful replantation.

Wounds are inspected to determine the extent of tissue injury. All wounds are irrigated with saline and debrided of foreign material and devitalized tissue. Depending on the extent of injury and degree of contamination; wounds may be closed primarily with sutures, left open to be closed later (delayed primary closure), or left open to be closed by secondary intention. Wounds may also be skin grafted, or closed with a cutaneous or myocutaneous flap. Tetanus prophylaxis is essential and is given based on established criteria. The risk of infection is considered, and appropriate antibiotics are given as indicated.

Fractures can cause significant blood loss. For example, a femur fracture can account for the loss of 1500 mL blood into the thigh. The larger the number of fractures, the greater is the associated blood loss and the greater is the risk of hemorrhagic shock. Dislocations should be reduced as soon as possible. The longer the delay in reducing a dislocated hip, the greater is the risk of avascular necrosis of the femoral head. If an open wound is associated with a fracture, then it is assumed that the wound communicates with the fracture. Therefore, this type of fracture is treated as an open fracture. An open fracture is, by definition, contaminated, and it requires immediate treatment to avoid infection. Open fractures are optimally managed by administration of intravenous antibiotics, as well as irrigation, debridement, and reduction in the operating room.

Compartment syndrome is associated with conditions that increase fascial compartmental pressure. This increase, in turn, causes interstitial tissue pressure to become higher than capillary perfusion pressure. The result is ischemia of the muscles and nerves within the fascial compartment. The syndrome usually takes hours to develop, but may develop rapidly (e.g., when there is an arterial bleed into a compartment). It typically occurs in the calf and forearm, but can also occur in the thigh, arm, foot, and hand. Muscular swelling and compartmental bleeding are the usual etiologic factors. Inciting events include arterial injuries, crush injuries, fractures, prolonged compression, and restoration of blood flow to a previously ischemic extremity. An early sign is decreased sensation, caused by neural ischemia, in the distribution of peripheral nerves traveling within the affected compartment. Other signs and symptoms include pain, especially pain that is exacerbated by passive stretch of the involved muscles, a tense swollen compartment, and weakness of the involved muscle. Decreased pulses and capillary filling are not reliable findings because they usually do not occur until late in the evolution of this condition. The diagnosis is usually made clinically; however, compartmental pressures can be measured whenever there is a question about the diagnosis (e.g., a comatose patient unable to provide a reliable exam). Compartmental pressures greater than 35 to 40 mm Hg confirm the diagnosis. Treatment is surgical **fasciotomy.** With decreased compartmental pressures and reestablishment of capillary blood flow, there is a general outpouring of acidic blood, potassium, myoglobin, and other cellular metabolites into the systemic circulation. Adequate renal function is necessary to clear these ischemic byproducts from the circulation. Myoglobin-induced acute renal failure is of great concern whenever there is severe muscle injury. Myoglobin exerts its toxicity in acid urine through direct tubular cell injury and through precipitation, which causes obstruction of the renal tubules. Treatment requires the maintenance of a high urine output (100 mL/hr or 1 mL/kg/hr) by aggressive fluid administration. Osmotic diuresis with mannitol and alkalinization of the urine by administration of sodium bicarbonate are adjunctive measures that may provide some benefit.

TRANSFER OF THE INJURED PATIENT

Outcome is enhanced when patients are cared for at designated regional trauma centers. It is no longer appropriate for trauma patients to be taken to the closest hospital; instead, transportation to the closest trauma center is the standard. In most major metropolitan areas, trauma patients are transported by emergency medical services to designated trauma facilities. However, circumstances arise when severely injured victims arrive at facilities not designed for such patients. For example, patients may be brought by friends or family to the nearest facility, or a rural location may necessitate initial evaluation at a nontrauma hospital. Additionally, prehospital circumstances may arise that necessitate paramedic transport to the closest facility, regardless of trauma designation (e.g., inability to maintain an airway). Therefore, it is essential for the physicians involved in initial management to recognize patients whose needs exceed the capability of the institution and to arrange for early transfer to a regional trauma center. Before transfer is considered, the physician should complete the primary and secondary surveys and initiate resuscitation. If the decision is made to transfer a patient to another hospital, direct physician-to-physician communication is necessary before the transfer occurs. In general, once the primary and secondary surveys are completed and the need for transfer identified, no further diagnostic or therapeutic maneuvers should be undertaken until after the patient arrives at the trauma center. Additional radiographs, CT scans, angiograms, and other maneuvers obtained prior to transfer are rarely in the patient's best interest and frequently serve to use up the "golden hour" when the most effective trauma care can be given. Satisfactory transfers are based on the principle of "do no further harm." In other words, the patient's level of care should never decline from one step to the next.

SUMMARY

Care of the injured patient begins with the primary survey. Identifying and treating all immediately life-threatening injuries is the first priority. Resuscitation is begun simultaneously with the primary survey. The secondary survey follows the rapid initial evaluation and involves a detailed head-to-toe assessment. In the definitive care phase, all injuries are prioritized and treated. The patient's ultimate outcome is directly related to the length of time between injury and definitive care.

SUGGESTED READINGS

American College of Surgeons. *Advanced Trauma Life Support Program for Doctors.* Chicago, IL: American College of Surgeons, 1997.

Bell RM. *ATLS: Advanced Trauma Life Support Compendium of Changes.* Chicago, IL: American College of Surgeons, 1997.

Biffl WL, Moore EE, Rehse DH, et al. Selective management of penetrating neck trauma based on cervical level of injury. *Am J Surg* 1997;174(6):678–682.

Chesnut RM. Management of brain and spine injuries. *Crit Care Clin* 2004;20(1):25–55.

Dolich MO, Varela JE, Compton RP, et al. 2576 ultrasounds for blunt abdominal trauma. *J Trauma* 2001; 50(1):108–112.

Eastridge BJ, Starr A, Minei JP, et al. The importance of fracture pattern in guiding therapeutic decision-making in patients with hemorrhagic shock and pelvic ring disruptions. *J Trauma* 2002;53(3):446–450.

Eddy VA, Morris J, Rozycki G. Trauma and pregnancy. In: Ivatury R, Cayten C, eds. *The Textbook of Penetrating Trauma.* Media, PA: Williams & Wilkins, 1996.

Esterra A, Mattox KL, Wall MJ. Thoracic aortic injury. *Semin Vasc Surg* 2000;13(4):345–352.

Kendall JL, Anglin D, Demetriades D. Penetrating neck trauma. *Emerg Med Clin North Am* 1998;16(1):85–105.

Kraus JF, Sorenson SB. Epidemiology. In: Silver JM, Yudofsky SC, Halea RE, eds. *Neuropsychiatry of Traumatic Brain Injury.* Washington, DC: American Psychiatric Press, 1994:3–41.

LeBlang SD, Dolich MO. Imaging of penetrating thoracic trauma. *J Thorac Imaging* 2000;15(2):128–135.

Mattox KL, Feliciano DV, Moore EE, et al. *Trauma.* 5th Ed. Columbus, OH: McGraw-Hill, 2004.

McGahan JP, Richards J, Gillen M. The focused abdominal sonography for trauma scan. *J Ultrasound Med* 2002;21(7):789–800.

Mirvis SE. Diagnostic imaging of acute thoracic injury. *Semin Ultrasound CT MR* 2004;25(2):156–179.

Narayan RK, Wilberger JE, Povlishock JT. *Neurotrauma.* New York, NY: McGraw-Hill, 1996.

Shatz DV, Kirton OC, McKenney MG, et al. *Manual of Trauma and Emergency Surgery.* Philadelphia, PA. WB Saunders Company, 2000.

Sievers EM, Murray JA, Chen D, et al. Abdominal computed tomography scan in pediatric blunt abdominal trauma. *Am Surg* 1999;65(10): 968–971.

Web-based Injury Statistics Query and Reporting System (WISQARS), National Center for Injury Prevention and Control, 2004. Available at: http://www.cdc.gov/ncipc/wisqars/.

Wilson RF, Walt AJ. *Management of Trauma: Pitfalls and Practice.* Baltimore, MD: Williams & Wilkins, 1996.

11

JEFFREY R. SAFFLE, MD ■ TINA L. PALMIERI, MD

Burns

OBJECTIVES

1. List the classification of burns by depth of injury, and indicate the anatomic and pathophysiologic differences between these injuries.
2. List the initial steps in the acute care of the patient with a burn injury.
3. List three types of inhalation injury, and describe their pathophysiology.
4. List the general indications for referral of a patient to a burn center.
5. Define burn shock, and outline its treatment.
6. List the advantages and disadvantages of fascial and tangential excision of burn wounds.
7. In addition to fluid resuscitation and surgery, list three other general areas of care that are important in the management of patients with burns.

Major burns hold a unique position in the public imagination as the most horrifying of all injuries, a perception that is often correct. To patients, acute burns are the "ultimate agony," and their long-term consequences present enormous psychological, social, and physical challenges to meaningful recovery. To the treatment team, burns are labor-intensive injuries that involve every facet of surgical care. Major burns are often used as paradigms for the most severe physiologic derangements that accompany trauma.

Burns are a major public health problem as well. Approximately 1.25 million Americans require medical care for burns annually. More than 5500 people die each year of burn-related injuries, primarily from house fires, and approximately 51,000 patients are hospitalized. This chapter describes the basic pathophysiology of burns and provides practical guidelines for their treatment.

PATHOPHYSIOLOGY OF BURN INJURY

The skin can be burned by a variety of agents, including direct heat from flames or scalding liquids, contact with hot objects or corrosive chemicals, and electrical current. Burns are classified according to the depth of injury. Figure 11-1 shows these injuries in relation to the structures of the skin. This knowledge provides a basic understanding of both the physiologic effects of burns of various depths and the findings seen on examination.

Epidermal Burns

Epidermal burns ("first-degree burns") involve only the epidermis. Within minutes of injury, dermal capillaries dilate. As a result, these burns are red, moderately painful areas that blanch with direct pressure. Blistering is absent from true epidermal injuries. Epidermal burn injuries have limited physiologic effects, and even extensive burns usually require only supportive care. This care usually consists of pain control (i.e., oral analgesics), adequate oral fluid intake, and application of a soothing topical compound (e.g., Neosporin ointment). Healing occurs within a few days as the injured epidermis peels off, revealing new skin. Because scarring occurs in the dermis, epidermal burns do not form scar tissue. Figure 11-2 shows a patient with primarily epidermal burns and some superficial dermal burns.

Partial-Thickness Burns

Partial-thickness burns ("second-degree burns") extend into, but not through, the dermis. These injuries vary greatly in both appearance and significance, depending

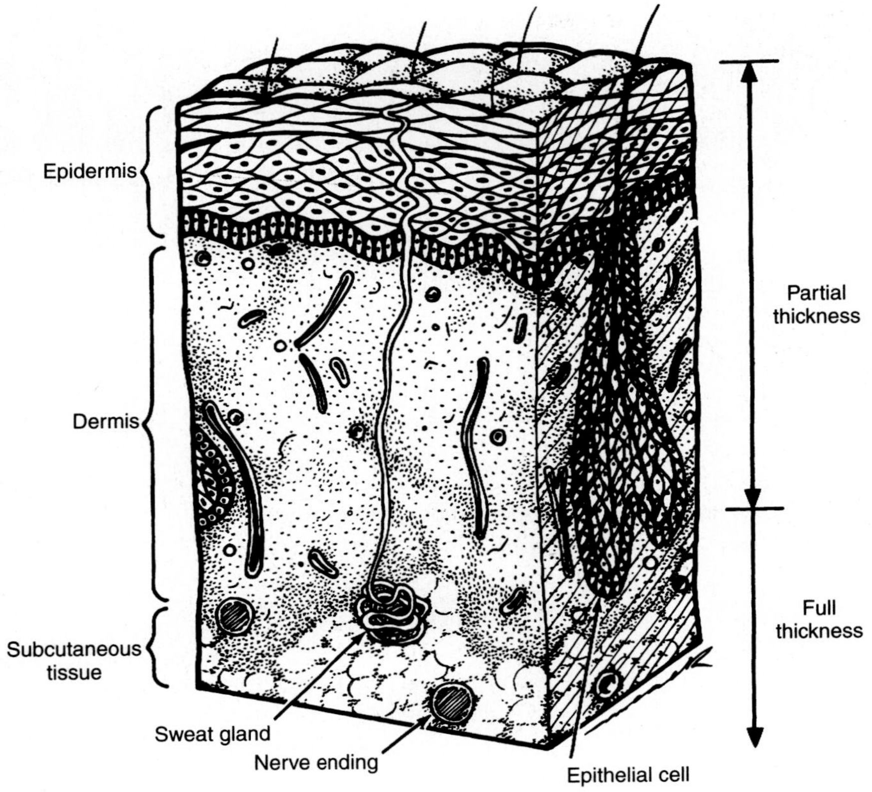

Figure 11-1 Anatomy of the skin, showing major skin structures and their relation to partial- and full-thickness burns. Epithelial cells make up the lining of hair follicles, and these structures penetrate deeply within the dermis. Even very deep partial-thickness burns can heal if these "epidermal appendages" survive. Dermal capillaries and nerve endings also reside in the deep dermis and survive most partial-thickness burns.

on their exact depth. Superficial partial-thickness burns (see Fig. 11-2) typically are reddened areas of skin. These burns form distended blisters, which consist of epidermis filled with proteinaceous fluid that escapes from damaged capillaries. The underlying dermis is moist, blanches on direct pressure, and is usually very painful because the cutaneous nerves, which reside in the deeper dermis, are intact. During the first 24 to 48 hours after the burn occurs, a coating of dead tissue, coagulated serum, and debris develops. This coating is called **eschar.** The appearance of the wound changes dramatically as eschar develops; it changes again as eschar separates during wound healing. In superficial partial-thickness burns, eschar usually separates within 10 to 14 days. As this separation occurs, punctate areas of new epidermal growth, called skin "buds," develop from the epidermal lining of hair follicles and sweat glands (Fig. 11-3).

Deep partial-thickness injuries look very different from more superficial burns. Coagulation necrosis of the upper dermis gives these wounds a dry, leathery texture. Erythema is usually absent, and the wounds may be a variety of colors, most often waxy white. Because epidermal appendages penetrate far into, and sometimes through, the dermis, even a very deep dermal burn can heal if it is followed long enough. These wounds also vary in the amount of pain that they produce; very deep wounds cause destruction of many dermal nerve endings and are less painful than more superficial injuries. Such wounds heal badly, however, because damaged dermis does not regenerate; instead, it is replaced by scar tissue that is often rigid, tender, and friable. For this reason, many deep dermal burns are best treated with excision of the burned tissue and skin grafting. The exact depth of partial-thickness burns is often difficult to judge, particularly after eschar forms. Burns of "indeterminate" depth (those that have some features of both partial- and full-thickness injuries) can be treated conservatively for 10 to 14 days; wounds that remain unhealed should undergo grafting. Figure 11-4 shows this type of burn.

Full-Thickness Burns

Full-thickness burns ("third-degree burns") occur when all layers of the skin are destroyed (Fig. 11-5). These wounds are usually covered with dry, avascular coagulum that is relatively insensate, because nerve endings have been destroyed. The wound surface may be almost any color, from waxy white (chemical burns) to completely black and charred (flame injury). In addition, as dermal proteins are coagulated, they contract, often forming a tight, tourniquet-like constriction that can cause circulatory compromise in the extremities. Very small full-thickness burns can heal by contraction, but larger injuries require skin grafting because even the deepest epidermal appendages are destroyed.

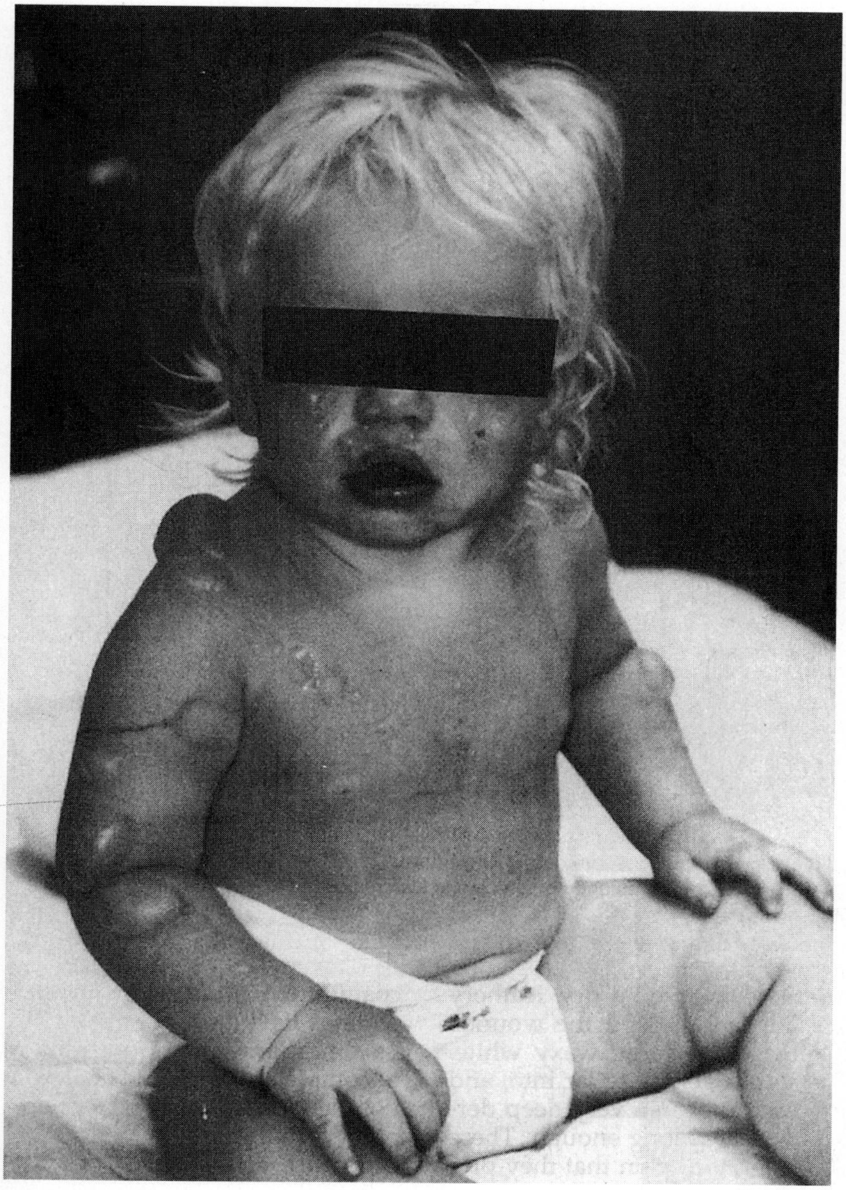

Figure 11-2 Superficial burn wounds. This child had extensive sunburn as a result of playing outdoors unattended. Most of his wounds are reddened, blanch easily, and show no blistering. These are epidermal, or first-degree, burns. Some areas on the right shoulder, right arm, and face show elevated blisters filled with fluid. They are characteristic of a superficial partial-thickness, or second-degree, burn. Although this child required only supportive care, this figure serves as a reminder that sunburns can be deep and serious injuries.

INITIAL CARE OF THE PATIENT WITH BURNS

Patients with burn injuries should be considered victims of multiple trauma, and many of the same treatment priorities and algorithms apply to their care. Familiarity with the principles of Advanced Trauma Life Support (see Chapter 9) is essential. This chapter focuses on the aspects of care that are unique to burn injuries.

Stop the Burning Process

A special problem associated with burn trauma is the tendency for burns to continue to produce tissue damage for minutes to hours after the initial burn occurs. This process can further injure the patient as well as endanger medical personnel. For example, if an oxygen mask is placed on a victim of flame injury, smoldering clothing may reignite. For this reason, it is critically important to stop the burning process before proceeding with any other measures. Flame burns should be extinguished completely by dousing with water, smothering, or rolling patients on the ground. Hot liquids, especially viscous liquids (e.g., tar, plastic), can remain hot enough to burn for some time; they should be cooled immediately with cool water or moist compresses. Once cooled, these compounds can be left in place on the patient if necessary. Caustic chemicals must be diluted immediately and completely with large amounts of water. Victims of electrocution can conduct current to rescue workers. These patients cannot be approached until the source of current is removed.

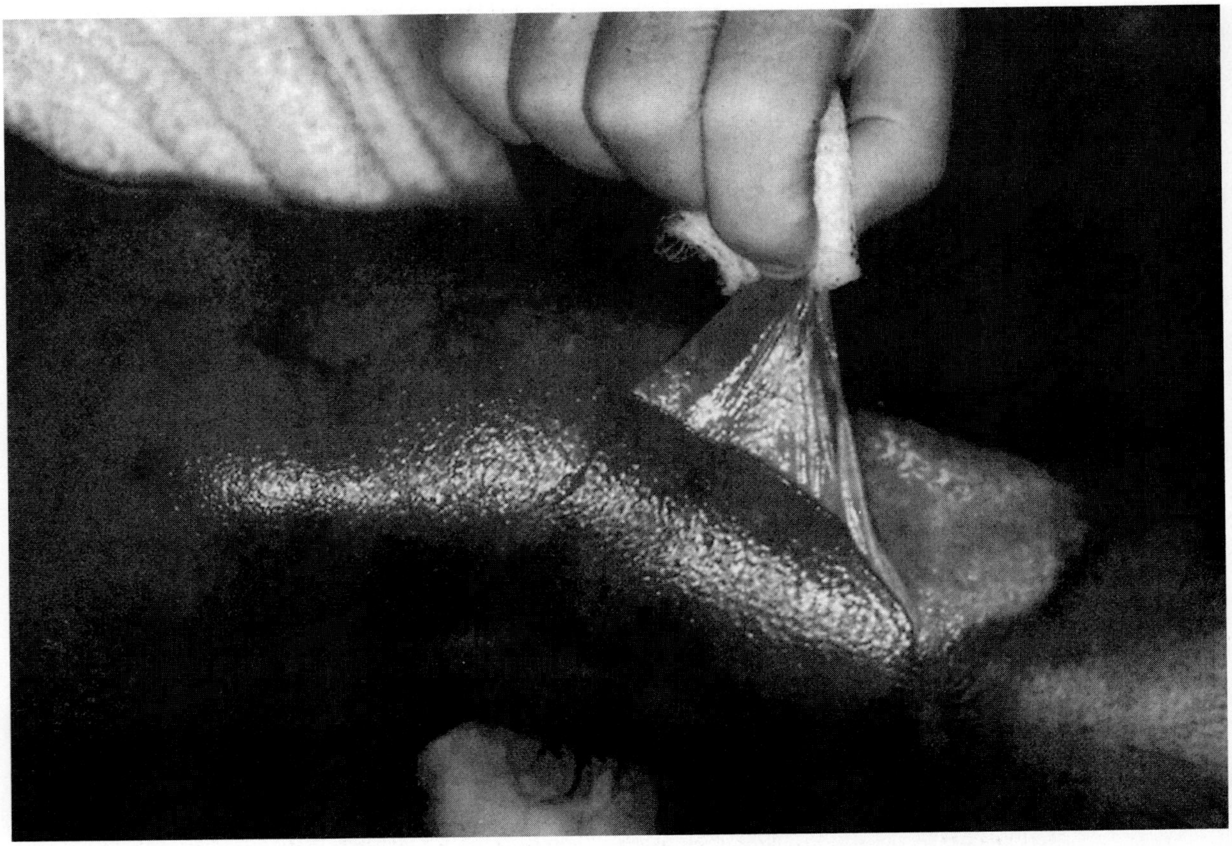

Figure 11-3 Separation of eschar in a superficial partial-thickness burn, approximately 5 days after injury. The yellowish, filmy eschar separates easily with gentle debridement, revealing an irregular surface of epidermal buds. Formation of an overlying eschar complicates the diagnosis of burn depth, but once eschar separates, the depth of injury can be determined accurately. This type of gentle debridement is performed at least twice daily on all open burn wounds.

Primary Survey

The primary survey is a quick examination that is designed to detect and treat immediately life-threatening conditions. It begins with evaluation of the patient's airway, breathing, and circulation (the "ABCs" of resuscitation). When the primary survey is performed on burn victims, special attention is paid to the possibility of smoke **inhalation injury,** which is a major source of both immediate and long-term morbidity and mortality. Inhalation injury should be suspected whenever the patient has been exposed to smoke. Table 11-1 lists the major types of inhalation injury and their treatment. The most common killer of victims of house fires is carbon monoxide, which displaces oxygen from hemoglobin and causes severe tissue hypoxemia. Smoke inhalation also produces airway swelling and obstruction or severe pulmonary edema. Even in the absence of smoke exposure, patients with severe facial burns can have massive swelling that leads to obstruction of the supraglottic airway. Because edema is progressive, signs of airway compromise may be absent for several hours after injury. Patients should be followed and reexamined regularly to detect this complication. Also during the primary survey, the examiner should note evidence of circulatory compromise in the extremities, which can be caused by severe edema and constricting burn wounds. Chapter 22 provides a more detailed review of the signs and symptoms of vascular compromise.

Resuscitation

The initial resuscitation of burn victims is similar to that of other patients. If injuries appear to be major, two large-bore intravenous lines are secured. A Foley catheter is placed to aid in resuscitation, and blood is drawn for laboratory studies. Formal calculation of fluid requirements is not performed, however, until the secondary survey is completed. Fluid resuscitation is an important, ongoing part of the definitive treatment of burn injuries and is discussed in detail later.

Secondary Survey

Often, the presence of a dramatic burn wound distracts the examiner from detecting other, more urgent injuries.

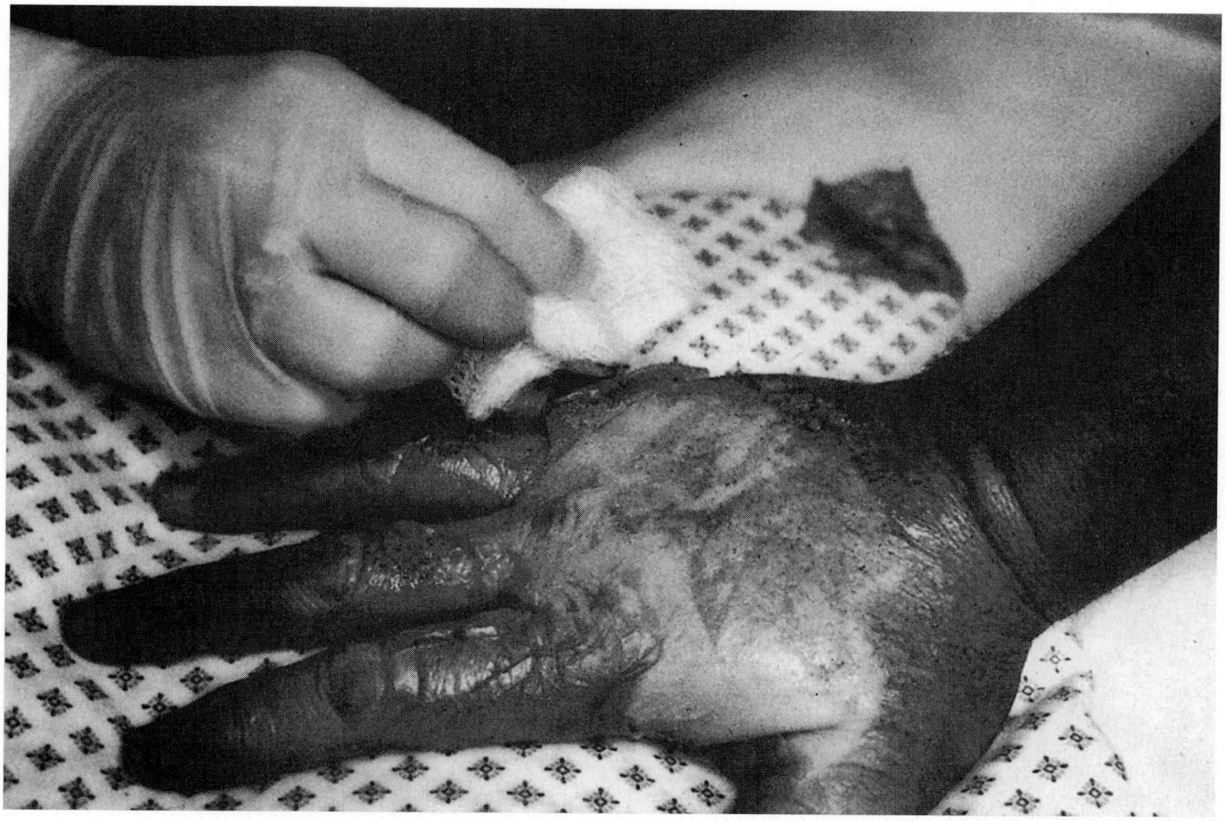

Figure 11-4 Deep partial-thickness burn. This man burned his hand with hot grease while cooking bacon. Loose, blistered skin is seen on the dorsal hand and fingers, but there is very little fluid beneath the blisters because of coagulation of the upper dermis. As the wound is debrided, a dry, pale, relatively insensate dermis is revealed. Although this wound has a deceptively unimpressive appearance, it is actually a far more serious injury than the wound shown in Figure 11-2.

In addition, the swelling, discoloration, and pain that accompany burns can obscure underlying abdominal tenderness, extremity fractures, or cyanosis. For these reasons, it is imperative that a comprehensive, head-to-toe examination of every burn patient be conducted. Only after the secondary survey is completed should burns be debrided by removing blistered skin and washing the burn wound thoroughly. The location, extent, and depth of burn wounds should be documented with a diagram such as the Lund and Browder chart (Fig. 11-6). This chart is used to calculate the total burn size, which is expressed as percentage of total body surface area (% TBSA). Only partial-thickness (second-degree) and full-thickness (third-degree) burn wounds are included in this estimate of burn size. This estimate is used to guide fluid resuscitation, nutrition, and other aspects of care. Wounds should not be dressed with antibiotic creams or ointments, or wrapped with dressings, until secondary assessment is completed and the burn is evaluated.

Burn Center Referral

Over the last 50 years, specialized burn care facilities have been developed to treat patients with serious burns. The American Burn Association and the American College of Surgeons have defined criteria for **burn centers,** similar to those developed for trauma centers. These criteria require that institutions maintain significant, multidisciplinary expertise in all phases of burn treatment. They also must commit space, resources, and personnel to the care of patients with burns. In addition, specific guidelines for the referral of patients to burn centers have been developed (Table 11-2). These guidelines are not absolute, but are widely used as standards for treatment. As a general rule, surgeons who do not work in burn centers should treat only patients with burn injuries that they are experienced in treating. They should consult a burn center with any questions about patient management.

DEFINITIVE CARE OF BURN INJURIES

After the initial assessment, patients with burn injuries require treatment for a number of physiologic consequences of injury. Support for several different problems may be required simultaneously, although the importance and magnitude of these problems may change. To help in or-

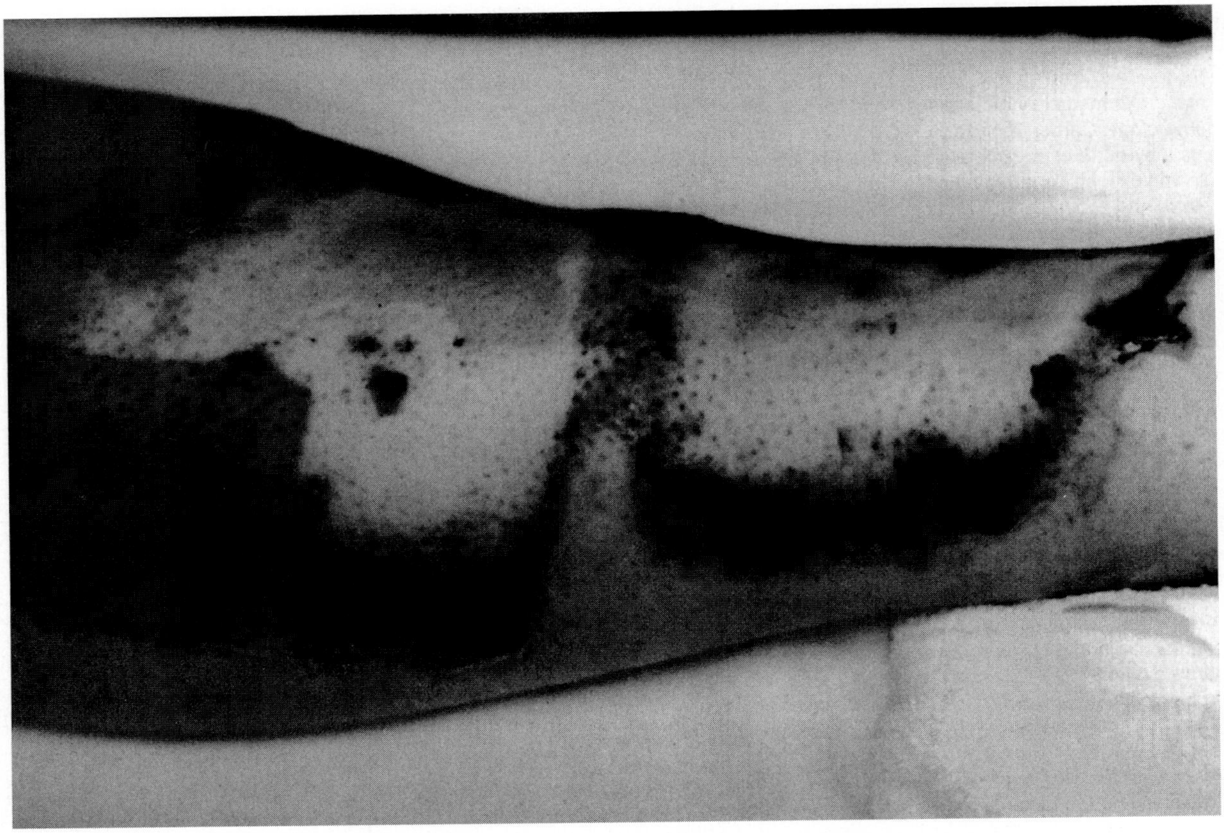

Figure 11-5 Full-thickness burn on the leg of a man whose pants caught fire while he was burning weeds. After debridement, the entire wound is dry, leathery, and painless. The wound is a variety of colors—white, brown, red, and black—because of areas of scorching of the dermis. When viewed tangentially, the contracture produced by coagulation of dermal proteins is seen. There is no need to follow a burn this deep conservatively; this wound was skin-grafted the day after the patient's admission.

ganizing treatment priorities and protocols, many physicians divide burn care into three periods: (1) resuscitation, (2) wound closure, and (3) rehabilitation. These distinctions are somewhat artificial, however, and many aspects of care overlap these periods. Careful attention to the individual patient's needs is essential at all stages of treatment.

Resuscitation Period

This period lasts for the first 24 to 48 hours after injury. After an acutely burned patient is evaluated and stabilized as described previously, fluid resuscitation is the most important goal of initial treatment. Burn injury produces a loss of capillary integrity, which results in edema formation. With large (≥ 15% to 20% TBSA) injuries, capillary leakage becomes systemic, producing total body edema and severely depleting circulating volume, a phenomenon known as **burn shock.** All patients who have burns of 10% to 15% TBSA or greater require formal fluid resuscitation. Remarkable amounts of fluid may be required for successful resuscitation of patients with very large burn injuries.

Many algorithms have been developed for burn resuscitation, but most successful regimens share several basic concepts. These are shown in Table 11-3 by the **Parkland formula,** a widely used, simple, and relatively generous resuscitation formula. It calls for isotonic crystalloid fluid (lactated Ringer's solution) to be given at an initial rate that is determined from burn size and body weight. Edema formation occurs throughout the first 24 hours postburn, but because it is most pronounced during the first 8 hours, one-half of the total fluid is given during that period. However, inhalation injury, multiple trauma, and other factors can influence an individual's fluid requirements. For this reason, regimens such as the Parkland formula really only indicate where to begin resuscitation, which should be guided thereafter by frequent and repeated evaluation of the patient. Maintenance of adequate urine output (> 30 mL/hr in adults; 1–2 mL/kg/hr in children) is an indicator of appropriate fluid intake and an important goal of treatment. The infusion rate is adjusted according to urine output. It is gradually decreased until a maintenance rate is reached. Vital signs, hematocrit, and other laboratory test results are carefully monitored as well.

Table 11-1 Types of Inhalation Injury

Carbon Monoxide Poisoning

Presentation: Immediately after exposure to flames and smoke.

Pathophysiology: Carbon monoxide (CO), a colorless, odorless gas, is a byproduct of *incomplete* combustion. It acts by displacing oxygen bound to hemoglobin molecules, producing carboxyhemoglobin (COHb) and causing tissue hypoxemia.

Diagnosis: Patients may have cherry-red coloration. Neurologic dysfunction is common, progressing from headache to confusion to coma. CO poisoning should be *strongly suspected* in any patient who is found unconscious at a fire scene or is trapped in a smoke-filled enclosure. Definitive diagnosis requires measurement of blood COHb levels, but treatment should not be postponed while the diagnosis is confirmed.

Treatment: Because oxygen competes with CO for hemoglobin binding, anyone who is suspected of having CO poison ing should be treated *immediately* with high-flow oxygen. Unconscious patients should be intubated. Hyperbaric oxygen helps to clear COHb more quickly, but should not supersede more immediate treatment.

Note: CO does not affect arterial oxygen tension. PO_2 is usually normal, but SaO_2 is greatly affected by CO poisoning.

Upper-Airway Obstruction

Presentation: Immediately up to 24 hours postburn.

Pathophysiology: Smoke contains hot gases, particulate matter, and chemicals, all of which can damage the orophary geal mucosa. This damage causes edema, mucosal sloughing, and gradual airway obstruction.

Diagnosis: Patients with burns of the mouth, nose, or pharynx may display singeing of nasal hairs or eyebrows, carbonaceous material on the lips or tongue, and blistering on the palate. Hoarseness, cough, and increasing stridor signal impending loss of airway.

Treatment: Early endotracheal intubation, high-flow oxygen, and meticulous pulmonary toilet (coughing, suctioning, and clearing of secretions). *Note:* Edema increases during the first 24 hours after injury, so airway obstruction can develop hours after the burn event, even in patients with no burns of the face or exposure to smoke.

Pulmonary Injury (True Inhalation Injury)

Presentation: Can be immediate, but symptoms may be entirely absent until days after injury.

Pathophysiology: Smoke contains a host of toxic chemicals, including formaldehyde, formic and hydrochloric acids, and acrolein, which are activated on contact with moist airways. The resulting damage causes mucosal sloughing, airway collapse, bronchiectasis, and hypoxemia, and predisposes damaged segments to the development of pneumonia.

Diagnosis: Patients present with hypoxia, respiratory distress, and infiltrates on chest radiograph. The most important clue to diagnosis is a history of prolonged exposure to smoke. Other signs and symptoms that are suggestive (but not diagnostic) of inhalation injury include burns of the face, nose, or lips; singeing of the nasal hairs or eyebrows; carbonaceous sputum or saliva; hoarseness or "crowing" respirations; bronchorrea; and tachypnea. Bronchoscopic find ings of carbonaceous deposition, swelling, or erythema of the tracheobronchial tree are diagnostic.

Treatment: Early, elective intubation should be considered. Patients should be treated with high-flow, moisturized oxygen and given meticulous pulmonary toilet, as described previously. Pneumonia should be identified and treated immediately, but prophylactic antibiotics have not proven helpful. *Note:* All three types of inhalation injury—CO poisoning, upper-airway obstruction, and "true" pulmonary injury—can occur individually or may be present simultaneously.

Fluid resuscitation does not stop the leakage of fluid into the interstitium; it is intended only to keep up with ongoing losses, which decrease over time. As resuscitation proceeds, therefore, so does tissue swelling. Fluid accumulating beneath the constricted eschar of a deep burn increases tissue hydrostatic pressure, sometimes to the point at which circulation is compromised. Frequent evaluation of extremity pulses, sensory and motor function, and pain is essential to the diagnosis of progressive ischemia. The treatment of this problem is **escharotomy**, an incision made through the rigid, leathery eschar to relieve the compression that is produced by ongoing edema and, thus, to restore distal circulation. Compression by edema can also affect the chest and abdomen, resulting in respiratory compromise and even arrest. Escharotomies can be performed on the torso and should provide immediate relief (Fig. 11-7). Because escharotomies are always made within surrounding burn wounds, they are repaired during wound excision and skin grafting, and they usually leave no additional scars.

Wound Coverage Period

This phase of treatment begins immediately after fluid resuscitation and lasts for days to weeks, until the burn wound either heals primarily or is successfully replaced with skin grafts. This period constitutes most of the patient's hospital care, and is the period of most intensive treatment. Patients who attain successful wound closure usually survive, although they may face prolonged rehabilitation.

Excision and Skin Grafting

Deeply burned skin is a great liability to the patient. Burn eschar serves as a site for infection. In addition, the loss of skin integrity causes increased evaporative fluid losses,

BURN ESTIMATE AND DIAGRAM
AGE vs AREA

Area	Birth 1 yr.	1-4 yr.	5-9 yr.	10-14 yr.	15 yr.	Adult	2^0	3^0	Total	Donor Areas
Head	19	17	13	11	9	7				
Neck	2	2	2	2	2	2				
Ant. Trunk	13	13	13	13	13	13				
Post. Trunk	13	13	13	13	13	13				
R. Buttock	2½	2½	2½	2½	2½	2½				
L. Buttock	2½	2½	2½	2½	2½	2½				
Genitalia	1	1	1	1	1	1				
R. U. Arm	4	4	4	4	4	4				
L. U. Arm	4	4	4	4	4	4				
R. L. Arm	3	3	3	3	3	3				
L. L. Arm	3	3	3	3	3	3				
R. Hand	2½	2½	2½	2½	2½	2½				
L. Hand	2½	2½	2½	2½	2½	2½				
R. Thigh	5½	6½	8	8½	9	9½				
L. Thigh	5½	6½	8	8½	9	9½				
R. Leg	5	5	5½	6	6½	7				
L. Leg	5	5	5½	6	6½	7				
R. Foot	3½	3½	3½	3½	3½	3½				
L. Foot	3½	3½	3½	3½	3½	3½				
						TOTAL				

Cause of Burn________________________

Date of Burn__________

Time of Burn__________

Age__________

Sex__________

Weight__________

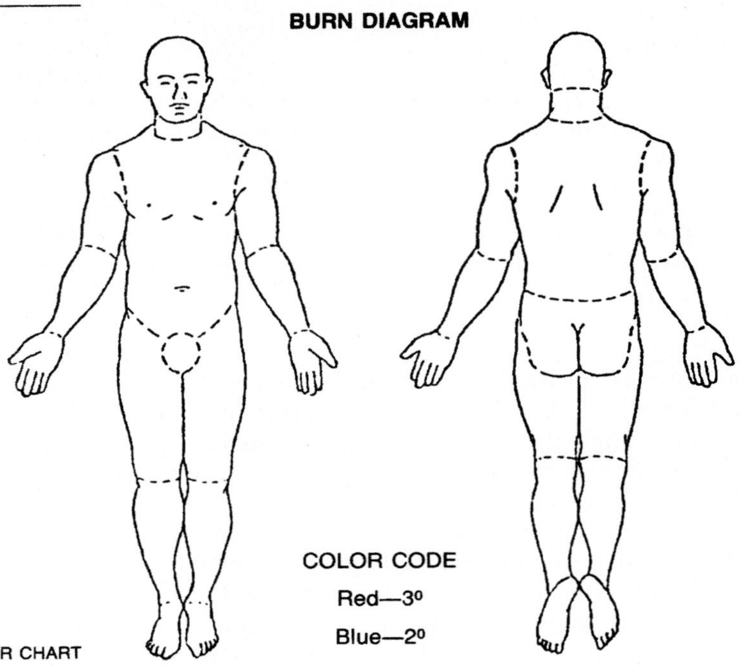

LUND AND BROWDER CHART

Figure 11-6 Lund and Browder chart. This chart is used to diagram the location and extent of burn wounds. The chart divides the body into its component parts and indicates the size of each part, expressed as percentage of total body surface area (% TBSA). Burned areas are indicated and also expressed as % TBSA. Accuracy is increased if burns are charted after the initial cleansing and debridement. The estimate of total burn size is used to guide initial fluid resuscitation, nutritional support, and surgical treatment. (Reprinted from Lund CC, Browder NC. The estimation of areas of burns. *Surg Gynecol Obstet* 1944;79:352–358).

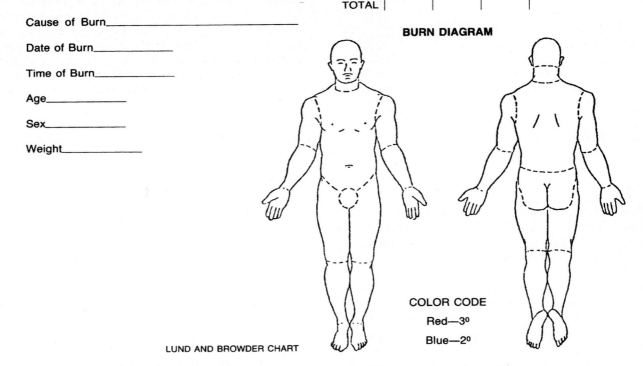

Table 11-2 Criteria for Referral to a Burn Center

1. Partial thickness burns greater than 10% total body surface area (TBSA).
2. Burns that involve the face, hands, feet, genitalia, perineum, or major joints.
3. Third-degree burns in any age group.
4. Electrical burns, including lightning injury.
5. Chemical burns.
6. Inhalation injury.
7. Complicated patients: Burn injury in patients with preexisting medical disorders that could complicate management, prolong recovery, or affect mortality (e.g., diabetes, HIV infection, etc.).
8. Burns and trauma: Any patients with burns and concomitant trauma (such as fractures) in which the burn injury poses the greatest risk of morbidity or mortality. In such cases, if the trauma poses the greater immediate risk, the patient may be initially stabilized in a trauma center before being transferred to a burn unit. Physician judgment will be necessary in such situations and should be in concert with the regional medical control plan and triage protocols.
9. Children: Burned children in hospitals without qualified personnel or equipment for the care of children.
10. Special care: Burn injury in patients who will require special social, emotional, or long-term rehabilitative intervention.

Adapted with permission from Committee on Trauma, American College of Surgeons. *Resources for Optimal Care of the Injured Patient: 1999.*

severe pain, and an intense inflammatory response that can escalate, leading to multiple organ failure and death. If followed conservatively, deep eschar eventually separates spontaneously, but this process can take weeks. During this time, the patient is exposed to ongoing stress and risk of infection. For these reasons, most burn centers now employ **early excision,** in which burned skin is cut off of the underlying tissue. Two techniques are used: **fascial** and **tangential excision.** In fascial excision, the scalpel or cautery is used to excise the entire skin and subcutaneous tissue, usually to the level of the underlying fascia. This procedure is easy to perform, is relatively bloodless, and permits good skin graft "take." Fascial excision is disfiguring, however, and the removal of subcutaneous fat leads to joint stiffness and poor mobility. During the last 2 decades, the technique of "layered," or tangential, excision has gained popularity. With this technique, sequential thin slices of skin are removed with a dermatome until viable tissue is encountered. This technique requires skill, and it produces significant bleeding. However, the cosmetic and functional results of grafting this type of wound are often superior to those of fascial excision. Tangential excision of deep partial-thickness burns permits salvaging of intact dermal elements, which improves the results of

Table 11-3 Principles of Fluid Resuscitation for Burns: The Parkland Formula

Principles

- Resuscitation should use primarily isotonic crystalloid solution because it is inexpensive and readily available, and can be given in large quantities without harmful side effects. Because injured capillaries are porous to proteins for the first several hours after injury, colloid-containing fluids are not used during this period.
- Resuscitation requirements are proportional to burn size and patient's body weight.
- Edema formation is most rapid during the first 8 hours postburn. It continues for 24 hours.
- Resuscitation must be guided by patient response (e.g., urine output, vital signs, mental status).

Practice: The Parkland Formula

- The formula:
- 4 mL lactated Ringer's × Body weight (kg) × % TBSA burned = Total fluid for 24 hr
- First 8 hours postinjury: Give one-half the calculated total.
- Second 8 hours postinjury: Give one-fourth the calculated total.
- Third 8 hours postinjury: Give one-fourth the calculated total.

Example:

A 220-lb (100-kg) man is burned while filling the gas tank on his boat. He is wearing a swimming suit and is burned over all of both legs, his chest, and both arms. Calculated burn size is 65% TBSA.

Calculated fluid requirements:

Total 4 mL lactated Ringer's × 100 kg × 65% TBSA burned = 26,000 mL in 24 hr
- First 8 hours = 13,000 mL or 1625 mL/hr
- Second 8 hours = 6500 mL or 812 mL/hr
- Third 8 hours = 6500 mL or 812 mL/hr

TBSA, total body surface area.

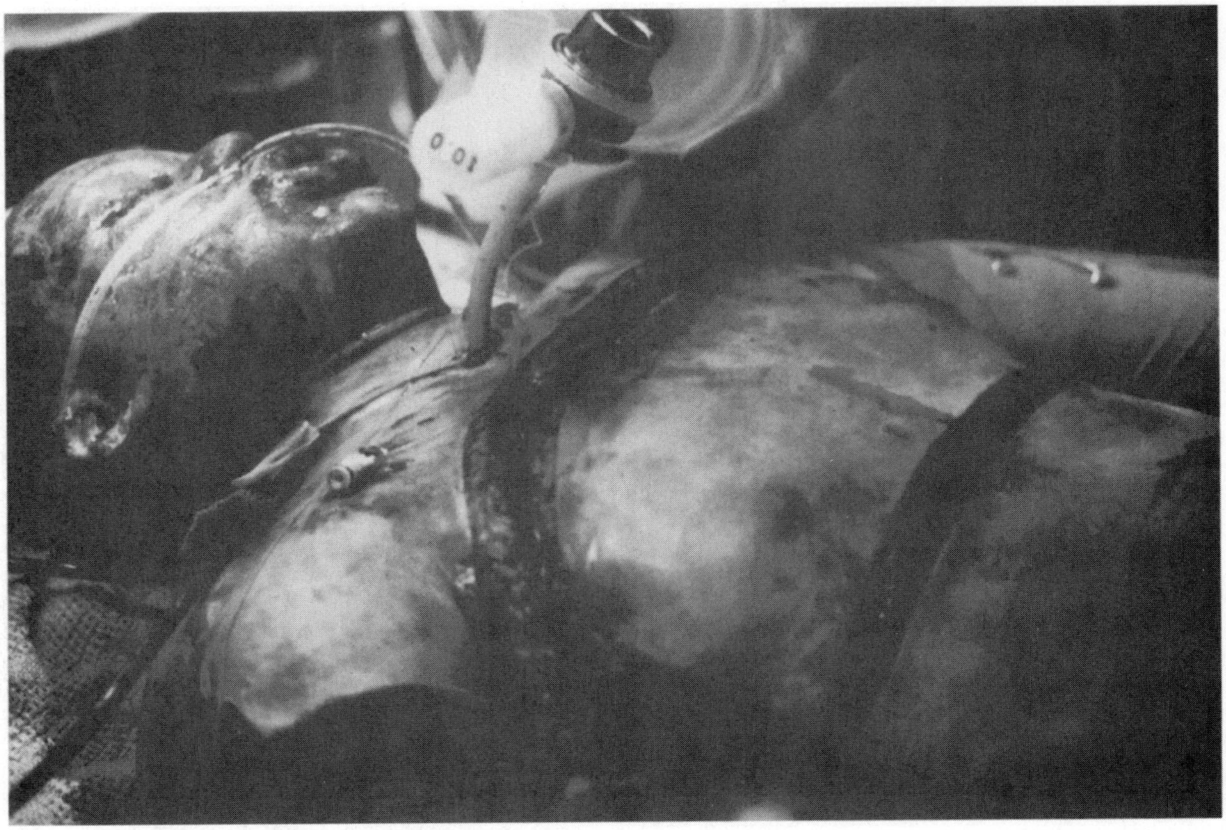

Figure 11-7 Massive edema and torso escharotomy. This man had a 75% full-thickness burn as the result of a gasoline fire. He is shown here approximately 24 hours after injury. Massive facial edema made oral intubation impossible; the patient required emergent cricothyroidotomy because of airway obstruction. As fluid resuscitation proceeded, edema accumulating beneath the rigid eschar of the torso created progressive compression and compromised ventilation. Chest escharotomy relieved this compression and improved ventilation. The escharotomy wound spread apart with progressive swelling.

skin grafting. To permit stabilization of cardiovascular function and intravascular volume (which can be further compromised by surgical blood loss), most surgeons wait until fluid resuscitation is completed before they begin excisional therapy. Limited burns of mixed or indeterminate depth can be followed for 10 to 14 days before the decision to proceed with surgery must be made.

Skin grafting is usually performed at the same time as excision. Currently, permanent coverage of an excised wound can be achieved only with the patient's own skin (**autograft**). Autografting can be performed with **full-thickness** or **split-thickness grafts.** Full-thickness grafts are obtained by excising an ellipse of skin from the groin or flank, which is closed with sutures. Split-thickness grafts use a dermatome to harvest intact skin at the level of the superficial dermis, typically 0.004 to 0.015 inch deep. This process yields a graft with sufficient dermis to provide secure coverage of the excised burn and leaves a wound that is superficial enough to heal spontaneously in 7 to 14 days. Figure 11-8 shows tangential excision and split-thickness skin grafting of a burned hand. In the treatment of very large burns, the urgency to remove eschar often requires that excision be performed, even if no donor sites are available for grafting. When insufficient autograft is available, several techniques are used to obtain skin coverage. First, skin can be expanded by meshing, or cutting multiple small slits in the skin. Widely meshed autografts cover larger areas, although the interstices of the mesh are prone to desiccation. For this reason, widely meshed autografts are usually covered with one of several skin substitutes, which can also be used alone to attain temporary closure of burn wounds. The most widely used skin substitute is cadaver **allograft** skin, obtained from tissue banks. Other skin substitutes include freeze-dried pig's skin, human amniotic membrane, and various synthetic materials, including a matrix of collagen and glycosaminoglycan called Integra. In recent years, considerable research has been devoted to the development of a man-made "artificial der-

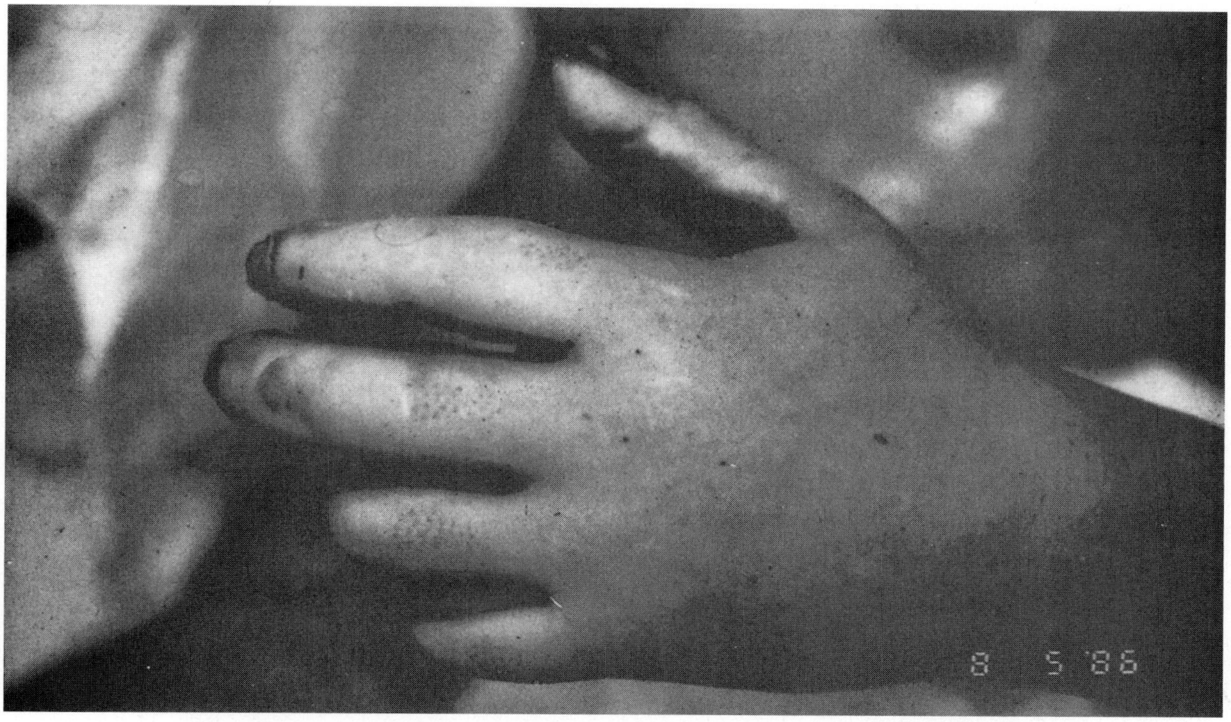

A

Figure 11-8 Excision and skin grafting. **A,** A 36-year-old man had a deep partial-thickness burn of the dorsal hand and fingers. (*continues*)

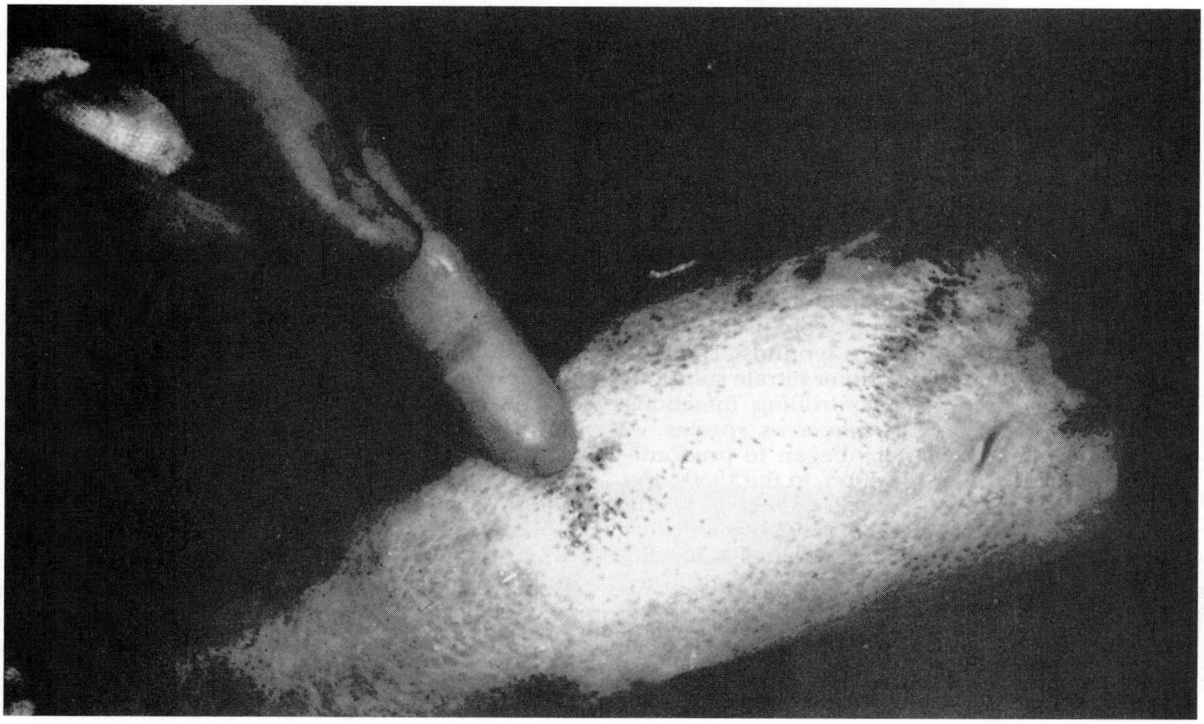

B

Figure 11-8 (*continued*) **B,** Under tourniquet control, the eschar is excised until only pale, intact dermis is seen. An area of residual discoloration is shown, indicating damaged tissue; this tissue will also be excised.

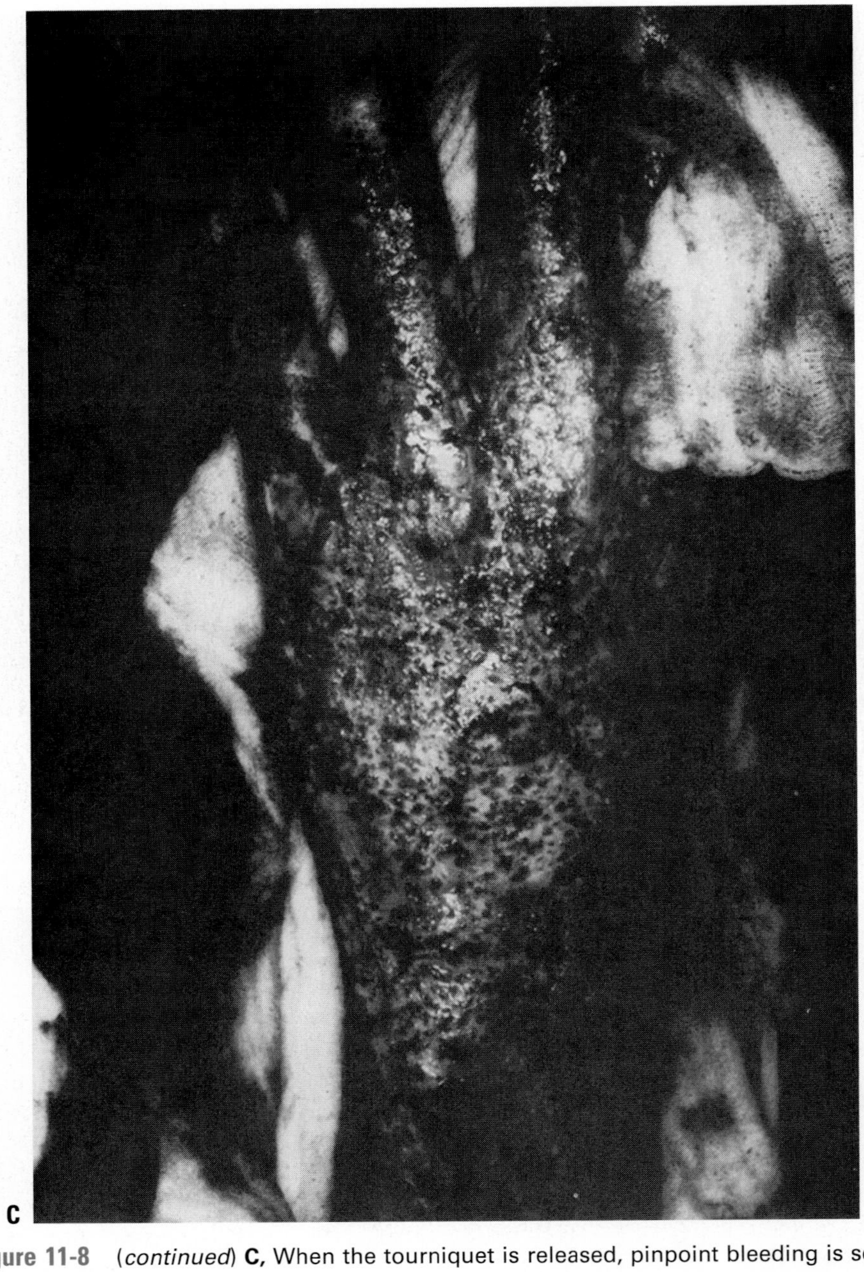

Figure 11-8 *(continued)* **C,** When the tourniquet is released, pinpoint bleeding is seen in all areas.

mis," which could be taken off the shelf and used to cover large burn wounds. A number of products are undergoing clinical testing, but it is too early to predict how effective they will be. Finally, it is possible to grow a patient's own epidermal cells in culture. These cultured epidermal allografts are expensive, fragile, and easily lost as a result of infection. Nonetheless, they have proved lifesaving in some patients with massive burns.

Infection Control

Immediately after burning, the skin surface is virtually sterile for 24 to 48 hours. Then it gradually becomes repopulated with bacteria. Burn eschar, especially the thick, avascular eschar of deep burns, is an ideal culture medium for bacteria, which multiply rapidly on such a surface. These bacteria may colonize burn eschar harmlessly. On the other hand, by penetrating through the burn wound, they may invade intact tissues and overwhelm local defenses, producing an invasive infection known as **burn wound sepsis.** Infection is also favored by the immunosuppression that accompanies severe burn injury. Burn wound sepsis is frequently fatal and, until recently, was the most common cause of death in hospitalized burn victims. With modern methods of wound

D
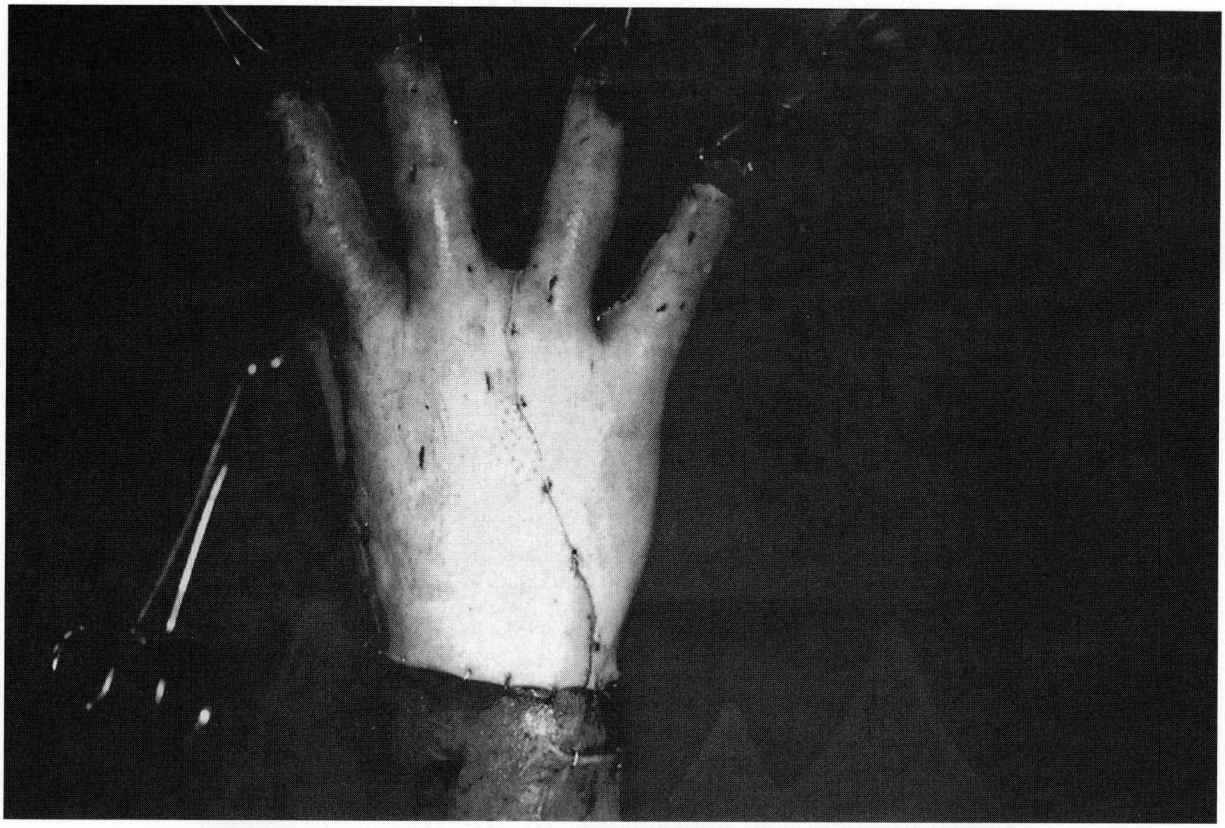

Figure 11-8 (*continued*) **D,** The hand is suspended with towel clips to facilitate placement of a split-thickness skin graft harvested from the patient's back. The graft is secured with skin staples and sutures.

management, however, it is now an uncommon occurrence in burn centers.

Much of the increased survival in patients with burns achieved in the last 50 years is the result of improved understanding and treatment of burn wound infections. Beginning in the 1940s, systemic antibiotics (e.g., penicillin) as well as many topical agents were used to control microbial contamination of burn wounds. The first widely used topical antimicrobial, silver nitrate solution, proved particularly effective in controlling infections caused by *Staphylococcus* and *Streptococcus* species. A variety of Gram-negative infections began to predominate as causes of burn wound infection. In the 1960s, the development of two powerful topical agents, mafenide acetate (Sulfamylon) and **silver sulfadiazene** (Silvadene, Thermazene, and SSD, among others), helped to control many Gram-negative bacteria, which were then replaced by resistant *Pseudomonas* as a leading cause of infection. More recently, a host of powerful systemic antibiotics and numerous other topical agents have helped to control *Pseudomonas* infections. This success has been followed by (and, to some extent, caused) the emergence of multiply resistant bacteria (e.g., methicillin-resistant *Staphylococcus aureus*, *Acinetobacter*, and vancomycin-resistant *Enterococcus*), as well as fungi and other exotic organisms, as important clinical pathogens in burn victims. This problem is multiplied by the development in many burn centers of entrenched, endemic microbial populations that are difficult to eradicate. Thus, as the medical community has developed increasingly powerful antimicrobials for burn care, the microbial fauna has adapted and continued to present new problems.

The most effective technique in the battle against burn wound infection is early burn excision and skin grafting (discussed previously). Meticulous wound care also remains an essential part of burn treatment during the repair phase. Beginning immediately postburn, wounds must be washed regularly and debrided carefully of old topical creams and ointments, dried serum, and bits of loose eschar (see Fig. 11-3). Topical antimicrobials are effective for only a few hours, and most experts agree that their replacement, as well as regular and thorough **debridement,** should be performed at least twice daily. These requirements also apply to freshly grafted burn wounds and to skin graft donor sites.

As the prevention and treatment of burn wound infection has become more successful, other problems have gained prominence as causes of morbidity and mortality

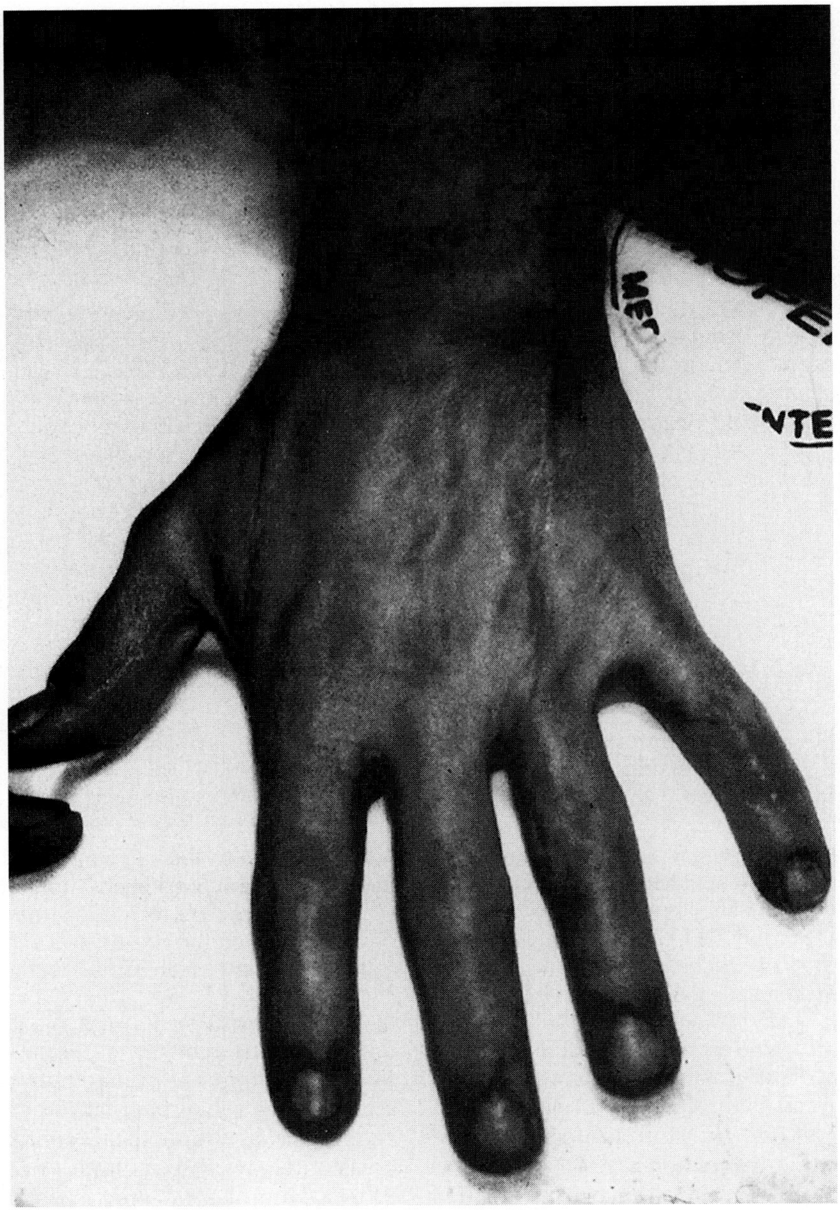

E

Figure 11-8 (*continued*) **E,** The hand several months later. The cosmetic result is excellent, and function is perfect. This result is far superior to the result expected with spontaneous healing.

in burn victims. In particular, pneumonia has emerged as the most common, and often the most troublesome, infection seen in burn patients. As outlined in Table 11-2, smoke inhalation causes chemical injury to the small airways of the lung, leading to bronchiectasis and mucous plugging. These effects permit infections to develop and render them difficult to clear. Pneumonia, in turn, often serves as a stimulus for systemic inflammation and infection, leading to the development of multiple organ failure. A host of other infectious complications can occur in burn victims. Septic thrombophlebitis can occur in veins that are cannulated for vascular access. When central veins are involved, systemic sepsis, endocarditis, and death can result. Localized infections can also develop in exposed bone or cartilage, the urinary tract, salivary glands, gallbladder, and other areas. Happily, these complications are rarely seen in burn treatment.

Nutritional Support

As part of the hormonal response to burn trauma, the metabolic rate rises dramatically. It can exceed twice the normal rate for prolonged periods, with a corresponding increase in nitrogen excretion. This change is the most severe metabolic response seen with any type of illness or injury, and the resulting catabolism can cause a fatal degree of inanition within a few weeks. In these patients, protein malnutrition causes both wasting of respiratory muscles and immune compromise, with resulting pulmonary infection and death. For this reason, burn patients require aggressive nutritional support and close monitoring throughout the wound closure phase of treatment, and sometimes longer. Enteral feeding is clearly superior to intravenous nutrition in burn victims. For this reason, patients with large injuries should undergo placement of enteral feeding tubes as soon as possible. A high-protein liquid diet should be infused until oral intake is adequate. Various formulas have been used to predict the caloric requirements of burn patients. None are entirely satisfactory, however, partially because of the wide variation seen among individuals and the fluctuations in energy expenditure that occur during the post-burn course. Many experts recommend the routine measurement of energy expenditure with indirect calorimetry and measurement of protein use with nitrogen-balance determinations, at least weekly. The technique of indirect calorimetry calculates the energy requirements of an individual by measuring the oxygen consumed during normal breathing. In recent years, improved understanding of the role of nutrition in trauma management has led to the development of "customized" nutritional products aimed at the specific needs of burn and trauma patients. The advantages of these products remain to be proven; a basic high-protein diet (1.5 to 2.0 g protein/kg body weight daily), in quantities sufficient to satisfy caloric requirements, is the most important principle in the nutritional management of these patients.

Rehabilitation Period

After burn wounds are closed, major emphasis is shifted to rehabilitation. However, it is incorrect to infer that rehabilitation should await wound closure. In practice, rehabilitation begins at the time of injury. As burn wounds heal, they contract because of the presence of myofibroblasts that begin to accumulate within wounds shortly after injury and continue to proliferate within scar tissue. If unopposed, burn scar contractures can immobilize extremities completely and produce hideous disfigurement. Much of the therapy provided during burn rehabilitation is aimed at preventing and correcting contractures. This therapy is more effective if it is begun quickly, while the scar tissue is still pliable and before it can "set" into significant contractures. Scar tissue remains inflamed and continues to remodel and reshape itself for at least a year after injury. Burn patients are usually followed for at least that long. In addition to motion and stretching exercises, tight-fitting antiburn scar garments are frequently used to retard the growth of hypertrophic scars. These custom-made garments are worn until the scar tissue softens and erythema fades. The process of recovering completely from a major burn is long and labor-intensive, but most burn victims can return to active and useful lives with appropriate therapy. Most patients return to work or school, even after burns of 70% TBSA or greater.

Reconstructive surgery may be needed to correct particularly difficult contractures, resurface areas of unstable wound coverage, or improve cosmetic appearance. This surgery is usually postponed until the burn scars mature and soften. However, many reconstructive procedures can be avoided with early and continued application of physical therapy and other rehabilitative techniques.

SUGGESTED READINGS

American Burn Association Practice Guidelines Group: practice guidelines for burn care. Published as a supplement to the *Journal of Burn Care and Rehabilitation. J Burn Care Rehabil* 2001.

Heimbach D. What's new in general surgery: burns and metabolism. *J Amer Coll Surg* 2002;194:156–164.

Monafo WW. Current concepts: initial management of burns. *N Engl J Med* 1996;225:1581–1586.

Pruitt BA, McManus AT. The changing epidemiology of infection in burn patients. *World J Surg* 1992;16:57–67.

Sheridan RL. Burns. *Crit Care Med* 2002;30:S500–S514.

Sheridan RL. Comprehensive treatment of burns. *Curr Prob Surg* 2001; 38:657–756.

Warden GD. Burn shock resuscitation. *World J Surg* 1992;16:16–23.

Williams JG, Herndon DN. Modulating the hypermetabolic response to burn injuries. *J Wound Care* 2000;9:115–119.

12

LEIGH NEUMAYER, MD, MS ■ D. BYRON MCGREGOR, MD
BARRY MANN, MD

Abdominal Wall, Including Hernia

OBJECTIVES

1 Know the relations of the layers of the abdominal wall and their pertinent reflections into the groin.
2 Define indirect inguinal hernia, direct inguinal hernia, and femoral hernia.
3 List the factors that predispose to the development of inguinal hernias.
4 Define and discuss the relative frequency of indirect, direct, and femoral hernias by age and sex.
5 Define incarcerated inguinal hernia, strangulated hernia, sliding hernia, and Richter's hernia.
6 Outline the principles of management for patients with groin hernias, including the surgical treatments for repair and the indications for their use.
7 Discuss the appropriate use of prosthetic materials in hernia repair.
8 Discuss the embryology of an umbilical hernia.

The abdominal wall is of obvious importance in keeping our insides inside. Knowledge of its anatomy is vital to plan transgressions for access to the enclosed viscera and to understand the common clinical problem of groin **hernias.** These hernias are the most common clinical problem addressed by surgeons, with more than 700,000 repairs performed annually. As many as 10% of these hernias eventually recur and require additional therapy. This chapter emphasizes anatomy and embryologic development because only with that knowledge can the surgeon plan structural changes to correct symptomatic defects. The chapter reviews the pertinent anatomy and discusses the most common hernias and their repair.

ANATOMY OF THE ABDOMINAL WALL

Surface Relations

The abdominal wall has few anatomic landmarks. Only the costal margins, anterior superior iliac spines, and umbilicus break the otherwise flat plane. Where anatomy failed, verbiage was substituted. Hypochondriacal (below the ribs), periumbilical (around the belly button), and epigastric (high abdominal) are examples of colorful, but imprecise, terms. Other attempts were made to define abdominal regions by drawing imaginary lines across the abdominal wall. Thus, the abdomen was halved, trisected, and even divided into as many as nine imaginary compartments in attempts to provide reliable topographic characteristics. The most useful of these is the creation of simple vertical and horizontal lines through the umbilicus, dividing the abdomen into four imaginary quadrants (Fig. 12-1). In this format, the right upper quadrant covers such disease-prone intraabdominal organs as the gallbladder, duodenum, right pleura, and liver. The left upper quadrant covers the spleen, stomach, left pleura, and tail of the pancreas. The left lower quadrant obscures the sigmoid colon and left ureter. The right lower quadrant overlies the right ureter, cecum, Meckel's diverticulum, and that common cause of right lower quadrant pain, the appendix.

Cutaneous Nerves

Cutaneous nerves arising from the intercostal nerves (T7 to L1) supply the sensation of the anterior abdominal wall. At each level, posterior divisions supply sensation to the

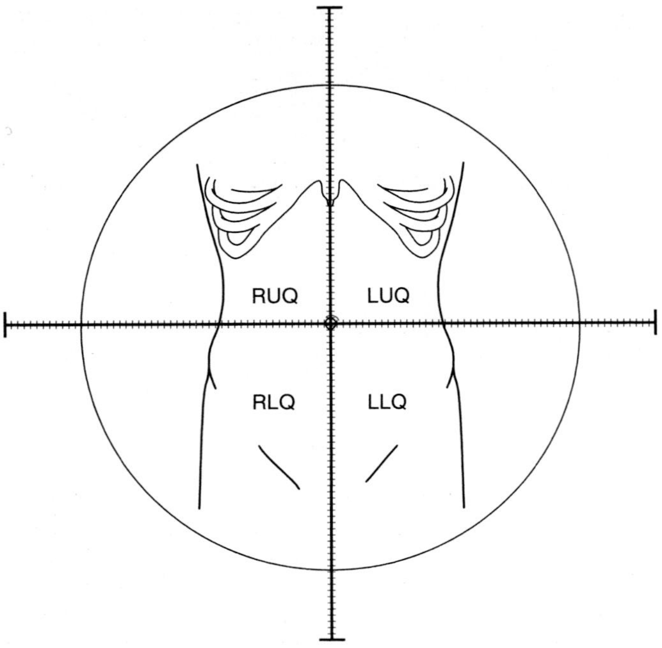

Figure 12-1 View of the anterior abdominal wall defining the descriptive sectors of anatomy. *RUQ,* right upper quadrant; *LUQ,* left upper quadrant; *RLQ,* right lower quadrant; *LLQ,* left lower quadrant.

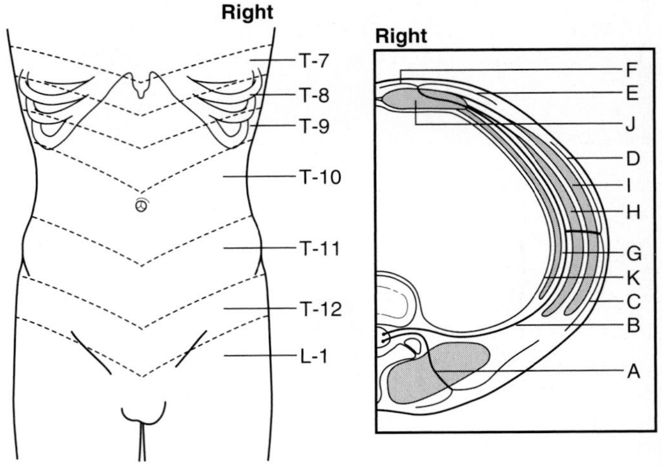

Figure 12-2 *Left,* Cutaneous nerve distribution to the anterior abdominal wall. *Right,* Schema of the cutaneous nerves. **A,** Posterior primary division. **B,** Anterior primary division. **C,** Posterior division of the lateral cutaneous nerve. **D,** Anterior division of the lateral cutaneous nerve. **E,** Lateral division of the anterior cutaneous nerve. **F,** Medial division of the anterior cutaneous nerve. **G,** Transversus abdominus muscle. **H,** Internal oblique muscle. **I,** External oblique muscle. **J,** Rectus abdominus muscle. **K,** Peritoneum.

back and flank. The anterior primary division, running between the transversus abdominus and the internal oblique, gives off the lateral cutaneous nerve, which traverses the internal and external oblique muscles at about the anterior axillary line. It then branches into anterior and posterior divisions. The anterior primary division continues its course beyond the lateral cutaneous branch; anteriorly it pierces the rectus sheath, supplies the rectus muscle, and proceeds anteriorly to innervate the midline and contribute to the segmental pattern started by the lateral cutaneous branches (see Fig. 12-2, *Right*). These nerves supply the anterior and posterior abdominal walls in a dermatome-like fashion, with a relatively transverse distribution in the upper abdomen and a more oblique pattern in the groin (Fig. 12-2, *Left*). The result of this rich cutaneous innervation is a series of dermatome-related clues to intraabdominal diagnoses. For example, visceral afferent fibers from the appendix follow the same nerve distribution as the small intestine, back to their T10 origins. Therefore, early in its course, appendicitis causes central abdominal pain in the T10 dermatome distribution. Later in the course of the disease, if the inflammatory process from the appendix develops anteriorly and irritates the peritoneum beneath the right lower quadrant of the abdomen, this irritation is sensed by somatic afferent fibers of the T12 nerve route. It is reflected back in the appropriate lower cutaneous distribution as hyperesthesia. The disease is often well described by abdominal pain findings alone. Despite this apparent degree of segmental precision, considerable overlap of cutaneous nerves exists. Because of this overlap, the sacrifice of any single cutaneous nerve usually causes no permanent sensory loss. This safety factor is less pronounced in the lower sensory nerves (ilioinguinal and iliohypogastric). The ilioinguinal and iliohypogastric nerves both arise variably from the lower thoracic (usually T12) and upper lumbar roots. The ilioinguinal nerve pierces the internal oblique muscle just superior and lateral to the internal (abdominal) ring and then runs with the spermatic cord. The iliohypogastric nerve is usually encountered just under the external oblique fascia, superior to the cord structures, often lying near the tendinous portion of the internal oblique muscle. The genitofemoral nerve usually travels with the spermatic cord. Injury to these nerves can leave permanent numbness in the groin, scrotum, and anterior thigh. Entrapment of these nerves in scar tissue or sutures can result in chronic pain for the patient. The incidence of chronic pain after inguinal hernia repair appears to be between 6% and 13%.

Layers of the Abdominal Wall

A brief review of the seven individual layers that make up the abdominal wall is helpful before any discussion of the use of these layers to explain surgical disease or design surgical repairs. The following discussion describes the anatomy of the seven individual layers, with particular attention to the origins and reflections of fascial continuity for each. The most notable reflection occurs in the groin, where all of the layers of the abdominal wall are reflected into the scrotum, much as the layers of a shirt, jacket, and overcoat are reflected off the chest wall and onto a sleeve, while maintaining constant relation to each other.

Skin

As elsewhere, Langer's lines of cleavage transgress the skin over the abdominal wall. The course of fibrous bundles and the disposition of elastin fibers in the corium produce these lines of skin tension. Across the anterior abdominal walls, these lines are dispersed transversely. In the lower abdomen, like the cutaneous nerves, Langer's lines assume a slightly more oblique pattern as they course into the groins. The skin, its cleavage lines, and its superficial cutaneous innervation all are continuous onto the scrotum in the male and the labia in the female.

Subcutaneous Tissue

The subcutaneous tissue of the abdominal wall has two layers. The more superficial and fatty of the two is Camper's fascia. The deeper, more fibrous, denser layer is Scarpa's fascia. There is considerable disagreement about the precise definition and fascial connection of these two adipose layers. In general, they can be incised in any plane, with little adverse effect. They are generally considered to be contiguous into the perineum as the superficial perineal fascia of Colles of the penis and the tunica dartos of the scrotum. It is from this continuity that infections and urinary extravasations proceed out of the perineum and into the abdominal wall.

External Oblique Muscle

The major functioning muscles of the abdominal wall are broad, flat, constricting layers. In general, these layers overlap throughout their course and join symmetrically in the midline. The most superficial of these is the external abdominal oblique muscle. This muscle arises broadly from the lower six ribs and interdigitations of the serratus anterior muscle. In the flank, it forms a thick, broad muscle, the fibers of which run obliquely downward. However, as it courses over the anterior aspect of the abdominal wall, the fibers of its **aponeurosis** run essentially transversely. High in the abdomen, this aponeurosis fuses with half of the aponeurosis of the internal oblique muscle at the lateral margin of the rectus abdominus muscle to form the anterior rectus sheath (Fig. 12-3). Lower in the abdomen, this fusion occurs near the midline.

In the groin, the aponeurotic fibers of the external oblique muscle angle downward, taking the direction of your fingers if they are placed comfortably in your jean pockets. Further laterally, this aponeurosis rolls on itself to form the inguinal ligament. This ligament is a free margin suspended between the anterior superior iliac spine and the pubic tubercle, with no muscular origins or insertions. Medially, the fibers of the inguinal ligament rotate and attach onto the most medial portion of **Cooper's ligament** as the lacunar ligament, which forms the final medial containment of a femoral hernia. The external oblique aponeurosis is contiguous into the scrotum as the external spermatic fascia and onto the anterior thigh as the fascia lata. Finally, near the medial attachment of the external oblique aponeurosis onto the pubic tubercle, the aponeurosis divides, forming a triangular orifice through which the spermatic cord and testicle descend. This aperture persists as the external or superficial inguinal ring.

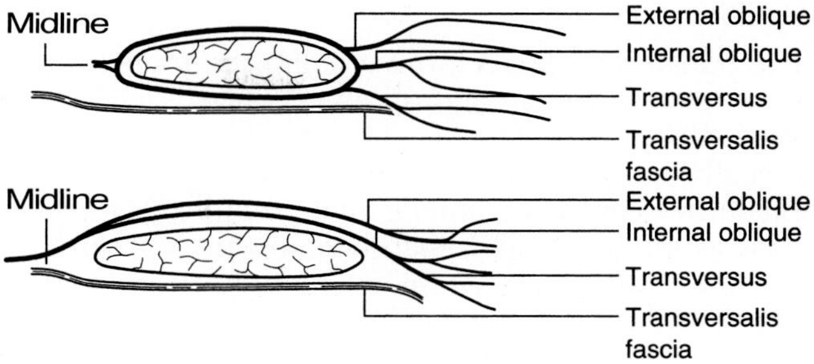

Figure 12-3 Cross-section showing midline fascial relations above *(top)* and below *(bottom)* the semicircular line of Douglas.

Internal Oblique Muscle

The internal oblique muscle arises broadly from the iliac crest, lumbodorsal fascia, and psoas fascia, as well as from continuity with its homologue, the internal intercostal muscles of the lower chest wall. Its fibers are directed obliquely upward in the high flank, transversely in the midflank, and slightly downward in the low flank. Like the external oblique muscle, the internal oblique forms a broad aponeurosis that fuses into the midline and contributes to the anterior rectus sheath throughout the abdomen as well as the posterior rectus sheath in the upper abdomen (see Fig. 12-3). The internal oblique remains muscular in the groin, where it has no attachments, and its fibers continue onto the spermatic cord as the cremasteric muscle.

Transversus Muscle

The transversus abdominus muscle, the deepest of the three muscular layers, has similar origins and attachments to the internal oblique, arising from the lower six ribs, the thoracolumbar fascia, and the iliac crest. It fuses medially to form the rectus sheaths and the linea alba. The fibers of its aponeurosis again run transversely, except in the groin, where they curve medially and downward to attach onto the pubic tubercle, the pectineal (Cooper's) ligament, and continue down the thigh as the anterior femoral sheath. In the groin, the aponeurosis of the transversus abdominus is fused to the underlying transversalis fascia to form the posterior inguinal wall. The spermatic cord descends through this wall (through its triangular orifice, the "abdominal," "deep," or "internal" inguinal ring). It is through this layer that all groin hernia pathology develops.

Transversalis Fascia

The transversalis fascia forms a complete, uninterrupted envelope of fascia around the interior of the abdominal cavity. Because it is a true fascial layer, it has little intrinsic strength, but through its fusion to aponeurotic layers it establishes continuity among such seemingly unrelated areas as the diaphragm, the obturator internus, and the aforementioned layers of the anterior abdominal wall. It is separated from the underlying peritoneum by a variable layer of preperitoneal connective tissue and fat. With the descent of the testicle, the transversalis fascia establishes continuity with the internal spermatic fascia of the spermatic cord.

Peritoneum

The peritoneum is a serous membrane that lines the entire peritoneal cavity and invests the intraabdominal structures. Details of the intraabdominal reflections of the peritoneum and the formation of the greater and lesser peritoneal sacs are discussed in Chapter 14, Stomach and Duodenum; Chapter 15, Small Intestine and Appendix; and Chapter 16, Colon, Rectum, and Anus. The peritoneum is best described as the exquisitely sensitive final lining layer of the anterior abdominal wall. With the descent of the testicle, a portion of the peritoneum is also advanced into the scrotum (Fig. 12-4). With complete development, this peritoneal remnant remains as the tunica vaginalis of the testicle. In normal development, the remainder of the peritoneal connection is obliterated and the peritoneal cavity is once again a sealed space within the abdominal cavity (with the exception of the fallopian tube orifices). If this obliteration process is not completed, the result is varying degrees of persistence of an open communication between the peritoneal cavity and the tunica vaginalis. These varying degrees of patency result in either an indirect hernia, a communicating or a noncommunicating hydrocele, or a mere persistent patency of the processus vaginalis, inviting herniation.

Midline Structures

All of the layers of the abdominal wall are continuous across the anterior midline. The skin, subcutaneous tissues, transversalis fascia, and peritoneum are simple continuations, but the fusions and attachments of the abdominal muscles, umbilicus, and umbilical cord remnants deserve special attention.

To understand these midline structures, the sheaths and locations of the rectus abdominus muscles must be described. In comparison to the other abdominal muscles, the rectus abdominus muscle consists of narrow, thick bands of muscle that parallel the midline from the costal cartilages to the pubic symphysis. Each muscle is divided along its course by a variable number of tendinous inscriptions that essentially divide the muscle into a series of interconnected muscles. Above the umbilicus, they are separated in the midline by a condensation of the aponeuroses of the other abdominal muscles (linea alba). The formation of the linea alba and of the rectus sheaths is of some anatomic interest and surgical importance (see Fig. 12-3). Approximately midway between the umbilicus and the symphysis pubis is an anatomic landmark, the semicircular line of Douglas. Above this line, the external oblique aponeurosis and the anterior leaf of the internal oblique aponeurosis fuse to form the anterior sheath. The posterior leaf of the internal oblique aponeurosis and the aponeurosis of the transversus fuse to form the posterior sheath in this position. Below the semicircular line, all three aponeuroses cross anterior to the rectus muscle, leaving only the peritoneum and the transversalis fascia between the rectus muscles and the abdominal contents. Below the semicircular line, the exact point of fusion of the aponeurotic layers to form the rectus sheath is variable. The external oblique usually joins far medially. The internal oblique and transversus fuse near the lateral edge of the rectus muscle. Wherever the latter fusion occurs, the anterior rectus sheath is born. No fusion of these layers occurs along the inguinal canal; therefore, the often mentioned, but seldom present, "conjoined tendon" normally (95% of cases) does not exist.

Umbilicus

By the start of the second trimester, the omphalomesenteric duct disappears, the gut rotates and reenters the peritoneal cavity, and the body walls form, with the exception of a ring of variable size in the middle of the abdomen. Through this ring pass the umbilical arteries, left umbilical

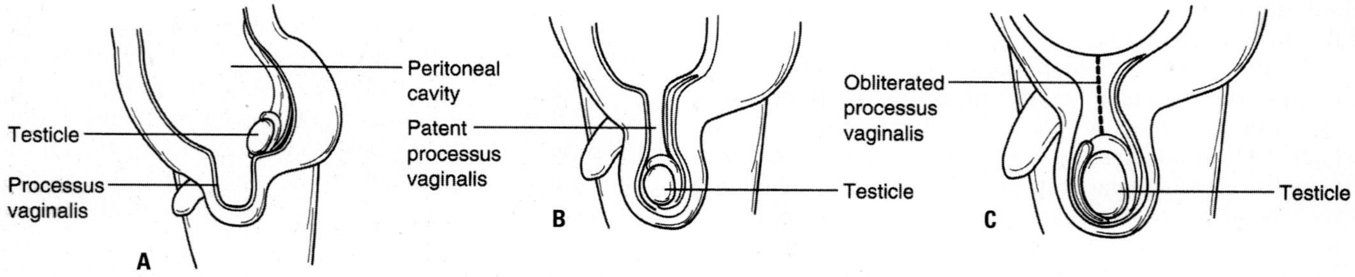

Figure 12-4 Peritoneal accompaniment of testicular descent. **A,** Before descent. **B,** Full patency of the processus vaginalis after descent. **C,** Patent remnant or noncommunicating hydrocele.

vein, and allantois, a tubular diverticulum of the embryonic hindgut. At birth, these three atrophy into fibrous cords. With healing of the transected cord, the force of retraction of those vessels modifies the formation of the umbilical ring scar. These forces result in weak portions of the scar, usually at the superior portion of the umbilical defect, where later herniations can develop.

Remnants of this physiologic closure yield structures that are of occasional surgical interest. The left umbilical vein persists as the ligamentum teres of the liver, coursing in the falciform ligament from the umbilicus to the hepatic margin. Although it physiologically closes and fibroses after birth, this vessel is frequently available for cannulation in the newborn (and even occasionally in the adult) for venous access. Remnants of the omphalomesenteric duct persist as vitelline duct cysts, duct patency with stooling at the umbilicus, or Meckel's diverticulum. Finally, failure of allantois closure may result in urachal cysts or total urachal fistula, with urinary soiling at the umbilicus.

ABDOMINAL INCISIONS

Access to the abdominal cavity is obtained by surgical incisions. The ideal incision provides adequate access to the intraabdominal organ under investigation, reestablishes the strength and form of the abdominal wall postoperatively, and leaves a cosmetically acceptable surgical scar. The commonly used surgical incisions are few (Fig. 12-5), but they deserve individual mention.

Midline vertical incisions are the most widely used. They are directed through the fused aponeurotic midline, anywhere from the xiphoid to the pubic tubercle. This incision has multiple advantages, including the speed at which it can be made (because no vascular structures cross the midline), its ability to provide access to all portions of the abdomen, and its extendibility. It is the incision of choice in trauma or when lack of a preoperative diagnosis requires exposure of all portions of the abdomen.

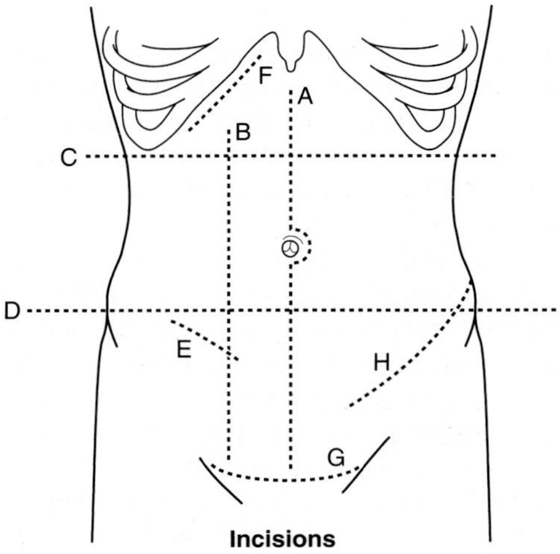

Figure 12-5 Common incisions across the anterior abdominal wall. **A,** Midline incision. **B,** Paramedian incision. **C** and **D,** Two of the multiple planes of transverse incisions. **E,** McBurney incision. **F,** Subcostal incision. **G,** Pfannenstiel incision. **H,** Kidney transplant incision.

Transverse incisions are preferred by some surgeons as being more "physiologic." The skin incisions are made in line with Langer's lines, resulting in more cosmetic scars. More important, they are made in line with the direction of muscle tension, so postoperative coughing or exercise tends to close the incision rather than open it (as occurs in vertical incisions). As a result, the incidence of wound dehiscence and late herniation is minimized. Transection of the rectus abdominus muscle is not a significant problem because a fibrous union that is the equivalent of an additional tendinous inscription results. Extension of this incision may not gain the access needed, and a second incision could be needed after the diagnosis is established.

Retroperitoneal incisions for access to the aorta and vessels, kidneys, and anterior spine are increasingly being used. In the lower quadrants, a chocky stick skin incision is used to access the iliac vessels and bladder for kidney transplantation.

Paramedian incisions have fallen into disrepute in recent years. They add very little to the exposure provided through a midline vertical incision. In addition, they have several disadvantages: (1) they are time consuming to create and close; (2) they may denervate medial portions of the rectus muscle and overlying skin; and (3) because of their inherent weakness, they are the most prone to herniation or disruption. The farther lateral a paramedian incision is fashioned, the more detrimental it is.

Subcostal incisions are advocated because they improve visibility for certain diseases in the upper abdomen. Although they combine some of the better features of the previous incisions, they offer the disadvantages of both. Lines of muscular pull, cutaneous innervation, and skin tension are all traversed, as with a vertical incision, whereas the possibility of extension in the case of misdiagnosis is compromised, as with a horizontal incision. A subcostal incision can be extended for liver transplants and exposure of the pancreas (a chevron incision).

Specific incisions are occasionally useful for specific diseases. The best example is the right lower quadrant McBurney incision for approach to the appendix. When a localized preoperative diagnosis is made, all of the benefits of this well-planned surgical incision can be realized. The transverse skin incision is in line with Langer's lines, and none of the cutaneous nerves, including the ilioinguinal and iliohypogastric, is disturbed. The precise location of McBurney's point, two-thirds of the distance from the umbilicus to the anterior iliac spine, allows the placement of a small incision immediately over the disease. The muscle layers are divided bluntly in line with their direction of pull, so herniation and disruption are rare. Once the peritoneum is closed, some claim that no further approximation of soft tissues is necessary for strong and cosmetic healing.

HERNIAS OF THE ABDOMINAL WALL

A hernia is the protrusion of any organ, structure, or portion thereof through its normal anatomic confines. In the abdominal wall, a hernia is the protrusion of all or part of any intraabdominal structure through any congenital, acquired, or iatrogenic defect. Whenever a hernia originates through a relatively small aperture, there is a risk of **incarceration**, which occurs when the contents of a hernia become entrapped and cannot be reduced back into the abdominal cavity. Incarceration of a hernia is the most common cause of bowel obstruction in people who have not had previous abdominal surgery. It is the second most common cause of small bowel obstruction (see Chapter 15, Small Intestine and Appendix, and Chapter 16, Colon, Rectum, and Anus). This entrapment can become so severe that the blood supply to or from the bowel is compromised (**strangulation**). The result is bowel necrosis. Strangulation should be suspected when there is erythema of the overlying skin or fever and elevated white blood cell count; this represents a true surgical emergency. Omentum or loops of bowel can remain incarcerated outside the abdominal wall for months or years without proceeding to strangulation; in general, chronic incarcerations are not painful nor do they cause an acute bowel obstruction. Acute incarcerations, on the other hand, are more troublesome, since they are more likely to result in strangulation. When a patient presents with an acute incarceration, one should attempt reduction and proceed with surgery urgently (or emergently if reduction is not possible).

Inguinal Hernias

Indirect Inguinal Hernia

Anatomy and Pathophysiology

An indirect inguinal hernia occurs when bowel, omentum, or another intraabdominal organ protrudes through the abdominal ring lateral to the epigastric vessels within the continuous peritoneal coverage of a patent processus vaginalis (Fig. 12-6). An indirect inguinal hernia is a congenital lesion; if the processus vaginalis does not remain patent, an **indirect hernia** cannot develop. Because 20% of male cadaver specimens retain some degree of processus vaginalis patency, patency of the processus vaginalis is necessary, but not sufficient, for hernia development. The medical history often yields the immediate reason for herniation (lifting a heavy object or coughing vigorously).

The indirect hernia has two close cousins in the groin, the hydroceles. The communicating hydrocele differs from the indirect hernia only in that no bowel has yet protruded into the groin. Instead, serous peritoneal fluid fills this peritoneal peninsula to whatever level the patency exists. Because there is free communication between the hydrocele and the peritoneal cavity, the fluid collection is greater after standing and less after recumbency, and it is significantly augmented by pathologic formation of ascites within the abdominal cavity. The noncommunicating hydrocele occurs when a small portion of the processus vaginalis adjacent to the testicle is not obliterated, but the remainder of the processus vaginalis between it and the peritoneal cavity is obliterated (Fig. 12-4). This results in a fluid-filled mass (hydrocele) in the scrotum that is unchanged by position or pressure.

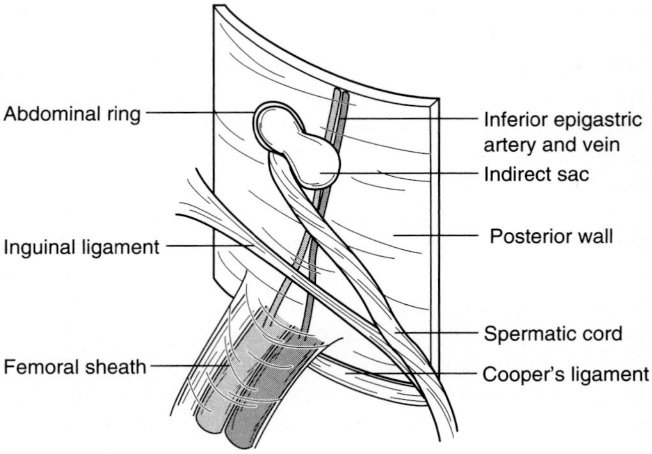

Figure 12-6 Indirect inguinal hernia. The posterior inguinal wall is intact. A hernia develops in the patent processus vaginalis (sac) on the anteromedial aspect of the cord. (In this figure and in Figures 12-7 and 12-8, the external oblique and internal oblique layers are not shown because they have no role in the development or repair of inguinal hernias.)

Clinical Presentation

Indirect hernias usually cause a bulge in the groin, typically as a result of increased abdominal pressure. A 20-year-old workman hoisting a refrigerator has adequate cause for making a previously undetected patent processus apparent. On the other hand, a 60-year-old man presenting with a new onset of a hernia should raise questions as to why this congenital lesion would appear at this late date. Often, chronic coughing from lung disease, straining at micturition from prostatism, or straining at defecation from a sigmoid obstruction causes an inguinal hernia. When obtaining a history from this patient, a thorough review of systems should be undertaken. Should he report any new symptoms such as cough or constipation, these symptoms should be investigated further. In the absence of related symptoms, most believe that extensive investigation of these organ systems at the time of hernia diagnosis is not warranted. Indirect hernias are the most common hernias in both sexes and all age groups (Table 12-1). They occur more commonly on the right because of delayed descent of that testicle.

Direct Inguinal Hernia

Anatomy and Pathophysiology

Unlike the serpentine course of the indirect hernia, the direct inguinal hernia proceeds directly through the poste-

Table 12-1 Approximate Relative Incidence of Hernia Type

	Direct	Indirect	Femoral
Men	40%	50%	10%
Women	Rare	70%	30%
Children	Rare	All	Rare

rior inguinal wall (Fig. 12-7). As opposed to indirect hernias, **direct hernias** protrude medial to the inferior epigastric vessels and are not associated with the processus vaginalis. The portion of the posterior inguinal wall through which a direct hernia occurs is **Hesselbach's triangle.** Its classic boundaries are the rectus sheath, inferior epigastric vessels, and inguinal ligament. They tend not to protrude with the cord into the scrotum and are generally believed to be acquired lesions, although there is considerable congenital variation in the strength of the posterior walls. Because they are acquired lesions, they are more common in older men. They occur over time as a result of pressure and tension on the muscle and fascia.

Clinical Presentation

Direct hernias, like indirect hernias, cause bulges in the groin. A spectrum of abnormality exists from very small-necked pedunculated herniations of preperitoneal fat (diverticular direct hernias) to large, bulging protrusions that destroy the entire posterior inguinal wall. As with all hernias, the larger the defect, the less likely the hernia is to incarcerate or strangulate.

Femoral Hernia

Anatomy and Pathophysiology

The third category of herniation in the groin is the **femoral hernia.** Like the direct hernia, it is an acquired lesion. Its etiology lies in a short medial attachment of the transversus abdominus muscle onto Cooper's ligament that results in an enlarged femoral ring that invites herniation (Fig. 12-8).

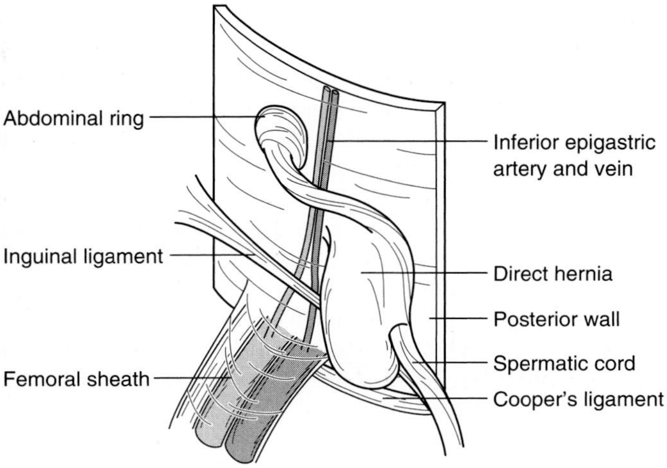

Figure 12-7 Direct inguinal hernia. The abdominal ring is intact. A hernia defect is a diffuse bulge in the posterior inguinal wall medial to the inferior epigastric vessels.

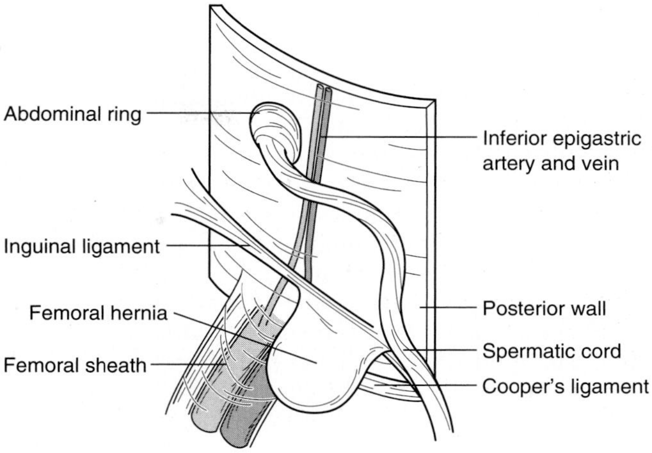

Figure 12-8 Femoral hernia. The defect is through the femoral canal, but otherwise involves similar structures and insertions as a direct inguinal hernia.

Clinical Presentation

On physical examination, femoral hernias cause bulges much lower in the groin than other hernias (below the inguinal ring and onto the anterior thigh). Despite maximal dilation from repeated protrusion, the femoral hernia ring is limited by rigid structures (the inguinal ligament, its lacunar attachments, and Cooper's ligament). Therefore, this hernia is very susceptible to incarceration and strangulation. Femoral hernias are often mistaken for lipomas or enlarged lymph nodes in the groin because they present as a mass inferior to the inguinal ligament.

Treatment

Groin hernias (direct, indirect, or femoral) are not curable by medical therapy, although palliation is sometimes sought with the use of a truss (not indicated for femoral hernias). A truss is a fist-sized ball of leather, rubber, or fabric that is positioned by the patient over the protruding hernia bulge and strapped in place with variously designed belts and straps. Hernia defects never close spontaneously, and the use of a truss can increase scarring. Given that inguinal hernias will not resolve on their own and have a perceived significant risk of strangulation, for several hundred years the teaching has been that the presence of a hernia is indication for repair. An in-depth review of the literature reveals a paucity of data on the risk of strangulation; it actually appears to be quite low (well below 0.1%). A careful risk–benefit analysis of hernia repair is therefore warranted. Some patients are at such high risk for complications from any invasive procedure that a truss may be the best approach. A patient with a small asymptomatic hernia may be best served by observation until the hernia becomes more symptomatic, given the known risk of chronic pain in 6% to 13% of patients undergoing hernia repair. A young patient whose livelihood depends on heavy lifting will likely need repair.

When an incarceration is encountered, a few gentle manual attempts at reduction (i.e., returning the entrapped organ to the confines of the abdominal cavity) are warranted. The patient should be placed in the Trendelenburg position (head-down) and given some pain medication for relaxation if necessary. Gentle steady pressure should be applied to the incarcerated hernia. The pressure should be applied in a cephalad, lateral, and slightly dorsal direction, understanding the course of the spermatic cord through the inguinal canal. Although these attempts are successful in only 60% to 70% of cases and are associated with some risk to the entrapped structure, they are justified by the potential benefits of patient comfort, relief of obstruction, and prevention of strangulation, and by the diagnostic information obtained.

The surgical repair of hernias is conceptually simple: (1) reduce any abdominal viscus to the abdominal cavity; (2) create a new, tension-free inguinal floor; (3) recreate a snug abdominal (internal) ring. Additionally, for indirect hernias, obliterate the processus vaginalis by either reduction back into the abdominal cavity or ligation of the processus at a point high against the abdominal wall; for femoral hernias, the femoral space must also be obliterated or covered with tissue or mesh.

Repair of Inguinal Hernias

In 2002, the Cochrane Group reviewed the literature regarding nonmesh (generally tension producing) and mesh repairs. This review of 20 randomized trials concluded that the use of mesh repair is associated with a 50% to 75% reduction in the risk of recurrence when compared to nonmesh repairs. There is also some evidence of quicker return to work and of lower rates of persisting pain among patients undergoing mesh repairs. In 2003, the Cochrane Group reviewed studies evaluating laparoscopic groin hernia repair. There were insufficient data to recommend one over the other, although the data suggest that pain is less and return to work is faster among patients undergoing laparoscopic repair. However, operation times were longer and there appeared to be a higher risk of serious (visceral or vascular injury) complications with laparoscopic repairs. Two large randomized trials in groin hernia repair are concluding at the time of this writing; however, data are not yet available. One trial evaluated laparoscopic versus open tension-free repair of groin hernias in nearly 2200 adult men. In this trial, laparoscopic repairs were associated with a 10% recurrence rate while open repairs had a 4% recurrence rate. The other trial is evaluating watchful waiting versus open tension-free repair in over 700 men; results will be available in early 2005. The current recommendations follow findings of the Cochrane review: in adult men, hernias should be repaired with mesh, whether the approach be laparoscopic or open. In women, since the round ligament can be ligated and the abdominal ring closed, the use of mesh can be reserved for those women with weak floors. In children with inguinal hernias, the hernia is repaired by high ligation (elimination) of the sac without muscle/fascia repair.

Mesh Repairs

There are many types of mesh repairs, but they differ by only two basic factors: (1) whether the mesh is placed on the "inside" (preperitoneally) or on the "outside" (anteriorly, i.e., on top of the internal oblique, but beneath the external oblique) and (2) how the space is accessed. The most commonly used mesh for groin hernia repairs is polypropylene (permanent). Of the many types of mesh repairs, only the most common ones are listed below.

Anterior Repairs

Lichtenstein Repair (Open). The Lichtenstein repair consists of placing a piece of mesh (currently recommended to be 3×6 inches in size) to repair the hernia. A slit is cut in the mesh to accommodate the spermatic cord. The mesh is sewn with a nonabsorbable running suture to the inguinal ligament, starting 2 cm medial to the pubic tubercle. Two interrupted sutures are used to tack the mesh superiorly and superior-laterally. A third interrupted suture is used to recreate the abdominal ring, suturing the inferior edge of each mesh tail to the inguinal ligament just lateral to the level of the abdominal ring. At least 6 cm of mesh tail are then tucked up underneath the external oblique fascia laterally.

Mesh-Plug Repair (Open). This repair uses a plug that looks a bit like a partially opened umbrella. The plug is placed in the defect (tip of the umbrella goes in first) and sewn in place. The plug can be used with or without an onlay piece of mesh similar to the Lichtenstein repair.

Preperitoneal Repairs

Stoppa Repair (Open). The Stoppa or preperitoneal repair places a very large piece of mesh in the preperitoneal space. The access to this space is through a transverse incision above the groin. This is the same repair as the extraperitoneal laparoscopic repair, aside from the access (through big incision for this repair, through several small incisions for the laparoscopic repair).

Kugel Repair (Open). This repair uses a piece of mesh that has been reinforced around the edges so that it will open and stay open once in place. The preperitoneal space is accessed through a small incision over the abdominal ring. The preperitoneal space is dissected using blunt finger dissection. The oval piece of reinforced mesh is then placed into this space. It does not require suturing because the pressure of the abdominal contents holds it in place against the posterior lower abdominal wall.

TEP Repair (Laparoscopic). The TEP (totally extraperitoneal) repair is a laparoscopic repair wherein the entire repair is done without entering the peritoneal cavity. The preperitoneal space is accessed by opening the ante-

THE HERNIA TEACHER

BARRY D. MANN, MD
Anne Seidman
Medical College of Pennsylvania
and Hahnemann University

First take Pretest below.
Then fold along fold A
Fold along fold B
Cut along dotted lines C & D until "Stop Cut".

To perform a right inguinal hernia repair, turn to Frame **1** and follow directions.

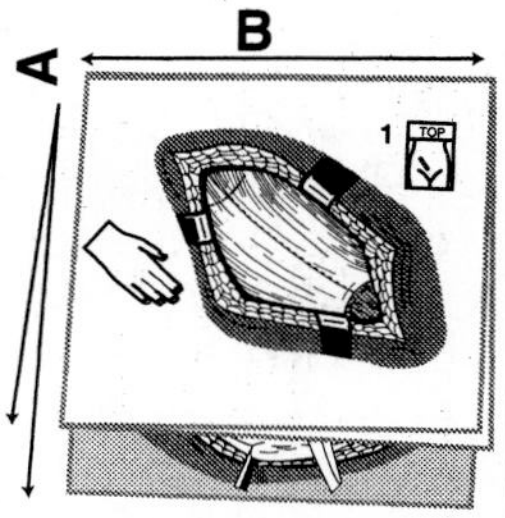

8

Circle T or F	Pre-test	Post-test
1. The fibers of the "conjoined tendon" separate to form the external (superficial) ring.	T F	T F
2. The cremasteric fibers invest the structures of the spermatic cord.	T F	T F
3. The illoinguinal nerve innervates the lateral thigh.	T F	T F
4. A direct sac is more closely adherent to the spermatic vessels than an indirect sac.	T F	T F
5. A finger placed through an indirect hernia sac should slip into the peritoneal cavity.	T F	T F
6. High ligation of a direct hernia sac is required for proper hernia repair.	T F	T F
7. A synthetic mesh sutured in place underneath the cord yields a satistactory hernia repair.	T F	T F
8. The origin of an indirect hernia is medial to the epigastric vessels.	T F	T F
9. The inguinal ligament is actually an extension of the external oblique aponeurosis.	T F	T F
10.Cooper's lig. is part of the "conjoined tendon".	T F	T F

FOLD B

1

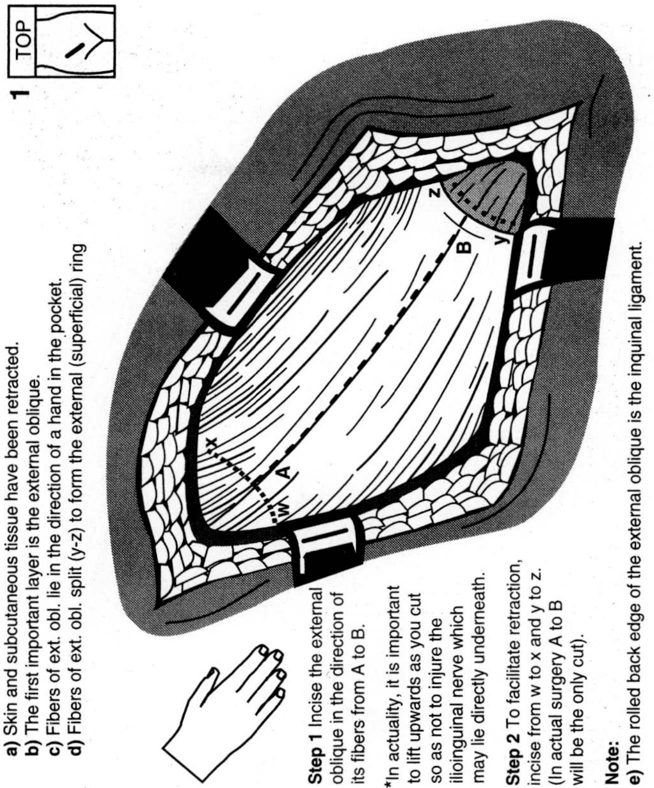

Note:
a) Skin and subcutaneous tissue have been retracted.
b) The first important layer is the external oblique.
c) Fibers of ext. obl. lie in the direction of a hand in the pocket.
d) Fibers of ext. obl. split (y-z) to form the external (superficial) ring

Step 1 Incise the external oblique in the direction of its fibers from A to B.

*In actuality, it is important to lift upwards as you cut so as not to injure the ilioinguinal nerve which may lie directly underneath.

Step 2 To facilitate retraction, incise from w to x and y to z. (In actual surgery A to B will be the only cut).

Note:
e) The rolled back edge of the external oblique is the inguinal ligament.

stop cut C

FOLD A

stop cut D

4

k) In this drawing, your finger has replaced the penrose drain. You are now teasing away the cremasteric fibers with a scissors. When this maneuver is complete (Frame **5**), you will have "skeletonized" the cord revealing ① *the vessels to the testicle*, ② *the vas deferens* (white), and ③ an *indirect sac* if one is present.

Turn to Frame **5**, orient to **TOP** and identify these items.

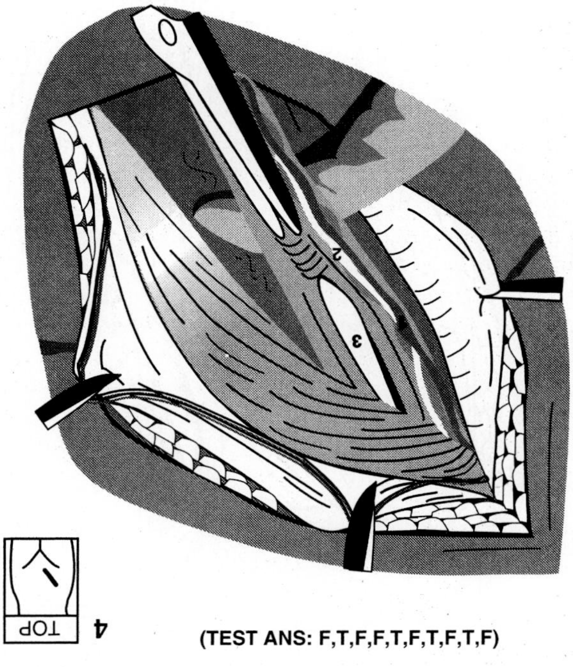

5

l) The Penrose drain now retracts the vessels and vas deferens (white)

Step 5 Mobilize the indirect sac which lies antero-medial to the cord by incising dotted line from **G** to **H**

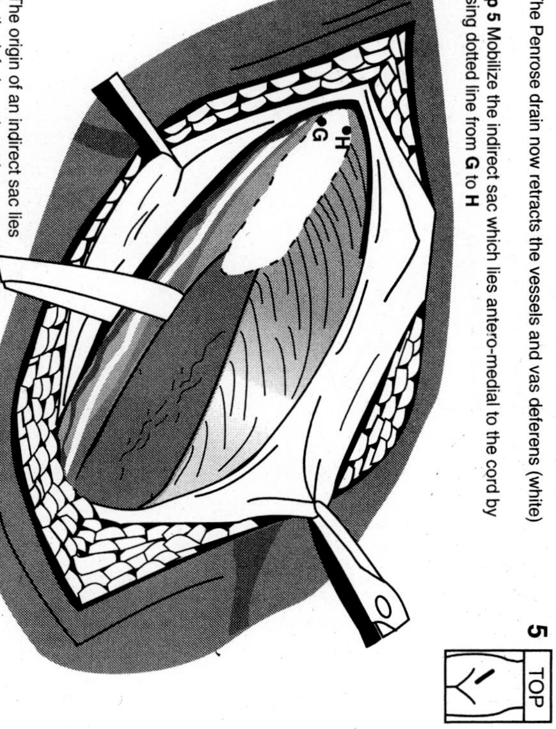

Note: The origin of an indirect sac lies lateral to the inferior epigastric vessels seen underneath (in Frame **7**)

Turn to Frame **6** and orient to TOP

(TEST ANS: F,T,F,F,T,F,T,F,T,F)

Figure 12-9 The Hernia Teacher. *continues*

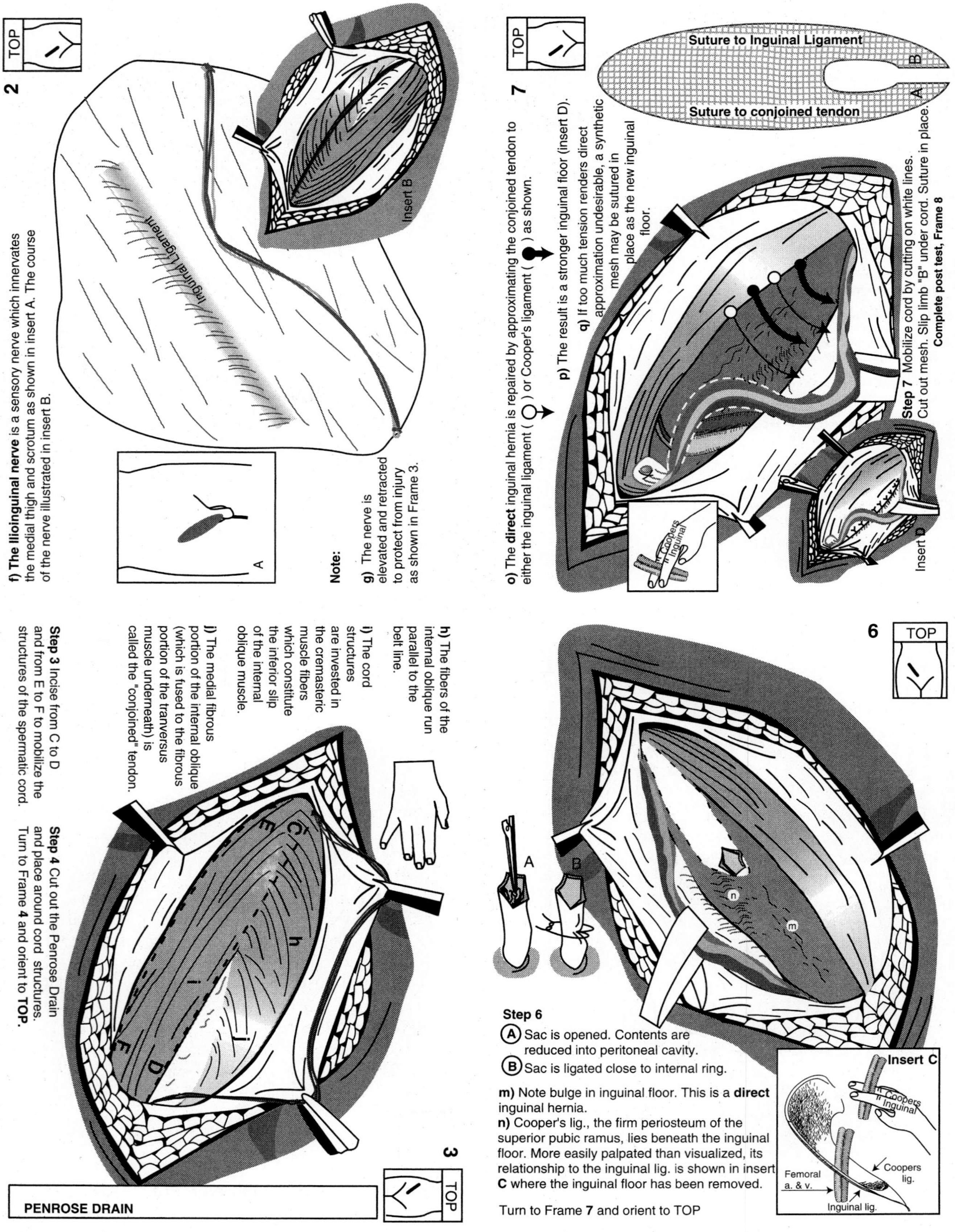
2
TOP
f) The Ilioinguinal nerve is a sensory nerve which innervates the medial thigh and scrotum as shown in insert A. The course of the nerve illustrated in insert B.
Inguinal Ligament
Insert B
A
Note:
g) The nerve is elevated and retracted to protect from injury as shown in Frame 3.
3
TOP
h) The fibers of the internal oblique run parallel to the belt line.
i) The cord structures are invested in the cremasteric muscle fibers which constitute the inferior slip of the internal oblique muscle.
j) The medial fibrous portion of the internal oblique (which is fused to the fibrous portion of the tranversus muscle underneath) is called the "conjoined" tendon.
Step 3 Incise from C to D and from E to F to mobilize the structures of the spermatic cord.
Step 4 Cut out the Penrose Drain and place around cord structures. Turn to Frame 4 and orient to TOP.
PENROSE DRAIN
6
TOP
A
B
n
m
Step 6
(A) Sac is opened. Contents are reduced into peritoneal cavity.
(B) Sac is ligated close to internal ring.
m) Note bulge in inguinal floor. This is a direct inguinal hernia.
n) Cooper's lig., the firm periosteum of the superior pubic ramus, lies beneath the inguinal floor. More easily palpated than visualized, its relationship to the inguinal lig. is shown in insert C where the inguinal floor has been removed.
Turn to Frame 7 and orient to TOP
Insert C
Coopers
Inguinal
Femoral a. & v.
Coopers lig.
Inguinal lig.
7
TOP
o) The direct inguinal hernia is repaired by approximating the conjoined tendon to either the inguinal ligament ( ) or Cooper's ligament ( ) as shown.
p) The result is a stronger inguinal floor (insert D).
q) If too much tension renders direct approximation undesirable, a synthetic mesh may be sutured in place as the new inguinal floor.
Suture to Inguinal Ligament
Suture to conjoined tendon
A
B
Coopers
Inguinal
Insert D
Step 7 Mobilize cord by cutting on white lines. Cut out mesh. Slip limb "B" under cord. Suture in place.
Complete post test, Frame 8

Figure 12-9 *continued*

rior rectus fascia just to one side of midline (usually the side to be repaired). The muscle is retracted laterally, and sliding a finger inferiorly along the posterior aspect of the rectus gives access to the preperitoneal space. The space is further developed using a balloon that is inflated in the space. A laparoscope camera is then placed through this incision. Trochars are placed through two other incisions; these then serve as working ports. Laparoscopic instruments are used to reduce the hernia sac back into the preperitoneal space, and then a large piece of mesh is placed and tacked with metal clips to prevent slippage.

TAPP Repair (Laparoscopic). The TAPP (transabdominal preperitoneal) repair is similar to the TEP except that the access to the preperitoneal space is gained by incising the peritoneum after placing a laparoscope into the peritoneal space. The peritoneum is reflected down and the hernia sac is reduced. The mesh is placed and tacked in the same locations, and then the peritoneum is brought back up over the mesh.

Classic Repairs

The following section is presented only for the sake of completeness. Most classic repairs are no longer performed. All are open repairs.

Marcy Repair. The Marcy repair is popular in very small or early indirect hernias. Because these hernias represent only a dilation of the abdominal ring, the Marcy repair simply makes snug that aperture by sewing the transversus aponeurosis on the lateral side of the ring to the transversus aponeurosis on the medial side of the ring until that layer is snug around the cord.

McVay (Cooper's Ligament) Repair. The McVay procedure is an anatomic repair, like the Marcy operation, that is used for larger indirect hernias and direct hernias. The principle of this repair is that when the posterior inguinal wall is destroyed by the hernia, the surgical repair of that wall should be as close as possible to the original anatomy. The strong transversus aponeurosis is sewn to Cooper's ligament, along that tendon's natural insertions and the anterior femoral sheath.

Bassini Repair. The Bassini repair is a more superficial repair in which margins of transversus and internal oblique muscles are anchored inferiorly to the inguinal ligament.

Halsted Repair. The Halsted repair is similar to a McVay repair except that the external oblique fascia is closed underneath the spermatic cord. It is important to know this when reoperating on these patients from an anterior approach. The cord will be in the subcutaneous tissue, literally unprotected by the external oblique fascia.

Shouldice Repair. The Shouldice repair incorporates a series of four running suture lines that approximate and imbricate the transversus aponeurosis to several lateral structures. In a sense, this procedure combines a deep repair similar to McVay's with a superficial repair similar to Bassini's.

Cut-Out Exercise

The authors of this chapter recognize that inguinal anatomy is complicated. Traditionally, an "open" hernia repair is considered a junior-level case. However, this classification seems to be based on the relatively low risk to vital structures, not the anatomic simplicity of the operation.

The cut-out exercise included in this chapter (Fig. 12-9) is an attempt to simplify the three-dimensional aspects of inguinal anatomy, which are important as surgical considerations. The exercise illustrates the concept of primary repair and allows the student to cut out a mesh and place it under the cord as in the basic Lichtenstein repair. All terms and concepts used within the exercise are compatible with the information delivered in this chapter.

We recommend that you carefully remove from the book the page containing the exercise, take the pretest, and then fold and cut the page as directed. Taking the posttest should convince you that you have improved your understanding. (The correct answers are listed on the obverse side of the "Penrose Drain.") We believe that working through this exercise, particularly before scrubbing on a hernia repair, will be of great benefit.

Umbilical Hernias

Anatomy and Pathophysiology

Like groin hernias, **umbilical hernias** are of three types. By far the most common is fortunately of least significance and threat to the patient. It is the small (usually < 1 cm) defect in the abdominal wall that results from incomplete umbilical closure. Through this fascial defect can protrude small portions of omentum, bowel, or other intraabdominal organs. In adults, even if umbilical closure occurred, the umbilical scar is subject to stretching and defects that can enlarge and produce a hernia. The other two types of abdominal wall herniation are much more severe, affect only the newborn, and, fortunately, are very uncommon. An omphalocele occurs when, after incomplete closure of the abdominal wall by the time of birth, a portion of the abdominal contents herniates into the base of the umbilical cord. Unlike the simple umbilical hernia, which is covered by skin, in omphalocele the abdominal contents are separated from the outside world by only a thin membrane of peritoneum and the amnion. Gastroschisis is an even more severe failure of abdominal wall development. It causes a full-thickness abdominal wall defect lateral to the umbilicus. The hernia of gastroschisis is into the amniotic cavity, so there is no sac. There is no covering of any kind over the intestinal contents, which protrude from the lateral edge of the umbilicus. (See Chapter 3, Pediatric Surgery, in Lawrence et al., eds., *Essentials of Surgical Specialties*, 3rd Ed.)

Clinical Presentation

Because the developmental process of the abdominal wall continues into extrauterine life, small protrusions of this type are very common in infants. Unless incarceration occurs, they are best ignored until the preschool years, and most resolve spontaneously. Despite their innocuous nature in infancy, however, umbilical hernias are some threat in adulthood. The rigid surrounding walls of the linea alba predispose the patient to incarceration and strangulation of protruded organs. Omphaloceles and gastroschisis, however, are perinatal emergencies that require immediate surgical attention. (See Chapter 3, Pediatric Surgery, in Lawrence et al., eds., *Essentials of Surgical Specialties*, 3rd Ed.)

Treatment

Commonly used folk remedies (e.g., stuffing cotton balls into the umbilicus, taping coins over it to prevent protrusion) only delay developmental closure or complicate the hernia with necrosis of the overlying skin. The treatment of umbilical hernia is as straightforward in concept as that of groin hernia: (1) reduce the abdominal contents and (2) establish the continuity of the abdominal wall. The surgical procedures for a simple umbilical hernia are as straightforward in execution as they are in concept. In adults with defects less than 1.5 cm in diameter, a primary repair (placing sutures to close the defect) is generally recommended. For defects larger than 1.5 cm, a mesh repair is recommended, since the recurrence rate for mesh repairs when the defect is larger is about half that of nonmesh repairs.

By necessity, surgical therapy for omphalocele and gastroschisis is intricate and complex, including bowel resection and the formation of extraanatomic compartments fashioned of prosthetic materials. Despite these efforts, the mortality rate for these lesions remains high. (See Chapter 3, Pediatric Surgery, in Lawrence et al., eds., *Essentials of Surgical Specialties*, 3rd Ed.)

Incisional (Ventral) Hernias

Anatomy and Pathophysiology

Incisional hernias can develop through any prior fascial incision. Deep wound infection is the most common cause of incisional hernias, although other factors such as obesity, steroid dependence, and number of prior operations may play a role. Incisional hernias are usually diagnosed by visualization of a bulge with an associated palpable fascial defect. In obese patients, an abdominal computed tomography (CT) scan may be needed to diagnose an incisional hernia. The patient may complain of the bulge, pain, or discomfort at the site. The patient can also present with a bowel obstruction if the hernia becomes acutely incarcerated. The risk of incarceration and strangulation is higher with smaller defects. Some patients develop extremely large incisional hernias, often after a prolonged hospital course with multiple abdominal operations. Their defects can be classified as "loss of the abdominal domain." These defects present a challenge to repair.

Treatment

Most incisional hernias will require repair with mesh. As with groin hernias, this repair can be performed via either an open or a laparoscopic approach. The "best" approach in terms of recurrence and patient-centered outcomes is yet to be determined. Whether the repair is open or laparoscopic, several principles are important: (1) avoid injury to intraabdominal structures, (2) create a tension-free repair, (3) overlap mesh onto fascia by 2 to 3 cm. If mesh is used, it can be placed either preperitoneally (between peritoneum and muscle) or on top of the muscles layers. The mesh is often secured around the periphery with tacking sutures placed through stab incisions in the skin. These tacking sutures are brought through all layers of the abdominal wall, through the mesh, then back through mesh and abdominal wall and tied (Fig. 12-10). The stab wounds are closed with surgical adhesive tape strips (Steri-Strips).

Component separation is an alternate to mesh repair of incisional hernias. There are several variations, but most involve making incisions through one or two fascial layers of the lateral abdominal wall. This allows approximation of the midline fascia medially. Defects less than 5 cm wide

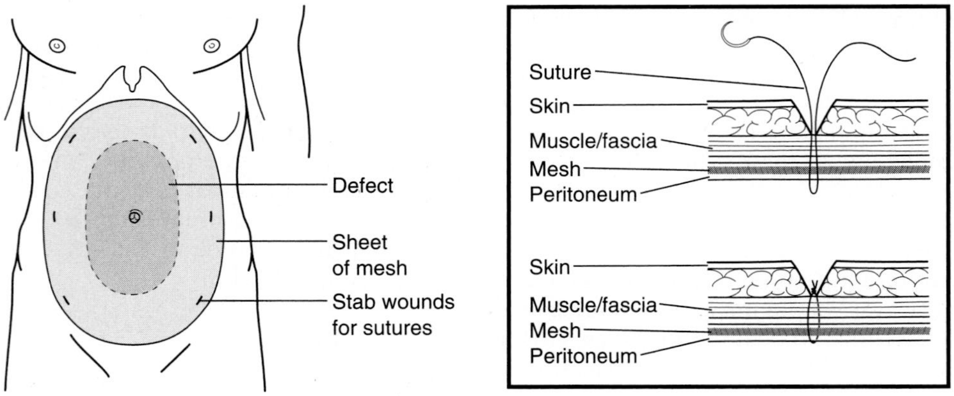

Figure 12-10 Incisional hernia repair. The mesh is secured around the periphery with tacking sutures placed through stab incisions in the skin and is brought through all layers of the abdominal wall, through the mesh, and then back through the mesh and abdominal wall. The sutures are then tied.

in the upper and lower abdomen and 10 cm wide in the midabdomen are amenable to closure with component separation. Larger defects will require mesh because there is a limit on how far the muscles and fascia can be mobilized without causing a defect elsewhere.

Repairs of incisional hernias are associated with a recurrence rate of about 10%. The risk of recurrence increases with each subsequent repair.

Other Hernias

Spigelian Hernia

Spigelian hernias are herniations through the semilunar line, which is the lateral margin of the rectus muscle, at or just below the junction with the semicircular line of Douglas. Unlike groin hernias, these hernias lie cephalad to the inferior epigastric vessels. The tight aponeurotic defect predisposes them to incarceration.

Grynfelt's Hernia

Grynfelt's hernia is a wide-mouthed hernia that protrudes through the superior lumbar triangle, which is bounded by the sacrospinalis muscle, the internal oblique muscle, and the inferior margin of the 12th rib. Diagnosis is hampered by the protrusion of these hernias under the latissimus dorsi muscle.

Petit's Hernia

Petit's hernia protrudes through the inferior lumbar triangle, which is bounded by the lateral margin of the latissimus dorsi, the medial margin of the external oblique, and the iliac crest. Like the superior lumbar hernia, these hernias are broad, bulging hernias that usually do not incarcerate.

Richter's Hernia

Richter's hernia is a hernia at any site through which only a portion of the circumference of a bowel wall, usually the jejunum, incarcerates or strangulates. Because the entire lumen is not compromised, symptoms of bowel obstruction can be absent, despite gangrene of the strangulated portion.

Littre's Hernia

Any groin hernia that contains a Meckel's diverticulum is Littre's hernia. This type of hernia is usually incarcerated or strangulated.

Armand's Hernia

Any groin hernia that contains the appendix is an Armand's hernia. Appendicitis can develop and presents a confusing clinical picture.

Obturator Hernia

Obturator hernias are deceptive hernias, often of Richter's type, that protrude through the obturator canal. They are much more common in women and usually occur in the seventh and eighth decades. An obturator hernia is classically diagnosed by the symptoms of intermittent bowel obstruction and paresthesias on the anteromedial aspect of the thigh as a result of compression of the obturator nerve (Howship-Romberg sign). The hernia can sometimes be palpated as a mass on rectal exam.

Hesselbach's Hernia

Like a femoral hernia, Hesselbach's hernia protrudes onto the thigh beneath the inguinal ligament, but courses lateral to the femoral vessels

Pantaloon Hernia

The **pantaloon hernia** is the simultaneous occurrence of a direct and an indirect hernia. The pantaloon hernia causes two bulges that straddle the inferior epigastric vessels.

Sliding Hernia

A **sliding hernia** is any hernia in which a portion of the wall of the protruding peritoneal sac is made up of some intraabdominal organ (usually sigmoid, cecum, ovary, or bladder). As the sac expands, the organ is drawn out, into the hernia. Its repair involves the careful return of the organ to the abdominal cavity, followed by the traditional sequence of obliteration of the sac and closure of the fascial defect.

Epigastric Hernia

An epigastric hernia, which is due to congenital or acquired weakness of the midline linea alba, protrudes through the crossing fibers of the linea alba above the umbilicus. It is more common in men than in women, and 20% of epigastric hernias are multiple.

Diastasis Recti

Diastasis recti is not a true hernia because it is only a fascial weakness, not a fascial defect. It occurs when the rectus muscles separate in the upper midline, making a wide linea alba. When the patient contracts the recti (for instance, when trying to sit up), this widening can be mistaken for a hernia because it does cause a bulge. Because the rate of recurrence after hernia repair is so large, these patients should just be reassured.

SUGGESTED READINGS

Anson BJ, McVay CB. The anatomy of the inguinal region. *Surg Gynecol Obstet* 1960;111:707.

Bassini E. Sulla cura radicale dell'ernia inguinale. *Arch Soc Ital Chir* 1887a;4:380. [Summarized by G Lusena in *La Societa Italiana di Chirurgia Nei Suio 30 Congressi (1883–1923)*. Rome, Italy: Manuzio, 1934:284.]

Lichtenstein IL, Shulmen AG, Amid PK, et al. The tension-free hernioplasty. *Am J Surg* 1989;157(3):188–193.

McCormack K, Scott NW, Go PM, et al. Laparoscopic techniques versus open techniques for inguinal hernia repair. *Cochrane Database Syst Rev* 2003;(1):CD001785.

McVay CB, Chapp JD. Inguinal and femoral hernioplasty: the evaluation of a basic concept. *Ann Surg* 1958;148:499.

Scott NW, McCormack K, Graham P, et al. Open mesh versus non-mesh repair of femoral and inguinal hernia. *Cochrane Database Syst Rev* 2002;(4):CD002197.

Shouldice EE. Surgical treatment of hernia. *Ont Med Rev* 1945;4:43.

Stoker DL, Spiegelhalter DJ, Singh R, et al. Laparoscopic versus open hernia repair. *Lancet* 1994;343:1243.

Toy F, Smoot R. Laparoscopic hernioplasty update. *J Laparoendosc Surg* 1992;2(5):197–205.

13

HIRAM C. POLK, JR., MD ■ MARY C. MANCINI, MD, PHD
JAMES A. MCCOY, MD

Esophagus

OBJECTIVES

1. Describe the anatomic and physiologic factors that predispose to reflux esophagitis.
2. Describe the techniques for examining the esophagus.
3. Describe esophageal hiatal hernia with regard to anatomic type (sliding and paraesophageal) and the relative need for treatment.
4. Describe the symptoms of reflux esophagitis, and discuss the diagnostic procedures needed to confirm the diagnosis.
5. List the indications for operative management of esophageal reflux. Discuss the physiologic basis for the antireflux procedure used.
6. Describe the pathophysiology and clinical symptoms associated with achalasia of the esophagus. Briefly outline the management options.
7. Describe the radiologic findings that characterize motility disorders of the esophagus, including achalasia. Discuss manometric evaluation of the lower esophageal sphincter.
8. List the common esophageal diverticula in terms of their location, symptoms, and pathogenesis.
9. List the two major cell types of esophageal cancers.
10. List the known etiologic factors for esophageal cancers.
11. List the symptoms that suggest esophageal malignancy.
12. Describe the natural history of a malignant lesion of the esophagus, and list the treatment options in the order of preference.
13. Outline a plan for diagnostic evaluation of a patient with a suspected esophageal tumor.
14. List the diagnostic modalities that are helpful in staging esophageal neoplasms.
15. Describe the etiology and presentation of traumatic perforation of the esophagus and the physical findings that occur early and late after this type of injury.
16. Describe the risk factors for spontaneous perforation of the esophagus.
17. Describe the diagnostic and management strategies for spontaneous esophageal perforations.

The esophagus provides a conduit for the passage of orally ingested material from the mouth and into the upper stomach. An important secondary function is to permit emesis of material, either because it is toxic or because the distal alimentary tract cannot provide for timely prograde passage. The esophagus also provides a conduit for endoscopic evaluation of the upper alimentary tract, including the biliary and pancreatic ducts. It also allows evaluation of the heart and thoracic aorta by transesophageal ultrasound and echocardiography. Common problems that affect the esophagus and require a physician's attention are hiatal hernia and **reflux esophagitis**, esophageal motility disorders, cancer, and occasional esophageal disruption. Esophageal atresia is addressed in the Pediatric Surgery chapter (See Chapter 3, Pediatric Surgery, in Lawrence et al., eds., *Essentials of Surgical Specialties*, 3rd Ed.).

ANATOMY

The esophagus is a muscular tube that originates at the cricoid cartilage and pharynx in the neck. It traverses the posterior mediastinum behind the aortic arch and left

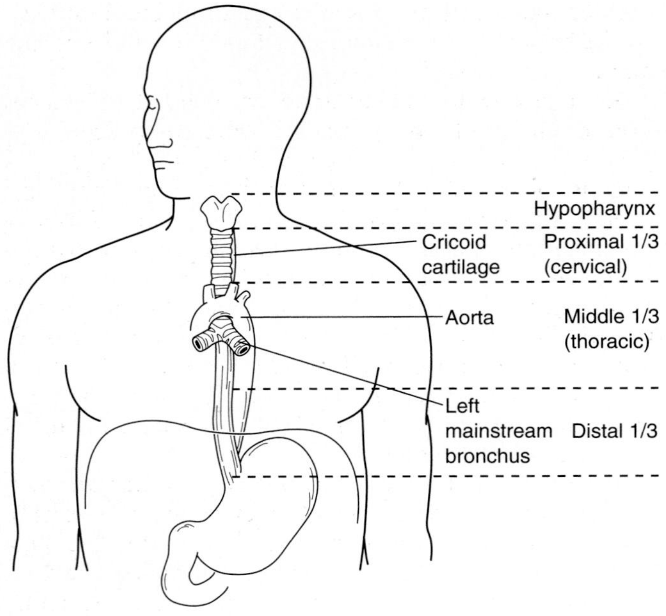

Figure 13-1 Clinical divisions of the esophagus.

mainstem bronchus to enter the abdominal cavity through the esophageal hiatus of the diaphragm. In most adults, a very short (< 3 cm) segment of true esophagus lies within the abdominal cavity before it joins with the fundus of the stomach (Fig. 13-1).

The esophagus has a mucosal layer, which consists of stratified squamous epithelium and occasional mucous glands, and two muscular layers. The inner muscular layer is oriented in a circular fashion, and the outer layer is oriented longitudinally. In contrast to the remainder of the gastrointestinal tract, there is no serosal layer. The significance of this anatomic relationship is apparent when considering the extension of neoplasms that originate in the esophagus, the relative ease with which the esophagus can be perforated during instrumentation, and the difficulty associated with surgical reconstruction after resection. The musculature of the upper one-third of the esophagus is skeletal, and that of the lower two-thirds is smooth muscle. Although the division between striated and smooth muscle cannot be determined precisely by histologic examination, the entire esophagus functions in a coordinated and sophisticated fashion. One physiologic sphincter is located in the neck (**upper esophageal sphincter**). The other is located at the level of the diaphragm (**lower esophageal sphincter**). Distinct muscle fibers with specialized sphincter function cannot be identified at this lower position. However, the peritoneal reflection that surrounds the esophageal hiatus and the phrenoesophageal ligament function together to produce an area of relatively high pressure with respect to the remainder of the esophagus and the stomach, which is located just distally.

PHYSIOLOGY

The motility of the distal esophageal sphincter has been studied widely, and the understanding thereof is growing rapidly. The esophagus is an active organ rather than a passive tube. When food enters the upper esophagus, it is

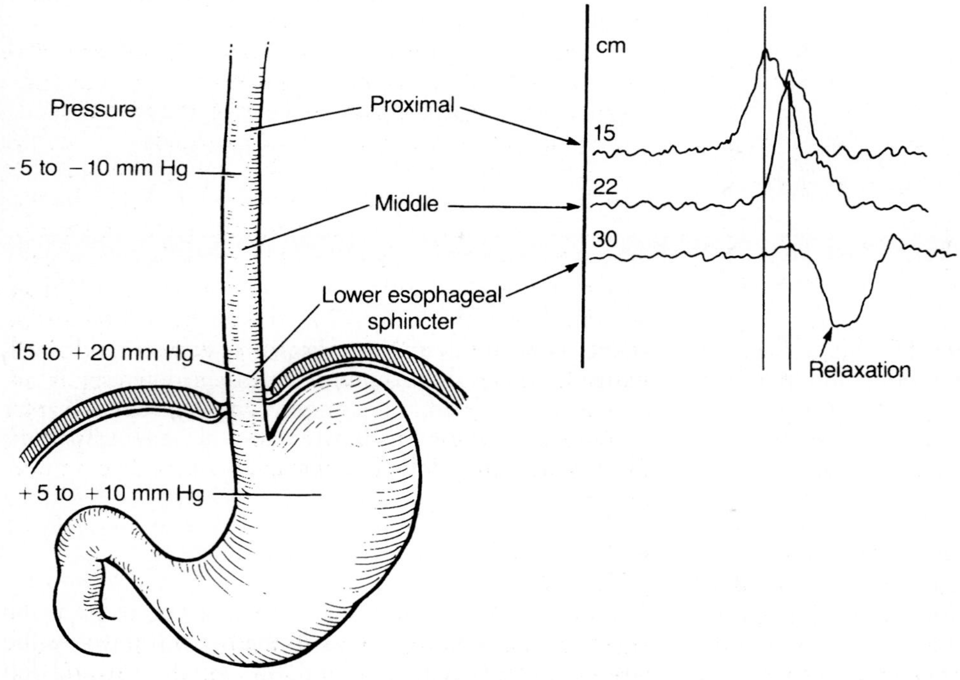

Figure 13-2 Manometry of a normal swallow. Note the progression of the primary peristaltic wave and the appropriate "relaxation" of the lower esophageal sphincter.

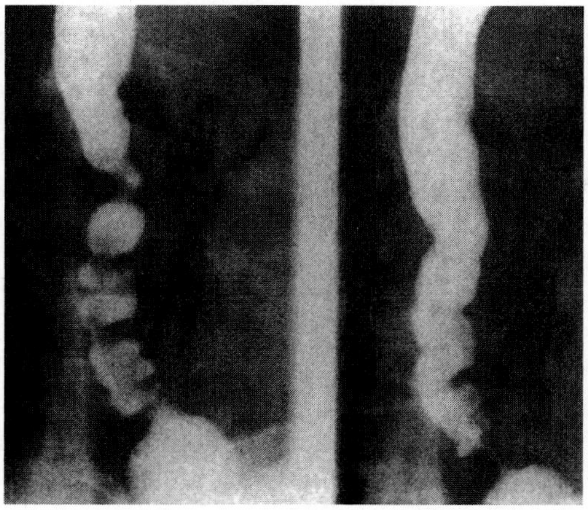

Figure 13-3 Barium swallow showing severe esophageal dysmotility with tertiary contractions in association with sliding hiatal hernia.

propelled down the esophagus by a peristaltic wave. Figure 13-2 shows the coordination of contraction and relaxation in the esophagus. The lower esophageal sphincter relaxes in anticipation of the food bolus, allowing the food to enter the stomach. The lower esophageal sphincter then returns to its normal high resting pressure of 15 to 25 cm H_2O greater than the pressure in the stomach to prevent reflux. Normally, swallowing a bolus of food causes a primary **peristaltic wave**. Secondary waves occur if the food is not cleared from the esophagus. Tertiary waves are abnormal and represent nonpropulsive "fibrillation" of the esophagus (Fig. 13-3).

PATHOPHYSIOLOGY

The purpose of the lower esophageal sphincter is to prevent the reflux of gastric content. However, unlike other sphincter mechanisms with well-defined circular muscle fibers (e.g., pylorus), this sphincter relies on a special anatomic relationship to accomplish this goal. Disturbances of this rather precarious relationship allow for the reflux of acid gastric content onto a sensitive, unprotected epithelial surface that is rich in sensory innervation. Conversely, failure of this lower sphincter to "relax" appropriately can result in proximal dilation of this muscular tube, which is not confined by a serosal layer, and can result in disordered contractility.

CLINICAL PRESENTATION AND EVALUATION

Detecting esophageal disorders requires meticulous attention to the symptoms described by the patient, because they may be manifestations of disease in other organ systems (e.g., angina pectoris or asthma) or signs of a systemic problem (e.g., collagen vascular or neurologic disorders). To better assess the patient, the student should become familiar with several terms.

Difficulty with the transition of ingested substances from the mouth to the stomach is called **dysphagia**. The patient usually complains that food becomes "stuck" and often is able to define the point of obstruction. Dysphagia occurs with both liquids and solids, and pain is usually not a component of the process. **Odynophagia** is painful swallowing. It may occur secondary to esophageal infection (e.g., *Candida* esophagitis, Cytomegalovirus, or herpesvirus infection), a foreign body in the esophagus, or injury to the esophagus. **Globus hystericus** is a "lump in the throat"; these patients must be evaluated carefully because the sensation may represent a mass lesion and not a psychological symptom.

Heartburn is also known as **pyrosis** or **water brash.** It is associated with gastroesophageal reflux disease (GERD), achalasia, and esophageal strictures. In exploring the diagnosis of GERD, it is best to allow patients to describe their symptom complex in their own words. Heartburn that spontaneously disappears over a period of months without therapy may be a sign of a severe disease process (e.g., esophageal stricture or carcinoma).

Regurgitation is the passive return of ingested material into the oropharynx. **Vomiting** is the active return of stomach contents to the oropharynx.

Recurrent episodes of bronchitis or pneumonia, particularly in the very young and the elderly, may be signs of recurrent aspiration of esophageal or gastric contents because of esophageal obstruction, congenital malformation, diverticula, or esophageal motility disorders. Esophageal disease must also be considered in the differential diagnosis of anemia and bleeding. Ulcerative esophagitis is the most common cause of esophageal bleeding and usually causes occult blood in the stool.

Hiccup, or **singultus,** is a sign of diaphragmatic irritation and may indicate a diaphragmatic hernia, acute gastric dilation, or subendocardial myocardial infarction.

Esophageal disease may cause signs and symptoms that are often indistinguishable from those of angina pectoris. Some historical features may help to differentiate between the two disease processes. Symptoms related to the esophagus are typically aggravated by changes in body position, particularly bending over. The symptoms are relieved by belching and only marginally relieved by nitroglycerin. Nitroglycerin relieves the symptoms of diffuse esophageal spasm. Usually, other symptoms related to the esophagus can be elicited from the patient. In any case, cardiac and esophageal evaluation must proceed simultaneously since myocardial ischemia and esophagitis are both common diseases.

EXAMINATION OF THE ESOPHAGUS

After a careful history is obtained, a physical examination is performed. Particular attention is paid to the oropharynx, neck, and supraclavicular regions. The stool is checked for occult blood. Subsequent diagnostic studies are directed by the patient's symptoms and the differential diagnosis. Posteroanterior and lateral chest radiographs are obtained to eliminate other thoracic pathology. Contrast studies with barium (e.g., barium swallow, cine-esophagram) are safe, highly cost-effective, and efficient methods for evaluating esophageal anatomy and function. Computed tomography (CT) scan of the chest is useful in examining the esophagus in relation to other anatomic structures in the thorax and in assessing the status of the mediastinum, particularly in esophageal cancer. Magnetic resonance imaging (MRI) provides no advantage over CT imaging in esophageal disease. Esophagoscopy allows for direct visualization of the esophageal lumen and is an indispensable diagnostic and therapeutic tool. With esophagoscopy, tumor specimens may be obtained for biopsy and varices may be occluded with sclerosing agents or devices.

Manometry and fluoroscopy are used to diagnose uncommon abnormalities in esophageal motility. Esophageal manometry measures changes in pressure of the upper and lower esophageal sphincters as well as in the body of the esophagus, providing a quantitative assessment of esophageal motility. In addition to assessing peristalsis, manometry can identify the normal cricopharyngeal and lower esophageal sphincters and determine whether they function normally. To determine the chemical basis of GERD, pH monitoring may be used, but it is not often needed clinically.

HIATAL HERNIA AND GASTROESOPHAGEAL REFLUX DISEASE

The two major types of hiatal hernia are type I, "sliding," and type II, paraesophageal or "rolling" (Fig. 13-4). Sliding hiatal hernias are 100 times more common than paraesophageal hernias. A sliding hernia allows the gastroesophageal junction and a portion of the stomach to "slide" into the mediastinum. A true sliding hernia involves the retroperitoneal portion of the proximal stomach. This type of hernia is physiologically significant only when it is associated with the reflux of gastric acid into the lower esophagus. With a paraesophageal hiatal hernia, the esophagogastric junction is in a normal position, and pure reflux is uncommon. The portion of the gastric fundus that herniates alongside the esophagus is prone to **incarceration** or **strangulation**, much like inguinal hernias. Like a true **hernia**, the fundus of the stomach is inside a sac of peritoneum. The medical treatment or surgical repair of a type I hiatal hernia depends on the degree of acid reflux and the resulting symptoms. In contrast, like any other hernia, a paraesophageal (type II) hiatal hernia should be surgically repaired on discovery to preclude incarceration or strangulation. A type III hiatal hernia is a combination of the elements of types I and II. It is usually a very large defect in the esophageal hiatus. Other abdominal organs may be found in the mediastinum with the stomach. Surgical repair is usually indicated.

In Western society, hiatal hernia occurs predominantly in women who have been pregnant and in men and women with increased intraabdominal pressure. Type I hiatal hernia with reflux is often found in patients who are overweight. Most investigators believe that increased intraabdominal pressure predisposes patients to reflux of gastric acid into the distal esophagus.

Although it is tempting to ascribe reflux to the presence of hiatal hernia, they are truly separate conditions. Although 80% of patients with reflux have demonstrable hiatal hernia, some do not. Qualitative investigation of reflux and the quantitation of its severity are relatively sophisticated processes that require several independent invasive tests. These tests include prolonged pH monitoring of the distal esophagus, with correlation of patient symptoms and delays in acid clearance (Fig. 13-5). These tests are expensive and are seldom needed in the case of the typical patient. Their use should be the exception rather than the rule. These investigations suggest that the symptoms of reflux are not exclusively related to an acidic environment and that alkaline reflux may occur as well. Pressures are recorded manometrically from three positions. Perfusion of the distal esophagus with hydrochloric acid alternating

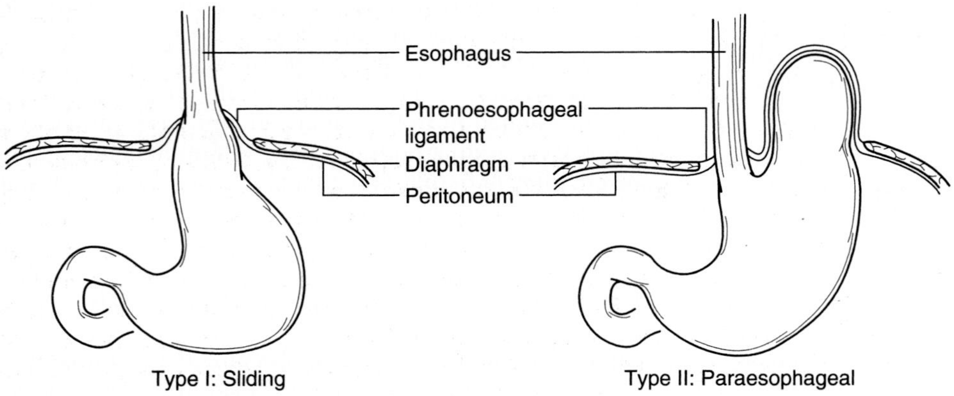

Figure 13-4 The two most common types of hiatal hernia. Note the relationships of each to the phrenoesophageal ligament and the peritoneum.

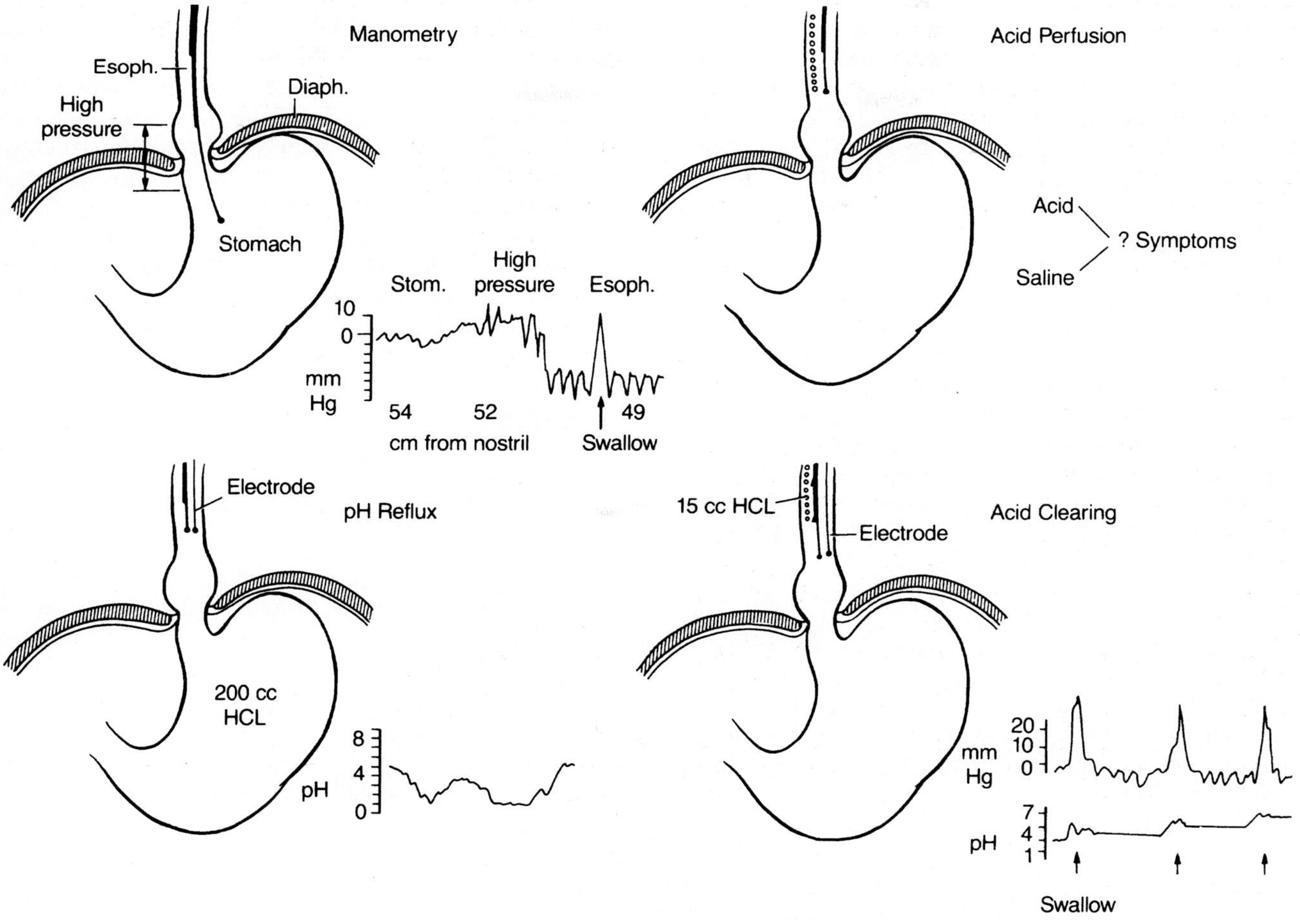

Figure 13-5 Various esophageal function tests. Catheters are passed into the esophagus through the nose or mouth. Pressure measurements are then made, or the catheters are used to infuse hydrochloric acid or saline to reproduce symptoms of acid reflux. To determine the presence of endogenous acid reflux, pH electrodes can also be inserted. Manometry and pH reflux are the most commonly performed tests. (Reprinted with permission from Skinner DB, Booth DJ. *Ann Surg* 1970;172:627–637.)

with normal saline is correlated with the patient's symptoms. Additionally, the rate of clearance of acid from the esophagus can be measured. A normal individual restores the pH to normal with fewer than 10 swallows. Manometry and pH testing are of value when barium studies show abnormal peristalsis, when periodic dysphagia occurs, or when esophagitis is not confirmed on endoscopy. Other uses may not be cost-effective.

Pathophysiology

The loss of the anatomic relationship between the diaphragmatic hiatus and the esophagus disrupts the mechanism of the lower esophageal sphincter, rendering it incompetent. Reflux of gastric acid produces a chemical burn of the susceptible esophageal mucosa. The degree of mucosal injury is a function of the duration of acid contact, not a product of excessive gastric acidity. It is caused by normal acid in the wrong place. Continued inflammation of the distal esophagus may cause mucosal erosion, ulceration, and eventually scarring and stricture. Chronic reflux may also transform the epithelium to columnar cells (**Barrett's esophagus**), which in turn may become cancerous (adenocarcinoma).

The subject of acid reflux into the lower esophagus deserves special comment because an understanding of the concept began to emerge only recently. The length of the intraabdominal segment of the esophagus may play a significant role in limiting reflux. A shortened intraabdominal segment correlates with symptomatic reflux. Further, after surgical antireflux procedures or esophageal replacement with reversed gastric tubes or colonic segments, a high-pressure zone can be measured that functions, both quantitatively and qualitatively, as the normal distal esophagus. The law of Laplace may have some bearing on reflux. Simply stated, the pressure required to distend a pliable

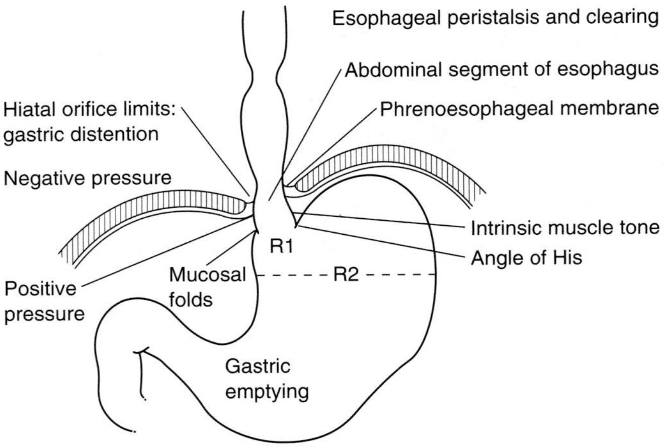

Figure 13-6 A summary of the anatomic and physiologic factors that are thought to prevent reflux of gastric content into the lower esophagus. (Modified with permission from Skinner DB. *Ann Surg* 1985;202:553.)

tube is inversely related to the diameter of the tube. Applied to the problem of reflux, it is easy to see how the larger-diameter stomach distends more than the small esophagus in response to pressure, unless the anatomic relation is altered. Consider this difference in view of the anatomic relation shown in Figures 13-2 and 13-6. Other considerations in the pathophysiology of reflux include other anatomic relations involving the angle of His and gastric mucosal folds, and a role for gastric emptying. Figure 13-6 shows a summary of these mechanisms.

Clinical Presentation

Many patients with type I hiatal hernia have no symptoms. Those with significant reflux classically have burning epigastric or substernal pain or tightness. This pain may radiate to the jaw. It may be described as tightness in the chest and can be confused with the pain of myocardial ischemia in 10% of patients. The intensity of the pain is positional, becoming worse when the patient is supine or leaning over. Antacid therapy often improves the symptoms. Patients may also complain of a lump or feeling that food is stuck beneath the xiphoid. This sensation is generally caused by muscular spasm of the esophagus. All common gastric irritants and stimulants (e.g., alcohol, aspirin, tobacco, caffeine, chocolate) exacerbate the symptoms. Occasionally, the only indication of reflux is chronic aspiration pneumonitis or asthma, or chronic laryngitis. Late symptoms of dysphagia and vomiting usually suggest stricture formation. Even in this case, nearly all patients have reflux symptoms before the onset of dysphagia. Type II hernias generally produce few symptoms until they incarcerate and become ischemic. Dysphagia, bleeding, and, occasionally, respiratory distress are the presenting symptoms.

Diagnosis

The diagnosis of hiatal hernia and reflux esophagitis can be confirmed by fluoroscopy during a barium swallow (Fig. 13-7). Sometimes barium reflux from the stomach into the distal esophagus is not observed radiographically, but is inferred by the presence of other anatomic abnormalities (e.g., dysmotility, stricture, ulceration). In addition, local signs of esophageal irritation or ulceration are often present. The diagnosis of reflux esophagitis is usually suspected based on the patient's history. Physical examination is generally unrewarding, unless significant weight loss suggests cancer. The diagnosis of reflux esophagitis can also be made by esophagogastroduodenoscopy (EGD) and biopsy of the inflamed esophagus. Most experienced endoscopists recognize esophagitis visually, and biopsy is seldom necessary to confirm the clinical findings. The basic evaluation for most patients is barium swallow and EGD. EGD can be deferred if the response to nonoperative therapy is satisfactory.

Bile reflux (duodenogastroesophageal reflux [DGER]) may complicate GERD, with the reflux of both bile and pancreatic enzymes adding to the esophageal mucosal injury. Ambulatory pH monitoring and ambulatory bilirubin monitoring may be helpful in evaluating GERD patients with Barrett's esophagus. Simultaneous acid reflux and DGER is most common in these patients.

The symptoms of GERD may be nonspecific and may mimic those of other disease processes (Table 13-1). Angina of cardiac origin must be evaluated if the patient has a sensation of substernal pressure that is not relieved by

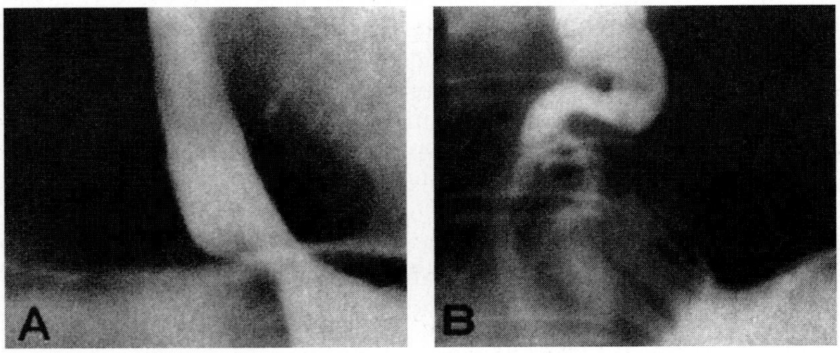

Figure 13-7 **A,** Normal distal esophagus shown by barium swallow. **B,** Small sliding hiatal hernia shown by barium swallow.

Table 13-1 Gastroesophageal Reflux Disease: Symptoms, Diagnosis, and Therapy

Symptoms	Diagnosis	Pathology	Therapy	Followup
Heartburn	Endoscopy	Erythema with or without ulcers	Eliminate coffee, tobacco, alcohol, constricting garments; administer antacids, H_2 blockers, or proton pump inhibitors; elevate head of bed	Repeat endoscopy 6–8 weeks
Heartburn, odynophagia, angina	Endoscopy, barium study	Linear ulcers	Medical therapy as above	Repeat endoscopy after 6–8 weeks; if unimproved, consider laparoscopic surgery
Cessation of symptoms, aspiration	Cardiac workup, barium study, endoscopy with biopsy	Stricture, carcinoma	Benign biopsy findings; biopsy equivocal for cancer	Dilation and antireflux; resection

belching or antacids. Occult blood in the stool may be secondary to erosive esophagitis, but peptic ulcer disease and colon cancer must be included in the differential diagnosis. A curious variant of reflux disease is Schatzki ring formation, which appears as a muscular constriction of the distal esophagus, presumably due to irritation of circular muscle by the refluxed acid. Ten percent of these formations become fibrotic and require dilation and/or excision. Treatment of the underlying reflux acid injury is essential. Dysphagia may be a sign of oropharyngeal carcinoma or esophageal motility disorders secondary to achalasia or stroke. A history of recurrent pneumonia may point to advanced GERD accompanied by distal esophageal stricture. In immunocompromised patients, the symptoms of GERD may indicate *Candida* esophagitis, Cytomegalovirus, or herpesvirus infection.

Treatment

Approximately 80% of patients respond to medical treatment, and half of them respond so completely that surgery is never necessary. Approximately 20% of patients do not respond to initial medical treatment, and half of those who initially respond ultimately relapse and require surgery.

Medical Treatment

Primary treatment for esophagitis is medical and includes all of the following:

1. Avoidance of gastric stimulants (coffee, tobacco, alcohol, chocolate).
2. Elimination of tight garments that raise intraabdominal pressure (e.g., girdles, abdominal binders).
3. Regular use of antacids, particularly those that coat the esophagus (e.g., Gaviscon), as well as the use of antacid mints (e.g., Tums, Rolaids) to provide a steady stream of protection. H_2 blockers may also be beneficial because they increase the pH of the refluxed gastric juices. In selected cases, metoclopramide is helpful when poor gastric emptying is a component of the symptom complex.
4. Abstinence from drinking or eating within several hours of sleeping.
5. Elevating the head of the bed at least 6 inches to reduce nocturnal reflux.
6. Weight loss in obese patients.

With the advent and popularity of the ION or proton pump inhibitors (PPI), second-line medicinal therapy has been altered. A proton pump inhibitor, ideally in combination with the measures described earlier, is effective in reversing severely symptomatic reflux esophagitis, but it is dose-dependent and is most effective relatively briefly. This treatment is very popular and very expensive.

Surgical Treatment

The principles of surgical treatment are relatively straightforward—to correct the anatomic defect and prevent the reflux of gastric acid into the lower esophagus by reconstruction of a valve mechanism (Fig. 13-8). There are several eponyms for the common surgical procedures for reflux esophagitis (i.e., Nissen, Hill, Belsey). Each one has its advocates, and each varies in its approach to repairing the defect and creating the valve. However, all procedures combine these two principles. The route of repair may be accomplished with a transthoracic or transabdominal approach. The abdominal approach allows access to other intraabdominal pathology that might require repair at the same time. On the other hand, esophageal shortening is best approached with a transthoracic exposure.

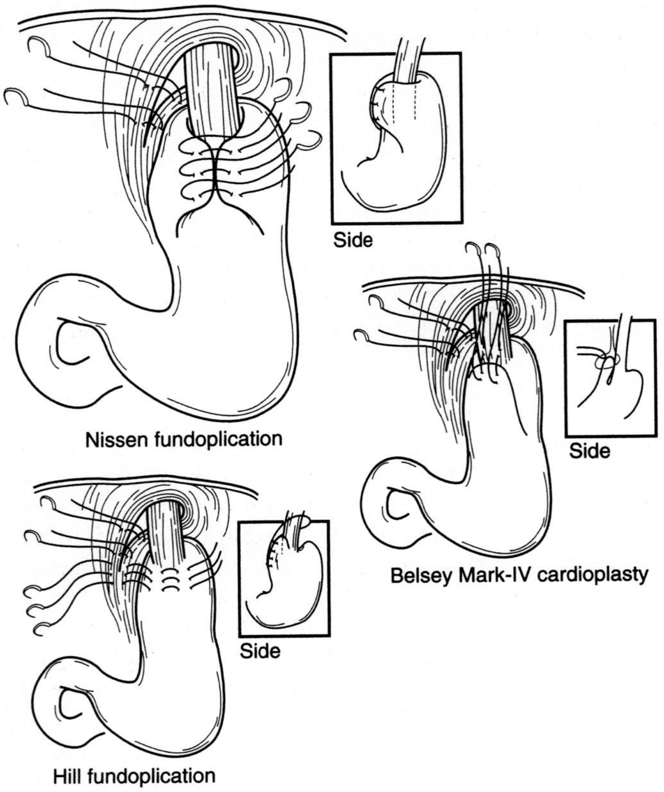

Figure 13-8 Three common hiatal hernia repairs. In each case, the defect at the esophageal hiatus is repaired and a valve mechanism is constructed using all or part of the gastric fundus. A partial form of the 360° Nissen fundoplication has become popular with laparoscopists (Thal or Toupet) and may be effective.

The acceptance of laparoscopic techniques for transabdominal fundoplication altered the face of surgical care in the United States. Clearly, this procedure can now be done reasonably simply and with an acceptable learning curve for the laparoscopically skilled surgeon. Interestingly, the effectiveness of proton pump inhibitors has now been matched (or more than matched) by the ease and success of minimal access surgery for reflux esophagitis. Significantly shorter hospital stays and convalescent periods are offset by the greater operating room expense of laparoscopy. Many such surgeries are now performed on an outpatient basis. Relaxation of the indications for surgery led to a rapid increase in antireflux surgery in the United States. The popularity of this surgery has become an attractive alternative to expensive medical therapy that can last for years. Furthermore, there is a growing recognition that an effective antireflux operation is associated with measurable regression of Barrett's in a significant number of these patients. The wisest course remains to be seen. New, endoscopically inserted devices or procedures are also under active study for the management of severe reflux.

Complications

Postoperative complications include the inability to belch or vomit (**gas-bloat syndrome**). This complication is minimized by the use of intraoperative calibration of the size of the gastroesophageal junction with a mercury bougie. Chewable simethicone tablets minimize gas bloating in the early postoperative period. Dysphagia may result from making the gastroesophageal junction too narrow. Disruption of the repair with recurrent symptoms, intraabdominal infection, and esophageal perforation are also complications. Finally, splenic injury is always a possibility for procedures in this area.

Prognosis

The common surgical procedures relieve symptoms in more than 90% of patients. The surgical mortality rate is less than 1%, and the morbidity rate is typical for clean, major abdominal procedures. With the laparoscopic approach, symptoms appear to be controlled at both short- and long-term followup. Many patients who were operated on laparoscopically also seemed to have less severe esophagitis initially, reflecting a likely decrease in the extent of esophagitis required to justify an operation.

ESOPHAGEAL MOTILITY DISORDERS

Esophageal motility disorders occur because of abnormalities of peristalsis at various levels in the esophagus. They may also lead to other disorders (e.g., diverticula) as a result of distal obstruction.

Achalasia

The most common motility disorder affecting the esophagus is **achalasia,** which literally means "failure to relax."

Pathophysiology

The pathophysiology of achalasia is located at the distal esophageal circular muscle segment. Contrary to common belief, it is not caused by spasm, but rather by failure of the high-pressure-zone sphincter to relax. The result is painless dysphagia and slow, progressive dilation of the proximal esophagus. The precise mechanism for the distal circular muscle abnormality is not known. A very rare cause of a similar illness is American *trypanosomiasis* (Chagas disease).

Clinical Presentation and Evaluation

Dysphagia, regurgitation of undigested food, and minimal weight loss are the symptoms of achalasia. Unlike reflux esophagitis, achalasia is seldom accompanied by pain. Patients often report consuming large quantities of liquids to force their food down. Aspiration pneumonia is common. Patients frequently complain of spitting up foul-smelling secretions when they simply lean forward. The diagnosis of achalasia is generally first confirmed roentgenographically by contrast studies of the esophagus, frequently with cineradiography. Dilation of the proximal esophagus is associated with a bird-beak deformity at the hiatus. In complicated cases, esophageal manometry may be extremely helpful, particularly in patients who have undergone previous operations. The manometric pressures are characteristic, showing tertiary waves with diffuse spasm and evidence of hypertonic activity of the esophagus at the high-pressure zone of the distal esophagus.

Treatment

Medical treatment is generally not helpful, although calcium channel blockers have not been adequately studied in proper trials. Surgical treatment is the most reliable, and more than 95% of patients have complete relief of symptoms.

Medical Treatment

Medical treatment involves an invasive endoscopic procedure in which a balloon is placed at the region of high pressure in the esophagogastric junction. The balloon is rapidly inflated ("forceful dilation") to rupture the distal esophageal circular muscle, without rupturing the full thickness of the mucosa. The response to forceful dilation is variable. Approximately 80% of patients are cured by this procedure, but the complications, when they occur, are severe. The procedure is now neither widely practiced nor readily learned.

Surgical Treatment

Esophageal myotomy (Heller myotomy) is carried out over the distal 5 cm of the esophagus and extended 1 cm onto the stomach, producing the same result as forceful dilation. The procedure, which is now performed laparoscopically, involves a surgical incision in the muscular layer of the lower esophagus (myotomy). Its only disadvantage is the occasional development of reflux as a result of an overly lengthy myotomy. Consequently, some surgeons accompany the myotomy with a modified **fundoplication**. A complete 360° wrap of the lower esophagus occasionally exacerbates dysphagia and therefore should be avoided.

Esophageal Diverticula

The second most common manifestation of esophageal motility disorders is the development of **diverticula** (outpouching of all or part of the wall of the organ). Diverticula are classified as either pulsion or traction, depending on the mechanism that leads to their development. **Esophageal diverticula** may occur at any level. Although endoscopy is frequently performed, it is important to avoid diverticular perforation because it is sometimes easier to pass the endoscope into the diverticulum than into the main channel of the esophagus.

Pathophysiology

Cervical Zenker's diverticula (Fig. 13-9) are classified as pulsion diverticula. They are closely related to dysfunction

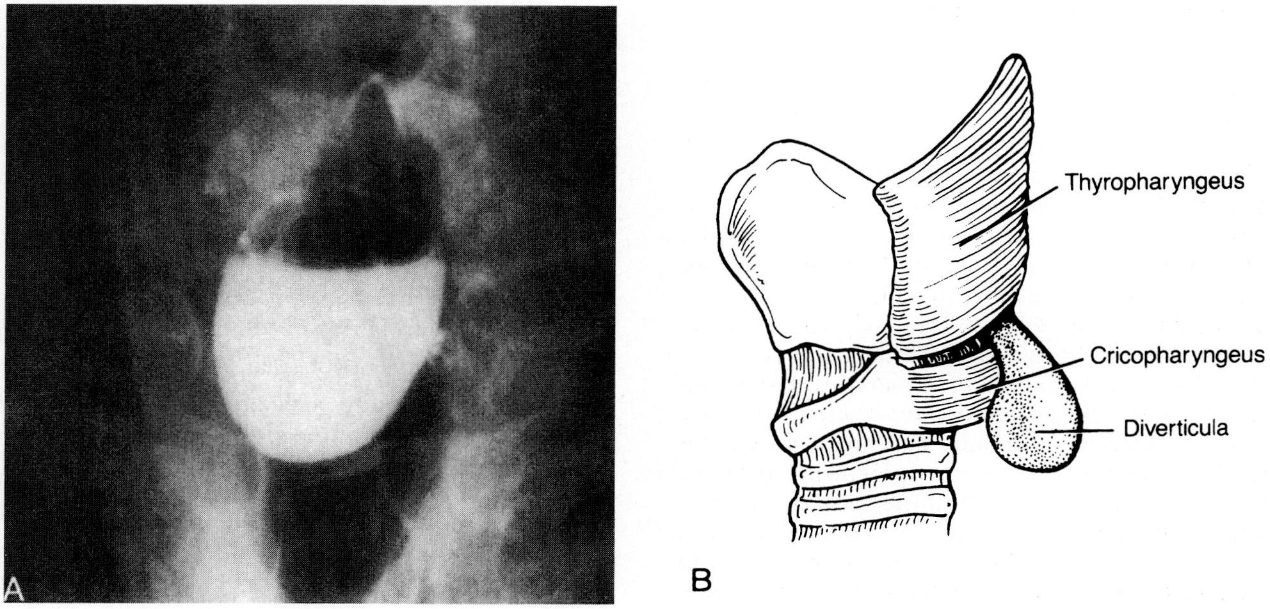

Figure 13-9 **A,** Barium retained after barium swallow shows a large pharyngealesophageal diverticulum, also known as Zenker's diverticulum. **B,** Diverticulum is a mucosal hernia between the two muscles of the pharyngeal constrictor mechanism. The diverticulum is false because it does not contain all of the layers of the esophagus, only mucosa.

of the cricopharyngeal muscle, although the precise abnormality of motility is unknown. Anatomically, they occur between the oblique fibers of the thyropharyngeal muscle and the more horizontal fibers of the cricopharyngeus, an area of potential weakness. Patients are typically elderly and may have some swallowing disorders associated with previous transient ischemic attacks or strokes.

Pulsion diverticula of the distal one-third of the esophagus are generally associated with dysfunction of the esophagogastric junction. They are caused by chronic stricture from acid reflux, antireflux surgical procedures, achalasia, or other uncommon disorders.

Middle-third esophageal diverticula are almost always traction diverticula and therefore are not related to an intrinsic abnormality in esophageal motility. They are usually caused by mediastinal inflammation (usually inflammatory nodal disease from tuberculosis or sarcoidosis) or histoplasmosis. This inflammation results in scar formation and subsequent contracture that places traction on the esophagus.

Clinical Presentation and Evaluation

Patients with symptomatic Zenker's diverticula have regurgitation of recently swallowed food or pills, choking, or a putrid breath odor. Patients with traction diverticula are asymptomatic and seldom require treatment.

Treatment

Patients with Zenker's diverticula are best treated by myotomy of the cricopharyngeal muscle and excision or elevation of the diverticulum. Patients with diverticula of the distal third of the esophagus should also have the diverticula excised and the underlying pathologic process corrected. This therapy relieves symptoms in more than 90% of patients. Surgical morbidity and mortality rates are less than 1%.

Other Disorders

Esophageal motility disorders are commonly found in association with a number of collagen vascular diseases, most notably scleroderma, a disease in which systemic smooth muscle is replaced by fibrosis. Although the etiology of scleroderma is not understood, its diagnosis depends in large part on the determination of esophageal abnormalities; as many as 70% of patients with scleroderma have esophageal involvement. Patients show marked abnormalities of esophageal motility, with a progressive decline in muscular contractility toward the lower esophageal sphincter. At this level, ineffective, poorly coordinated simultaneous contractions are recorded. These findings occur before the classic changes are noted by standard barium swallow radiographs. Patients have the constitutional symptoms of general malaise and fatigue. If the esophagus is involved, they may also have dysphagia or may need to force down their food with large volumes of liquids. With progressive reflux, extensive ulceration of the distal esophagus may occur. Medical therapy with antacids and H_2 blockers or proton pump inhibitors may offer only partial relief. **Stricture** formation is common. Although there is no known cure for the disease, surgical therapy to relieve severe esophageal symptoms in selected patients may offer significant palliation. Diffuse esophageal spasm, often confused with angina pectoris, is a painful process of multiple areas of circular muscle spasm throughout the length of the esophagus. It is often called "nutcracker esophagus." Dysphagia is associated with segmental spasm and is often due to stress and/or other psychological factors.

ESOPHAGEAL NEOPLASMS

Benign tumors of the esophagus are exceedingly rare and are mentioned only for the sake of completeness. However, malignant tumors affect 2.6 per 100,000 population in the United States, with a male:female ratio of 3 to 4:1 and an increased incidence among African-American men. Squamous cell carcinoma, with a dismal prognosis, is three to four times more common in African-American men than in white men. Worldwide, the incidence of esophageal cancer varies tremendously, from an extremely low incidence in many Western societies to endemic proportions in certain regions of China and Africa.

Benign Tumors

Benign tumors of the esophagus arise from the various anatomic layers of this organ. They are most common in the middle and distal thirds. Leiomyomas are the most common intramural tumors, and the potential for malignant degeneration appears quite low. They have a characteristically smooth surface that is seen to indent the lumen of the esophagus on contrast radiography. Although the tumors are usually asymptomatic, many surgeons recommend excision to eliminate progressive tumor growth, which causes dysphagia, and to exclude the possibility of malignancy.

Malignant Tumors

Squamous carcinoma makes up approximately 85% of all primary esophageal neoplasms. Adenocarcinoma occurs in approximately 10% of esophageal cancers and is increasing in frequency, especially among individuals with recalcitrant reflux. Sarcomas account for 0.8% of all esophageal tumors. Primary esophageal lymphoma is rare, but potentially curable. Tumors of the amine precursor uptake and decarboxylation system (APUDomas) make up 0.8% to 2.4% and usually have metastatic spread on initial presentation.

Epidemiology

The high incidence of esophageal cancer in various geographic areas (i.e., Coastal South Carolina; Washington,

DC; Linxian County, China; Transkei, South Africa) suggests that environmental factors are important in the etiology. For example, low dietary levels of ascorbic acid, alpha-tocopherol, retinol, and riboflavin, and high levels of nitrosamines in fungus-infected food are associated with endemic areas of esophageal cancer in Linxian County, China. In the United States and other Western countries, alcohol, tobacco, achalasia, Barrett's esophagus, and caustic esophageal injury all seem to play a role in the pathogenesis of most esophageal cancer, whether squamous or adenocarcinoma.

In the high-risk areas of the United States, tobacco and alcohol were identified as major risk factors for esophageal cancer, particularly when the daily consumption of alcohol is equivalent to greater than 9 g ethanol in any form and when the patient smokes more than 20 cigarettes per day. In other parts of the world, the etiology is related to diet, vitamin deficiency, poor oral hygiene, surgical procedures, and a number of premalignant conditions (e.g., caustic burns, Barrett's esophagus, radiation, Plummer-Vinson syndrome).

Adenocarcinoma develops in approximately 10% of patients with Barrett's esophagus. Tylosis, an autosomal dominant disorder characterized by hyperkeratosis of the palms and soles, is the only verified genetic disorder known to be associated with esophageal cancer. It is estimated that affected family members have a 95% chance of esophageal cancer if they live long enough.

Pathophysiology

Carcinoma of the esophagus usually arises from squamous epithelium. Occasionally, adenocarcinoma occurs in the esophagus, but more commonly, these tumors originate in the fundus of the stomach and extend upward into the esophagus. Submucosal extension is common and frequently occurs over an extended distance. Because there is no serosal layer, invasion of adjacent structures is common. Adenocarcinomas may be the result of malignant transformation of the columnar epithelium that replaces the normal squamous lining of the distal esophagus as a result of chronic acid reflux. This metaplasia is known as Barrett's esophagus and seems to be increasingly widely recognized.

Clinical Presentation and Evaluation

Unfortunately, the symptoms of esophageal malignancy are often insidious at the onset, precluding early diagnosis and effective treatment. Dysphagia is the most common symptom. It usually begins with solid foods and then, over a period of weeks to months, progresses to include liquids. Retrosternal pain with swallowing (odynophagia) is the second most common symptom. Constant pain in the mid-back or midchest may be an ominous symptom of mediastinal invasion. Patients seem to ignore these symptoms and seek medical evaluation only after anorexia or weight loss occurs. Hoarseness may occur with local invasion in upper esophageal or midesophageal cancer. Some patients with cervical or upper thoracic esophageal cancer have acquired tracheoesophageal fistula as a result of erosion of the tumor into the trachea or bronchus. They may also have frequent episodes of pneumonia as a result of recurrent aspiration. Frequently, the disease is so advanced that patients cannot swallow their own saliva.

The presentation of carcinoma of the esophagus ranges from early carcinoma that is limited to the mucosa to more advanced forms that extend through the muscle layers and beyond. It infiltrates locally and involves the adjacent lymph nodes after spreading along the numerous submucosal lymphatics. The absence of a serosal layer allows earlier extension into adjacent mediastinal structures (e.g., tracheobronchial tree, pericardium, aorta), and 75% of patients have positive nodes at initial presentation.

The presumptive diagnosis of esophageal cancer is made by the typical ragged edge, shelf, or apple core appearance on barium contrast studies of the esophagus (Fig. 13-10). An upper gastrointestinal series is often followed by endoscopy and biopsy of the lesion. Few esophageal cancers remain occult after barium and endoscopic studies of the esophagus are completed.

Screening esophagoscopy with Lugol's solution is used with some success to detect abnormal areas that represent malignancy. Lugol's solution contains iodine, which reacts with the high content of glycogen in normal esophageal mucosa, producing a black or green-brown color. Unstained areas are abnormal and are likely malignant. This is obviously most applicable in areas where the cancer is endemic.

CT is commonly used to stage esophageal cancer. However, CT is more reliable in detecting extranodal metastases or recurrent cancer. Endoscopic ultrasound (EUS) is being used with some success in pretreatment staging and continues to improve the evaluation of esophageal cancer by allowing the endoscopist to assess the length of the primary tumor and aid in fine-needle aspiration of mediastinal nodes. Three-dimensional EUS will permit further advances. The positron emission tomography (PET) scan is useful in staging mediastinal and distant metastatic esophageal disease.

Laparoscopy is the most accurate modality (96%) for detecting intraabdominal metastasis, and it allows biopsy confirmation. Video-assisted thoracic surgery, when performed by a skilled thoracoscopist, will offer similar results for mediastinal and intrathoracic metastatic diseases (Fig. 13-11).

Abrasive brush cytology is of value in detecting early esophageal cancer in high-risk areas in China and in South Africa. Brush biopsy is performed by having the patient swallow a capsule that contains the brush attached to a long thread. The predictive value of the brush cytology screening program in South Africa was 90%.

Treatment

Approximately 7% to 10% of esophageal malignancies arise in the cervical esophagus. When feasible, surgical treatment includes removal of all tumor-containing tissue.

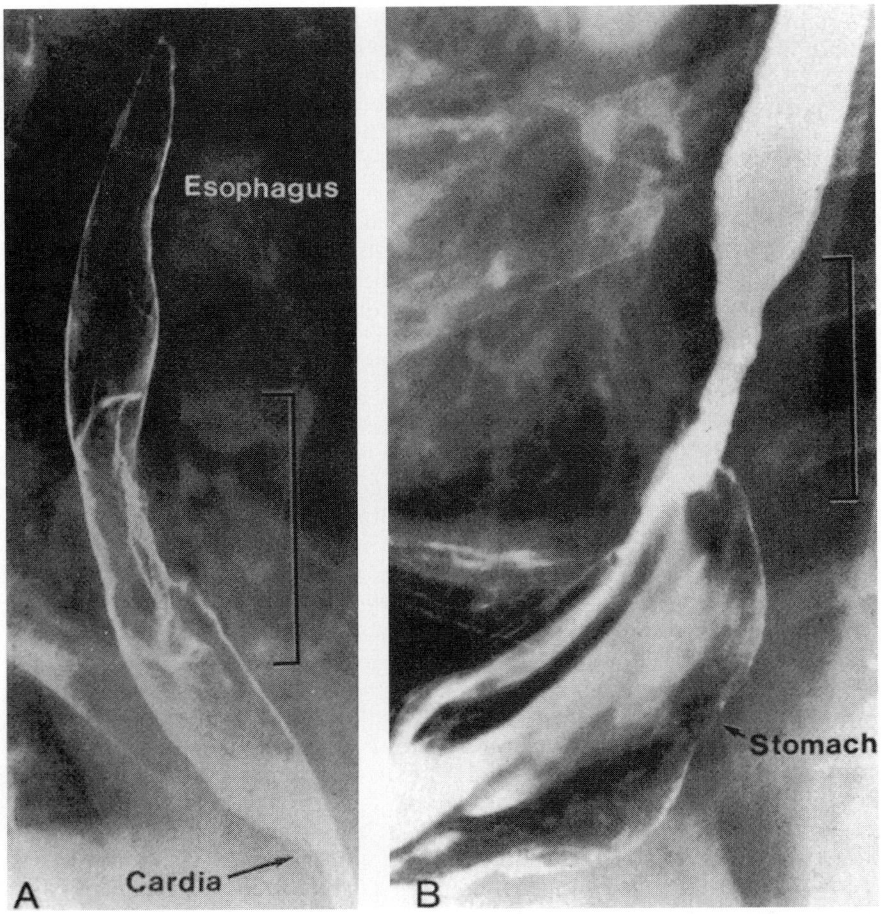

Figure 13-10 **A,** Contrast radiograph showing the typical "apple core" lesion of carcinoma of the middle one-third of esophagus. **B,** Ragged edge seen in carcinoma of the distal esophagus.

This treatment may involve cervical esophagectomy with en bloc laryngectomy and esophageal replacement with stomach, colon, or jejunum. If en bloc bilateral lymph node dissection is included, the jugular veins are spared.

Tumors in the upper and middle thirds of the thoracic esophagus are managed by resection with a transthoracic approach and by reestablishing continuity with esophagogastrostomy. If an adequate amount of stomach is not available, colon and jejunal grafts may be used. For patients with lesions of the distal esophageal and gastric cardia, resection is traditionally carried out with a left thoracoabdominal esophagogastrectomy and either pyloroplasty or pyloromyotomy to prevent delayed gastric emptying.

Transhiatal total esophagectomy without thoracotomy is increasingly popular, regardless of the level of the tumor. Gastrointestinal continuity is reestablished by bringing up the stomach through the posterior mediastinum and performing an anastomosis between the fundus and the cervical esophagus. Pyloromyotomy and feeding jejunostomy are also performed. This procedure avoids the morbidity associated with making a major thoracic incision and performing a gastrointestinal anastomosis in the chest.

Because patients with squamous cell carcinoma or adenocarcinoma of the esophagus have a very poor prognosis, treatment should be directed toward restoring effective swallowing. Palliation in patients with a disease that has a life expectancy of 100 days is especially important; at first thought, feeding and nutritional strategies seem most attractive. In fact, they tend to prolong a very poor quality of life. Radiation and/or intubation (see below) may be the most humane options. Treatment of patients with favorable tumors (small, possibly curable lesions and those without evidence of overt lymph node dissemination) should be aggressive and based on tumor location. Radiation therapy is the primary mode of treatment for cancer that arises in the upper esophagus. Surgical treatment at this level usually requires removal of the esophagus en bloc with the larynx, permanent tracheostomy, and restoration of swallowing by a free microsurgically constructed vascular pedicle of jejunum or colon into the neck. Tumors that involve the middle third of the esophagus are usually treated by a staged procedure with total thoracic esophagectomy and bypass. Reconstructive options include pulling the stomach into the neck and interposing a segment of colon. Cancer involving the lower third of the esophagus or proximal stomach is best treated by esophagogastric resection and an end-to-end anastomosis in the midchest.

At a small number of centers, expertise and success is increasing in managing localized carcinoma of the esophagus and Barrett's metaplasia with high-grade dysplasia

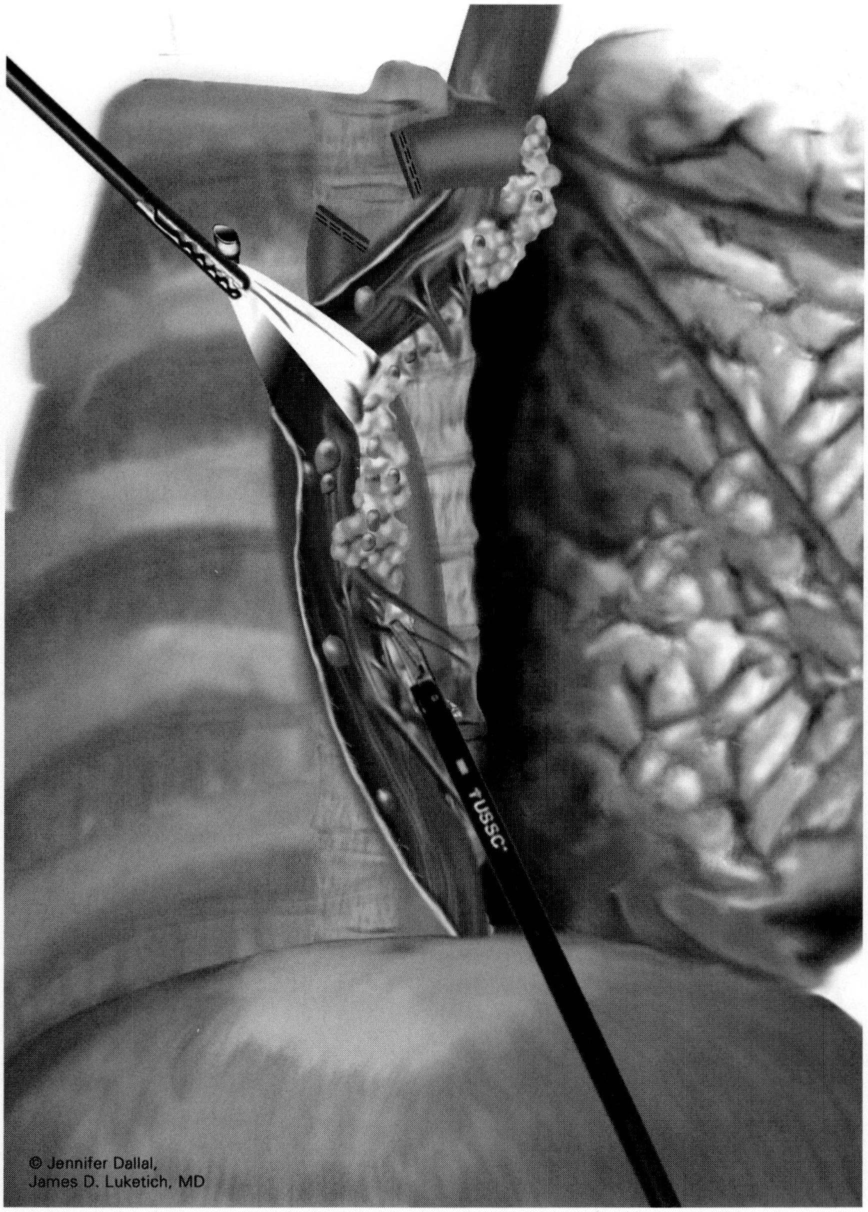

Figure 13-11 Thoracoscopic mobilization of the esophagus. (Reprinted with permission from Nguyen NT, Schauer PR, Luketich JD. Combined laparoscopic and thoracoscopic approach to esophagectomy. *J Am Coll Surg* 1999;188: 328–332.)

using a minimally invasive procedure that involves a combined thoracolaparoscopic approach (Fig. 13-12).

Controlled clinical trials of multimodality therapy (neoadjuvant, preoperative chemoradiation, or chemoradiation without surgery) for advanced esophageal carcinoma are being conducted, but the benefits remain unclear. As the incidence of adenocarcinoma increases in younger patients, the benefits from preoperative chemoradiation could become important.

Prognosis

Squamous cell carcinomas and adenocarcinomas of the esophagus have a very poor prognosis. The cure rate for the most favorable cases seldom exceeds 20%, and, in general, the overall cure rate for all esophageal cancer is only 5%. In theory, combined preoperative chemotherapy and radiation therapy may be helpful in some patients. Palliation is available with a number of endoesophageal tubes (Celestin, Souttar, Mousseau-Barbin). The placement of these tubes is often associated with high morbidity, and the average survival is less than 3 months. Expansive metal stents for palliation are being tried, with lower operative morbidity and better palliation. Endoscopic laser provides temporary relief of obstruction, but must be repeated frequently. Photodynamic therapy with laser ablation decreases the overt incidence of adenocarcinoma in some patients with Barrett's esophagus. Whether this eliminates or delays ultimate transition to invasive adenocarcinoma remains to be shown.

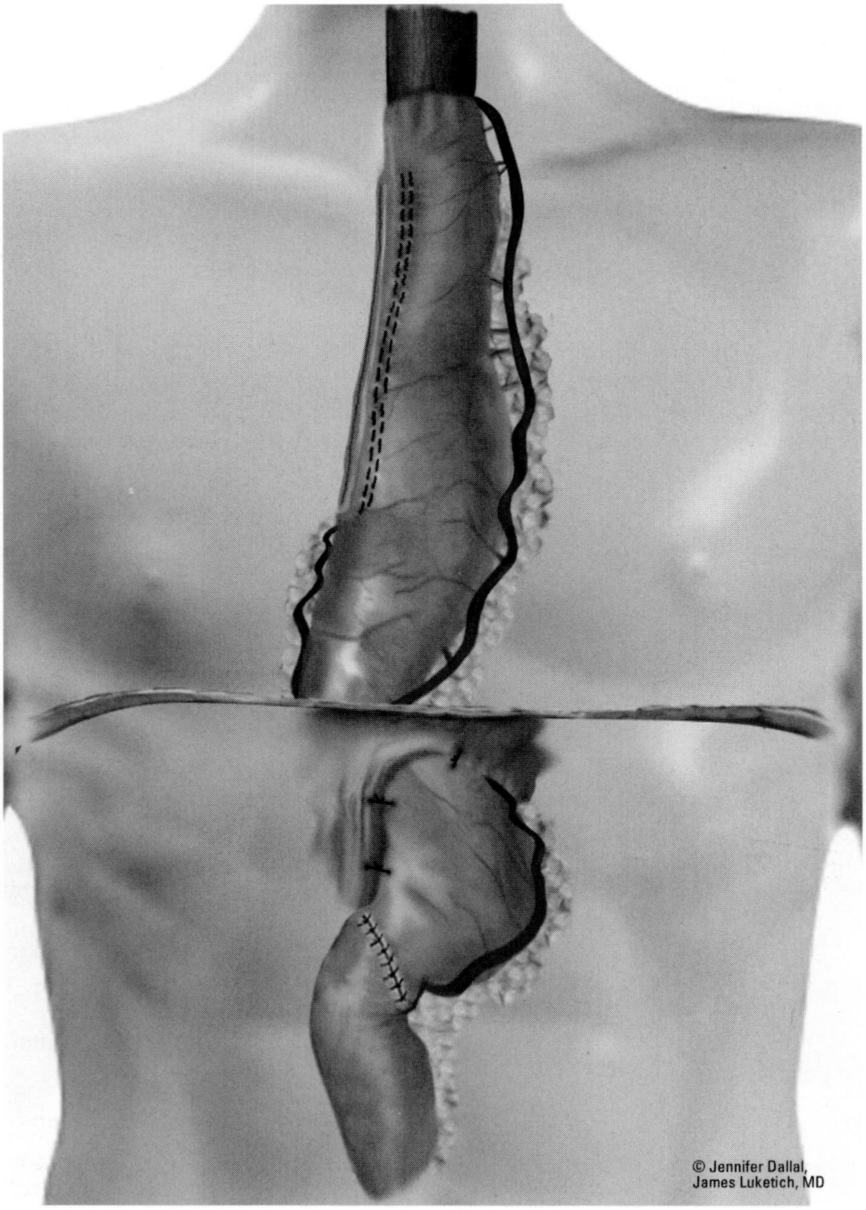

Figure 13-12 Completed laparoscopic thoracoscopic operation. (Reprinted with permission from Luketich JD, Schauer PR, Christie NA, et al. Minimally invasive esophagectomy. *Ann Thorac Surg* 2000; 70:906–912.)

TRAUMATIC ESOPHAGEAL DISORDERS

Because of their frequent occurrence and because of the morbidity and mortality associated with their lack of recognition and aggressive management, three traumatic injuries of the esophagus deserve brief mention: disruption or perforation of the esophagus, foreign body ingestion, and ingestion of caustic substances.

Esophageal Perforation

Esophageal perforation is usually the result of instrumentation. Causes include endoscopic or biopsy procedures, the passage of nasogastric tubes or instruments designed to dilate strictures, and the occasional inflation of devices used to tamponade bleeding varices in the esophagus (e.g., Sengstaken-Blakemore tubes, balloon dilation for achalasia). Spontaneous perforation of the esophagus also occurs, usually after an episode of forceful vomiting or retching that dramatically increases intraesophageal pressure (**Boerhaave's syndrome**). In this condition, the lack of a serosal layer makes perforation more common in the esophagus than at any other location in the alimentary tract. Perforation by external trauma is discussed in Chapter X, Trauma.

Clinical Presentation and Evaluation

The symptoms of esophageal perforation may be dramatic or occult, depending on the location of the perforation and its etiology. Perforation by nasogastric tube or EGD may be insidious, and only after several hours will the patient be found in extremis and in profound shock from mediastinal sepsis. At other times, the event is catastrophic from the onset, with severe chest or abdominal pain, hypotension, diaphoresis, nausea, and vomiting to suggest the diagnosis in relation to interventions that preceded the collapse.

Treatment

Treatment requires aggressive surgical intervention because the mortality rate is directly related to the interval between occurrence and intervention. Surgical drainage and repair, if possible, are necessary. Patients who present or are recognized late and are stable can occasionally be managed by tube thoracostomy and systemic antibiotics.

Foreign Body Ingestion

Foreign body ingestion is common in toddlers and mentally ill adults. The history must be confirmed with appropriate imaging studies. Once the diagnosis is confirmed and appropriate general anesthesia has been administered, the patient is best treated with gentle extraction using a rigid esophagoscope. A contrast study to exclude esophageal perforation should be performed before the patient is discharged. Irrespective of the cause, underlying esophageal disease should be considered (e.g., foreign body lodged on an acid-induced structure).

Ingestion of Caustic Materials

Ingestion of caustic materials, either accidentally (as by children) or intentionally (as by an adult in a suicide attempt), is a medical emergency. The most ominous is the ingestion of alkaline-containing products (e.g., Drano, Liquid-Plumr). These solutions can destroy the tissue to varying degrees, from the lips well into the small intestine. Ingestion of acidic material is only slightly less injurious.

Evaluation

The most important aspect of treatment is the early identification of the etiologic agent (e.g., acid, alkaline, specific toxin), because each agent requires a different approach. Second, careful physical examination of the oropharyngeal cavity is required to estimate the severity of injury. Invasive endoscopic procedures are usually urgently necessary.

Treatment

Induced vomiting and neutralization of caustic substances are not suggested because they are potentially harmful and ineffective. Airway maintenance is the first priority, followed by maintenance of patency of the esophagus. Antiinflammatory agents are generally recommended for alkaline or acid burns if they are used within the first 24 hours.

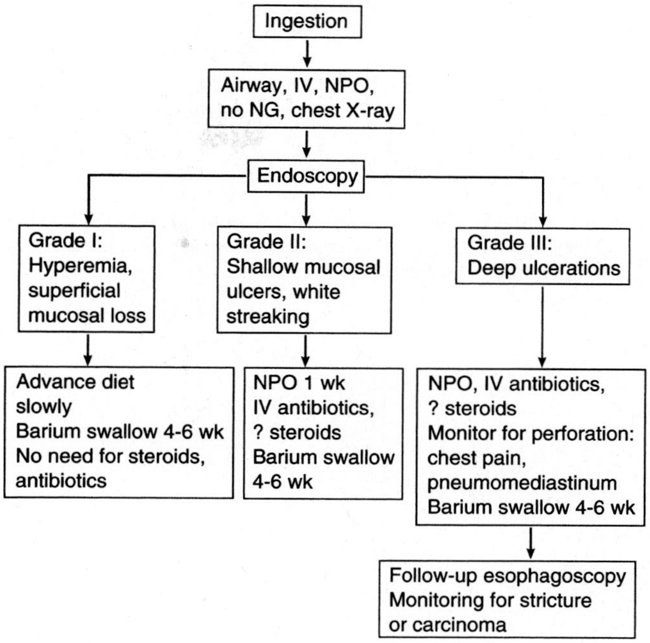

Figure 13-13 Algorithm for caustic ingestion. IV, intravenous; NG, nasogastric tube; NPO, nothing by mouth.

Steroids should not be used when perforation has occurred. Long-term therapy is directed toward the prevention, by dilation and ultimate surgical management, of stricture formation. The use of antibiotics as adjuvant therapy is controversial. Figure 13-13 shows an algorithm for caustic ingestion.

SUMMARY

In summary, diseases that affect the esophagus are quite common and represent disabling problems for some patients. The diagnosis can be accomplished with a careful barium study of the upper gastrointestinal tract and skilled endoscopic examination and biopsy. CT scans of the chest are useful in examining the esophagus in relation to other anatomic structures in the thorax and in assessing the status of the mediastinum, particularly in esophageal cancer. MRI provides no advantage over CT imaging in esophageal disease. An occasional patient whose disease is not clarified by these studies will require manometric study of the esophagus. Treatment of benign diseases of the esophagus is usually successful, unless distal esophageal inflammation progresses to stricture. The treatment of cancer of the esophagus at the time of clinical presentation is usually for palliation. Most recent efforts to improve cure rates for esophageal cancer have focused on modifying risk factors and diagnosing the disease earlier. Traumatic injury of the esophagus requires prompt, aggressive management, with surgical consultation from the onset.

SUGGESTED READINGS

Bais JE, Bartelsman JFWM, Bonjer HJ, et al. Laparoscopic or conventional Nissen fundoplication for gastro-oesophageal reflux disease: randomised clinical trial. *Lancet* 2000;355;170–174.

Bousamra M, Haasler GB, Parviz M. A decade of experience with transthoracic and transhiatal esophagectomy. *Am J Surg* 2002;183: 162–167.

Brown LM, Blot WJ, Shuman SH, et al. Environmental factors and high risk of esophageal cancer among men in Coastal South Carolina. *J Natl Cancer Inst* 1988;80:1620–1625.

DeCamp MM Jr, Swanson SJ, Jaklitsch MT. Esophagectomy after induction chemoradiation. *Chest* 1999;116:466S–469S.

Ferguson MK, ed. General thoracic surgery part II. *Surg Clin North Am* 2002;82(Aug):683–883.

Haddad NG, Fleischer DE. Neoplasms of the esophagus. In: Castell DO, ed. *The Esophagus*. Boston. MA: Little Brown and Company 1995:269.

Luketich JD, Schauer PR, Christie NA, et al. Minimally invasive esophagectomy. *Ann Thorac Surg* 2000;70:906–912.

Rao YG, Pal S, Pande GK, et al. Transhiatal esophagectomy for benign and malignant conditions. *Am J Surg* 2002;184:136–142.

14

JOHN PAIGE, MD ■ J. PATRICK O'LEARY, MD

Stomach and Duodenum

OBJECTIVES

1 Describe the clinical significance of aspects of gastric and duodenal anatomy in the pathophysiology and therapy of peptic ulcer disease.

2 Review the physiology of gastric acid secretion and its role in the development and treatment of gastric and duodenal ulcer disease.

3 Understand how the physiology of vitamin B_{12} absorption can lead to deficiency after certain gastric operations.

4 Compare and contrast the pathophysiology, evaluation, and treatment of gastric and duodenal ulcer disease.

5 Discuss the presentation, classification, and treatment of adenocarcinoma of the stomach.

6 List the diagnostic options for identifying the location and etiology of benign ulcer disease.

7 Describe the common operations performed for the treatment of complicated ulcer disease and discuss their complications.

8 Identify the clinical and biochemical features of Zollinger-Ellison syndrome (gastrinoma) that aid in differentiating it from benign ulcer disease and discuss therapeutic options in its treatment

9 Review the classification, pathophysiology, and therapy of obesity.

10 Describe the advantages and disadvantages of common procedures performed for the treatment of severe obesity and list their complications.

ANATOMY

The Stomach

The stomach is a pliable, saccular organ that is located in the left hypochondrium and epigastrium. Its major function is to prepare ingested food for digestion and absorption. The stomach is separated from the rest of the gastrointestinal tract by two distinct regions. The proximal one, located in the distal esophagus near the gastroesophageal (GE) junction, is a functional high-pressure zone known as the lower esophageal sphincter (LES). It is marked histologically by a mucosal change from squamous to columnar epithelium. In healthy individuals, the LES is greater than 2 cm in length with a resting pressure above 6 mm Hg. This elevated resting pressure prevents reflux of caustic gastric contents into the esophagus. With swallowing, a reflex relaxation of the LES occurs, facilitating entrance of food into the stomach. The distal region is located at the junction of the distal portion of the stomach, or antrum, with the duodenum. At this point, a definite mucosal change is seen histologically, and a well-defined sphincter of smooth muscle known as the pylorus is present. The restricted lumen of the pylorus, or pyloric channel, is 1 to 3 cm long. The pylorus prevents the reflux of duodenal contents into the stomach and, in association with the antral pump, controls the rate of gastric emptying. After ingestion of a meal, particles larger than 3 to 5 mm are not allowed to leave the stomach until the final "cleansing" wave of peristalsis occurs several hours later.

The stomach can be divided into three distinct regions based on physiologic and histologic differences. The most proximal portion is the fundus. This area plays a crucial role in accommodating the entrance of food into the stomach by undergoing receptive relaxation. As a food bolus moves past the pharynx and into the esophagus, vagal stimulation causes relaxation of the fundus, preventing an increase in the intragastric pressure and allowing food to pass and be stored. The fundus also houses the gastric pacemaker responsible for initiating motor activity. It is centered on the greater curvature, near the short gastric vessels. The middle portion of the stomach is the corpus. Most of the acid-producing **parietal cells** as well as the pepsinogen-producing chief cells are located here. Another important cell in the corpus is the enterochromaffin-like (ECL) cell. It plays an important indirect role in hydrochloric acid secretion. The corpus assists in the storage of gastric contents as well as in their peristaltic grinding against the pylorus. The most distal stomach is the antrum. It contains the G cells, which produce gastrin. Care must be taken to completely remove this section of the stomach when performing an **antrectomy** and vagotomy for ulcer disease to prevent hypersecretion of gastrin. The simplest way to differentiate antral tissue from other gastric tissue is to demonstrate the absence of the brightly eosin-staining parietal cells that are present in the corpus and fundus. Finally, mucus-secreting goblet cells are found throughout the entire stomach.

The wall of the stomach has four layers: the mucosa, submucosa, muscularis, and serosa. The mucosa is arranged in a coarse rugal pattern and has a complex glandular structure. It is separated from the submucosa by the muscularis mucosa. Its abundant blood supply arises from the rich vascular network of the submucosa. The muscularis surrounds the submucosa. It has three layers of smooth muscle: the outermost longitudinal muscle, the middle circular muscle, and the innermost oblique muscle. The autonomic pacemaker in the fundus is located in the circular muscle layer. The serosa overlies the muscularis and is the outermost covering.

The arterial blood supply to the stomach includes the right and left gastric arteries, right and left gastroepiploic arteries, short gastric arteries, and gastroduodenal arteries (Fig. 14-1). Because of this abundant blood supply, surgical devascularization of the stomach rarely occurs. Sympathetic innervation parallels arterial flow. Parasympathetic innervation passes through the vagus nerves. A clear understanding of the course of these parasympathetic nerves is essential, since they stimulate the parietal cell mass to secrete hydrochloric acid. In addition, they control the motor activity of the stomach. As the vagus nerves traverse the mediastinum, the left trunk rotates so that it enters the abdomen anterior to the esophagus (Fig. 14-2). The right trunk rotates so that it enters the abdomen posterior to the

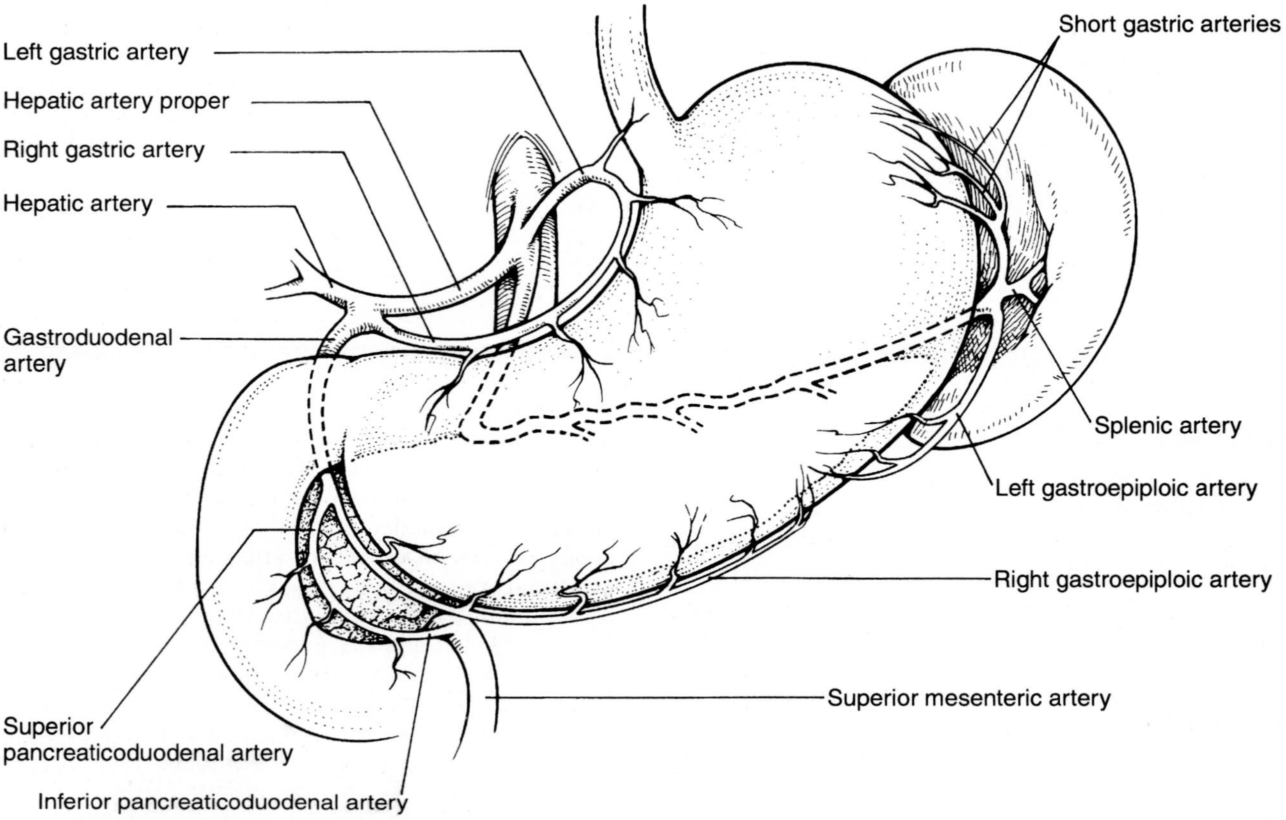

Figure 14-1 The major arteries that supply the stomach. The gastroduodenal artery is located behind the duodenum. Posterior penetrating duodenal ulcers may erode into this artery and cause hemorrhage.

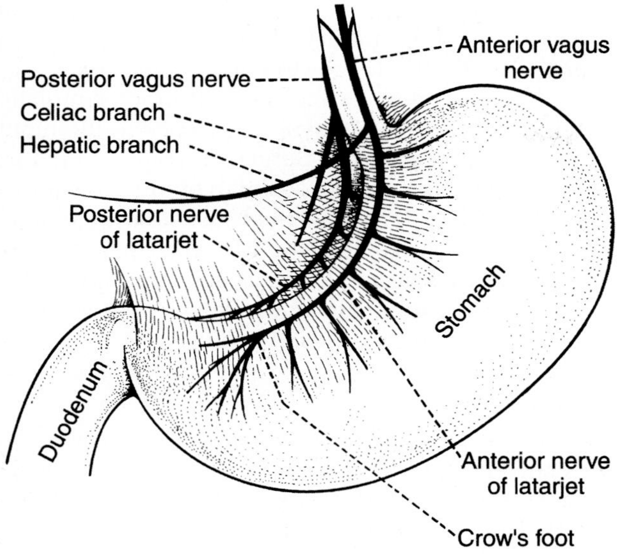

Figure 14-2 Branches of the vagus nerve innervate the stomach, pylorus, and duodenum. If the distal nerve of Latarjet is denervated, the pylorus does not relax in response to normal stimuli.

esophagus. Both nerves innervate the stomach from the lesser curvature. The right vagus gives off a posterior branch to the celiac plexus, from which nerves pass to the midgut (pancreas, small intestine, and proximal colon). Also, the right vagus occasionally gives off a small branch that travels behind the esophagus to innervate the stomach. This branch is referred to as the criminal nerve of Grassi. When it is not properly identified and divided during a parietal cell or **truncal vagotomy**, it will continue to stimulate acid secretion in the stomach, leading to recurrent peptic ulcer disease. The left vagus gives off a hepatic branch that passes through the gastrohepatic ligament and innervates the gallbladder, biliary tract, and liver.

The Duodenum

The duodenum is a metabolically active organ that receives chyme from the stomach. In addition, it is the site of drainage of bile from the liver and secretions from the pancreas. The duodenum produces myriad hormonally active agents. Anatomically, it has four regions: the duodenal bulb (first part), the descending duodenum (second part), the transverse duodenum (third part), and the ascending duodenum (fourth part). The duodenum becomes the jejunum as it enters the peritoneum at the ligament of Treitz. The descending duodenum is the site of the intestinal pacemaker. Additionally, the ampulla of Vater enters the duodenum at the posteromedial aspect of the descending portion. Through this sphincter, bile and pancreatic secretions are released into the gastrointestinal tract. The Brunner's glands in the duodenum are the site of mucus secretion, protecting the duodenal mucosa from gastric acid injury.

The blood supply to the duodenum comes primarily from the gastroduodenal artery and the superior mesenteric artery, although other smaller vessels are contributors. The gastroduodenal artery is the first branch of the proper hepatic artery. It courses immediately posterior to the duodenal bulb and divides into the superior pancreaticoduodenal arcades. A **duodenal ulcer** that penetrates through the posterior wall of the duodenal bulb does so in the vicinity of the gastroduodenal artery. If the vessel wall is exposed to the gastric digestive enzymes and acid, erosion and massive bleeding may occur. The superior mesenteric artery arises from the descending aorta and supplies the inferior pancreaticoduodenal arcades.

PHYSIOLOGY

Hydrochloric Acid Secretion

The human is the only mammal that secretes hydrochloric acid in the fasting state. This finding prompted some investigators to hypothesize that duodenal ulcer disease is an affliction of civilization. Gastric acid secretion is a complex, highly regulated process in which multiple specialized gastric and duodenal cells play an essential role. A well-developed mucosal defensive mechanism is also present in the stomach to protect it from caustic injury. The parietal cell rests at the heart of this elaborate system.

The parietal cell is responsible for creating the concentrated acid environment within the lumen of the stomach. It accomplishes this task by actively secreting hydrogen ion against a 1,000,000:1 concentration gradient. A H^+/K^+-ATPase (proton) pump within the cell exchanges hydrogen ions for potassium ions in a 1:1 ratio. Adenosine triphosphate (ATP) is the source of energy. Chloride ion is transported into the lumen in conjunction with this process. Water and bicarbonate are byproducts of this reaction, and they passively diffuse into the plasma and extracellular space. These proton pumps are stored within intracellular membrane compartments just below the apical (luminal) surface of the parietal cell. When the cell is stimulated, these compartments fuse with the apical membrane, and hydrogen ion is released into the stomach lumen. The proton pump, therefore, is critical for active secretion of hydrochloric acid. Direct blockage of this fundamental step inhibits gastric acid production. Proton pump inhibitors (PPIs), developed by the pharmaceutical industry, work in this manner. They have dramatically altered the therapy of duodenal ulcer and gastric reflux disease.

The parietal cell membrane has three important receptors involved in hydrochloric acid secretion: a cholecystokinin B (CCK_B) **gastrin** receptor, a muscarinic 3 (M_3) acetylcholine receptor, and a histamine 2 (H_2) receptor (Fig. 14-3). These receptors engage in a synergism in which simultaneous activation of two or more of them by

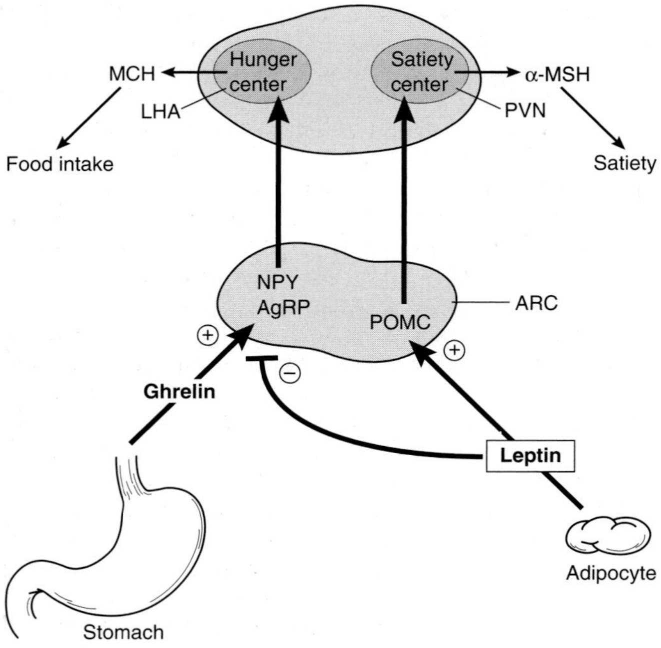

Figure 14-3 Hormonal axis controlling energy homeostasis. Ghrelin and leptin activate first-order neurons in the arcuate nucleus (ARC) of the hypothalamus, leading to stimulation of the hunger and satiety centers. NPY, neuropeptide Y; AgRP, agouti-related protein, POMC, propiomelanocortin; LHA, lateral hypothalamic area; PVN, paraventricular nucleus; MCH, melanin-concentrating hormone; and αMSH, α-melanocyte-stimulating hormone.

the appropriate ligand augments acid secretion. Conversely, when any one of these sites is blocked, the other sites become less responsive to stimulation. Thus, when vagal innervation is interrupted, the parietal cell response to gastrin becomes blunted.

Mechanisms of Acid Stimulation

Hydrochloric acid secretion by the parietal cell mass occurs in a sequential order divided into three general phases. Each phase has distinct mechanisms of activation. The initial cephalic phase is mediated by the central nervous system (CNS). The subsequent gastric phase involves the release of ligands by the stomach. Finally, the intestinal phase completes the process by releasing various gastrointestinal neuropeptides as well as histamine.

Cephalic Phase

The sight, smell, or thought of food activates afferent neural pathways to the CNS. Efferent activity proceeds from the hypothalamus to the stomach via the vagus nerve. Acetylcholine release by the vagus stimulates the parietal cell directly by binding to its M_3 receptor. Activation of the receptor leads to an intracellular cascade resulting in the release of hydrochloric acid. Acetylcholine also indirectly stimulates acid secretion by activating antral cells that produce gastrin-releasing protein (GRP). GRP then promotes gastrin secretion from antral G cells. Finally, acetylcholine can stimulate the ECL cells to release histamine.

In addition to food's visual and olfactory stimulation of acid release, its actual physical presence in the mouth activates the vagal pathway. Surgical division of the vagal nerves supplying the parietal cell mass blunts this parasympathetic response, decreasing acid secretion. In addition, anticholinergic blockade of the M_3 receptor can inhibit the response. Such agents, however, are not nearly as effective as other acid inhibitors now available, have multiple side effects, and are not used clinically.

Gastric Phase

The gastric phase commences with food entering the stomach. Stretch receptors within the stomach activate intragastric parasympathetic reflex pathways that promote further acetylcholine release. In addition, chemical and stretch receptors within the antrum detect alkalinization, antral distension, and the presence of amino acids. In response, the G cells release gastrin. The gastrin enters the venous circulation and exerts both a direct and indirect effect. Some gastrin binds the CCK_B receptors on the parietal cells, promoting hydrochloric acid secretion. This direct mechanism of action is the weaker of the two. Gastrin promotes acid secretion mainly via the ECL cells. Here, gastrin activates receptors, causing histamine release from the ECL cells. The histamine then binds the H_2 receptors on the parietal cells, stimulating acid release.

Gastrin appears to be the most influential of the three ligands (acetylcholine, histamine, and gastrin) responsible for acid secretion by the parietal cell. It exhibits marked heterogeneity, being processed into multiple fragments from the initial preprogastrin produced by the G cells. Three main forms include 14-, 17-, and 34-amino acid species. Of these, the 17-amino-acid gastrin is the most biologically active in stimulating acid secretion. It has a short half-life of only 2 to 3 minutes, and, like all fragments, is neutralized in the small intestine and kidney.

Certain foods can also stimulate acid secretion. Both alcohol and caffeine act directly on the mucosa to increase hydrochloric acid release. Proteins also seem to promote acid secretion indirectly via their breakdown products as described above.

Intestinal Phase

The intestinal phase of gastric acid production occurs with the arrival of the products of digestion in the small intestine. Although knowledge regarding this phase is somewhat limited, it is associated with substantial elevations in various serum peptides. Some of them, like enterooxyntin, stimulate gastric acid output. Other peptides are inhibitory (see the section on mechanisms of acid suppression and mucosal protection below). The parietal cell H_2 (histamine) receptor may play an important role in this phase of acid secretion.

Mechanisms of Acid Suppression and Mucosal Protection

When stimulated, the parietal cell mass in the stomach can drop the pH to as low as 1.0. In this acidic environment, pepsinogen is activated to pepsin and begins to hydrolyze proteins into peptones and amino acids. Unchecked, this process would lead to severe caustic injury and autodigestion of the stomach. Fortunately, several mechanisms exist to suppress acid secretion and protect the gastric mucosal lining.

Endocrine-Mediated Acid Suppression

The release of acidic chyme into the duodenum stimulates the secretion of numerous hormones that help suppress gastric acid production. **Secretin**, a 27-amino-acid peptide released by duodenal S cells, plays an important role in this suppression. Luminal acidity, biliary salts, and fatty acids stimulate its secretion. In turn, secretin inhibits gastrin release, gastric acid secretion, and gastric motility. Somatostatin, a tetradecapeptide, is another important mediator. It is released with a drop in gastric pH and acts directly on the parietal cells to inhibit acid secretion. In addition, it inhibits gastrin release when gastric luminal pH drops to less than 1.5. Finally, somatostatin reduces histamine release from ECL cells. Cholecystokinin and gastric inhibitory polypeptide (GIP), both released by cells in the duodenum, also act to suppress gastric acid production. Thus, an enterogastric feedback mechanism exists in which duodenal peptides help suppress acid production in the stomach once food enters the intestines.

Gastric Mucosal Protection

Within the stomach is a sophisticated, highly efficient barrier system that protects the gastric mucosal lining from caustic injury and digestion. The goblet cells are central to this process. They produce a mucopolysaccharide that attaches to the luminal surface of the gastric mucosa, creating a protective barrier. The gastric glandular epithelium also secretes bicarbonate in exchange for chloride ions. The amount of bicarbonate produced by the stomach can only neutralize a small portion of the maximum acid output. The gastric lining, however, is preserved because the gel-like mucosal barrier traps the secreted bicarbonate. Any back-diffusion of hydrogen ions into it, therefore, leads to their rapid neutralization and clearance. As a result, even though the pH in the stomach may drop to as low as 1.0, the pH at the luminal surface of the mucosal cells rarely falls below 7.0. When this mechanism is not functioning adequately, as seen in *Helicobacter pylori* infection, damage to the mucosa can occur. **Gastritis** or **gastric ulcers** can result.

Vitamin B_{12} (Cobalamin) Absorption

The stomach and duodenum play an important role in vitamin B_{12} (cobalamin) absorption. To be properly absorbed in the terminal ileum, vitamin B_{12} must be complexed to intrinsic factor (IF). This glycoprotein is produced by the parietal cells in the stomach and binds to vitamin B_{12} after pancreatic proteases have isolated it in the proximal small bowel. Failure of any step in this sequence can result in vitamin B_{12} deficiency with the subsequent development of megaloblastic anemia, irreversible sensory neuropathy, and dementia.

The Schilling test is an effective means of determining the cause of vitamin B_{12} deficiency. In the first part of the test, a patient is given an oral dose of radiolabeled cobalamin followed by an intramuscular injection of unlabeled vitamin. The excretion of cobalamin in the urine is then determined by collecting a 24-hour urine sample. An abnormal value corresponds to less than 10 % excretion of vitamin. Abnormal results are followed by a repeat Schilling test using radiolabeled cobalamin bound to IF. Urinary excretion in this case will be normal if IF deficiency, as seen in pernicious anemia, is responsible for the poor vitamin B_{12} absorption. It will remain abnormal in cases of bacterial overgrowth or ileal disease causing the vitamin deficiency. Finally, the Schilling test can also be administered using radiolabeled cobalamin bound to proteins in scrambled eggs. An abnormal result in this situation would suggest failure of the vitamin to dissociate from the ingested food, as occurs in patients with achlorhydria.

Duodenal Bicarbonate Secretion

Like the stomach, the duodenum has several mechanisms of mucosal protection. Mucus is produced by Brunner's glands, helping to create a protective barrier over the mucosa. In addition, the duodenal cells secrete sodium bicarbonate via a transmucosal electrical gradient. This production is up to six times greater than that of the stomach. As a result, the sodium bicarbonate can neutralize all of the hydrogen ions that are normally presented to the duodenal bulb. Additional bicarbonate comes from the pancreas. It, however, only neutralizes a small amount of the total acid load.

Duodenal bicarbonate is stimulated locally by mucosal irritation. Pancreatic bicarbonate is released in response to secretin stimulation. It increases the volume of pancreatic secretions of bicarbonate and water. The cells of origin of these secretions are the centroacinar cells.

BENIGN GASTRIC DISEASE

Gastric Ulcer Disease

Benign gastric ulceration is often lumped with benign duodenal ulceration under the term *peptic ulcer disease* (PUD). This grouping is useful since both forms of ulceration have important similarities in pathophysiology, presentation, evaluation, and treatment. Certain types of gastric ulcer behave much like duodenal ulcers. Additionally, both gastric and duodenal ulceration have uncomplicated and complicated manifestations. Finally, medical therapy and indications for surgical intervention are similar. Key differences, however, do exist in presentation, evaluation, and treatment. Subtle nuances in the symptoms of uncomplicated disease can exist between the two types of ulceration. Most importantly, the risk of underlying malignancy in gastric ulceration changes aspects of evaluation and management. This chapter, therefore, discusses each entity in separate sections to emphasize such differences. Because much overlap does exist, however, similarities will be covered in the sections on duodenal ulcer disease.

Although the exact pathogenesis of benign gastric ulceration is still poorly understood, *H. pylori* and nonsteroidal antiinflammatory drugs (NSAIDs) are recognized as important ulcerogenic agents. Each promotes ulcer formation by altering the balance between the protective and potentially harmful components of the gastric environment. In the case of *H. pylori* infection, this imbalance occurs due to a diffuse gastritis, dysregulation of acid secretion, and damage to the mucosal defensive barrier. Chronic infections can result in achlorhydria and loss of the mucopolysaccharide coating of the mucosa, leading to ulcerogenesis. NSAIDs, on the other hand, cause injury by inhibiting prostaglandin synthesis. This decrease alters local blood flow, mucus production, and bicarbonate secretion in the stomach. As a result, the gastric mucosal defensive mechanisms are diminished, exposing the lining to damage. Taken together, *H. pylori* infection and NSAID use, either alone or in combination, are thought to be the etiology of most benign gastric ulcer disease worldwide. Tobacco use is also an important risk factor. The role of alcohol in ulcerogenesis is unclear.

Classification

Gastric ulcers can be classified into four types according to their anatomic location. Type I gastric ulcers occur along the lesser curvature of the stomach in the transition zone between the antrum and cardia. Type II gastric ulcers arise in combination with duodenal ulcers. Type III gastric ulcers develop in the prepyloric region. Finally, type IV gastric ulcers occur high on the lesser curve near the gastroesophageal junction.

The classification of a gastric ulcer has important implications in terms of its frequency, pathophysiology, and treatment. Type I gastric ulcers are the most frequent, whereas type IV gastric ulcers are relatively infrequent. Both types, however, are associated with normal or low acid output. In contrast, both type II and type III gastric ulcers are associated with gastric acid hypersecretion. In fact, they behave much like duodenal ulcers. Their treatment, therefore, follows guidelines similar to duodenal ulcer disease.

Knowing the pathophysiology of *H. pylori* infection is helpful in understanding the distribution and characteristics of many gastric ulcers. *H. pylori* are small, curved, microaerophilic Gram-negative rods with multiple flagella. They are spread from person to person via gastro-oral or fecal-oral transmission. Once ingested, these urease-producing bacteria colonize the antrum of the stomach, causing local mucosal inflammation. In an individual with a high gastric acid output, this colonization spreads distally into the duodenal bulb as the duodenal mucosa in this region undergoes gastric metaplasia. In a person with a low gastric acid output, it spreads more proximally into the cardia. Colonization is particularly dense at the transition zone between the stomach antrum and cardia. Such observations help explain why most benign gastric ulcers are type I (within a few centimeters of the gastric transition zone) and why these ulcers are associated with low acid output. Also, they help explain why type II ulcers are associated with duodenal ulcers. Finally, they reveal why type II and type III ulcers are associated with acid hypersecretion.

NSAID-induced ulcers are a caveat for the above classification. They can occur anywhere in the stomach, and, therefore, do not always fall neatly into the above classification scheme. Additionally, treatment can be somewhat different. Consequently, some authors have proposed an additional type V classification for gastric ulcerations due to NSAIDs.

Clinical Presentation and Evaluation

The clinical presentation of benign gastric ulcer depends on the severity of the disease process. In uncomplicated gastric ulceration, patients typically complain of a characteristic gnawing epigastric pain that can radiate to the back. Often, this pain is associated with ingestion of food, producing anorexia and weight loss. Complicated gastric ulcers can produce such antecedent symptoms. Some, however, remain asymptomatic until the development of the complication. Up to 10% of NSAID-induced ulcers behave in this fashion. The presentation, evaluation, and initial treatment of complicated gastric ulceration follow guidelines similar to complicated duodenal ulcer disease.

Evaluation of a patient suspected of having an uncomplicated gastric ulcer begins with a thorough history and physical examination. In addition to determining the duration and character of symptoms, risk factors are sought. In particular, the patient should be questioned regarding current tobacco or NSAID use, prior PUD, or history of *H. pylori* infection. Physical examination should focus on searching for signs of a malignant process (see adenocarcinoma of the stomach below).

Upper endoscopy confirms the diagnosis. This study involves the passage of a fiberoptic scope from the mouth into the esophagus, stomach, and duodenum. The mucosa is examined in detail. If an ulcer is present, it can usually be seen. Photographs of any lesion may be taken for documentation. Additionally, they can be used for evaluation of subsequent healing.

Because of the risk of underlying malignancy, all gastric ulcers require multiple biopsies at the time of endoscopy to establish the presence or absence of carcinoma. Endoscopic features suggestive of malignancy include a bunched-up ulcer border or large (> 3 cm) ulcer size.

Biopsy specimens should include samples incorporating the margin of the ulcer. Cytology and brushings are also helpful as an adjunct to biopsy. Despite such guidelines, false-negative results are still common due to the small sample size of the biopsy specimens. The presence of achlorhydria in a patient with gastric ulceration is also suggestive of a malignant process. Finally, all patients with gastric ulcers, like those with duodenal ulcers, require testing to determine the presence or absence of *H. pylori* infection. Samples can be obtained for this purpose at endoscopy.

Medical Treatment

First-line therapy for uncomplicated gastric ulcer disease is medical and follows guidelines similar to those for uncomplicated duodenal ulcer disease. In brief, this regimen includes cessation of all ulcerogenic agents (tobacco, NSAIDs, aspirin, steroids, and even alcohol), treatment of *H. pylori* infection with appropriate antibiotics, and acid suppression therapy. Additional options for gastric ulcer treatment include the administration of cytoprotective agents such as sucralfate and misoprostol. Sucralfate is an aluminum salt containing sulfated sucrose. On ingestion, the sucrose polymerizes, coating the gastric ulcer with a protective barrier that prevents further injury. Misoprostol is a prostaglandin E analogue that promotes gastric mucosal protection by enhancing the defensive mechanisms of the gastric lining. Even with the best of medical care, however, the nonhealing and recurrence rates of gastric ulcer disease can be high.

Repeat endoscopy is mandatory after medical treatment of a gastric ulcer. Usually, it is performed 6 weeks after diagnosis. By this time, the ulcer should show evidence of substantial (> 50%) healing. If it does not, medical therapy may be continued, depending on the index of suspicion for malignancy and the overall condition of the patient. After another 4 to 6 weeks of treatment, endoscopy is again undertaken. If the ulcer is still present, elective operative intervention is indicated unless a compelling reason exists to preclude the patient as an operative candidate. At each endoscopy, multiple biopsy specimens of the margin of the ulcer are taken. It is only after appropriate histologic review of these specimens that an ulcer can be said to be benign. Even so, despite the best efforts of pathologists, false-negative results do occur. The failure of a gastric ulcer to heal after adequate medical therapy is highly suggestive of an underlying malignant process.

Surgical Treatment

Operative intervention is reserved for complicated gastric ulcer disease. As in complicated duodenal ulcer disease, four main indications exist: bleeding, perforation, **gastric outlet obstruction**, and intractability. Additionally, a high index of suspicion for coexistent malignancy can be an indication. The mainstay of operative therapy is excision of the ulcer. For type I, II, and III ulcers, a generous antrectomy (50% gastrectomy) is performed. Gastrointestinal continuity is then restored using one of three options. In a **Billroth I** reconstruction, the duodenum is reanastomosed to the remaining stomach (Fig. 14-4). In a **Billroth II** reconstruction (Fig. 14-5), the anastomosis is between the remaining stomach and a loop of jejunum. Finally, a Roux-en-Y gastroenterostomy (Fig. 14-6) can be performed, but this procedure is often associated with delayed gastric emptying. Type II and III ulcers also require truncal vagotomies to decrease gastric acid secretion. Type IV ulcers may require near total gastrectomy with Roux-en-Y reconstruction. Another option for type IV ulcers is local excision of the ulcer. Every resected gastric ulcer must undergo histologic review to verify that a gastric carcinoma is not hidden in the depths of the crater. For this reason, complete excision of the ulcer is always required. If a gastric carcinoma is present, appropriate evaluation and treatment should be instituted. The recurrence rate after surgical treatment for a gastric ulcer is often very low.

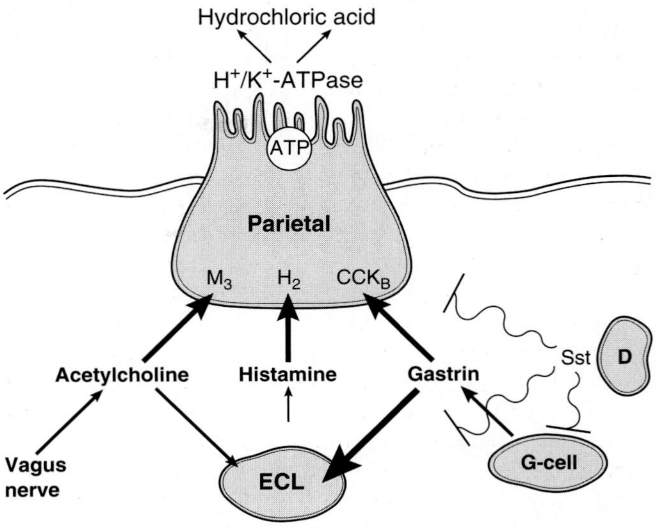

Figure 14-4 Gastric acid secretion by the parietal cell. The interplay between the vagus nerve, G-cell, and enterochromaffin-like (ECL) cell leads to parietal cell stimulation and hydrochloric acid secretion via three hormonal receptors. Somatostatin (Sst) release inhibits this acid secretion. M_3, muscarinic 3; H_2, histamine 2; CCK_B, cholecystokinin B; D, D-cell; ATP, adenosine triphosphate.

Acute Gastritis

Acute gastritis produces an inflammation of the stomach mucosa that can be associated with erosions and hemorrhage. Patients can present with many symptoms, including nausea, vomiting, hematemesis, melena, blood per rectum, or hematochezia. *H. pylori* infection, NSAID or aspirin use, bile reflux, alcohol ingestion, irradiation, and local trauma can all contribute to an inflammatory response. Treatment involves acid suppression, removal of the noxious agent, occasional gastric decompression, and nutritional support.

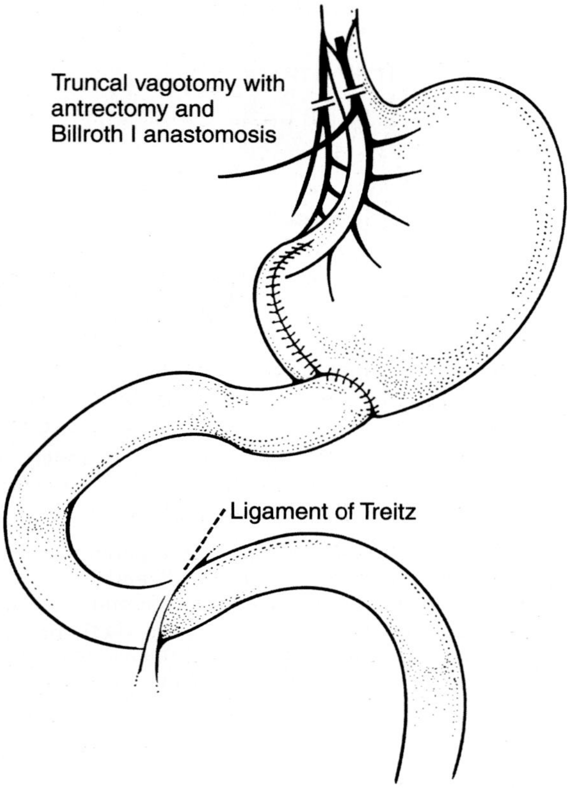

Figure 14-5 An antrectomy removes the distal portion of the stomach, where gastrin is produced. In addition, it removes the pylorus, thus allowing gastric emptying after vagotomy. In a Billroth I reconstruction, the duodenum is anastomosed to the stomach in continuity.

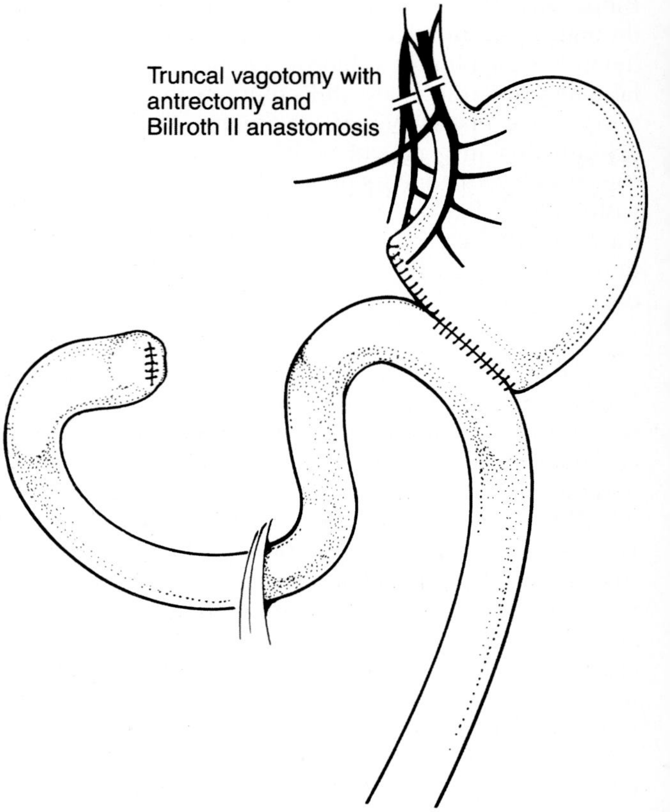

Figure 14-6 In a Billroth II reconstruction, the duodenum is not attached to the stomach; the stomach is anastomosed to a proximal loop of jejunum. This procedure is particularly useful when the duodenum is extensively scarred.

Stress Gastritis

Stress gastritis is another important cause of acute inflammation. It typically occurs in patients suffering from severe physiologic stress, and, if not properly recognized and treated, it can lead to significant morbidity and mortality. Patients develop mucosal erosions beginning in the proximal stomach and progressing rapidly throughout the rest of the organ. Classic presentations include ulcer formation in major burn victims (Curling's ulcer) and patients with CNS injury (Cushing's ulcer). This form of gastritis also occurs in other critically ill patients, such as those with severe trauma or organ failure. Medical prophylaxis is the best therapy, and its use in the intensive care unit has dramatically improved outcomes. PPIs, H_2-receptor blockers, antacids, sucralfate, and misoprostol all are effective agents. Prophylaxis should be started as soon as possible, since stress gastritis typically develops within 48 hours from the onset of physiologic stress.

Once stress gastritis is present, aggressive acid suppression is essential. Intraluminal pH should not decrease below 4.0. Treatment includes intravenous administration of PPIs or H_2 blockers. Alternately, antacids can be directly delivered into the stomach via a nasogastric tube. Sucralfate and misoprostol are also helpful adjuncts.

Hemorrhage is the most common complication of stress gastritis. In critically ill patients, it can be life threatening. Patients can present with blood per rectum or in the nasogastric tube, a drop in hematocrit, or hemodynamic instability. Nasogastric aspiration of bloody fluid often suggests the diagnosis. Upper endoscopy confirms it. Gastric lavage with either water or saline beforehand can help clear the stomach of blood clots and aid in visualization. Treatment should focus on initial fluid resuscitation and stabilization. Such therapy is instituted immediately, before any diagnostic interventions. Acid suppression is also started, if not already begun. A blood type and crossmatch is obtained, and the serial hematocrits are followed. At the time of upper endoscopy, isolated sites of bleeding can be treated with electrocautery, heater probe, injection of vasoconstrictive agents, or laser therapy.

In cases of persistent bleeding, more aggressive interventions are required. Selective visceral angiography (typically of the left gastric artery) with remobilization is one such option. Operative therapy is another. Of the several possible surgical interventions, vagotomy and pyloroplasty (see complicated duodenal ulcer disease), with oversewing of the bleeding erosions, is a quick, conservative procedure that controls hemorrhage in approximately 50% of patients. If bleeding recurs, total gastrectomy is considered.

Hypertrophic Gastritis (Menetrier's Disease)

Hypertrophic gastritis, also known as Menetrier's disease, is a rare disorder of the lining of the stomach characterized by massive hypertrophy of the gastric rugae. The exact etiology of the disease is unknown, but it is believed to be autoimmune in character. In particular, tumor necrosis factor (TNF)-β overexpression is thought to play a role. The thickening of the mucosal folds occurs as a result of hyperplasia of the mucus-secreting cells in the corpus and fundus. Patients can present with epigastric pain, nausea, vomiting, occult hemorrhage, anorexia, weight loss, and diarrhea. Progression of disease is associated with a protein-losing gastropathy that can lead to hypoproteinemia and peripheral edema. Diagnosis requires upper endoscopy with mucosal biopsy. On occasion, a full-thickness gastric biopsy is required to confirm the diagnosis.

Treatment is typically nonoperative. Acid suppression therapy with antacids, H_2-receptor antagonists, or PPIs should be initiated. A high-protein diet and careful monitoring of nutritional status is essential. Anticholinergic medications can sometimes help decrease protein loss due to the gastropathy. In rare instances, total gastrectomy may be required. Menetrier's disease is a risk factor for the development of adenocarcinoma of the stomach.

Mallory-Weiss Syndrome

An upper gastrointestinal hemorrhage secondary to linear tearing at the GE junction is a well-described phenomenon known as the Mallory-Weiss syndrome. Typically, these tears form after episodes in which a strong Valsalva maneuver causes mechanical stress on the mucosa in this region. Retching (often from acute alcohol intoxication), heavy lifting, childbirth, vomiting, blunt abdominal trauma, and seizures have all been associated with the syndrome. Patients typically present with hematemesis, melena, or hematochezia after such an antecedent history. Evaluation focuses on hemodynamic assessment and verification of a tear as the bleeding source. A nasogastric tube is placed, and gastric lavage performed. The presence of blood should prompt endoscopic evaluation. The tears are visualized on retroflexion. Nuclear scintigraphy or selective angiography can also provide a diagnosis if endoscopy is unavailable. Laboratory investigations should include determination of coagulation parameters and serial hematocrits. A blood type and crossmatch is obtained.

Initial therapy is nonoperative. Fluid resuscitation and stabilization is foremost. Acid suppression is then instituted with either PPIs or H_2-receptor blockers. Most bleeding will stop without any further intervention. If bleeding persists, endoscopy can be repeated and the tear treated with electrocautery, heater probe, or injection therapy. Selective angiography with embolization is another option. Surgery is a last resort. The presence of subserosal staining along the lesser curve at the time of exploration is pathognomonic. Gastrotomy with oversewing of all tears is undertaken. Rebleeding after any of the above interventions typically occurs within 24 hours.

Gastric Polyps

Gastric polyps are rare, but greater numbers are being diagnosed as more patients are undergoing upper gastrointestinal endoscopy. The polyps are either hyperplastic or adenomatous. Hyperplastic polyps are more common and are typically benign, although some can develop into cancers. Adenomatous polyps have a more substantial risk of malignant degeneration. If the polyp measures less than 0.5 cm, the risk of malignancy is low. A polyp that is greater than 1.5 cm in diameter has a considerably greater risk. When a gastric polyp is diagnosed, the physician may evaluate the patient for the presence of other polyps.

The presence of multiple benign polyps in the small intestine and melanous spots on the lips and buccal mucosa is known as Peutz-Jeghers syndrome. Peutz-Jeghers syndrome is an autosomal dominant trait that has a high degree of penetrance. In these patients, conservative therapy is indicated because the tumors are hamartomas and are infrequently malignant.

Bezoar

The accumulation of a large mass of indigestible fiber within the stomach is known as a **bezoar.** If the material is made up of vegetable fiber, it is called a phytobezoar. If it is predominantly hair, the mass is called a trichobezoar. Trichobezoars are more common in children and among inmates of mental institutions. Patients with large bezoars can sometimes present with gastric outlet obstruction. Although most bezoars may be broken up using the endoscope, some require surgical removal.

MALIGNANT GASTRIC DISEASE

Adenocarcinoma of the Stomach

Almost 95% of stomach cancers are adenocarcinomas. Worldwide, adenocarcinoma remains a leading cause of cancer-related death. Its overall incidence, however, has been steadily declining over the last 50 years. Additionally, marked regional variability exists. While the frequency of adenocarcinoma in the United States and Europe remains relatively low, it is considerably higher in Asia, particularly Japan and China. High rates are also seen in Russia, Chile, and Finland. Environmental factors, especially diet, are thought to account for this discrepancy, since émigrés from these high-risk areas who settle in the United States have a lower incidence of disease.

Important risk factors of gastric adenocarcinoma include *H. pylori* infection, pernicious anemia, achlorhydria, and chronic gastritis. A history of caustic injury from lye ingestion also increases the risk of malignant degeneration. Finally, the presence of adenomatous polyps in the stomach is considered a risk factor.

Classification of Gastric Adenocarcinoma

Adenocarcinoma of the stomach can be divided into various classification schemes related to its clinical and histologic appearance. In the United States, cancers are often categorized into ulcerative, polypoid, scirrhous, and superficial spreading subtypes based on their endoscopic appearance. Of these, ulcerative carcinomas are by far the most frequent. Even though some differences in prognosis do exist between certain subtypes, the usefulness of this classification system is somewhat limited.

Two distinct histologic types of gastric adenocarcinoma exist: intestinal and diffuse. The intestinal type is well differentiated with glandular elements. It is more common in regions with a high incidence of disease. Typically, it occurs in older patients and spreads hematogenously. The diffuse type is poorly differentiated with characteristic signet ring cells. It occurs in younger patients and has an association with blood type A. It spreads via the lymphatics and local extension.

Linitis plastica is the term used to describe the complete infiltration of the stomach with carcinoma. In this situation, the stomach can look like a leather bottle. Patients with this variant of gastric cancer have a particularly poor prognosis.

Clinical Presentation and Evaluation

The clinical presentation of gastric adenocarcinoma depends on its stage. Early cancers are usually asymptomatic. As a result, in the United States they often go unrecognized until later in their progression. In Japan these early cancers are more frequently diagnosed because of an aggressive endoscopic screening protocol. The low incidence of gastric carcinoma in the United States, however, makes the cost of such a program prohibitive.

More advanced disease leads to the development of symptoms. Patients can complain of vague epigastric pain similar to that produced by gastric ulceration. Often, it can be present for an extended period of time. Unexplained weight loss is another early complaint. As the disease progresses, patients begin to have more specific symptoms. Dysphagia, hematemesis, melena, nausea, or vomiting develops. Patients may also present with new onset iron deficiency anemia or guaiac-positive stools.

The initial evaluation for a patient suspected of having gastric carcinoma begins with a thorough history and physical examination. Risk factors are determined, and the patient is queried regarding lack of energy and unintentional weight loss. Physical examination should focus on signs of advanced disease. An enlarged left supraclavicular lymph node (Virchow's node) or a palpable umbilical node (**Sister Mary Joseph's node**) indicates distant lymphatic spread. Additionally, a palpable rectal ridge (Blumer's shelf) or the presence of ascites suggests peritoneal dissemination. All these findings are ominous signs and worrisome for extensive disease. On abdominal exam, the presence of an epigastric mass may indicate a locally advanced tumor.

Diagnostic workup and clinical staging should follow the National Comprehensive Cancer Network consensus guidelines. Upper endoscopy is essential to characterize the location and extent of disease. Additionally, multiple biopsies of the lesion are required to obtain a histologic diagnosis. Often, endoscopic ultrasound is undertaken to determine the depth of tumor invasion, an important aspect of staging. Metastatic spread to the lungs, liver, and ovaries (Krukenberg's tumor) does occur. Imaging studies to rule out such involvement are therefore necessary. A chest radiograph and computed tomography of the abdomen and pelvis are adequate screening modalities. Laboratory investigations include a complete blood cell count, electrolytes, creatinine level, and liver function tests. Upper gastrointestinal series are not necessary and can miss some cancers, especially the superficial spreading subtype.

Because gastric carcinoma can spread intraabdominally, metastasis to the peritoneum and the omentum do occur. Such lesions are difficult to identify using conventional computed tomography. As a result, laparoscopy has become a key component of staging. Patients who do not have any evidence of metastatic disease on initial workup now undergo laparoscopic staging. During this procedure, the abdomen is carefully explored for evidence of peritoneal, hepatic, or omental disease. Any suspicious lesions are biopsied. Abdominal washings are typically taken as well, and the local extent of tumor determined. The presence of metastatic disease precludes curative resection and can help avoid an unnecessary laparotomy.

Treatment

Complete surgical resection in an attempt to cure gastric adenocarcinoma should only be undertaken in the presence of localized disease. Considerable debate exists regarding the extent of such a resection. For most distal lesions, many surgeons favor a radical subtotal gastrectomy. In this procedure, approximately 85% of the stomach is removed, including the omentum. The proximal portion of the resected specimen is then immediately examined by the pathologist to verify that it is free of tumor involvement. Only after such verification is gastrointestinal continuity restored by means of a Roux-en-Y gastrojejunostomy. Total gastrectomy is reserved for either large distal lesions or more proximal tumors. Splenectomy or pancreatectomy may also need to be included in the operative procedure. They should, however, be avoided unless absolutely necessary.

Another controversial topic is the extent of lymph node dissection at the time of resection. The Japanese favor a radical lymphadenectomy. In the United States, a less extensive dissection is undertaken. Comparisons between the two approaches in Japan point toward improved survival in those patients having the radical lymph node removal. These results have not been duplicated in Western countries. In fact, the more extensive dissections seem to cause higher morbidity without a survival benefit. The reason for such a discrepancy is poorly understood.

The role of adjuvant therapy following surgical resection is also somewhat controversial. Although several studies have shown little difference in survival compared to surgery alone, a recent randomized trial in the United States did. As a result, patients in the United States now receive postoperative 5-fluorouracil and leucovorin with radiation therapy. Several randomized trials are currently underway to evaluate the efficacy of neoadjuvant therapy as well. The results of these trials employing preoperative chemotherapy and radiation may alter current practice patterns.

As mentioned earlier, the best cure rates are reported in Japan, where there is a high percentage of the superficial spreading type. Even with this type of tumor, the 5-year survival rate is less than 50%. In most studies from English-speaking countries, curative resection is associated with a 5-year survival rate of less than 10%. Pathologic staging of the resected specimen is the best predictor of survival (Fig. 14-7). The case for early diagnosis is made in studies that evaluated the 5-year survival rate in patients who had an incidental carcinoma found during stomach surgery for supposed benign disease. Some studies report that the 5-year survival rate in this highly selected cohort approaches 75%.

Patients with metastatic disease cannot be cured. Palliative therapy should focus on quality of life. Because the morbidity and mortality associated with palliative surgery can be high, it should be undertaken with caution. In selected patients with good preoperative status, it may be beneficial. The resection should include the lesion, with an adequate cephalic margin, and the entire stomach distal to the tumor. Clear indications for palliative surgical intervention include proximal or distal tumor obstruction and bleeding. Endoscopic stent placement and laser therapy are also palliative options. Chemotherapy and radiation offer little help.

Gastric Lymphoma

The stomach is the primary source of almost two-thirds of all gastrointestinal lymphomas. Patients with gastric lymphoma tend to be older, and the non-Hodgkin's variant predominates. Patients typically present with symptoms similar to those seen in gastric adenocarcinoma. Upper abdominal pain, unexplained weight loss, fatigue, and bleeding are all encountered. Diagnosis can often be made with tissue biopsies during upper endoscopy. Sometimes, however, the presence of lymphoma is only determined at the time of surgical exploration. If the diagnosis is made preoperatively, the workup should follow that undertaken for any lymphoma to determine its stage. Chest radiography, abdominal computed tomography, and bone marrow biopsy all should be undertaken.

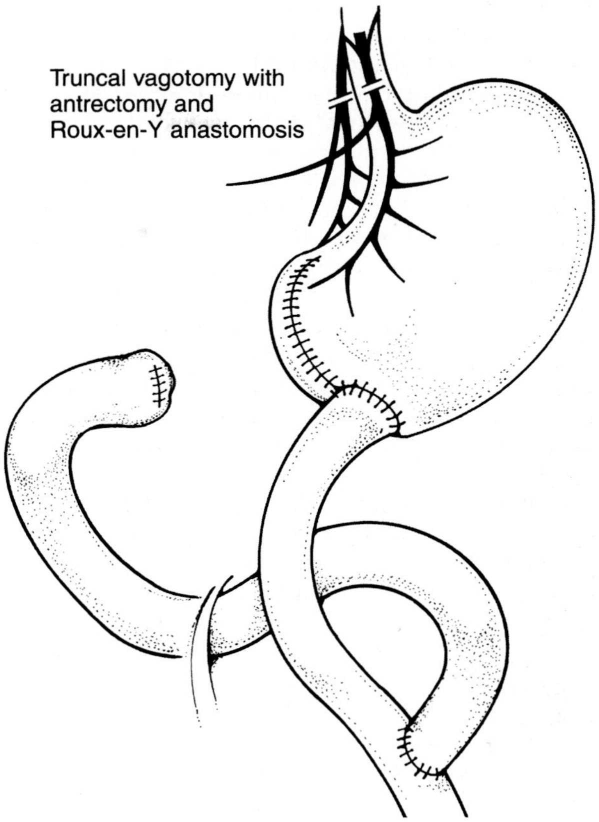

Figure 14-7 A Roux-en-Y anastomosis reduces the reflux of small bowel contents into the stomach. Peristalsis in the small bowel carries food and fluid away from the stomach. This procedure is particularly useful when a patient has a history of alkaline reflux gastritis.

The treatment of primary gastric lymphoma is somewhat controversial. Some specialists advocate chemotherapy alone, citing high 5-year survival rates in early stage disease. Such treatment, however, does run the risk of causing gastric perforation or hemorrhage, necessitating surgical intervention. Other physicians believe that operative resection of grossly involved tissue is the best option. Such treatment can be followed with chemotherapy or radiation treatment. When the lesion is confined to the stomach, the 5-year survival of such a resection can approach 75%.

Gastrointestinal Stromal Tumor (GIST)

Formerly known as leiomyomas and leiomyosarcomas, gastrointestinal stromal tumors (GISTs) are submucosal growths of the gastrointestinal tract arising from a variety of cell types. The stomach is the most common site for these masses. GISTs can be either benign or malignant, but, unless direct invasion is present, differentiation between the two is often difficult. Large tumor size (> 6 cm) and tumor necrosis suggest malignancy. Typically, such a determination is made only after the pathologist has counted the number of mitotic figures under high-powered field. The finding of more than 10 such figures per 50 fields is considered evidence of malignancy.

The clinical presentation of GISTs is similar to other gastric tumors. Many patients are asymptomatic. Nonspecific abdominal pain can occur. Bleeding and obstruction can be manifestations. Finally, some patients present with an abdominal mass. Evaluation typically involves upper endoscopy, which reveals a submucosal mass. Central ulceration may be present. Biopsy is usually nondiagnostic. Endoscopic ultrasound may be employed. Abdominal computed tomography should be performed to determine the tumor size, presence of invasion, and evidence of metastasis. The liver is the most common site for disseminated disease.

Treatment of a stomach GIST involves local excision. A margin of 2 to 3 cm should be included in the resection specimen. Enucleation is avoided because of the risk of malignancy in the tumor. Likewise, the tumor capsule should not be disrupted to avoid spillage. Depending on the extent of the tumor, a more extensive gastric resection may be needed. Patient survival following resection depends on the presence of malignancy. The prognosis for a benign lesion is excellent. Malignant GIST, however, can be quite aggressive. In such cases, chemotherapy using imatinib mesylate has been effective.

BENIGN DUODENAL DISEASE

Uncomplicated Duodenal Ulcer Disease

In the United States, PUD accounts for billions of dollars in health care expenditures. Nearly 500,000 new cases are diagnosed annually. As a result, the number of adult Americans having active disease remains relatively constant at approximately 2 million. Duodenal ulcers constitute the majority of this disease burden. They typically form in the duodenal bulb. *H. pylori* and NSAIDs are important ulcerogenic agents. An association with tobacco also exists. In contrast to gastric ulcers, duodenal ulcers rarely harbor any underlying malignancy. Their workup and treatment, therefore, differ somewhat from the evaluation and therapy of gastric ulcers.

Most duodenal ulcer disease is uncomplicated. Dramatic changes in the understanding and treatment of this disorder have occurred over the last 2 decades. The identification of *H. pylori* as a potential ulcerogenic agent and the development of effective acid suppression medications are now recognized as seminal events in the evolution of care. In the process, the treatment of PUD shifted from the domain of the surgeon to that of the internist.

Clinical Presentation and Evaluation

The clinical presentation of uncomplicated duodenal ulceration has features similar to that of uncomplicated gastric ulcer disease. Patients often complain of a burning epigastric abdominal pain that is gnawing in character. It may radiate to the back, especially if the ulcer is located in the posterior aspect of the duodenal bulb. Certain aspects of presentation, however, are different from uncomplicated gastric ulceration. The pain typically occurs 1 to 3 hours after food ingestion and is accentuated by fasting. It may awaken patients from sleep. Relief from pain typically occurs after use of over-the-counter acid suppressants. Food intake can also improve pain. In such a situation, a recent history of weight gain may be noted.

A thorough history and physical examination remain important components of the initial evaluation of the patient suspected of having uncomplicated duodenal ulceration. In addition to characterizing the nature of the pain, risk factors are determined. They include a history of PUD, prior *H. pylori* infection, NSAID ingestion, or tobacco use. Physical exam focuses on the abdomen. Mild epigastric tenderness on palpation may be present. Finally, signs of occult blood loss are sought. Pallor, orthostasis, and guaiac-positive stools are significant findings.

Traditional Diagnostic Testing

Classically, the diagnosis of uncomplicated duodenal ulcer disease was made by means of an upper gastrointestinal contrast study using barium (upper gastrointestinal series). Although it is now infrequently used for making such a diagnosis, an understanding of its mechanics is helpful. In this examination, barium and air are swallowed. The esophagus, stomach, and duodenum are then observed fluoroscopically. Finally, radiographs are made for permanent documentation. During the procedure, care is taken to observe swallowing mechanics, peristaltic activity, gastric distensibility, and pyloric function; the mucosal pattern is noted; evidence of organ displacement is sought, and the pyloric sphincter size and shape are determined.

The upper gastrointestinal series is still a widely available, inexpensive, and safe exam. Unfortunately, it tends to miss many acute lesions of the duodenum. In such cases, ancillary findings such as duodenal spasm, deformity, or mucosal swelling may suggest the diagnosis. Even so, it is no longer a useful primary diagnostic modality for PUD given current practice patterns.

Gastric acid analysis is another classic evaluative study for uncomplicated duodenal ulcer disease. In this test, a nasogastric tube is placed into the stomach for collection of gastric aspirates. Samples are obtained over a 1-hour period before and after the administration of an intravenous acid secretagogue, usually pentagastrin. Most patients with uncomplicated duodenal ulceration have a high ($>$ 4.0 mEq/hr) basal acid output. Over two-thirds have an elevated stimulated acid output.

Gastric acid analysis is particularly useful in identifying the rare patient who develops duodenal ulceration due to an occult gastrinoma (see the discussion under Zollinger-Ellison syndrome below). In such an individual, the basal acid output may be 10 times the upper limit of normal. The parietal cell mass is often maximally stimulated by elevated baseline serum gastrin levels. Accordingly, the stimulated acid output increases only minimally compared to basal output values. Due to evolutions in the care of both PUD and gastrinoma, however, gastric acid analysis has also fallen into disuse.

Current Diagnostic Testing

Today, the diagnosis of uncomplicated duodenal ulceration is often made empirically. In the patient with typical signs and symptoms, noninvasive testing for the presence of *H. pylori* infection is undertaken. Both quantitative and qualitative serologic antibody testing exists. These studies have the advantage of low cost and wide availability. Their accuracy, however, depends on the probability of infection. In developed countries, they are particularly useful at identifying active *H. pylori* infection among younger patients, because of its low incidence. The presence of antibody in older individuals, however, is a less reliable indicator of active disease, since it can persist for years after the infection has been successfully eradicated.

Other useful noninvasive diagnostic studies are the urease tests. They identify the presence of *H. pylori* infection by indirectly detecting the organism's urease activity. Urease hydrolyzes urea into ammonia and carbon dioxide. The increased carbon dioxide can be detected in either the blood or breath of the patient. PPIs and bismuth compounds must be withheld several weeks prior to such testing to prevent false-negative results. The main advantage of the urease tests is that they identify only active disease. They are also useful in documenting successful eradication of the bacteria.

A final noninvasive study is the fecal antigen test, which identifies the presence of *H. pylori* using antibodies. Like the urease tests, it is positive only during an active infection. Again, care must be taken when interpreting results in patients on PPIs and bismuth compounds. It is helpful in verifying eradication of the bacteria after therapy. Upper endoscopy is usually reserved for patients who have failed initial therapy or for those with worrisome symptoms (presence of gastric ulceration). In such cases, endoscopy provides a means of direct visualization and characterization of the ulceration. Additionally, it can also identify concomitant disease or suggest an alternative diagnosis. Finally, it provides a means of obtaining biopsies. Rarely, samples are taken from a mass associated with the duodenal ulceration. More typically, gastric tissue is obtained to test for the presence of *H. pylori*. Since this infection is typically confined to the distal stomach in duodenal ulcer disease, these samples should be taken from the antrum. Both tissue culturing and histologic review can detect the organism. These methods are, however, time consuming and expensive. An alternative method is the rapid urease test. A tissue biopsy (usually antral) is placed on a pH-sensitive indicator containing a large amount of urea. In the presence of *H. pylori*, the urease produces ammonia and carbon dioxide, altering the media pH and producing a color change. Like its noninvasive counterparts, it is positive only during active infection. Because these studies are inexpensive and quick, they have become a popular means of bedside screening for the presence *H. pylori* after routine endoscopy. Finally, they are useful in verifying complete eradication of infection after appropriate therapy.

Treatment

The treatment of uncomplicated duodenal ulcer disease is nonoperative. It is aimed at promoting ulcer healing and preventing its recurrence. Such goals are best achieved by the removal of all ulcerogenic agents and the institution of acid suppression therapy. To this end, tobacco and NSAID (including aspirin) use should be discontinued indefinitely. Additionally, *H. pylori* infection must be eradicated. Unfortunately, this organism is tenacious, and antibiotic resistance is growing. As a result, two or more antibiotics are required to treat adequately any infection. Currently, antibiotic therapy is combined with acid suppression using PPIs or H_2-receptor antagonists.

Recommendations are similar to those in the Maastricht-2 2000 consensus report. First-line therapy involves a minimum of 7 days of treatment involving acid suppression with dual antibiotic therapy using clarithromycin and amoxicillin or clarithromycin and metronidazole. Second-line regimens include repeating first-line treatment interchanging amoxicillin and metronidazole or instituting traditional quadruple therapy. This regimen consists of an acid-suppression drug, bismuth, metronidazole, and tetracycline for a minimum of 7 days (14, classically). Due to increasing antibiotic resistance, patients should undergo some form of testing for the presence of *H. pylori* after treatment. Eradication of *H. pylori* leads to more rapid healing of duodenal ulcers, resolution of gastritis, and lower recurrence rates for both duodenal and gastric ulcers.

Acid-suppression therapy should be continued until the ulcer is healed. If the etiology of the ulcer is apparent, PPIs or H_2-receptor antagonists can usually be discontinued after a relatively short time interval. If the etiology of the ulcer is unclear, they should be continued until its cause is determined and treated.

Complicated Peptic Ulcer Disease

Complicated peptic ulcer disease has four main manifestations: perforation, hemorrhage, gastric outlet obstruction, and intractability. As a result, the presentation, evaluation, and initial treatment of complicated duodenal ulcer disease and complicated gastric ulcer disease are the same. Differences in care can arise at the time of surgical intervention.

Clinical Presentation and Evaluation

The type of complication determines the clinical presentation and evaluation. Patients with perforated ulcers present with acute onset of severe epigastric pain. Often, they are able to report the exact time of day that the symptoms began. Physical examination usually reveals tachycardia and evidence of a rigid (surgical) abdomen resulting from diffuse chemical peritonitis. Occasionally, however, a more localized peritonitis may develop as gastric acid drains into the right paracolic gutter. In such cases, the patient presents with right lower quadrant rebound tenderness very similar to that seen in acute appendicitis. Evaluation should include an upright chest radiograph. Evidence of free intraperitoneal air (**pneumoperitoneum**) outlining the diaphragm or liver is diagnostic of a perforated intraabdominal viscus (Fig. 14-8). Patients should also have a complete blood count and basic metabolic panel drawn.

A patient presenting with a bleeding ulcer will report hematemesis, melena, or blood per rectum. Massive bleeding can occur, and some patients may exhibit signs of early or late shock. Physical examination may reveal hypotension, tachycardia, pallor, mental status changes, and active bleeding. In such cases, volume resuscitation with crystalloid or whole blood should be immediately instituted. Evaluation of any gastrointestinal hemorrhage should focus on determining the site of bleeding. A nasogastric tube is placed, and gastric lavage performed. The presence of blood suggests an upper gastrointestinal source. Endoscopy is confirmatory. Additionally, it allows characterization of the ulcer and determination of *H. pylori* status. Patients with bleeding ulcers should have serial hematocrits followed and coagulation parameters determined. Finally, blood type and crossmatch should be ready at all times.

Patients with gastric outlet obstruction resulting from chronic ulcer scarring will complain of inability to tolerate oral intake. In particular, they may report projectile vomiting of food shortly after eating, much like infants with pyloric stenosis. (See Chapter 3, Pediatric Surgery, in Lawrence et al., eds., *Essentials of Surgical Specialties*, 3rd Ed.). A history of weight loss is common. These patients often delay seeking medical attention. As a result, they suffer from varying degrees of dehydration. Physical examination may reveal upper abdominal fullness, decreased skin turgor, dry mucus membranes, or epigastric peristaltic waves. Evaluation should focus on assessing the extent of metabolic derangement. Electrolyte and creatinine levels are informative. Often, these patients develop a hypokalemic, hypochloremic metabolic alkalosis. In severe cases, they will have evidence of paradoxical aciduria as the distal renal tubules sacrifice hydrogen ions for potassium (see Chapter 3, Fluids and Electrolytes).

Finally, patients with intractable ulcers will have symptoms of persistent disease after adequate nonoperative therapy. Often, these individuals will have undergone multiple treatments for ulceration without relief or healing. Additionally, they may develop recurrence of disease after an apparently successful initial therapy. Fortunately, such patients are becoming less frequent. Physical examination in these patients mirrors findings seen in uncomplicated PUD. Intractability should alert the clinician to the possibility of rarer causes of ulceration (see the section on Zollinger-Ellison syndrome below). Evaluation should be directed accordingly.

Treatment

The treatment of complicated PUD typically involves an initial stabilization phase. During this period, the patient is resuscitated and nonoperative therapies are instituted. Depending on a patient's complication and response to

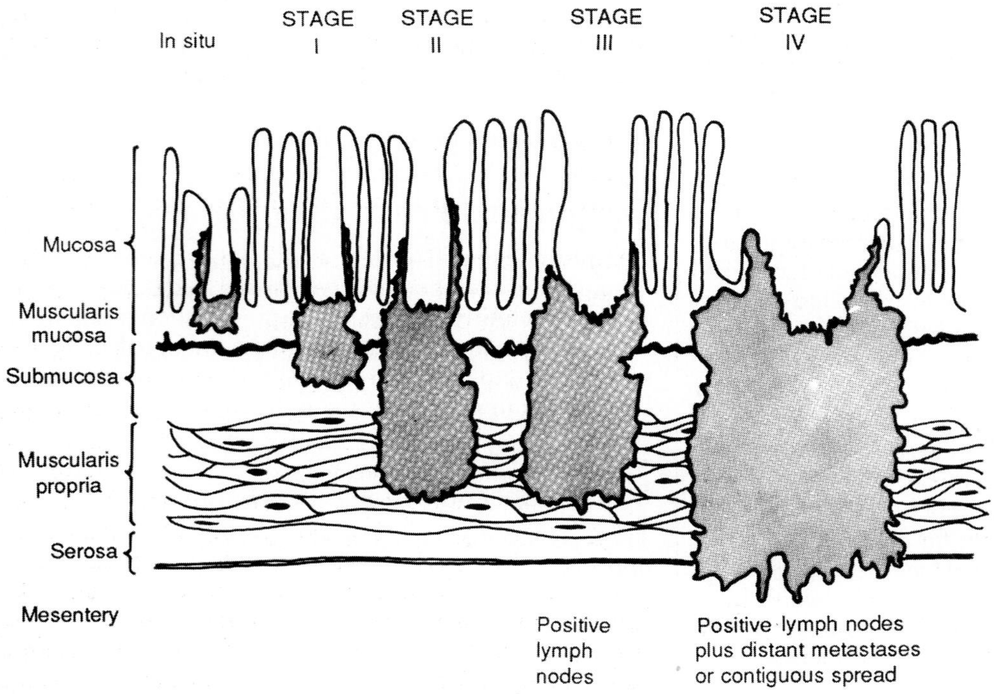

Figure 14-8 As tumor penetration of the bowel wall progresses, so does stage. The staging is important because with advanced stages, survival is severely limited.

treatment, this phase can be definitive. Otherwise, the patient will require operative intervention. At the time of surgery, two objectives should be met. First, the complication should be properly treated. Second, a definitive antisecretory procedure should be performed. In this way, ulcer recurrence is minimized. Antisecretory procedures are discussed more fully under the intractability section below.

Perforation

A perforated ulcer is a surgical emergency. Patients should be prepared for the operating room with fluid resuscitation and nasogastric decompression. At the time of surgical exploration, the site of perforation is identified. Typically, this is an ulcer located on the anterior aspect of the duodenal bulb. If the perforation is less than 6 hours old, the ulcer is plicated (oversewn), and an acid-reducing procedure is performed. The plication is often buttressed with a tag of omentum (Graham patch). If the perforation is more than 6 hours old, the acid-reducing procedure is not performed. Both open and laparoscopic repair of simple perforated duodenal ulcers have been described.

Complex perforated duodenal ulcers can be therapeutic challenges. Large, friable ulcers are difficult to close. In such circumstances, more extensive procedures are required. They focus on patching the opening or excluding it from the flow of gastrointestinal contents. Adequate drainage of the duodenal region is essential.

In rare cases, patients with a perforated ulcer may be treated nonoperatively. Typically, the patient is a clinically stable elderly individual with multiple medical problems who presents relatively late (12 or more hours) after the onset of symptoms. Because of the high operative risk, these patients are treated with nasogastric decompression, volume resuscitation, nothing by mouth, and serial abdominal exams with blood laboratories. If the perforation has sealed off, they will improve and avoid operation. Surgical intervention, however, is indicated if any clinical deterioration occurs.

Hemorrhage

In patients who have upper gastrointestinal hemorrhage, initial stabilization is necessary. At least two large-bore intravenous lines are inserted. Volume resuscitation then follows American Trauma Life Support (ATLS) guidelines: 2 L of crystalloid is followed by whole blood. The stomach is decompressed using a nasogastric tube. High-dose PPI therapy is instituted. Finally, any coagulation abnormalities are corrected.

Hemorrhage is initially treated by upper endoscopy. Options include electrocautery, heater probe, or injection therapy. Using such techniques, most bleeding can be successfully stopped. Endoscopic signs worrisome for risk of rebleeding include active hemorrhage at the time of endoscopy, a visible vessel in the ulcer crater, and fresh clot on the ulcer. Endoscopy may be repeated if rebleeding occurs. Angiography and selective embolization is sometimes employed in patients who have a very high operative risk.

Surgical intervention is reserved for refractory bleeding. In general, a transfusion requirement of six or more units of blood over the first 12 hours is an indication for surgery. Elderly patients or those who are hemodynamically unstable may require earlier operative therapy. Younger, more stable patients can be resuscitated longer. At the time of laparotomy, the bleeding artery is ligated. In the case of a posterior duodenal ulcer, duodenotomy with three-point U-stitch fixation of the ulcer bed is necessary. In a type IV gastric ulcer, left gastric artery ligation may be necessary. An acid-reducing procedure is also performed.

Gastric Outlet Obstruction

In patients with gastric outlet obstruction, the stomach is decompressed with a nasogastric tube for 5 or 6 days, or until it returns to near-normal size. During this time, the patient is allowed nothing by mouth. Nutrition and fluids are administered intravenously. Because most patients are hypochloremic and alkalotic, initial resuscitation should be with normal saline crystalloid solution. Malnutrition is ameliorated by total parenteral nutrition. Careful monitoring for electrolyte abnormalities is undertaken.

Most cases of gastric outlet obstruction require operative intervention because of the cicatricial scarring around the site of the ulcer. Such procedures require either removal of the obstruction or its bypass. Typically, antrectomy can be performed with appropriate reconstruction. If this cannot be done, a gastroenterostomy to drain the stomach must be created. An acid-reducing procedure is also necessary.

In some cases, the gastric outlet obstruction develops due to mucosal edema rather than scarring. The prolonged nasogastric decompression helps decrease the swelling and provides resolution of the obstruction. Endoscopy, however, is still required to characterize the extent of scarring, biopsy any suspicious lesions, and screen for *H. pylori*. Occasionally, an operation can be avoided.

Intractability

Patients with ulcers unresponsive to conventional medical management have intractable disease. They may require surgical intervention to decrease acid secretion. The surgeon can alter such secretion through interruption of the vagal neural pathway with or without removal of the gastrin-producing cells in the antrum.

The most straightforward approach to vagal interruption is by means of a truncal vagotomy. In this procedure, all vagal trunks at or above the esophageal hiatus of the diaphragm are completely transected. As a result, the entire parietal cell mass is denervated. Unfortunately, truncal vagotomy also denervates the antral pump, the pyloric sphincter mechanism, and most of the abdominal viscera. Gastric motility is disrupted, and a gastric drainage procedure is required to facilitate gastric emptying. Otherwise, gastric antral dilation occurs, stimulating gastrin release. The most common complementary drainage procedure is pyloroplasty, which is performed by incising the pylorus

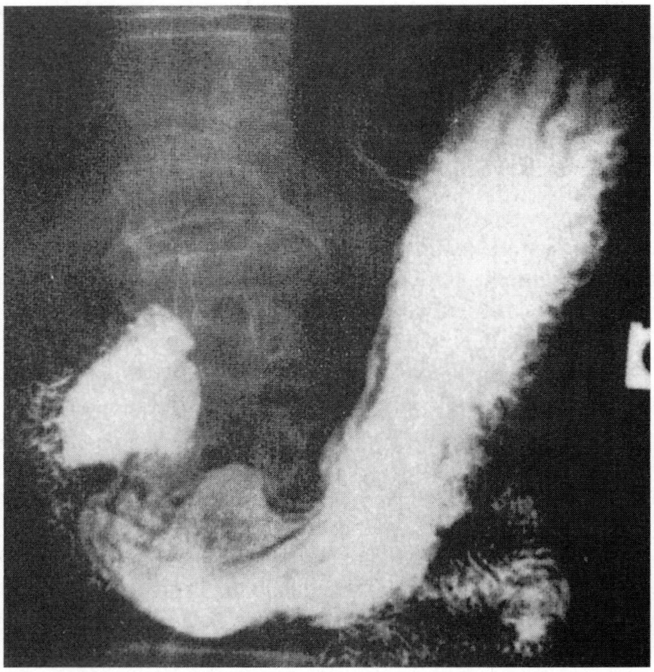

Figure 14-9 An upright posteroanterior chest radiograph often shows subdiaphragmatic air in patients with a perforated ulcer.

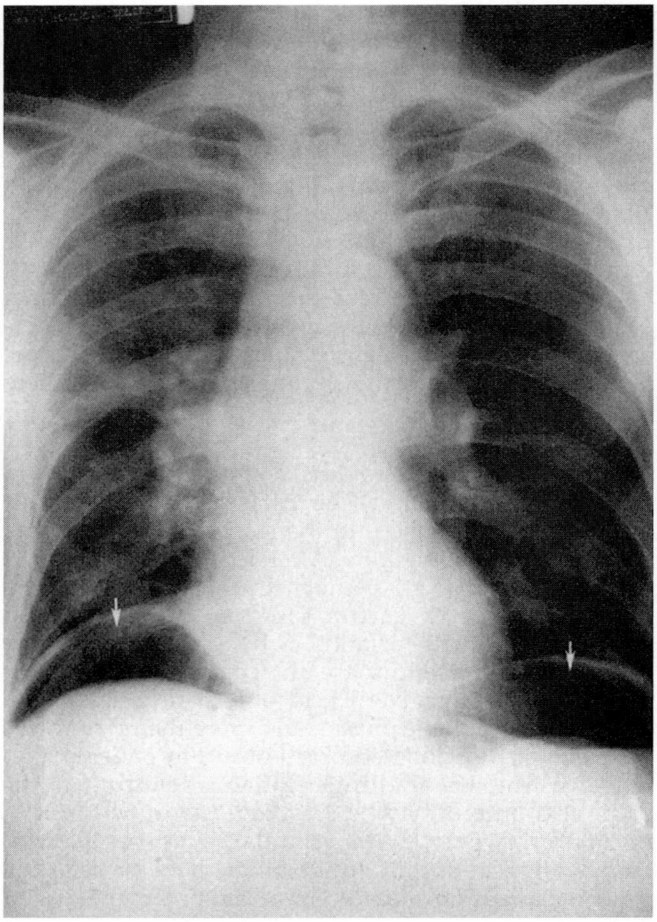

Figure 14-10 When the trunk of the vagus nerve is divided, a pyloroplasty is also performed to allow gastric emptying. This pyloroplasty is the most common type performed.

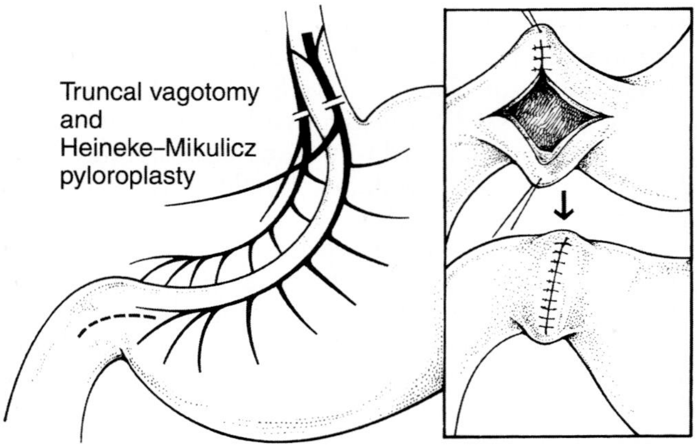

Figure 14-11 Because a selective vagotomy denervates the pylorus, a pyloroplasty is performed to allow gastric emptying.

horizontally and closing it vertically (Fig. 14-9). Various modifications of pyloroplasty have been proposed, and most are known by eponyms. If pyloroplasty is not possible, gastroenterostomy is an alternative. Many surgeons add distal gastrectomy (**antrectomy**) to the truncal vagotomy (Fig. 14-4). Antrectomy augments the effect of vagotomy by removing the bulk of the gastrin-producing cells (G cells). In this way, both the cephalic phase and the gastric phase of acid stimulation are interrupted. Truncal vagotomy with antrectomy is associated with a lower recurrence rate than truncal vagotomy with pyloroplasty (1.5% versus 10%).

Selective vagotomy provides total denervation of the stomach, from above the crus of the diaphragm down to and including the pylorus (Fig. 14-10). This procedure spares the parasympathetic innervation of the abdominal viscera. Like truncal vagotomy, however, it denervates the antral pump and pylorus, necessitating some type of drainage procedure. Most surgeons employ pyloroplasty. Advocates of this type of vagotomy claim that it more completely denervates the stomach compared to a truncal vagotomy. They also emphasize that the parasympathetic innervation to other abdominal organs (liver, gallbladder, pancreas, small intestine, and proximal colon) is spared. Finally, proponents note the similar frequency of postgastrectomy syndromes (see section on postgastrectomy syndromes below) between the two forms of vagotomy.

The most recent approach to vagal interruption to gain popularity is **proximal gastric vagotomy** (Fig. 14-11). It is also known as parietal cell vagotomy or highly selective vagotomy. In this procedure, the vagus nerve is identified as it courses along the lesser curvature of the stomach. The branches innervating the parietal cell mass are then individually divided. Near the level of the antrum, the nerves forming the "crow's foot" are preserved. This maneuver maintains the normal innervation and functioning of the antral pump and pyloric sphincter mechanisms, obviating the need for a drainage procedure. Patients with gastric outlet obstruction as a result of peptic ulcer disease are not candidates for this procedure. Proximal gastric vagotomy has the lowest incidence of postgastrectomy syndromes. The ulcer recurrence rate is greater than 10%, but the morbidity and mortality rates are relatively low. Patients with ulcer recurrence after proximal gastric vagotomy can now be relatively easily managed with antisecretory medications.

The decision about which procedure to perform on an individual patient is complicated. It is based on the age of the patient, the likelihood of ulcer recurrence, the severity of symptoms, and the patient's sex and weight. The procedures that have the highest cure rate (i.e., truncal vagotomy and antrectomy) also have the highest incidence of postgastrectomy side effects, such as **dumping syndrome** (see Table 14-1). Likewise, procedures with the lowest cure rate have the lowest incidence of side effects. Therefore, the surgeon's responsibility is to select the procedure for each patient that is likely to be effective in treating the ulcer diathesis while minimizing the likelihood of side effects. It is possible to predict which patients are at high risk for postgastrectomy complications; young, thin women are particularly vulnerable. In these patients, it may be advantageous to avoid performing truncal vagotomy, especially with the availability of proximal gastric vagotomy, which is an excellent alternative.

Duodenal Polyps

Duodenal polyps typically arise as a part of an inherited familial disorder. One of the more well known of these genetic conditions is familial adenomatous polyposis. Patients having this autosomal dominant syndrome develop multiple adenomatous polyps in the colon and gastroduodenal region. Because of the possibility of malignant degeneration of these polyps, close monitoring is required. Most patients require early prophylactic removal of the colon. All patients need routine endoscopic surveillance of the stomach and duodenum with removal of any polyps. The presence of cancer or villous adenoma in a duodenal polyp requires surgical excision. Another important condition is Peutz-Jeghers syndrome (see section on gastric polyps above).

MALIGNANT DUODENAL DISEASE

Zollinger-Ellison Syndrome

Although very rare, **Zollinger-Ellison syndrome** is perhaps the most well-known endocrine tumor disorder. It is the direct result of a gastrin-producing neoplasm (gastrinoma). The resultant hypergastrinemia causes near maximal stimulation of the parietal cell mass. Hydrochloric acid is constantly secreted, leading to the well-described clinical manifestations of the syndrome. Over two-thirds of these tumors are located in the anatomic triangle whose apices include the junction of the cystic duct with the common bile duct, the junction of the second and third portion of the duodenum, and the neck of the pancreas.

Gastrinomas can occur sporadically or as part of an inherited familial disorder. A strong association exists with the multiple endocrine neoplasia type 1 (MEN-1) syndrome. This disorder is characterized by the clinical constellation of pituitary adenomas, hyperparathyroidism, and pancreatic islet cell tumors (of which gastrinomas are the most common). Approximately 60% of all gastrinomas are malignant. Unfortunately, about half of the patients with the malignant variant of the disease die within 5 years of diagnosis. Because of its slow growth pattern, however, long-term survival up to 15 years is seen in some patients.

Table 14-1 Relative Incidence of Recurrence and Operative Mortality Rate Expressed as Percentages

	Recurrence Rate (%)	Operative Mortality Rate (%)	Dumping		Afferent Loop Syndrome	Blind Loop Syndrome	Alkaline Reflux Gastritis	Metabolic Sequelae
			Early	Late				
Vagotomy/pyloroplasty	5–10	1–2	2+	2+	0	0	1+	1+
Vagotomy/antrectomy Billroth I	1–2	1–4	2+	2+	0	0	1+	1+
Vagotomy/antrectomy Billroth II	1–3	1–4	3+	3+	2+	2+	2+	2+
Selective vagotomy	5–10	1–2	2+	2+	0	0	0	1+
Proximal gastric vagotomy	10–15	1	0	0	0	0	0	0
Total gastrectomy	0	2–5	3+	2+	0			2+

[a] These numbers are averages taken from the larger series published in the literature. The relative incidences of the postgastrectomy syndromes are expressed on a scale of 0 to 4+, with 0 indicating relative absence of symptoms and 4+ indicating frequent profound symptoms.

Clinical Presentation and Evaluation

A high degree of suspicion is necessary to identify patients with Zollinger-Ellison syndrome. Often, the diagnosis is suggested by unusual clinical presentations. One such manifestation is the patient complaining of ulcer-like symptoms with concomitant chronic or severe diarrhea. Additionally, patients may present with extremely virulent ulcer diathesis. In such cases, they will have multiple duodenal ulcers or ulceration in atypical locations (jejunum or ileum). Finally, patients may report a personal or family history of refractory PUD or endocrine disease.

Evaluation begins with a thorough history and physical examination focused on establishing the presence of any of the above-mentioned associations. In particular, a personal or family history of MEN-1 diseases is sought. Diagnosis rests on establishing the presence of hypergastrinemia with hypersecretion of acid. A fasting serum gastrin level is therefore necessary. Care, however, must be taken to make sure that the patient has discontinued any PPIs for at least 1 week prior to testing. PPI use increases gastrin levels. The presence of elevated gastrin levels above 1000 pg/mL is often considered diagnostic. Abnormal values less than 1000 pg/mL should prompt further confirmatory testing. The investigation of choice is the secretin stimulation test. In addition to being safe, it has a high specificity and sensitivity. Fasting serum gastrin levels are obtained at 2, 5, 10, 15, 30, 45, and 60 minutes after the intravenous infusion of secretin. An elevation in the baseline gastrin value is seen in patients with Zollinger-Ellison syndrome. For most laboratories, this increase must be greater than or equal to 200 pg/mL. The presence of acid hypersecretion is established by measuring the gastric pH. A value of 2.5 or less is considered positive. Gastric acid analysis can also be performed.

Once the diagnosis of Zollinger-Ellison syndrome has been established, further evaluation should focus on tumor localization and clinical staging. Commonly used imaging modalities include computed tomography, magnetic resonance imaging, and ultrasonography. Somatostatin receptor scintigraphy and endoscopic ultrasound are also popular. These neoplasms are often quite small and, as a result, their preoperative localization can be quite difficult. A thorough search should be undertaken, however, because knowing the site of the primary tumor helps with operative planning. The liver is the most common site for metastatic disease.

Finally, all patients with newly diagnosed Zollinger-Ellison syndrome should undergo some form of screening for MEN-1 syndrome. Although genetic testing is available, it requires thorough pretest counseling. A more straightforward screen is to obtain a serum calcium level. If it is elevated, a parathyroid hormone level should be determined. The presence of hyperparathyroidism is highly suggestive of concomitant MEN-1 (see Chapter XX, Surgical Endocrinology).

Treatment

Traditional therapy for Zollinger-Ellison syndrome involved total gastrectomy with esophageal anastomosis in an effort to treat the often virulent ulcer diathesis. Although this procedure provided absolute protection from recurrent ulcer disease, it was associated with a high mortality. Additionally, significant aberrations in metabolism could occur. Pernicious anemia, malnutrition, and weight loss were all encountered. Fortunately, advances in the surgical and medical treatment of the disorder have made total gastrectomy a very rare intervention.

Because of these same advances, however, some controversy exists regarding current therapeutic interventions. Most experts now agree that patients with Zollinger-Ellison syndrome should be placed on high-dose PPIs to lower the production of hydrochloric acid. By doing so, they help prevent ulcer diathesis and improve the hypersecretory diarrhea. H_2-receptor antagonists have become second-line agents. Surgical exploration is indicated in patients having sporadic gastrinoma without metastasis. At the time of laparotomy, a proximal gastric vagotomy is performed to decrease acid secretion. In addition, a thorough search is made for the tumor. If it is found, it is resected. Cure is possible with successful removal of the neoplasm.

The role of surgery in patients having gastrinoma in association with MEN-1 is more controversial. If hyperparathyroidism is present, a parathyroidectomy is indicated because it helps attenuate gastrin release. Because cure is rarer in patients with MEN-1, some experts do not recommend surgical exploration in patients without metastasis. Other specialists contend it is helpful, especially in the hands of experienced surgeons.

The presence of metastatic disease decreases survival. Some experts recommend surgical debulking. Other options include chemotherapy and hepatic embolization. Hormonal manipulation using long-acting synthetic analogues of somatostatin (octreotide) can also be effective. Octreotide suppresses the elevated gastrin concentrations and may help in slowing tumor growth. All patients with metastatic disease, as well as those whose tumors could not be found at surgical exploration, require continued PPI therapy.

Adenocarcinoma of the Duodenum

The duodenum is the most common site for adenocarcinoma in the small bowel. Approximately two-thirds of these lesions are located in the second part of the duodenum, usually in the periampullary region. Fortunately, it is a rare disease because patients typically present late in its course. Symptoms can range from nonspecific abdominal pain with weight loss to those of intestinal or gastric outlet obstruction. Some patients will present with melena or hematochezia due to ulceration of the lesion. Physical examination often is unremarkable. Diagnosis is often made by means of upper endoscopy with tissue biopsy. Computed tomography is helpful to determine evidence of local invasion or metastatic spread.

Surgical excision is indicated in resectable disease. Pancreaticoduodenectomy is typically performed if the tumor is present in the first or second portion of the duodenum. An extended small bowel resection with duodenojejunostomy is an option if tumor is limited to the third or fourth portion of the duodenum. Patients with unresectable disease or evidence of metastasis at the time of exploration should have a diverting gastroenterostomy. Postoperative radiation therapy may be helpful. In patients with positive lymph nodes, prognosis is very poor, with 5-year survivals below 15%.

Duodenal Lymphoma

Lymphoma of the duodenum is also relatively rare; most small bowel primaries occur in the ileum. The clinical presentation is similar to that for duodenal adenocarcinoma. Abdominal pain, weight loss, and fatigue are common. Complications include perforation, bleeding, or obstruction. Endoscopy may be helpful in diagnosing duodenal lymphomas. Computed tomography assists in determining disease extent. If the diagnosis is made prior to surgical exploration, complete clinical staging is performed, following guidelines similar to those for gastric lymphoma. Wide surgical excision with staging should be performed if disease appears resectable. Adjuvant chemotherapy can be employed postoperatively. Patients with disseminated disease receive chemotherapy and local radiation.

POSTGASTRECTOMY COMPLICATIONS

Postgastrectomy Syndromes

The innervated intact stomach is a careful guardian of the gastrointestinal tract. When the stomach is denervated, and especially when the pyloric mechanism is ablated, the exquisite control of gastric emptying is abolished. This change, in association with the anastomotic characteristics of many reconstructions, is the reason for most common postgastrectomy syndromes. Several reconstructions produce a defunctionalized limb of intestine or place the duodenum or jejunum at risk for obstruction or bacterial overgrowth. Others allow easy ingress of bile and duodenal secretions into the gastric pouch. These aberrations in normal anatomy produce the various postgastrectomy syndromes.

In the evaluation of a patient with a complicated postoperative course, an upper gastrointestinal series may be performed. This series is used to document the extent of gastric resection and type of reconstruction, to determine the cause of vomiting (if present), and to assess gastric emptying and motility. Gastric emptying can also be defined more physiologically by administering a radionuclide-labeled meal followed by sequential imaging. Clues to the diagnosis can also be acquired by examination with an endoscope, which allows direct visualization and biopsy.

Early Dumping Syndrome

Early dumping syndrome is characterized by a select set of symptoms that occur after the ingestion of food of high osmolarity. This type of meal may contain a large quantity of simple and complex sugars (e.g., milk products). Approximately 15 minutes after the meal is ingested, the patient has anxiety, weakness, tachycardia, diaphoresis, and, frequently, palpitations. The patient may also describe feelings of extreme weakness and a desire to lie down. Crampy abdominal pain may also be present. Often borborygmi are heard, and diarrhea is not uncommon. Gradually, the symptoms clear.

The patient with early dumping has uncontrolled emptying of hypertonic fluid into the small intestine. Fluid moves rapidly from the intravascular space into the intraluminal space, producing acute intravascular volume depletion. As the simple sugars are absorbed and as dilution of the hypertonic solution occurs, symptoms gradually abate. Intravascular volume is replenished as fluid shifts from the intracellular space and is absorbed from the intestinal lumen. Fluid shifts, however, do not explain all of the symptoms associated with early dumping. The release of several hormonal substances, including serotonin, neurotensin, histamine, glucagon, vasoactive intestinal peptide, kinins, and others, is believed to contribute to the symptom complex. The use of a somatostatin analogue to block these hormonal substances may be of benefit to some patients.

This problem is best treated by avoiding hypertonic liquid meals, altering the volume of each meal, and ingesting some fat with each meal to slow gastric emptying. Liquids are ingested either before the meal or at least 30 minutes after the meal. Some authors claim that beta-blockers (10 to 20 mg propranolol hydrochloride) taken 20 minutes before a meal are helpful in approximately 50% of cases. In some patients with Billroth I or II anastomoses and recalcitrant symptoms, surgical construction of a Roux-en-Y gastrojejunostomy may be necessary. This procedure works by delaying gastric emptying.

Late Dumping Syndrome

As in early dumping, the patient suddenly has anxiety, diaphoresis, tachycardia, palpitations, weakness, fatigue, and a desire to lie down. In late dumping, the symptoms usually begin within 3 hours after the meal. This variant of dumping is not associated with borborygmi or diarrhea. The physiologic explanation for late dumping involves rapid changes in serum glucose and insulin levels. After the meal, a large bolus of glucose-containing chyme is presented to the mucosa of the small intestine. Glucose is absorbed much more rapidly than when the intact pylorus is present to meter gastric emptying. Extremely high serum glucose levels may occur shortly after the meal and may elicit a profound outpouring of insulin. The insulin response exceeds what is necessary to clear the glucose from the blood, and subsequently, hypoglycemia results. The symptoms in late dumping are the direct result of rapid fluctuations in serum glucose levels.

Nonoperative therapy for this syndrome includes the ingestion of a small snack 2 hours after meals. Crackers and peanut butter make an excellent supplement to abort or ameliorate the symptoms. If symptoms cannot be controlled by nonoperative management, then either conversion of the previous procedure to a Billroth I (if not already present) or construction of a Roux-en-Y gastrojejunostomy is considered. Surgical intervention is considered only in patients who do not respond to aggressive nonoperative therapy.

Postvagotomy Diarrhea

Almost half the patients who undergo truncal vagotomy experience a change in bowel habits (i.e., increased frequency, more liquid consistency). In most cases, the symptoms improve or disappear with time. However, a small percentage of patients ($< 1\%$) have severe diarrhea that does not relent with time. These patients may experience diarrhea that is explosive in onset, is not related to meals, and occurs without warning.

The pathophysiology of postvagotomy diarrhea is not entirely known. Gastric hypoacidity and the effects of vagal denervation on intestinal motility are possible etiologies. A diminished bile salt concentration secondary to biliary dysfunction may also be a contributing factor. In most patients with postvagotomy diarrhea, fluid intake is restricted and the intake of foods that are low in fluid content is increased. Antidiarrheal agents such as codeine, diphenoxylate hydrochloride, or loperamide may be of benefit. Cholestyramine, which binds bile salts, or somatostatin analogues may also be used. If the postvagotomy diarrhea is severe or is refractory to medical management, a reversed 10-cm segment of jejunum is inserted 100 cm distal to the ligament of Treitz. This procedure delays small bowel transit time, but has many inherent problems.

Afferent Loop Obstruction

Afferent loop obstruction occurs only after gastrectomy with a Billroth II reconstruction. It is usually associated with a kink in the afferent limb adjacent to the anastomosis. Pancreatic and biliary secretions are trapped in the afferent limb, where they cause distension. Symptoms usually include severe cramping abdominal pain that occurs immediately after the ingestion of a meal. Patients often characterize the pain as crushing. Within 45 minutes, the patient feels an abdominal rush that is associated with increased pain, followed by nausea and vomiting of a dark brown, bitter-tasting material that has the consistency of motor oil. These symptoms result from the spontaneous, forceful decompression of the obstructed limb. Classically, no food is present. The symptoms resolve with vomiting. These patients often have profound weight loss because they stop eating to prevent the pain. The best treatment is exploration of the abdomen and conversion of the Billroth II anastomosis to either a Roux-en-Y gastrojejunostomy or a Billroth I gastroduodenostomy.

Blind Loop Syndrome

Blind loop syndrome is more common after a Billroth II procedure than after a Roux-en-Y procedure. It also occurs in patients who underwent bypass of the small intestine secondary to radiation injury or morbid obesity. Blind loop syndrome is associated with bacterial overgrowth in the limb of intestine that is excluded from the flow of chyme. This excluded limb of intestine harbors bacteria that proliferate and interfere with folate and vitamin B_{12} metabolism. A deficiency of vitamin B_{12} leads to megaloblastic anemia. The bacterial overgrowth may cause deconjugation of bile salts and lead to steatorrhea. Patients often have diarrhea, weight loss, and weakness, and they are often anemic. A Schilling test using cobalamin bond to intrinsic factor is often abnormal. Treatment consists of orally administered, broad-spectrum antibiotics that cover both aerobic and anaerobic bacteria (e.g., tetracycline). After successful therapy, a repeat Schilling test will be normal. Unfortunately, regrowth of bacteria can occur. As a result, antibiotic therapy is often only a temporizing step. Many of these patients require conversion to a Billroth I gastroduodenostomy.

Alkaline Reflux Gastritis

Alkaline reflux gastritis is seen in patients in whom duodenal, pancreatic, and biliary contents reflux into the denervated stomach. These patients have weakness, weight loss, persistent nausea, and epigastric abdominal pain that often radiates to the back. In addition, they are often anemic. Upper endoscopy will reveal an edematous, bile-stained gastric epithelium that is atrophic and erythematous. Mucosal biopsies should be taken away from the anastomosis. They demonstrate inflammatory changes with a characteristic corkscrew appearance of submucosal blood vessels. Nuclear scintigraphy will often demonstrate delayed gastric emptying.

Although a variety of medical regimens have been proposed to treat alkaline reflux gastritis (e.g., oral ingestion of cholestyramine, antacids, H_2 blockers, or metoclopramide), none is uniformly satisfactory. Surgical correction consists of diverting the duodenal contents away from the stomach with a long-limb Roux-en-Y gastrojejunostomy. The minimum distance between the gastrojejunostomy and the entry point of the biliopancreatic limb draining the digestive juices into the intestine is 40 cm (18 inches). Such a reconstruction is effective therapy in most patients.

Recurrent Ulcer Disease

Recurrent ulcer disease following surgical intervention is most commonly due to incomplete vagotomy. Often, the posterior vagal trunk or a branch of the right posterior nerve (criminal nerve of Grassi) is left intact. Each operation has its accepted recurrence rate. Truncal vagotomy and antrectomy has one of the lowest rates at around 2%. Proximal gastric vagotomy has the highest at approximately 12%. Traditionally, confirmation of an incomplete vagotomy was made by means of the Hollander test, in which gastric acid output was measured after creating an insulin-induced hypoglycemia in the patient. This rather dangerous diagnostic procedure was abandoned and replaced by one in which gastric acid output was determined after sham feeding. Currently, upper endoscopy is used to help confirm persistent vagal innervation to the stomach. Congo red is used to demonstrate areas of pH drop in the gastric mucosa after the administration of an acid secretagogue (pentagastrin). Such regions have intact vagal innervation. Treatment options include long-term PPIs versus reoperative vagotomy.

For patients with recurrent ulceration and verified complete vagotomy, a more thorough evaluation is required. In particular, a search for an endocrine etiology should be initiated. A family history of MEN-1 should be sought. Calcium and parathyroid hormone levels should be obtained to look for hyperparathyroidism. Gastrin levels should be drawn to rule out the presence of a gastrinoma. Therapy should follow guidelines described in the Zollinger-Ellison syndrome section.

Gastric Atony

Many gastric reconstructions result in the denervation of the stomach and ablation of the pylorus. As a result, gastric motility is altered. Rapid emptying of liquids is common and can result in both early and late dumping syndrome (see above). Additionally, delayed emptying of solids due to gastric atony can occur. This phenomenon is poorly understood. Over half of all patients with a Roux-en-Y gastrojejunostomy demonstrate substantial delays in gastric emptying on ^{99m}Tc-labeled egg albumin scintigraphy. Only about half of these patients with delayed emptying, however, exhibit any symptoms. Frequently, such symptoms will improve with time and not require intervention. If medication is required, urecholine may prove beneficial. Promotility agents, such as metoclopramide or erythromycin, are also useful.

Metabolic Disturbances

Although a variety of metabolic abnormalities are identified after gastric resection, anemias are the most common. Vitamin B_{12} or folate deficiency from decreased absorption can lead to megaloblastic anemia in up to 20% of patients. Treatment involves appropriate supplementation. Iron deficiency secondary to altered absorption or chronic blood loss can produce a microcytic anemia in as many as 50%. Iron replacement therapy is often required. In the case of chronic bleeding, the source (often reflux gastritis) must be identified and treated.

Altered bowel function is common following gastric reconstructions. Approximately one in four patients has frequent, loose stools postoperatively. The increased intestinal transit can have detrimental side effects. If rapid enough, steatorrhea can develop. Calcium and magnesium can chelate to the intestinal fats, leading to decreased absorption with resultant osteomalacia. Supplemental calcium as well as bisphosphonates can prevent such bone loss.

SURGICAL TREATMENT OF OBESITY

Obesity

With well over half the U.S. population overweight and nearly one-third obese, weight and its effect on health have become important topics of research and concern. Obesity is now a well-recognized risk factor for a multitude of comorbid conditions responsible for early mortality and billions of dollars in health care expenditures. Because of a dearth of effective nonoperative therapies, bariatric surgery has become a mainstay of treatment for the severely obese. As a result, it has experienced a rapid rise in use over the last decade.

Obesity is the result of an imbalance in energy homeostasis. A positive caloric accumulation leads to the storage of excess energy as fat. This positive balance can be due to either increased energy intake or decreased energy expenditure. A mere 10 kcal/day (one saltine cracker) of extra energy can result in a 1-lb weight gain over the course of a year. Both genetic and environmental influences are responsible for the development of obesity. For example, energy intake may increase secondary to altered appetite regulation, a genetic influence, or as a result of greater food availability, an environmental cause. Likewise, energy expenditure can be decreased due to a genetically determined low body metabolism or from an environmentally related sedentary lifestyle. Such a plethora of potential sources for weight gain emphasizes the multifactorial nature of obesity. An understanding of the classification, evaluation, and treatment of obese patients is essential for providing quality care to this often-marginalized group of people.

Physiology of Appetite Regulation

Appetite regulation has become an area of intense research over the last decade, increasing our understanding of energy homeostasis. The hypothalamus, stomach, and adipocyte all play important roles in this complex process (see Fig. 14-12). Food intake is triggered by the release of the hormone ghrelin from gastric oxyntic cells. This compound stimulates the release of neuropeptides in the "hunger center" of the hypothalamus, increasing caloric consumption. To signal adequate caloric load, the adipocyte releases the hormone leptin, which activates the "satiety center" of the hypothalamus. In this manner, food intake is decreased.

The stomach, adipocyte, and hypothalamus, therefore, constitute an intricate hormonal axis that helps to control energy homeostasis via regulation of appetite. Defects within this axis can lead to energy imbalance with important metabolic consequences. For example, leptin-receptor deficiency results in loss of the satiety signal and the development of obesity. It is one of the few disorders for which exogenous leptin administration is potentially curative. Likewise, ghrelin overproduction is thought to con-

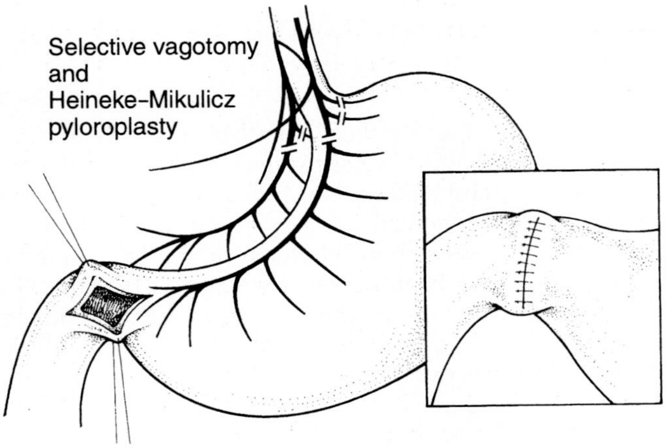

Figure 14-12 A proximal gastric vagotomy (highly selective vagotomy) denervates the acid-producing parietal cells without interfering with the antral pump or pylorus.

tribute to the hyperphagia and obesity seen in patients with Prader-Willi syndrome.

Classification of Obesity

By definition, obesity is an excess of total body fat. By contrast, overweight is an excess of body weight. An individual can therefore be overweight but not have excess body fat. Obesity can occur in the setting of increased (hypermuscular), normal, or decreased (sarcopenic) lean body mass. Multiple techniques exist to measure total body fat. Each, however, has its drawbacks, making none ideal. Hydrostatic weighing, in which an individual is immersed in water, is very accurate, but costly and cumbersome. Anthropometry comparing skinfold thickness is easier, but very operator-dependent. Bioelectrical impedance analysis provides a useful indirect measurement by determination of resting energy expenditure. It, however, requires overnight fasting.

Given the difficulties with determining total body fat, the body mass index (BMI) has become a useful surrogate marker. It is calculated by dividing an individual's weight in kilograms by the square of his or her height in meters:

$$\text{BMI} = \text{weight (kg)} / [\text{height (m)}]^2$$

Using the BMI, a person can be classified into various weight categories reflecting total body fat (see Table 14-2). Even though very helpful, the BMI can occasionally overestimate (as in body builders) or underestimate (as in the elderly) total body fat. The classification system based on BMI provides the basis by which individuals are treated for overweight and obesity. Surgical intervention is reserved for two groups of people: those having a BMI between 35 and 40 with concomitant significant comorbid conditions and those with a BMI of 40 or more.

Table 14-2 Weight Classification and Risk of Illness Based on Body Mass Index (BMI)

BMI Range	Weight Classification	Risk of Illness
Less than 18.5	Underweight	Increased
18.5 to 24.9	Ideal weight	Normal
25.0 to 29.9	Overweight	Increased
30.0 to 39.9	Obese	High/very high
40.0 or greater	Severely obese	Extremely high

Adapted from Bessesen DH, Kushner R. *Evaluation and Management of Obesity*. Philadelphia, PA: Hanley and Belfus, Inc., 2002.

Clinical Presentation and Evaluation

Severely obese patients can present in a variety of ways. Some patients are "healthy" without any recognized illnesses. They are unhappy, however, with either the restrictions that severe obesity places on their daily activities or its psychological consequences. As a result, they seek medical attention in an effort to lose weight, improve their quality of life, and help their self-image. Other patients are already being treated for one or more of the comorbid conditions arising from obesity. Such illnesses may stem from the metabolic changes related to excess fat. Insulin resistance, atherosclerosis, dyslipidemia, vein thrombosis, and cholelithiasis result from such metabolic alterations. Other conditions arise from the physical strains that obesity places on the body. Sleep apnea, degenerative joint disease (DJD), gastroesophageal reflux disease (GERD), and urinary stress incontinence are such physical manifestations. Finally, some disorders have a combined metabolic and physical etiology. Hypertension, infertility, psychosocial illnesses, and heart failure fall into this category. Patients with these preexisting comorbid conditions are often referred to the bariatric surgeon in an effort to induce weight loss and improve associated diseases.

The evaluation of a severely obese patient for surgical intervention requires a multidisciplinary approach. Foremost, potential bariatric patients should undergo a thorough medical assessment including a complete history and physical. Important comorbid conditions should be identified, and appropriate treatment should be initiated. Particular attention should be paid to the cardiopulmonary status of the patient to exclude significant disease. In particular, evidence of coronary artery disease or obesity hypoventilatory syndrome (daytime hypercapnea) should be carefully sought. Additionally, treatable endocrine causes of obesity, such as Cushing's disease or syndrome, need to be ruled out. Finally, terminal diseases, including severe liver disease and certain cancers, must also be excluded.

In addition to a medical evaluation, the bariatric patient should undergo other assessments. An extensive psychological profile should be performed by a mental health professional. In this manner, any psychiatric disorders, such as depression, can be identified, and appropriate therapy started. Also, any history of physical or mental abuse that might interfere with postsurgical recovery and adaptation can also be addressed. If a serious condition is found, any surgical intervention should be postponed until satisfactory improvement following treatment. A dietician should conduct a full nutritional assessment. Such an evaluation aids in determining caloric intake and identifying detrimental eating habits. It also provides an opportunity for preintervention education regarding required dietary changes. Finally, a fitness evaluation to stratify conditioning is useful. It also allows for education and the development of an exercise program.

After completion of all the evaluations, the individual's case should be discussed in a treatment team setting. It provides an opportunity for a comprehensive review of the patient in which each discipline presents pertinent findings and concerns. In this manner, any potential impediments to a successful outcome can be identified and addressed prior to intervention. Such an approach fosters a sense of team interaction in the treatment of the patient, allows for optimization of the patient before treatment, and improves quality of care.

Treatment

Treatment for overweight and obese people falls into three broad categories: behavior modification, pharmacotherapy, and surgical intervention. All three therapies are able to induce a degree of weight loss. Only bariatric surgery, however, has been successful in helping people lose a significant amount of weight *and* keep it off. In 1998, the National Institutes of Health (NIH) developed guidelines based on BMI for appropriate weight loss interventions (see Table 14-3). These criteria help health care workers in determining the best weight loss approach for a person of any given size.

Table 14-3 National Institutes of Health Guidelines for Treatment of Overweight and Obesity

BMI Range	Behavior Modification	Pharmacotherapy	Surgery
25.0 to 26.9	Yes*	No	No
27.0 to 29.9	Yes*	Yes*	No
30.0 to 34.9	Yes	Yes	No
35.0 to 39.9	Yes	Yes	Yes*
40 or more	Yes	Yes	Yes

* Comorbidities present.
BMI, body mass index.
Adapted from 1998 National Institutes of Health clinical guidelines.

Behavior Modification

Behavior modification for weight loss is a multibillion-dollar commercial industry in the United States. The 1998 NIH guidelines recommend it for any patient who is obese and for those individuals who are overweight with comorbid conditions. Two main forms of modification exist: reduction in energy intake (diet) and augmentation in energy expenditure (exercise). Dietary modification is an effective means of inducing weight loss. The most common form is the low-calorie diet (LCD), which aims for an energy deficit ranging from 500 to 1000 kcal/day. For women, this negative energy balance is reached on 1000 to 1200 kcal/day. For men, it requires an intake of 1200 to 1500 kcal/day. Following such guidelines, patients will lose about 1 to 2 lb per week. The goal of such therapy is a 10% weight loss over 6 months. A very low calorie diet (VLCD) limits energy intake to fewer than 800 kcal/day. It often consists of high-protein liquid meals supplemented with essential vitamins, minerals, fatty acids, and electrolytes. Short-term weight loss can be dramatic, with some individuals losing up to 20 kg in as little as 3 months. The long-term weight loss from VLCDs, however, is not different from that produced by LCDs. Additionally, VLCDs require close physician supervision because of the increased risk of complications. Hyperuricemia, gout, cardiac complications, and cholelithiasis all can occur. As a result, they are not recommended as therapies in the 1998 NIH guidelines. They should only be considered for obese individuals with severe concomitant comorbid conditions or for the severely obese.

Many commercial programs emphasize the macronutrient composition of their diets as an important component in losing weight. Such diets are either reduced carbohydrate or reduced fat. Reduced carbohydrate diets have increased in popularity recently. They are based on the belief that increased carbohydrate consumption is responsible for weight gain. They therefore focus on severely limiting carbohydrate intake in an attempt to lose weight. Even though these diets can cause a decrease in weight, it is often due to diuresis from depletion of glycogen stores. Furthermore, ketogenesis resulting from the low availability of carbohydrates leads to appetite suppression. Weight, therefore, is often regained when the diet is abandoned and carbohydrates reintroduced. Finally, to keep carbohydrate intake low, protein and fat content are increased. The high fat exposes the individual to the risk of atherosclerotic changes and its sequelae. The high protein is potentially detrimental to renal function, especially in borderline cases. Care should be taken, therefore, in pursuing these reduced carbohydrate programs.

Reduced fat diets focus on fat consumption as the major contributor to weight gain, and they limit its intake. Since fat is the most energy-dense macronutrient (having 9 kcal/g), its reduction is useful in decreasing the total energy consumption. In fact, both reduced carbohydrate and reduced fat diets are really only effective in the setting of decreased caloric intake. The macronutrient composition, therefore, is not the most important aspect of the diet.

Instead, decreasing energy intake is the essential feature. A reduced fat diet provides the additional benefit of decreasing atherosclerotic risk. It is therefore the recommended approach in promoting weight loss.

Unlike decreasing energy intake, increasing energy expenditure is much less effective in causing weight loss. It results in minimal reductions, both alone and in combination with dietary restriction. Typical recommendations suggest increasing activity to reach an energy expenditure of 1000 kcal/week. Such an energy deficit can be obtained in a single day of dietary restriction, showing why increased activity does not lead to significant weight loss. It is, however, very effective in preventing weight regain after successful loss because of its role in long-term weight maintenance.

Energy expenditure comes from three main sources. The resting metabolic rate produces the most energy. A small contribution comes from the thermic effect of the digestion of food. Physical activity produces the rest. Of the three, physical activity is modifiable. It can be increased by adjusting lifestyle habits, such as taking stairs instead of an elevator, or engaging in structured exercise. The latter is the most useful in reaching recommended energy expenditure goals. For example, walking two miles a day for 5 days a week will produce an expenditure of 1000 kcal/week.

Although often effective over the short term, behavior modification fails to result in many long-term successes. Maintaining a dietary restriction or structured exercise protocol can be difficult, and people often lapse. The lost weight is regained with additional pounds. Unfortunately, only a small fraction of individuals who lose weight by behavior modification are able to keep it off.

Pharmacotherapy

Pharmacotherapy for the treatment of obesity has a rather checkered history. The association of fenfluramine and dexfenfluramine with cardiopulmonary complications (valvular disease and pulmonary hypertension) resulted in their rapid removal from the market in the late 1990s. Several short-term, centrally acting noradrenergic agents are available, but they have an addictive potential. Additionally, U.S. Food and Drug Administration (FDA) approval limits their use to 3 months' duration. Weight regain is common after their cessation. Currently, only two long-term weight reduction agents are FDA approved. The 1998 NIH guidelines recommend pharmacotherapy for obese individuals. Additionally, anyone with a BMI of 27 to 30 and concomitant comorbid conditions can be considered for drug treatment.

Sibutramine is one of the two drugs approved by the FDA for long-term weight loss. It is an appetite suppressant whose mechanism of action is as a combined serotonin and norepinephrine uptake inhibitor. Patients are started on an initial dosage of 10 mg a day. Important side effects include tachycardia, hypertension, headache, and insomnia. The former two can result in cessation of the drug. Sibutramine can produce an approximately 5% to 10% weight loss, but weight regain occurs when the drug is stopped.

Orlistat is the second FDA-approved drug. This pentaenoic acid ester is a potent inhibitor of pancreatic lipase activity. It promotes weight loss by reducing intestinal fat digestion. The higher the fat content of the ingested food, the more effective is the drug. Side effects, however, also increase. Fecal leakage, bloating, and increased flatulence can result. A patient's diet, therefore, should be limited to about 30% fat calories. Long-term use results in about a 10% weight loss. Initial dosing is 120 mg three times a day. Multivitamins are sometimes given in conjunction with orlistat to ensure against a theoretical reduction in fat-soluble vitamins.

Surgical Intervention

Because of the limited success of both behavior modification and pharmacotherapy in weight loss therapy, surgical intervention has increased in popularity as a treatment modality for obesity. It is reserved, however, for severe cases, given the inherent risks of operative intervention. In 1991, an NIH Consensus Development Conference established criteria by which patients should be considered for operative treatment of obesity. In addition to the previously mentioned BMI thresholds (reiterated in the 1998 NIH guidelines), potential surgical candidates must have failed at nonoperative attempts at weight loss. They also must be psychologically stable and willing to follow postoperative diet instructions. Finally, they must not have any medical (i.e., endocrine) cause for their obesity. Operative therapy should be pursued only after these criteria have been met.

Bariatric procedures induce weight loss by decreasing energy intake. Two major mechanisms are responsible for this decrease. Restrictive operations limit food intake by forcing the patient to eat smaller portions. Vertical banded gastroplasty (VBG) and adjustable gastric banding (AGB) are the two most common examples of such interventions. Malabsorptive operations alter food processing by limiting its absorption in the intestines. Biliopancreatic diversion (BPD) with or without duodenal switch (BPD/DS) is the most popular of these procedures. The Roux-en-Y gastric bypass (RNYGB) is considered a combined restrictive and malabsorptive operation. In general, restrictive procedures are less extensive than malabsorptive ones, but they result in less overall weight loss and cure of comorbid conditions. Malabsorptive procedures, on the other hand, have better weight loss but increased risk of problems with malnutrition. Both types of operations can be performed by either open or laparoscopic approach. Laparoscopic procedures decrease the rate of wound infection and incisional hernia formation. Overall morbidity and mortality, however, is similar between the two approaches.

At one point, VBG was one of the most commonly performed bariatric procedures in the United States. Initial enthusiasm, however, has waned with the realization that it is not as effective as other operations in maintaining weight loss. Currently, its use is in decline. The critical aspects of performing a VBG include the creation of a proximal gastric pouch by stomach partitioning and the reinforcement of the stoma with banding (see Fig. 14-13).

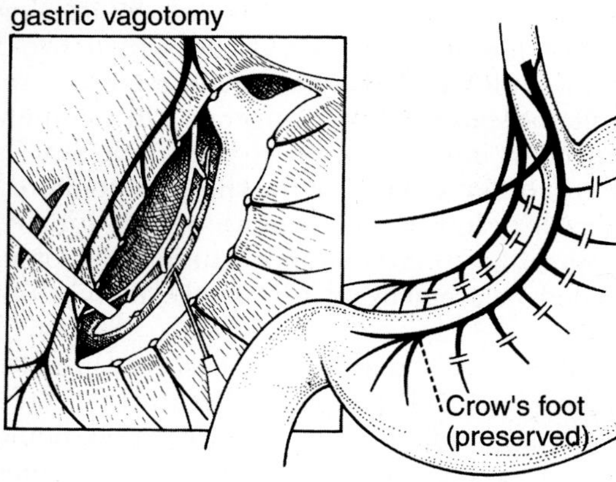

Figure 14-13 Vertical banded gastroplasty (VBG). In a VBG, a small gastric pouch is created by partitioning the stomach. The stoma into the distal stomach is then reinforced with a mechanical band. Fistulae formation at the partition site can lead to weight regain.

Partitioning is usually via gastric stapling, and Marlex is a popular banding material. Patients typically lose between 30% to 50% excess body weight (EBW) within the first couple of years. Weight regain, however, can occur due to staple line breakdown. Additionally, revisional operations can be frequent. Such results will likely lead to the abandonment of VGB as a first-line bariatric procedure in the near future.

In contrast to VBG, AGB has increased in frequency as a viable surgical alternative for severe obesity. The advent of laparoscopic variations of AGB has contributed to this trend. Key aspects of this procedure include creation of a proximal gastric pouch using an inflatable band and placement of an access port (see Fig. 14-14). A pars flaccida technique is used to create a posterior gastric tunnel from the lesser curve to the angle of His. The band is then positioned and secured by imbricating its anterior aspect. The distal fundus is sutured to the proximal gastric pouch. The port is placed on the abdominal muscle fascia. Adjustments of the band are made by instilling sterile solution percutaneously via the access port. If adjustments are not done under fluoroscopic guidance, incremental increases in the band size are undertaken to avoid overfilling it. Patients with the adjustable band lose between 45% to 55% EBW over the first few years. Long-term U.S. data do not exist, since FDA approval occurred only in 2001.

BPD and BPD/DS are more complex procedures. BPD is basically a subtotal gastrectomy with a very distal Roux-en-Y reconstruction. BPD/DS involves sleeve gastrectomy, duodenal transection with duodenojejunostomy creation, and very distal jejunoileostomy (see Fig. 14-15). Both operations can result in 70% to 90% EBW loss within the first few years, but nutritional problems can be severe. Given their complexity and issues with malnutrition, the BPD and BPD/DS have not enjoyed in the United States the same popularity as other bariatric procedures.

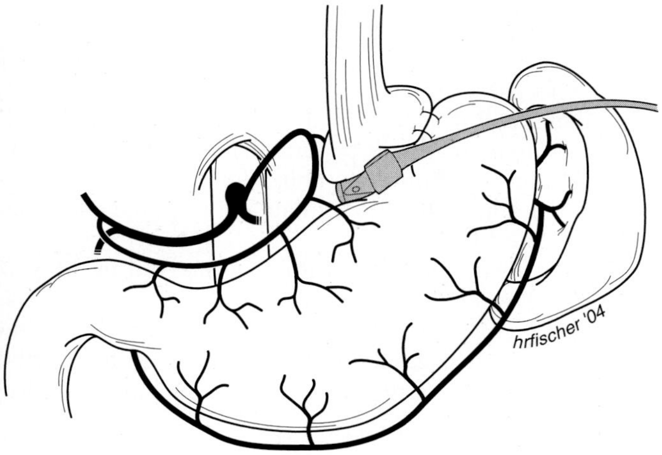

Figure 14-14 Adjustable gastric banding (AGB). An inflatable band is placed around the proximal portion of the stomach, creating a small pouch and restricting food intake. The stoma size into the distal stomach can be adjusted by inflating or deflating the band.

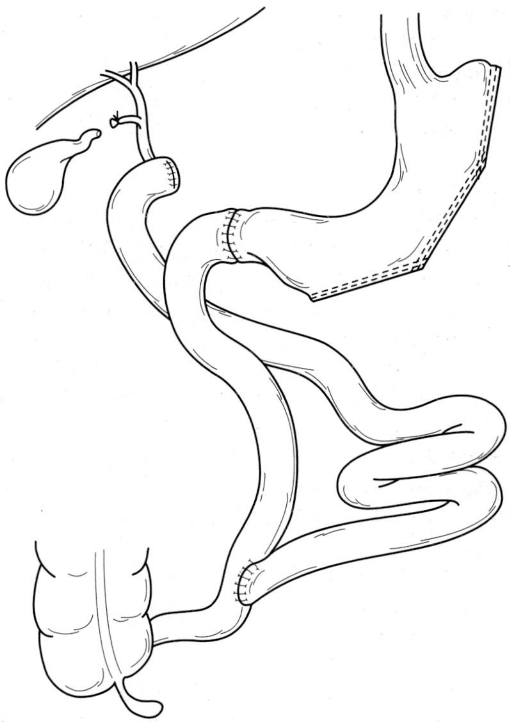

Figure 14-15 Biliopancreatic diversion with duodenal switch (BPD/DS). In a BPD/DS, the stomach is reduced in size, the gallbladder is removed, the proximal duodenum is divided and reanastomosed to more distal small bowel, and a short common channel is created via a jejunoileostomy. Weight loss is predominantly secondary to malabsorption, and complications related to malnutrition are more frequent in this procedure.

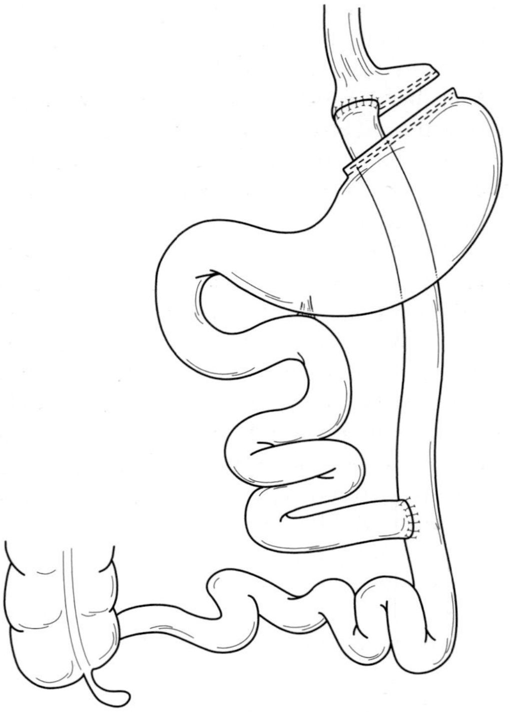

Figure 14-16 Roux-en-Y gastric bypass. In a gastric bypass, the stomach is transected unevenly, creating a small proximal pouch. A Roux-en-Y gastrojejunostomy is then created. Weight loss occurs due to decreased food intake as well as some malabsorption. Gastric bypass is currently the most common bariatric procedure performed in the United States.

RNYGB is currently the most common operative intervention for severe obesity in the United States. Important features include the creation of a small proximal gastric pouch with a Roux-en-Y gastrojejunostomy (see Fig. 14-16). The pouch is typically created by transecting the stomach. The Roux limb measures from 75 to 100 cm in length. Although more complex than VBG and AGB, it is more straightforward than BPD or BPD/DS. Weight loss averages between 75% to 85% EBW within a couple years. Nutritional problems tend to be less severe than BPD or BPD/DS. Long-term weight loss of 60% EBW at up to 15 years is documented.

Complications of Bariatric Operations

Approximately 100,000 bariatric procedures will be performed in the United States in 2004. This explosion in surgical interventions for severe obesity mirrors the epidemic spread of the disorder throughout the world. An understanding of certain complications encountered following bariatric operations is important.

Anastomotic Leak

Unrecognized anastomotic leaks following RNYGB, BPD, and BPD/DS can have devastating consequences. Because of the extreme size of severely obese patients, typical signs of intraabdominal peritonitis are often masked, delaying diagnosis. A high index of suspicion is necessary to avoid such a situation. In RNYGB, the gastrojejunostomy is frequently the site of leakage. Some surgeons will routinely test the connection intraoperatively to ensure no leak is present. Often, a drain is placed at the site and monitored for evidence of leak in the postoperative period. Finally, routine postoperative contrast swallow studies are sometimes performed before starting oral intake to rule out leakage.

Bariatric patients with anastomotic leakage will often have nonspecific signs. Persistent tachycardia ($>$ 120 beats/min) or tachypnea in the postoperative period should alert the surgeon to the possibility of a leak. A swallow study using water-soluble contrast is the most helpful diagnostic test. If a leak is present, surgical reexploration with repair of the leak and drainage of the area is usually required. Often, if the suspicion of leak is high, reexploration is performed without further investigation.

Deep Vein Thrombosis and Pulmonary Embolus

Morbidly obese individuals are at increased risk for developing deep vein thrombosis (DVT) and pulmonary embolus (PE). The increased adipose tissue causes metabolic changes that predispose them to thrombogenesis. Combined with the venous stasis due to general anesthesia and decreased postoperative mobility, bariatric patients are particularly susceptible to developing venous thrombosis. Aggressive prophylaxis is important to help minimize risk. Combination therapy including low–molecular-weight heparin, sequential compression devices, and early ambulation is most helpful.

PE can manifest as severe hypoxia and tachypnea. Cardiovascular collapse can occur with saddle emboli. Aggressive supportive therapy is essential. Oxygen supplementation and maintenance of blood pressure are important. Helical computed tomography is quickly replacing ventilation–perfusion scintigraphy as the diagnostic procedure of choice. Heparin anticoagulation remains the initial standard therapy. It is often started before completion of diagnostic evaluation. Some patients have vena caval filters placed to prevent further embolization from the lower extremities. Long-term anticoagulation is required after resolution of the PE.

DVT typically manifests with asymmetrical swelling of a lower extremity. Diagnosis is made using Doppler ultrasound of the affected extremity. Treatment consists of initial heparin anticoagulation. Patients will require a period of continued anticoagulation during postoperative followup.

Stricture

Patients undergoing RNYGB can develop a stricture at the gastrojejunostomy as it heals. They typically complain of progressive intolerance of solids and liquids about 1 to 2 months after undergoing the procedure. Additionally, they can describe food as "getting stuck" in their pouch. Upper endoscopy is the diagnostic procedure of choice. If a stricture is present, pneumatic balloon dilation can be performed to open the anastomosis. The endoscope should be able to enter into the Roux limb after dilation. Multiple sessions are sometimes necessary.

Nutritional Disturbances

Nutritional disturbances are more frequently encountered in patients undergoing malabsorptive procedures. Patients who have undergone BPD and BPD/DS are particularly susceptible to such complications. Protein energy malnutrition (see the protein needs section in Chapter XX, Nutrition) can occur due to inadequate intake or severe malabsorption. Additionally, various vitamin and mineral deficiencies can occur. Of these, vitamin B_{12} deficiency is the most important, especially in patients with RNYGB. Because the distal stomach is bypassed, intrinsic factor can no longer combine with vitamin B_{12}. As a result, it cannot be absorbed in the ileum. Patients, therefore, may require periodic administration of intramuscular or sublingual vitamin B_{12} to avoid the hematologic and neurologic complications brought on by deficiency.

Partly because of the potential nutritional disturbances, bariatric patients require lifelong followup. Such care usually involves yearly checkups to make sure that the patient is eating properly and getting adequate vitamins and minerals. Any pertinent laboratory investigations can be obtained at this time.

Gallbladder Disease

One in three severely obese individuals will develop cholelithiasis with rapid weight loss. This statistic has prompted some experts to recommend routine cholecystectomy at the time of any bariatric procedure to eliminate this risk. Ursodeoxycholic acid is another option. It decreases the risk of developing cholelithiasis following bariatric surgery to around 2%. Patients take the medication for approximately 3 to 9 months after their operation. This time interval corresponds to the period of greatest weight loss. Most surgeons will perform cholecystectomy at the time of initial operation if patients have preexisting cholelithiasis or symptoms of biliary colic.

Adjustable Gastric Band Complications

AGB complications include gastric prolapse and band erosion. Gastric prolapse can occur in both the immediate and late postoperative period. The stomach below the band herniates through it, creating an asymmetric, enlarged proximal pouch. Food can become lodged in this region, causing nausea and vomiting. Additionally, patients can begin to complain of reflux symptoms. In severe cases, gastric outlet obstruction occurs and the stomach can become strangulated. Contrast swallow study can provide the diagnosis by showing an asymmetric proximal pouch with poor emptying. Initial treatment includes complete deflation of the band. Occasionally, the prolapse will resolve, and the band can be slowly reinflated. Operative reduction of the prolapse with band repositioning or replacement is often necessary. Patients with upper abdominal pain and symptoms suggestive of prolapse should undergo operative exploration to rule out strangulation.

Band erosion into the stomach is a relatively rare (about 1%) long-term complication. Patients will present months to years after operation. Some may notice loss of restriction with eating. Others will suddenly develop an infection or fluid collection at their port site. Contrast swallow study usually provides the diagnosis. Confirmation can be made with endoscopy. Patients with erosion usually require operative exploration, removal of the adjustable band, and closure of any openings. Patients can undergo a second bariatric procedure after healing.

ACKNOWLEDGMENTS

We thank the following colleagues for their contributions to this chapter: Daniel J. Jurusz, MD; Glen Steeb, MD; James F. Lind, MD; Raymond J. Joehl, MD; Edwin C. James, MD; Talmadge A. Bowden Jr., MD; Mary McCarthy, MD; Rudy G. Danzinger, MD; Guy Legros, MD; Gordon Telford, MD; Ajit K. Sachdeva, MD, FRCS(C), FACS; Thomas A. Miller, MD, FACS; and Steven T. Ruby, MD.

SUGGESTED READINGS

Abdalla EK, Ahmed SA, Pearlstone DB, et al. Gastric cancer. In: Feig BW, Berger DH, Fuhrman GM, eds. *The M.D. Anderson Surgical Oncology Handbook*. 3rd Ed. Philadelphia, PA: Wolters Kluwer Company, 2003.

Baron RB. Nutrition. In: Tierney LM Jr, McPhee SJ, Papadakis MA, eds. *Current Medical Diagnosis and Treatment*. 42nd Ed. New York, NY: The McGraw-Hill Companies, Inc., 2003.

Byrne TK. Complications of surgery for obesity. *Surg Clin North Am* 2001;81:1181.

Cheung LY, Delcore R. Stomach. In: Townsend CM, Beauchamp RD, Evers BM, Mattox KL, eds. *Sabiston Textbook of Surgery*. 16th Ed. Philadelphia, PA: WB Saunders Company, 2001.

Cottam DR, Mattar SG, Schauer, PR. Laparoscopic era of operations for morbid obesity. *Arch Surg* 2003;138:367.

Hwang RF, Robinson EK, Cusack JC, et al. Small-bowel malignancies and carcinoid tumors. In: Feig BW, Berger DH, Fuhrman GM, eds. *The M.D. Anderson Surgical Oncology Handbook*. 3rd Ed. Philadelphia, PA: Wolters Kluwer Company, 2003.

Jensen RT. Zollinger-Ellison syndrome. In: Doherty GM, Skögseid B, eds. *Surgical Endocrinology*. Philadelphia, PA: Wolters Kluwer Company, 2001.

Korner J, Leibel RL. To eat or not to eat—how the gut talks to the brain. *N Engl J Med* 2003;349:926.

Kral JG. Morbidity of severe obesity. *Surg Clin North Am* 2001;81:1039.

Livingston EH. Stomach and duodenum. In: Norton JA, Bollinger RR,

Chang AE, Lowry SF, Mulvihill SJ, Thompson RW, eds. *Surgery Basic Science and Clinical Evidence*. New York, NY: Springer-Verlag New York Inc., 2001.

Madura JA. Postgastrectomy problems: remedial operations and therapy. In: Cameron JL, ed. *Current Surgical Therapy*. St. Louis, MO: Harcourt Health Sciences Company, 2001.

Samuelson LC, Hinkle KL. Insights into the regulation of gastric acid secretion through analysis of genetically engineered mice. *Annu Rev Physiol* 2003;65:383.

Shiotani A, Graham DY. Pathogenesis and therapy of gastric and duodenal ulcer disease. *Med Clin North Am* 2002;86:1447.

Zollinger RM, Ellison EH. Primary peptic ulcerations of the jejunum associated with islet cell tumors of the pancreas. *Ann Surg* 1955;142:709.

15

JOHN D. MELLINGER, MD ■ BRUCE V. MACFADYEN, JR., MD
DAVID W. MERCER, MD ■ JOHN R. POTTS, III, MD

Small Intestine and Appendix

OBJECTIVES

1 Discuss the location, frequency, size, and various clinical presentations of a patient with a Meckel's diverticulum.

2 Describe the treatment of Meckel's diverticulum that is incidentally found at surgery and the treatment of one that is symptomatic.

3 Describe the various clinical presentations of a patient with Crohn's disease, and explain how they can differ from the presentation of a patient with ulcerative colitis.

4 Outline a diagnostic approach to a patient with Crohn's disease.

5 Discuss the medical and surgical treatment plans for patients with Crohn's disease. Describe the complications associated with the disease process, and explain when surgery is indicated.

6 Discuss the relative frequency of the most common benign and malignant small bowel tumors.

7 Discuss the clinical presentation and diagnostic approach to the following types of small bowel tumors: adenocarcinoma, carcinoid, and lymphoma.

8 Describe the carcinoid syndrome, and list the features of a carcinoid tumor that suggest it may be malignant. List the features that must be present for carcinoid syndrome to occur.

9 Discuss the role of surgery in the management of patients with small bowel tumors.

10 Describe the common etiologies, signs, and symptoms of small bowel mechanical obstruction, and contrast them with those of paralytic ileus.

11 Discuss the complications of small bowel obstruction, including fluid and electrolyte shifts, vascular compromise of the small bowel, and sepsis.

12 Outline the appropriate laboratory tests and radiographs that are used in the diagnostic evaluation of a patient with a suspected small bowel obstruction.

13 Discuss the clinical appearance of small bowel strangulation and the potential difficulty of making that diagnosis.

14 Compare and contrast mechanical small bowel obstruction with colon obstruction.

15 Outline a treatment plan for a patient with small bowel obstruction. Discuss the indications for operative therapy.

16 Discuss the signs, symptoms, and differential diagnosis of acute appendicitis, and describe how diseases that mimic it may be differentiated.

17 Outline the diagnostic workup of a patient with suspected appendicitis, and describe the laboratory findings that would confirm the diagnosis.

18 List and discuss the common complications of appendicitis and subsequent appendectomy, and explain how each can be prevented or managed.

19 Describe the presentation and management of appendiceal carcinoid and its significance as an incidental finding.

Diseases of the small intestine and appendix constitute some of the most common surgical emergencies. Acute appendicitis, mechanical small bowel obstruction, paralytic ileus, and Crohn's disease are particularly frequent problems encountered in the care of the patient with abdominal complaints. In normal settings, the small bowel is an amazingly prolific organ with regard to its physiology, having digestive, nutritional, immunologic, and endocrine functions. Alteration of these functions by disease and iatrogenic intervention can have profound implications for patient management. A thorough understanding of the physiology and pathophysiology of these organs is thus fundamental to the care of the surgical patient.

This chapter will focus on the anatomy, physiology, and pathophysiology of the small intestine and appendix. Diseases including those mentioned above, as well as neoplastic and diverticular diseases of these organs, will be reviewed. Medical and surgical management, including important differential diagnostic considerations, will be detailed.

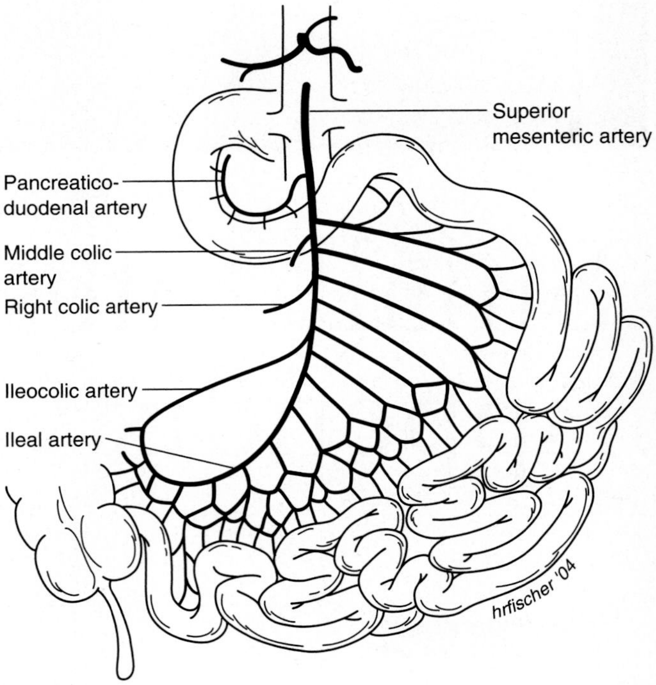

Figure 15-1 Anatomy of the small intestine demonstrating vascular anatomy of the varying segments. Note longer vasa recta in jejunum versus ileum.

ANATOMY

The small intestine is composed of three segments: the duodenum, jejunum, and ileum. The duodenum extends from the pylorus to the **ligament of Treitz.** The jejunum consists of the first 40% of small bowel distal to the duodenum. The ileum consists of the remaining 60%. The duodenum is retroperitoneal, whereas the jejunum and ileum are tethered on a mesentery that extends from the left upper quadrant to the right lower quadrant. The duodenum itself is divided into four segments, including the bulb (first portion) and descending duodenum (second portion), which harbors the major and minor duodenal papillae. In 90% of cases, the minor papilla allows drainage of the dorsal pancreatic duct (accessory **duct of Santorini**), and the major papilla drains the common bile duct and the main pancreatic duct (**duct of Wirsung**). The third and fourth portions are defined by their respective proximal and distal relation to the superior mesenteric vessels, as these structures course anterior to the duodenum. The jejunum has more prominent plica circulares and longer vasa recta than the ileum (Fig. 15-1). The blood supply to the small intestine is primarily via the superior mesenteric artery, with the duodenum also being supplied by the gastroduodenal artery, originating from the celiac axis via the common hepatic artery. Venous drainage parallels the arterial supply, with the majority of the venous effluent coursing through the superior mesenteric vein, which is joined by the splenic and inferior mesenteric veins to constitute the portal vein. Lymphatic drainage is via lacteals and lymphatic channels paralleling the venous drainage, ultimately joining at the cisterna chyli in the upper abdomen below the aortic hiatus of the diaphragm.

The terminal ileum has an abundance of lymphatic tissue known as **Peyer's patches** and terminates at the ileocecal valve. In addition to these concentrations of lymphatic tissue, the gut also possesses prominent populations of lymphatic cells in the lamina propria and the mucosa. Together these populations comprise what is termed gut-associated lymphoid tissue (GALT). Follicular B cells from the periphery of Peyer's patches and similar lymphoid nodules throughout the gut may migrate to mesenteric nodes and from there to the bloodstream via the thoracic duct. These cells can then return to the mucosa adjacent to their area of origin as B2 memory cells, forming a population of cells known as mucosa-associated lymphoid tissue (MALT). The nerve supply to the small intestine and appendix is mediated through the autonomic nervous system. Parasympathetic fibers originate from the vagus nerve and traverse to the gut via the celiac plexus. Sympathetic fibers travel via the splanchnic nerves from ganglion cells in the superior mesenteric plexus. Pain fibers activated by intestinal distension communicate primarily via sympathetic visceral afferent fibers.

The appendix arises from the cecum at the confluence of the taenia coli and is accompanied by an adjacent mesentery, the mesoappendix, in which courses the appendiceal artery as a terminal branch of the ileocolic artery. It is also rich in lymphatic tissue and may be positioned variably in relation to the cecum, including retrocecal and, rarely, truly retroperitoneal locations.

PHYSIOLOGY

The primary function of the small intestine is digestion of food and absorption of the ingested water, electrolytes, and nutrients into the bloodstream. This is accomplished through a complex set of processes that include intestinal motility, the activity of digestive enzymes, the secretion of digestive juices, and absorptive processes predicated on both simple diffusion and active transport. Autonomic and endocrine regulation of all these processes is abundant and critical to their coordination.

Intestinal motility allows for mixing, propulsion, and storage of enteric contents. The enteric nervous system, which includes intrinsic neural plexuses and autonomic extrinsic neural pathways, governs this motility. Submucosal (Meissner's) and myenteric (Auerbach's) plexuses help perform intrinsic regulatory functions and receive input from local receptors in the mucosa and smooth muscle of the gut. Acetylcholine functions as the primary excitatory neurotransmitter at the myenteric plexus level, and vasoactive intestinal peptide and somatostatin are the prominent inhibitory neurotransmitters. Extrinsic control is exerted from the central nervous system through parasympathetic, primarily excitatory, pathways via the vagal and pelvic parasympathetic nerves, and through sympathetic, primarily inhibitory, channels networked via sympathetic ganglia. In general, the enteric nerves determine whether contraction occurs, and intrinsic myogenic control determines the pattern of contraction. Several dozen additional peptides, often referred to generically as gastrointestinal hormones, provide an additional level of control and coordination through endocrine and paracrine effects on the gut itself, as well as the biliary tract and pancreas (see below). Segmenting contractions allow for mixing function, and peristaltic contractions for propagative function. Tonic contractions are also seen and help to preserve baseline muscle tonicity.

A cyclic pattern of digestive activity is observed during fasting, which involves muscular contractions that migrate from the duodenum to the terminal ileum. This is referred to as the migrating motor complex (MMC), or interdigestive myoelectric complex (IDMEC). The MMC has four distinct phases, which are characterized by differing levels of electrical depolarization activity and corresponding intestinal contraction. Phase 1 is quiescent, with no spikes (larger electrical fluctuations) or contractions. Phase 2 has accelerating and intermittent spike and contractile activity. Phase 3 is characterized by a sequence of high-amplitude spiking activity and corresponding strong, rhythmic gut contractions. Phase 4 is a subsequent brief period of intermittent spike activity before the return to quiescence. The duration of the entire cycle is 90 to 120 minutes, and the migration, which begins in the foregut, takes 2 hours to migrate down the small intestine. Eating abolishes the cycle and induces intermittent contractile activity. This fasting cycle may have a role in "housecleaning" the gut during the interdigestive period and preventing stasis and bacterial overgrowth in the distal small bowel. The ileocecal valve itself facilitates normal emptying phases and limits bacterial overgrowth that otherwise could occur secondary to reflux of colonic contents.

The secretion of 5 to 10 liters a day of digestive fluid by the salivary glands, stomach, biliary tree, pancreas, and intestine itself is handled primarily by the small intestine, which absorbs 80% of the resulting succus entericus on a daily basis. The small bowel does this isosmotically, without concentrating the enteric contents intraluminally. In the jejunum, fluid is resorbed following the gradient created by Na-coupled nutrient absorption, and it is here that the majority of small intestinal fluid is absorbed. Na is the major ion that dictates osmotic gradients favorable for water absorption, and Cl is the usual driving force for secretion. Hormones, peptides, drugs, toxins, and immunologic factors may all impact this delicate isosmotic balance and foster increased delivery of succus to the colon, with resulting diarrhea.

The major nutrient substrates absorbed by the small intestine are fats, carbohydrates, and proteins. Each has its own digestive and absorptive requirements. Fat digestion involves a crucial intraluminal phase, which allows the eventual delivery of a water-insoluble nutrient into an aqueous environment. Ingested fat (triglycerides and cholesterol esters) is mechanically broken down into small droplets that are then digested intraluminally by lingual and pancreatic lipase into free fatty acids and monoglycerides complexed with calcium. Bile salts then act as a detergent to allow formation of micelles containing these smaller substrates as well as fat-soluble vitamins. The micelle dissociates at the enterocyte apical membrane, delivering the free fatty acids, cholesterol, and monoglycerides to the cell membrane, where they can permeate the lipid regions of the membrane into the cell without requirement for specific carriers. Inside the enterocyte, triglycerides are reconstituted from the absorbed constituents and packaged into chylomicrons suitable for subsequent lymphatic transport. Only medium-chain triglycerides are capable of being absorbed directly into the portal system without going through the chylomicron–lymphatic pathway. The majority of fat absorption occurs in the duodenum and upper jejunum, although the bile salts that facilitate fat digestion are resorbed primarily in the terminal ileum.

Carbohydrate digestion begins with salivary amylase. The process is completed in the jejunum and is accomplished by the intraluminal breakdown of complex starch into oligosaccharides, primarily by pancreatic amylase, and the subsequent breakdown of oligosaccharides by brush border enzymes into glucose, galactose, and fructose. Glucose and galactose are then absorbed via Na-coupled carrier transport, and fructose by facilitated diffusion. This system of digestion, which limits the osmotic load of the smaller monosaccharides to a step accomplished at the border of the enterocyte membrane just prior to absorption, serves to minimize osmotic pressure in the intestinal lumen.

Dietary proteins are, like fat, absorbed primarily in the duodenum and jejunum. Digestion begins in the stomach via the action of gastric pepsin, although protein digestion is still efficient in the absence of this step. Cholecystokinin secretion by proximal intestinal endocrine cells is stimulated by the presence of polypeptides in the intestinal lumen, and in turn stimulates pancreatic secretion of peptidases (including precursors of trypsin, chymotrypsin, elastase, and carboxypeptidase), which break the polypeptides down further to oligopeptides and amino acids. These compounds are polar and require specific carrier proteins to be absorbed across the enterocyte membrane. This absorption is coupled to Na transport, which is driven by a favorable electrochemical gradient, thus allowing the amino acids to be accumulated against a concentration gradient.

In addition to the above general mechanisms controlling the absorption of fluid and nutrients from the small intestine, several important substances are absorbed in specific areas of the digestive tract. Vitamin B_{12}, complexed with gastric intrinsic factor, is absorbed in the terminal ileum. The fat-soluble vitamins A, D, E, and K, as well as bile salts, are also absorbed primarily in this area. Calcium and iron are absorbed primarily in the duodenum and proximal small bowel. Knowledge of these specific patterns of specialized absorption can facilitate a comprehension of disease states that can result from segmental intestinal disease or resection.

The small intestine is the largest endocrine organ in the body. A variety of hormonal signals act in endocrine, paracrine, autocrine, and neurotransmitting functions. Collectively, these substances help to regulate intestinal secretion and motility, and provide trophic influences on the gastrointestinal organs, including the gut mucosa, liver, and pancreas. Secretin, cholecystokinin, motilin, gastric inhibitory peptide (GIP), vasoactive intestinal polypeptide (VIP), gastrin-releasing peptide, somatostatin, neurotensin, peptide YY (PYY), and glucagon-like peptide 2 (GLP-2) are prominent among the agents elaborated by the small bowel that impact these processes. Secretin is produced by duodenal S cells in response to acid or bile and stimulates pancreatic production of bicarbonate and water. Cholecystokinin is released by proximal small bowel mucosa in response to fatty acids and certain amino acids and facilitates gallbladder emptying and pancreatic enzyme secretion (formerly also called pancreozymin). Motilin is produced in the jejunum and helps coordinate stomach and lower esophageal sphincter function with small intestinal activity during fasting. GIP is produced by jejunal K cells and stimulates insulin release in response to luminal carbohydrate and fat. VIP stimulates pancreatic and intestinal secretion, inhibits gastric secretion, and functions primarily as a neuropeptide. Neurotensin is secreted in response to fat, stimulates pancreatic exocrine secretion, facilitates fat absorption, and has important mucosal trophic effects. Gastrin-releasing peptide stimulates release of all intestinal hormones except secretin, helps regulate gastric acid and gastrin secretion (enterogastrone function), and has important mucosal trophic effects as well. Somatostatin is found in many organs, including the small bowel, and acts as an "off" switch for intestinal hormone, gastric, and pancreatic secretion, as well as intestinal motility. Peptide YY is found in the distal small bowel and proximal colon; it affects gastric and pancreatic secretion and provides trophic influences on the intestinal mucosa. GLP-2 is one of a family of peptides previously termed enteroglucagon and is a potent small intestinal trophic hormone. Our understanding of the various roles of these agents and their interactions with other regulatory systems, including the gut neural system, continues to expand and offers the potential for therapeutic manipulation. Examples of the latter include the use of somatostatin to suppress pancreatic and gastrointestinal fistula output, or to regulate neuroendocrine tumors of the intestinal tract, and the use of erythromycin as a motilin agonist to stimulate gastric motility.

The immune function of the small intestine is significant in protecting the body against a host of pathogens that gain access via the gastrointestinal tract. Antigen processing and the development of cellular and humoral immunity, coordinated via the gut-associated lymph tissue (GALT), plays a complementary role to the functions of peristalsis, enzyme and mucus secretion, and competitive influences of the intestinal microflora in protecting against disease. The synthesis and secretion of immunoglobulin A (IgA), in particular by plasma cells in the lamina propria, is a paramount function of the gut immune system. Such IgA is secreted into the intestinal lumen and serves to suppress bacterial growth and adherence to epithelial cells. IgA also can neutralize bacterial toxins and viruses.

DISEASES OF THE SMALL INTESTINE

Meckel's Diverticulum

Significance and Incidence

Meckel's diverticulum is the most common congenital anomaly of the small intestine and represents a remnant of the embryonic vitelline, or omphalomesenteric, duct. It is present in approximately 2% of the population, has a 2:1 male:female predominance, has two types of mucosae, and is typically located within 2 feet of the ileocecal valve ("rule of twos"). Symptoms due to Meckel's diverticula are rare, and are increasingly so as the patient harboring the diverticulum ages. Accordingly, symptoms may develop in 5% of infants harboring the diverticulum, in only 1.5% of individuals at age 40, and extremely rarely in elderly patients, with an overall lifetime risk of symptomatic disease in not more than 4% of the affected population.

Anatomy

Meckel's diverticula evolve when there is incomplete obliteration of the vitelline duct, which arises from the midgut and typically closes between the eighth and 10th

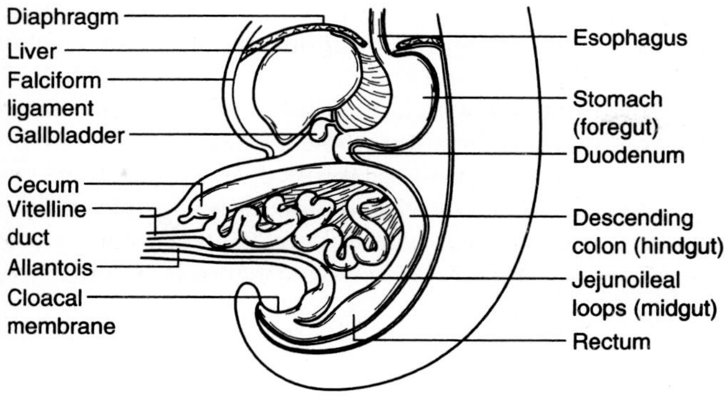

Figure 15-2 Embryonic development of Meckel's diverticulum.

week of gestation (Fig. 15-2). The diverticulum arises from the antimesenteric border of the ileum, usually within 60 cm of the ileocecal valve (Fig. 15-3). Its blood supply is from the vitelline vessels, arising from the ileal blood supply.

Pathophysiology

The cells lining the vitelline duct have pluripotential capabilities. As a result, it is not uncommon to find heterotopic mucosa within the diverticulum. The most common type of such mucosa is gastric (50%). Less frequently, pancreatic and colonic mucosa may be found in the diverticulum. Gastric mucosa in particular, because of its capacity to produce acid in direct proximity to small bowel mucosa, may cause ulceration of the adjacent small intestinal mucosa and hemorrhage. Benign tumors including lipomas, leiomyomas, neurofibromas, and angiomas have been described in diverticula as well. Such tumors may act as a lead point for intussusception and bowel obstruction.

Persistence of the vitelline duct itself can also cause a variety of problems. If there is complete persistence, a sinus from the umbilicus to the ileum may result, presenting as an enteric fistula at the umbilicus itself. If the umbilical end of the duct only remains patent, an umbilical sinus may result. If the duct obliterates but leaves a fibrous cord remnant, this remnant may act as a point of fixation of the small intestine to the abdominal wall and facilitate bowel obstruction. The diverticulum may also become occluded with fecal material and become inflamed, presenting in a fashion very similar to acute appendicitis.

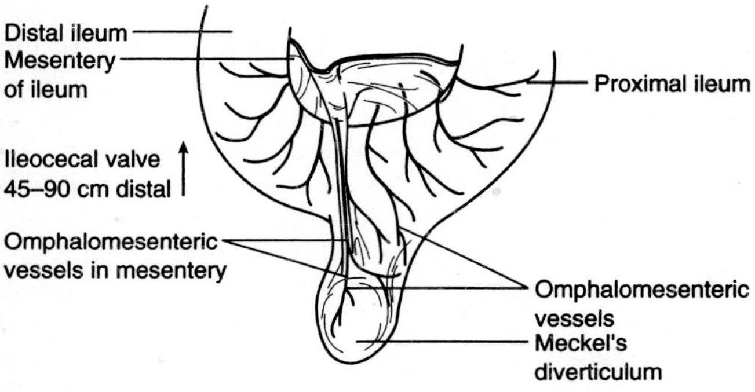

Figure 15-3 Anatomy of Meckel's diverticulum.

Clinical Presentation and Evaluation

The most common presenting illnesses related to Meckel's diverticula are listed in Table 15-1 and include obstruction, hemorrhage, inflammation, and umbilical fistula. Hemorrhage presents with bright red or maroon blood per rectum, is usually painless, and is most common in infants under 2 years of age. Diagnosis can be made 90% of the time with radionuclide scanning using technetium 99m pertechnetate, which is taken up by the ectopic gastric mucosa and delineates the presence of the diverticulum. The positivity of this test may be enhanced by cimetidine or pentagastrin administration, but this is not usually required.

Intestinal obstruction can occur because of volvulus of the small bowel around the diverticulum, or the constrictive effect of a mesodiverticular band (Fig. 15-4). Intussusception may also occur, with the diverticulum acting as a lead point. The latter may present with a palpable right-sided mass and the passage of "currant jelly" stool. Air or contrast enema, particularly in the pediatric population, can facilitate reduction of the intussusception in the acute setting if no bowel compromise has evolved, but subsequent resection of the diverticulum and release of any fibrous attachments should be accomplished.

Diverticulitis closely mimics acute appendicitis, and hence a Meckel's diverticulum should be sought if a patient, especially a younger one, is being explored for suspected appendicitis and is found to have a normal appendix. Less common complications can include iron deficiency anemia, malabsorption, foreign body impaction, perforation, and incarceration in a hernia (Littre's hernia), including inguinal, femoral, and umbilical herniae.

Table 15-1 Clinical Presentation in Meckel's Diverticula[a]

Clinical Presentation	Frequency (%)
Hemorrhage	23
Ileus	31
Intussusception	14
Diverticulitis	14
Perforation	10
Miscellaneous (e.g., fistula, tumor)	8

[a] Occurrence in 1044 cases of Meckel's diverticula compiled from previously published reports.

Adapted with permission from Scharli AF. In: Freeman NV, Burge DM, Griffiths DM, Malone PSJ, eds. *Surgery of the Newborn.* Edinburgh, Scotland: Churchill Livingstone, 1994.

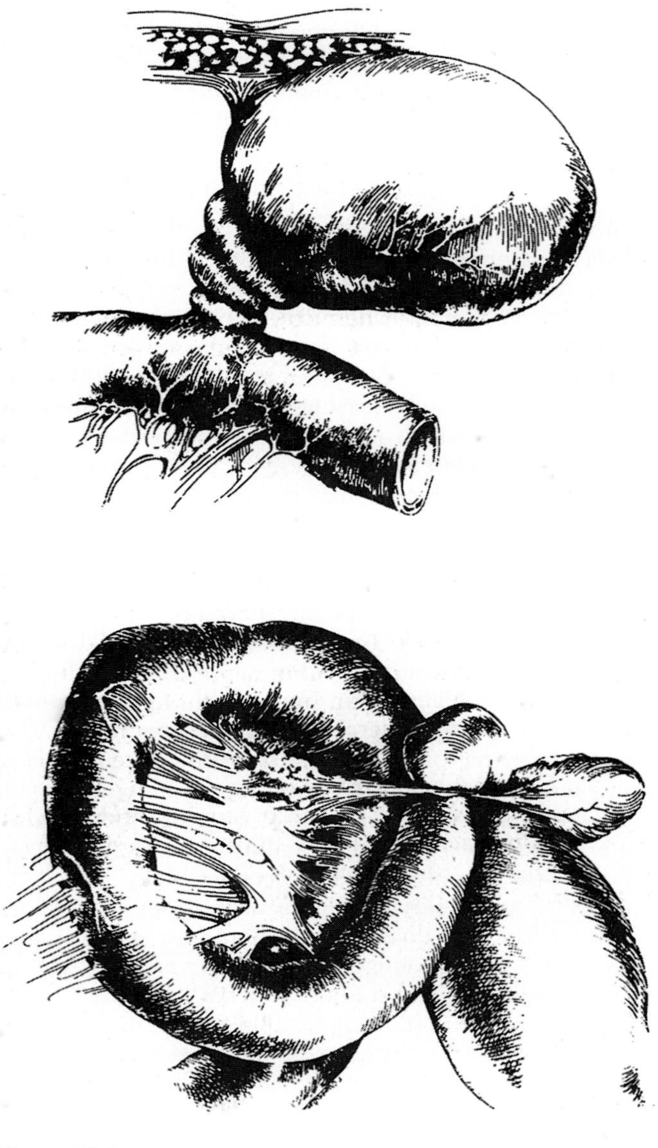

Figure 15-4 Obstruction caused by a mesodiverticular band.

Differential Diagnosis

Acute appendicitis, small bowel obstruction from other causes, and regional enteritis present similarly to, and are more common than, disease related to Meckel's diverticulum. Lower gastrointestinal bleeding, except in the very young patient, is much more commonly due to other pathologies including diverticular disease of the colon and angiodysplastic lesions. Meckel's diverticulum is accordingly appropriately considered in small children presenting with lower abdominal pain, obstruction, lower gastrointestinal bleeding, or umbilical drainage, and should be regarded as a consideration of secondary priority in older patients, in whom other pathologies are far more likely. Studies oriented toward the identification and exclusion of such processes, particularly in the older patient, may help in excluding more common pathologies and may include endoscopic and contrast studies of the gastrointestinal tract. Patients with acute obstructive and inflammatory presentations dictating surgical intervention will typically have the diagnosis established at surgery. Patients with atypical, subacute presentations and negative workup for other processes may benefit from Meckel's scans, small bowel contrast studies, or even laparoscopy to establish the diagnosis.

Treatment

Resection of the diverticulum is curative and appropriate for the patient presenting with complications related to it. When the diverticulum is broad based, segmental bowel resection may be required to adequately remove all ectopic tissue. Laparoscopic resections are being accomplished and are an option when a Meckel's diverticulum is found to be the source of disease during laparoscopic exploration for suspected appendicitis or obstruction. There is continued controversy regarding the most appropriate management when an asymptomatic diverticulum is found incidentally at the time of surgery for other purposes. In the younger patient, especially, the low morbidity of resection may be justified as a preventive measure. However, this potential benefit is small and clearly diminishes as the patient ages and the likelihood of symptomatic disease decreases. Settings in which resection may be considered in patients outside the pediatric age range include when the diverticulum has a narrow base, when a mesodiverticular band is present, or when heterotopic tissue is evident. Incidental resection may also be appropriate in patients with hostile abdomens who would be difficult to reexplore, for example in the setting of multiple adhesions and recurring small bowel obstruction or pending radiation therapy. Ideally, the base of the diverticulum is closed transversely so as to minimize luminal narrowing.

Crohn's Disease of the Small Intestine

Significance and Incidence

Crohn's disease, first described in 1932, has a worldwide prevalence of 10 to 70 cases per 100,000 population. A detailed understanding of its underlying cause remains elusive. It occurs primarily in industrialized nations and appears to be related to underlying genetic as well as environmental factors. First-degree relatives of affected patients have a demonstrably higher risk of the disease than the general population, and disease concordance is significantly higher in monozygotic than dizygotic twins, suggesting a genetic correlation. The *IBD1* locus on chromosome 16 has been identified as a consistent linkage in kindreds with high incidences of Crohn's disease. It is likely that multiple genomic regions may be involved, and the precise genes and gene products that may predispose to the disease continue to be elucidated. Environmental factors that have been implicated include nonsteroidal antiinflammatory drug use and smoking. Current understanding would suggest that, under the influence of predisposing genetic and environmental factors, sustained mucosal immune responses to luminal microflora are responsible for the disease.

The timing of onset of disease has a bimodal distribution, with an early peak in the late teens and early twenties, and a later one in the sixth and seventh decades. The distribution of the disease can be anywhere from the mouth to the anus, although small intestinal and colonic involvement are most common. The ileocecal area is involved in 40% to 50% of patients, the small intestine only in 30% to 40%, and isolated colonic involvement is seen in 20%. The disease may go into prolonged remission but tends to have a recurring course with intermittent flares or exacerbations, and is not curable. As such, it is a significant public health problem.

Pathophysiology

Crohn's disease is a chronic, transmural inflammatory condition of the alimentary tract and may include extraintestinal manifestations affecting the skin, eyes, mouth, joints, and biliary system (see also clinical presentation below). Inflammatory bowel disease patients, including those with Crohn's disease, appear to have an increased number of surface-adherent and intracellular bacteria in the bowel epithelium, and may have genetically determined abnormal host immune responses that allow for continued immune activation and changes in the epithelial mucosal barrier. The end result of this sustained immune and inflammatory response, mediated by a wide range of cytokines, arachidonic acid metabolites (including prostaglandins), and reactive oxygen metabolites (including nitric oxide), is tissue destruction and clinically manifest disease. As outlined above, it appears likely, based on current understanding, that a combination of genetic, environmental, and microflora-induced events leads to the evolution of disease in a complex, synergistic fashion. No specific genetic alteration, infectious agent, or environmental stimulus single-handedly explains this process.

Crohn's disease can be distinguished from ulcerative colitis in a number of its clinical features, although approximately 10% of cases remain "indeterminate" after careful investigation. Common distinguishing features are detailed in Table 16-6, Chapter 16, Colon, Rectum, and Anus. Recognized distinctions include the tendency of Crohn's to involve segments of the gastrointestinal tract other than the colon, with areas of sparing ("skip areas") between affected areas. Transmural involvement and the associated tendency to develop fistulae, as well as the presence of noncaseating granulomata on histology, are also characteristic of Crohn's. Ulcerative colitis, on the other hand, is a mucosal disease, always involves the rectum, and may spread in confluent fashion proximally in the colon, but without skip areas. It does not affect the small intestine (except as so-called backwash ileitis). Because of its transmural nature and tendency to have periods of remission and exacerbation, Crohn's also may lead to the development of fibrotic strictures and obstructive symptomatology.

On gross inspection, the bowel involved with Crohn's may demonstrate fat wrapping or creeping of the mesenteric fat up onto the bowel serosa, and the bowel itself may appear thickened (Fig. 15-5) and erythematous. The mesentery itself is often thickened and shortened and harbors lymphadenopathic nodes. Adherence of inflamed loops of bowel to the parietes, bladder, and other loops of intestine, with or without frank fistula formation, may be seen. If fistulization occurs, abscesses may also be noted, including retroperitoneal and intraabdominal abscesses. Perianal fistulae are a particularly vexing manifestation of Crohn's and are more common in patients with colorectal involvement than in patients with isolated small bowel disease.

The bowel mucosa may exhibit aphthoid ulceration, fissures, and crypt abscesses on endoscopic and histologic review. Noncaseating granulomata are characteristic and are seen in 60% of cases histologically, although they may be missed on endoscopic biopsy, which typically samples only the mucosa.

Clinical Presentation

The common presenting triad of Crohn's includes abdominal pain, diarrhea, and weight loss. The symptoms are typically gradual in onset and progressive over time, although a waxing and waning of symptom severity is common. The pain can be related to partial obstruction due to edema and, in more established cases, fibrosis. In such settings, patients may have associated nausea and vomiting, and may notice increased symptoms when higher residue foods are consumed. Right lower quadrant pain is frequent, based on the frequency of ileocecal involvement, although other areas may well be affected depending on

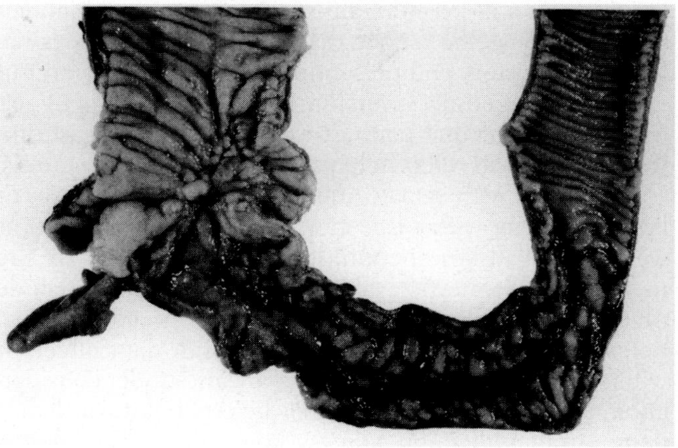

Figure 15-5 Right colon and terminal ileal specimen from Crohn's patient demonstrating narrowing of the diseased segment related to chronic transmural inflammation.

disease distribution. Bleeding is uncommon with Crohn's, in contradistinction to ulcerative colitis, in which bloody diarrhea is a relatively frequent presentation. As the disease progresses, constitutional symptoms including malaise, fatigue, fever, weight loss, and anorexia are common.

Perianal involvement, particularly irregular and multiple anal fistulae, should heighten the concern of Crohn's disease. Fissures and abscesses may also occur. Perianal manifestations are most common in patients with colonic involvement, although they can be seen in patients who otherwise appear to have isolated small bowel disease. Occasionally, intervention on what appears to be a simple perianal abscess or fistula will lead to poor wound healing or incomplete response to treatment, which may be a harbinger of Crohn's.

Extraintestinal manifestations of Crohn's are more common when colonic disease is present, and may include ocular (conjunctivitis, iritis, uveitis, iridocyclitis, episcleritis), skin (pyoderma gangrenosum, erythema nodosum multiforme), joint (ankylosing spondylitis, hypertrophic osteoarthropathy, arthritis), and biliary manifestations (sclerosing cholangitis, pericholangitis, granulomatous hepatitis), as well as vasculitis and aphthous stomatitis. Often these manifestations will respond to control of the underlying bowel disease.

Nutritional losses frequently accompany Crohn's disease due to diminished oral intake and impaired absorption, particularly with terminal ileal disease. Hypoalbuminemia, deficiencies of fat-soluble vitamins (A, D, E, and K), and deficiencies of vitamin B_{12} may be seen. Gallstones are frequent in longstanding disease, due to lithogenic bile brought on by loss of terminal ileal bile salt reabsorption. Growth retardation and developmental delays are accordingly common in younger patients. Nutritional support, given parenterally or enterally depending on the patient's presentation, can correct these deficits and is a critical part of early treatment in the patient with more advanced disease.

While some patients present with urgent issues such as acute bowel obstruction or abscess, the majority of patients present with a more indolent course. There are no laboratory studies specific for the diagnosis, and careful evaluation of the history and presenting findings is important in triggering diagnostic suspicion. In the nonemergent setting, endoscopic and contrast evaluations of the gastrointestinal tract will often help establish the likely diagnosis. Colonoscopy with visualization of the terminal ileum, or barium enema with inspection of the terminal ileum as well, and small bowel contrast studies (Fig. 15-6) are the most useful diagnostic evaluations. Findings may include ulceration, edema, stricture, or fistula formation. In patients with signs or symptoms of abscess or mass effect, or when other diagnostic possibilities are also under consideration, computed tomography may be very helpful and may demonstrate phlegmon, abscess, bowel thickening, partial obstruction, and, occasionally, fistulae. Enteroclysis study of the small intestine may be helpful when standard small bowel follow-through is inconclusive. This test involves intubation of the small intestine with injection of air and contrast to allow mucosal detail to be outlined more precisely than can be achieved with standard small bowel contrast examination. Endoscopic biopsies may be helpful, but because they sample primarily mucosa, often fail histologically to prove the diagnosis of Crohn's. Esophagogastroduodenoscopic examination and/or upper gastrointestinal contrast examination may also be important in the patient suspected of having foregut involvement. Cystography or cystoscopy, and detailed vaginal examination, may also be helpful in the patient with suspected urinary or vaginal fistulae.

Differential Diagnosis

Crohn's disease and ulcerative colitis may be hard to distinguish, particularly when the involvement is primarily colonic and diffuse. Other colitides may also be hard to differentiate in the acute setting, although they generally lack the prodromal illness common in the Crohn's patient. Acute appendicitis, acute regional ileitis due to Yersinia infection, pelvic inflammatory disease, and tuberculosis of the bowel may also be confounding diagnostic possibilities.

Treatment

Medical Therapy

Medical management of Crohn's disease can include a variety of measures that control symptoms, compensate for side effects of the disease, and impact the underlying inflammatory process. Symptom management can include analgesic therapy and suppression of bowel motility, as well as wound care measures for patients with fistulae. Compensatory therapy typically includes fluid, and often nutritional, management, preferably using enteral approaches, although parenteral administration and complete bowel rest are not uncommonly required for severe disease. Control of the inflammatory diathesis can often be achieved with an expanding array of pharmacologic agents.

Antidiarrheal agents including loperamide, diphenoxylate, codeine, and cholestyramine may help in symptom management. They should be used with care and have their greatest utility in patients with chronic diarrhea related to short bowel from prior resections or chronic diarrhea not associated with obstructive features. They can lead to paralytic ileus, bacterial overgrowth, and even toxic megacolon if used injudiciously. Cholestyramine has its greatest efficacy in patients with bile-salt–induced diarrhea due to ileal disease and/or resection. Simple lactose avoidance and/or use of lactase supplementation may also help with diarrheal symptomatology.

Nutritional support is often required in patients with chronic and subacute presentations. Enteral nutrition, with its capacity to preserve mucosal and hepatic cellular structural integrity and function, its lower cost, and its superior safety profile, is preferable. Elemental diets have not been demonstrated to be superior to standard enteral

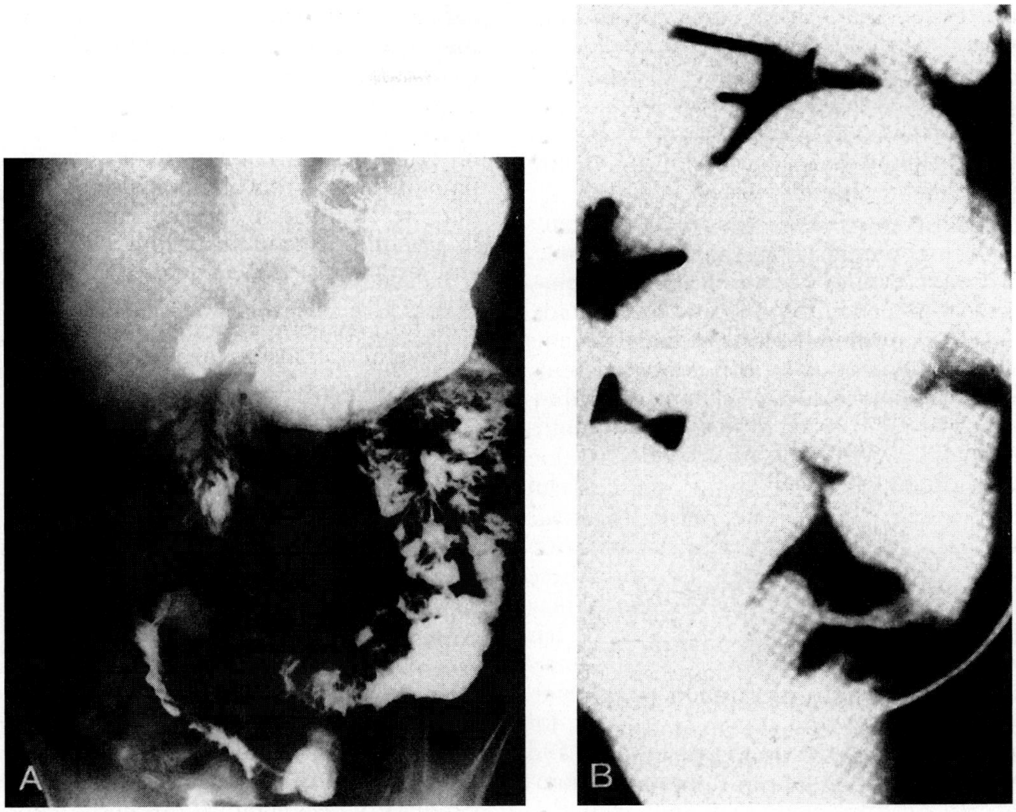

Figure 15-6 **A,** Small bowel study showing a narrowed segment of distal small bowel and a similar change in the antrum of the stomach. The mucosal pattern of the bowel is altered by pseudopolyps, and the valvulae conniventes are absent. The upper small bowel suggests skip areas of Crohn's involvement, whereas the distal bowel is narrowed and contiguously involved with Crohn's disease. **B,** Small bowel study showing the "string sign of Kantor" in the terminal ileum adjacent to the cecum, with proximal dilation of the ileum.

formulae, and while they have the theoretical appeal of minimizing the work of digestion, are generally not palatable and require tube administration. Patients with obstructive features, severe disease, and fistulae (especially proximal small bowel fistulae) will often require parenteral administration. Replacement of vitamins including those absorbed in the terminal ileum as outlined above is frequently necessary. In severely malnourished patients, refeeding syndrome should be anticipated as feedings are commenced. Particular attention to the serum phosphate and potassium levels is necessary in this regard, since chronic depletion becomes taxed by the sudden need to process and store intracellular energy substrates.

A broad array of pharmacologic agents can assist in inducing and maintaining disease remission. Sulfasalazine was one of the first agents recognized to have efficacy, particularly for colonic disease, when it was noted that patients taking this drug for arthritic complaints would often note improvement if they had concomitant colitis. In the distal ileum and colon, intestinal bacteria remove the sulfonamide moiety of sulfasalazine, and the 5-aminosalicylate component is thereby released where it may exert antiinflammatory effects. It appears this effect may be due to the inhibition of nuclear factor kappa B, which is a potent inflammatory cytokine. It may also limit production of prostaglandins and leukotrienes and assist as a scavenger of reactive oxygen metabolites. Newer preparations of 5-aminosalicylic acid (mesalamine) allow delivery of this agent without the sulfonamide moiety to the more proximal small bowel based on pH-dependent or slow-release matrices.

Corticosteroids have significant efficacy in Crohn's disease, particularly when it is unresponsive to 5-aminosalicylate compounds. Topical agents are useful for disease limited to the distal colon, but do not impact small bowel disease. Prednisone in doses up to 60 mg/day can be used orally for more severe disease. A clinical response is seen in the majority of patients within 7 to 10 days of treatment. Intravenous steroids such as hydrocortisone or methylprednisolone can be used for patients unable to tolerate enteral dosing. Budesonide, which is 90% eliminated on first-pass metabolism in the liver, has recently become available, offering the hope of luminal steroid benefit while minimizing systemic toxicities. The latter correlate with the dose and duration of therapy and include hypertension, cataracts, osteoporosis, weight gain, striae, and adrenal suppression. Budesonide has its greatest effect on terminal ileal and right-sided colonic disease and is slightly less efficacious, overall, than conventional corticosteroids.

Immunosuppressive and immune-modulating agents including azathioprine, 6-mercaptopurine, methotrexate, cyclosporine, tacrolimus, and mycophenolate mofetil may be useful, particularly in patients unresponsive to steroids, or as part of a strategy to minimize steroid requirements and toxicity in patients remaining dependent on the same. Azathioprine and 6-mercaptopurine, to which azathioprine is metabolized in red blood cells, take 3 to 6 months to achieve effect. They have been shown to be of value in preventing relapse of disease once remission has been medically or surgically induced, a benefit that steroids lack. Gastrointestinal side effects including liver function abnormalities and pancreatitis may be seen with these agents, as may bone marrow toxicity. Methotrexate may also have remission-sustaining benefits. Cyclosporine has been found to be of use in fistulous Crohn's disease unresponsive to other therapies including steroids and antibiotics (especially metronidazole). Particular concern for nephrotoxicity is required with cyclosporine therapy, and prophylaxis for *Pneumocystis carinii* pneumonitis is recommended in patients on continued treatment with this agent.

Infliximab, a chimeric monoclonal antibody directed against tumor necrosis factor-α, has been shown in recent prospective studies to have significant efficacy in patients with steroid-resistant, moderate to severe Crohn's disease. This agent also has documented effectiveness in the management of enterocutaneous fistulae associated with Crohn's disease (including perianal fistulae) and is effective, although expensive, as maintenance therapy.

While a number of other agents are also being investigated as potential treatments for Crohn's, including growth hormone and thalidomide, one class in particular is worthy of brief mention. Probiotics, living organisms as an oral supplement facilitating intestinal microbial balance, have been shown to reduce relapse rates in conjunction with mesalamine therapy and to reduce pouchitis in patients with inflammatory bowel disease who have undergone colectomy and ileal pouch reconstruction. Given the current understanding of microbial stimuli triggering sustained mucosal inflammatory responses as a pathophysiologic mechanism in Crohn's patients, these nonimmunosuppressive agents may offer hope in future management strategies.

Surgical Therapy

Surgical therapy in Crohn's patients is reserved for complicated disease and disease refractory to medical management. Complications that may require surgical management can include enteric fistulae, obstruction, and perforation. Hemorrhage is rarely an indication for surgical intervention in Crohn's disease. Many fistulae can be managed medically, but enterovesical fistulae usually require surgical management to prevent recurring urosepsis and eventual renal dysfunction. Because of the likelihood of recurrence of Crohn's disease after surgery (as high as 40% within 5 years and 75% within 15 years of operation), the basic surgical strategy is one of disease management rather than radical extirpation. Thus, with small intestinal disease, limited bowel resection to grossly normal bowel is typically accomplished. There is no need to achieve microscopically normal margins, and indeed overly aggressive resection may predispose the patient long term to short bowel syndrome, given the propensity for recurrent disease. When recurrence is seen, it is most commonly proximal to the site of prior disease, although this is not always the case. In the setting of fibrotic, chronic strictures, strictureplasty may be employed to relieve obstructive symptoms and minimize bowel resection.

Because patients with Crohn's often have bacterial colonization of the small intestine and at least partial obstructive pathology, mechanical bowel preparation (when possible) and antibiotic prophylaxis are advisable. Septic, anastomotic, and wound complications are not uncommon. Primary anastomosis is usually possible, although temporary stomas may be required in the setting of advanced peritonitis or the septically complicated patient on immunosuppressive medical therapy. Removal of the appendix to prevent future diagnostic confusion has traditionally been recommended at the time of management of small intestinal Crohn's disease, provided the base of the appendix at the insertion to the cecum is not itself involved, in which case fecal fistula may complicate the appendectomy.

Patients with fistulae who fail to respond to medical management can be managed with resection of the communicating bowel and simple debridement or limited excision of the communicating cutaneous or nonenteric visceral tract. For patients with established abscesses, percutaneous drainage and optimization of medical management, with delayed surgical intervention if necessary, is appropriate. If perianal fistulae fail to respond to medical management, options can include simple drainage of abscesses and placement of setons to ensure ongoing drainage versus more aggressive strategies including fecal diversion or even proctectomy. As a general rule, surgical intervention is limited and conservative for the patient with minor perianal disease, and aggressive incisions or debridements are avoided because of the potential for nonhealing of larger postsurgical wounds. Diversion is reserved for the patient with recurring septic insults or perineal soiling despite medical and limited surgical management, and proctectomy for end-stage disease unresponsive to other measures. Nearly all patients coming to surgical therapy will require perioperative nutritional support. At the time of any operative intervention, inspection of the entire bowel for skip lesions should be made, and careful documentation of the length of bowel resected and length of small intestine remaining should be made for future reference. As a general rule, patients who maintain 100 cm of small intestine will be able to sustain themselves on oral intake, although the absorptive health of the remaining intestine and presence of an intact ileocecal valve can impact this significantly.

Complications

The complications of Crohn's disease frequently dictate changes in medical or surgical management strategies, indeed define the clinical behavior of the disease, and are therefore substantially outlined in the preceding section. Malnutrition, obstruction, fistulous disease, and electrolyte disturbances are all in this category. The most frequent complications of medical management include medication side effects, particularly with steroids and immunosuppressive agents, and progression of the disease when resistant to medical therapy. Surgical treatment can be complicated by wound infection, short bowel syndrome (see below), wound healing problems (particularly in patients on preoperative immune suppression), and fistulae, which may result from anastomotic leaks following resection. Anal incontinence can complicate advanced perianal disease or be a consequence of overly aggressive surgical approaches that compromise sphincter integrity. Given the chronicity of the illness and the frequent requirement for repeated surgical intervention and care, the surgeon often forms a close and ongoing relationship with the patient suffering from recurring and complicated Crohn's disease.

Short bowel syndrome is worthy of specific mention at the close of this section, since Crohn's disease of the small intestine can lead to this problem, along with neonatal necrotizing enterocolitis, mesenteric vascular catastrophes, midgut volvulus, and trauma. Overall, Crohn's disease accounts for approximately one-fourth of cases, typically due to recurring disease and repeated surgical interventions over a period of years. As mentioned previously, the syndrome is rare if at least 100 cm of adult intestinal length can be maintained, particularly if the terminal ileum, due to its specialized absorptive functions, and the ileocecal valve as a brake and guard against bacterial overgrowth in the small intestine are preserved. The small bowel and, to a limited extent, colon can undergo adaptive change in response to decreased small bowel length and absorptive capacity. Accordingly, in the initial phases, pharmacologic suppression of gastric secretion, bile salt binding with cholestyramine, and use of isosmolar, low-fat, easily absorbed enteral formulae may help to facilitate management. Trophic stimulation to the remaining gut mucosa with some degree of enteral support, even if insufficient to meet caloric and nutritional needs, is valuable. Pharmacologic motility suppression is often utilized. Glutamine-enriched formulae appear to facilitate maintenance and adaptation of the residual intestinal epithelium, and other enterotrophic agents (including recombinant growth hormone, epidermal growth factor, and glucagon-like peptide 2) continue to be investigated for their potential benefit. Parenteral nutrition is often required, at least during the adaptive phase. In patients who become dependent on parenteral nutrition because of extensive small bowel resection and disease, long-term deficiencies that are not seen with short-term nutritional support can evolve. Examples include essential fatty acid deficiency, vitamin deficiencies, and deficiencies of trace elements. Venous access problems and access-related septic complications are also frequent in these patients. Gallstones, due to interruption of the enterohepatic circulation and the development of lithogenic bile, and nephrolithiasis are common. The latter is due to fat malabsorption and resulting fat binding with calcium, leading to increased intraluminal, noncomplexed, absorbable oxalate and hyperoxaluria. Operations to attempt to improve absorptive surface (lengthening procedures) or decrease transit time (valve construction, interposition) have met with varying success. Small bowel transplantation is an option for the patient who remains dependent on parenteral nutrition, with 1-year survivals reported in the 70% range, and a similar percentage of patients so treated achieving enteral independence (see Transplantation chapter).

Small Bowel Tumors

A variety of tumors can arise from the epithelial and mesenchymal components of the small intestine. Tumors are much less common in the small intestine than in the colon and rectum, despite the greater length and absorptive surface area of the small bowel. Small bowel tumors may present with obstructive symptoms, bleeding, or symptoms of metastatic disease. They may also act as lead points for intussusception. Diagnosis is most commonly made by contrast evaluation, enteroclysis in particular.

Endoscopic evaluation of the duodenum and proximal jejunum, as well as of the terminal ileum, has also been used to diagnose these lesions. Until recently, endoscopic evaluation of the intervening small intestine has been difficult, often requiring specialized instruments, which are tedious to employ, or operative assistance. Capsule endoscopy has recently emerged as a technology that may assist greatly in the diagnosis of small bowel lesions including tumors. With this technique, the patient swallows a capsule-sized device equipped with light-emitting diodes, batteries, and a complementary metal-oxide-semiconductor (CMOS) chip that transmits two images per second to a unit worn on the waist, where images are stored for later downloading and interpretation. Early experience with this technology has demonstrated its potential to document small bowel pathology, including the presence of otherwise occult tumors, in a minimally invasive fashion.

Benign Tumors

Benign small intestinal tumors are much more common than malignant lesions. The majority are asymptomatic. Both sexes are equally affected, with a peak incidence in the sixth decade. The most common of these lesions have traditionally been referred to as **leiomyomas**, which occur most commonly in the jejunum. Many of these lesions, which can occur anywhere in the digestive tract, are on the benign end of a spectrum of mesenchymal tumors of the gastrointestinal tract and are now referred to as gastrointestinal stromal tumors (GISTs). These lesions arise from the interstitial cells of Cajal. Lesions in this category can be diagnosed by immunohistochemical determination of their expression of the c-kit proto-oncogene protein, also known as CD117. Benign lesions in this category show fewer mitoses than their malignant counterparts, generally are of smaller size, and lack features such as necrosis, nuclear pleomorphism, and invasive or metastatic behavior. If c-kit expression is negative, the lesion may be classified as a true leiomyoma rather than as a GIST. Even benign-appearing lesions may cause overlying mucosal ulceration or obstructive symptoms, particularly if they reach a large size, and may manifest delayed local recurrence. Lipomas may also rarely demonstrate these features, are more common in men, and occur most commonly in the duodenum or ileum.

Other nonepithelial, benign small bowel lesions may include **hemangiomas**, **hamartomas**, lymphangiomas, and neurogenic tumors such as schwannomas and neurofibromas. Hemangiomas are an important potential cause of occult bleeding and constitute 5% of benign small bowel lesions. These lesions are often multiple, as can be seen in Osler-Weber-Rendu syndrome. Capsule enteroscopy may offer particular promise in delineating hemangiomas, given their potential for multiplicity and the fact that they do not show up on standard contrast studies. For actively bleeding lesions, angiography may also be useful. Hamartomas are usually isolated and typically asymptomatic. They can be a cause of bleeding or intussusception, particularly in the pediatric population. Multiple hamartomas may be seen in association with Peutz-Jeghers syndrome, an autosomal dominant trait also associated with mucocutaneous hyperpigmentation.

Epithelial benign lesions of the small intestine include tubular, villous, and Brunner's gland **adenomas**. Brunner's gland adenomas occur primarily in the duodenum and are usually asymptomatic, as are most tubular adenomas. Adenomas with villous histology are more likely to harbor malignancy (overall risk 30%—increasing with lesion size), and should be excised for this reason (Fig. 15-7). Duodenal carcinoma of the periampullary region, typically arising from a preexisting benign adenoma, is the most common malignancy affecting individuals with familial polyposis after proctocolectomy, and the duodenum and papilla should be endoscopically surveilled in patients with this diagnosis.

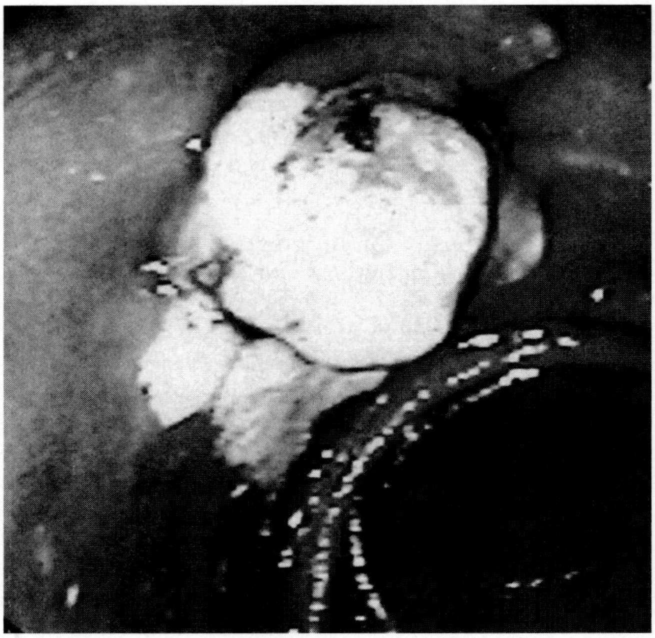

Figure 15-7 Ampullary villous adenoma. Reconstruction of the biliary and pancreatic ducts was necessary after local excision of the tumor.

Malignant Tumors

A variety of malignant tumors can affect the small intestine, although these constitute only 2% of all gastrointestinal tract malignancies. Overall, malignant tumors are slightly more common in males than females, and the average age at presentation is in the sixth decade.

Adenocarcinomas

Adenocarcinomas account for approximately half of all small intestinal malignancies. They are most common in the duodenum, with decreasing incidence as one moves distally in the small bowel. Obstruction, often associated with weight loss, is the most common presentation. Small intestinal obstruction in the absence of hernia or prior abdominal surgery and associated adhesions should heighten one's concern that a small intestinal neoplasm may be present. Occult bleeding and anemia may also be noted. In a younger individual, occult small intestinal bleeding is frequently due to small bowel neoplasia. Massive bleeding is rare. Lesions in the periampullary region may present with painless jaundice and, rarely, otherwise unexplained pancreatitis. Nearly half of small intestinal adenocarcinomas are diagnosed at the time of operation.

Surgical intervention should include wide resection of the involved bowel with margins to facilitate removal of the associated mesenteric lymphatic drainage pathways. Adjuvant therapies have little demonstrated efficacy, and 5-year survival is generally poor, in the 10% to 30% range, reflecting the tendency toward delayed diagnosis predicated on advanced, symptomatic disease. As mentioned above, endoscopic screening of the periampullary region in particular may allow earlier diagnosis in patients with genetic polyposis syndromes and known associated risk.

Carcinoid Tumors

Carcinoid tumors arise from the Kulchitsky cells in the crypts of Lieberkühn. These cells are part of the amine precursor uptake and decarboxylation (APUD) system. They are sometimes called argentaffin cells because of their histologic staining characteristics. Malignant behavior correlates with lesion size; metastasis occurs in only 2% of patients with primary tumors less than 1 cm in size, but in 90% of those with primary tumors larger than 2 cm. Between 40% and 50% of all gastrointestinal carcinoids originate in the appendix, with the small intestine being the second most common gastrointestinal site. Small intestinal carcinoids are most common in the ileum and may be multicentric in as many as 30% of patients.

Obstruction is the most common presenting finding in patients with small intestinal carcinoid. This is usually not due to the size of the primary lesion, but rather an intense desmoplastic reaction that characteristically occurs in the adjacent bowel mesentery. Bleeding and intussusception are less common. Many patients do experience nonspecific symptoms including anorexia, fatigue, and weight loss. The diagnosis is often made at laparotomy. Surgical treatment consists of wide excision of the bowel and adjacent mesentery, which may require right hemicolectomy with terminal ileal lesions. If resectable liver metastases are noted at the time of operation, they should also be removed.

The **carcinoid syndrome** is a complex of manifestations that metastatic intestinal carcinoids may demonstrate. Episodic cutaneous flushing (especially of the head and trunk), bronchospasm, intestinal cramping and diarrhea, vasomotor instability, pellagra-like skin lesions, and right-sided valvular heart disease may be seen (Fig. 15-8). These attacks may be spontaneous or may be triggered by exer-

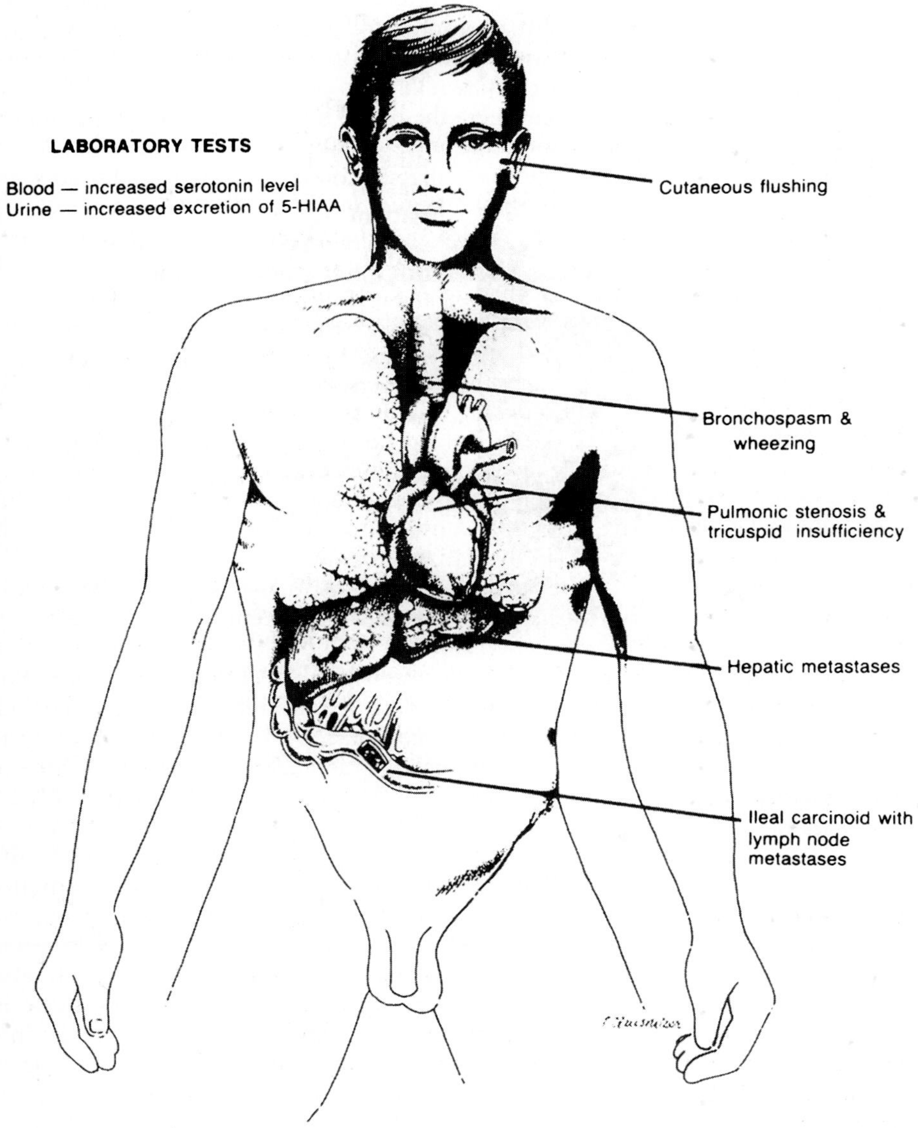

Figure 15-8 Clinical manifestations of malignant carcinoid syndrome.

tion, excitement, alcohol, anesthesia, or tumor manipulation. These manifestations are related to the elaboration of 5-hydroxytryptamine (serotonin) by the tumor. This substance is degraded on delivery to the liver via the portal vein into 5-hydroxyindole acetic acid (5-HIAA), as well as other vasoactive peptides including 5-hydroxytryptophan, kallikrein, histamine, and adrenocorticotropic hormone (ACTH). It is not entirely clear which combination of these substances is responsible for the syndrome. The liver is highly effective in clearing serotonin and its metabolites from the bloodstream when delivered via the portal vein. Thus, for the syndrome to occur, the bowel lesion must have metastasized to the liver to allow delivery to the venous circulation in a postportal location, or the primary lesion must be in another location not draining via the portal system, such as the lungs, gonads, or rectum. The syndrome is confirmed, when suspected, by urinary measurement of 5-HIAA. Treatment is via resection, when this is possible.

Lymphoma

The small intestine is the most common site of extranodal **lymphoma**, although only 5% of all lymphomas are found there. Lymphoma accounts for 10% to 15% of all small bowel malignancies. Again, the fifth and sixth decades are the periods of highest incidence. The ileum is the most common site of involvement, given the concentration of lymphoid tissue in Peyer's patches in that region. Although more commonly described in the stomach in association with chronic gastritis associated with *Helicobacter pylori* infection, so-called MALT lymphomas may occur in the small intestine and are found in a subset of patients with small intestinal lymphoma. While the majority of patients present with nonspecific symptoms such as vague abdominal pain, weight loss, fatigue, and malaise, up to one-fourth may declare as abdominal emergencies (perforation, hemorrhage, obstruction, intussusception). Nodularity and thickening of the bowel wall on contrast studies or computed tomography (CT) scan, often with associated mesenteric adenopathy on CT, may allow preoperative suspicion of the diagnosis. Surgical resection is usually accomplished, often with subsequent chemotherapy and/or radiation, depending on the type of lymphoma and stage of disease. Overall 5-year survival is in the 20% to 40% range. Patients diagnosed prior to laparotomy and treated with chemoradiation without surgical resection may experience bowel perforation from tumor lysis, particularly when there is extensive involvement of the bowel wall.

Gastrointestinal Stromal Tumors/Leiomyosarcoma

As mentioned above, most mesenchymal tumors of the gastrointestinal tract, formerly referred to as leiomyosarcomas, are now referred to as GIST lesions. They can have a spectrum of clinical behaviors from benign to malignant, may occur anywhere in the small intestine, have a peak incidence in the sixth decade, and can present with obstruction, bleeding, or perforation. GIST lesions universally exhibit c-kit protein expression, as noted above in the discussion of benign tumors. Malignant mesenchymal lesions that do not exhibit this expression may still be classified as true leiomyosarcomas. Small bowel GISTs appear to have a worse prognosis than similar lesions of the esophagus and stomach. Wide excision with adjacent mesentery is performed, and malignant behavior is predicted from mitoses, evidence of invasive behavior, and tumor necrosis. Overall, approximately 50% of patients will demonstrate recurrence within 2 years. For patients with metastatic GIST lesions, impressive responses may be seen with imatinib, a tyrosine kinase inhibitor used also in patients with chronic myelogenous leukemia.

Small Bowel Obstruction

Significance and Incidence

The most frequent indication for operation on the small intestine is bowel obstruction. The most common cause for obstruction worldwide is hernia, usually inguinal or incisional (in an area of prior abdominal intervention). Rarely, small bowel obstruction (SBO) can be caused by internal hernias related to mesenteric defects or recesses in an area where the bowel transfers from a retroperitoneal to an intraperitoneal location (e.g., paraduodenal). In Western industrialized nations, postsurgical adhesions are the most frequent cause of SBO. Adhesions are present in at least two-thirds of patients who have undergone prior intraperitoneal surgery and in more than 90% of patients who have had two or more prior intraabdominal operations. Overall, 5% to 10% of patients who have had prior abdominal surgery will subsequently have symptoms of SBO. Adhesions may less frequently be the cause of obstruction during or following acute inflammatory illnesses of the peritoneal organs managed without surgery, such as acute diverticulitis, cholecystitis, appendicitis, pelvic inflammatory disease, or endometriosis. Postsurgical, adhesive SBO thus constitutes a significant public health problem in industrialized countries.

Other causes of SBO include intestinal volvulus and intussusception. Volvulus may occur because of postsurgical adhesive fixation of the bowel, or as a function of congenital malrotation or bands. A closed loop of intestine results, causing the obstruction. Intussusception, in which a portion of the intestine telescopes on itself leading to obstruction, can occur spontaneously in small children or due to the effect of intestinal peristalsis acting on a "lead point" such as a polyp or tumor in older patients. As outlined above, intestinal tumors can also be a cause of SBO and should always be suspected in patients with obstructive presentation who lack herniae or a history of prior surgical intervention. Crohn's disease, particularly with acute edema or chronic stricture formation, can also be responsible, as previously discussed. So-called **gallstone ileus**, in which a large gallstone erodes through the gallbladder into an adjacent loop of adherent intestine in the setting of cholecystitis, can also be an etiology for SBO, particularly in the elderly population. The stone typically migrates to the distal small bowel and causes obstruction of the intestinal lumen. Air in the biliary tree on plain film (due to the cholecystenteric fistula), in combination with features of SBO, can raise the suspicion of the diagnosis. Multiple stones may be present in the small intestine in this setting and should be sought for at the time of exploration. Finally, a proximal, duodenal obstruction may be seen in patients with the superior mesenteric artery (SMA) syndrome. In this setting, typically evolving in a setting of rapid and significant weight loss, the third portion of the duodenum may be compressed by the acute angle between the SMA at its takeoff from the aorta and the aorta itself. Diagnosis often is made with lateral arteriography or other imaging studies, which, in the appropriate clinical setting, document the point of obstruction at this specific location.

Pathophysiology

Fluid deficits frequently evolve as a function of emesis, decreased absorption, and hormonally stimulated secretion triggered by luminal distension. As the process progresses, "third space" losses due to bowel wall edema and transudation of fluid into the peritoneal cavity may also occur. Electrolyte abnormalities can vary with the location of the obstruction and duration of illness.

The most serious complication of SBO is strangulation of the involved intestine. In this setting, more common with closed loop and high-grade obstructions, the bowel becomes ischemic and eventually infarcts as edema and kinking of the mesentery impact mesenteric vascular patency. Local or systemic sepsis, and frank perforation of the affected bowel, may supervene. A number of clinical and laboratory parameters have been used in an attempt to predict progression of obstruction to the point of strangulation. Fever, tachycardia, leukocytosis, and localized abdominal tenderness have most commonly been cited as indicators of a higher risk of strangulation. In some series, the risk of strangulation has increased from 7% when one of these signs is present to 67% when all four are noted. However, it is critical to recognize that bowel infarction may evolve even in the absence of these signs, and all four can be present without infarction having occurred. The risk of infarction also appears to rise in patients with high-grade obstruction who are managed nonoperatively for more than 24 to 48 hours, assuming there are no signs of resolution in that time frame.

Clinical Presentation and Evaluation

History

A detailed past medical history, including notation of prior abdominal surgeries or illnesses, is of utmost importance. Patients should also be asked about prodromal bulges or focal pain that may herald the presence of a hernia. Individuals with vague and chronic symptomatology prior to the onset of frank obstructive symptoms may have underlying disease states, such as inflammatory disease or neoplasia. The typical onset of acute SBO is marked by colicky abdominal pain in the periumbilical region, given the midgut autonomic innervation pathways of the majority of the small intestine. Pain may become more steady as peristaltic activity lessens and generalized bowel distension progresses with the diathesis. As mentioned above, pain and tenderness that begin to localize in a more somatic pattern should heighten concern for bowel ischemia and peritonitis with attendant parietal peritoneal irritation. Nausea and vomiting are prominent complaints in many patients, although the onset of these symptoms may be delayed in more distal obstructions due to small bowel capacitance. Abdominal distension is also more prominent with distal obstruction for the same reason and may be unimpressive with very proximal obstructions. Constipation, and in particular the lack of any flatus (obstipation), is a particularly ominous sign for higher-grade obstruction, but may not be immediate given the potential for passage of air and stool already in the colon at the onset of illness. Conversely, in partial SBO, passage of stool, including even loose stools, and some flatus may persist despite the obstructive process.

Examination

Patients with SBO typically present after a period of pain, often associated with nausea and vomiting, and attendant fluid and electrolyte disturbance. Patients may appear acutely distressed in the early, colicky phases of the illness or may appear lethargic as dehydration and electrolyte disturbances ensue. Tachycardia, dry mucous membranes, decreased skin turgor, and even relative hypotension may be seen in more advanced cases. The abdomen is frequently distended, again depending on the location of the obstruction, and may be tympanitic if the intestine is distended with air or dull to percussion if the bowel loops are fluid-filled or ascites has evolved. On auscultation, high-pitched sounds and rushes may be noted early in the illness, and a dearth of bowel activity is characteristic as distension progresses or peritonitis ensues. Surgical scars and areas of potential herniation should be carefully examined. In obese patients, areas of focal contour change, erythema, or tenderness near a surgical scar may be the only clue to bowel incarceration within an otherwise occult hernia. Diffuse mild tenderness is frequent and often will improve after acute decompression via a nasogastric tube, assuming bowel ischemia has not already occurred. Patients with impressive persistent tenderness or more advanced peritoneal signs such as percussion tenderness, rebound tenderness, and fear of movement may have already progressed to advanced disease, and such findings should prompt more urgent surgical intervention.

Radiographic Studies

An abdominal series including supine and upright abdominal films and an upright chest radiograph are the most valuable initial studies. These studies may document other processes, which can mimic the presentation of SBO. Specific inspection should be made for renal or biliary calculi, pneumoperitoneum ("free air"), pneumatosis intestinalis, and pneumonia. In the absence of confounding illness, typical findings would include bowel distension proximal to the point of obstruction and collapse of the bowel, manifest by nonvisualization on the radiograph, distal to the same point (Fig. 15-9). Air fluid levels may be seen on upright films and denote lack of normal propulsive activity in affected loops of intestine. Focal loops of intestine that are persistently abnormal on serial films may represent closed-loop obstruction. It is important to recognize that fluid-filled loops of obstructed bowel may blend with other soft tissue densities on radiography and mislead the clinician who doesn't see a "typical" obstructive pattern. On the other hand, if the bowel is massively distended with air, it may be difficult to distinguish the small and large bowel. In such settings, water-soluble contrast enema may help to exclude the possibility of a large bowel obstructive mechanism.

Computed tomography may be very useful in settings of diagnostic confusion, given its ability to delineate confounding illnesses such as nephrolithiasis, diverticulitis, and pancreatitis, or mesenteric vascular disease. It also has the capacity to demonstrate dilated, fluid-filled small intestinal loops, which as noted above can be missed on plain films and may even demonstrate a transition zone between dilated and decompressed small intestine, documenting SBO as the source of illness. It can accomplish many of these goals even without administration of oral contrast and is assuming a more prominent role in evaluating the patient with suspected SBO.

Contrast studies of the small intestine are useful in the patient with persistent partial obstructive symptoms, or when it is difficult to distinguish paralytic ileus from mechanical obstruction. It is important before pursuing such studies to be confident one does not need to exclude colonic obstruction or mesenteric occlusive disease, since the contrast enema and angiogram used to evaluate for these entities may be obscured by the contrast used for the small bowel follow-through study. Small bowel contrast studies are usually not necessary in the acute, high-grade setting, in which clinical findings, plain film results, and computed tomography are typically adequate to guide management.

Laboratory Data

Laboratory data are not specific in SBO but may be of value in excluding other pathologies and guiding resuscitation. Leukocytosis, particularly if it persists despite nasogastric decompression and fluid resuscitation, may be a sign of progression toward ischemia. Electrolytes should be closely monitored. A hypokalemic, "contraction" alkalosis is common in patients with advanced dehydration. Hyperamylasemia may be seen with SBO, but if it is marked in degree, it may heighten the suspicion for acute pancreatitis as a confounding illness. Urinalysis is important in exclud-

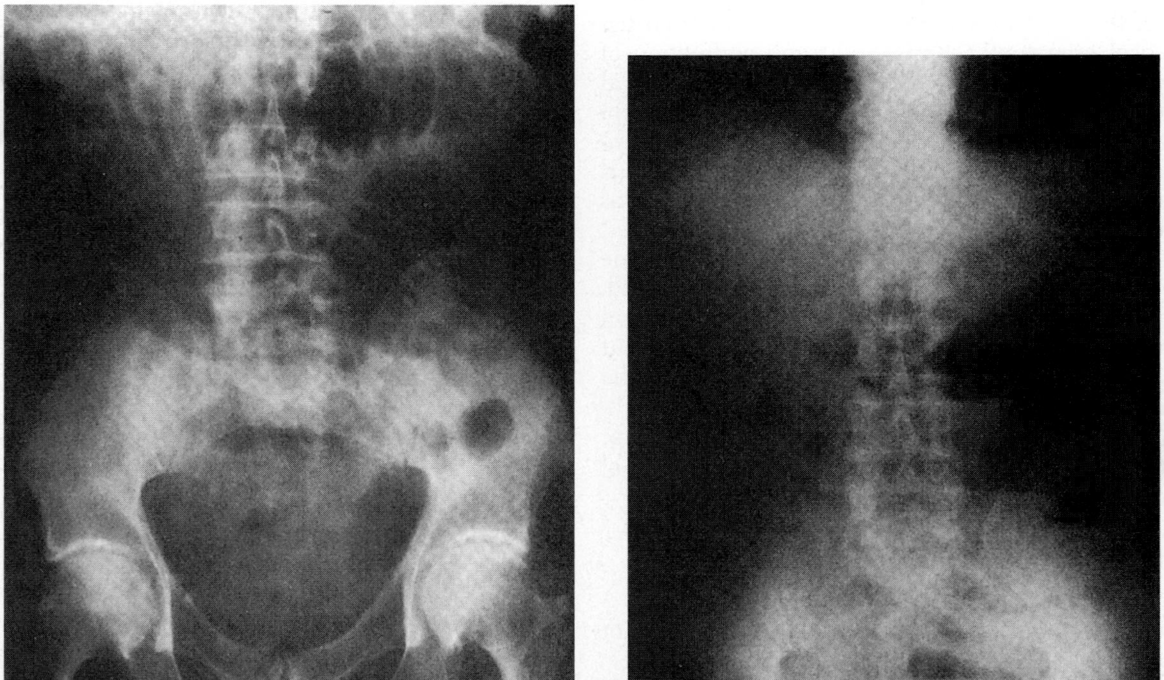

Figure 15-9 Mechanical small intestinal obstruction. **A,** Decubitus abdominal radiograph. There are many centrally located loops of air-filled small intestine and no gas at the periphery of the abdomen. Valvulae conniventes are shown. **B,** Upright abdominal radiograph. Multiple air-filled levels are seen.

ing evidence for urinary infection or stone disease as a source of symptoms. Lactic acidosis, particularly in the setting of adequate volume administration, may signal bowel ischemia, although frank infarction may be seen without acidosis and its absence should not be overinterpreted in the patient who is failing to resolve with appropriate conservative measures.

Differential Diagnosis

Paralytic Ileus

Paralytic ileus is the most frequent differential diagnostic entity considered in the setting of possible SBO. In this process, bowel motility is suppressed as a consequence of systemic or inflammatory illness, and the bowel may become distended and the patient obstipated in a pattern not unlike that of SBO, despite the lack of a mechanical obstruction. Narcotics, bed rest, trauma, hypothyroidism, electrolyte deficiencies (especially potassium, calcium, magnesium, and phosphate), anesthesia, psychotropic medication, and systemic or peritoneal inflammatory illnesses or sepsis are all common causes of ileus. Pain, nausea and emesis, and abdominal distension may all be seen similar to the pattern of SBO, although subtle differences may be noted in the pattern of these symptoms (Table 15-2). Typically, plain films will demonstrate diffuse bowel dilation, including both the small and large intestine, without evidence of a transition zone (Fig. 15-10). Contrast enema to exclude colonic obstruction, and, if this condition is excluded, small bowel contrast study may be required in cases where the distinction between ileus and mechanical obstruction remains difficult.

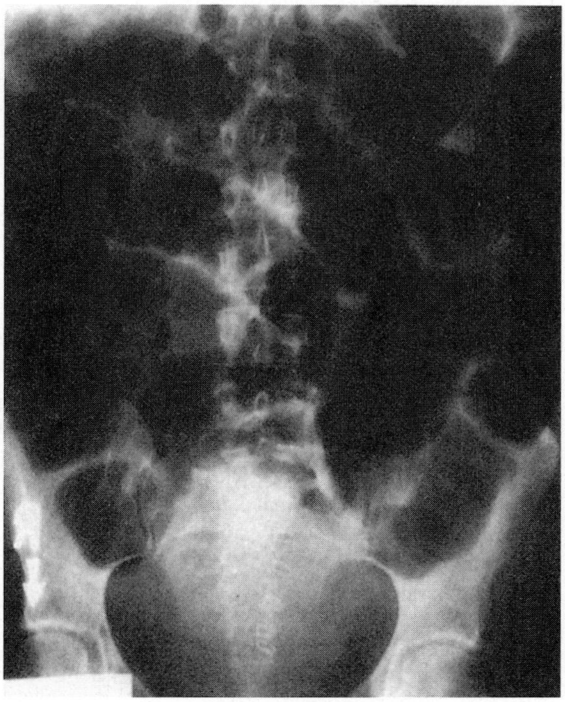

Figure 15-10 Abdominal radiograph showing paralytic ileus of the small bowel. This condition is differentiated from mechanical small bowel obstruction and colonic obstruction by air in the distal sigmoid colon and rectum.

Treatment

Treatment for SBO begins with resuscitation. Correction of fluid and electrolyte deficits should commence even as initial diagnostic studies are being accomplished. Typically, this will include intravenous volume replacement with isotonic solutions, tailored and supplemented as dictated by any specific electrolyte abnormalities encountered. It is important to establish euvolemia before aggressively replacing electrolytes such as potassium, since rapid rises in the serum level may be encountered if renal perfusion has not been restored. Frequent assessment of urine output via a Foley catheter is the best simple tool for assessing adequacy of volume replacement and may be supplemented in the setting of complicated cardiac disease by invasive central pressure monitoring, if necessary. In adults, an hourly urine output of at least 0.5 mL/kg is usually indicative of adequate volume resuscitation. Nasogastric decompression is commenced via nasogastric tube placement to control emesis, relieve intestinal distension proximal to the obstruction, lower the risk of aspiration, and allow monitoring of ongoing fluid and electrolyte losses. The patient is given nothing per mouth and followed closely for response to initial resuscitation.

If the obstruction is partial or low grade and there is a history of prior abdominal surgery with no palpable hernia, the obstruction is likely adhesive in nature, with an approximately 80% chance of resolution if the above measures are followed. Patients who have incarcerated herniae should have reduction of the same, if possible, and close observation thereafter to ensure that the obstructive process resolves. An unsuccessful reduction may manifest as persistent pain or tenderness, with or without inflammatory examination or laboratory signs. Repair of the hernia following resolution of any obstructive signs should then be accomplished to prevent recurrence. Nonreduceable herniae should be urgently repaired following rapid volume resuscitation and correction of any severe electrolyte

Table 15-2 Characteristics of Paralytic Ileus and Small Intestinal Obstruction

Paralytic Ileus	Small Intestinal Obstruction
Minimal abdominal pain	Crampy abdominal pain
Nausea and vomiting	Nausea and vomiting
Obstipation and failure to pass flatus	Obstipation and failure to pass flatus
Abdominal distension	Abdominal distension
Decreased or absent bowel sounds	Normal or increased bowel sounds
Gas in the small intestine and colon on radiograph	Gas in the small intestine only on radiograph

disturbances. Individuals who have no prior surgery or externally demonstrable herniae on which to blame the obstruction should be prepared for surgery, provided the diagnosis seems clear, since a high percentage of such patients will have conditions such as neoplastic lesions or internal herniae that will require operative management. Similarly, patients with complete or high-grade obstructions should generally be prepared for prompt surgical intervention, since in this setting the likelihood of resolution is diminished and the risk of bowel ischemia heightened. Patients in whom conservative therapy is initially justified should be taken to surgery if there is not definite clinical and radiologic improvement within 24 to 48 hours, or sooner if there is evidence of deterioration as manifest by exam changes, fluid requirements, radiologic signs, or laboratory parameters. The risk of bowel compromise increases after that time frame, provided there is no evidence of improvement. Settings in which a longer period of observation and conservative, nonsurgical management may be appropriate include early postoperative obstructions, the majority of which may resolve within 2 weeks as acute, bulky adhesions and associated postoperative bowel edema begin to mature and resolve, respectively. Patients with known carcinomatosis, or recurrent obstructions in the setting of multiple prior operations and a known hostile abdomen, may also be candidates for a longer period of nonoperative management. Long intestinal tubes (Baker, Miller-Abbott), which can be manipulated under radiologic guidance into the more distal small bowel, may have utility in such settings as a means to achieve decompression and relief of obstruction without surgical intervention, although their management is often laborious to achieve this benefit.

If surgery is required, preoperative antibiotics are given to cover Gram-negative aerobes and anaerobes, which may proliferate in the normally sterile, but now obstructed and stagnant, small bowel. At laparotomy, adhesions are mobilized, herniae reduced and repaired, and the bowel carefully inspected to ensure integrity of its blood supply. If there is question in regard to bowel viability, intraoperative assessment with fluorescein dye or Doppler ultrasound to assess perfusion may augment clinical evaluations of bowel viability such as color, bleeding, and peristalsis. No test is foolproof, and if the surgeon has significant concern, a second-look operation in 24 hours may be appropriate. Care to not be overly aggressive in resection is especially important in patients with underlying Crohn's disease, or when the amount of remaining small intestine is approaching the 100 cm range, after which there would be a high likelihood of dependence on long-term parenteral nutrition. Clearly compromised bowel should be resected. If neoplasia is found, an appropriate resection is accomplished. In general, it is possible to reanastomose the small bowel primarily, although delay of this until a second-look operation in the acute and questionably viable setting, or following temporary stoma diversion in complicated situations, is occasionally necessary. If intussusception is found in the adult, resection because of the high likelihood of a lead point lesion should be accomplished. In children, spontaneous intussusception is often able to be managed nonoperatively with pneumatic or contrast enema reduction.

A number of series have now been published evaluating the use of laparoscopy in SBO. While success with this approach in a modest number of cases is well documented, hazards with laparoscopic access and bowel manipulation in the face of distension limit the widespread application of this technique, particularly in the multiply reoperated and surgically hostile abdomen. Interest in this area, and successful use particularly with uncomplicated adhesive obstructions, will likely continue to evolve in the future.

Complications

Wound infection, anastomotic leak, abscess, peritonitis, and fistula formation may all complicate operative intervention for SBO, especially when bowel infarction and/or resection have occurred. Overall, mortality is less than 1% for laparotomy in the setting of uncomplicated SBO but may exceed 25% when strangulation has occurred. With extensive resection, short bowel syndrome can eventuate and necessitate long-term parenteral access and nutritional support. Recurrent obstruction may also be seen, as in any postlaparotomy patient. Interest in prevention of recurrent obstruction with chemical or barrier devices intended to limit adhesion formation continues, although to date there is insufficient evidence of efficacy to justify routine use. Currently, a commercially available barrier composed of sodium hyaluronate and carboxymethylcellulose has been shown to be effective in decreasing adhesions after laparotomy. However, it has not been proven to diminish the incidence of recurrent bowel obstruction in prospective studies.

DISEASES OF THE APPENDIX

Acute Appendicitis

Significance and Incidence

Acute appendicitis is the most common emergent surgical illness, affecting approximately 5% of the population. The majority of patients are between the ages of 5 and 35 and typically present in the first 24 to 48 hours of illness. Atypical presentation and delayed diagnosis are more common in children and the elderly, with an attendant higher risk of perforation, as high as 15% to 25%, in those settings.

Anatomy

The vermiform appendix is located in the right lower quadrant at the confluence of the taenia coli on the cecal apex. It can be in a variety of positions in relation to the cecum, including in a retrocecal position. The location of the appendix determines the location of tenderness as the disease progresses. The appendiceal artery travels in the mesoappendix and originates from the ileocolic artery.

The appendix is lined by columnar epithelium and is rich in lymphatic follicles, which are most numerous in people between 10 and 20 years of age. Individuals in this age group may harbor as many as 200 such follicles in the organ. The presence of this lymphatic tissue correlates closely with the predominant ages affected by acute appendicitis. In the United States, approximately 10,000 deaths per year are attributable to diseases of the appendix.

Pathophysiology

Acute appendicitis develops as a consequence of obstruction of the appendiceal lumen. Lymphoid hyperplasia, seen in 60% of patients with appendicitis, is the most common etiology of luminal obstruction. An accumulation of fecal material, or fecalith, is noted histologically in 35% of patients. Viral illnesses that elicit lymphoid hyperplasia are a frequent prodrome to the onset of appendicitis in the young. As the appendiceal lumen becomes compromised, mucus secretion by the epithelium leads to distension of the appendix distal to the narrowed lumen, with eventual compromise of venous outflow as the organ becomes increasingly turgid, and ultimately, ischemic. Necrosis and bacterial proliferation in the stagnant, ischemic environment may supervene. Bacterial toxins can lead to further mucosal damage. As the swelling, infection, and ischemia progress, they may become transmural and lead to gangrene and perforation. If perforation occurs, the resulting peritonitis may be walled off by omentum or other adjacent visceral structures. Diffuse peritonitis can also develop if the process is not localized, as may more frequently be the case in younger children who lack well-developed omentum. If the process is not controlled, spread of infection into the portal system via the venous effluent (pylephlebitis) may result, giving rise to air in the portal system or liver abscesses.

Clinical Presentation and Evaluation

The above pathophysiology correlates closely with the historical pattern of pain classically described by the patient with acute appendicitis. Initial discomfort is due to luminal distension and is perceived as poorly localized, periumbilical pain, consistent with the midgut origin of the appendix and its corresponding pattern of autonomic innervation. As the disease progresses to the point of transmural inflammation, irritation of the adjacent parietal peritoneum occurs, which is innervated somatically rather than autonomically and is perceived in localized fashion at the point of irritation, most commonly in the right lower quadrant. The initial pain may be associated with anorexia, nausea, and, in some cases, vomiting. Repetitive vomiting and diarrhea may be harbingers of a mimicking illness such as gastroenteritis. Low-grade fever and leukocytosis are common, but not universal, and may be more pronounced as the disease progresses.

On examination, the patient will classically exhibit tenderness in the region of **McBurney's point**, located one-third of the distance from the anterior superior iliac spine to the umbilicus. If the appendix lies inferior to the cecum, pain on rectal and/or pelvic examination may also be present. Signs of peritoneal irritation including rebound tenderness, percussion tenderness, and, in advanced cases, involuntary guarding and hyperesthesia may be present. Pain in the right lower quadrant on palpation of the left lower quadrant (**Rovsing's sign**) is another sign of a focal right lower quadrant process, as is perceived pain in that area with gentle movement such as heel tap or, historically, jostling during transport. Other physical signs that may be present, depending on the position of the appendix, may include pain with right hip extension (**psoas sign**), which suggests an inflamed retrocecal appendix lying against the iliopsoas muscle, and pain with passive rotation of the flexed right hip (**obturator sign**), suggesting inflammation adjacent to the obturator internus muscle in the pelvis.

If the appendix perforates, there may be temporary improvement in visceral pain due to decompression of the turgid organ, but increasing peritonitis soon follows. Peritonitis becomes more likely as the duration of symptoms extends beyond 24 hours and may be associated with high fever and leukocytosis with left shift.

In the pregnant patient, the appendix is often displaced into a more cephalad position and may confuse the diagnostician. The leukocytosis of pregnancy may further confuse the picture. A high level of suspicion is warranted in this setting, since progression to perforation and peritonitis is associated with a fetal death rate of 35% or more.

Radiologic studies may aid in the diagnosis of acute appendicitis, particularly in atypical settings. Plain abdominal films are rarely helpful, although a right lower quadrant fecalith may be seen in a minority of cases and supports diagnostic suspicion. Barium enema has been used historically, with nonvisualization of the appendix being interpreted as presumptive evidence of luminal obstruction and possible appendicitis, but there is a 10% to 15% false-positive and false-negative rate with this study. More recently, ultrasound has been found to be quite sensitive, with the classic finding being the presence of a noncompressible tubular structure with corresponding focal tenderness in the right lower quadrant. Computed tomography (CT) can also provide evidence for the diagnosis and help exclude other confounding pathology. Findings on CT scan may include distension of the appendix, nonfilling of the appendix with enteral contrast, inflammatory changes in the surrounding fat, abscess formation, and free fluid. In the patient with fairly classic symptoms and findings, additional tests such as these are unnecessary and not cost-effective. However, in the setting of less typical findings, such studies can be useful in guiding therapy.

Differential Diagnosis

The differential diagnosis of right lower quadrant pain includes a variety of enteric, urologic, musculoskeletal, and gynecologic conditions. Common entities that may mimic acute appendicitis include pelvic inflammatory disease, pyelonephritis, gastroenteritis, inflammatory bowel disease, endometriosis, ovulatory pain (Mittelschmerz), and ruptured or hemorrhagic ovarian cyst. Meckel's diverticulitis, cecal or sigmoid diverticulitis, acute ileitis, cholecystitis, and perforated peptic ulcer disease may also have features similar to appendicitis in some settings. It is particularly important to consider and exclude entities in the differential diagnosis that are managed nonoperatively, which may include urinary tract infections or stones, hepatitis, pelvic inflammatory disease, right lower lobe pneumonia, and ovulatory or menstrual pain. Conversely, in cases of diagnostic uncertainty, close observation and/or operative intervention may be necessary to prevent progression of appendicitis into its more advanced and complicated stages. Accordingly, it has traditionally been deemed appropriate to find a normal appendix in 10% to 20% of explored patients to minimize the chance of missing a progressing appendicitis until it has reached the point of perforation. With increased use of the CT scan in equivocal cases, the incidence of false-positive appendicitis should be reduced to 5%.

Given the above differential diagnosis, all patients should have a careful history taken and a physical examination performed to exclude confounding illnesses. A careful urinary and gynecologic evaluation especially should be included. Laboratory studies including a complete blood count (CBC) with differential and a urinalysis should be routinely carried out. Abdominal films, chest radiography, and more advanced studies such as CT or ultrasound should be used selectively when they will impact patient management by excluding other pathology or documenting disease that the clinician suspects but cannot confirm.

Treatment

Appendectomy is the primary treatment for acute appendicitis. Appropriate preoperative preparation should include intravenous fluid resuscitation and antibiotic coverage suitable for colonic flora. A second-generation cephalosporin, broad-spectrum penicillin, or combination of a fluoroquinolone and anaerobic coverage with metronidazole are frequently employed antimicrobial strategies. If the appendix has not ruptured, antibiotics may be discontinued within the first 24 hours postoperatively. If frank peritoneal perforation and contamination or abscess are found, antibiotics are typically continued until the patient is afebrile, has a normal white blood cell count, and has regained gastrointestinal function.

Once the decision to operate has been made, it should be accomplished expeditiously, since the possibility of perforation increases after the first 24 to 36 hours of illness. Appendectomy may be appropriately accomplished either via an open or laparoscopic approach (see Chapter 26, Surgical Procedures, Techniques, and Skills). The former is commonly done through a muscle-splitting incision centered on McBurney's point in the right lower quadrant. If appendicitis is found, the appendix is mobilized into the wound and the mesoappendix taken down, allowing isolation of the base of the appendix where it joins the cecum. The appendix is removed after ligature control of its base. The stump may be left or inverted, with the latter approach being used when there is concern over the viability of the tissue at the appendiceal base. If the patient presents with more advanced peritonitis and/or significant diagnostic uncertainty, a lower midline incision may be more appropriate to allow wider access to the pelvic peritoneal cavity. Laparoscopic appendectomy is also a well-attested option. In most series it has been associated with slightly less postoperative pain and lower wound infection rates than standard appendectomy. Conversely, some studies have suggested higher postoperative abscess rates with laparoscopy in perforated appendicitis. Equipment costs, particularly if a stapler is used to control the appendiceal base, make it typically more expensive than standard appendectomy. Laparoscopy may be a particularly attractive option in the setting of diagnostic uncertainty, since it allows inspection of the peritoneal cavity before committing to a given operative exposure. If the appendix is normal with either open or laparoscopic evaluation, possible confounding pathology should be sought for and excluded. Typically this would include inspecting the gynecologic organs, the terminal ileum for Meckel's diverticulum or Crohn's disease, and inspecting or palpating the sigmoid, gallbladder, and right colon for pathology that would explain right-sided abdominal complaints.

Occasionally, the patient presenting with advanced findings may be found to have a palpable mass on examination and corresponding localized abscess on computed tomography or ultrasound. Such patients may be treated nonoperatively with percutaneous radiologic drainage of the abscess and antibiotics. The subject of subsequent interval appendectomy is controversial; historically this has been advised at a 6- to 8-week interval after the acute episode. More recent evaluations of this strategy have documented that most patients do not go on to have recurrent acute appendicitis, and in view of this, so-called interval appendectomy may not be necessary.

Complications

Postoperative wound infection is the most common complication of appendectomy. Pelvic abscess is not uncommon, particularly when there has been frank perforation and peritoneal soilage. Fecal fistula can also be seen and should raise the concern of Crohn's disease at the cecal base. If, in the setting of advanced inflammation, the surgeon is not careful to clearly delineate the appendiceal base, appendiceal remnants may be left and be a source of recurrent problems in rare instances. In settings of significant contamination, wound infection can be minimized by leaving the skin open to heal by secondary intention or delayed primary closure (see Chapter X Wounds and Wound Healing).

Appendiceal Tumors

Appendiceal tumors may include carcinoid, carcinoma, and mucocele. Carcinoid tumors of the appendix account for approximately half of gastrointestinal carcinoids. The vast majority of appendiceal carcinoids are benign, although they can be a source of luminal obstruction and appendicitis. Lesions less than 2 cm in size are usually treated adequately by simple appendectomy. As the size of the carcinoid increases, the possibility of malignancy and lymphatic spread also increases. For lesions larger than 2 cm in diameter, a formal right hemicolectomy to allow wider removal of the lymphatic drainage pathway is accordingly recommended.

Mucoceles are often a consequence of luminal obstruction and may be related to underlying carcinoma of the appendix, which constitutes less than 1% of all appendiceal disease. Symptoms of acute appendicitis often are associated with these lesions at presentation. Patients who have unusual or unexpected findings at the time of surgery may have such underlying neoplasia, and a formal oncologic resection (right hemicolectomy) should be considered if the suspicion warrants. Perforated mucoceles and carcinomas, and some such lesions that have not grossly perforated, may be associated with pseudomyxoma peritonei either at the time of presentation or during subsequent followup. The overall cure rate for appendiceal adenocarcinoma is in the 50% to 60% range at 5-year followup.

SUGGESTED READINGS

Cullen JJ, Kelly KA, Moir CR, et al. Surgical management of Meckel's diverticulum: an epidemiologic, population-based study. *Ann Surg* 1997;220:564–569.

Davila RE, Faigel DO. GI stromal tumors. *Gastrointest Endosc* 2003; 58:80–88.

Leon EL, Metzger A, Tsiotos GG, et al. Laparoscopic management of small bowel obstruction: indications and outcome. *J Gastrointest Surg* 1998;2:132–140.

Long KH, Bannon MP, Zietlow SP, et al. A prospective randomized comparison of laparoscopic appendectomy with open appendectomy: clinical and economic analyses. *Surgery* 2001;129:390–400.

Memon MA, Nelson H. Gastrointestinal carcinoid tumors: current management strategies. *Dis Colon Rectum* 1997;40:1101–1118.

Michelassi F, Block GE. Surgical management of Crohn's disease. *Adv Surg* 1993;26:307–322.

Neugut AI, Marvin MR, Rella VA, et al. An overview of adenocarcinoma of the small intestine. *Oncology (Huntingt)* 1997;11:529–536.

Podolsky DK. Inflammatory bowel disease. *N Engl J Med* 2002;347: 417–429.

Sosa J, Gardner B. Management of patients diagnosed as acute intestinal obstruction secondary to adhesions. *Am Surg* 1993;59:125–128.

Temple LK, Litwin DE, McLeod RS. A meta-analysis of laparoscopic versus open appendectomy in patients suspected of having acute appendicitis. *Can J Surg* 1999;42:377–383.

16

MERRIL T. DAYTON, MD

Colon, Rectum, and Anus

OBJECTIVES

1 Describe the clinical findings of diverticular disease of the colon.
2 Discuss five complications of diverticular disease and their appropriate surgical management.
3 List the differential diagnosis, initial management, diagnostic studies, and indications for medical versus surgical treatment in a patient with left lower quadrant pain.
4 Identify the common symptoms and signs of carcinoma of the colon, rectum, and anus.
5 Discuss the appropriate laboratory, endoscopic, and x-ray studies for the diagnosis of carcinoma of the colon, rectum, and anus.
6 Using the TNM (tumor, node, metastasis) and Dukes' classification systems, discuss the staging and 5-year survival rate of patients with carcinoma of the colon and rectum.
7 Differentiate ulcerative colitis from Crohn's disease of the colon in terms of history, pathology, x-ray findings, treatment, and risk of cancer.
8 Discuss the role of surgery in the treatment of patients with ulcerative colitis and Crohn's colitis.
9 List the signs, symptoms, and diagnostic aids for evaluating presumed large bowel obstruction.
10 Discuss at least four causes of colonic obstruction in adults, including the frequency of each cause.
11 Outline a plan for diagnostic studies, preoperative management, and treatment of volvulus, intussusception, impaction, and obstructing colon cancer.
12 Given a patient with mechanical large or small bowel obstruction, discuss the potential complications if the treatment is inadequate.
13 Discuss the anatomy of hemorrhoids, including the four grades encountered clinically, and differentiate internal from external hemorrhoids.
14 Describe the symptoms and signs of patients with external and internal hemorrhoids.
15 Outline the principles of management of patients with symptomatic external and internal hemorrhoids, including the roles of nonoperative and operative management.
16 Outline the symptoms and physical findings of patients with perianal infections.
17 Outline the principles of management of patients with perianal infections, including the role of antibiotics, incision and drainage, and primary fistulectomy.
18 Describe the symptoms and physical findings of patients with anal fissures.
19 Outline the principles of management of patients with anal fissures.
20 Name the two most common cancers of the anal canal and describe their clinical presentation.
21 Describe the recent changes in the approach to the treatment of anal canal cancers.
22 Describe the presentation and treatment of anal condyloma.
23 Name the diagnostic test of choice for lymphogranuloma venereum. How is this condition treated?
24 Name the causative agent in herpetic proctitis.

The colon and rectum are the terminal portion of the alimentary tract. Although the colon and rectum are biologically nonessential, it is important to understand their physiology, anatomy, and pathophysiology because of the high incidence of disease originating in them. Conditions such as diverticulosis coli, colonic polyps, adenocarcinoma of the colon and rectum, and ulcerative colitis affect a large number of patients in the United States, and the economic, social, and personal costs are enormous. Paradoxically, although the colon is much less vital for nutrition, fluid maintenance, and overall homeostasis than the small intestine, disease is far more common in the colon and rectum.

The anus, anal canal, and sphincters play a critical role in continence, a function that is important for comfortable social interaction. Benign conditions (e.g., hemorrhoids, anal fissures) are common and result in frequent visits to the physician as well as a large expenditure for nonprescription medications.

ANATOMY

The large intestine may be divided into several parts (Fig. 16-1). The cecum is the largest part and is the site where the small bowel enters the colon. There is no distinct division between the cecum and the ascending colon, which is partially fixed posteriorly in the right gutter of the posterior abdominal cavity and is therefore a retroperitoneal structure. The hepatic flexure is the bend in the ascending colon where it becomes the transverse colon, which is suspended freely in the peritoneal cavity by the transverse mesocolon. The transverse colon bends again at the spleen (splenic flexure) and again becomes partially retroperito-

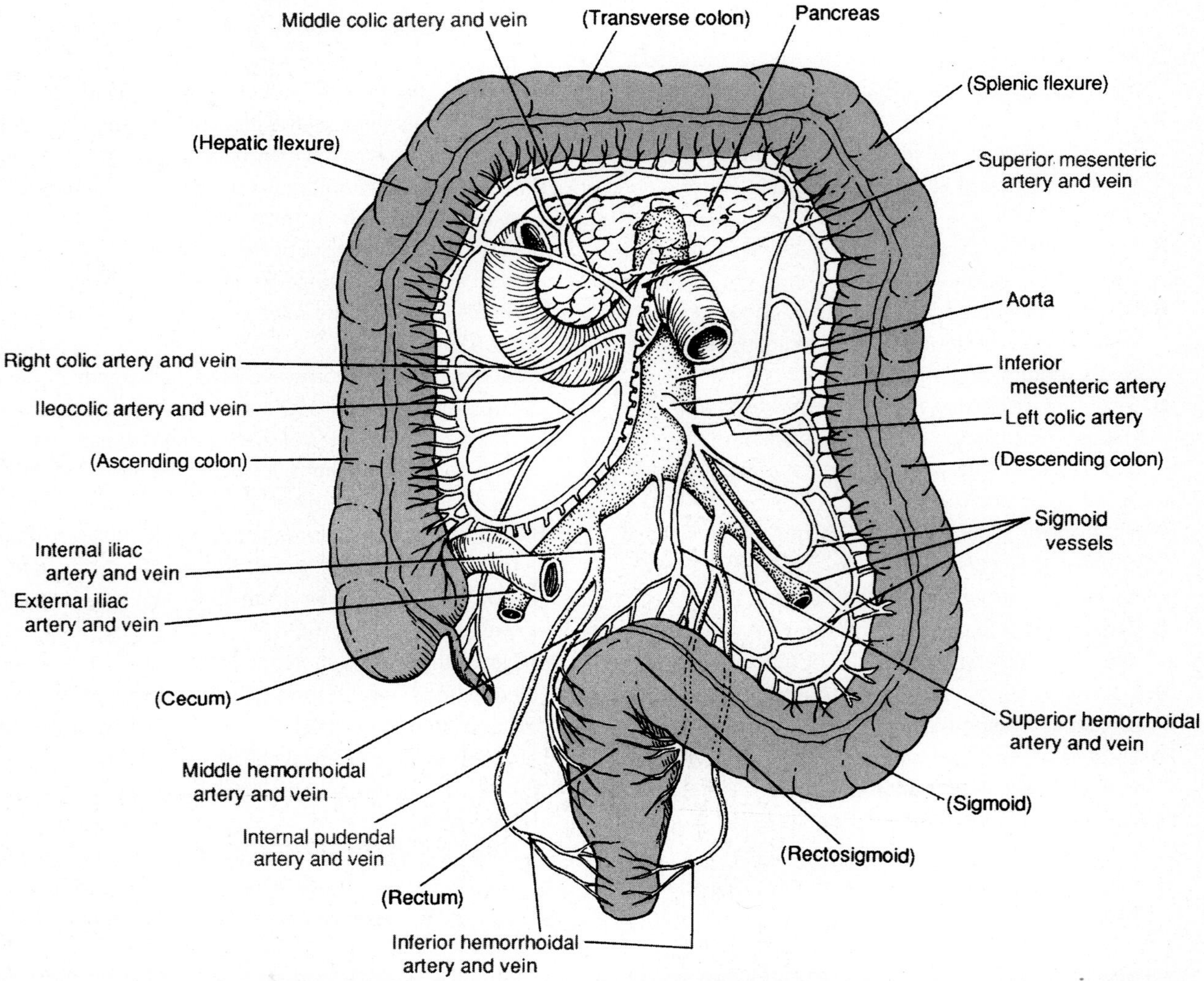

Figure 16-1 Normal anatomy and blood supply of the colon and rectum.

neal. The descending colon remains retroperitoneal up to the sigmoid colon, which is a loop of redundant colon in the left lower quadrant. The distal sigmoid colon, which is intraperitoneal, becomes the rectum at the sacrum and becomes partially retroperitoneal. The rectum continues to the sphincters that form the short (3 cm) anal canal.

The rectum is 15 cm long. Its origin is marked by anatomic change from the colon. The teniae coli disperse at approximately the level of the sacral promontory. As a result, the longitudinal muscle layer becomes a continuous, homogeneous layer. In addition, the proximal rectum is covered by peritoneum anteriorly, but not posteriorly, down to approximately 10 cm above the anal verge, where the rectum becomes an extraperitoneal structure. Rectal biopsy higher than 8 to 9 cm above the anal verge is more hazardous on the anterior wall because of the risk of perforation into the peritoneal cavity.

The anal canal is approximately 3 to 4 cm long and extends from the anorectal junction (dentate, or pectinate, line) to the anal verge (Fig. 16-2). The dentate line marks the junction between the columnar rectal epithelium, which is insensate, and the squamous anal epithelium, which is richly innervated by somatic sensory nerves. For this reason, pathologic conditions that arise below the level of the dentate line cause severe pain. Immediately proximal to the dentate line are longitudinal folds called the columns of Morgagni (rectal columns). Perianal glands normally discharge their secretions at the base of these columns, at the level of the anal crypts. Perirectal abscesses usually originate in this area.

The blood supply to the colon (see Fig. 16-1) is more complex than that to the small bowel. Like the small intestine, the ascending colon and proximal half of the transverse colon are supplied by branches of the superior mesenteric arteries, whereas the distal half of the transverse colon, descending colon, and sigmoid colon are supplied by branches of the inferior mesenteric artery. The importance of understanding this complex arterial blood supply is that in certain areas of the colon (e.g., splenic flexure) that are at the junction of two separate blood vessel systems, the blood supply may be relatively poor. For this reason, anastomoses in this region would carry a higher risk of ischemic compli-

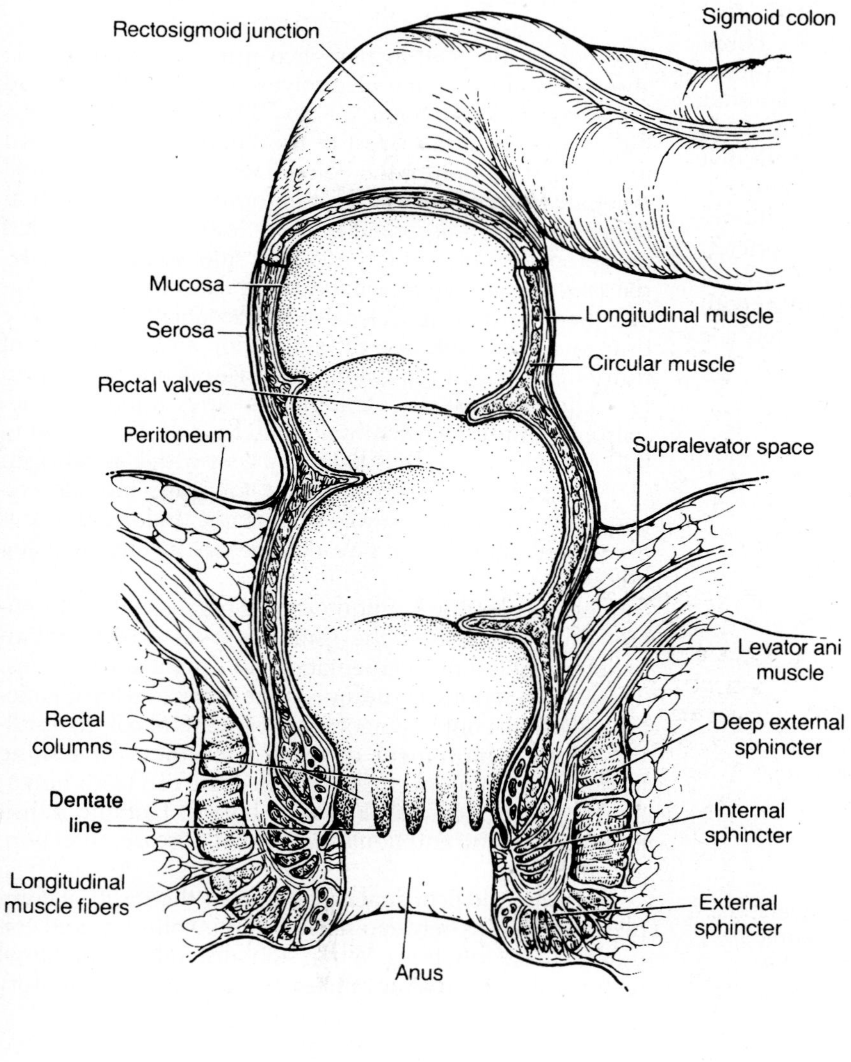

Figure 16-2 Normal anatomy of the anorectal canal.

cations. The venous drainage of the large bowel is less complex because most branches accompany the arteries and eventually drain into the portal system.

The arterial supply to the rectum is derived from a branch of the inferior mesenteric artery (superior hemorrhoidal artery) for the upper rectum, and from branches of the internal iliac arteries (middle hemorrhoidal arteries) and the internal pudendal arteries (inferior hemorrhoidal arteries) for the middle and lower rectum. Veins from the upper rectum drain into the portal system through the inferior mesenteric vein. The middle and inferior rectal veins drain into the systemic circulation through the internal iliac and pudendal veins. Hemorrhoids are physiologic venous cushions that connect the two systems. They may become distended or thrombose, leading to symptoms of hemorrhoid disease.

Lymphatic drainage of the large intestine parallels the arterial blood supply, with several levels of lymph nodes as one moves toward the aorta. In general, tumor metastases move from one level to another in an orderly progression, with the paracolic lymph nodes involved first, followed by the middle tier of lymph nodes, and last by the periaortic lymph nodes.

The bowel wall of the colon has the same layers as the small intestine: mucosa, submucosa, muscularis, and serosa (Fig. 16-3). The major difference is that the colon has no villi (i.e., the mucosal crypts of Lieberkühn form a more uniform surface with less absorptive area). Another major difference is that the outer longitudinal smooth muscle layer is separated into three bands (teniae coli) that cause outpouchings of bowel between the teniae (haustra).

The anal sphincter mechanism resembles a tube enclosed in a funnel. The tube is the internal sphincter, which is a continuation of the circular muscular layer of the rectum. This involuntary sphincter is made of smooth muscle. The funnel is the external sphincter, which is a striated voluntary muscle. The external sphincter has three parts: the subcutaneous, superficial, and deep portions. The deep portion is in continuity with the levator ani muscles, which form the base of the pelvic floor. The anatomy of the sphincters must be kept in mind in the diagnosis and treatment of perirectal pathology.

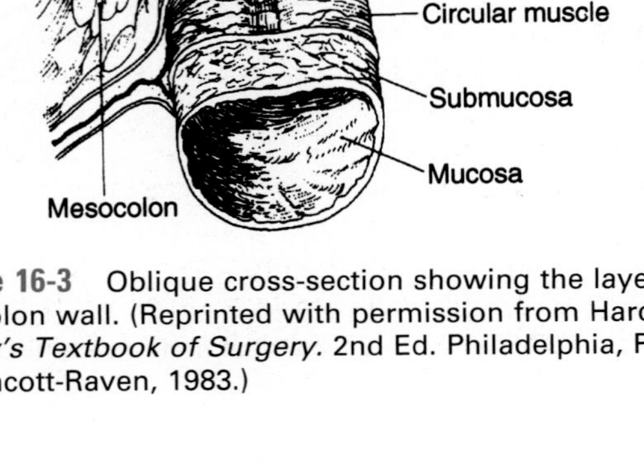

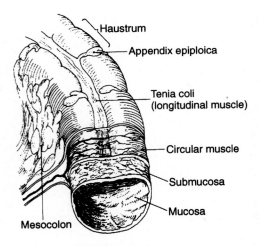

Figure 16-3 Oblique cross-section showing the layers of the colon wall. (Reprinted with permission from Hardy JD. *Hardy's Textbook of Surgery*. 2nd Ed. Philadelphia, PA: Lippincott-Raven, 1983.)

Innervation of the colon is primarily from the autonomic nervous system. Sympathetic nerves pass from the spinal cord through the sympathetic chains and sympathetic ganglia to postganglia that end in Meissner's and Auerbach's plexuses in the bowel wall. Sympathetic stimulation causes inhibition of colonic muscular activity. Parasympathetic innervation comes through the vagus nerve for the first half of the colon. The second half (distal transverse and beyond) is innervated by branches from the second through the fourth sacral cord segments. Parasympathetic activity results in stimulation of colon muscle activity. However, the most important control of colon activity appears to be mediated by regional reflex activity that occurs in the submucosal plexuses (patients with spinal cord transection continue to have relatively normal bowel function).

PHYSIOLOGY

The colon and rectum have two primary functions: (1) absorption of water and electrolytes from liquid stool and (2) storage of feces. Some 600 to 700 mL of chyme enters the cecum each day. Most of the stool water is absorbed in the right portion of the colon, leaving 200 mL of stool evacuated as solids daily. This amount is a small fraction of the total water absorbed in the intestinal tract. The left portion of the colon and the rectum store solid fecal material, and the anorectal apparatus regulates the evacuation of solids, permitting defecation at a socially acceptable time and place. Because little digestion and absorption of nutrients occur in the colon, the organ is not essential to life. The composition of colonic gas varies among individuals and is influenced substantially by diet. Some 800 to 900 mL/day is passed as flatus, 70% of which is nitrogen (N_2) derived from swallowing air. Other gases include oxygen, carbon dioxide, hydrogen, methane, indole, and skatole. Indole and skatole give colonic gas its characteristic odor.

Colonic motility is unique among organs of the alimentary canal because of the multiple types of contraction patterns, including segmentation and mass contractions. These contractions are unique to the colon and are characterized by the contraction of long segments of colon, resulting in mass movement of stool. Movement of residue through the colon occurs at a slower rate (18 to 48 hours) than through the small bowel (4 hours). Colonic transit is accelerated by emotional states, diet, disease, infection, and bleeding.

The physiology of anal continence is the result of complex interactions between sensory and involuntary and voluntary motor functions. When stool distends the proximal rectum, the internal sphincter relaxes, allowing sensory sampling of the rectal contents. This very sensitive mechanism allows, among other things, the passage of gas without incontinence to stool. Defecation involves a complex interplay among the pelvic floor muscles, rectum, and distal colon.

The normal frequency of defecation is approximately every 24 hours, but it may vary from 8 to 72 hours. Any patient who has a significant change in bowel habits should be evaluated for the possibility of serious disease. Severe constipation (ability to pass flatus, but not stool) and obstipation (inability to pass stool or flatus) are examples of changes that should be evaluated.

The colon harbors a greater number and variety of bacteria than any other organ in the body. Most of these organisms are anaerobes; *Bacteroides fragilis* is the most common. The most common aerobes are *Escherichia coli* and enterococci. Although the bacteria perform a number of important functions for the host (e.g., degradation of bile pigments, production of vitamin K), their high number and variety increase the risk of infection during colon surgery. Some studies show postoperative infection rates as high as 25% to 30% after surgery on colon that was not "prepared" (cleaned out) before operating.

COLON AND RECTUM

Diagnostic Evaluation

Patients who have signs or symptoms that are referable to the colon or rectum may be evaluated by several modalities. The digital examination is an important means of detecting many disease processes, including tumors or polyps, abscesses, ulcers, hemorrhoids, and colorectal bleeding. The tendency to defer the digital rectal examination because of patient discomfort or physician inconvenience is a serious error.

Although rigid sigmoidoscopy was the standard method of visualizing the distal colon and rectum for many years, it has largely been replaced by fiberoptic flexible sigmoidoscopy. This method provides a higher diagnostic yield and is much less uncomfortable for the patient. This examination allows visualization of the last 30 to 65 cm of the colorectal complex and results in detection of 60% of colorectal neoplasms. In addition to detecting polyps and neoplasms, it can aid in detecting sites of hemorrhage, ascertaining the etiology of obstruction, evacuating excessive colonic gas, and removing foreign bodies from the rectum. Because of the frequency of colorectal disease, this examination should be an integral part of the routine examination of patients who are older than 50 years of age. In the absence of other symptoms, flexible sigmoidoscopy should be performed every 3 to 5 years.

An abdominal series (flat plate and upright radiograph) should be obtained on any patient who has significant abdominal pain. This series is helpful in detecting pneumoperitoneum, large bowel obstruction (e.g., volvulus, tumor), paralytic ileus, appendicolith, and less common diseases. Both of these radiographs should be obtained, not simply an abdominal flat plate.

Barium enema remains an important diagnostic modality in detecting disease in this region. After the colon and rectum are prepared, contrast medium is introduced under mild pressure to fill the entire organ. Air insufflation, with some intraluminal barium remaining, allows particularly sensitive detection of polyps and small lesions (Fig. 16-4). Barium enema is particularly helpful in diagnosing tumors, diverticulosis, volvulus, and sites of obstruction.

The most accurate diagnostic tool is fiberoptic **colonoscopy**. This instrument allows visualization of the entire colon and rectum and the last few centimeters of terminal ileum. It also provides diagnostic and therapeutic options that were not previously available without surgery (e.g., polyp removal, colonic decompression, stricture dilation, hemorrhage control, foreign body removal). After the patient undergoes thorough bowel preparation and mild sedation, the device is inserted into the anus and advanced with a steering mechanism located on the handle (Fig. 16-5). Although this instrument was initially used primarily to evaluate ambiguous findings on barium enema studies, more physicians are using it for diagnostic purposes and postoperative followup. Colonoscopy is now a primary diagnostic modality to evaluate lower gastrointestinal bleeding of unknown etiology, inflammatory bowel disease, stricture, equivocal barium enema findings, posttumor removal, pseudo-obstruction, and polyps (Fig. 16-6).

Angiography is useful in detecting the source of moderate or rapid colonic bleeding. It is not helpful in patients with slow, chronic blood loss. A promising new diagnostic modality called virtual colonoscopy, which uses a recently developed technique that combines computed tomography (CT) scan capability and computer virtual reality software, may make future surveillance easier, less painful, and quicker. The technique is being thoroughly evaluated in clinical studies but is still less accurate than colonoscopy and cannot be recommended over colonoscopy at this time.

Terminology

Understanding the treatment of colonic diseases requires familiarity with terms that are unique to this organ. **Colostomy** is the surgical procedure in which the colon is divided and the proximal end is brought through a surgically created defect in the abdominal wall (Fig. 16-7). Its purpose is nearly always to divert stool from a diseased segment distally in the colon or rectum or to protect a distal anastomosis. The distal segment is either oversewn and placed in the peritoneal cavity as a blind limb (**Hartmann's procedure**) or brought out inferiorly to the colostomy through the abdominal wall (mucous fistula). A loop colostomy is created by bringing a loop of colon through a defect in the abdominal wall, placing a rod underneath, and making a small hole in the loop to allow stool to exit into a colostomy bag. Ileostomy is a similar procedure in which ileum is brought through the abdominal wall to divert its contents from distal disease or, in proctocolectomy, to serve as a permanent stoma.

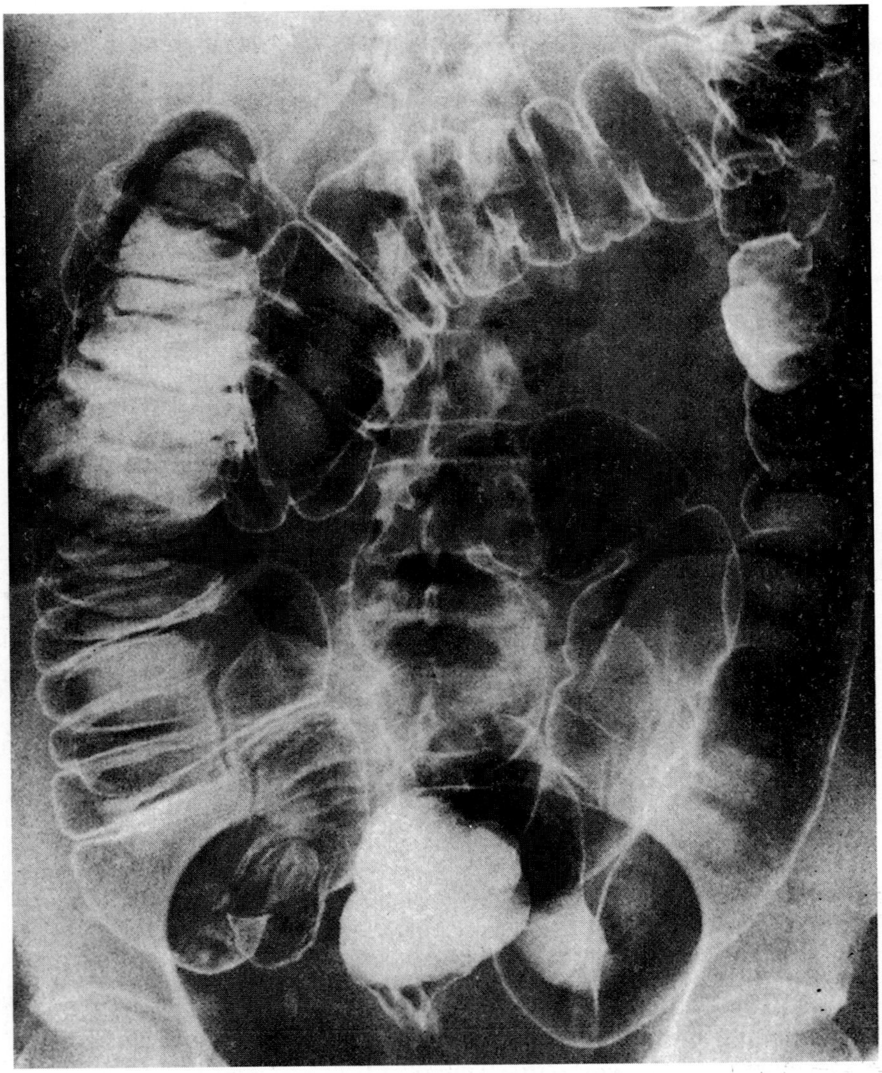

Figure 16-4 Normal air-contrast barium enema.

Other terms that often confuse medical students include **proctocolectomy, abdominoperineal resection,** and **low anterior resection**. Proctum is a synonym for rectum. Proctocolectomy is operative removal of the entire colon and rectum (e.g., for ulcerative colitis or polyposis syndromes). Abdominoperineal resection, which is used in the surgical treatment of low rectal cancers, is the operative removal of the lower sigmoid colon and the entire rectum and anus, leaving a permanent proximal sigmoid colostomy (e.g., for low rectal cancer). Low anterior resection, which is used to surgically treat cancers in the middle and upper sections of the rectum, is removal of the distal sigmoid colon and approximately one-half of the rectum, with primary anastomosis of the proximal sigmoid to the distal rectum.

Diverticular Disease

Diverticular disease develops at different rates in different countries with widely varying dietary habits, suggesting the probable influence of diet on the development of this condition. The incidence of diverticular disease is progressive from the fifth to the eighth decade of life, and 70% of elderly patients may have asymptomatic diverticula. Clearly, there is some influence of the aging process on the incidence, but whether it is related to general relaxation of the colonic tissue or to lifelong dietary habits is not clear. Dietary influences have been implicated based on comparative geographic epidemiology; these studies implicate the lower-fiber diet found in Western Europe and the United States. Some postulate that lower stool bulk results in higher generated luminal pressures for propulsion. The resultant increased work causes hypertrophy that leads to diverticulosis.

Two types of diverticula are found in the colon. **Congenital,** solitary, **"true" diverticula** (full-wall thickness in the diverticular sac) are uncommon, but when present, are found in the cecum and ascending colon. **Acquired (false) diverticula** are very common in Western countries, and 95% of patients with the condition have involvement

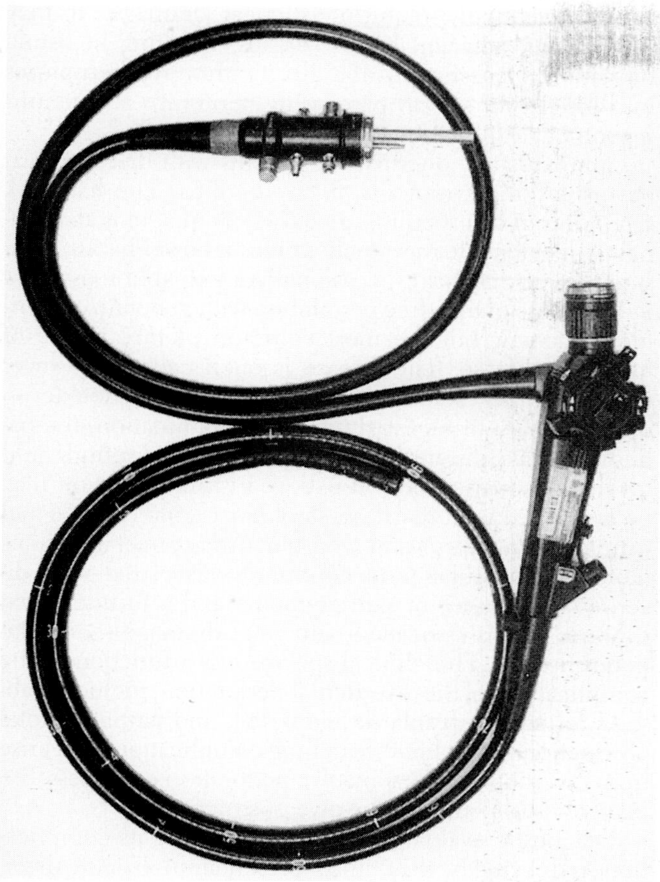

Figure 16-5 Fiberoptic colonoscope used for diagnostic and therapeutic maneuvers in the colon.

of the sigmoid colon. These diverticula are mucosal herniations through the muscular wall. The muscles of the colon have an inner circular smooth muscle layer and a thinner outer layer, which includes three longitudinal bands, the teniae. The most favorable area for herniation occurs where branches of the marginal artery penetrate the wall of the colon (Fig. 16-8). The etiology of herniation is probably related to the colon's exaggerated adaptation for fecal propulsion. One theory suggests that diverticular disease results from higher than normal segmental contractions of the sigmoid colon that lead to high intraluminal pressure. These high intraluminal pressures are confined to the segments that have diverticula. Specifically, the sigmoid colon has localized pressure increases because of segmentation between contraction rings. Contraction of the wall generates high-pressure zones within the segment. As a result, herniation occurs at the weakest point, near the vascular penetration of the bowel wall.

Diverticulosis

General use of the term diverticulosis is reserved for the presence of multiple false diverticula in the colon. This condition is most often an asymptomatic (80%) radio-

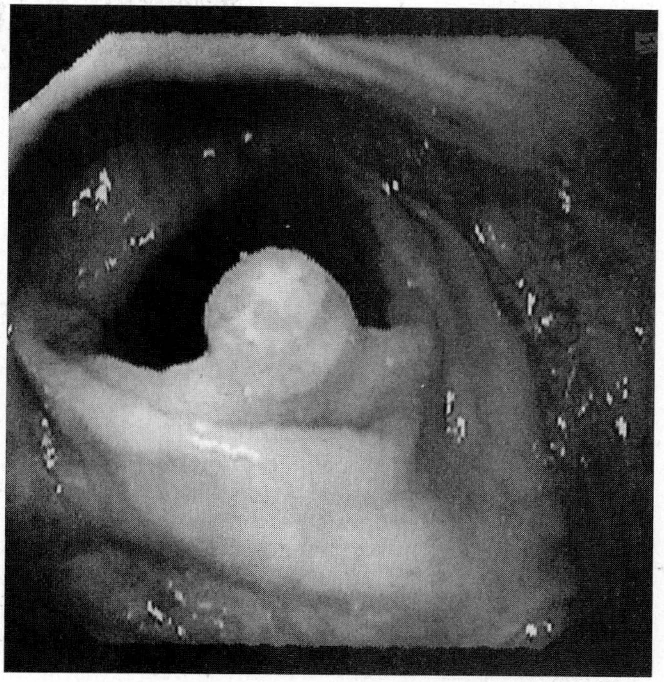

Figure 16-6 A polyp detected during colonoscopy.

graphic finding when a barium enema is performed for some other diagnostic purpose (Fig. 16-9). Nevertheless, certain symptoms are attributed to diverticula in the absence of either inflammation or bleeding.

Clinical Presentation and Evaluation

Symptoms include recurrent abdominal pain, often localized to the left lower quadrant, and functional changes in bowel habits, including bleeding, constipation, diarrhea,

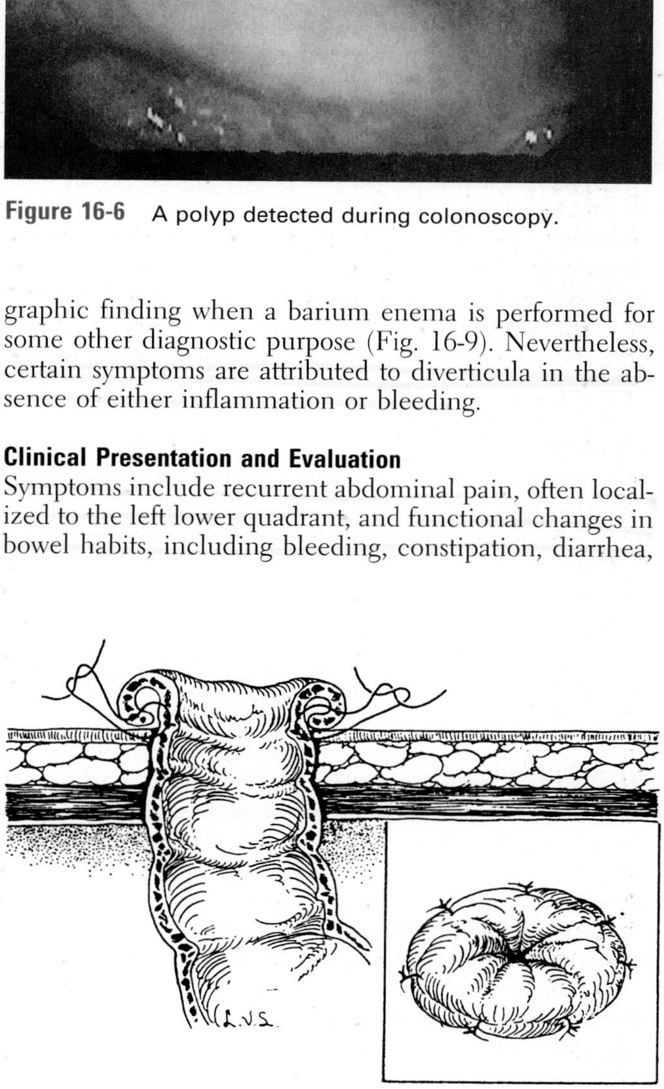

Figure 16-7 Lateral and anterior appearance of an end colostomy. (Reprinted with permission from Way L. *Current Surgical Diagnosis.* 7th Ed. Stamford, CT: Appleton & Lange, 1985.)

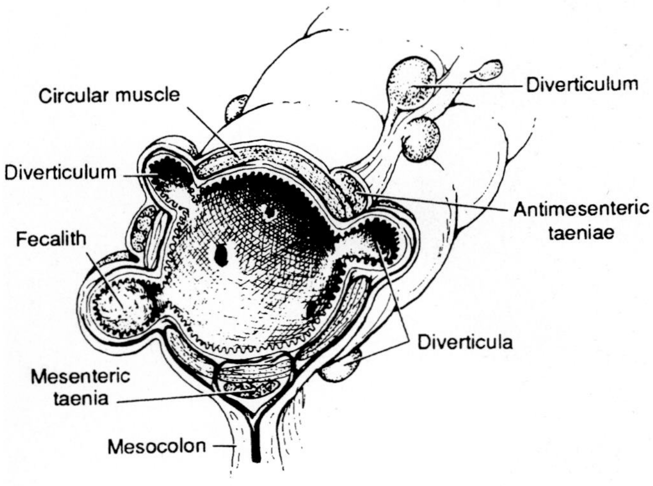

Figure 16-8 Mucosal herniation characteristic of diverticulosis. Most herniations occur at a site where the blood vessel penetrates the bowel wall.

or alternating constipation and diarrhea. The physical examination is most often unremarkable, or it shows mild tenderness in the left lower quadrant. By definition, fever and leukocytosis are absent. Additional roentgenographic findings may include segmental spasm and luminal narrowing. Endoscopic evaluation of the lumen generally does not show anything except the openings of the diverticula.

Treatment

Management of asymptomatic patients with diverticular disease is controversial. Although certain public health organizations recommend a diet with increased fiber content, no specific definition of fiber dietary content has been given for the normal adult. Patients are encouraged to consume fresh fruits and vegetables, whole-grain breads and cereals, and bran products. Pharmacologic preparations of fiber (e.g., psyllium seed products) are more expensive but are more likely to be taken by patients.

Diverticulitis

Diverticulitis describes a limited infection of one or more diverticula, including extension into adjacent tissue. The condition is initiated by obstruction of the neck of the diverticulum by a fecalith. The obstruction leads to microperforation that results in swelling in the colon wall or macroperforation that involves the pericolic tissues.

Clinical Presentation and Evaluation

The clinical presentation depends on the progression of infection after the perforation. If the perforation is small, it may spontaneously regress. If it is large, it may be confined to pericolic tissues and abate after treatment with antibiotics. The process may enlarge to form an extensive abscess in the mesenteric fat that remains contained, eventually requiring surgical drainage. It may burrow into adjacent hollow organs, resulting in fistula formation. Occasionally, the diverticulum freely ruptures into the peritoneal cavity, causing peritonitis and requiring urgent exploration.

Approximately one-sixth of patients with diverticulosis have signs and symptoms of diverticulitis. The hallmark symptoms of diverticulitis are left lower quadrant abdominal pain (subacute onset), alteration in bowel habits (constipation or diarrhea), occasionally a palpable mass, and fever. Occasionally, free perforation with generalized peritonitis occurs, but the most common picture is one of localized disease. The disease is often called left lower quadrant appendicitis. When cicatricial obstruction develops secondary to repeated bouts of inflammation, the patient will have distension, high-pitched bowel sounds, and severe constipation or obstipation. Fistula formation may be associated with diarrhea, stool per vagina (colovaginal fistula), pneumaturia and recurrent urinary tract infections (colovesical fistula; most commonly associated with diverticular disease), or skin erythema and a furuncle that ruptures and is associated with stool drainage (colocutaneous fistula). The clinical spectrum is a function of the complications of the diverticular perforation, including abscess formation, fistula development, and partial or total obstruction. Of all life-threatening complications that arise from diverticulitis, 44% involve perforation or abscess, 8% involve fistula, and 4% involve obstruction.

Diagnostic evaluation of diverticulitis or its complications is directed by the clinical presentation. If acute diverticulitis is suspected, abdominal radiographs are obtained; a barium enema is contraindicated in the acute phase. Barium enema may be obtained 2 to 3 weeks after the episode to confirm the clinical impression. If the patient has obstructive symptoms or evidence of a fistula (e.g., pneumaturia), a contrast enema is indicated. If free perforation has occurred, upright abdominal radiographs show pneumoperitoneum.

Colovesical fistula is the most common type of fistula encountered in diverticulitis, with a complication occurring in approximately 4% of cases. The differential diagnosis includes carcinoma of the colon, cancer of other organs (e.g., bladder), Crohn's disease, radiation injury, and trauma as a result of foreign bodies. Some patients are symptom-free or mildly symptomatic. However, others have refractory urinary tract infections, fecaluria, and pneumaturia. The most common physical finding is a palpable mass, and leukocytosis secondary to urinary tract infection is frequently found. The diagnostic triad includes barium enema, cystography, and intravenous pyelogram. However, in a patient with no demonstrable lesion, a dye marker (e.g., methylene blue) can be instilled into the bladder or rectum.

Treatment

Treatment of the complications of diverticular disease is directed at the specific complication (Table 16-1). Treatment of acute diverticulitis is initially medical in 85% of

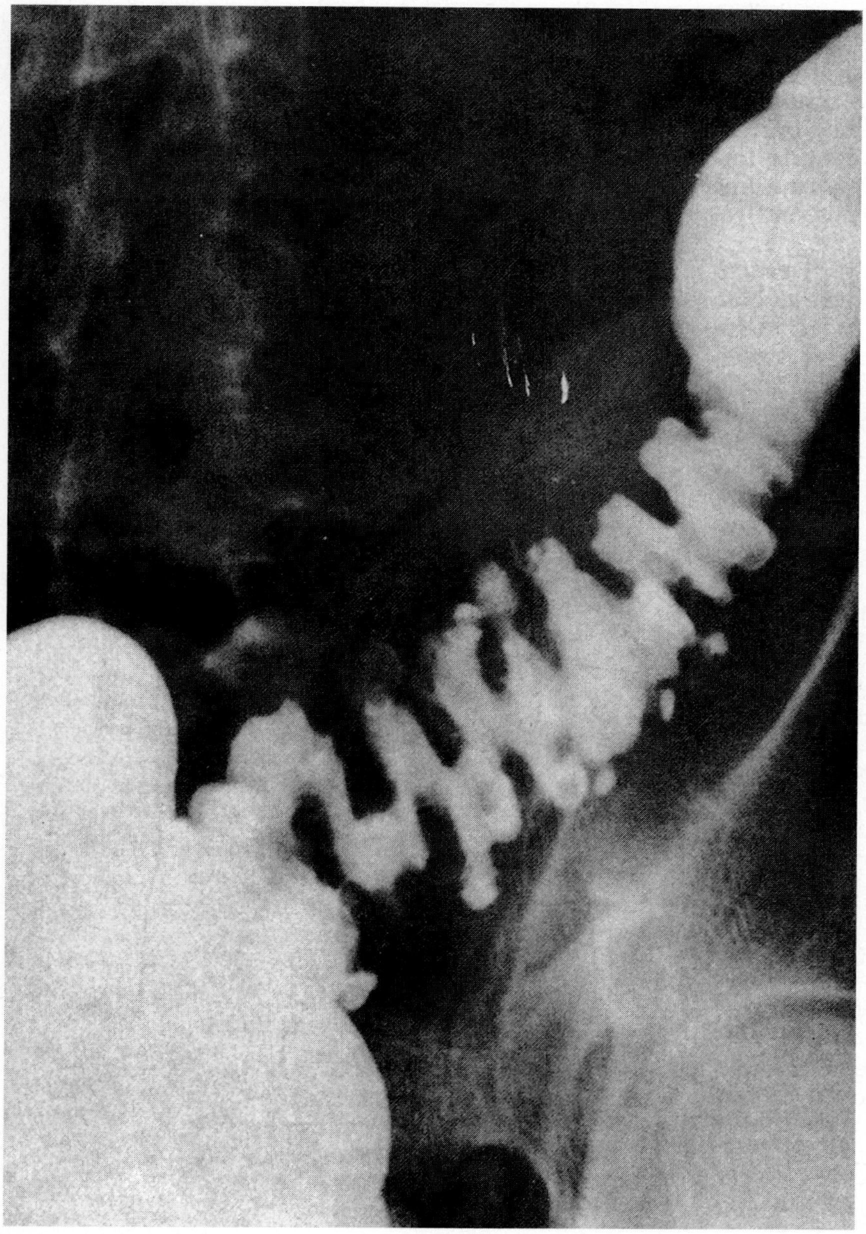

Figure 16-9 Sigmoid diverticulosis shown on barium enema.

cases. It consists of admitting the patient to the hospital, instituting intravenous hydration, giving the patient nothing by mouth, and administering intravenous antibiotics (usually broad coverage of Gram-negative coliforms as well as coverage for anaerobes, particularly *B. fragilis*) for 5 to 7 days. Most patients respond to nonoperative treatment and do not require further therapy. However, a subsegment of this group has repeated bouts of acute diverticulitis, requiring hospitalization. The natural history of diverticulitis in those who have repeated bouts is gradual progression to one of the serious complications. For this reason, most surgeons believe that any patient who has had two severe bouts of diverticulitis requiring hospitalization

Table 16-1	Indications for Surgery of Diverticular Disease
Perforation Obstruction Intractability Bleeding Fistula	

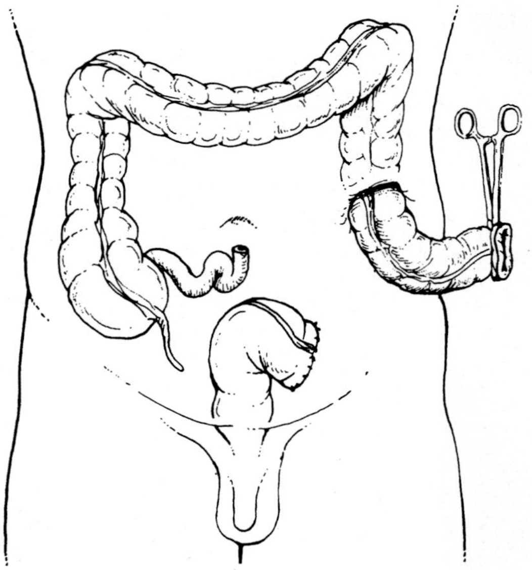

Figure 16-10 Operative therapy for diverticular disease usually involves resection of the sigmoid portion of the colon. If the operation is done for acute perforation or obstruction, the segment may be resected, a diverting colostomy brought to the abdominal wall, and the distal rectal stump oversewn (Hartmann procedure). A second stage of the operation involves colostomy takedown and anastomosis to the rectal stump.

should be scheduled for elective sigmoid colectomy (the site of the problem in 95% of cases). In the case of perforation, obstruction, or abscess, immediate surgical resection of the diseased sigmoid colon is indicated, with a temporary diverting colostomy and a Hartmann procedure (Fig. 16-10). No attempt at a primary reanastomosis should be made in this setting of unprepared bowel because of the high risk of infection and bowel leak. If the disease is refractory or a fistula is present, the patient may undergo bowel preparation and formal sigmoid colectomy with primary anastomosis.

The treatment for colovesical fistula is surgery. Primary closure of the bladder and resection of the sigmoid colon with primary anastomosis is the usual treatment. However, in the presence of severe infection, the colon anastomosis may be delayed and a temporary colostomy performed. Generally, the operation is successful, and recurrence is rare.

Diverticular Bleeding

Diverticulosis is occasionally associated with gastrointestinal hemorrhage. Bleeding is the primary symptom in 5% to 10% of all patients with diverticular disease. Bleeding from diverticula is occasionally massive (diverticulosis is the most common cause of massive lower gastrointestinal bleeding) and may be lethal. Massive bleeding is defined as bleeding that is sufficient to warrant transfusion of more than four units of blood in 24 hours to maintain normal hemodynamics. Of all patients with bleeding distal to the ligament of Treitz, approximately 70% have diverticulosis as the source of the bleeding. Approximately 25% of the time, the bleeding is massive.

Clinical Presentation and Evaluation

The patient generally has profuse bright or dark red rectal bleeding and hypotension. Unfortunately, the age, sex, and symptoms of patients with bleeding diverticular disease are the same as those with cancer and other lesions. Patients with cancer are unlikely to bleed as severely as patients with diverticulosis, but carcinomas bleed more frequently.

After the history, physical examination, and resuscitation with volume expanders and blood transfusions, the diagnostic approach to the patient with lower gastrointestinal hemorrhage includes insertion of a nasogastric tube with aspiration (to rule out an upper gastrointestinal source) and rectal examination to rule out severe hemorrhoidal bleeding (e.g., portal hypertension) or ulcer. The diagnostic procedure of choice to rule out lower gastrointestinal (GI) sources of bleeding is colonoscopy. Before a colonoscopy can be performed, a mechanical bowel prep using lavage must be completed to clear the colon of stool and old blood. If massive bleeding continues, angiography is the next diagnostic procedure of choice. If the bleeding is intermittent or angiography is indeterminate, colonoscopy after rapid colonic lavage is the preferred modality. In addition to diverticulosis, the differential diagnosis includes angiodysplasia, solitary ulcers, varices, cancer, and, rarely, inflammatory bowel disease.

Treatment

If the bleeding does not cease spontaneously, surgical resection of the involved segment is indicated.

Polyps and Carcinoma of the Colon and Rectum

Colorectal Polyps

Polyp is a morphologic term that is used to describe small mucosal excrescences that grow into the lumen of the colon and rectum. A variety of polyp types have been described, all with different biologic behaviors (Table 16-2). Approximately 5% of all barium enema studies show polyps. Approximately 50% occur in the rectosigmoid region, and 50% are multiple.

Distinguishing among polyp types is important because some types are clearly associated with carcinoma of the colon. Inflammatory polyps (pseudopolyps) are common in inflammatory bowel disease and have no malignant potential. Hamartomas (juvenile polyps and polyps associated with Peutz-Jeghers syndrome) similarly have very low malignant potential and often spontaneously regress or autoamputate. They may be safely observed. However, polyps that fall into the general category of “adenoma” are clearly

Table 16-2 Comparison of Colonic Polyps

Type	Frequency	Location	Malignant Potential	Treatment
Tubular	Common: 10% of adults	Rectosigmoid in 20%	7% malignant	Endoscopic excision
Villous	Fairly common, especially in the elderly	Rectosigmoid in 80%	33% malignant	Surgical removal
Hamartoma	Uncommon	Small bowel	Low; uncommon	Excise for bleeding or obstruction
Inflammatory	Uncommon, except in IBD	Colon and rectum	None	Observation
Hyperplastic	Fairly common	Stomach, colon, and rectum	None	Observation

IBD, inflammatory bowel disease.

premalignant, and appropriate vigilance is indicated. Three subdivisions of adenomas are described: (1) tubular (Fig. 16-11), (2) tubulovillous, and (3) **villous adenoma.** Most polyps are either **sessile** (flat and intimately attached to the mucosa) or **pedunculated** (rounded and attached to the mucosa by a long, thin neck; Fig. 16-12). Tubular and tubulovillous adenomas are more commonly pedunculated, whereas villous adenomas are more commonly sessile. Evidence for malignant potential includes (1) the high incidence of cancer associated with the polyps in familial polyposis syndrome or Gardner's syndrome, (2) simultaneous occurrence of cancers and polyps in the same specimen, (3) carcinogens that experimentally produce both adenomas and cancers in the same model, and (4) lower cancer risks associated with those who have polyps removed. Approximately 7% of tubular, 20% of tubulovillous, and 33% of villous adenomas become malignant. Villous adenomas greater than 3 cm in diameter have a greater probability of malignancy.

Clinical Presentation and Evaluation

Polyps are usually asymptomatic, but occasionally bleed enough to cause the patient to seek medical evaluation. They are most commonly detected during routine endoscopic surveillance. Occasionally, a family history of polyps causes the patient to seek endoscopic screening.

Treatment

Treatment of adenomatous polyps involves colonoscopic polypectomy of pedunculated polyps where possible. If some cannot be safely removed colonoscopically, biopsy should be performed and a segmental resection of the colon done if the lesion is a villous adenoma or is large, ulcerated, or indurated. For disease conditions that are characterized by extensive polyposis (familial polyposis syndrome or Gardner's syndrome), the treatment most commonly performed is total abdominal colectomy, mucosal proctectomy, and **ileoanal pullthrough**.

Carcinoma of the Colon and Rectum

Cancer of the colon and rectum is a major cause of death in the United States. The American Cancer Society estimates that over 55,000 people die of this disease annually. Approximately 140,000 to 145,000 new cases are identified each year. Although a large number of factors are associated with the development of this disease, theories about its etiology center on the impact of intraluminal chemical carcinogenesis. There are various theories as to whether these carcinogens are ingested or are the result of biochemical processes that occur intraluminally from existing substances that are found normally in the fecal stream. Geographic epidemiologic studies show that certain populations have a very low incidence of cancer of the colon and rectum, apparently as a result of identifiable dietary factors (e.g., high fiber, low fat), although social customs and a lack of environmental carcinogens cannot be excluded. Certain health agencies promote a low-fat, high-fiber diet as protective against cancer of the colon and rectum. Chemoprevention by ingestion of such agents as carotenoids and other antioxidants has been suggested, but the efficacy of this measure is unproven. There is good evidence that prostaglandin inhibitors such as aspirin and sulindac significantly lower the risk of polyp formation and colon cancer when taken on a regular basis.

Most large bowel cancers occur in the lower left side of the colon, near the rectum (Fig. 16-13), although recent studies suggest a slow shifting to right-side lesions. Synchronous (simultaneously occurring) tumors develop in 5% of patients, whereas 3% to 5% of patients have metachronous tumors (a second tumor developing after resection of the first).

Familial polyposis syndrome, Gardner's syndrome, and the cancer family syndrome (hereditary nonpolyposis colon cancer or HNPCC) clearly show that certain patient subsets are genetically predisposed to cancer of the colon. Other predisposing diseases include ulcerative colitis, Crohn's colitis, lymphogranuloma venereum, and certain polyps (described previously).

The peak incidence of colon cancers occurs at approximately 70 years of age, but the incidence begins to increase in the fourth decade of life. Rectal cancer is more common in men, and colon cancer appears to be more common in women.

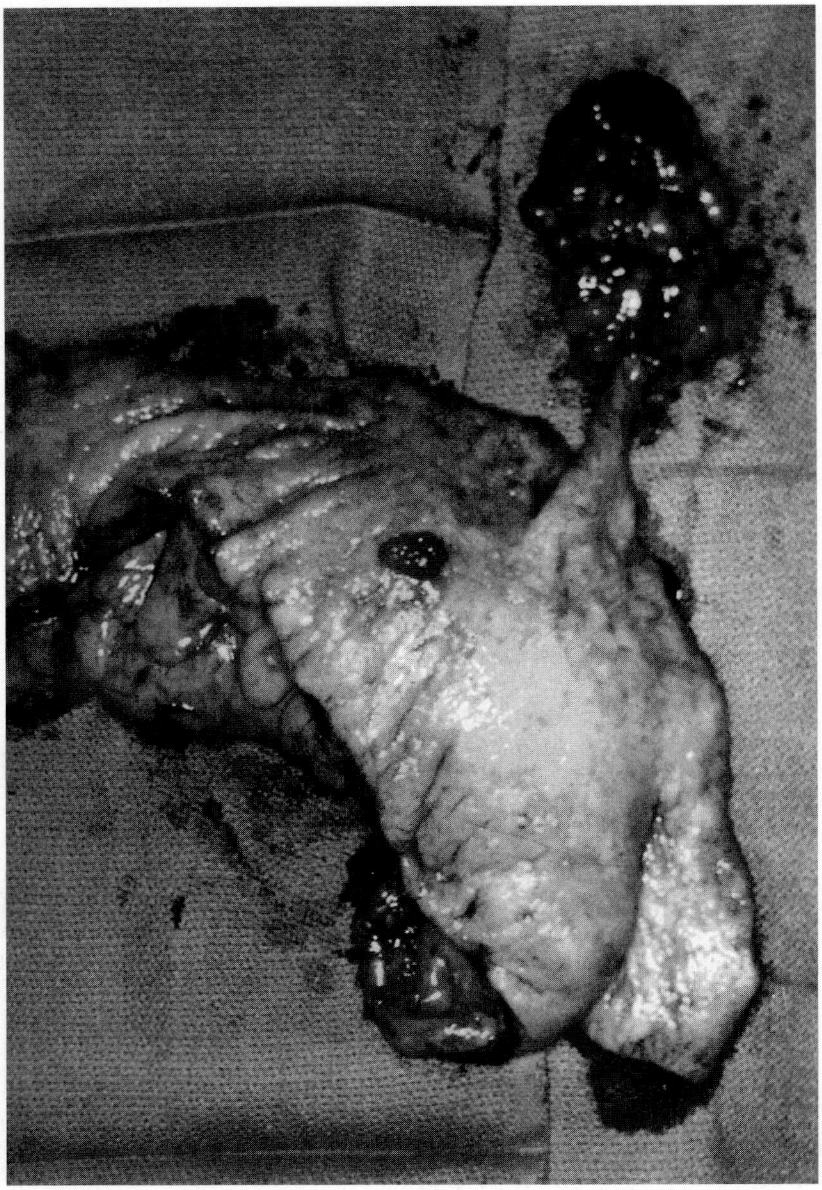

Figure 16-11 Large tubular adenoma in a resected segment of the sigmoid colon.

Screening

Of all gastrointestinal cancers, more progress has been made in improving cure rates in colorectal cancer than any other; currently, the 5-year survival rate is 60%. There is little question that this improvement is the direct result of two factors: (1) an effective screening instrument, colonoscopy, and (2) effective strategies for screening based on risk factors. Mild risk factors include age, diet, physical inactivity, obesity, smoking, race, and alcohol. Intermediate risk groups include those with a personal history of colorectal cancer or adenoma, as well as those with a strong family history. Followup studies have revealed that individuals with one first-degree relative with colorectal cancer have a twofold increased risk of colorectal cancer, and those with two first-degree relatives have a sixfold increased risk. Patients at high risk for developing colorectal cancer are those with familial colorectal cancer syndromes (familial polyposis, Gardner's, and HNPCC) and patients who have had ulcerative or Crohn's colitis for more than 10 years.

For patients with normal or mild risk, the American Cancer Society recommends that, beginning at age 50, both men and women should follow one of these five screening options:

1. Yearly fecal occult blood test plus flexible sigmoidoscopy every 5 years
2. Flexible sigmoidoscopy every 5 years
3. Yearly fecal occult blood test
4. Colonoscopy every 10 years
5. Double contrast barium enema every 5 years

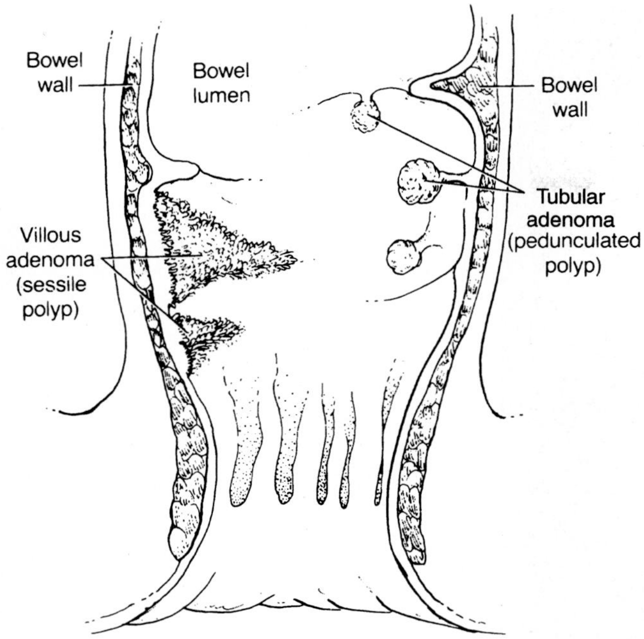

Figure 16-12 Characteristic appearance of a villous adenoma (sessile polyp) compared with a tubular adenoma (pedunculated polyp). Sessile polyps tend to be more difficult to manage because they are difficult to remove endoscopically and because their malignant potential is greater.

If the patient is intermediate risk, the screening should begin at age 40 and be done more frequently than every 10 years (e.g., every 3 to 5 years). In the high-risk group, screening is a function of duration of disease. In inherited polyposis groups, blood tests are now available to rule out the disease in familial polyposis and HNPCC. For patients unable to access the blood tests, screening should begin in the teen years, since full expression of the disease can occur by age 20. Patients who have had ulcerative or Crohn's colitis for 10 years or more should begin annual colonoscopic surveillance with biopsies. Serious consideration should be given to prophylactic total colectomy with ileoanal pullthrough in both high-risk groups before an invasive cancer develops.

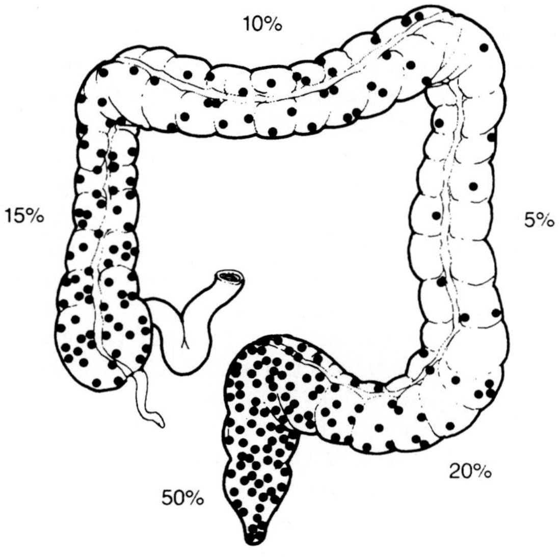

Figure 16-13 Frequency distribution of adenocarcinoma of the colon and rectum.

Clinical Presentation and Evaluation

The clinical signs and symptoms of colorectal cancer are determined largely by the anatomic location. Cancers of the right colon are usually exophytic lesions associated with occult blood loss, resulting in iron deficiency anemia (Table 16-3). At advanced stages of the disease, patients may have a palpable right lower abdominal mass. Recent retrospective studies indicated that the incidence of right colon cancers is increasing at a greater rate than that of left colon cancers. Right-sided lesions may account for as many as one-third of all new cases seen, with most diagnosed at a late stage. Cancers that arise primarily in the left and sigmoid colon are more frequently annular and invasive, resulting in obstruction and macroscopic rectal bleeding (see Table 16-3). Cancers of the rectum also cause a symptom complex of rectal bleeding, obstruction, and, occasionally, alternating diarrhea and constipation. Tenesmus occurs with far advanced disease.

Any patient with a change in bowel habits, iron deficiency anemia, or rectal bleeding should undergo the following studies: (1) a digital rectal examination with testing to rule out occult blood and (2) a barium enema study (Fig. 16-14) or complete colonoscopy. If rectal bleeding occurs, workup for a possible malignancy should be initiated, even if the apparent source is a benign lesion (e.g., hemorrhoid).

Bright red rectal bleeding should always be evaluated by an examination of the perianal region, digital rectal examination, and flexible sigmoidoscopy. The value of preoperative total colonoscopy lies in its ability to detect the 3% to 5% of patients with synchronous colon cancers,

Table 16-3 Symptoms of Colon and Rectal Cancers

	Site of Cancer		
Symptom	**Right Colon**	**Left Colon**	**Rectum**
Weight loss	+	+/0	0
Mass	+	0	0
Rectal bleeding	0	+	+
Tympany	0	0	+
Virchow's node	+	0	0
Blumer's shelf	+	+	0
Anemia	+	0	0
Obstruction	0	+	+

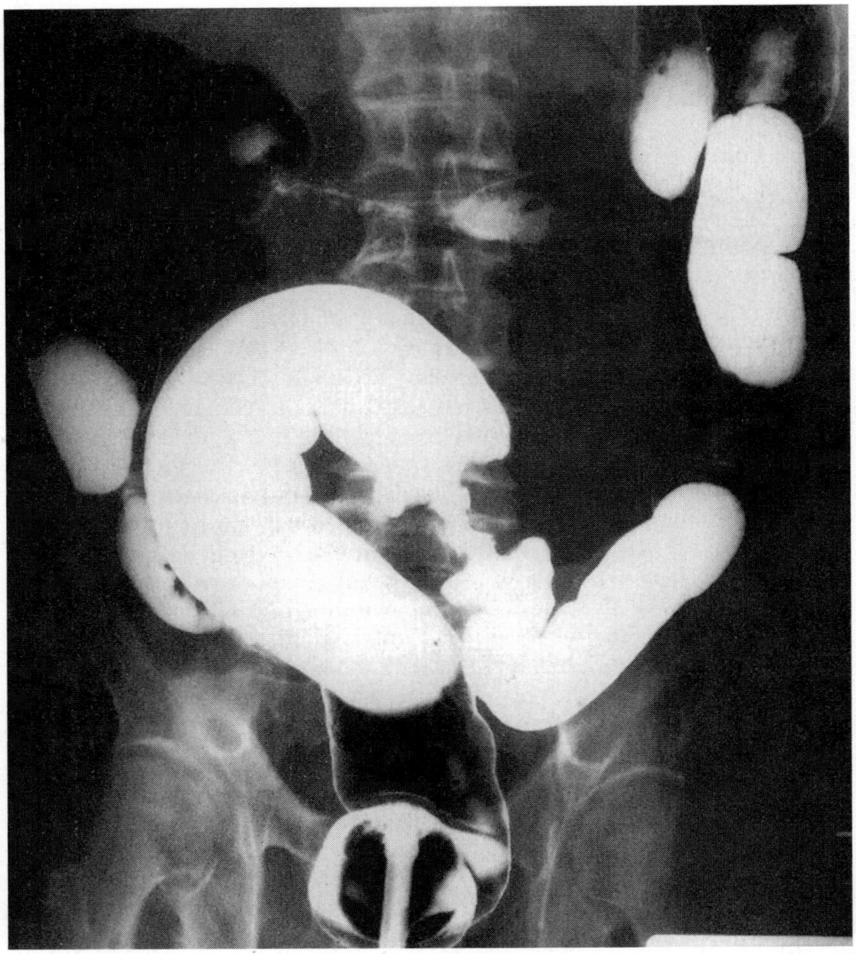

Figure 16-14 Carcinoma of the sigmoid colon causing high-grade obstruction and showing a classic "apple core" lesion.

allowing better planning of surgical therapy. Computed tomography of the abdomen is not routinely indicated before surgery. Preoperative blood tests should evaluate the patient's overall nutritional status and should include liver function tests and a **carcinoembryonic antigen** study. Results of the antigen study are elevated in many gastrointestinal malignancies and, although it is not specific for colorectal cancer, it may be useful in following patients after resection to detect recurrence.

Diagnostic studies often show an obstructing lesion in the sigmoid colon that occurs in the presence of diverticula but is suspicious for malignancy. Because both conditions may coexist and it is occasionally impossible to distinguish between the two, the surgeon should proceed with a "cancer operation," which includes a wide lymph node resection, whenever there is any question. Diverticular stricture, polyps, benign tumors, ischemic structure, and Crohn's colitis are included in the differential diagnosis.

Treatment

The surgical treatment used by most surgeons includes adequate local excision of the tumor, with a length of normal bowel on either side, and resection of the potentially involved lymph node draining basin found in the mesentery that is determined by the vascular supply. Removal of the lymphatics that drain the tumor region should be part of the operation because nodal involvement is present in more than 50% of specimens. A certain subset of patients with carcinoma of the colon and rectum and lymph node metastasis at a site that is fairly distant from the primary lesion, but is included in the resected specimen, may be rendered disease-free by the surgical resection. Colorectal cancer may also spread hematogenously, intraluminally, or by direct extension or peritoneal seeding (Blumer's shelf on rectal examination). The most common organ involved in distant colorectal metastases is the liver.

Patients whose tumors are no longer confined to the bowel and are adherent to extraperitoneal structures in the pelvis, upper abdomen, or other area should have en bloc resections (which include resection of the tumor and any other invaded structure) whenever possible, with the area being subsequently marked with metal clips to identify it as a site of potential recurrence. When the small bowel is involved, it should be included en bloc in the resection. Studies indicate that small bowel involvement does not change the stage-for-stage prognosis. Similarly, a partial cystectomy or total hysterectomy should be performed with the resection if the tumor is adherent to these organs. Bilateral oophorectomy is recommended by some in menopausal or postmenopausal women to remove occult ovarian metastasis and improve staging.

Tumors of the cecum and ascending colon are treated with right hemicolectomy that includes resection of the distal portion of the ileum and the colon to the midtransverse colon with an ileomidtransverse colon anastomosis (Fig. 16-15). Hepatic flexure lesions are best treated by an extended right colectomy that includes resection to or beyond the level of midtransverse colon. Lesions in the transverse colon require a transverse colectomy with complete mobilization and anastomosis of ascending to descending colon. Splenic flexure and left-sided lesions are treated with a left hemicolectomy that includes resection from the level of the midtransverse colon to the sigmoid. Sigmoid colon lesions are treated with sigmoid resection. However, obstructing sigmoid lesions may require left hemicolectomy and sigmoid colectomy. Obstructive or perforating tumors that prevent bowel preparation and primary anastomosis should be treated with resection, diverting colostomy, and Hartmann's pouch or mucous fistula.

Tumors in the upper and middle one-third of the rectum are treated with low anterior resection with primary anastomosis. Tumors in the lower one-third of the rectum require specialized procedures (e.g., abdominoperineal resection with permanent end-sigmoid colostomy; Fig. 16-16). When the expertise and equipment are available, selected high-risk patients with rectal lesions that are smaller than 2 cm, exophytic, mobile, and well differentiated may be treated with transanal full-thickness resection of the lesion or local laser ablation.

Recent developments in minimally invasive surgery involving the use of the laparoscope suggest that laparoscopic

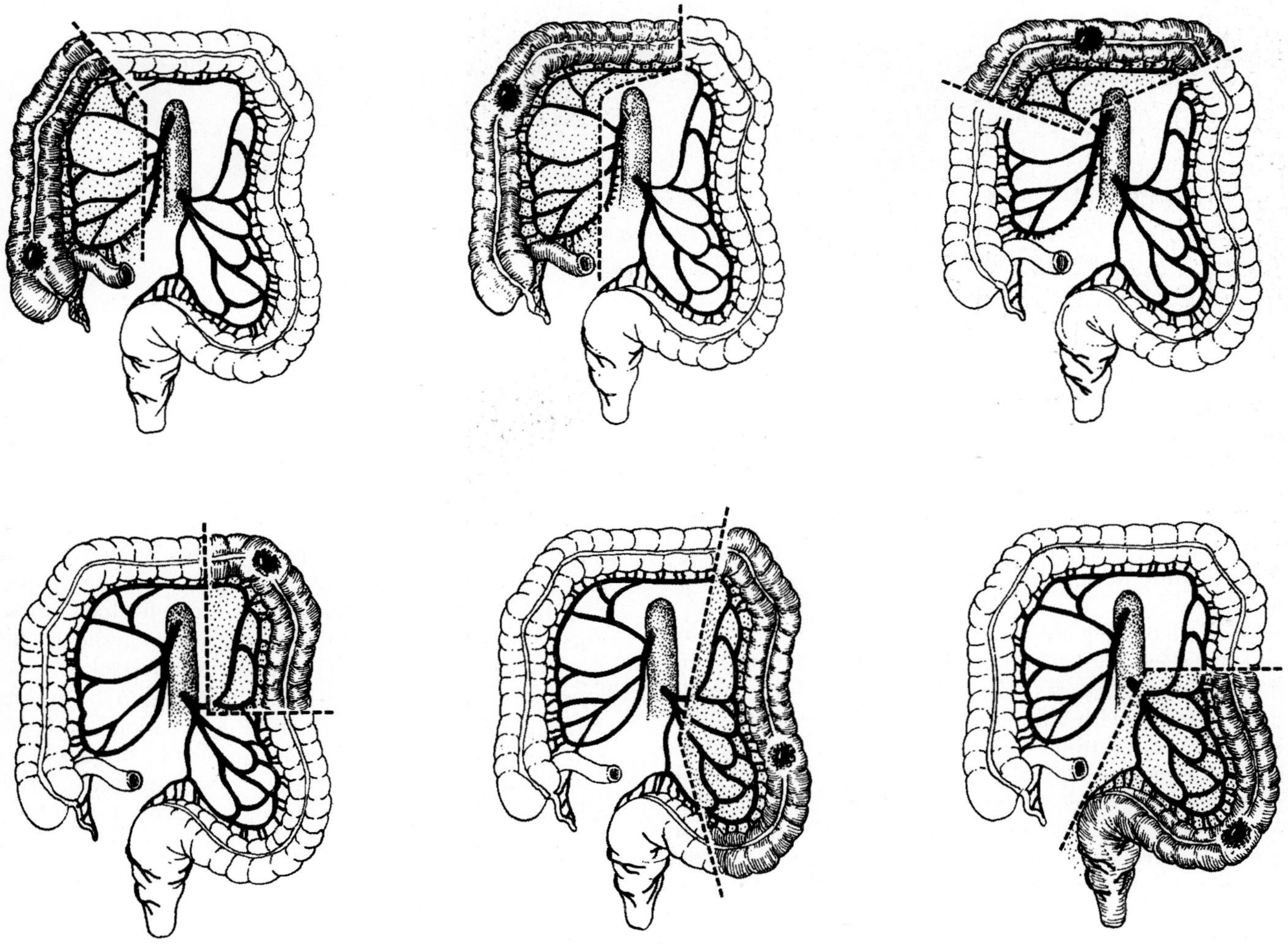

Figure 16-15 Indicated operative resection for colon cancer in different sites. The boundaries of the resection are dictated by lymphatic drainage patterns that parallel the blood supply.

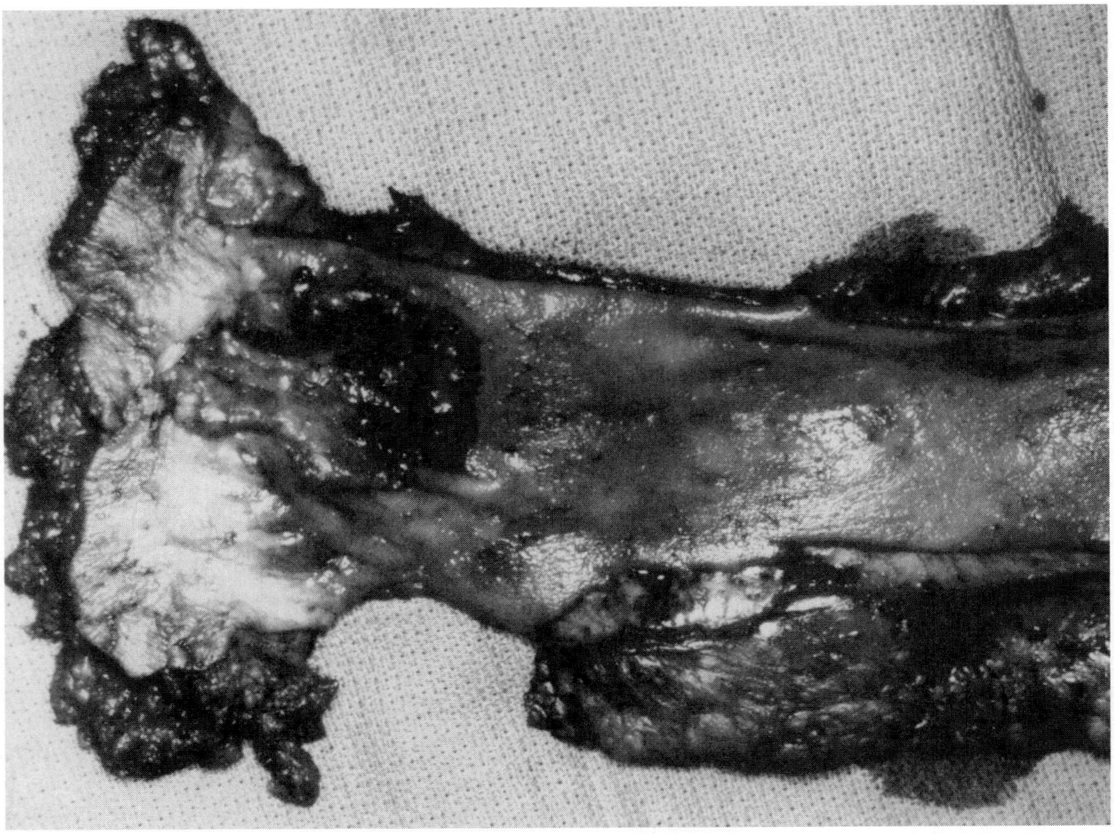

Figure 16-16 Adenocarcinoma of the low rectum invading the anal canal and requiring abdominoperineal resection.

resection of colon cancers can be done safely and effectively. A number of preliminary studies show that the operation can be done technically with resection of an acceptable number of lymph nodes in the lymphadenectomy specimen. The procedure is usually done with a small abdominal incision to facilitate removal of the bowel containing the tumor and to assist in the anastomosis. Further experience is needed to determine whether laparoscopy can continue to be safely used for resection of colorectal tumors.

The use of adjuvant therapies in the treatment of colon and rectal carcinoma generated considerable research in the last several decades. The main outcome from the randomized trials with 5-fluorouracil (5-FU) as a single agent in an adjuvant setting was that no improvement occurred in the disease-free interval, nor was there an increase in cure rate compared with surgery alone. However, subsequent studies showed conclusively that 5-FU used in combination with levamisole or leucovorin lowers the mortality rate in patients with **Dukes'** stage C tumors. The recent development of a new chemotherapeutic agent, oxaliplatin, has excited GI oncologists because it appears to be twice as effective as 5-FU in reducing cancer recurrence in high-risk patients as well as treating patients with metastatic colorectal cancer.

Because of their significant rate of recurrence (20%) despite the most radical surgical procedure, rectal tumors that have completely penetrated the rectal wall, with or without lymph node metastases, are treated additionally by radiation combined with 5-FU. The question of whether to use preoperative or postoperative radiation seems to be strictly a matter of choice. However, postoperative radiation seems more widely applicable because it permits a selection based on the final pathologic staging and prevents treating patients who are not at risk for local recurrence. It also eliminates those who are not candidates because of distant disease. The usual tumoricidal doses of approximately 50 to 60 cGy can be tolerated in the postoperative period if the surgeon and the radiation oncologist plan the adjuvant radiation therapy before surgery, even if it is to be given postoperatively. Well-conducted trials indicate that postoperative radiation therapy prevents recurrence, increasing disease-free intervals and survival rates.

Prognosis

Dukes first proposed a system of staging large bowel cancer more than 50 years ago. Subsequent modifications have been made, particularly those by Astler and Coller

Table 16-4 Dukes-Astler-Coller System

Stage	Description	5-Year Survival Rate (%)
A	Confined to the mucosa	85–90
B1	Negative nodes; extension into, but not through, the muscularis propria	70–75
B2	Negative nodes; extension through the muscularis propria	60–65
C1	Same level of penetration as B1, but with positive nodes	30–35
C2	Same level of penetration as B2, but with positive nodes	25
D	Distant metastases	< 5

(Table 16-4). The American Joint Committee on Cancer developed the TNM (tumor, node, metastasis) system (Table 16-5). Other attempts have been made to look at clusters of prognostic factors (e.g., tumor markers, size of the lesion) and elements that are not included in Dukes' original classification, which was based on the depth of invasion. The most important prognostic variable is lymph node involvement.

For patients who have had curative resection and for whom no adjuvant therapy is appropriate, the question of followup surveillance is of maximal importance. Certain large centers recommend monthly physical examination, bimonthly measurement of carcinoembryonic levels, and either endoscopy or barium enema study every 6 months for the first 2 years of followup because most recurrences occur in the first 18 to 24 months. The use of carcinoembryonic antigen is well established, with recurrence suggested not by the absolute level of this antigen, but rather by a progressive rise. A progressive rise mandates a complete evaluation of the patient, including computed tomography or magnetic resonance imaging, and possible second-look surgical procedure. A potentially important new diagnostic modality used to detect widespread metastases in colorectal cancer is the positron emission tomography (PET) scan. This technique relies on administering radioactive positrons, which collide with electrons in diseased tissue that then emit gamma rays sensed by a color monitor. Although the number of patients who benefit from this thorough survey is not large, a sufficient number benefit to make it worthwhile. The prognosis of colon and rectal carcinoma depends on the classification detailed in Table 16-4. For patients who have recurrences, the effective management of liver metastases, pelvic and anastomotic recurrences, and solitary pulmonary metastases has been demonstrated.

Ulcerative Colitis and Crohn's Disease of the Colon

Ulcerative colitis is an idiopathic inflammatory bowel disorder that involves the mucosa and submucosa of the large bowel and rectum. It has a bimodal distribution with regard to age. The first, and largest, peak (two-thirds of all cases) includes ages 15 to 30, whereas the second, smaller peak (one-third of all cases) occurs at approximately age 55. The disease is slightly more common in Western countries, and its annual incidence is 10 per 100,000 popula-

Table 16-5 TNM Staging System

Primary Tumor (T)	
TX	Primary tumor cannot be assessed
TO	No evidence of primary tumor
Tis	Carcinoma in situ; intraepithelial tumor or invasion of the lamina propria
T1	Tumor invading the submucosa
T2	Tumor invading the muscularis propria
T3	Tumor invading through the muscularis propria into the subserosa, or into nonperitonealized pericolic or perirectal tissues
T4	Tumor directly invading other organs or structures or perforating the visceral peritoneum
Regional Lymph Nodes (N)	
NX	Regional lymph nodes cannot be assessed
NO	No regional lymph node metastasis
N1	Metastasis in 1–3 pericolic or perirectal lymph nodes
N2	Metastasis in ≥4 pericolic or perirectal lymph nodes
N3	Metastasis in any lymph node along the course of a named vascular trunk or metastasis to ≥1 apical node (when marked by the surgeon)
Distant Metastasis (M)	
MX	Presence of distant metastasis cannot be assessed
MO	No distant metastasis
M1	Distant metastasis

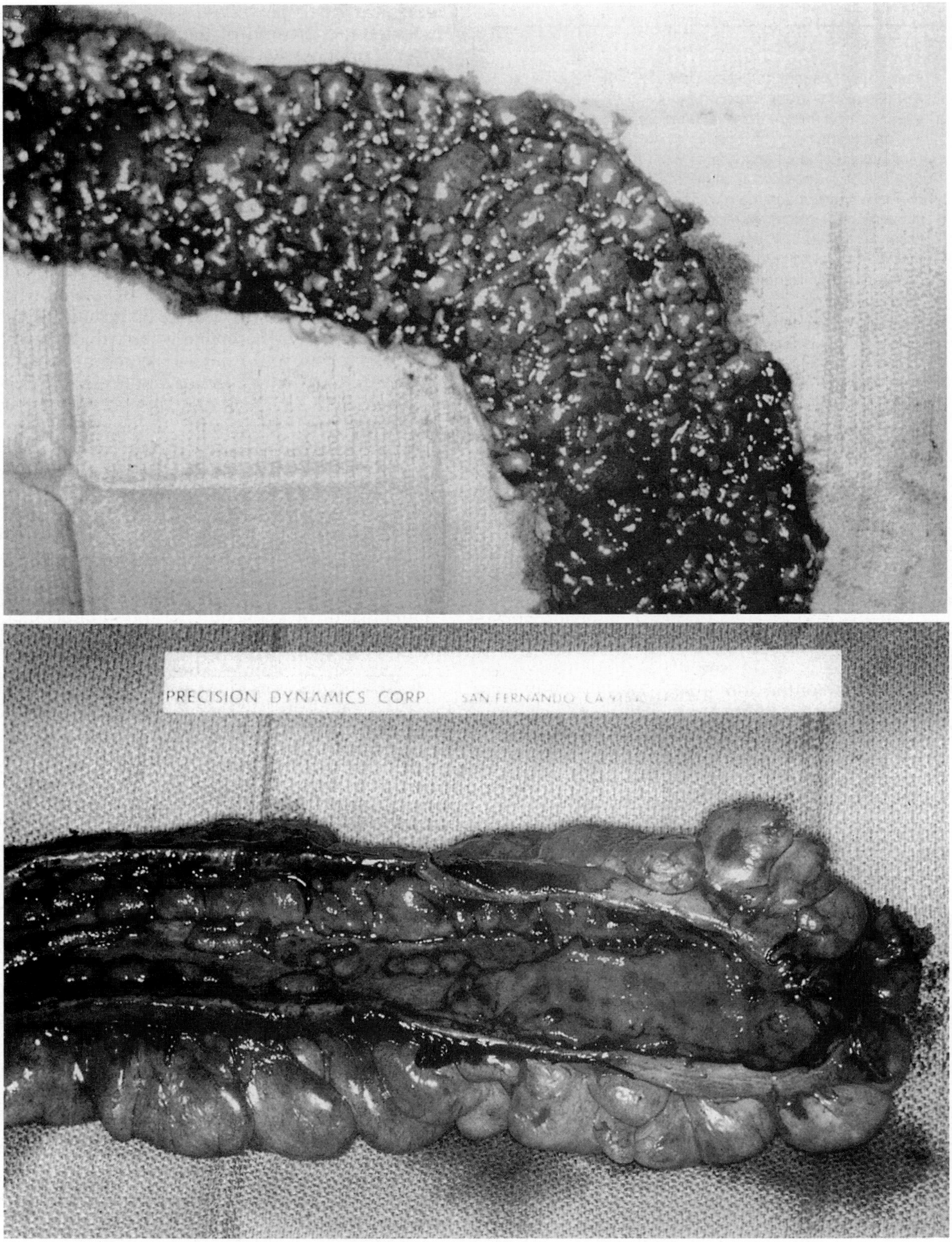

Figure 16-17 **A,** Severe ulcerative colitis showing pseudopolyps, deep ulceration, and friability. **B,** Severe Crohn's colitis showing linear ulcers and "cobblestoning."

tion. A family history of ulcerative colitis is positive in 20% of patients, suggesting a genetic predisposition.

Crohn's disease is a transmural disease that can involve any portion of the alimentary canal. In a minority of patients, disease is limited to the colorectal region. Like ulcerative colitis, it occurs in a bimodal distribution. Although it more commonly occurs in the region of the terminal ileum, when it occurs exclusively in the colorectum, it is often confused with ulcerative colitis. Gross differences that may be used to distinguish it from ulcerative colitis include rectal sparing, skip lesions (in which diseased segments alternate with normal segments), aphthous sores, and linear ulcers. Crohn's disease is discussed in greater detail elsewhere. This section focuses on ulcerative colitis.

The exact etiology of ulcerative colitis is unknown. Infectious, immunologic, genetic, and environmental factors are implicated, but none is proven. The female:male occurrence ratio among patients with ulcerative colitis is 5:4. There is an increased incidence of the disease among Jews, but it is uncommon among blacks and Native Americans.

Pathologic findings include invariable involvement of the rectum (> 90%) with variable proximal extension. Occasionally, the rectum alone is involved (ulcerative proctitis). In contrast to Crohn's disease, skip areas of normal bowel between diseased segments are not seen. The mucosa is initially involved, with lymphocyte and leukocyte infiltration that then involves the submucosa with microabscess formation. The crypts of Lieberkühn are commonly affected (crypt abscesses), but muscle layers are rarely involved. The coalescing of these abscesses and erosion of the mucosa lead to pseudopolyp formation, which is identified readily on endoscopic examination. Approximately one-third of the patients affected with ulcerative colitis have pancolitis, in which the entire colon is severely involved.

In addition to the material contained here, the student should refer to Chapter 15 for a discussion of ulcerative colitis and Crohn's disease.

Clinical Presentation and Evaluation

The clinical presentation of ulcerative colitis is variable. The disease may have a sudden onset, with a fulminant, life-threatening course, or it may be mild and insidious. Patients often have watery diarrhea that contains blood, pus, and mucus, accompanied by cramping, abdominal pain, tenesmus, and urgency. To varying degrees, patients have weight loss, dehydration, pain, and fever. Fever is usually indicative of multiple microabscesses or endotoxemia secondary to transmural bacteremia. Approximately 55% of patients have a mild, indolent course; 30% have a moderately severe course that requires large doses of prednisone or sulfasalazine (Azulfidine); and 15% have a fulminant, life-threatening course. The fulminant presentation is often associated with massive colonic dilation secondary to transmural progression of the disease and destruction of the myenteric plexus (toxic megacolon). Patients have severe constitutional symptoms related to sepsis, malnutrition, anemia, acid–base disturbances, and electrolyte abnormalities.

Extraintestinal manifestations occur in a small percentage of patients, including ankylosing spondylitis, peripheral arthritis, uveitis, pyoderma gangrenosum, sclerosing cholangitis, pericholangitis, and pericarditis. The amount of information obtained on physical examination depends on the acuteness and severity of the disease process at the time of examination. If the patient is seen in a quiescent phase, there may be few or no findings; if the patient is seen in an acute phase, there may be a finding of an acute abdomen.

The mainstay of diagnosis is endoscopy with biopsy. Typical endoscopic findings include friable, reddish mucosa with no normal intervening areas, mucosal exudates, and pseudopolyposis (Fig. 16-17*A* and *B*). A secondary diagnostic study is barium enema, in which mucosal irregularity may be seen. Frequently, shortening of the colon, loss of normal haustral markings, and a "lead-pipe" appearance may be seen (Fig. 16-18). No specific laboratory tests are diagnostic for ulcerative colitis; however, leukocytosis and anemia may be present.

The differential diagnosis includes other inflammatory or infectious disorders, including Crohn's disease, bacte-

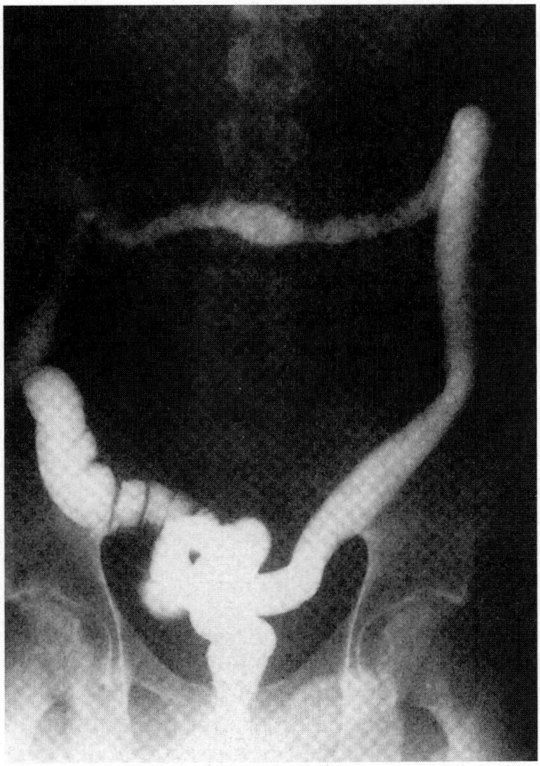

Figure 16-18 Barium enema showing the characteristic changes associated with chronic ulcerative colitis. Shown are loss of the haustral pattern, ulcerations, and foreshortening. Because of these changes, the colon is said to resemble a "lead pipe."

Table 16-6 Comparison of Ulcerative Colitis and Crohn's Colitis

	Ulcerative Colitis	Crohn's Colitis
Symptoms and signs		
Diarrhea	Severe, bloody	Less severe, bleeding infrequent
Perianal fistulas	Rare	Common
Strictures or obstruction	Uncommon	Common
Perforation	Free, uncommon	Localized, common
Pattern of development		
Rectum	Virtually always involved	Often normal
Terminal ileum	Normal	Diseased in majority of patients
Distribution	Continuous	Segmented, skip lesions
Megacolon	Frequent	Less common
Appearance		
Gross	Friable, bleeding granular exudates, pseudopolyps, isolated ulcers	Linear ulcers, transverse fissures, cobblestoning, thickening, strictures
Microscopic	Inflamed submucosa and mucosa, crypt abscesses; fibrosis uncommon	Transmural inflammation, granulomas, fibrosis
Radiologic	Lead-pipe, foreshortening, continuous, concentric	String sign in small bowel; segmental, asymmetric internal fistulae
Course		
Natural history	Exacerbations, remissions, dramatic flare-ups	Exacerbations, remissions, chronic, indolent
Medical treatment	Initial response high (> 80%)	Response less predictable
Surgical treatment	Curative	Palliative
Recurrence	No	Common

rial colitis, and pseudomembranous colitis. The disease that is most commonly confused with ulcerative colitis is Crohn's disease of the colon. In approximately 10% of cases, there is an overlap of features; this type of colitis is called indeterminate colitis. Its clinical behavior appears to be more like ulcerative colitis than Crohn's disease, however. Table 16-6 shows distinguishing characteristics of both disease processes.

Treatment

Medical therapy is usually the initial treatment. It is successful in approximately 80% of cases. In mild disease, the treatment is primarily symptomatic, with the use of antidiarrheal agents that slow gut transit (e.g., loperamide) and bulking agents (psyllium seed products) that result in semiformed, less watery stools. In moderate disease, sulfasalazine or mesalamine-based preparations should be tried because they induce remission in approximately half of all patients initially. In severe disease, most patients respond dramatically to steroid administration. Unfortunately, because of severe side effects, the dose is tapered and minimized whenever possible. Recent studies demonstrate efficacy of an anti–tumor necrosis factor (anti-TNF) monoclonal antibody in treating patients with Crohn's disease, especially in the presence of fistulae. While this treatment is more effective in patients with Crohn's disease of the small bowel, patients with primary colonic involvement also have significant response rates. Elimination of milk from the diet is occasionally helpful. Supportive therapy, including physical and emotional support, is important.

Major complications are toxic megacolon, colonic perforation, massive hemorrhage, serious anorectal complications, and carcinoma development after years of disease. Initial therapy for toxic megacolon is aggressive medical care, including gastric decompression, antibiotics, intravenous administration of fluids, hyperalimentation, and elimination of all other medications, specifically anticholinergics.

Surgical therapy is indicated when medical therapy fails or surgically treatable complications ensue (e.g., hemorrhage, perforation, obstruction, carcinoma). Because of the increased risk of carcinoma, long-standing ulcerative colitis is also an indication for surgical intervention. The risk increases 1% to 2% per year after the initial 10 years of disease. In the past, the definitive operative procedure for ulcerative colitis was total proctocolectomy with permanent ileostomy. Recently, procedures were devised to maintain fecal continence, including an operation that involves constructing a reservoir with a continence-producing nipple valve out of the small intestine (Kock's continent ileostomy). This operation has met with limited success. Subtotal colectomy with ileoproctostomy is attempted in some patients who have less severe rectal involvement and absolutely no perianal problems. Unfortunately, this operation does not cure the disease and subjects the patient to the risks of recurrent disease or the development of a malignancy in the remaining remnant. Total colectomy with mucosal proctectomy and ileoanal pullthrough (Fig. 16-19A–*D*) is now the operation of choice. The procedure is performed with a surgically constructed ileal reservoir, thereby sparing the patient a per-

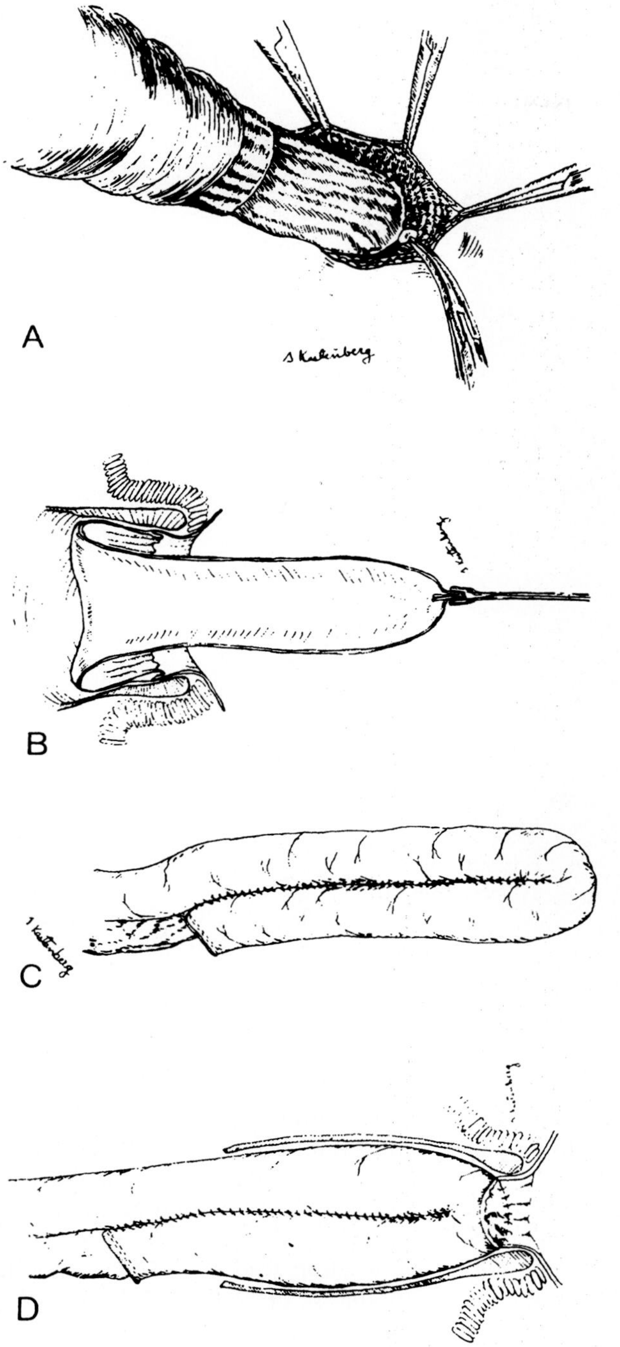

Figure 16-19 Ileoanal pullthrough is the operation of choice for definitive treatment of ulcerative colitis and familial polyposis syndrome. **A,** After removal of the entire colon, the mucosa is stripped away from the muscular layers of the rectum. **B,** This dissection is continued down to the dentate line, and the mucosa is everted out through the anus and resected. **C,** A small reservoir is constructed from the terminal ileum using a J-shaped configuration. **D,** This J-shaped pouch is then pulled through the muscular cuff and anastomosed to the dentate line to create a neorectum.

manent abdominal ileostomy. A recent variation of this procedure removes the colon and all but 2 cm of the rectum. The remaining rectal stump receives a stapled anastomosis. There is, however, significant concern that this operation does not represent a cure because diseased mucosa is left behind, raising the possibility of subsequent development of cancer in the retained rectal stump. The advantage of the stapled operation is that very often it can be done without a diverting ileostomy. Because patients with toxic megacolon, perforation, or other complications have much higher morbidity and mortality rates, early surgery may be indicated.

Colonic Obstruction and Volvulus

Obstruction of the Large Intestine

Only 10% to 15% of intestinal obstruction in adults is the result of obstruction of the large bowel. The most common anatomic site of colonic obstruction is the sigmoid colon. The three most common causes are adenocarcinoma (65%), scarring associated with diverticulitis (20%), and volvulus (5%). Inflammatory disorders, benign tumors, foreign bodies, fecal impaction, and other miscellaneous problems account for the remainder. Obstructive adhesive bands, which are often seen in the small bowel, are extremely uncommon in the colon.

Clinical Presentation and Evaluation

Signs and symptoms include abdominal distension; cramping abdominal pain, usually in the hypogastrium; nausea and vomiting; and obstipation. Radiologic findings show distended proximal colon, air–fluid levels, and no distal rectal air (Fig. 16-20).

Physical examination usually shows abdominal distension, tympany, high-pitched metallic rushes, and gurgles. On palpation, a localized, tender, palpable mass may indicate a strangulated closed loop or an area of inflamed diverticular disease.

An important element that affects the clinical expression of large bowel obstruction is whether the ileocecal valve is competent. If it is incompetent, the signs and symptoms produced are indistinguishable from those of routine small bowel obstruction. If the ileocecal valve is competent, as is the case in approximately 75% of patients, a "closed loop" obstruction occurs between the ileocecal valve and the obstructing point distally. Massive colonic distension results, and the cecum may reach a diameter of 12 cm, increasing the possibility of perforation, with or without gangrene. It is critically important for the clinician to distinguish between complete large bowel obstruction and partial large bowel obstruction. Patients with complete large bowel obstruction have obstipation that includes a history of no flatus or stool passage for 8 to 12 hours. On the other hand, patients with partial large bowel obstruction describe the passage of some gas or stool. Distinguishing between the two is important because a patient with complete bowel obstruction should undergo emergent opera-

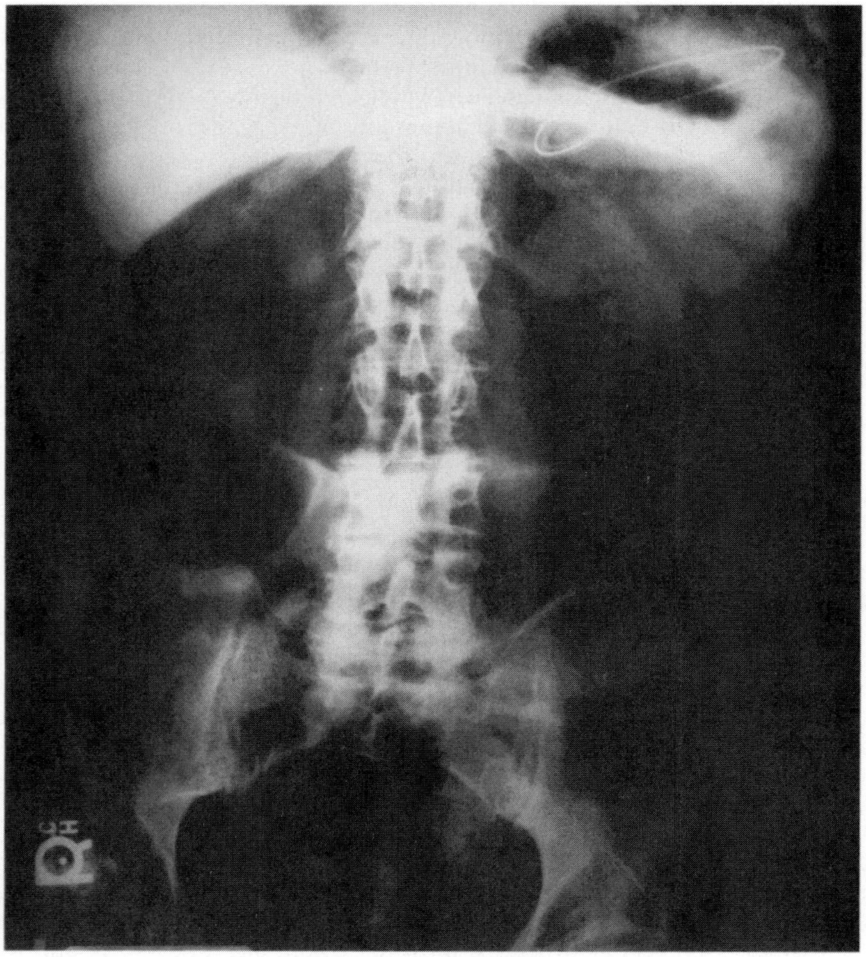

Figure 16-20 Massive colonic distension caused by a cecal volvulus.

tion. Those with partial large bowel obstruction may often be treated by nasogastric decompression and intravenous fluids with resolution of the acute obstruction. This distinction has important surgical ramifications because patients with partial large bowel obstruction can then be prepared for surgery by cleaning out the large intestine, thus avoiding a colostomy.

The appropriate diagnostic techniques include plain films of the abdomen. In patients in whom the cecum measures more than 12 cm and a definitive lesion cannot be delineated, laparotomy is undertaken. The use of barium enema confirms the diagnosis of colonic obstruction and identifies the exact location. If the obstruction is shown on plain abdominal films, barium enema is not necessary. Barium should never be given orally in the presence of suspected colonic obstruction because it may accumulate proximal to the obstruction and cause a barium impaction. Colonoscopic examination plays a major role in Ogilvie's syndrome (localized paralytic ileus of the colon without mechanical obstruction); otherwise, it is reserved for the occasional case of volvulus for decompression.

Treatment

All patients with large bowel obstruction should be treated with intravenous fluids, nasogastric suction, and continuous observation until the diagnosis is established and definitive therapy is undertaken. Potentially lethal complications of large bowel obstruction are perforation and abdominal peritonitis and sepsis. The major causes of severe colonic obstruction leading to these complications include carcinoma of the colon, with or without perforation; diverticulitis; sigmoid volvulus; and cecal volvulus.

Emergency laparotomy is undertaken for acute large bowel obstruction with cecal distension beyond 12 cm, severe tenderness, evidence of peritonitis, or generalized sepsis. Perforation caused by volvulus, obstructing cancers, or diverticular strictures usually requires laparotomy with the appropriate surgical procedures, usually resection and diverting colostomy.

For the occasional case of Ogilvie's syndrome in which there is idiopathic, enormous dilation of the right side of the colon without mechanical obstruction (pseudo-obstruction), the current therapy is fiberoptic colonoscopy, with decompression and placement of a long rectal decompression tube. Cecostomy may be necessary in cases of recurrence. If colonoscopic decompression is not successful, a high percentage of patients will respond to IV neostigmine administration (inhibits breakdown of acetylcholine), which results in contraction of the affected colon.

The various conditions that lead to large bowel obstruction result in differing prognoses, most of which depend on the patient's age and the comorbidity of existing diseases, particularly cardiovascular disease. Unfortunately, the overall death rate of patients who have a cecal perforation approaches 30%. Thus, prompt laparotomy is the mainstay of treatment.

Volvulus of the Large Intestine

Volvulus is rotation of a segment of the intestine on the axis formed by the mesentery (Fig. 16-21). The most common sites of occurrence in the large bowel are the sigmoid (70%) and cecum (30%). Volvulus accounts for 5% to 10% of cases of large bowel obstruction and is the second most common cause of complete colonic obstruction. Stretching and elongation of the sigmoid with age is a predisposing factor. The first occurrence of volvulus in more than 50% of cases is in patients 65 years of age or older. For unknown reasons, patients who are confined to mental institutions or nursing homes have an increased risk for this disease. Volvulus also occurs in patients who have a hypermobile cecum because of incomplete fixation of the ascending colon at the time of intrauterine development. This condition allows the cecum to twist about the mesentery, forming a closed-loop obstruction at the entry and exit points, with major pressure at the sites of the twist. The vessels are partially occluded, and circulatory impairment leads to prompt gangrene and perforation.

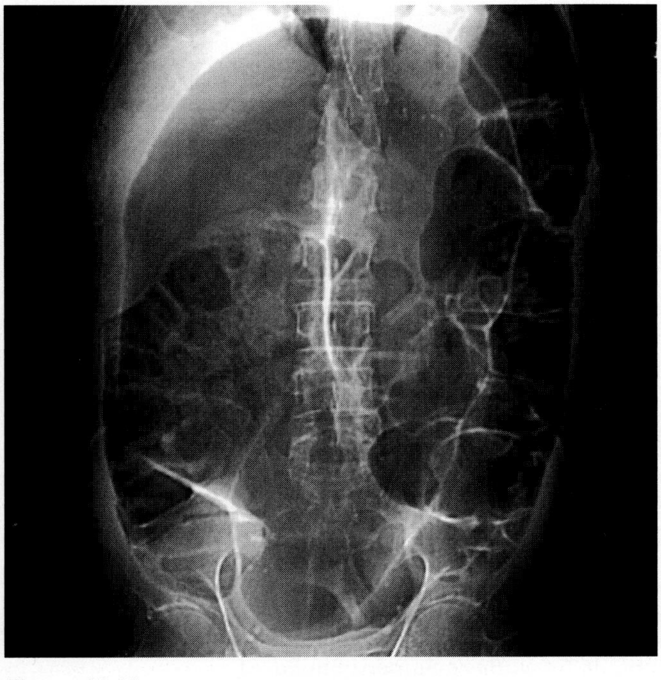

Figure 16-21 Volvulus of the sigmoid colon.

Clinical Presentation and Evaluation

The patient has abdominal distension, which is often massive; vomiting; abdominal pain; obstipation; and tachypnea. Physical examination shows distension, tympany, high-pitched tinkling sounds, and rushes. Diagnostic studies include abdominal x-ray films and barium enemas. Abdominal radiographs show a massively dilated cecum or sigmoid without haustra that often assumes a kidney bean appearance. Barium enema study shows the exact site of obstruction, with a characteristic funnel-like narrowing that often resembles a bird's beak or an ace of spades.

Treatment

Sigmoidoscopy with rectal tube insertion to decompress sigmoid volvulus is the recommended initial treatment for that location. Emergency operation is performed promptly if strangulation or perforation is suspected or if attempts to decompress the bowel are unsuccessful. Surgical therapy involves resection without anastomosis and the construction of a temporary colostomy. Most patients with sigmoid volvulus are easily decompressed and subsequently require elective resection, except for very high-risk elderly patients. Cecal volvulus is always treated surgically, either with cecopexy (suturing the cecum to the parietal peritoneum) or with right hemicolectomy with ileotransverse colostomy if the cecum is gangrenous.

ANUS AND RECTUM

Diagnostic Evaluation

The anus and rectum are the site of many conditions that cause pain, protrusion, bleeding, discharge, or a combination of these. Most people complain generally about their "hemorrhoid problem"; it is up to the physician to distinguish between various pathologies that may present similarly.

Examination of the perianal and rectal area is an integral part of every physical examination. The importance of gentleness and empathy cannot be overemphasized. A complete history must be obtained before the examination; this information alone suggests the diagnosis in more than 80% of the cases. Gentle parting of the buttocks allows inspection that may show fissures, skin tags, hemorrhoids, fistulae, tumors, and dermatologic or infectious conditions. Gentle digital examination may show tumors, polyps, fluctuation, and sphincter weakness.

Anoscopic examination is mandatory because many visible lesions are not palpable. It may be deferred, however, in the presence of acute pain. The anoscope is a beveled instrument devised to examine the anal canal. It allows detection of more subtle lesions (e.g., ulcers, villous adenomas, infectious disorders) than the rigid or flexible proctosigmoidoscope. The proctosigmoidoscope, however, is the instrument of choice for a proper evaluation of the rectum because it is the only instrument that allows exact localization of rectal lesions.

Rectal Prolapse (Procidentia)

Rectal prolapse is intussusception of a full-thickness portion of the rectum through the anal opening. This condition occurs most commonly in thin, asthenic women who have weak rectal attachments and may involve from 4 to 20 cm of rectum protruding through the anal opening. The entity must be distinguished from mucosal prolapse, which is eversion of 2 to 3 cm of rectal mucosa through the anal opening but which is not full thickness. They can be distinguished by the concentric, circumferential mucosal folds seen in true prolapse compared to the radial pattern of folds seen in mucosal prolapse (Fig. 16-22).

Clinical Presentation and Evaluation

Symptoms of prolapse include rectal pain, mild bleeding, incontinence, mucous discharge, and a wet anus. On rare occasions, the prolapse cannot be reduced and ischemia results. The prolapse commonly occurs after each bowel movement and must be manually reduced.

Treatment

Management of true rectal prolapse involves an intraabdominal procedure including sigmoid resection (redundant bowel) with rectopexy (suturing the bowel wall to the presacral fascia to immobilize it). Recurrence rates are less than 5% if the procedure is correctly performed. For very high-risk patients, a procedure can be done in which the entire resection is done through the perineum, but recurrence rates are much higher. Treatment of mucosal prolapse is a three-column hemorrhoidectomy.

Hemorrhoids

Hemorrhoids are vascular cushions located in the anal canal. Hemorrhoidal disease, which most often causes hemorrhoidal protrusion or bleeding, is usually precipitated by constipation and straining at stool. Pregnancy, increased pelvic pressure (ascites, tumors), portal hypertension, and excessive diarrhea may influence the development of hemorrhoidal symptoms.

Hemorrhoids are usually found in three constant positions: left lateral, right anterior, and right posterior. It is preferable to refer to the actual anatomic position of the anorectal processes because the old "o'clock" system referred to the findings when the examination was performed in the lithotomy position. In the modern ambulatory setting, most patients are examined either in the left lateral (Simm's) or the knee-chest position, which change the terms of reference by 90° to 180°.

Hemorrhoids are classified as either internal or external. **Internal hemorrhoids** originate above the dentate line; external hemorrhoids are located below the level of the dentate line. Because the rectal mucosa above the dentate line is insensate, bleeding from internal hemorrhoids is usually painless. Conversely, external hemorrhoids are covered by richly innervated anoderm and usually cause pain when thrombosis occurs.

Clinical Presentation and Evaluation

A patient with hemorrhoids has symptoms of hemorrhoidal protrusion or bleeding. In cases of protrusion, the hemor-

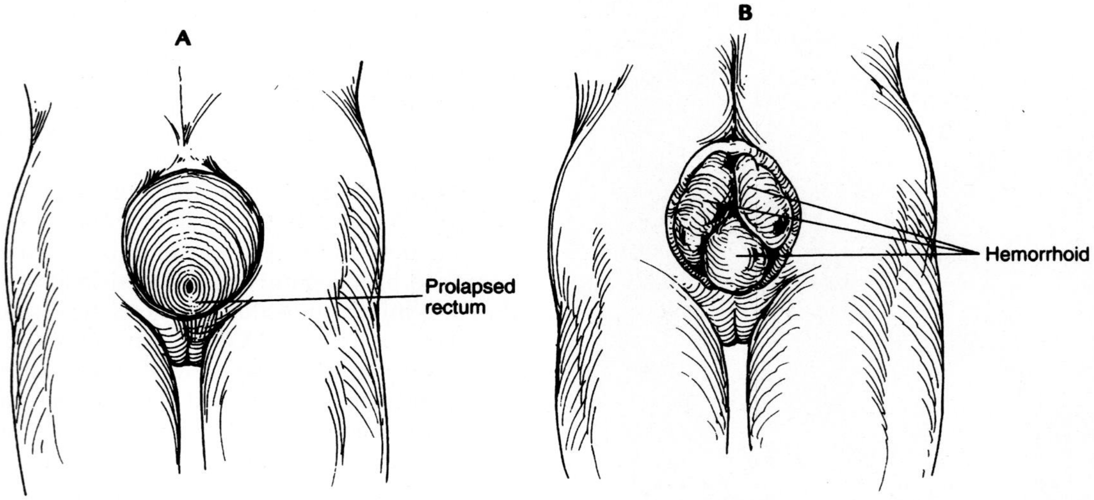

Figure 16-22 **A,** True rectal prolapse is characterized by concentric, circumferential mucosal folds. **B,** Mucosal prolapse is characterized by radial folds separating the mucosa. (Reprinted with permission from Polk HC Jr., et al. *Basic Surgery.* 5th Ed. St. Louis, MO: Quality Medical Publishing, 1995.)

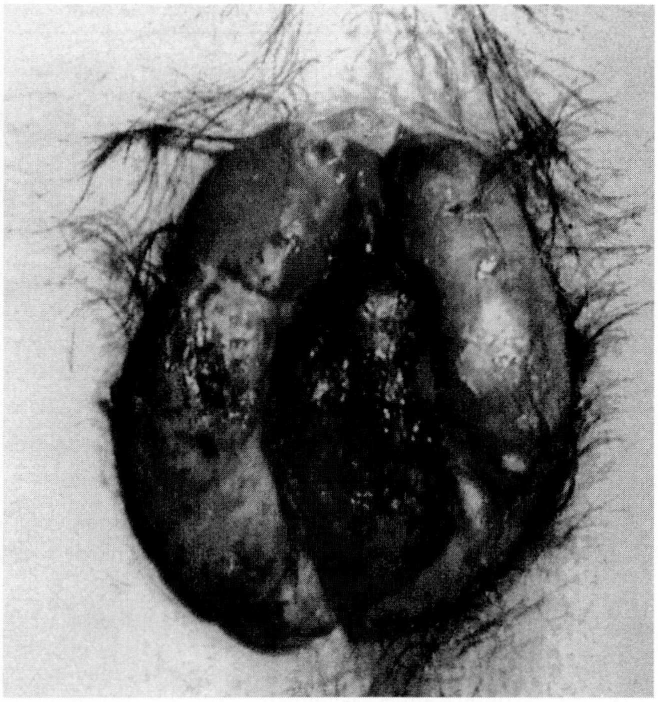

Figure 16-23 Fourth-degree hemorrhoids associated with thrombosis.

rhoids are graded according to the level of prolapse. First-degree internal hemorrhoids do not prolapse; the anoscope must be used to visualize them. Second-degree internal hemorrhoids prolapse with defecation and return spontaneously to their anatomic position. Third-degree internal hemorrhoids prolapse with defecation and require manual reduction. Fourth-degree hemorrhoids are not reducible (Fig. 16-23). There is no classification for external hemorrhoids; they are either present or absent. Mixed hemorrhoids are a combination of internal and external hemorrhoids.

Bleeding may be minimal, appearing only on toilet paper, or it may occasionally be severe enough to cause anemia. It is usually bright red, coats the stool (rather than being mixed with it), and is painless, unless there is thrombosis, ulceration, or gangrene.

Treatment

Treatment is based on the presence of symptoms and the degree of disease (Table 16-7). Asymptomatic hemorrhoids are best left alone; cosmetic treatment is not indicated. Bulk-forming agents (e.g., psyllium derivatives) and avoidance of constipation are recommended. First-degree internal hemorrhoids are treated similarly; rubber-band ligation (banding) or infrared coagulation may be indicated, depending on the size of the hemorrhoids on anoscopic examination. Most colorectal surgeons have abandoned sclerotherapy and cryosurgery. Second-degree internal hemorrhoids and some third-degree hemorrhoids are treated with banding. Formal surgical hemorrhoidectomy is used for fourth-degree hemorrhoids, for mixed third-degree hemorrhoids with a large external component, and in some emergency situations (e.g., gangrene, severe ulceration).

External hemorrhoids usually cause few problems. Contrary to popular belief, hemorrhoids do not itch or burn; it is the perianal skin that is the site of pruritus ani. However, large external hemorrhoids may interfere with perianal hygiene and thus be indirectly associated with pruritus. In these cases, excision may be indicated. It is usually done under local anesthesia.

Some patients may have severe perianal pain and a lump close to the anus after a bout of constipation or prolonged sitting. Examination shows an obvious thrombosed external hemorrhoid. This condition is self-limited and resolves progressively over 7 to 10 days; creams, suppositories, and topical adjuncts are useless. If the patient is seen early in the course of the disease (the first 24 to 48 hours), treatment consists of excision of the thrombosed hemorrhoid under local anesthesia. If the patient is seen later in

Table 16-7 Internal Hemorrhoids: Classification and Treatment

Degree	Definition	Treatment
First	Bulge in the anal canal lumen; does not protrude outside the lumen	*Asymptomatic:* take bulking agents; avoid constipation; increase water intake *Symptomatic:* same treatment as asymptomatic; rubber-band ligation; infrared coagulation
Second	Protrudes with defecation Reduces spontaneously	Conservative management (see above) or rubber-band ligation
Third	Protrudes with defecation Must be reduced manually	*Selected cases:* rubber-band ligation *Mixed:* surgical hemorrhoidectomy
Fourth	Protrudes permanently incarcerated	Surgical hemorrhoidectomy

the course of the disease, spontaneous resolution is usually underway and conservative treatment is indicated. Sitz baths and a mild nonnarcotic analgesic are recommended.

Perianal Infections: Abscess and Fistula-in-Ano

Abscess

Most anorectal abscesses are believed to start with obstruction of the perianal glands that are located between the internal and external sphincters (intersphincteric space). These glands normally discharge their secretions at the level of the anal crypts that are located at the base of the columns of Morgagni. The term "of cryptoglandular origin" describes the origin of perirectal abscesses. As the early intersphincteric abscess (Fig. 16-24, *left*) increases in size, it tends to spread along the planes of lesser resistance and to manifest fully as a perianal abscess (Fig. 16-24, *right*). It may also manifest as an ischiorectal abscess in the ischiorectal fossa, located outside the external sphincter mechanism and below the level of the levatores ani muscles (Fig. 16-25, *left*). If the infection spreads above the levators (Fig. 16-25, *right*), the supralevator abscess may be very difficult to diagnose clinically. Perianal and ischiorectal abscesses are the most common. They account for as many as 70% of perirectal abscesses.

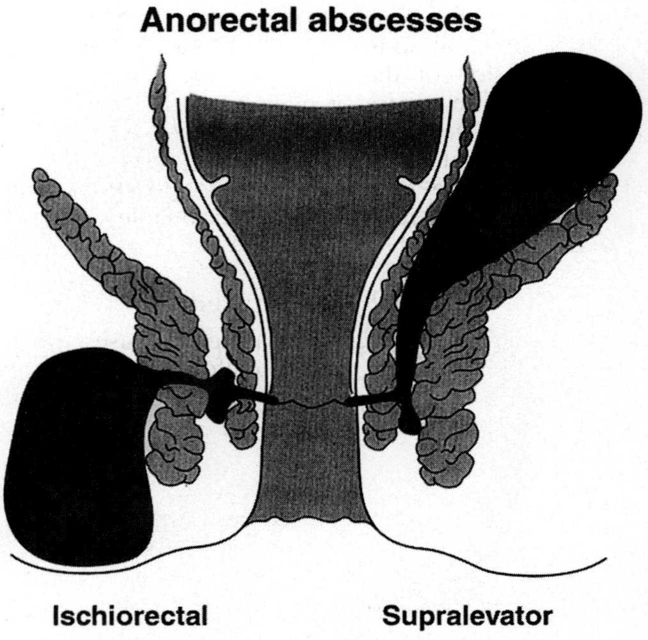

Figure 16-25 Simple intersphincteric abscesses may progress to more complex ischiorectal and supralevator abscesses.

Clinical Presentation and Evaluation

Except for early intersphincteric abscesses and supralevator abscesses, perianal pain and swelling are readily apparent in perirectal abscesses. Spontaneous drainage of pus may occur. The cardinal signs of infection (pain, fever, redness, swelling, and loss of function) are usually present.

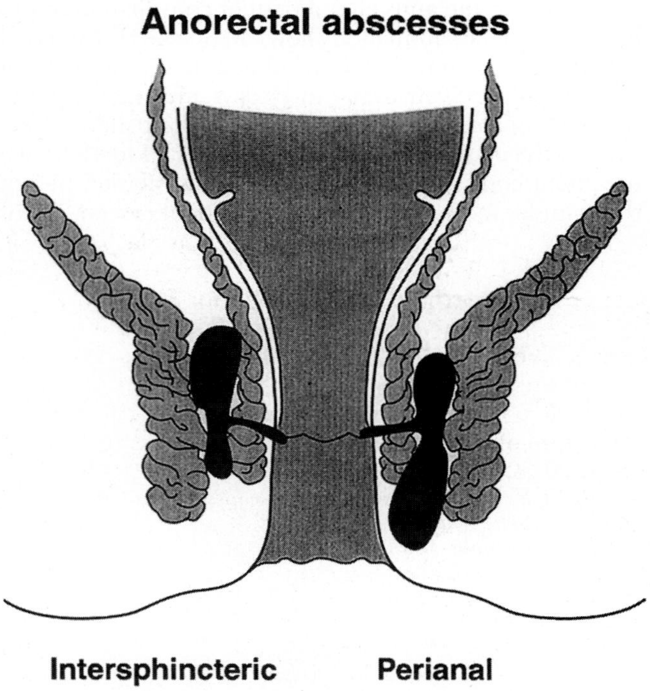

Figure 16-24 Progression of intersphincteric abscess to perianal abscess.

Treatment

Treatment is complete and thorough drainage of the abscess. Failure to adequately drain the abscess results in ongoing pain, sepsis, and overall treatment failure. Often, the most effective surgical drainage can best be done in the operating room with adequate anesthesia. Antibiotics alone have no role in the primary treatment of an abscess. However, antibiotics may be used in conjunction with surgical incision and drainage in patients who are immunocompromised; those who have diabetes, leukemia, or AIDS; or those who are undergoing chemotherapy.

Fistula-in-Ano

After drainage of a perirectal abscess, the patient has a 50% chance of having a chronic **fistula-in-ano**. An anorectal fistula is an abnormal communication between the anus at the level of the dentate line and the perirectal skin, through the bed of the previous abscess. Fistulae are named in relation to the sphincter mechanism (Table 16-8). Intersphincteric fistulae are the result of perianal abscesses; transsphincteric fistulae are the result of ischiorectal abscesses; suprasphincteric fistulae are the result of supralevator abscesses. Extrasphincteric fistulae bypass the anal canal and the sphincter mechanism and open high up in the rectum.

Table 16-8 Perianal Infections
Abscess: acute phase
Intersphincteric
Perianal
Ischiorectal
Supralevator
Fistula: chronic phase
Intersphincteric
Transsphincteric
Suprasphincteric
Extrasphincteric

Clinical Presentation and Evaluation

Fistulae manifest as chronic drainage of pus and sometimes stool from the skin opening. They never heal spontaneously, and surgical correction is indicated to eliminate the symptoms.

Goodsall's rule helps the examiner to predict the trajectory of the fistulous tract and the probable location of the internal anal opening (Fig. 16-26). With the patient in the lithotomy or the knee-chest position, an imaginary line is drawn at the level of the anus, parallel to the floor. For external openings located anterior to this line, the fistula tract usually goes radially straight into the anal crypt. For external openings located posterior to this imaginary line, the fistula tract generally curves around, and the internal opening is in a frank midline position. However, the greater the distance between the anus and the external opening, the less reliable and helpful Goodsall's rule becomes. The trajectory of complex anal fistulae is unpredictable.

Treatment

Fistulotomy consists of unroofing the fistula tract, allowing the fistula to heal slowly by secondary intention. Judgment must be exercised to avoid cutting a large portion of the sphincter muscle, which may precipitate incontinence.

Preliminary identification of the fistula tract by gentle insertion of a probe into the external skin opening, through the tract, until the internal anal opening is found, allows intraoperative evaluation of the structures that need division. Staged fistulotomy with a Seton stitch permits immediate division of all nonsphincteric structures. Then the sphincter muscle is progressively divided to avoid incontinence.

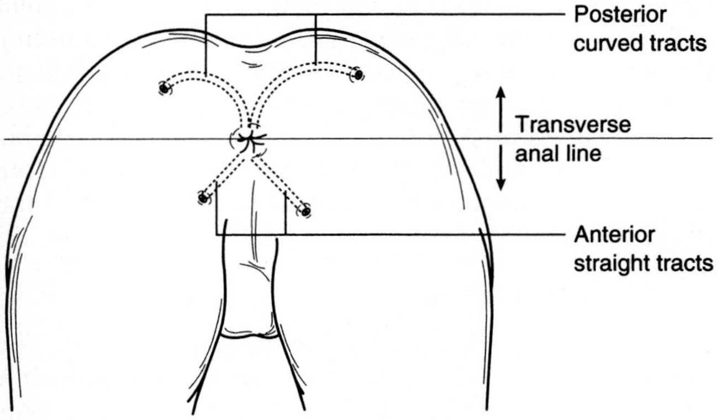

Figure 16-26 Goodsall's rule. (Reprinted with permission from Schwartz SI, et al. *Principles of Surgery.* 6th Ed. New York, NY: McGraw-Hill, 1994. Reproduced with permission of The McGraw-Hill Companies.)

Anal Fissures

The most common cause of severe localized anorectal pain is fissures. While hemorrhoids often cause discomfort and mild pressure symptoms, they rarely cause the severe pain associated with fissures. That pain is dramatically increased during bowel movements and is often associated with streaks of blood in the stool. **Anal fissures** are painful linear tears in the lining of the anal canal, below the level of the dentate line. They are most often located posteriorly in both sexes, but women also have anterior anal fissures. They occur in the posteroanterior plane because pelvic muscular support is weakest along this axis. Ectopic lateral fissures suggest an unusual diagnosis (e.g., Crohn's disease, leukemia, sexually transmitted disease, malignancy).

Clinical Presentation and Evaluation

Fissures are secondary to local trauma, either from constipation or excessive diarrhea. Pain typically starts with defecation and may persist from minutes to hours. It is disproportionate to the size of the lesion. If bleeding is present, it is usually minimal and bright red.

If the history suggests an anal fissure, gentle retraction of the buttocks will reveal the tear at the anal verge. Rectal examination is usually associated with severe pain and significant sphincter spasm. In cases of chronic recurrent anal fissures, the classic triad of an external skin tag, a fissure exposing the internal sphincter fibers, and a hypertrophied anal papilla at the level of the dentate line is pathognomonic.

Treatment

Treatment is based on the duration and severity of the symptoms. Acute anal fissures usually respond to conservative treatment, avoidance of diarrhea or constipation, bulk laxatives to keep bowel movements atraumatic, and a mild nonnarcotic analgesic. Sitz baths are helpful for comfort. If conservative treatment fails, or if the fissure is chronic, surgery is recommended. Several surgical options are available. In uncomplicated cases, the operation of choice is a lateral internal sphincterotomy. A small portion of the internal sphincter is cut, which releases the sphincter spasm, relieves pain, and allows the fissure to heal. The operation carries a small risk of minor incontinence.

Anal Malignancy

Perianal and anal canal malignancies are rare, accounting for only 3% to 4% of all anorectal carcinomas. There are essentially two types of anal cancers: epidermoid carcinoma (a generic type that includes squamous cell, basaloid, cloacogenic, mucoepidermoid, and transitional carcinomas) and malignant melanoma. The anus is the third most common site for malignant melanoma, after the skin and the eyes.

Clinical Presentation and Evaluation

Either type of malignancy may cause pain, bleeding, or a lump. Delay in diagnosis is often a consequence of both patient and physician neglect. In cases of malignant melanoma, lymph node involvement and widespread metastasis are common at presentation. The diagnosis is often delayed because of the lack of pigmentation of these lesions (amelanotic melanoma). Examination should include palpation of the inguinal lymph nodes, a site of potential metastasis.

Treatment

In the past, abdominoperineal resection and permanent colostomy were the mainstays of treatment for both types of cancer. This approach has been almost completely abandoned in epidermoid cancers in favor of combined modality chemotherapy and radiation therapy, using a protocol of pelvic radiation with infusion of 5-FU and mitomycin C. With this treatment, 5-year survival rates range from 82% to 87%. Surgery is indicated in cases in which residual tumor is present after radiation and chemotherapy. Abdominoperineal resection is indicated in this setting.

Prophylactic inguinal node dissection is not recommended unless clinically palpable nodes are present because of the high morbidity associated with this procedure. Synchronous inguinal node metastasis is an ominous sign, and survival rates are poor. Conversely, metachronous inguinal node involvement has a better prognosis. Inclusion of the groins in the radiated fields decreases the incidence of metachronous lymph node involvement without adding much morbidity.

For malignant melanoma, the prognosis is dismal, regardless of the treatment. For good-risk patients, abdominoperineal resection is a reasonable option to maximize survival.

Anorectal Sexually Transmitted Diseases

More than 20 sexually transmitted diseases can be present in the anorectal area. Therefore, it is important to inquire about a complete sexual history in patients with anorectal symptoms.

Anal Condylomas

Anal condylomas are caused by human papilloma virus. They are the most common anorectal infection affecting homosexual men, but may also be seen in heterosexual men and women and even children. Transmission at birth and by close contact with infected patients has been reported.

Anal condylomas are more common in homosexual men who practice anal-receptive intercourse. The lesions are found perianally, intraanally, on the penis, and in the urethra. In women, the lesions may be found in the vagina, vulva, cervix, or urethra. Condylomas acuminata are pink or white papillary lesions. They vary in size from less than 1 mm to large cauliflowerlike lesions. They bleed easily, and difficulty in maintaining perianal hygiene leads to pruritus ani. Discomfort and pain are often present.

Various topical caustic agents (bichloracetic acid, podophyllin) and local destructive therapies (electrocoagulation, cryotherapy, laser excision) have been tried with mitigated success. Regardless of the technique, the recurrence rate is high (10% to 50%). Persistent causative sexual behavior obviously increases the recurrence rate.

Chlamydia and Lymphogranuloma Venereum

Chlamydial infections are among the most common sexually transmitted diseases. Chlamydial proctitis is increasing in both men and women who practice anal-receptive sex. The disease usually begins as vesicles and progresses to an ulcer. Inguinal adenopathy is a prominent sign. The rectal symptoms are tenesmus and pain. Patients who have lymphogranuloma venereum usually have hematochezia. Sigmoidoscopy may show a friable, ulcerating, erythematous mucosa. Biopsy findings are not definitive. The microimmunofluorescent antibody titer is the test of choice; however, the complement fixation test is still used. Most patients are successfully treated with tetracycline or doxycycline. Erythromycin is reserved for those who are insensitive to tetracyclines.

Gonorrhea

Neisseria gonorrhoeae infections of the rectum account for as many as 50% of the cases of gonorrhea in homosexual men. Evaluation and followup of patients with rectal gonorrhea require cultures of the urethra, rectum, and pharynx. Most patients have nonspecific complaints, including pruritus, tenesmus, and hematochezia. Sigmoidoscopy shows a thick, yellow mucopurulent discharge. The rectal mucosa ranges from normal to erythematous and edematous. Culture and Gram stain are used for organism identification. Treatment is ceftriaxone 250 mg given once intramuscularly.

Herpes Simplex Virus

Herpes simplex virus type 2 causes herpetic proctitis. The infection is acquired by direct inoculation. Approximately 15% of homosexual men with rectal symptoms have only this virus identified by rectal culture. The symptoms begin 4 to 28 days after inoculation. The majority of patients have pain and burning worsened by bowel movements. Some patients have a syndrome that is characterized by lumbosacral radiculopathy associated with sacral paresthesias. Symptoms include impotence; lower abdominal, buttock, and thigh pain; and urinary dysfunction. Lesions include vesicles with red areolae, ruptured vesicles, and aphthous ulcers. The usual locations include the perianal skin, anal canal, and lower rectum. Patients who are seen in the relapsing stage may report a history of crusting lesions followed by healing. Scrapings for cytologic examination show intranuclear inclusion bodies and giant cells. Treatment is aimed at relieving symptoms: sitz baths, topical anesthetics, and analgesics. Acyclovir has benefit in the acute and relapse phases. Continuous suppressive therapy is warranted only in the most severe cases.

SUGGESTED READINGS

American Society of Colon and Rectal Surgeons Standards Task Force. Practice parameters for the management of anal fissure. American Society of Colon and Rectal Surgeons, 1993.

American Society of Colon and Rectal Surgeons Standards Task Force. Practice parameters for the treatment of hemorrhoids. *Dis Colon Rectum* 1993;36:1118.

Becker JM, Soper NJ. Problems in general surgery. *Inflamm Bowel Dis* 1999;16(2):1–166.

Boulis-Wassif S, Gerard A, Loygue J, et al. Final results of a randomized trial on the treatment of rectal cancer with preoperative radiotherapy alone or in combination with 5-fluorouracil, followed by radical surgery. Trial of the European Organization on Research and Treatment of Cancer Gastrointestinal Tract Cancer Cooperative Group. *Cancer* 1984;53:1811–1818.

Cirocco WC. Lateral internal sphincterotomy remains the treatment of choice for anal fissures that fail conservative therapy [letter; comment]. *Gastrointest Endosc* 1998;47(2):212–214.

Fazio VW, Marchetti F, Church M, et al. Effect of resection margins on the recurrence of Crohn's disease in the small bowel. A randomized controlled trial. *Ann Surg* 1996;224(4):563–571; discussion 571–573.

Gordon PH. Current status—perianal and anal canal neoplasms. *Dis Colon Rectum* 1990;33(9):799–808.

Hanauer SB. Drug therapy: inflammatory bowel disease. *N Engl J Med* 1996;334:841–848.

Kelly CP, Pothoukas C, LaMont JT. *Clostridium difficile* colitis [see comments]. *N Engl J Med* 1994;330(4):257–262.

MacRae HM, McLeod RS. Comparison of hemorrhoidal treatment modalities. A meta-analysis. *Dis Colon Rectum* 1995;38(7):687–694.

Mandel JS, Bond JH, Church TR, et al. Reducing mortality from colorectal cancer by screening for fecal occult blood. Minnesota Colon Cancer Control Study [published erratum appears in *N Engl J Med* 1993;329(9):672] [see comments]. *N Engl J Med* 1993;329(19):1365–1371.

Mangiante EC, Croce MA, Fabian TC, et al. Sigmoid volvulus. A four-decade experience. *Am Surg* 1989;55(1):41–44.

McGuire HH Jr. Bleeding colonic diverticula. A reappraisal of natural history and management. *Ann Surg* 1994;220(5):653–656.

Moertel CG, Fleming TR, Macdonald JS, et al. Fluorouracil plus levamisole as effective adjuvant therapy after resection of stage III colon carcinoma: a final report. *Ann Intern Med* 1995;122(5):321–326.

O'Brien MJ, Winawer SJ, Zauber AG, et al. The National Polyp Study. Patient and polyp characteristics associated with high-grade dysplasia in colorectal adenomas. *Gastroenterology* 1990;98(2):371–379.

Present DH, Rutgeerts P, Targan S, et al. Infliximab for the treatment of fistulas in patients with Crohn's disease. *N Engl J Med* 1999;340(18):1398–1405.

Ritchie JK. The results of surgery for large bowel Crohn's disease. *Ann R Coll Surg Engl* 1990;72(3):155–157.

Roberto PL, Veidenheimer MC. Current management of diverticulitis. *Adv Surg* 1994;27:189–208.

Russell MGVM, Stockbrugger RW. Epidemiology of inflammatory bowel disease: an update. *Scand J Gastroenterol* 1996;31:417–424.

Wexner SD. Managing common anorectal sexually transmitted disease. *Infect Surg* 1990;9:9.

Wexner SD, Reissman P, Pfeifer J, et al. Laparoscopic colorectal surgery: analysis of 140 cases. *Surg Endosc* 1996;10(2):133–136.

Williamson PR, Hellinger MD, Larach SW, et al. Twenty-year review of the surgical management of perianal Crohn's disease. *Dis Colon Rectum* 1995;38:389–392.

Winawer SJ, Zauber AG, Ho MN, et al. Prevention of colorectal cancer by colonoscopic polypectomy. The National Polyp Study Workgroup [see comments]. *N Engl J Med* 1993;329(27):1977–1981.

17

RUDY G. DANZINGER, MD ■ RUSSELL NAUTA, MD ■ JASON PARK, MD

Biliary Tract

OBJECTIVES

1 Outline the factors that contribute to the formation of the three most common types of gallstones.
2 Describe the epidemiology of gallstone disease as it relates to patient evaluation and management.
3 Discuss the most useful laboratory tests and imaging studies to evaluate patients with diseases of the biliary tract.
4 Describe the management of asymptomatic gallstones found incidentally on radiologic studies or at celiotomy.
5 Compare and contrast the (1) clinical presentation, (2) laboratory and radiologic findings, and (3) management of a patient with chronic cholecystitis (biliary colic) and a patient with acute cholecystitis.
6 List the differences in the clinical presentation and evaluation of a jaundiced patient with choledocholithiasis and a jaundiced patient with biliary obstruction secondary to malignancy.
7 Describe the clinical presentation, evaluation, and management of a patient with (1) acute cholangitis and (2) acute suppurative cholangitis. Highlight the differences between the two conditions.
8 Describe the clinical presentation, evaluation, and management of a patient with acute biliary (gallstone) pancreatitis.
9 Outline the clinical presentation, evaluation, and management of a patient with gallstone ileus. Contrast these with the corresponding features of other types of small bowel obstruction.
10 Outline the epidemiology, clinical presentation, evaluation, and management of carcinoma of the gallbladder.
11 Outline the clinical presentation, evaluation, and management of carcinoma of the extrahepatic biliary ducts.
12 List the common causes of benign strictures of the common bile duct, and describe the clinical features of patients who have such strictures.
13 Outline the various options available to treat stones in the gallbladder and the extrahepatic biliary ducts.
14 Outline the indications for cholecystectomy. Discuss the advantages of the laparoscopic approach over open cholecystectomy.
15 Compare and contrast the complications associated with laparoscopic cholecystectomy with those associated with open cholecystectomy.
16 Outline the postoperative management of a patient after (1) cholecystectomy and (2) common bile duct exploration.

Diseases of the gallbladder and bile ducts are common in the adult population of North America. Approximately 10% of adults have gallstones, and more than 600,000 cholecystectomies are performed annually in the United States, accounting for more than $5 billion in health care costs. In Canada, approximately 50,000 cholecystectomies are performed each year. Accurate clinical assessment, including pertinent history and accurate physical examination, yields valuable information about the diagnosis of common diseases of the biliary tract. Laboratory tests are helpful in distinguishing among various causes of jaundice, and imaging studies play a pivotal role in confirming the diagnosis of biliary tract disease. To minimize the risk of iatrogenic injury, the surgeon must possess the skills to recognize common variations in the anatomy of the biliary tract and to perform careful dissection of the vital structures during surgery. This dictum was reemphasized in recent years with the meteoric rise in the popularity of **laparoscopic cholecystectomy,** which has replaced open cholecystectomy as the preferred operation for most patients with gallstone disease.

ANATOMY

The anatomy of the extrahepatic biliary system varies considerably from individual to individual, and many anomalies are reported. To prevent inadvertent injury to the extrahepatic bile ducts and related structures during cholecystectomy, anticipation of anomalous anatomy and careful, bloodless dissection are vitally important.

The gallbladder is a thin-walled, contractile saclike organ attached to the undersurface of the liver at the anatomic division of the right and left lobes. It is usually tubular, approximately 10 cm long, and 5 cm in diameter. Most commonly, 75% of the gallbladder is covered by peritoneum, and the remainder is intimately attached to the liver. In some patients, the gallbladder is completely covered by peritoneum and is suspended by a mesentery. In others, it is almost completely embedded in the liver. In general, the less the gallbladder is attached to the liver, the easier is its surgical removal. The gallbladder consists of the fundus, body, neck, and cystic duct, which is lined by the spiral valves of Heister. Surgical synonyms for the neck are the *infundibulum* or *Hartmann's pouch*.

The cystic duct joins the common hepatic duct (formed by the confluence of the left and right hepatic ducts) to form the common bile duct. The hepatocystic triangle (triangle of Calot) is the anatomic area that is bounded by the inferior margin of the liver superiorly, the common hepatic duct medially, and the cystic duct laterally. A number of important normal (i.e., right hepatic artery) and anomalous structures traverse this triangle. The common bile duct passes through the head of the pancreas, usually joins the pancreatic duct within 1 cm of the wall of the duodenum, and then empties into the second portion of the duodenum, through the ampulla of Vater. Bile flow into the duodenum is regulated in part by the sphincter of Oddi, which encircles the distal bile duct. The most common anatomic configuration of this region is shown in Figure 17-1, which demonstrates the usual relations of the important ductal and arterial structures.

The bile ducts and gallbladder, which are embryologic outgrowths of the duodenum, have *bilateral* visceral (autonomic nervous system) innervation. Subsequently, pain generated in these structures is dull in character and can be felt in a band encircling the upper abdomen—T7 and T8 dermatomes (see the discussion on biliary colic below).

PHYSIOLOGY

The liver secretes 500 to 1000 mL of bile per day under physiologic conditions. The volume of bile secretion is

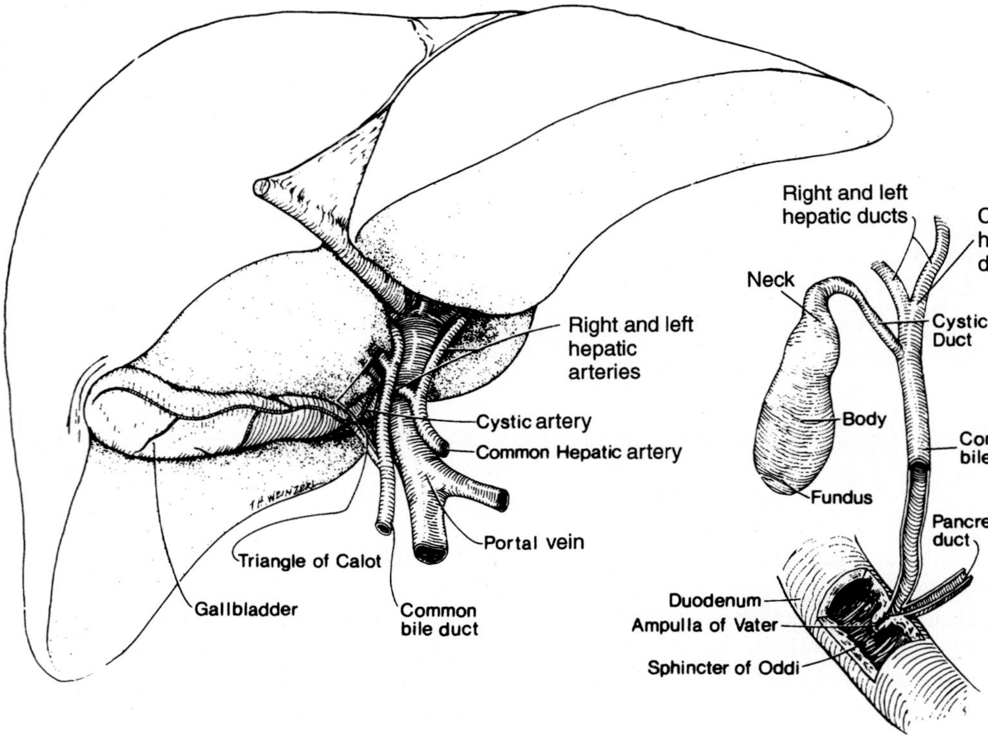

Figure 17-1 Anatomy of the gallbladder, porta hepatis, and extrahepatic bile ducts.

highest during gastric emptying and lowest during prolonged fasting. When the sphincter of Oddi is closed, most hepatic bile is diverted into the gallbladder for storage and concentration. The gallbladder concentrates the bile by absorbing Na^+, Cl^-, and water. Throughout gastric emptying, cholecystokinin and autonomic neural activity cause contraction(s) of the gallbladder along with relaxation of the sphincter of Oddi. The result is a slow, sustained emptying of most of the gallbladder bile into the duodenum. Simultaneously, hepatic bile flow is increased because of the addition of (a) water and bicarbonate secretion and (b) the continuous return of bile acids through the enterohepatic circulation—most of which have just been emptied into the duodenum from the gallbladder.

The electrolyte composition of hepatic bile is similar to that of plasma. Bile also contains cholesterol, bile acids, phospholipid (primarily lecithin), conjugated bilirubin, and protein. Primary bile acids are synthesized from cholesterol in the liver and are conjugated with glycine or taurine before they are excreted in the bile. Conjugated bile acids and lecithin form vesicles and micelles, which bring the cholesterol into solution in bile. The relative concentrations of cholesterol, bile acids, and lecithin must be maintained within a fairly limited range to maintain the cholesterol in solution. A change in their relative concentrations may favor the formation and precipitation of cholesterol crystals (Fig. 17-2). Cholesterol is most soluble in a mixture that contains at least 50% bile acids and smaller amounts of lecithin. Once in the duodenum, bile acids traverse the small intestine; most are returned to the liver through the portal blood where they are reconjugated

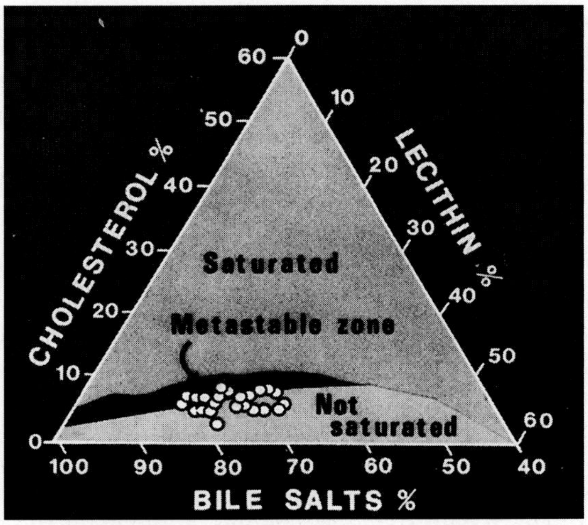

Figure 17-2 The molar percentages of cholesterol, lecithin, and bile salts in bile plotted on triangular coordinates. A relative change in the concentrations of these components can lead to supersaturation of the bile with cholesterol, increasing the likelihood of gallstone formation. In the metastable zone, there is supersaturation of cholesterol, but its precipitation occurs extremely slowly. (Copyright, American Gastroenterological Association, Bethesda, MD. Used with permission.)

and promptly reexcreted. Small amounts of bile acids are reabsorbed passively throughout the small intestine, but most of the reabsorption occurs actively at the level of the terminal ileum. Thus, there is an effective mechanism for enterohepatic circulation of bile acids. Depending on the duration of gastric emptying (e.g., quantity of the meal, fat content), the same bile acid molecules may recirculate two or three times after a meal. Normally, approximately 5% of bile acids escape reabsorption in the ileum. They are deconjugated or dehydroxylated by intestinal bacteria, rendering them less water soluble, or are adsorbed to intraluminal particulate matter. To keep the bile acid pool relatively constant, the lost bile acids are replaced by hepatic synthesis of new bile acids through a negative feedback mechanism. The liver can compensate for a loss of as much as 20% of the bile acid pool by the synthesis of new bile acids. Greater losses lead to a diminished bile acid pool, hence decreasing bile acid concentration and making the bile more lithogenic (prone to stone formation).

Bilirubin is actively excreted by hepatocytes into bile as a conjugated water-soluble diglucuronide (direct bilirubin). This mechanism is responsible for the green-brown color of bile and the brown color of stool. Extrahepatic obstruction to the flow of bile by benign or malignant diseases leads to the accumulation of predominantly conjugated (direct) bilirubin, which is water soluble and is excreted in the urine, making it dark. In contrast, hemolytic diseases, which cause excessive breakdown of heme, and hepatocellular diseases, which preclude adequate conjugation of bilirubin, lead to the accumulation of predominantly unconjugated (indirect) bilirubin, which is fat soluble and is not excreted in the urine.

Bile in the duodenum is important for alkalinizing acid gastric chyme, making luminal contents isoosmolar, and digesting and absorbing fats and the fat-soluble vitamins (A, D, E, and K). Hence, obstructive jaundice or external bile diversion may cause problems with fat assimilation (steatorrhea) and blood coagulation (prolonged prothrombin time secondary to vitamin K malabsorption).

GALLSTONE DISEASE

Pathogenesis of Gallstones (Cholelithiasis)

The most common types of gallstones in the Western population are of the mixed variety, which contain a high proportion of cholesterol. These stones account for approximately 75% of all types of gallstones. Precipitation of cholesterol as crystals tends to occur if the bile is lithogenic and supersaturated with cholesterol. These crystals, in the presence of enucleating factors (an imbalance between nucleation-inhibiting and nucleation-promoting proteins), may agglomerate to form gallstones and entrap other components of bile (e.g., bilirubin, mucus, Ca^{++}) in the process. Most mixed stones do not contain enough calcium to render them radiopaque; thus, they are usually not seen on plain radiographs. Occasionally, a single large stone forms and is composed almost entirely of cholesterol (cholesterol solitaire). Incomplete emptying of the gallbladder (a normal phenomenon) affords ideal conditions for agglomeration; for this reason, most stones form in the gallbladder.

Pigment stones are of two types, black and brown. Black pigment stones account for approximately 20% of all biliary stones and are generally found in the gallbladder. They typically form in sterile gallbladder bile and are commonly associated with hemolytic diseases and cirrhosis. In chronic hemolysis, there is hypersecretion of bilirubin conjugates in the bile and greater secretion of monoglucuronides compared with diglucuronides, which favors the precipitation of pigment stones. In contrast, brown stones are associated with infected bile. They are found primarily in the bile ducts and are soft. Pigment stones often contain enough calcium to render them radiopaque.

Gallbladder sludge is amorphous material that contains mucoprotein, cholesterol crystals, and calcium bilirubinate. It is often associated with prolonged total parenteral nutrition, starvation, or rapid weight loss. Gallbladder sludge may be a precursor of gallstones.

The source of most stones found in the biliary ducts (**choledocholithiasis**) is the gallbladder. However, bile stasis and infection involving the bile ducts predispose to the formation of primary bile duct calculi within the ducts.

Epidemiology of Gallstones

Both genetics and the environment appear to influence the incidence of gallstones. The incidence increases with age, and women are affected approximately three times as often as men are. The prevalence of gallstone disease among white women who are younger than 50 years of age is 5% to 15%; in older women, it is approximately 25%. Among white men who are younger than 50 years of age, the prevalence is 4% to 10%; in older men, it is 10% to 15%. Gallstone disease also tends to cluster in families. Native Americans have an extremely high prevalence of gallstones; more than 50% of men and 80% of women have mixed stones by the age of 60 years. Obesity (excessive cholesterol biosynthesis), multiparity (altered steroid metabolism, lithogenic bile, gallbladder hypomotility), high-dose estrogen oral contraceptives, some cholesterol-lowering agents (alteration of cholesterol and bile acid biosynthesis), rapid weight loss (increased bile saturation index and gallbladder stasis), and prolonged total parenteral nutrition (hyperconcentration of bile and gallbladder stasis) all predispose to the formation of stones. Diseases that diminish the bile acid pool (e.g., Crohn's disease involving the terminal ileum or resection of the terminal ileum) increase the incidence of stones. Patients with hemolytic disorders and alcoholic cirrhosis tend to form pigment stones.

Theoretically, the following manipulations may help to decrease the risk of gallstone formation: avoiding obesity (see above); following a high-fiber diet (to diminish the enterohepatic circulation of dehydroxylated bile acids); eating meals at regular intervals (to diminish gallbladder storage time); and eating foods with low levels of saturated fatty acids (to diminish the nucleation of lithogenic bile).

Diagnostic Evaluation

History and Physical Examination

In patients who have symptoms that suggest biliary tract disease, the differential diagnosis can be narrowed by obtaining the pertinent history and performing an accurate physical examination. The history may provide valuable clues that point to either an acute or a chronic condition. If the patient is jaundiced, the history can suggest either obstructive or hepatocellular disease and may indicate an underlying malignancy. Specific physical findings may also yield useful information that can help with the differential diagnosis.

The hallmark of chronic gallstone disease is pain, described as **biliary colic.** The pain is usually steady, fairly severe, and located in the epigastrium or the right upper quadrant of the abdomen sometimes going through to the back at the same level. The pain is visceral, often described as dull or aching, poorly localized, and may last from 1 to 4 hours. The cause of the pain is transient obstruction of the cystic duct by a gallstone. The pain is secondary to increased pressure in the gallbladder that results from contraction against a stone that is impacted in the cystic duct (ball-valve effect). Typical biliary colic is caused by obstruction and is not associated with acute inflammation or infection. The pain tends to occur postprandially, but it may have no relation to meals, and may awaken the patient at night. The pain can occur after any meal, but larger meals and those that contain fat are most likely to cause pain. Biliary pain is seldom relieved by anything but time or potent analgesics. Nausea and vomiting may accompany this episodic pain. The patient is well before the onset of pain and then again within minutes to a few hours after the pain subsides.

Acute inflammation or infection involving the gallbladder causes sharp, steady, well-localized pain in the right upper quadrant of the abdomen or in the epigastrium. The pain lasts longer than 3 to 4 hours and may continue for several days. It is mediated by somatic sensory nerves, with cortical localization. It is often accompanied by nausea, vomiting, and systemic manifestations of an inflammatory process.

In patients with jaundice, the presence of light-colored stools and dark, tea-colored urine suggests extrahepatic biliary obstruction. In the presence of this combination, severe or sharp pain suggests a benign etiology for the jaundice (e.g., calculous disease of the biliary tract). In contrast, patients with malignancies (e.g., carcinoma of the pancreas) generally have dull, vague, or insignificant upper abdominal pain. A history of marked weight loss is often present in patients with malignant conditions. Pruritus is believed to be caused by high tissue concentrations of reabsorbed conjugated bile acids and is often present in patients with obstructive jaundice.

On examination, a patient with biliary colic appears doubled-up or restless, whereas a patient who has pain associated with inflammation tends to be still because the pain is aggravated by movement. The pulse rate may be high secondary to pain, inflammation, or infection. Fever often accompanies inflammatory conditions, and high fever may be present if complications (e.g., gangrene of the gallbladder, abscess) are present or if the patient has cholangitis. Low blood pressure signifies severe dehydration or septic shock. The abdomen of patients with biliary colic is soft, but some tenderness may be found in the right upper quadrant. Once the pain subsides, the abdomen is nontender between episodes of colic. In **acute cholecystitis,** examination of the abdomen may show a positive **Murphy's sign** (cessation of inspiration because of pain on deep palpitation of the right upper quadrant) when the visceral peritoneum overlying the gallbladder is inflamed. Once the inflammation spreads to the adjacent parietal peritoneum, abdominal examination shows localized guarding and rebound tenderness. A tender mass representing the inflamed gallbladder may also be palpable in the right upper quadrant of the abdomen in acute cholecystitis. The presence of a nontender, palpable gallbladder with jaundice suggests underlying malignant disease, such as carcinoma of the pancreas (**Courvoisier's law**) (see Chapter 18, Pancreas). In such conditions, the gallbladder is passively distended as a result of back pressure caused by the distal malignant obstruction. If a stone is the cause of the distal ductal obstruction, the site of origin of the stone is generally a diseased thick-walled gallbladder, which is incapable of passive distension.

Laboratory Tests

A number of laboratory tests aid in the diagnosis and management of biliary tract disease. The hemoglobin or hematocrit may be elevated if the patient is dehydrated. Leukocytosis with a shift to the left suggests acute inflammation and infection. Serum amylase and lipase may be slightly elevated in both acute cholecystitis and acute cholangitis, but marked elevations suggest acute pancreatitis. Liver function tests are helpful in detecting hyperbilirubinemia and providing information about the underlying disease process. The serum level of unconjugated (indirect) bilirubin increases in hemolytic disorders, whereas the conjugated (direct) fraction is elevated with extrahepatic biliary obstruction or cholestasis. Alkaline phosphatase (ALP) is synthesized by the biliary tract epithelium. Serum alkaline phosphatase levels increase as a result of overproduction in conditions that cause extrahepatic biliary obstruction or, less commonly, from cholestasis resulting from a drug reaction or primary biliary cirrhosis. The serum level of this enzyme is moderately elevated in hepatitis, and it may also be elevated as a result of bone disease. Alkaline phosphatase of hepatobiliary origin may be differentiated from that originating from bone by confirming its heat stability. The concomitant elevation of 5′-nucleotidase or glutamyltranspeptidase (GGT) also indicates that the source of the elevated alkaline phosphatase is the biliary tract. Aspartate aminotransferase (AST) and alanine aminotransferase (ALT) are released from hepatocytes, and serum levels of both enzymes are increased significantly in various types of hepatitis. AST and ALT are also often elevated with biliary obstruction, particularly when it is acute. As a rule, however, the increase in alkaline phosphatase and GGT are greater than the increase in the levels of AST and ALT in biliary obstruction. The converse suggests hepatitis. If the biliary ductal system is partially obstructed (e.g., by a primary or metastatic neoplasm), alkaline phosphatase is released into the serum from the obstructed ducts, but the serum bilirubin may be normal. International normalized ratio (INR) is often elevated (prothrombin time is often prolonged) in patients with obstructive jaundice as a result of the malabsorption of vitamin K. In obstructive jaundice, the water-soluble conjugated (direct) bilirubin is excreted in the urine. On the other hand, urobilinogen is produced in the intestine as a result of bacterial metabolism of bilirubin. Then it is reabsorbed from the intestine and secreted in the urine. Bile duct obstruction leads to the reduction of urobilinogen in the urine because the excretion of bilirubin into the intestine is blocked.

Imaging Studies

Imaging studies are very helpful in establishing the definitive diagnosis in patients who have clinical features that suggest biliary disease. They are also useful in a variety of therapeutic interventions. Table 17-1 lists commonly used imaging studies and their diagnostic and therapeutic potential.

Approximately 10% to 15% of gallstones contain sufficient calcium to render them radiopaque. These stones are visible on plain radiographs of the abdomen (Fig. 17-3). Air in the biliary system may be seen as a result of communication between the biliary and gastrointestinal (GI) tracts secondary to a pathologic fistula or a connection created by a previous surgical procedure. Also, air in the lumen or wall of the gallbladder may be seen in **acute emphysematous cholecystitis.**

Ultrasonography is the initial study of choice in most patients with suspected biliary tract disease. For stones in the gallbladder, both the sensitivity and the specificity of this study are approximately 95%. Ultrasonography can successfully detect stones as small as 3 mm in diameter, and sometimes even smaller stones may be seen (Fig. 17-4). However, the study is less helpful for visualizing stones in the bile ducts. Ultrasonography is highly sensitive for detecting dilation of the bile ducts and may provide information on whether the site of biliary obstruction is intrahepatic or extrahepatic. If the gallbladder is distended and the ducts are dilated, the site of obstruction is likely to be distal to the junction of the cystic duct and the common hepatic duct. The finding of a thickened gallbladder wall or a pericholecystic collection of fluid supports the diagnosis of acute cholecystitis. Additionally, ultrasonography provides information about the liver and pancreas. The study is noninvasive,

Table 17-1 Imaging Studies Commonly Used in the Diagnosis and Management of Biliary Disease

Imaging Procedure	Diagnostic or Therapeutic Potential
Plain abdominal radiograph	Calcified gallstone Air in the biliary tree Air in the gallbladder wall or lumen
Ultrasonography	Stones in the gallbladder (possibly in duct) Thickened gallbladder wall Dilation of intrahepatic and extrahepatic ducts Liver lesion Pancreatic mass
Radionuclide scan (HIDA scan)	Filling of gallbladder Filling of bile ducts Passage of bile into the duodenum
Computed tomography (CT)	Pancreatic mass Dilation of intrahepatic and extrahepatic ducts Liver lesion Stones in the gallbladder or bile ducts
Magnetic resonance cholangiography (MRC)	Stones in gallbladder or bile ducts Dilated or structured bile ducts Masses in liver, pancreas, or ducts
Transhepatic cholangiogram (PTC)	Detecting bile duct obstruction Draining obstructed bile duct Bypassing bile duct obstruction with stent Obtaining cytology specimen Detecting bile leak from ducts Extracting bile duct calculus
Endoscopic retrograde cholangiopancreatography (ERCP)	Detecting bile duct obstruction Draining obstructed bile duct Inserting stent to bypass obstruction or control bile leak Detecting pancreatic duct obstruction Obtaining cytology specimen Detecting bile leak from ducts Extracting bile duct calculus Obtaining biopsy of a neoplasm Performing sphincterotomy

quick, relatively inexpensive, and does not entail the use of radiation. The **oral cholecystogram** has been replaced by ultrasonography for routine workup of patients with biliary colic.

Radionuclide biliary scanning (HIDA scan) involves the intravenous injection of a ^{99m}technetium-labeled derivative of iminodiacetic acid. The radionuclide is excreted by the liver into the bile in high concentrations. Then it enters the gallbladder (if the cystic duct is patent) and duodenum. The normal gallbladder begins to fill within 30 minutes. Visualization of the common bile duct and duodenum without filling of the gallbladder after 4 hours indicates cystic duct obstruction, which supports the diagnosis of acute cholecystitis (Fig. 17-5). The sensitivity and specificity of the HIDA scan for diagnosing acute cholecystitis are 95% to 97% and 90% to 97%, respectively. False-positive results may occur in patients who are receiving total parenteral nutrition or those who have hepatitis. The scan is also of value in identifying a suspected bile leak after surgery. However, the HIDA scan is not useful for showing stones in either the gallbladder or the common bile duct. The study can be successfully performed even when the serum bilirubin level is moderately elevated.

In patients with jaundice, particularly with dilated ducts and evidence of extrahepatic obstruction on ultrasonography, detailed radiographic visualization of the biliary ductal anatomy may be helpful in confirming the diagnosis and planning therapy. Direct injection of contrast agent into the ducts is necessary in these cases. This may be achieved by performing a **percutaneous transhepatic cholangiogram (PTC)** or an **endoscopic retrograde cholangiopancreatogram (ERCP)**. PTC involves inserting a thin needle through the skin and body wall, into the liver parenchyma, and injecting contrast medium directly into the intrahepatic bile ducts. Dilated bile ducts facilitate this procedure, yielding a success rate of more than 95%. If

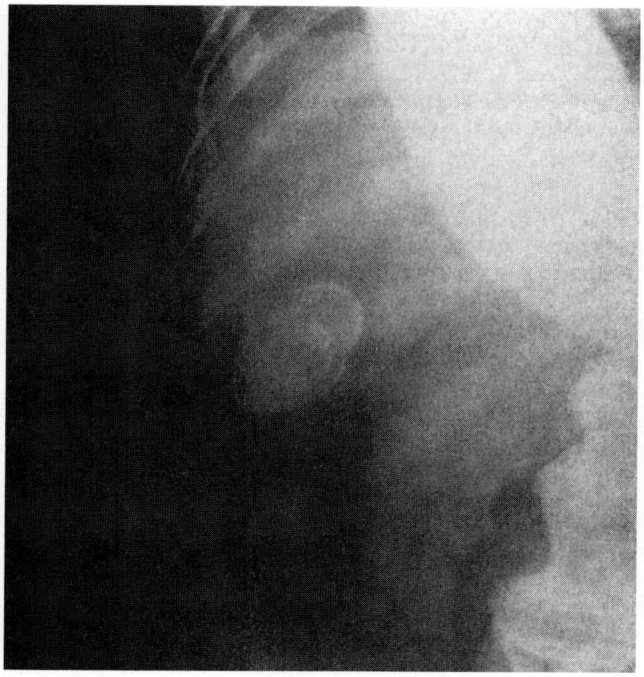

Figure 17-3 Plain radiograph of the abdomen showing gallstones (frequency < 10%).

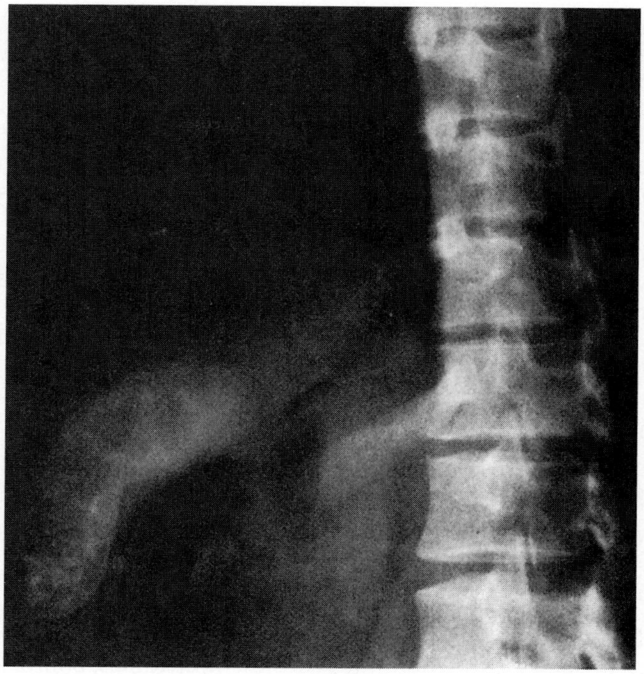

Figure 17-5 Oral cholecystogram showing gallstones.

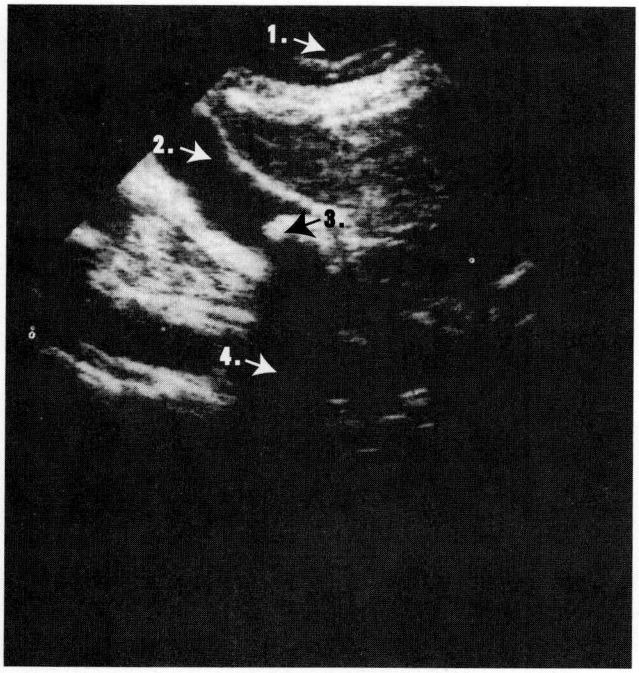

Figure 17-4 Ultrasound of the gallbladder showing gallstones. 1. Anterior abdominal wall; 2. Gallbladder; 3. Stones; 4. Acoustic shadow.

the ducts are of normal caliber, the test is successful only 70% to 80% of the time. PTC is particularly valuable for visualizing the proximal ductal system. It can also be used to obtain a cytologic diagnosis, extract stones, and aid in the placement of a biliary drainage catheter into the obstructed bile ducts. ERCP requires a skilled endoscopist, who cannulates the sphincter of Oddi and injects contrast medium to obtain a picture of the biliary and pancreatic ductal anatomy. This study is particularly valuable in patients who have bile ducts of normal size and in those with suspected ampullary lesions because a diagnostic biopsy specimen can also be obtained in the latter situation. Further, endoscopic brushing of an obstructed site may provide a cytologic diagnosis. In addition, ERCP can be used to perform a sphincterotomy, which involves cutting the sphincter of Oddi with an electrosurgical current through a wire attached to the ERCP catheter. This facilitates the extraction of biliary calculi and placing a stent through an area of bile duct obstruction. If coagulopathy is present, it must be corrected before either PTC or ERCP.

Computed tomography (CT) scan is especially helpful in identifying the level and cause of a biliary obstruction and in imaging neoplasms. Specific anatomic definition of their size, position, and spread by the CT scan greatly assists in planning curative or palliative therapy. Also, percutaneous needle aspiration (cytology) or small-core needle biopsy (histology) performed with the aid of a CT scan can help in establishing a definitive diagnosis. CT scan is not the preferred test for the diagnosis of cholelithiasis because of its lower sensitivity in detecting gallstones, its higher cost compared with ultrasonography, and its use of radiation.

Magnetic resonance cholangiography (MRC) refers to selected MR imaging of the biliary and pancreatic ducts, which is helpful in demonstrating common duct stones and other biliary tract abnormalities. It is beginning to replace diagnostic PTC and ERCP for this purpose. Open field MR technology may allow therapeutic manipulations, presently performed by PTC, in the future. The obvious advantages of this diagnostic procedure are that it is noninvasive and does not involve the use of radiography.

Intravenous cholangiography (IVC) has been replaced by more modern tests.

Figure 17-6 shows an algorithm for the evaluation of a jaundiced patient.

Clinical Presentation and Treatment of Gallstone Disease

Asymptomatic Gallstones

Many individuals have asymptomatic gallstones that remain silent throughout life. Of these individuals, approximately 1% to 2% per year will develop symptoms or complications of gallstone disease. Thus, two-thirds of these people remain free of symptoms or complications after 20 years. Although complications secondary to gallstones may occur at any time, most patients experience symptoms for some time before a complication develops. Thus, in adults, prophylactic cholecystectomy is not indicated for asymptomatic gallstones. However, after patients have symptoms of biliary colic, they are at increased risk for complications and should consider elective cholecystectomy. The risk of gallbladder carcinoma in patients with gallstones is too low to justify cholecystectomy for asymptomatic gallstones.

Chronic Cholecystitis

Biliary colic is the classic and most common symptom associated with chronic calculous cholecystitis. Characteristic features of biliary colic were described earlier. Nausea and vomiting may accompany this pain. Other associated symptoms include intolerance to fatty foods, flatulence, belching, and indigestion. These symptoms are encompassed by the collective term dyspepsia. However, the symptoms of dyspepsia are nonspecific and may be second-

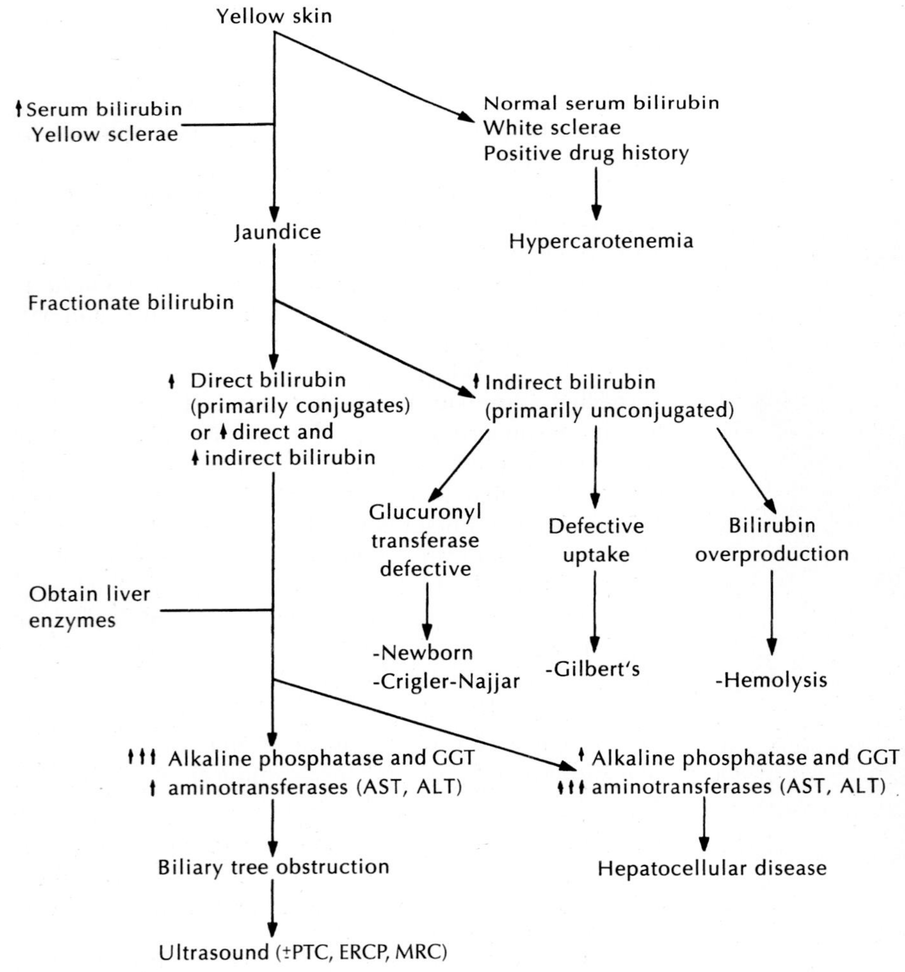

Figure 17-6 Algorithm for the evaluation of a jaundiced patient. PTC, percutaneous transhepatic cholangiogram; ERCP, endoscopic retrograde cholonagiopancreatogram.

ary to other diseases. Because the condition is not associated with acute infection, fever and chills are absent. In contrast to patients who have acute inflammatory conditions, patients with biliary colic are typically not still and are often doubled-up or writhing during the episode of pain. Palpation of the abdomen during the episode of biliary colic may elicit tenderness in the right upper quadrant or the epigastrium, but there are no clinical signs of peritoneal irritation. The abdomen is generally soft, and bowel sounds are active. Between episodes of biliary colic, the abdomen shows no specific abnormality. The differential diagnosis includes angina pectoris, peptic ulcer disease, gastroesophageal reflux, ureteral obstruction, and irritable bowel syndrome.

Because biliary colic is not associated with acute inflammation, the total and differential leukocyte counts are within the normal range. In addition, liver function tests may be entirely normal. Typically, biliary colic is distinguished from acute cholecystitis by the presence of the characteristic clinical features described previously and by the absence of leukocytosis or a "shift to the left." Ultrasonography is the preferred study for evaluation of the biliary tract in these patients. If the results of ultrasonography are equivocal, it should be repeated at an interval. ERCP with collection of bile for examination of microlithiasis is recommended for the very occasional patient who presents with a clinical picture of biliary colic but has negative findings on ultrasonography.

Management of the episode of biliary colic includes administration of parenteral analgesics, for severe pain, and observation. After cholelithiasis is confirmed, the optimum treatment is elective cholecystectomy. In most cases, the laparoscopic approach is used. An intraoperative **cholangiogram** may be added to evaluate the biliary ducts for stones (if these are suspected). If the operative cholangiogram performed during the laparoscopic cholecystectomy shows common duct calculi, the duct should be explored, or the patient may be referred subsequently for ERCP and sphincterotomy to extract the stones.

In patients with comorbid conditions that preclude the performance of safe cholecystectomy and in those who refuse surgery, oral dissolution therapy may be considered. Ursodeoxycholic acid is the most desirable agent. However, the stones should be small and composed mainly of cholesterol (floating, radiolucent stones), within a functioning gallbladder. Oral dissolution therapy, which may take 6 to 12 months to dissolve the stones, yields a dissolution rate of 90% for stones smaller than 5 mm and a dissolution rate of 60% for calculi smaller than 10 mm. However, in approximately 50% of these patients, the gallstones recur within 5 years of discontinuing the therapy. **Extracorporeal shock wave lithotripsy (ESWL)** has been used to manage gallstone disease in selected patients, but support for this procedure has waned with the rise in popularity of laparoscopic cholecystectomy.

Acute Cholecystitis

The underlying pathology in acute cholecystitis is similar to that of biliary colic associated with chronic cholecystitis, except that there is sustained obstruction of the cystic duct in this condition. Thus, the gallbladder becomes progressively more distended and inflamed. As the disease progresses, inflammation extends beyond the visceral peritoneum overlying the gallbladder to involve the parietal peritoneum. Complications of empyema, gangrene, or perforation of the gallbladder may result from progression of the disease process and bacterial involvement. Most patients with acute cholecystitis have a history of biliary colic or dyspepsia. The pain of acute cholecystitis is constant. It is located in the right upper quadrant of the abdomen or the epigastrium and may radiate to the back. Nausea and vomiting are common. The patient is usually febrile, but the fever rarely exceeds 38.3°C (101°F) unless a complication has supervened. On examination, the patient has tenderness in the right upper quadrant and a positive Murphy's sign. Once inflammation progresses to involve the parietal peritoneum, the patient has rebound tenderness and guarding. A tender mass is palpable in the right upper quadrant in approximately 20% of cases. Generalized peritonitis with rebound tenderness may be present if the disease has progressed to free perforation. Free uncontained perforation with spillage of the gallbladder contents into the peritoneal cavity occurs in fewer than 1% to 2% of patients with acute cholecystitis.

The differential diagnosis includes acute pancreatitis, penetrating peptic ulcer (erosion into the pancreas), perforated peptic ulcer, and acute appendicitis. A careful history and physical will lead to an accurate diagnosis in most patients. Laboratory studies show leukocytosis (with a total leukocyte count of approximately 12,000 to 15,000/mL), and a "shift to the left." Many patients with acute cholecystitis have mild hyperbilirubinemia. If the patient has high levels of serum bilirubin, stones in the common bile duct should be suspected; mild increases in serum AST, ALT, and alkaline phosphatase are usually present, and the serum amylase and lipase levels may also be moderately elevated.

Radiologic studies should include plain radiographs of the chest and abdomen. Upright views are necessary to exclude pneumoperitoneum from another underlying cause of the acute abdomen. Plain radiographs may also show gallstones if they are radiopaque. However, the finding of stones does not in itself establish the diagnosis of acute cholecystitis. Ultrasonography is very helpful in making a definitive diagnosis. In addition to detecting gallstones with a high degree of accuracy, the study often shows specific characteristic findings of acute cholecystitis, such as a distended gallbladder, thickened gallbladder wall (> 3 to 4 mm), pericholecystic fluid collection, and ultrasonographic Murphy's sign. This sign is elicited by demonstrating the presence of the most tender spot directly over the sonographically localized gallbladder with the ultrasound probe. This sign is present in 98% of patients with acute cholecystitis. Ultrasonography can also provide additional information about the liver, intrahepatic bile ducts, common bile duct, and pancreas.

HIDA scan is very useful in confirming the diagnosis

of acute cholecystitis in cases in which ultrasonography shows gallstones, without other ultrasonographic evidence to support the diagnosis. Nonvisualization of the gallbladder after 4 hours of the study indicates cystic duct obstruction and is interpreted as positive for acute cholecystitis. However, certain patients (e.g., individuals receiving total parenteral nutrition, those who have fasted for a long time) may demonstrate nonvisualization of the gallbladder on HIDA scan, yielding a false-positive result. Therefore, ultrasonography is preferred over HIDA scanning as the initial definitive radiologic study to confirm acute cholecystitis.

The initial management of acute cholecystitis includes a regimen of nothing by mouth, administering intravenous fluids, and starting antibiotic therapy. The bacteria commonly associated with acute cholecystitis are *Escherichia coli, Klebsiella pneumoniae, Streptococcus faecalis,* and *Clostridium welchii* or *Clostridium perfringens.* Severe cases require broad antibiotic coverage, sometimes with multiple agents, to cover a wide spectrum of Gram-negative aerobes and enterococcus. Parenteral analgesics may be administered judiciously after the diagnosis is confirmed and further plans for therapy are made. A nasogastric tube is inserted if the patient has abdominal distension (with paralytic ileus) or is vomiting.

The optimum approach to treatment includes early cholecystectomy within 3 days of the onset of symptoms. This approach prevents complications (e.g., perforation, gangrene) and makes the surgical procedure easier than if it were performed later in the course of the disease, when the inflammatory reaction and edema are more severe. However, the timing of the operation must be based on other factors as well. It should be delayed if major medical problems must be addressed and performed earlier if perforation or abscess is suspected. The cholecystectomy may be performed laparoscopically, but this approach should be converted to an open one if bleeding or poor definition of the anatomy leads to technical difficulty. Overall, operations for acute cholecystitis are associated with slightly higher mortality and morbidity rates compared with those for chronic cholecystitis, often as a result of underlying cardiovascular, pulmonary, or metabolic disease.

Patients with acute cholecystitis who are too ill to undergo cholecystectomy may require **cholecystostomy**. This procedure involves the removal of the gallbladder contents with continuous drainage of the gallbladder. Percutaneous cholecystostomy under radiologic or ultrasound guidance is preferred to the surgical approach.

Acute gangrenous cholecystitis is associated with a morbidity rate of 16% to 25% and a mortality rate of 20% to 25%. Patients with this condition tend to be older and generally have more serious comorbid conditions than patients with nongangrenous cholecystitis. These patients usually present with a more serious systematic illness with a higher leukocytosis. Local perforation may be seen on ultrasound or HIDA scan. Treatment includes stabilization of the medical condition, administration of broad-spectrum antibiotics, and performance of emergency cholecystostomy or cholecystectomy.

Acute emphysematous cholecystitis results from gas-forming bacteria and is associated with a higher risk of gangrene and perforation compared with nonemphysematous cholecystitis. It generally affects older individuals, and diabetes mellitus is present in 20% to 50% of these patients. The classic findings on plain radiographs include air within the wall or lumen of the gallbladder, air–fluid level within the lumen of the gallbladder, or air in the pericholecystic tissues. Air in the bile ducts may also be seen. Patients with acute emphysematous cholecystitis should receive broad-spectrum antibiotics, including coverage for anaerobes. In addition, they should undergo emergency cholecystectomy.

Although most patients with acute cholecystitis have associated calculi, acute cholecystitis can occur without calculi. **Acute acalculous cholecystitis** may complicate the course of a patient who is being treated for other conditions in a medical or surgical intensive care unit. Many patients are receiving total parenteral nutrition and mechanical ventilatory support and have received blood transfusions. Establishing the diagnosis of acute acalculous cholecystitis can present significant difficulty. The clinical features resemble those of acute calculous cholecystitis; however, the patient often cannot give a coherent history, and the associated conditions result in complex physical findings that are less revealing and more difficult to interpret. Ultrasonography or CT scan are helpful in establishing the diagnosis. Ultrasonography may show gallbladder distension, thickened gallbladder wall, pericholecystic fluid, and a sonographic Murphy's sign. HIDA scan may help to establish the diagnosis, but it often yields a false-positive result and is associated with a specificity of only 38% in such cases. After the diagnosis is established, the management is similar to that of patients with acute calculous cholecystitis. However, patients with acute acalculous cholecystitis are more likely to be candidates for percutaneous or operative cholecystostomy (instead of cholecystectomy) in view of their associated medical problems and higher risk for perioperative complications.

Choledocholithiasis and Acute Cholangitis

In approximately 15% of patients with gallstones, the stones pass through the cystic duct and enter the common bile duct, resulting in choledocholithiasis. Although the smaller stones that enter the common bile duct can progress further into the duodenum, choledocholithiasis may lead to sequelae associated with significant morbidity and mortality (e.g., cholangitis, pancreatitis).

Patients with choledocholithiasis often have a history of previous episodes of biliary colic. The characteristic feature in the clinical presentation is jaundice accompanied by light-colored stools and dark, tea-colored urine. The jaundice associated with choledocholithiasis typically fluctuates in intensity compared with the progressive jaundice caused by malignant disease. If infection supervenes,

acute cholangitis will develop. It is characterized by jaundice, right upper quadrant abdominal pain, and fever associated with chills (**Charcot's triad**). The condition can become further complicated with the presence of pus in the biliary ducts, resulting in **acute suppurative cholangitis**. In this condition, the patient may also have hypotension and mental confusion in addition to Charcot's triad. These five features together constitute **Reynold's pentad**.

On examination, a patient with choledocholithiasis appears deeply jaundiced if a stone is obstructing the duct. Fever is characteristically associated with acute cholangitis and acute suppurative cholangitis; however, septic and debilitated patients may have hypothermia. Examination of the abdomen may be unremarkable in a patient with choledocholithiasis or may reveal tenderness (without a palpable mass) in the right upper quadrant if cholangitis is present. Rebound tenderness is not usually found, even in the presence of acute cholangitis. Bowel sounds are generally audible and may even be normal.

The differential diagnosis in patients with obstructive jaundice or cholangitis includes choledocholithiasis, malignancy (e.g., carcinoma of the pancreas, bile ducts, or gallbladder), and stricture.

The diagnostic workup of jaundice associated with probable choledocholithiasis starts with laboratory studies described previously. In patients with cholangitis, the leukocyte count is elevated, with a shift to the left. Bile duct obstruction leads to elevation in total bilirubin, with a predominance of the direct fraction, marked elevation of serum alkaline phosphatase and GGT, and mild elevations of AST and ALT. Serum amylase and lipase may also be moderately elevated. Ultrasonography is the best initial imaging study in patients with choledocholithiasis and cholangitis. It often shows dilated intrahepatic and extrahepatic ducts along with the presence of gallbladder stones, suggesting that stones are the likely cause of the common duct obstruction. As stated previously, stones in the common bile duct are frequently missed on ultrasonography. PTC, ERCP, and MRC are the best studies to define the specific site and determine the source of the bile duct obstruction. Figure 17-7 shows a PTC demonstrating the typical meniscus sign in the distal common bile duct, indicating that the obstruction is secondary to stones. ERCP may be very useful for extracting stones from the common bile duct.

The management of patients with choledocholithiasis varies with the clinical situation. A patient with choledocholithiasis without evidence of cholangitis should undergo elective extraction of stones from the common duct. Extraction may be achieved endoscopically (through ERCP and sphincterotomy) or operatively. The management of acute cholangitis, especially acute suppurative cholangitis, requires urgent intervention, and septic shock (if present) necessitates prompt resuscitation. A patient with cholangitis is started on a regimen of nothing by mouth, administration of intravenous fluids, and antibiotic therapy after blood cultures are obtained. The broad spectrum of aerobic and anaerobic bacteria listed in the section

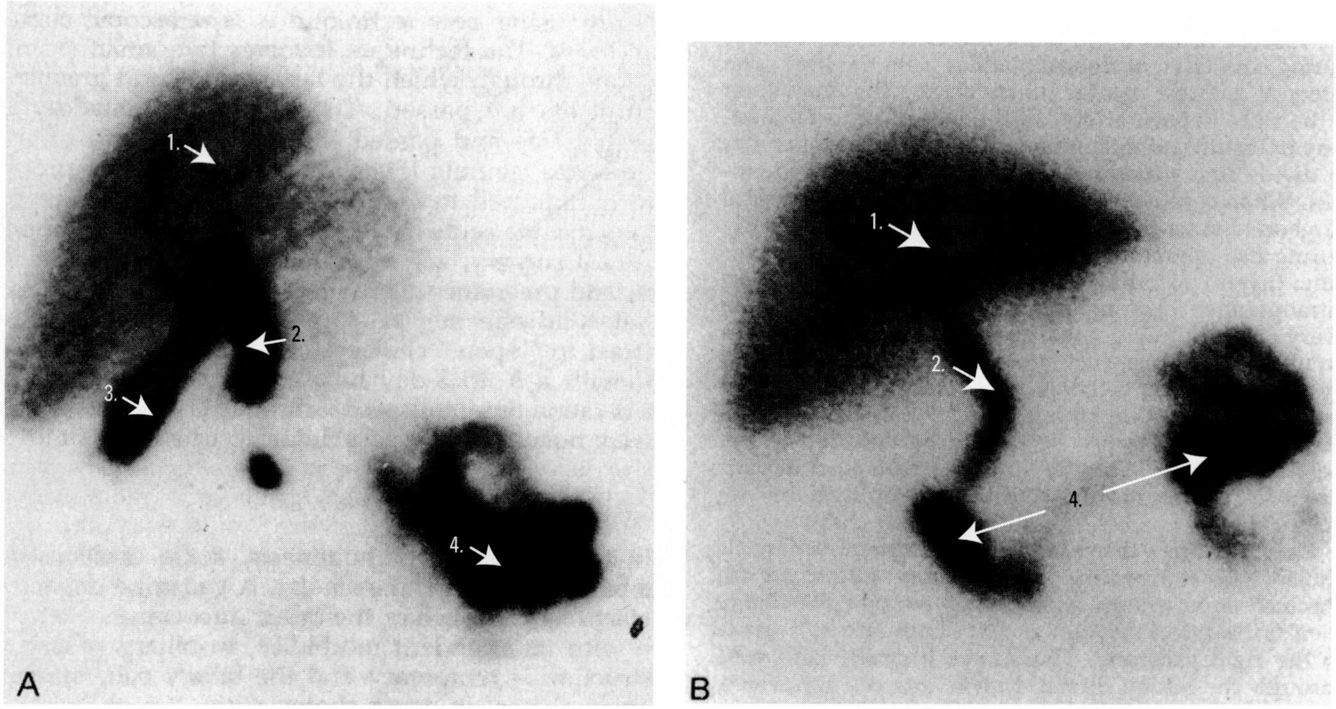

Figure 17-7 Radionuclide biliary (HIDA) scans. **A,** With and **B,** without visualization of the gallbladder. 1. Liver; 2. Common bile duct; 3. Gallbladder; 4. Activity in intestine.

on acute cholecystitis as well as *Enterobacter* and *Pseudomonas* species must be considered in selecting the appropriate antibiotic coverage. Any clotting abnormalities should be corrected by giving parenteral vitamin K or administering fresh frozen plasma before an invasive procedure. Vomiting or abdominal distension resulting from paralytic ileus necessitates the insertion of a nasogastric tube. More than 70% of patients with cholangitis respond to this regimen, thus allowing for completion of the workup and adequate planning for the definitive treatment, which includes extraction of stones from the common bile duct and cholecystectomy. If a patient does not respond to this therapy, urgent decompression of the bile duct through ERCP, PTC, or open surgery can be lifesaving. Patients with acute suppurative cholangitis require urgent decompression of the common bile duct after the initial resuscitation and administration of broad-spectrum antibiotics.

When stones are detected in the bile duct by any type of cholangiography before cholecystectomy, the calculi can be removed by ERCP and sphincterotomy, and the patient can then undergo elective laparoscopic cholecystectomy. The success rate with ERCP and sphincterotomy in these cases is greater than 90%, with a complication rate of approximately 10%. If the surgeon is experienced in advanced laparoscopic biliary surgery, laparoscopic cholecystectomy and extraction of the bile duct calculi through the cystic duct or choledochotomy is an option. Open bile duct exploration is still a good option, but endoscopic or laparoscopic stone removal is becoming the procedure of choice. If the gallbladder was previously removed, the bile duct calculi should be removed endoscopically with ERCP and sphincterotomy. Lithotripsy can be used to break large stones. The fragments can then pass spontaneously or be removed with ERCP and sphincterotomy or PTC. If the stones cannot be removed by these methods, an open procedure is necessary.

Acute Biliary (Gallstone) Pancreatitis

Approximately 60% of nonalcoholic patients with acute pancreatitis have associated gallstones. Although the occurrence of **acute biliary (gallstone) pancreatitis** may be attributed to transient or persistent obstruction of the ampulla of Vater by a large stone, passage of small stones and biliary sludge, rather than the impaction of a large stone, is often the cause of the pancreatitis. Patients with acute biliary pancreatitis have the classic clinical picture of pancreatitis; however, the serum amylase and lipase levels may be very high compared to patients with alcoholic pancreatitis, who may have less functioning pancreatic tissue because of chronic alcohol consumption.

Management of patients with acute biliary pancreatitis includes initial resuscitation and supportive care, with correction of any existing fluid deficits and treatment of respiratory insufficiency, if present. Antibiotics are added for severe pancreatitis and for the management of septic complications. Parenteral analgesics may be administered once the diagnosis is made and treatment is initiated. Determination of the severity of the disease and estimation of prognosis are carried out using the same criteria as for alcoholic pancreatitis. A definitive operation should be performed after the patient improves clinically, preferably during the same hospitalization. This procedure includes cholecystectomy, cholangiography, and extraction of stones from the common bile duct if any are detected on the cholangiogram. Acute pancreatitis recurs in 25% to 60% of patients if a definitive operation is not performed at this time. However, the operation should be delayed in patients with very severe pancreatitis unless infected pancreatic necrosis or cholangitis is present, both of which occur infrequently in patients with acute biliary pancreatitis. Progression of the disease despite conservative management may necessitate urgent ERCP and sphincterotomy.

Gallstone Ileus

Although **gallstone ileus** accounts for only 1% to 3% of all cases of intestinal obstruction, the condition is the cause of nonstrangulated small intestinal obstruction in approximately 25% of patients older than 70 years of age. It occurs more commonly in women than in men (3.5:1 ratio). Gallstone ileus results from the erosion of a large stone through the gallbladder directly into the small intestine, creating an internal fistula between the gallbladder and the intestinal tract, usually at the level of duodenum. Passage of the stone along the length of the small intestine may cause episodes of partial small bowel obstruction until the stone becomes impacted in a narrow portion of the intestine, usually in the distal ileum just proximal to the ileocecal valve. A history of biliary colic or gallstone disease suggests the diagnosis. Patients present with the clinical picture of small intestinal obstruction; however, the intermittent nature of the obstruction in the early stages (before impaction of the stone) often results in delay in the diagnosis.

Plain radiographs of the abdomen show findings of small intestinal obstruction and may show air in the biliary tree. Occasionally, a large stone has sufficient calcium to be seen in the intestine. Ultrasonography is useful in detecting gallstones and may even reveal the offending stone, although it may be difficult to visualize because of the overlying gas-containing loops of intestine. Barium study of the small intestine may demonstrate the biliary-enteric fistula and confirm the distal small intestinal obstruction. CT with oral contrast is becoming the preferred diagnostic test, because it can demonstrate all the features best: air in the biliary tree, biliary-enteric fistula, site of obstruction, and the obstructing stone. However, even with the availability of imaging studies, the correct diagnosis of gallstone ileus as the cause of small intestinal obstruction is made preoperatively in less than one-half of patients.

Appropriate management of gallstone ileus includes celiotomy and enterolithotomy (extraction of the stone from the small intestine to relieve the obstruction). In a few selected patients who are otherwise healthy, cholecystectomy and definitive correction of the internal fistula may also be performed. Because most patients with gallstone ileus are elderly and have other comorbid conditions, cholecystectomy and correction of the fistula are dangerous and unnecessary. The mortality rate remains high because of the frequent coexistence of medical problems (e.g., cardiac disease, diabetes mellitus, obesity). There is also a high risk of postoperative wound infection.

GALLBLADDER CANCER

Gallbladder cancer accounts for less than 2% of all malignant tumors. It generally occurs in the elderly and is more common in women than in men. Gallbladder cancers tend to spread early through direct ingrowth into the liver and adjacent structures in the porta hepatis, and by metastasizing to the regional lymph nodes and liver. Histologically, most such cancers are adenocarcinomas.

Early-stage disease is asymptomatic. Most early-stage tumors are found incidentally by the pathologist on histologic review of a gallbladder removed for gallstone disease. An association with such chronic inflammatory conditions as chronic cholecystitis or gallstone ileus has been postulated. However, as most chronically inflamed gallbladders do not go on to become malignant, cholecystectomy should not be offered as prophylaxis against malignancy. Indeed, even the presence of a calcified gallbladder wall on plain film or CT (the porcelain gallbladder)—once thought to be highly associated with future malignancy—has been found to have this consequence much less often than initially described.

Patients with more advanced gallbladder cancer may have vague right upper quadrant pain, weight loss, and malaise. Jaundice is present in approximately 50% of such patients. Physical examination may show a mass in the right upper quadrant of the abdomen.

Because of its rarity, however, gallbladder cancer is seldom suspected preoperatively, since these symptoms overlap substantially with those of calculous disease.

Disease localized to the peritonealized surface of the gallbladder is effectively treated with cholecystectomy. Larger tumors, or those that abut the liver parenchyma, are treated with wedge resection of the gallbladder fossa and liver bed, with regional lymphadenectomy. Porta hepatis lymphadenectomy lacks the standardization associated with other abdominal lymphadenectomies, because of the proximity of vital structures and the organ's lack of a mobile mesentery. Moreover, despite radical approaches, the 5-year survival rate remains poor (less than 5% at 5 years) unless the cancer is detected incidentally as a small focus within a gallbladder removed for symptomatic stone disease.

EXTRAHEPATIC BILE DUCT MALIGNANCIES

Cancer of the extrahepatic bile ducts is uncommon, with an autopsy incidence of 0.01% to 0.5%. It occurs with equal frequency in both sexes, usually affecting individuals between 50 and 70 years of age. As with gallbladder cancer, chronic inflammatory processes often precede the development of overt malignancy. The risk of bile duct malignancy is significantly higher in patients with ulcerative colitis and sclerosing cholangitis. Other risk factors include choledochal cyst and parasitic disease. Approximately one-third of patients with bile duct carcinoma have associated gallstones. Bile duct tumors are usually well circumscribed, and two-thirds of these carcinomas are located above the junction of the cystic duct with the common hepatic duct. Histologically, the lesions are usually mucin-producing adenocarcinomas. In general, bile duct cancers are slow-growing, locally advanced tumors that rarely metastasize to distant sites. However, because of the anatomic relationships of the extrahepatic ducts to the liver, portal vein, and hepatic artery, curative resection of these lesions is the exception rather than the rule.

Common symptoms relate to local growth, impingement on the liver, and obliteration of the ductal lumina. They include jaundice, weight loss, abdominal pain, and pruritis; fever is less common. In contrast to the fluctuating jaundice that is often seen in patients with common duct calculi, the jaundice associated with bile duct cancers is progressive. On physical examination, hepatomegaly may be found. A palpable, nontender gallbladder in a jaundiced patient indicates that the site of the obstructing tumor is distal to the junction of the cystic duct with the common duct (**Courvoisier's law**) (see Chapter 18, Pancreas). Distal bile duct malignancies presenting in this manner thus mimic the symptoms of pancreatic tumors.

Laboratory studies show a typical picture of obstructive jaundice, making ultrasound and measurement of fractionated bilirubin good initial studies. Most patients have dilated intrahepatic ducts. However, the absence of intrahepatic ductal dilation does not rule out obstruction, since ducts may be of normal caliber because of incomplete obstruction, tumor ingrowth, or sclerosing cholangitis. Ultrasound, CT scanning, and MR imaging are helpful in determining the extrahepatic extent of the tumors and providing information about their resectability and invasion of adjacent structures. PTC and ERCP are very helpful in demonstrating lesions, assessing intraductal tumor extent, and obtaining cytologic specimens. PTC is particularly useful for evaluation of the proximal lesions and establishing antegrade access for stenting of operative ductal reconstructions (e.g., choledochojejunostomy).

Tumors in the proximal one-third of the ductal system may require resection of both the left and right hepatic ducts with a Roux-en-Y hepaticojejunostomy. If resection is not possible, the tumor may be percutaneously traversed with a guide wire and a hollow stent passed through it to relieve the biliary obstruction. Resection of bile duct cancers offers the best chance of survival, although the prognosis after resection of these proximal lesions is poor, with 5-year survival rate of only 5% at best.

Middle-third tumors are best treated by resection and Roux-en-Y hepaticojejunostomy. The 5-year survival rate after resection of middle-third lesions is approximately 10%. Like proximal lesions, unresectable tumors may be bypassed operatively or the lumen held open with a stent placed via a percutaneous or retrograde approach. The operation of choice for distal common duct tumors is the Whipple procedure, which involves resecting the distal common duct (with the tumor), the pancreatic head, and the entire duodenum. Three anastomoses, connecting pancreatic remnant, hepatic duct, and proximal GI tract in sequence to a mobilized length of jejunum, must be performed after the resection. The 5-year survival rate after a Whipple procedure for a lesion of the distal third of the common bile duct is approximately 30% to 40%. If resection is not possible, palliation can be achieved through an internal surgical bypass (Roux-en-Y choledochojejunostomy) or prosthetic stent insertion. If unresectability is determined at operation rather than through preoperative studies, the creation of an operative bypass obviates the need for an indwelling prosthesis and its potential occlusion.

CONGENITAL CHOLEDOCHAL CYSTS

Very uncommonly, cystic enlargements of the bile ducts occur that are thought to be congenital. These are more frequent in females (4:1 female:male) and often present in the late teens or early 20s as pain and jaundice or even as an upper abdominal mass. These enlargements should be diagnosed when imaging studies detect marked extrahepatic ductal dilation in young adults in the absence of any cause of obstruction. Recommended surgical management is total excision with Roux-en-Y hepaticojejunostomy. Continued followup of these patients is important, since anastomotic structures can occur and choledochal cysts are associated with an increased risk of bile duct cancer (see Chapter 3, Pediatric Surgery, in Lawrence et al., eds., *Essentials of Surgical Specialties*, 3rd Ed.).

BILE DUCT INJURY AND STRICTURE

Because bile ducts have a low elastin content, little redundancy, and a poor blood supply ascending through the hepaticoduodenal ligament, injury can be potentially disastrous. More than 90% of bile duct strictures result from iatrogenic injury during an operative procedure. Most severe injuries in current practice involve the common duct, the hepatic duct, or the confluence of the left and right hepatic ducts. Approximately 75% of injuries occur during simple cholecystectomy and involve division of the bile duct and its vasculature close to the duodenum. This underscores the importance of recognizing the anatomic variations of the biliary tree correctly and proceeding in a cautious systematic fashion, even during routine cholecystectomy. The incidence of bile duct injuries associated with laparoscopic cholecystectomy is higher than that associated with open cholecystectomy, a trend that should decrease with each surgeon's experience and with all new surgeons thoroughly trained in the laparoscopic approach. Unfortunately, many iatrogenic injuries go unrecognized until they declare themselves as a subhepatic collection, iatrogenic occlusion, or delayed stricture formation.

When bile duct injury or anomaly is suspected intraoperatively, cholangiography should be performed. Injuries to ducts smaller than 3 mm that drain a small amount of liver parenchyma may be ligated. If the injured duct is 4 mm or larger, laparotomy is performed, and immediate operative repair occurs. If there is no loss of length, avulsion, or devascularization, primary repair of a simple ductal injury may be performed. A T-tube stent is placed and brought out through another location in the common duct. A choledochoenteric anastomosis should be performed if there is significant loss of length or devascularization of the common duct.

In the early postoperative period, bile duct injury may cause atypically severe abdominal pain, jaundice, drainage of bile (from a drain or through the wound), signs of acute abdomen, and sepsis. HIDA scan is useful in confirming the presence of bile extravasation and assessing whether bile is pooling within the abdomen. Ultrasonography or CT scan may be obtained to detect or exclude an intraabdominal collection. Definition of the exact location of the ductal injury requires either PTC or ERCP. A minor leak from an accessory hepatic duct is likely to heal spontaneously and merely requires placement of a percutaneous drainage catheter in the subhepatic space under CT or ultrasound guidance. Leakage from a cystic duct may be treated with ERCP sphincterotomy alone or, more commonly, ERCP sphincterotomy and placement of a stent. If major ductal injury is detected postoperatively, reconstruction should be undertaken once the anatomy has been defined, the bile leak controlled, and the sepsis resolved.

Late development of stricture leads to obstructive jaundice and recurrent cholangitis. Long-standing strictures may result in biliary cirrhosis and portal hypertension. Diagnosis of strictures is confirmed by PTC/ERCP or MRC. Cholangitis should be managed with antibiotics and the stricture treated by anastomosing the dilated proximal bile duct to a Roux-en-Y loop of jejunum. In the hands of experienced surgeons, excellent outcome of the operative repair is achieved in 70% to 90% of patients. For poor-risk patients, in lieu of dilation, stenting is an option.

Table 17-2 summarizes the common clinical syndromes and complications that can result from cholelithiasis.

BRIEF DESCRIPTION OF SELECTED PROCEDURES

Laparoscopic Cholecystectomy

Laparoscopic cholecystectomy has replaced open cholecystectomy as the preferred approach to the management

Table 17-2 Summary of the Common Clinical Syndromes That Result From Cholelithiasis and the Complications of Cholelithiasis

Syndrome	Etiology	Findings
Biliary colic	Transient cystic duct obstruction	Episodes of upper abdominal pain Nonspecific physical findings Ultrasound: cholelithiasis
Acute cholecystitis	Sustained cystic duct obstruction	Constant, severe right upper quadrant pain
	Acute inflammation of gallbladder	Elevated temperature Murphy's sign Rebound tenderness Leukocytosis Mild hyperbilirubinemia Ultrasound: cholelithiasis, with or without other signs of gallbladder inflammation HIDA scan: nonvisualization of gallbladder
Choledocholithiasis	Stone in the common bile duct (can cause intermittent obstruction, "ball-valve" effect)	History of abdominal pain, jaundice, light stool, dark urine Laboratory findings: obstructive jaundice picture Ultrasound: cholelithiasis with dilated ducts CT, MRC, PTC, ERCP—ductal stones
Acute cholangitis	Infected bile; septicemia Stone impacted in the common bile duct Stricture of the common bile duct (previous biliary surgery)	History same as choledocholithiasis but acutely ill patient with abdominal pain, jaundice, fever, chills; may also have hypotension and change in mentation (in acute suppurative cholangitis)
	Tumor obstructing the common bile duct (especially after an invasive diagnostic procedure that might have seeded the bile with bacteria)	Laboratory findings: same as choledocholithiasis, plus elevated white blood cell count Ultrasound: same as choledocholithiasis, but gallbladder may have been removed previously if the etiology is a stricture
Biliary (gallstone) pancreatitis	Acute pancreatitis Passage of small stones or sludge through the sphincter of Oddi	Acutely ill, severe constant epigastric pain, with or without radiation through to the back With or without history of biliary colic
	Occasionally stones impacted in sphincter Oddi	Tenderness, guarding in upper abdomen Markedly elevated serum amylase/lipase Ultrasound, CT scan, MRC cholelithiasis, with or without inflammatory mass in pancreas
Gallstone ileus	Cholecystenteric fistula	Elderly debilitated patient
	Very large gallstone(s)	Incomplete bowel obstruction
	Stone obstructing intestine (usually distal ileum)	Radiograph shows bowel obstruction (usually distal small bowel) May show air in biliary tree and may see large stone obstructing Ultrasound: ± stone in gallbladder and air in biliary tree CT: all of the above

CT, computed tomography; ERCP, endoscopic retrograde cholangiopancreatography; HIDA, dimethyl iminodiacedic acid, a radionuclide biliary scan; MRC, magnetic resonance cholangiography; PTC, transhepatic cholangiogram.

of gallstone disease in most elective and many emergent situations. When performed electively in an otherwise healthy patient, most procedures can be done as day surgery. If the patient has serious comorbidities, postoperative hospital stay is usually only 24 to 48 hours (even after surgery for acute cholecystitis). The main reasons patients can undergo this surgery with such a short hospital stay is the greatly reduced postoperative incisional pain as compared to that with open cholecystectomy. (See Chapter 26, Surgical Procedures, Techniques, and Skills, for a description of the procedure).

The advantages of the laparoscopic approach are reduced postoperative pain, wound, and pulmonary complications; the possibility of a short hospitalization; and rapid recovery from the procedure with early return to normal activity. The main risks associated with the laparoscopic approach are related to injury to the bile ducts, intestine, and major vessels (usually resulting from blind trocar insertion or the injudicious use of electrocautery). With greater experience of the operating surgeon, the risk of complications diminishes significantly. If anatomy is obscured because of the pathologic process or technical difficulties encountered with the laparoscopic approach, the laparoscopic procedure is converted to a laparotomy. There is some controversy as to whether cholangiography should be performed routinely or selectively at the time of laparoscopic cholecystectomy. Increasingly, a selective approach, governed by the relative indicators for common duct exploration, is preferred. If stones are found in the common bile duct on cholangiography, they may be removed laparoscopically through the cystic duct during the same operation or the laparoscopic procedure can be converted to an open common bile duct procedure to extract the stones. Alternatively, ERCP and sphincterotomy may be performed postoperatively

Open Cholecystectomy and Common Bile Duct Exploration

Open cholecystectomy is generally performed through a right subcostal incision. After the abdomen is entered, the gallbladder is exposed by packing off the adjacent viscera. (See Chapter 26, Surgical Procedures, Techniques, and Skills, for a further description of an open cholecystectomy.) An intraoperative cholangiogram may be performed through the cystic duct at any time to define the anatomy and confirm or exclude suspected choledocholithiasis. A drain is not routinely placed after elective cholecystectomy.

There are absolute and relative indications for common bile duct exploration during open cholecystectomy. Absolute indications include a palpable common duct stone and common duct stones visualized on preoperative or intraoperative cholangiograms. Relative indications include jaundice, acute biliary pancreatitis, ductal dilation, small gallbladder stones (i.e., small cystic duct), and single-faceted gallbladder stones (facets on the gallstone require the presence of at least two stones; if one stone is found, a second one may have passed into the common bile duct). Operative cholangiogram is performed to confirm or exclude stones in the bile duct when only relative indications for bile duct exploration are present.

The procedure for open common bile duct exploration involves mobilizing the duodenum (Kocher maneuver) and making a small longitudinal incision in the common duct. Then the lumen is irrigated with saline using flexible catheters to help flush out stones and debris from the duct. Inflatable balloon catheters are passed both proximally and distally in an attempt to extract stones. A small endoscope (choledochoscope) may be advanced through the opening and the duct thus carefully visualized both proximally and distally to determine whether residual stones are present. A variety of instruments, including stone forceps and collapsible wire "baskets," are available to remove stones that remain impacted and resist removal by the previous maneuvers. All stones, mucus, and debris are removed from the bile duct, and the duct is irrigated with saline. A T-tube is then placed in the lumen of the duct, and the opening in the duct is closed around the T-tube. A completion cholangiogram is obtained to ensure that no stones remain in the duct and that contrast flows freely in the duodenum. A closed drainage catheter is often left in the subhepatic space. When there are multiple stones, or the physician believes that there are stones left in the bile duct, it is prudent to perform an anastomosis between the bile duct and the GI tract (choledochoduodenostomy or choledochojejunostomy), or to perform sphincterotomy so that residual stones may pass easily from the duct into the intestine.

The peritoneal drainage catheter is removed within 24 to 48 hours postoperatively if the drainage is minimal, but should be left in place longer if it is draining significant amounts of blood or bile. Such drainage requires an investigation of the source. The typical T-tube is placed for gravity drainage for 1 week, after which an injection of contrast material in the radiology department is obtained. If the dye flows freely into the duodenum and demonstrates no filling defects, the T-tube may be subsequently clamped or pulled. T-tubes are typically not pulled before the 10th postoperative day, and the established track typically drains 1 to 3 days after tube removal and then closes spontaneously. If there is any concern about interpretation of the cholangiogram, the T-tube is left in place for a longer period of time and the x-ray study is repeated.

Occasionally, despite thorough common duct exploration, a filling defect is noticed in the postoperative T-tube cholangiogram, indicating a missed or retained stone. In approximately 20% of patients, these stones pass spontaneously, especially if they are small. Under such circumstances, the T-tube is left in place for 4 to 6 weeks, and the cholangiogram is repeated. If retained stones remain, they may be extracted with one of four approaches. The usual approach is to remove the T-tube and advance a wire (Dormier) basket through the T-tube tract into the duct under fluoroscopy so that the stones might be retrieved. In the hands of skilled operators, this approach is successful in as many as 95% of cases. A flexible choledochoscope may also be advanced through this tract to assist with stone retrieval by direct vision using the basket. An alternative approach involves ERCP and sphincterotomy. The fourth approach utilizes lithotripsy to fragment larger stones in the bile duct to facilitate extraction. In the rare circumstances where none of these methods is successful, operative reexploration of the duct is necessary.

Endoscopic Extraction of Common Bile Duct Stones

Most common bile duct stones are removed by ERCP and sphincterotomy. Sphincterotomy of the sphincter of Oddi is performed by a special cautery wire passed through the duodenoscope into the sphincter. The common duct is then cleared of stones and debris using special balloon catheters or wire baskets also passed through the duodenoscope. When performed electively, this is usually an ambulatory procedure. If the patient is jaundiced, vitamin K–deficient coagulopathy must be corrected with parenteral vitamin K before this invasive procedure. If a stone cannot be extracted, jaundice can be relieved by inserting a stent with one end above the stone and the other in the duodenum. This stent is left in place, providing biliary decompression until ERCP extraction can be attempted again or surgical stone removal can be arranged. As well as the risks of ERCP, sphincterotomy and stone manipulation add the potential complications of postprocedure GI bleeding (1% to 2%) and duodenal or common duct perforation (0.3%).

Extracorporeal Shock Wave Lithotripsy

ESWL is used to fragment kidney stones so that they can pass through the urinary tract. Some believe that the same principle could be applied to the treatment of gallstones. The use of ESWL for stones in the gallbladder has not gained wide acceptance because of limited patient eligibility, a high failure rate, a high recurrence rate, the need for long-term use of a dissolution agent (e.g., ursodeoxycholic acid), and the need for expensive equipment that cannot be used as well for renal ESWL.

SUGGESTED READINGS

Afdhal, Nezam H. *Gallbladder and Biliary Tract Diseases*. New York, NY: Marcel Dekker, 2000.

Ahrendt SA, Nakeeb A, Pitt HA. Cholangiocarcinoma. *Clin Liver Dis* 2001;5(1):191–218.

Bartlett DL. Gallbladder cancer. *Sem Surg Oncol* 2000;19(2):145–155.

Hanau LH, Steigbigel NH. Acute (ascending) cholangitis. *Infect Dis Clin North Am* 2000;14(3):521–546.

Indar AA, Beckingham IJ. Acute cholecystitis. *BMJ* 2002;325(7365):639–643.

Lillemoe KD. Surgical treatment of biliary tract infections. *Am Surg* 2000;66(2):138–144.

Strasberg SM. Laparoscopic biliary surgery. *Gastroenterol Clin North Am* 1999;28(1):117–132.

Trowbridge RL, Rutkowski NK, Shojania KG. Does this patient have acute cholecystitis? *JAMA* 2003;289(1):80–86.

Wanebo HJ, Vezeridis MP. Carcinoma of the gallbladder. *J Surg Oncol Suppl* 1993;3:134–139.

18

KENNETH W. SHARP, MD ■ STEVEN B. GOLDIN, MD, PHD
KIMBERLY D. LOMIS, MD

Pancreas

OBJECTIVES

1 Classify pancreatitis on the basis of the severity of injury to the organ.
2 List four etiologies of pancreatitis.
3 Describe the clinical presentation of a patient with acute pancreatitis, including indications for surgical intervention.
4 Discuss at least five potential early complications of acute pancreatitis.
5 Discuss the criteria that are used to predict the prognosis for acute pancreatitis.
6 Discuss the mechanism of pseudocyst formation with respect to the role of the pancreatic duct, and list five symptoms and physical signs of pseudocysts.
7 Describe the diagnostic approach to a patient with a suspected pseudocyst, including the indications for and the sequence of tests.
8 Discuss the symptoms of a pancreatic pseudocyst as well as the medical and surgical treatment.
9 Discuss four potential adverse outcomes of chronic pancreatitis as well as the surgical diagnostic approach, treatment options, and management.
10 List four pancreatic neoplasms, and describe the pathology of each with reference to cell type and function.
11 Describe the symptoms, physical signs, laboratory findings, and diagnostic workup of a pancreatic mass on the basis of the location of the tumor.
12 Describe the surgical treatment of pancreatic neoplasms, exocrine or endocrine.
13 Discuss the long-term prognosis for pancreatic cancers on the basis of pathology and cell type.

Diseases of the pancreas are common and often require surgical intervention. The pancreas is subject to congenital, inflammatory, infectious, posttraumatic, and neoplastic diseases. Its exocrine role in digestion was not known until the 1800s, and its ability to modulate glucose metabolism was demonstrated in 1921 by Banting and Best. Inflammatory diseases of the pancreas were described in the late 1800s by a pathologist, Fitz, and surgery for pancreatic neoplasms was popularized by the work of Whipple et al. in the 1930s. As a result of our greater understanding of pancreatic anatomy, physiology, and pathophysiology, we can now identify those patients with pancreatic disease who will benefit from surgical intervention.

ANATOMY

The pancreas is a gland that lies in a transverse orientation in the retroperitoneum at the level of the second lumbar vertebra. It is usually between 12 and 18 cm long, and it weighs between 70 and 110 g. The gland is divided into four distinct parts: head, neck, body, and tail (Fig. 18-1). The head of the pancreas accounts for approximately 30% of the gland. It is surrounded by the "C-loop" of the duodenum. The head is the part of the gland that extends to the right of the superior mesenteric vein. Anteriorly, this section is marked by the gastroduodenal artery. The unci-

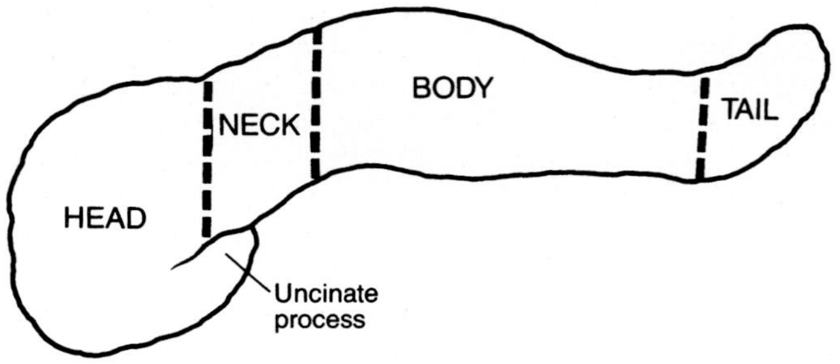

Figure 18-1 Regional anatomy of the pancreas.

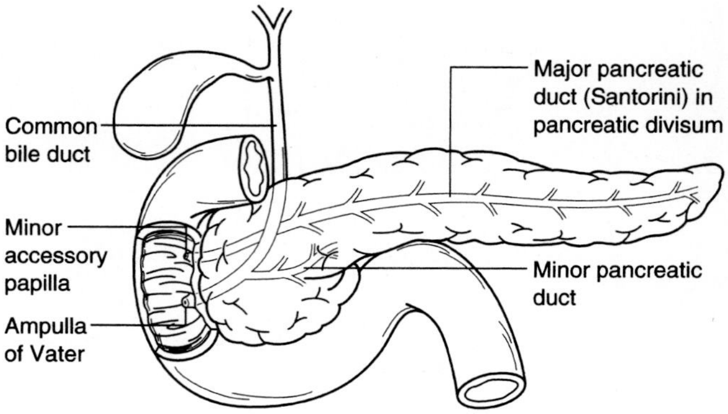

Figure 18-2 Anatomy of the pancreas divisum ductal system showing the ducts of Wirsung (main duct) and Santorini (accessory duct) and their relation to the common bile duct.

nate process is considered a portion of the head. The neck of the gland is the portion overlying the superior mesenteric vein and artery. The body extends from the left of the superior mesenteric vessels toward the splenic hilum. The tail is the most distal portion of the gland extending into the hilum of the spleen. The anatomic boundary between the body and the tail is vague and has little effect on the management of pancreatic disease. The anterior surface of the gland is in contact with the transverse mesocolon as well as the posterior wall of the stomach. Its posterior surface is devoid of peritoneum and is bounded by the common bile duct, superior mesenteric vessels, inferior vena cava, and aorta.

Ductal Anatomy

An understanding of pancreatic ductal anatomy necessitates familiarization with the embryology of pancreatic development. The pancreas begins as dorsal and ventral buds that arise from the duodenal tube. Because of differential growth and gut rotation, the ventral bud passes posteriorly to the duodenal tube and fuses with the larger dorsal bud. Fusion of the ducts of the ventral and dorsal buds forms the main pancreatic duct. The caliber of the pancreatic duct ranges from 3 to 4 mm in the head to 1.5 to 2 mm in the tail. In approximately 90% of cases, the main pancreatic duct (**duct of Wirsung**) drains through the major papilla (ampulla of Vater) into the second portion of the duodenum. The common bile duct often forms a common channel with the main pancreatic duct before it enters the ampulla and the sphincter of Oddi. Figure 18-2 represents the ductal anatomy of **pancreas divisum**, which occurs when the dorsal and ventral buds of the embryonic pancreas do not fuse their ducts, and develop separate entrances into the duodenum. In this anomaly, the accessory duct (Santorini) drains into the duodenum through a minor ampulla. The major ampulla always drains the common bile duct and the pancreatic duct of Wirsung.

Two important anomalies can occur during embryologic development of the pancreas. Pancreas divisum occurs when the ventral and dorsal ducts do not fuse. This condition, which is seen in 5% to 10% of the population, results in the drainage of most of the pancreatic secretions through the minor papilla. The drainage from the head and uncinate process is through the major papilla. This condition is a proposed etiology of idiopathic recurrent pancreatitis. The other anomaly, **annular pancreas,** is less common. Its exact etiology is unknown, but presumably it is caused by incomplete rotation of the ventral pancreatic bud, leading to a ring of pancreatic tissue around the second portion of the duodenum. Annular pancreas is one of the causes of duodenal obstruction in infants and children.

Arterial Blood Supply

The pancreatic head shares a blood supply with the duodenum, necessitating resection of both structures when the pancreatic head must be resected (e.g., cancer of the pancreatic head). The gastroduodenal artery arises from the common hepatic artery, marking the beginning of the proper hepatic artery, and passes posterior to the duodenal bulb. It divides to form the anterior and posterior superior pancreaticoduodenal arteries. These vessels anastomose with the anterior and posterior inferior pancreaticoduodenal arteries that arise directly from the superior mesenteric artery (Fig. 18-3).

The dorsal pancreatic artery is present in 90% of people, but has a variable origin. In most cases, it arises from the proximal splenic artery, but may be a branch of the celiac axis or superior mesenteric artery. It divides into a right branch, which passes along the upper margin of the uncinate process and joins the anterior arcade, and a left branch, which becomes the inferior pancreatic artery and supplies the pancreatic body and tail. The splenic artery is the source of multiple superior pancreatic branches that supply the body of the pancreas. The largest is the **pancreatic magna** (great pancreatic artery).

Venous Drainage

The venous drainage of the pancreas and duodenum corresponds to the arterial supply. The veins are immediately

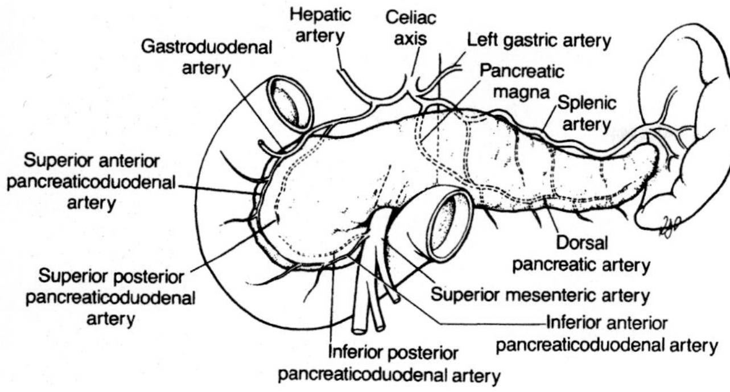

Figure 18-3 Blood supply of the pancreas.

superficial to the arteries. The anterior venous arcade drains into the superior mesenteric vein. The posterior venous arcade usually drains into the portal vein. The surgical neck of the pancreas overlies the junction of the splenic and superior mesenteric veins, which then constitute the portal vein lying behind and slightly medial to the common bile duct.

An important point in the surgical anatomy is the fact that venous tributaries enter the portal and superior mesenteric veins along their lateral borders. The anterior vascular plane allows dissection behind the neck of the pancreas, anterior to the portal and mesenteric veins. The venous drainage of the body and tail is through tributaries that enter the splenic vein and the inferior pancreatic vein, which enters either the inferior or superior mesenteric vein.

Innervation

Inflammatory and neoplastic diseases of the pancreas often cause pain that is mediated through the abundant supply of afferent sensory nerve fibers. The pancreas is also innervated by fibers of both the sympathetic (greater splanchnic nerve) and parasympathetic (vagus nerve) autonomic nervous systems. All fibers pass through the celiac or superior mesenteric plexus. Pain fibers accompany the sympathetic fibers and follow the blood vessels to the gland. The treatment of pancreatic pain is occasionally based on transthoracic division of the greater splanchnic nerve (often done thoracoscopically for the pain of pancreatic cancer or chronic pancreatitis) or ablation of the celiac plexus (permanent lytic blocks may be done percutaneously by experienced anesthesiologists or intraoperatively at the time of palliative surgical procedures in patients with unresectable malignancy).

PHYSIOLOGY

Exocrine

The exocrine pancreas secretes 1000 to 2000 mL/day of isotonic, alkaline fluid that contains electrolytes and digestive enzymes. Although the sodium and potassium concentrations are similar to those in plasma, the bicarbonate concentration is elevated, accounting for the alkaline pH (approximately 8.0). Many of the 20 different digestive enzymes that are synthesized by the pancreas are secreted as inactive precursors (e.g., trypsin and chymotrypsin are secreted as trypsinogen and chymotrypsinogen) and are activated by contact with the duodenal contents.

Two hormones play a central role in regulating pancreatic exocrine secretion: secretin and cholecystokinin (CCK). Duodenal acidification stimulates the release of secretin, which stimulates the secretion of pancreatic juice that is rich in bicarbonate. The intraluminal products of digestion, especially peptides, amino acids, and free fatty acids, stimulate the release of CCK, which stimulates the secretion of pancreatic digestive enzymes. In addition, CCK potentiates the action of secretin and causes gallbladder contraction so that bile is mixed with pancreatic secretions to digest fat, protein, and carbohydrate.

Endocrine

The islets of Langerhans make up 1.5% of the pancreas by weight. They are responsible for the endocrine functions of the gland. The islets measure 75 to 150 μm and are more abundant in the tail of the gland. Their major function is the control of glucose homeostasis. In response to low serum glucose, alpha cells secrete glucagon, a peptide that is composed of 20 amino acids. The resulting glycogenolysis releases glucose into the bloodstream. Beta cells, which constitute 60% of the islets, secrete insulin in response to increases in serum glucose. Insulin promotes the transfer of glucose across cell membranes. Delta cells, which constitute a small proportion of islet cells (5% to 10%), secrete somatostatin, the most potent known inhibitor of pancreatic exocrine secretion.

PATHOPHYSIOLOGY

Acute Pancreatitis

Acute pancreatitis is a diffuse inflammation of the pancreas that can range in severity from a mild self-limited attack to severe systemic inflammation and death. Several well-known factors are associated with acute pancreatitis, although the precise etiology is not well understood. The two most common causes, alcohol ingestion and biliary calculi, account for 85% of cases.

Acute pancreatitis is characterized by enzymatic destruction of the pancreatic substance by the release and activation of pancreatic enzymes into the glandular parenchyma. The microscopic (histologic) changes range from interstitial edema and inflammation in mild cases to hemorrhage and necrosis in severe cases.

Etiology

All causes of acute pancreatitis can be categorized into the following groups: metabolic, mechanical, postoperative

Table 18-1 Etiologic Factors of Pancreatitis

Metabolic	Mechanical	Postoperative and Traumatic	Vascular	Infectious
Alcohol	Cholelithiasis	0.8%–17% Gastric procedures	Periarteritis nodosa	Mumps
Hyperlipoproteinemia	Pancreas divisum	0.7%–9.3% Biliary procedures	Atheroembolism	Coxsackie B
Hypercalcemia	Duct obstruction (ascaris, tumor, etc.)	Direct pancreatic injury		Cytomegalovirus
Drugs	ERCP	Injury to pancreatic blood supply		Cryptococcus
Genetic	Ductal bleeding	Obstruction of the pancreatic duct at the duodenum		
Scorpion venom	Duodenal obstruction	Cardiopulmonary bypass—ischemia		

ERCP, endoscopic retrograde cholangiopancreatography.

and traumatic, and vascular (Table 18-1). The most common etiology within the metabolic group is alcohol, which accounts for as many as 40% of all cases of pancreatitis. Generally, the first episode is preceded by 6 to 8 years of significant alcohol ingestion and is often followed by recurring acute attacks. After multiple attacks of acute pancreatitis, the pancreas is permanently damaged, and the clinical syndrome of **chronic pancreatitis** develops. Exactly how alcohol causes pancreatitis is not known. A common theory is that alcohol induces changes in the secretory response of the pancreas and that these changes result in a higher protein content in the secretions. This higher content leads to the precipitation of protein and the blockage of small pancreatic ductules. Other metabolic causes of pancreatitis include hyperlipidemia and hypercalcemia. Although causative mechanisms are not clear, the drugs associated with acute pancreatitis include corticosteroids, thiazide diuretics, furosemide, estrogens, azathioprine, and dideoxyinosine.

The most common mechanical etiology of acute pancreatitis is gallstones. It is estimated that as many as 60% of nonalcoholic patients with pancreatitis have gallstones. Like the etiology of alcohol-induced pancreatitis, the etiology of gallstone-induced pancreatitis is not completely understood. In 1901, Halsted and Opie proposed the common channel theory based on the observation of severe pancreatitis in a patient with a common channel within the ampullae of Vater made up of the common bile duct and the pancreatic duct. They proposed that a gallstone could block the pancreatic duct within the ampulla, leading to reflux of bile into the pancreatic duct that results in acute pancreatitis. This theory is disputed by some who have shown experimentally that bile in the pancreatic duct at physiologic pressures does not cause pancreatitis. It has been suggested that transient obstruction of a common channel might lead to reflux of pancreatic juice into the common bile duct. The mixing of bile and pancreatic juice may lead to the formation of a substance that is highly toxic to the pancreas. Other mechanical causes of pancreatitis include blunt and penetrating trauma to the pancreas and malignant obstruction of the pancreatic duct by tumors of the distal common duct, pancreas, ampulla of Vater, and duodenum.

Ischemic injuries to the pancreas, secondary to hypotension or devascularization during upper abdominal surgery, may initiate pancreatitis or may play a role in the progression of pancreatic edema to pancreatic necrosis. Postoperative pancreatitis is seen after gastric surgery in as many as 15% of cases and after biliary surgery in 10% of cases. Pancreatitis following biliary procedures may be traumatic in etiology, especially in cases where instrumentation of the common bile duct is performed. Acute pancreatitis is a complication in 1% of patients who undergo endoscopic retrograde cholangiopancreatography (ERCP). This complication may be due to an acute increase in intraductal pressure. Approximately 8% to 10% of cases of pancreatitis have no recognizable etiology (idiopathic pancreatitis).

Clinical Presentation and Evaluation

Patients with acute pancreatitis have noncrampy, epigastric abdominal pain. The character of the pain is variable, and it frequently radiates to the left or right upper quadrant or the back. The pain may be alleviated by sitting or standing. It is associated with nausea and often a significant amount of vomiting. Physical examination is characterized by fever, tachycardia, and upper abdominal tenderness with guarding. Bowel sounds are generally absent because of the presence of an adynamic ileus. Generalized abdominal and rebound tenderness may also occur in severe pancreatitis. In hemorrhagic pancreatitis, blood may dissect into the posterior retroperitoneal soft tissue, causing a flank hematoma known as Grey-Turner's sign, or up the falciform ligament, resulting in a periumbilical ecchymosis called Cullen's sign. Laboratory evaluation shows leukocytosis and elevated serum amylase and lipase. Severe cases of pancreatitis can initiate systemic inflammatory response syndrome with activation of inflammatory mediators (cytokines, activated lymphocytes, and activation of the complement cascade), and this results in injury in many sites remote from the pancreas. In severe cases of pancreatitis, there may also be abnormal liver chemistries, hyperglycemia, hypocalcemia, elevated blood urea nitrogen (BUN) and creatinine levels, and hypoxemia as a result of injury to liver, lung, and kidney.

The differential diagnosis of acute pancreatitis includes acute cholecystitis, perforated peptic ulcer, mesenteric ischemia, esophageal perforation, and myocardial infarction. Table 18-2 contains a list of possible causes of hyperamylasemia, which should be considered in the differential of any patient with an elevated amylase level. Patients with suspected acute pancreatitis should be evaluated radiologically with (1) a chest radiograph to look for sympathetic pleural effusions, atelectasis, or hemidiaphragm elevation (suggestive of fluid sequestration) and to exclude free air; (2) plain and upright abdominal radiographs to evaluate for possible calcifications (indicating chronic pancreatitis), gallstones (though only about 15% of gallstones are radiopaque), local adynamic ileus (or signs of bowel obstruction), or a "cutoff sign" where gas in the transverse colon appears to end abruptly; and (3) ultrasonography to look for gallstones, common duct dilation, pancreatic enlargement, and peripancreatic fluid collections. Ultrasonography may be limited in its utility in obese patients or in patients with significant amounts of bowel gas overlying the pancreas. If complicated acute pancreatitis is suspected, computed tomography (CT) is preferred over ultrasound because of its greater sensitivity in detecting peripancreatic fluid, pancreatic edema, and pancreatic necrosis. CT scans are useful in cases of unclear clinical diagnosis but are not necessary in straightforward cases of mild pancreatitis. Magnetic resonance cholangiography (MRCP) can be additionally used in selected cases to noninvasively visualize the bile duct for gallstones.

Prognosis

Outcome after acute pancreatitis is directly proportional to the severity of the attack. Eighty percent of patients with pancreatitis will recover from the attack without sequelae, while 20% will experience some form of complication. Grading systems for the severity of pancreatitis are used to predict those at risk for complications. One of the first systems for grading severity was developed by Ranson. This system (**Ranson's criteria**) uses readily measured laboratory and clinical variables (Table 18-3). Five variables are measured at admission, and six additional variables are measured over the ensuing 48 hours. The presence of three or more criteria indicates severe pancreatitis and is associated with an increased incidence of local and systemic complications. It should be emphasized that the level of serum amylase is not of prognostic significance and is not reflective of the severity of the attack.

The other main prognostic index is the Acute Physiology and Chronic Health Evaluation II (APACHE II) score. Although it was first used to stratify intensive care unit patients, this scoring system was adapted to assess patients with acute pancreatitis. Although it is not as simple and straightforward as Ranson's criteria, the APACHE II system also uses readily obtainable variables (Table 18-4). Numeric scores are assigned to physiologic measurements, age, and preexisting organ insufficiencies to provide a score that reflects the severity of the disease. The main advantage of the APACHE II system is that a score can be derived at any time during the patient's hospital course. With Ranson's criteria, the variables that indicate severity are prognostic only during the first 48 hours after admission. Patients with APACHE II scores of 8 or greater are considered to have severe acute pancreatitis.

Finally, CT scans can yield prognostic information. The severity and complications of the attack are correlated to the amount of pancreatic necrosis and the size and location of peripancreatic and extrapancreatic fluid collections seen on abdominal contrast CT scans.

Treatment

Medical

The medical therapy of acute pancreatitis can be divided into general supportive therapy, which includes preven-

Table 18-2 List of Disease Processes That May Result in Hyperamylasemia

Perforated ulcer	Ovarian tumor or cyst
Ischemic bowel	Lung cancer
Small bowel obstruction	Prostate cancer
Renal failure	Diabetic ketoacidosis
Salivary gland infection	Macroamylasemia
Ectopic pregnancy	

Table 18-3 Prognostic Factors: Risk of Major Complications or Death (Ranson's Criteria)

At admission
Age > 55
WBC count > 16,000
Glucose > 200 mg/100 mL
LDH > 350
AST > 250
During 48 hr after admission
Hct > 10-point decrease
BUN > 5 mg/100 mL increase
Ca^{++} < 8.0
pO_2 < 60 mm Hg on room air
Base excess > 4 mEq/L
Estimated fluid sequestration > 6000 mL

AST, aspartate aminotransferase; BUN, blood urea nitrogen; Hct, hematocrit; LDH, lactate dehydrogenase; WBC, white blood cell.

Table 18-4 Variables Scored in the APACHE II Severity of Disease Classification System

Physiologic Variables	Age Ranges	Chronic Health Problems and Variables
Temperature	≤ 44	Liver
Mean arterial pressure	45–44	Cardiovascular
Heart rate	55–64	Respiratory
Respiratory rate	65–74	Renal
Oxygenation	≥ 75	Immunocompromised
Arterial pH		
Serum sodium		
Serum potassium		
Serum creatinine		
Hematocrit		
White blood cell count		
Glasgow Coma Score		

The actual physiologic ranges and points assigned are not indicated in this table; only the variables considered are listed. APACHE, Acute Physiology and Chronic Health Evaluation.

tion of complications such as deep vein thrombosis or peptic ulceration, and specific treatment of pancreatic inflammation or its complications. In patients with mild bouts of pancreatitis without complications, it is appropriate to maintain them strictly without food until the pain and tenderness has resolved. Since the level of serum amylase is not related to the severity of the attack, it is acceptable to base decisions regarding letting the patient eat or drink upon assessment of symptom resolution. In patients with more severe episodes of pancreatitis, it is important to maintain adequate tissue perfusion by monitoring cardiovascular parameters and also to maintain adequate intravascular volume. A massive amount of fluid can be sequestered in the retroperitoneal tissues because of the presence of activated enzymes and inflammation. Pancreatitis is often compared with a retroperitoneal "burn" because of the magnitude of fluid extravasation and third-space fluid loss that it causes. In severe cases, administration of several liters of isotonic solution may be required. Fluid management is aided by the use of a central venous line or even a pulmonary artery catheter in difficult cases to monitor cardiac function and a urinary catheter to measure urine output. Electrolytes (including calcium and magnesium) and blood glucose are carefully monitored.

Respiratory function is monitored carefully because severe hypocalcemia and respiratory failure can cause early death in severe pancreatitis. Oxygenation may be impaired by sympathetic pleural effusions, atelectasis, hemidiaphragm elevation, and fluid overload. Oxygenation is monitored with pulse oximetry or arterial blood gas measurements if necessary. Patients with severe pancreatitis can also have respiratory distress syndrome as part of their systemic inflammatory response syndrome that requires intubation and aggressive ventilatory support.

Specific inhibition of pancreatic secretions in an effort to decrease peripancreatic inflammation has been attempted with the use of nasogastric suction. Studies in patients with mild alcoholic pancreatitis do not show a benefit with this mode of therapy. However, nasogastric suction may be useful in patients with more severe forms of pancreatitis with ileus and vomiting. Anticholinergics, somatostatin analogues, inhibitors of the inflammatory cascade, specific enzyme inhibitors (e.g., aprotinin—a proteolytic enzyme inhibitor), and antacids have been used in an attempt to decrease the degree of pancreatic inflammation, but none has any significant benefit. Similarly, antibiotics do not decrease morbidity or mortality in patients with mild pancreatitis; however, they are used quite liberally in the treatment of **gallstone pancreatitis** because of concern that this condition might be confused with cholangitis—though data supporting this practice are lacking. Patients with severe pancreatitis (more than three positive Ranson's criteria) are often treated with prophylactic antibiotics to try to reduce infectious complications such as infected pancreatic necrosis. The use of broad-spectrum antibiotics early in the course of necrotizing pancreatitis has been supported by a meta-analysis of several prospective randomized controlled trials and may reduce mortality in this devastating illness.

Nutritional support must also be provided in the patient with preexisting nutritional deficits or in the patient with severe disease predicted to be unable to eat for over 7 to 10 days. A nasal duodenal feeding tube may be used to provide nutrients to the patient without potentially stimulating the pancreas and exacerbating the attack. Total parenteral nutrition may also be useful in those patients with a nonfunctional gastrointestinal tract.

Surgical

The surgical management of patients with pancreatitis is controversial. When the diagnosis is not clear, diagnostic laparotomy is recommended, not only to establish the diagnosis of pancreatitis but also to rule out other nonpancreatic lesions that may mimic pancreatitis (e.g., perforated ulcer, gangrenous cholecystitis, mesenteric infarction).

In some cases, patients with severe gallstone pancreatitis may be treated with early removal of an impacted stone at the ampulla of Vater. This procedure is considered only in severe cases and in cases with suspected cholangitis complicating the diagnosis. Endoscopic sphincterotomy is a procedure in which the ampulla of Vater and common bile duct are cannulated via a side-viewing duodenoscope, and a wire cautery sphincterotome is used to cut the ampulla and sphincter followed by stone extraction with a balloon catheter. Patients with mild to moderate gallstone pancreatitis should be allowed to recover from their pancreatitis. Cholecystectomy may be performed during the same hospital admission to reduce the length of convalescence or the probability of another episode of gallstone pancreatitis and to avoid another hospitalization. Patients with complicated pancreatitis (cyst, infection, fluid collections) generally should be allowed to completely recover from all complications prior to cholecystectomy.

Complications

Acute pancreatitis has many major and minor complications. Metabolic complications include hyperglycemia, hypocalcemia, and renal failure. Varying degrees of respiratory insufficiency and hypoxemia may also be present. Coagulopathy and hemorrhage may also occur as a result of the depletion of coagulation factors or erosion into a major vessel. The most common local complications are paralytic ileus and sterile peripancreatic fluid collections. Patients may have obstruction of the biliary tree or duodenum due to local edema. Inflammation and edema in the pancreatic body and tail may cause thrombosis of the splenic vein, which can lead to sinistral portal hypertension (left-sided portal hypertension) and gastric varices.

Necrosis of the gland and the peripancreatic tissues in the retroperitoneum is a common finding in patients with severe episodes. This finding may be present within the early stages of the attack and is determined by contrast-enhanced dynamic CT scan. In general, necrosis of less than 30% of the pancreas usually resolves without further sequelae. Patients with greater degrees of necrosis are at increased risk of tissue infection and organ dysfunction. The management of sterile necrosis has been debated in the past, but most groups currently advocate operative intervention only in cases of infection. Local infectious complications of acute pancreatitis markedly increase the mortality associated with a given attack. Infected pancreatic necrosis is associated with the highest mortality rate (> 40%). The risk of infection is directly proportional to the extent of necrosis. Typically, infection becomes manifest 2 to 3 weeks into the patient's illness. Frequently, patients have worsening of organ dysfunction. The diagnosis of infected necrosis is made by CT findings of air in the retroperitoneum or by CT-guided needle aspiration of necrotic pancreatic tissue, with demonstration of organisms by Gram's stain. Therapy for infected pancreatic necrosis is operative debridement with blunt dissection, antibiotics, and supportive care. Multiple operations may be needed to remove the infected debris without damaging adjacent structures. Percutaneous drainage usually fails because the large pieces of infected necrotic material cannot drain through small catheters. An example of the tissue removed from a pancreatic gland that became infected and necrotic is seen in Figure 18-4.

A pancreatic abscess is a discrete collection of pus adjacent to the pancreas, without underlying necrosis, and is much rarer than infected pancreatic necrosis. Typically, an abscess is an infected acute fluid collection, or an infected pseudocyst. Treatment is the same as for any intra-abdominal abscess: external drainage. Drainage can be accomplished by open operation or, in some cases, by nonoperative percutaneous drainage. The mortality risk for pancreatic abscess is less than that for infected necrosis.

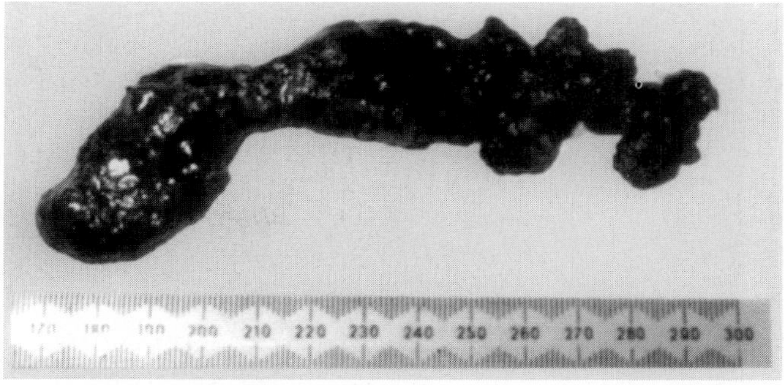

Figure 18-4 Photograph of infected necrotic pancreatic tissue.

Pseudocysts

The most common complication of pancreatitis is the development of an acute fluid collection in the peripancreatic area or, in more severe cases, at distant locations in the retroperitoneum. This complication is caused by ductal disruption during an episode of acute pancreatitis and pancreatic and peripancreatic tissue autolysis. Enzymatic fluid collects in and around the pancreas and is walled off by surrounding viscera. Most of these acute fluid collections resolve. Those that persist become **pseudocysts** — a collection of peripancreatic fluid in a cystlike structure that has no epithelial lining. Pseudocysts may be termed communicating or noncommunicating, based upon whether the cyst is connected to the pancreatic duct. Over the course of 4 to 6 weeks after the initial attack, the wall of these persistent fluid collections matures into a fibrotic scar.

Clinical Presentation and Evaluation

The most common symptoms of pseudocysts are epigastric pain, nausea, vomiting, and early satiety. On occasion, pseudocysts can create mechanical obstruction of either the stomach or duodenum, but this is uncommon. Jaundice secondary to biliary obstruction can occur as a result of pseudocyst formation, but this is also unusual.

A thorough history and a complete physical examination are essential in the evaluation of a pseudocyst. Obviously, obtaining a history of alcoholism and previous pancreatitis is important. Fever, weight loss, and a history of jaundice are other salient clinical features. Clinical features that lead to suspicion of a pseudocyst include persistent abdominal pain for longer than 1 week after an episode of pancreatitis, persistent elevations of serum amylase or lipase, and the development of a palpable abdominal mass.

Sonography and CT scans are the first-line noninvasive studies to assess an abdominal mass. Sonography is useful because it is relatively inexpensive and is quite accurate in distinguishing solid from cystic masses. Further delinea-

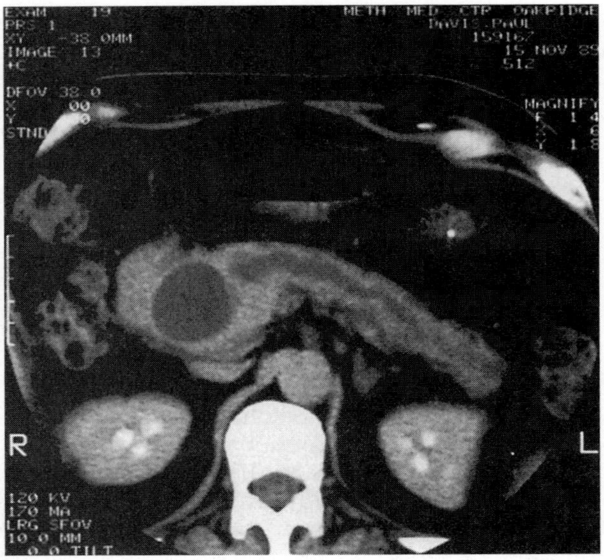

Figure 18-5 Computed tomography scan showing the pancreas of a patient with chronic pancreatitis. A pseudocyst is seen in the head of the pancreas, and a dilated pancreatic duct is seen distally.

in distinguishing solid from cystic masses. Further delineation of the mass and surrounding tissue structures is obtained with a CT scan (Fig. 18-5). Not only can the mass and its relation to surrounding structures be clearly outlined, but serial examinations can also show growth or shrinkage of the mass over time. Further, CT and sonography can be used in more invasive therapeutic techniques that permit direct needle or catheter aspiration or drainage of the fluid collection.

Treatment

Medical

The majority of acute peripancreatic fluid collections resolve spontaneously with conservative medical management. The conservative approach consists of allowing "pancreatic rest" by maintaining the patient on total parenteral nutrition and avoiding oral intake that would stimulate pancreatic secretion. During observation of the patient over a period of weeks, progressive decrease in size predicts that the pseudocyst will resolve. Once pain and nausea resolve, oral intake may be tried, but must be stopped if symptoms recur. Simple daily palpation of the mass should show reduced tenderness and diminished size. Ultrasound and, if necessary, CT can document the disappearance of the pseudocyst very accurately.

Medical management continues until the cyst resolves or a mature cyst wall forms. Maturation of the cyst wall, during which the cyst wall develops enough fibrosis to support suturing to the stomach or jejunum for internal drainage, generally requires 4 to 6 weeks.

Clearly, pseudocysts that occur suddenly in patients with acute pancreatitis are much more likely to resolve than long-standing masses in patients with a history of chronic pancreatitis. Complications from pseudocysts (e.g., infection, hemorrhage) can be catastrophic. A patient who has a pseudocyst and sudden onset of fever may have an infected pseudocyst that requires drainage. Hemorrhage from a pseudocyst is rare, but can be life threatening. Pseudocysts may abut large peripancreatic vessels (splenic, inferior and superior pancreaticoduodenal), and the digestive enzymes in the pseudocyst fluid may affect the vessel wall. Erosion into an artery can occur, with rapid onset of hypotension and severe abdominal pain. A patient with known pancreatitis who has sudden, severe abdominal pain (from sudden expansion of a pseudocyst with blood) or hypotension should undergo volume resuscitation and be taken promptly to angiography to search for a bleeding pseudoaneurysm. Embolization should be performed if possible.

Surgical

If the cyst does not resolve within 4 to 6 weeks and the patient is still symptomatic, the cyst is drained. Pseudocysts that communicate with the pancreatic duct on ERCP should be drained surgically since external drainage will likely result in a pancreatic fistula. If the pseudocyst does not communicate with the pancreatic duct and is approachable by CT-directed drainage, aspiration may be attempted, but recurrence rates are high. Newer endoscopic techniques are being developed to endoscopically drain pseudocysts via an endoscopic cyst-gastrostomy in selected cases. This decision is best made jointly by the radiologist, gastroenterologist, and surgeon. Two basic surgical techniques are used to drain pseudocysts: for internal drainage, the lumen of the pseudocyst is anastomosed to the lumen of a limb of the jejunum in a Roux-en-Y cyst-jejunostomy. For external drainage, if the cyst is fixed to the stomach by inflammation, a cyst-gastrostomy is performed. Internal drainage is preferred, but if it cannot be done because of technical problems, an immature cyst wall, or infection, then external drainage is used. Internal drainage is acceptable in more than 90% of cases. External drainage often requires a second operation because of pancreatic fistula. Biopsy of the cyst wall is recommended at the time of surgical drainage to confirm that the cyst is truly a pseudocyst rather than a cystadenoma or cystadenocarcinoma.

Chronic Pancreatitis

Etiology

Inflammation of the pancreas progresses to a chronic state for a variety of reasons. If the initial inflammatory insult is severe enough to cause permanent ductal damage, recurring pancreatitis can develop, usually because of ductal obstruction or stasis (Table 18-5). The causes of such a significant injury include trauma and cholelithiasis. The most important cause of **chronic pancreatitis** is persistent alcohol ingestion.

Congenital causes include cystic fibrosis, familial pancreatitis, and pancreas divisum. Pancreas divisum is con-

Table 18-5 Marseilles Classification of Pancreatitis

Category	Characteristics
I	Acute pancreatitis: a single episode of pancreatitis in a previously normal gland
II	Acute relapsing pancreatitis: recurrent attacks that do not lead to permanent functional damage; clinical and biologic normalcy in the interval between attacks
III	Chronic relapsing pancreatitis: progressive functional damage persisting between attacks; frequent pain-free intervals
IV	Chronic pancreatitis: inexorable and irreversible destruction of pancreatic function; constant pain

troversial as a cause of pancreatitis, since the developmental variation may be seen in many asymptomatic patients. The etiology in rare cases is probably related to inadequate drainage of the duct of Santorini via the minor papilla. It has been treated with endoscopic stent placement through the minor papilla or surgical sphincteroplasty of the minor ampulla. Repeated episodes of pancreatitis result in interruption and obstruction of large and small pancreatic ducts, with subsequent autodigestion. As a result of the edema and tissue destruction, the pancreas undergoes scarring and fibrosis, with loss of functional substance. The result of this process is pancreatic insufficiency, which manifests as exocrine and endocrine failure. Loss of exocrine function leads to malabsorption. When pancreatic secretion of enzymes decreases to 10% of normal, protein and fat cannot be adequately absorbed. The resulting steatorrhea is quantitated by measuring stool fat in a patient who is receiving a prescribed fat diet. Pancreatic endocrine dysfunction causes diabetes. Generally, these patients respond to insulin treatment and do not seem to be as vulnerable to small vessel disease as other diabetic patients. Nonetheless, insulin administration is difficult in this population because many continue their heavy alcohol intake.

Clinical Presentation and Evaluation

Pain is the most common symptom of chronic pancreatitis. The pain is usually intermittent, but with the development of subsequent attacks of pancreatitis and more scarring and fibrosis, the pain may become inexorable and unrelenting. Eating may be impossible because of the resulting pain. Patients often resort to increased alcohol intake and the use of painkilling drugs to obtain relief. Drug dependency, malnutrition, and vitamin B_{12} deficiency are common. Malabsorption as a result of exocrine insufficiency may cause steatorrhea and fat-soluble vitamin deficiency.

Patients with suspected chronic pancreatitis and those with known chronic pancreatitis who have new symptoms should be assessed by CT scan to search for surgically correctable causes or complications. CT has the greatest sensitivity for showing gland enlargement or atrophy, duct enlargement, calcifications, masses, pseudocysts, and inflammation (Fig. 18-6). The liver, gallbladder, and bile ducts are also visualized. Ultrasonography is less expensive than CT, but it is also less successful in showing the pancreas, especially in obese patients and those with gas-filled intestines. However, ultrasonography is the preferred diagnostic study for following changes in pseudocysts if they are clearly visualized. It is also the preferred method for the initial study of jaundiced patients, even if the jaundice has a pancreatic cause.

Treatment

Patients with chronic pancreatitis are managed conservatively, with the intention of reducing trauma to the pancreas. When necessary, surgery is considered for appropriate complications, such as pseudocysts. Because alcoholism is the leading cause of pancreatitis, abstinence is strongly advised. If other specific causes are identified, they are corrected to minimize further injury. Medical treatment of chronic pancreatitis is a low-fat diet (to minimize steatorrhea), enzyme replacement, and insulin for hyperglycemia. Medical treatment rarely resolves the pain of chronic pancreatitis.

Surgery is indicated in patients with chronic pancreatitis who have incapacitating pain that is resistant to medical therapy and in patients with anatomic abnormalities that cause recurrent bouts of acute pancreatitis. Preoperative delineation of pancreatic anatomy by CT, ERCP, or magnetic resonance cholangiopancreatography (MRCP) is necessary. These studies are used to map the ductal anatomy and to delineate obstructions, strictures, calculi, duct ectasia, and pseudocysts. ERCP is invasive and carries a small, but definite, risk of exacerbating pancreatitis, biliary or pancreatic sepsis, or pseudocyst infection. ERCP is very useful in identifying dilated pancreatic ducts, strictures,

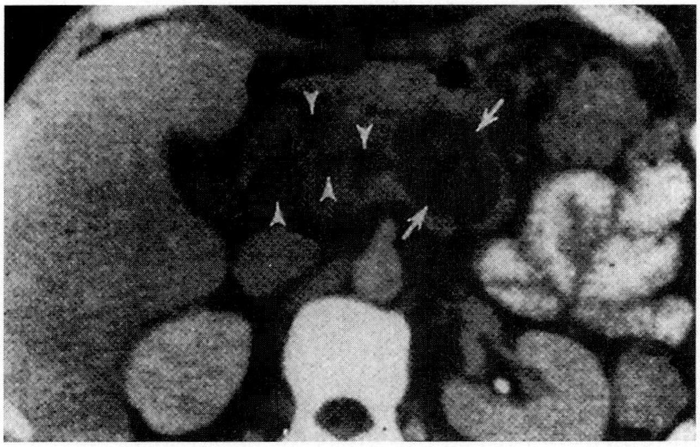

Figure 18-6 Computed tomography scan showing multiple pseudocysts (*arrows*) in a patient with chronic pancreatitis.

fistulas, and common bile duct obstruction. CT is noninvasive as is MRCP, but both rarely show the details of pancreatic ductal anatomy necessary to allow a plan for a surgical procedure.

The surgical options for treating chronic pancreatitis are ductal decompression (for patients with dilated pancreatic ducts) or pancreatic resection (for patients without dilated ducts). Patients with segmental ductal obstruction or alternating areas of stricture and dilation ("chain of lakes") are best treated by decompression of the duct into a loop of jejunum (lateral pancreaticojejunostomy, or modified Puestow or Partington-Rochelle procedure). Drainage procedures, when possible, are preferable to resectional procedures, because they preserve more glandular tissue and are more likely to delay the development of exocrine and endocrine insufficiency due to disease progression. The long-term results of the modified Puestow procedure are good, with approximately 70% of patients achieving lasting relief of pain. Pancreatic resection is reserved for patients without pancreatic duct dilation who have disease limited to a segment of the gland. Results are similar to those obtained with ductal decompression. As mentioned, a significant number of patients will have progression to exocrine insufficiency and diabetes after a surgical procedure. Near-total and total pancreatectomy is rarely indicated because these operations leave the patient with no exocrine or endocrine function. Of note, patients may still continue to have severe pain even after total pancreatectomy. Thoracoscopic splanchniecectomy has been used in selected cases of chronic pain with some success. Celiac blocks have not usually been successful for long-term relief of pain in chronic pancreatitis, though they have good success in patients with unresectable malignancy, as these patients have very short survival.

Surgical intervention is also indicated to treat several complications of chronic pancreatitis. Patients with biliary strictures and associated liver enzyme abnormalities benefit from biliary enteric decompression. Pseudocysts are common in patients with chronic pancreatitis; however, unlike acute fluid collections associated with acute pancreatitis, these are less likely to resolve. Operative drainage should be undertaken in patients with symptoms or a pseudocyst that is larger than 5 cm.

Pancreatic Neoplasms

General Considerations

Pancreatic adenocarcinoma is the fourth most common cause of cancer deaths in the United States, accounting for approximately 30,000 deaths per year. The male:female ratio in most series is approximately 2:1, and the annual incidence is approximately nine new cases per 100,000 population. The principal risk factors for pancreatic carcinoma appear to be increasing age and cigarette smoking. Although controversy exists over the etiologic role of diabetes and alcohol, cigarette smoking appears to double the risk of pancreatic carcinoma. The most common location for pancreatic carcinoma is in the head of the gland, accounting for approximately two-thirds of all cases, though the carcinoma may be multicentric. The most common malignancy of the pancreas is an adenocarcinoma originating from the ductal epithelium. The rest of the neoplasms that arise in the pancreas are islet cell tumors and cystadenocarcinomas, which account for fewer than 10% of pancreatic malignancies. Lymphomas are rarely encountered, but are important to consider since resection is not the preferred treatment (chemotherapy and radiation carry similar success, and the patient does not need the potential morbidity of a pancreatic resection).

Clinical Presentation and Evaluation

The signs and symptoms of pancreatic carcinoma are related to the anatomy of the region. Tumors that originate in the periampullary region may present relatively early with painless jaundice. However, most patients have a combination of weight loss, jaundice, and pain as a result of infiltration of the tumor in the peripancreatic region. Pain tends to be in the posterior epigastric region, with radiation to the back. The pain of pancreatic disease is constant, posterior, and radiating. In contrast, intermittent colic is usually associated with biliary tract disease. A palpable nontender gallbladder in a jaundiced patient is more commonly associated with malignancy than with cholelithiasis (**Courvoisier's sign**). This unusual sign is explained by the distensibility of a nonfibrotic gallbladder wall in a patient without gallstones, as opposed to a chronically scarred and inflamed gallbladder in a patient with chronic cholelithiasis.

The evaluation of patients with jaundice should begin with ultrasonography, which accurately shows biliary dilation, liver lesions, and, to a lesser degree, pancreatic lesions. In patients who have a history and physical findings that suggest pancreatic carcinoma, CT can be used as the initial diagnostic test. CT provides better detail of the periampullary region without sacrificing accuracy in detecting biliary dilation. It is also helpful in detecting liver metastases and assessing local tumor invasion. In many centers, a high-quality, contrast-enhanced CT scan is accurate for making the determination of tumor resectability. Three-dimensional CT scanning is now becoming commonplace and is replacing angiography for delineating the vascular anatomy. In Figure 18-7, a large pancreatic head mass is seen on CT scan. Radiographic features of unresectability include liver metastases, ascites, or vascular invasion (portal or superior mesenteric vein, superior mesenteric artery, hepatic artery, vena cava, or aorta). Endoscopic ultrasound is the newest modality for evaluating pancreatic lesions. Its sensitivity and specificity are similar to that of CT. However, unlike CT, endoscopic ultrasound is more invasive and is highly operator-dependent. MRCP, ERCP, and percutaneous transhepatic cholangiography can also be used to delineate the biliary and pancreatic ductal anatomy. Biliary drainage can also be achieved endoscopically or transhepatically. Preoperative tissue sampling or drainage of the biliary system is not

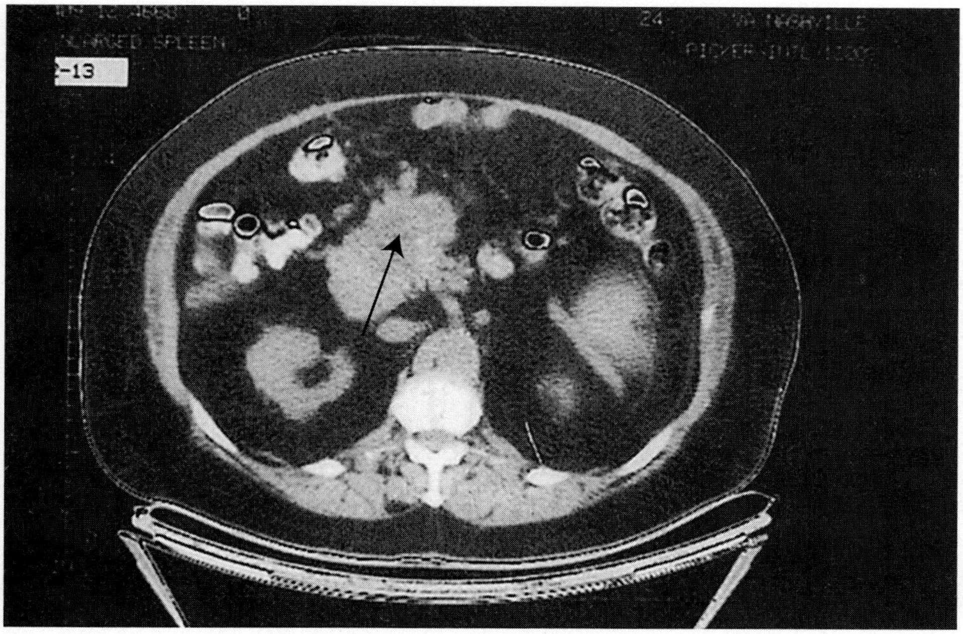

Figure 18-7 Computed tomography scan showing a large pancreatic head mass.

routinely indicated in patients whose imaging studies suggest a resectable pancreatic tumor. Tissue sampling to establish a diagnosis in patients in which imaging studies show unresectable lesions is valuable and may be obtained by percutaneous CT–guided biopsy or endoscopic ultrasound–guided biopsy. Endoscopic drainage of the biliary tract is the preferred palliative treatment of patients in whom the diagnosis can be established and in whom unresectability has been established.

Treatment

Patients with obstructive jaundice may develop vitamin K–related coagulopathies because of biliary obstruction, malnutrition, and liver injury and should be corrected. Baseline studies are recommended to evaluate hepatic function and nutritional status, including albumin, transferrin (or prealbumin), and prothrombin time. The operative approach to pancreatic cancer involves assessment for regional and local spread. Patients without preoperative evidence of systemic or regional dissemination (which makes the tumor unresectable) undergo exploration with curative intent. For lesions in the head of the pancreas and the periampullary region, a **pancreaticoduodenectomy (Whipple procedure)** is done. Lesions of the body and tail are treated with a distal pancreatectomy. With the advent of laparoscopic technology, many surgeons begin the procedure laparoscopically to avoid a laparotomy in patients whose lesion is found at exploration to be unresectable. At laparoscopy or laparotomy, incurable disease is defined by liver metastases or peritoneal seeding of tumor, both of which may be missed by all available preoperative imaging techniques. Invasion of the mesenteric root, celiac axis, or mesenteric vessels also constitutes unresectability. In patients with unresectable disease, palliation can be achieved with minimally invasive techniques. Biliary drainage is accomplished by endoscopic stenting in most cases. Patients with gastric outlet obstruction can be managed with gastrojejunostomy. Back pain can be improved with a celiac axis alcohol infusion or "block."

Pancreaticoduodenectomy involves resection of the distal common bile duct, duodenum, and head of the pancreas. Classically, an antrectomy has been done; however, many surgeons currently do a pylorus-preserving procedure. After resection, continuity is restored with choledochojejunostomy, pancreaticojejunostomy, and gastrojejunostomy (Figs. 18-8, 18-9, and 18-10).

Complications are common, due to the magnitude of the procedure. However, most complications are managed without reoperation, and the mortality rate of the procedure is less than 5% in modern series. A frequent complication is leakage from the pancreaticojejunostomy. This leakage may manifest as amylase-rich drainage from drains placed intraoperatively (a pancreatic fistula) or as abscess formation with overwhelming sepsis. The incidence of pancreatic fistula is approximately 20% in most series. Management includes assurance of adequate drainage of pancreatic secretions, provision of nutrition (often including total parenteral nutrition), and control of fistula output. Most of these leaks close with nonoperative therapy. Other complications that may occur include delayed gastric emptying and leak from the biliary anastomosis or gastrojejunostomy.

Prognosis

The majority of pancreatic cancer patients initially present with unresectable disease. Of those that undergo removal of all gross disease, the majority die from recurrence. Fac-

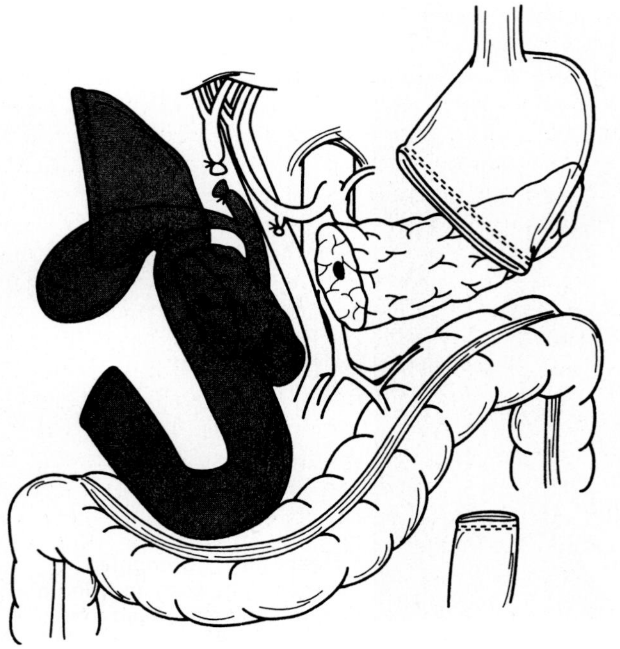

Figure 18-8 Details of Whipple resection (pancreaticojejunostomy) showing antrectomy, duodenectomy, cholecystectomy, distal common bile duct resection, and partial pancreatectomy. A vagotomy is also performed.

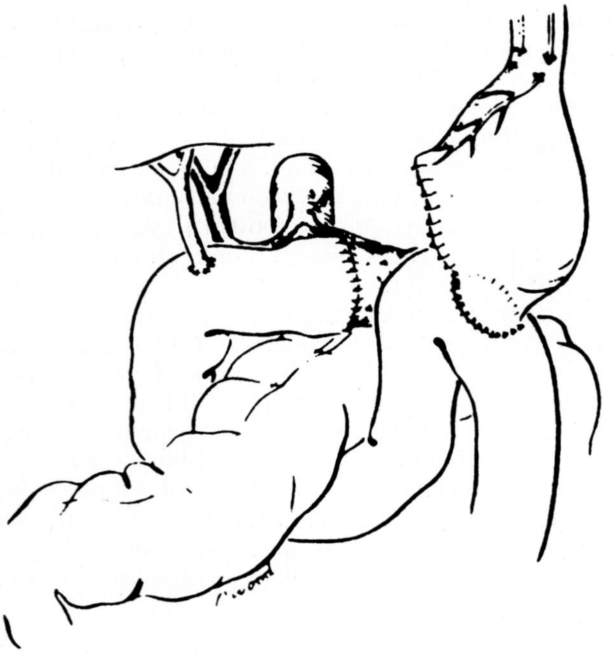

Figure 18-9 Reconstruction after a Whipple resection showing pancreaticojejunostomy, choledochojejunostomy, and gastroenterostomy.

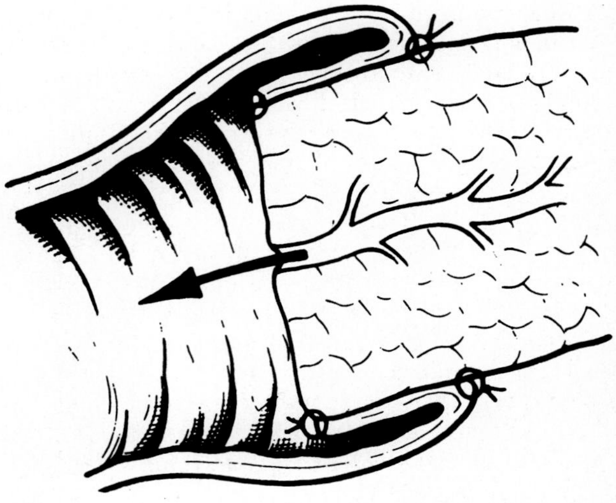

Figure 18-10 Detailed view of pancreaticojejunostomy. The pancreas inverts into the jejunum.

tors associated with a poor prognosis include lymph node metastasis, tumor size greater than 3 cm, and perineural invasion. Patients who undergo resection for cure have a median survival of approximately 19 months, with the majority of these patients receiving postoperative chemotherapy and radiation treatment. Patients with unresectable disease have a median survival of 6 months. Patients without lymph node metastases have a 5-year survival rate of approximately 20%. Although surgical therapy is the only curative modality, further advances in the treatment of pancreatic cancer will require the development of effective chemotherapeutic regimens and radiation protocols. Adjuvant radiation and chemotherapy after curative resection are common, but little data support their efficacy.

Cystadenoma and Cystadenocarcinoma

There are few benign pancreatic tumors. The most common are cystadenomas, which may be serous or mucinous. The serous varieties are also called microcystic adenomas and have a short, cuboidal cell lining. These are more common in women than men and usually are diagnosed in the seventh decade. Recently, there have been reports of serous cystadenocarcinomas, but these are very rare. Mucinous cystic neoplasms are much more common than serous cystadenomas and are also more common in women than men. They have an earlier mean age of diagnosis, which is the fifth decade. These tumors have a tall, columnar cell lining and are filled with mucus. Some have suggested that the majority of these benign lesions will eventually develop into a cancer. The treatment of a mucinous cystadenoma is resection, not drainage.

The prognosis for cystadenocarcinoma of the pancreas is much better than for the more common ductal (noncystic) adenocarcinomas, with approximately 50% of patients living 5 years. Aggressive surgical treatment is therefore indicated.

A final group of cystic tumors includes the solid and cystic papillary neoplasms of the pancreas. These have been termed "Hamoudi neoplasms" and occur primarily in young women in their 20s. Long-term survival is common following resection. Because of the possibility of malignancy, complete surgical resection is recommended.

Islet Cell Tumor of the Pancreas

The two most common functional islet cell neoplasms of the pancreas arise from the beta cells (insulinoma) and the delta cells (gastrinoma). Other islet cell neoplasms of the pancreas secrete glucagon, somatostatin, VIP, pancreatic polypeptide, and chromogranin A, but they are extremely rare. The most common type of islet cell tumor is the nonfunctional/nonsecretory tumor. Ninety percent of insulinomas are benign, while the majority of other islet cell tumors are malignant.

The classic symptoms of insulin-producing neoplasms are attacks consisting of palpitations, tremulousness, and tachycardia. These symptoms are precipitated by fasting. Whipple's triad includes fasting blood sugar levels less than 45 mg/100 mL, symptoms during fasting, and relief of symptoms with administration of glucose. Simultaneous measurement of serum insulin and blood glucose levels is diagnostic in showing an inappropriately high serum insulin level relative to blood glucose. Serum C-peptide and urinary sulfonylurea must also be measured to rule out factitious hypoglycemia. C-peptide is produced with insulin by the insulinoma or pancreas. If C-peptide levels are low and insulin levels are elevated, self-administration of exogenous insulin by the patient should be suspected. Likewise, if urinary sulfonylurea is elevated, the patient is likely ingesting oral hypoglycemic agents. Localization of the tumor is the goal of the preoperative evaluation. The majority of insulinomas are solitary and benign. Angiography shows hypervascular lesions in approximately one-half of patients. Percutaneous transhepatic sampling of portal and splenic vein blood for measurement of insulin levels may also be helpful in the detection of insulinoma. CT scans of the abdomen show the lesion less than 50% of the time. The most successful means to identify a tumor is careful exposure of the pancreas surgically for careful palpation. Intraoperative ultrasound is used to confirm the findings and establish the anatomic relation to the pancreatic duct.

Surgical resection is the preferred management for patients with insulinoma. Delay in treatment is associated with neurologic damage as a result of recurrent episodes of hypoglycemia. The surgical treatment is resection of the tumor if it can be found. Usually, the tumor is simply enucleated without major pancreatic resection. Medical treatment is reserved for patients with unresectable malignant lesions. Streptozotocin and diazoxide are used with limited success. Other islet cell neoplasms should undergo formal resection due to their higher malignant potential.

Zollinger-Ellison Syndrome

Zollinger-Ellison syndrome is severe peptic ulcer disease caused by a gastrin-secreting islet cell tumor. These tumors are most commonly found in the gastrinoma triangle defined by the junction of the cystic and common bile ducts superiorly, the junction of the second and third portion of the duodenum inferiorly, and the junction of the neck and body of the pancreas (where the superior mesenteric artery crosses under the pancreatic neck) medially. Gastrinomas have also been located outside the pancreatic and biliary system including in the heart, liver, lungs, ovary, bile ducts, kidney, mesentery, and bones. Hence, imaging studies done to localize these tumors should be done throughout the entire body.

The diagnosis of Zollinger-Ellison syndrome should be considered in patients with ulcers in unusual locations (distal duodenum or jejunum), recurrent duodenal ulcers, profuse watery diarrhea, or with large gastric rugal folds seen on endoscopy. Elevations of the fasting serum gastrin greater than 750 pg/dL are common, but not diagnostic. The most common false-positive elevation of serum gastrin is found in patients with atrophic gastritis and achlorhidria. These patients have no peptic ulcers on endoscopy and have a neutral gastric pH while they are not taking H_2 blockers or proton pump inhibitors. Patients with suspected gastrinomas and low levels of fasting serum gastrin should have a secretin-stimulation test to confirm the diagnosis before they undergo further imaging studies or an operation. A fasting gastrin level is obtained, followed by rapid intravenous administration of 2 units/kg secretin. Serum gastrin levels are obtained at 1, 3, 5, 7, 10, and 15 minutes. A positive test result is indicated by a doubling of the fasting level or an absolute increase of 200 pg/dL over the fasting level. Once diagnosed, it is important to determine whether this is part of a multiple endocrine neoplasia (MEN) syndrome (pituitary, pancreatic, parathyroid adenomas—see Chapter 21, Surgical Endocrinology) or sporadic.

CT scan and ultrasound of the abdomen are used to attempt preoperative localization of gastrinomas, but they fail in as many as 50% of cases. Selective angiography to look for vascular blush may detect gastrinomas in as many as 75% of cases. Patients with gastrinomas as part of a MEN syndrome are much more likely to have multicentric lesions than patients with sporadic gastrinomas; these lesions are difficult to localize. Octreotide-labeled nuclear medicine scans are highly sensitive and specific in detecting gastrinomas and metastatic disease, but precise correlation to the exact anatomic locations is difficult.

Surgical removal of gastrinomas should be attempted in good-risk surgical patients, especially if the lesion can be localized preoperatively and is not multicentric. Intraoperative ultrasound can be extremely useful in determining the location of tumors and the relation of the tumor to the bile duct, pancreatic duct, or major vessels. Many of these tumors can be removed with simple enucleation, but some require major pancreatic resection. Some tiny lesions located in the duodenal wall may be detected by transilluminating the duodenal wall with intraoperative endoscopy or direct duodenotomy.

Currently, blind subtotal pancreatic resection is rarely

used for gastrinomas. Historically, total gastrectomy was used to prevent fulminant complications of peptic ulceration for undetectable or metastatic gastrinomas but, with the availability of potent acid secretion inhibitors (e.g., proton pump inhibitors), it is rarely used today. Most gastrinomas are malignant, although histologic differentiation between benign and malignant tumors is extremely difficult. Clinical differentiation is based on the detection of metastatic disease with imaging studies or surgical exploration.

SUGGESTED READINGS

Abrams RA. Adjuvant therapy for pancreatic adenocarcinoma: what have we learned since 1985? *Int J Radiat Oncol Biol Phys* 2003;56:Supplement 3–9.

Baron TH, Morgan DE. Current concepts: acute necrotizing pancreatitis. *N Engl J Med* 1999;340:1412–1417.

Delcore R, Friesen SR. Gastrointestinal neuroendocrine tumors. *J Am Coll Surg* 1994;178:187–211.

Golub R, Siddiqi F, Pohl D. Role of antibiotics in acute pancreatitis: a meta-analysis. *J Gastrointest Surg* 1998;2:496–503.

Lillemoe KD. Current management of pancreatic carcinoma. *Ann Surg* 1995;221:133–148.

Park BJ, Alexander R, Libutti SK, et al. Operative management of islet-cell tumors arising in the head of the pancreas. *Surgery* 1998;124:1056–1062.

Ranson JHC, Rifkind KM, Roses DF, et al. Prognostic signs and the role of operative management in acute pancreatitis. *Surg Gynecol Obstet* 1974;139:69.

Sarr MG, Carpenter HA, Prabhakar LP, et al. Clinical and pathological correlation of 84 mucinous cystic neoplasms of the pancreas. *Ann Surg* 2000;231:205–212.

Soper NJ, Brunt LM, Caller MP, et al. Role of laparoscopic cholecystectomy in the management of acute gallstone pancreatitis. *Am J Surg* 1994;167:42–51.

Steer ML, Waxman I, Freedman S. Chronic pancreatitis. *N Engl J Med* 1995;332:1482–1490.

Steinberg W, Tenner S. Acute pancreatitis. *N Engl J Med* 1994;330:1198–1210.

Werner J, Uhl W, Hartwig W, et al. Modern phase-specific management of acute pancreatitis. *Dig Dis* 2003;21:38–45.

Yeo CJ, Sohn TA, Cameron JL, et al. Periampullary carcinoma: analysis of 5-year survivors. *Ann Surg* 1998;227:821–831.

Yousaf M, McCallion K, Diamond T. Management of severe acute pancreatitis *Br J Surg* 2003;90:407–420.

19

WILLIAM C. CHAPMAN, MD ■ JOHN R. POTTS, III, MD

Liver

OBJECTIVES

1. List at least three common benign tumors of the liver, and describe their appropriate treatment.
2. List four factors that favorably influence the prognosis after resection of hepatic metastasis from colorectal cancer.
3. List the two most common primary hepatobiliary malignancies and their relative frequency.
4. List the steps involved in diagnosing a hepatic mass.
5. Compare and contrast the clinical and pathologic features and the treatment of hepatic adenoma and focal nodular hyperplasia.
6. List the three major complications of portal hypertension.
7. List four forms of specific therapy for acute variceal hemorrhage in the order in which they are typically applied.
8. List at least three sites of portosystemic collateral formation in patients with portal hypertension.
9. List at least four causes of portal hypertension in addition to cirrhosis.
10. List three complications associated with ascites formation in the patient with portal hypertension.

In the liver, mass lesions (tumors, cysts, and abscesses), complications of **portal hypertension,** organ failure, and trauma constitute the vast majority of hepatic diseases for which surgical intervention is warranted.

ANATOMY

The liver is the largest single gland in the body. In the average adult, it weighs approximately 1500 g. It is located below the diaphragm, with its greatest mass to the right of the midline. It is covered by the tough, fibrous Glisson's capsule, which extends into its parenchyma along penetrating vessels. Except for the bare area over its posterior surface near the vena cava, the liver is invested in peritoneum. Reflections of the peritoneum (falciform, coronary, and triangular "ligaments") attach the liver to the diaphragm and abdominal wall. Another reflection of the peritoneum, the gastrohepatic ligament, attaches the liver to other abdominal viscera.

A plane passing from the left side of the gallbladder and through the left side of the vena cava divides the left and right lobes of the liver. Each lobe has four segments described by vertical passage of the major hepatic veins and horizontal passage of the major portal venous and hepatic arterial branches. This surgically important segmental anatomy is not visible on the surface of the liver (Figs. 19-1 and 19-2).

The liver enjoys a dual blood supply. In most individuals, the hepatic artery arises from the celiac axis. Occasionally, it comes from the superior mesenteric artery (i.e., "replaced hepatic artery"). The portal vein represents the confluence of drainage from the bowel and spleen. The portal vein supplies 70% of the blood flow to the liver. The right, middle, and left hepatic veins drain directly into the inferior vena cava.

PHYSIOLOGY

The functional unit of the liver is the lobule. On the periphery of each lobule lie hepatic arterial and portal venous branches. Centrally lies a draining vein. Blood from these

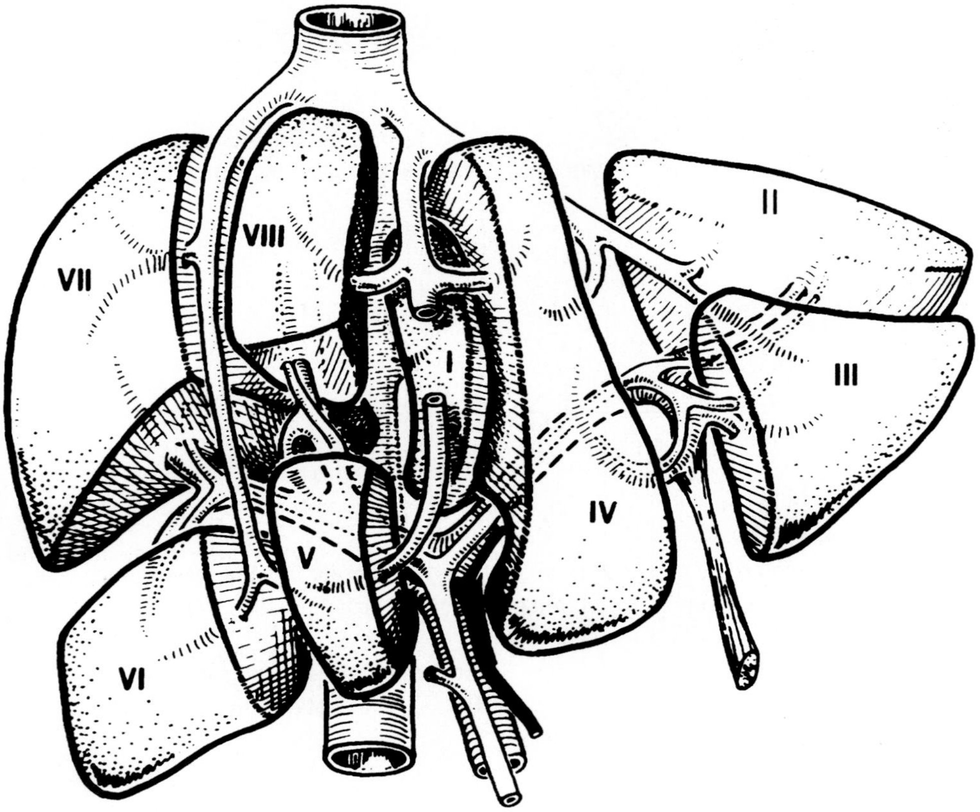

Figure 19-1 The functional division of the liver and liver segments according to Couinaud's nomenclature (segments *I–VIII*). (Reprinted with permission from Blumgart LH, ed. *Surgery of the Liver and Biliary Tract.* New York, NY: Churchill Livingstone, 1994:5.)

vessels converges in the hepatic sinusoids with which each hepatocyte has intimate contact.

The liver performs more than 2000 metabolic functions, including bile production and the metabolism of protein, carbohydrates, fats, vitamins, drugs, and toxins. The hepatocyte, which is the principal cell of the liver, accounts for the majority of metabolic activity. These cells continually divide and can potentially reproduce the entire cell mass of the liver every 50 days. The cells are aligned in a single layer along the hepatic sinusoids, and they transport essential substrates and hormones intracellularly. The hepatocytes then transport metabolic products either back into the plasma or into the bile canaliculus, which is positioned on the opposite side of this single layer of cells. In this way, the hepatocyte monitors and regulates plasma levels of proteins and ensures that metabolic requirements are met.

The liver also performs many important immunologic functions. **Kupffer cells** line the vascular endothelium and are in close proximity to hepatocytes. These macrophages represent 80% to 90% of the fixed macrophages of the body and are subject to frequent turnover. Their unique position within the liver allows them to interface directly with damaging agents (e.g., endotoxin) from the portal circulation. These cells secrete a variety of effectors on hepatocytes and other cells within the body, including tumor necrosis factor (TNF-α), interleukin-1 (IL-1), interleukin-6 (IL-6), and other important cytokines.

HEPATIC TUMORS, CYSTS, AND ABSCESSES

With the increased availability and use of abdominal imaging techniques, including computed tomography (CT) scanning, symptomatic and incidental liver abnormalities are discovered with greater frequency. An important role of the physician who is treating a patient with a newly discovered hepatic abnormality is to determine both the likely etiology of the abnormality and whether further diagnostic or therapeutic measures are needed. Careful patient assessment is needed because incidental benign liver tumors and cysts are common and usually require no specific therapy. On the other hand, some benign liver tumors are resected, if feasible, even in the asymptomatic patient. An important principle is to avoid liver biopsy early in the workup of a newly discovered liver mass in an otherwise asymptomatic patient. Needle biopsy is usually not necessary to determine the most likely diagnosis. It is subject to sampling error and may introduce additional risks of bleeding or tumor seeding in a patient who might undergo tumor resection regardless of the biopsy result.

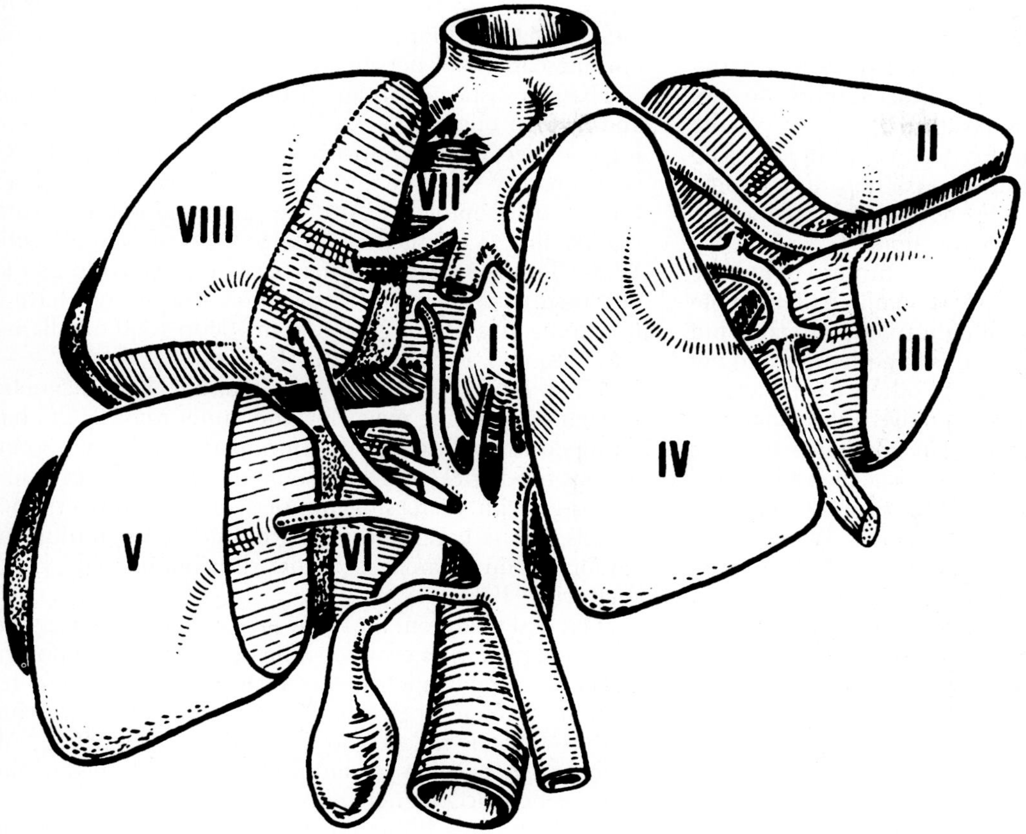

Figure 19-2 The biliary anatomy of the segments of the liver. The caudate lobe (segment *I*) drains into both the right and left ductal systems. (Reprinted with permission from Blumgart LH, ed. *Surgery of the Liver and Biliary Tract.* New York, NY: Churchill Livingstone, 1994:11.)

Benign Tumors

Hemangioma

Cavernous hemangioma of the liver is the most common benign liver tumor and occurs in as many as 8% of the general population. These are probably congenital lesions and are embryologic hamartomas (benign tumors with two distinct cell types). They may enlarge over the lifetime of an individual. Some reports suggest hormonal responsiveness, including enlargement during pregnancy. Cavernous hemangiomas that are larger than 4 cm are defined as giant hemangiomas. These lesions are often incidental findings and require no specific therapy. Ultrasonography is usually diagnostic, showing focal hyperechoic abnormalities that are characteristic of these lesions. Contrasted CT imaging usually shows a progressive peripheral-to-central prominent enhancement and a central hypodense region.

Most patients are asymptomatic at presentation and remain so in followup. Spontaneous rupture is extremely rare. Longitudinal studies assessing long-term (> 10 years) followup in patients with giant cavernous hemangiomas confirm the absence of spontaneous rupture. Occasionally, patients with very large hemangiomas have pain, and surgical resection may be considered. Microscopic evaluation shows endothelial vascular spaces separated by fibrous septa. Nonresectional strategies used in the past (e.g., radiation, high-dose steroid administration, hepatic artery ligation, embolization) did not show efficacy. These lesions may undergo spontaneous thrombosis, which causes transient pain, elevation in hepatic transaminases, and involution on imaging studies.

Hepatic Adenoma

A **hepatic adenoma** is a benign tumor that usually occurs in young women between 30 and 50 years of age. Most patients have a history of estrogen exposure, usually in the form of long-standing use of oral contraceptives and occasionally from estrogen replacement therapy. These tumors grossly appear as solitary, unencapsulated masses. Their cut surfaces have a smooth, soft appearance. Microscopically, they appear as sheets of hepatocytes without portal triads or bile ducts.

The usual treatment of hepatic adenoma is surgical resection, if it can be safely performed, because of the risk of subsequent growth and possible rupture. In approximately 20% to 35% of cases, patients have pain or shock as a result of spontaneous rupture of the tumor. Hepatocellular carcinoma occasionally develops within these tumors. This risk appears to be increased for larger lesions (> 5 cm).

The clinical presentation is often highly suggestive of hepatic adenoma, but definite preoperative diagnosis may not be possible. CT scanning usually shows a solid hypodense lesion, sometimes with evidence of adjacent hemorrhage. ^{99m}Tc sulfa colloid scanning usually shows a corresponding filling defect because these tumors do not contain Kupffer cells and do not take up this tracer. Needle biopsy may help to establish the diagnosis, but sampling errors can make it difficult to distinguish hepatic adenoma from focal nodular hyperplasia or hepatocellular carcinoma on the basis of needle biopsy alone.

The treatment of choice for these tumors is hepatic resection whenever possible. Occasionally, patients note tumor regression on withdrawal of hormonal therapy, but this situation is uncommon, and this treatment should not be used as primary therapy for an otherwise resectable tumor in a healthy patient. Intraoperative ultrasonography is performed in these patients, as in any patient with a hepatic neoplasm, to search for unsuspected additional tumors and to define the relation of the tumor to adjacent portal venous and hepatic arterial structures. Women with a history of hepatic adenoma should use alternative methods of contraception and avoid subsequent use of oral contraceptives. Avoidance of subsequent pregnancy is optimal, but if a patient becomes pregnant, she should undergo periodic surveillance ultrasound assessment of the liver.

Focal Nodular Hyperplasia

Focal nodular hyperplasia (FNH) is a well-circumscribed benign lesion. It usually has a central scar with fibrous septa and nodular hyperplasia. Unlike in hepatic adenoma, bile ducts are scattered throughout. These tumors do not have premalignant potential, and rupture or hemorrhage is extremely rare. These tumors are usually found incidentally when ultrasound or CT scanning is performed for some other cause.

The major difficulty in managing FNH lies in establishing a diagnosis. CT scanning does not differentiate this lesion from other solid liver masses but may sometimes demonstrate a classic central stellate scar, and ultrasonography may not provide assistance with the differential diagnosis. Arteriography may show a characteristic spoke-wheel pattern, but even needle biopsy may not distinguish this tumor from hepatic adenoma. For these reasons, FNH is often excised in the good-risk medical candidate who has a symptomatic tumor, but may be observed in the patient who is a poor operative candidate and in whom the diagnosis is strongly suspected based on imaging studies.

Malignant Tumors

Hepatocellular Carcinoma

Hepatocellular carcinoma (HCC), or hepatoma, accounts for more than 90% of all primary liver malignancies. This tumor usually occurs in patients with underlying liver disease (70% to 80%). It occurs at high rates in areas where hepatitis B is endemic. Although cirrhosis from any cause appears to be associated with the development of HCC, it is also found at increased rates in noncirrhotic chronic carriers of hepatitis B and C.

HCC is suspected in any patient with known cirrhosis and sudden clinical decompensation, including worsening jaundice, encephalopathy, or increasing ascites. HCC is also part of the differential diagnosis for any solid liver tumor. α-Fetoprotein (AFP) is an α_1-globulin serum marker that is elevated in 60% to 80% of patients with HCC. This tumor marker may also be elevated to 200 to 400 mg/dL in patients with cirrhosis who do not have a hepatoma. Elevations greater than 500 to 1000 mg/dL are almost always associated with HCC.

When HCC is suspected, ultrasound, CT, or magnetic resonance scanning may show the tumor mass. HCC has a propensity for vascular invasion, particularly into portal venous tributaries, and the likelihood of vascular invasion increases with increasing tumor size. This property accounts for the common finding of satellitosis (multifocal tumors within a similar segmental distribution in the liver) seen with HCC.

The best treatment for HCC is resection with clear surgical margins, whenever possible, in a patient with no evidence of extrahepatic disease. Unfortunately, surgical resection is often impossible because of the underlying cirrhosis that is so common in patients with HCC. Although it is possible to remove as much as 70% of the normal hepatic parenchyma at liver resection, the presence of cirrhosis limits the regenerative capacity of the liver. No specific studies conclusively determine the extent of hepatic parenchyma that can be safely resected in a cirrhotic patient, and most surgeons attempt only small peripheral wedge or segmental resections in this setting. When patients with HCC and cirrhosis undergo successful tumor resection, the remaining liver is the most common site of future recurrence ($\geq$ 50% of patients), probably because similar etiologic factors are present in the remaining liver (e.g., hepatitis with the formation of second primary lesions) and also from satellite lesions that were not detected at initial resection. Other sites of tumor metastasis include lung and bone. Brain and intraperitoneal metastases are less common.

Liver transplantation has theoretical appeal for patients with HCC because it not only removes the malignant tumor, but also eliminates possible sites of recurrence in the remaining diseased liver. It also provides hepatic replacement in patients who usually have severely limited hepatic reserve in addition to their tumor. Limitations to the use of liver transplantation in the treatment of patients with hepatoma include the limited number of donor livers for transplantation and the high cost of this treatment modality. Additionally, the results are poor when extrahepatic tumor is present. This tumor may undergo accelerated growth under the influence of the immunosuppression that is required to prevent rejection of the transplanted liver. Recent strategies used preoperative chemoembolization followed by posttransplant adjuvant chemotherapy in carefully selected patients. Chemoembolization involves the infusion of chemotherapy (usually doxorubicin [Adriamycin]) combined with gelatin foam particles. This process induces tumor ischemia while prolonging chemotherapy dwell times at the site of hepatic tumors. This procedure is possible for hepatic tumors because of the dual blood supply present for the liver. Further, because most hepatomas derive 85% or more of their blood supply from a hepatic arterial source, this treatment modality induces a much greater effect than on the surrounding nontumor hepatic parenchyma, where at least 50% of the oxygen and nutrient supply is derived from a portal venous source. In many centers, liver transplantation in combination with pretransplantation chemoembolization is the treatment of choice for patients with advanced cirrhosis and small (< 5 cm) but unresectable HCC, and such patients now receive accelerated listing priority by the United Network for Organ Sharing (UNOS).

The fibrolamellar variant of HCC occurs more often in younger patients and often is not associated with underlying cirrhosis. Patients with this tumor usually do not have elevated AFP levels and have a better long-term prognosis after resection than patients with standard HCC. It is unclear whether this improved prognosis is related to the less aggressive nature of the tumor or to the absence of underlying liver disease and a greater resectability rate.

Cholangiocarcinoma

Cholangiocarcinoma (see Chapter 17, Biliary Tract) usually causes obstructive jaundice and a bile duct stricture on endoscopic retrograde cholangiopancreatography. There is often no visible tumor mass on CT scanning. Occasionally, primary tumors of bile duct origin present as a solid tumor within the substance of the liver. These tumors are treated with liver resection. Other rare primary tumors of the liver include angiosarcoma and epithelioid hemangioendothelioma.

Metastatic Tumors

The most common malignant tumors found in the liver represent metastatic carcinoma, most commonly from a gastrointestinal source (probably because the hepatic sinusoids are the first capillary bed encountered for blood from a gastrointestinal source). In patients who die of malignant disease, 30% to 40% have hepatic metastases at autopsy. Although hepatic metastases usually are indicative of widespread metastatic carcinoma, in selected cases hepatic metastases may be the only residual disease and therefore can be treated with hepatic-only directed therapy. This approach is clearly established for colorectal carcinoma, where successful resection of metastatic foci can result in 5-year survival rates of 30% to 40% in properly selected patients.

Requirements for successful hepatic resection of colorectal metastases include the absence of extrahepatic disease and the ability to safely resect all hepatic disease. Patients who have hepatic metastasis more than 1 year after colon resection and those without regional lymph node involvement at the time of colon resection fare better than those with synchronous colon and metastatic liver lesions and those with mesenteric lymph node involvement. Patients with three or fewer liver lesions resected appear to fare better than those with more lesions. However, long-term survival is reported with resection of as many as five metastatic foci. Patients with multilobar metastases resected appear to do as well as those in whom all metastatic foci are confined to a single lobe.

Although resection of hepatic metastases may afford long-term survival, most of these patients (60% to 70%) have recurrence of colorectal carcinoma, and the residual liver is the most common site of recurrence. For this reason, resected patients require careful selection and close followup. It is unclear whether patients who undergo successful hepatic resection of colorectal metastases benefit from adjuvant systemic or regional chemotherapy after liver resection. Current clinical trials that address this question may provide results within the next several years.

Recently, ablative therapy techniques (cryoablation and radiofrequency ablation [RFA]) have become available for treatment of primary and metastatic tumors. This therapy is usually reserved for patients with liver-confined but unresectable tumors. Cryoablation is performed by passing a metal probe into the tumor and circulating liquid nitrogen through the probe to freeze-kill the tumor and a rim of nontumor liver parenchyma (usually at least a 1-cm rim to act as a "margin," if possible). RFA is performed by passing a needle guide into the tumor; radiofrequency energy is then used to heat the tumor and a surrounding rim of nontumor parenchyma. Cryoablation has been associated with significant complications when approximately 30% or more of the liver is treated, including coagulopathy, renal failure, and a systemic inflammatory response–like syndrome (SIRS). Similar complications have not been observed with RFA. Because RFA is able to be performed through a much smaller probe and can be performed laparoscopically, it is more frequently utilized than cryoablation. The precise role of ablative therapy in the management of hepatic tumors remains to be fully defined.

Hepatic Cysts

Simple Cysts and Polycystic Liver Disease

Cystic disease of the liver is a common finding, particularly with the increased use of CT to investigate many abdominal conditions. Simple cysts occur in as many as 10% of patients. They are usually small and asymptomatic. They usually contain clear serous fluid and do not communicate with the biliary tree. Although they may appear in multiples, they usually number fewer than three to four and are scattered throughout the liver.

Simple cysts are most often asymptomatic, but occasionally may become quite large and may be associated with pain or early satiety because of the mass effect. Needle

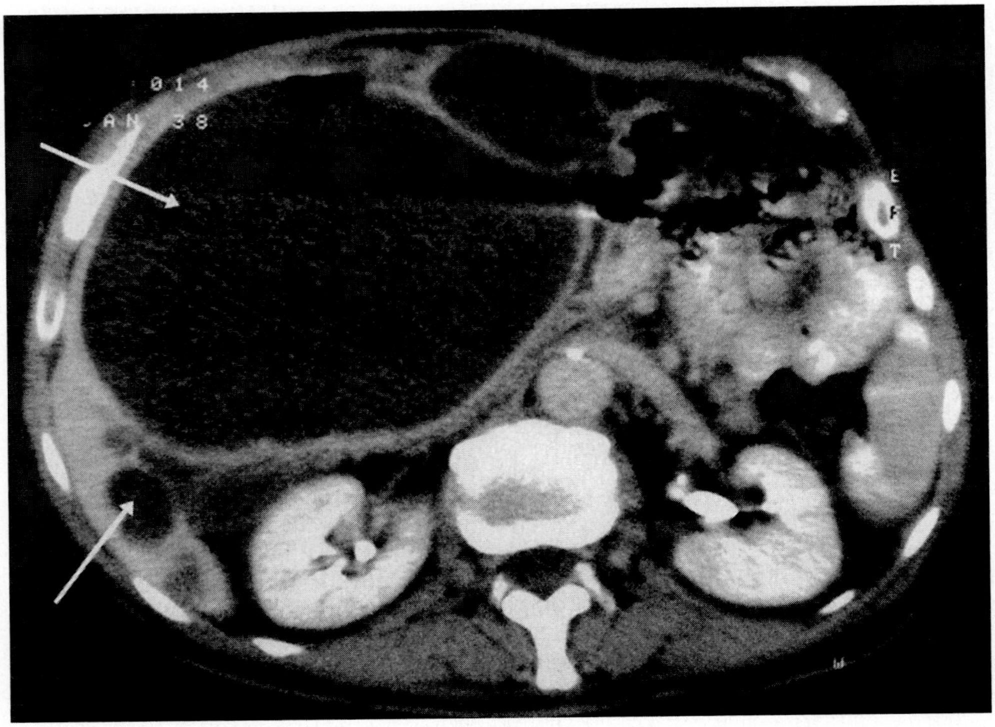

Figure 19-3 Computed tomography scan showing multiple large and small cysts within the liver (*arrows*) in a patient with polycystic liver disease.

aspiration provides temporary relief, but the cysts almost always recur. For this reason, standard treatment includes unroofing or fenestrating the cyst wall and allowing the cyst fluid to drain into and be resorbed by the peritoneal cavity. Surgical resection of simple cysts is not usually required and may be dangerous because large portal and hepatic venous branches may be compressed in the cyst-parenchyma interface and because there is usually no clear plane for resection of the cyst wall.

Polycystic liver disease (Figs. 19-3 and 19-4) is an autosomal dominant disorder that causes multiple cysts that are microscopically similar to simple cysts. Unlike simple cysts, however, these cysts are innumerable, and progressive enlargement is the norm. Additionally, patients with polycystic liver disease often have polycystic kidney disease that may progress to end-stage renal disease. The hepatic cysts in this condition may be treated with resection of the dominant area of cystic involvement, but simple cyst unroofing alone is rarely effective because of the extensive involvement. Some patients have extensive involvement of the entire liver, but even in this situation, it is rare for hepatic synthetic function to be significantly altered.

Cystic Neoplasms

Although most patients with liver cysts have nonneoplastic simple cysts that require treatment only if they are symptomatic, some cystic lesions are cystadenoma or cystadenocarcinoma. A clue to the neoplastic nature of these cysts is the presence of thick walls with multiple septations within the cyst. Unlike simple cysts and polycystic liver disease, which occur with similar frequency in men and women, cystadenoma occurs with a much higher frequency in women, usually in middle age. Calcifications in the cyst wall may also be noted and are more common in cystadenocarcinoma than in the benign variety. Because of the malignant potential of these lesions, the preferred treatment is surgical excision. Nonresectional procedures, including marsupialization (creation of a pouch), drainage into the peritoneal cavity, and drainage into the gastrointestinal tract, are associated with a high rate of cyst recurrence and the development of infected cysts. Therefore, they are not indicated.

Hydatid Cysts

Hydatid cystic disease occurs when humans become infected with echinococcal organisms and act as an accidental host. The normal life cycle of this parasite involves sheep and carnivores (wolves or dogs). Humans are infected by contact with dog feces. The most common infecting organism is *Echinococcus granulosis*, which forms unilocular cysts within the hepatic parenchyma that may grow as large as 10 to 20 cm. Within the larger cysts are multiple daughter cysts that contain innumerable protoscolices.

The diagnosis of hydatid cyst disease is suspected in any patient who has lived in an endemic region (Alaska, regions of the southwest United States, and many foreign countries) and who has cystic hepatic lesions that contain characteristic daughter cysts. Calcifications may also be present and are sometimes indicative of long-standing indolent infection. The diagnosis is confirmed with serologic

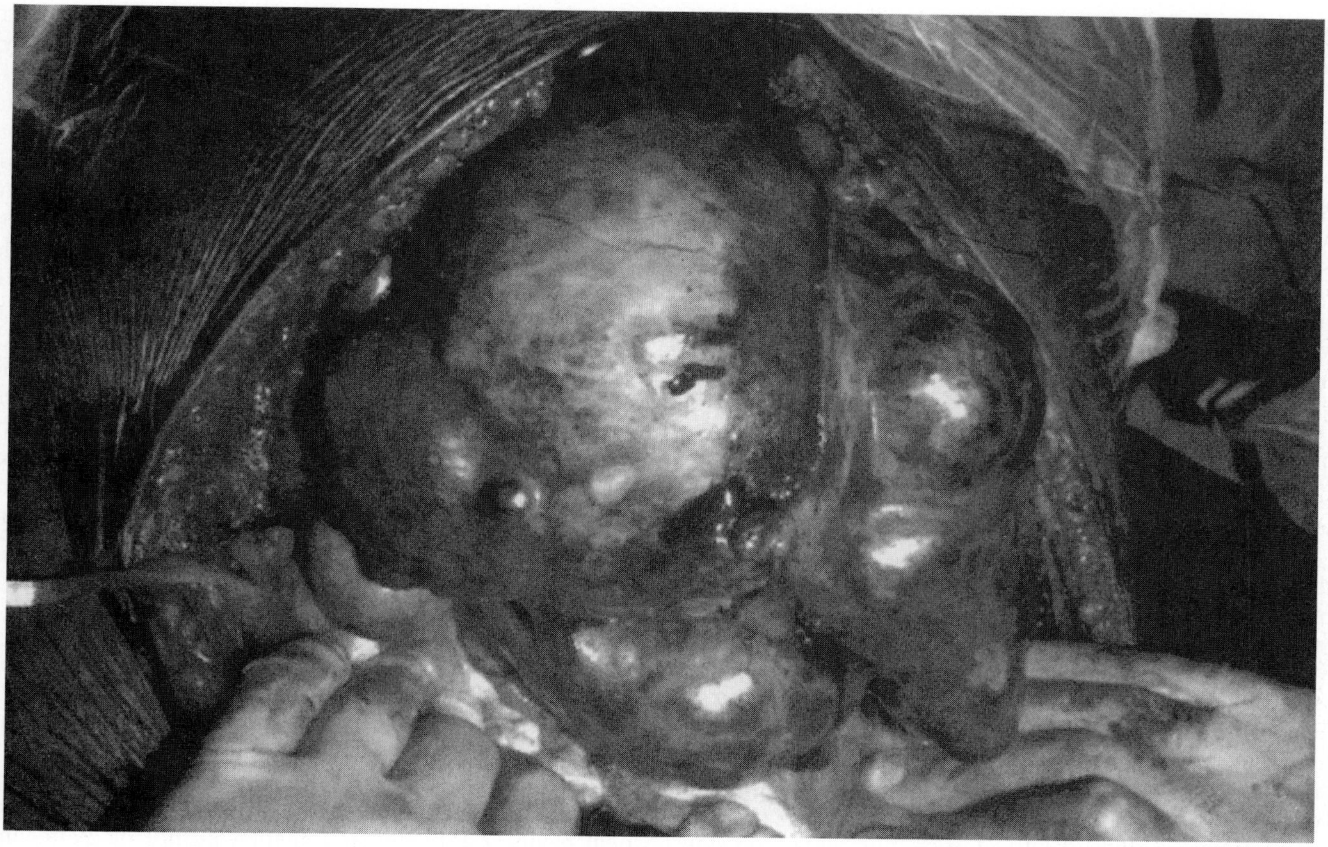

Figure 19-4 A polycystic liver.

testing. If the diagnosis is suspected, needle aspiration or biopsy must not be performed because it may produce disastrous results from seeding of protoscolices throughout the abdominal cavity and may also induce profound anaphylaxis. After the diagnosis is established, antiparasitic therapy with albendazole is initiated. In some cases, this therapy alone may be successful in controlling further growth and spread of the hydatid cystic disease. However, if antihelminthic therapy alone is unsuccessful, open exploration is performed, and the area of cystic involvement is walled off with a scolecidal agent (e.g., hypertonic saline). The cyst contents are then carefully removed, with care taken to dissect out the inner cyst lining, which may contain infective parasites. Extreme caution is used to avoid spillage of any of the cyst contents into the peritoneal cavity because spillage can lead to intraperitoneal recurrence of hydatid cyst disease.

Hepatic Abscesses

Pyogenic Abscess

Patients with bacterial liver abscess usually have right upper quadrant pain, fever, and leukocytosis. The alkaline phosphatase level is elevated in most patients, and CT and ultrasound imaging show a hypoechoic abnormality that sometimes is associated with a hyperechoic or hypervascular wall. Although hepatic abscess may develop as a consequence of hematogenous seeding from any site, this complication usually occurs from a gastrointestinal (i.e., diverticulitis) or biliary tract source.

Percutaneous aspiration and drain placement aid in the diagnosis and facilitate resolution of the infectious process. Antimicrobial therapy is directed by the results of blood and abscess cultures. Biliary stenting may be required if biliary obstruction contributed to the abscess formation. As part of the hepatic abscess workup, a source is sought and treated if indicated.

Amebic Abscess

Although rare in the United States, amebic hepatic abscess is relatively common in regions endemic for amebiasis, including Central and South America. For this reason, it should be considered in immigrants from these regions. Liver abscess occurs in as many as 10% of patients with amebiasis and is one of the most common sites of extraintestinal infection. Percutaneous aspiration shows a sterile fluid that has a characteristic "anchovy paste" appearance. These abscesses respond dramatically to metronidazole. Unlike pyogenic abscesses, they do not require percutaneous drainage.

PORTAL HYPERTENSION AND ITS COMPLICATIONS

Portal hypertension is simply abnormally high pressure in the portal vein or its tributaries. Figure 19-5 shows the normal portal circulation. One uncommon but relatively straightforward form of portal hypertension is sinistral, or left-sided, portal hypertension. In this disorder, thrombosis of the splenic vein (usually caused by pancreatitis or pancreatic tumor) leads to increased pressure in the spleen, which causes splenomegaly and secondary hypersplenism. Another consequence of this disorder is the development of isolated gastric varices because of the return of splenic blood flow to the portal vein through the short gastrics, the submucosal veins of the stomach, and the coronary vein. Splenectomy cures this compartmentalized form of portal hypertension.

Much more common is generalized portal hypertension, in which the portal vein and all of its tributaries are under high pressure. Cirrhosis causes approximately 90% of all portal hypertension in the United States. Approximately 70% of cases of cirrhosis are caused by chronic ethanol ingestion. Portal hypertension can also result from portal vein thrombosis (which accounts for 50% of portal hypertension in children, often related to umbilical vein catheter placement in infancy) and schistosomiasis (which, worldwide, is the most common cause of presinusoidal portal hypertension). In addition, portal hypertension occasionally results from excessive inflow (e.g., a large arteriovenous fistula to a portal vein tributary). Obstruction of hepatic venous outflow can transmit high pressure to the portal vein. The best-known example of this phenomenon is the Budd-Chiari syndrome of hepatic venous occlusion, which can result from various thrombotic states or from the formation of vascular webs in the vena cava. Rarely, congestive heart failure causes portal hypertension in adults. Regardless of the etiology, the increased pressure in the portal vein is compensated for in part by dilation of the portal venous tributaries and in part by the development of collateral channels to the systemic venous system. **Portosystemic collateral routes** form where portal and systemic veins normally meet (Fig. 19-6). These sites include the submucosal veins of the esophagus, which communicate with the azygous system cephalad; the hemorrhoidal veins, which communicate with the iliac system caudad; the umbilical vein, which communicates with veins of the anterior abdominal wall; and the retroperitoneum, which communicates with the vena cava. Adhesions to the abdominal wall can also carry large portosystemic collateral channels. With the development of portal hypertension, the patient may have three complications: ascites, **hepatic encephalopathy**, and variceal bleeding.

Ascites

Ascites is the accumulation of serous fluid in the peritoneal cavity. In portal hypertension, ascites forms as a result of increased hydrostatic pressure and decreased colloid oncotic pressure caused by deficient protein production. This situation favors transudation of fluid out of the vascular space, into the parenchyma, and ultimately into the peritoneal cavity. Clinically significant volumes of ascites are usually detected on physical examination by dependent dullness to percussion and by eliciting a fluid wave. Ultrasound or CT scan detects smaller amounts. A number of conditions other than portal hypertension can result in ascites accumulation, including hypoproteinemic states

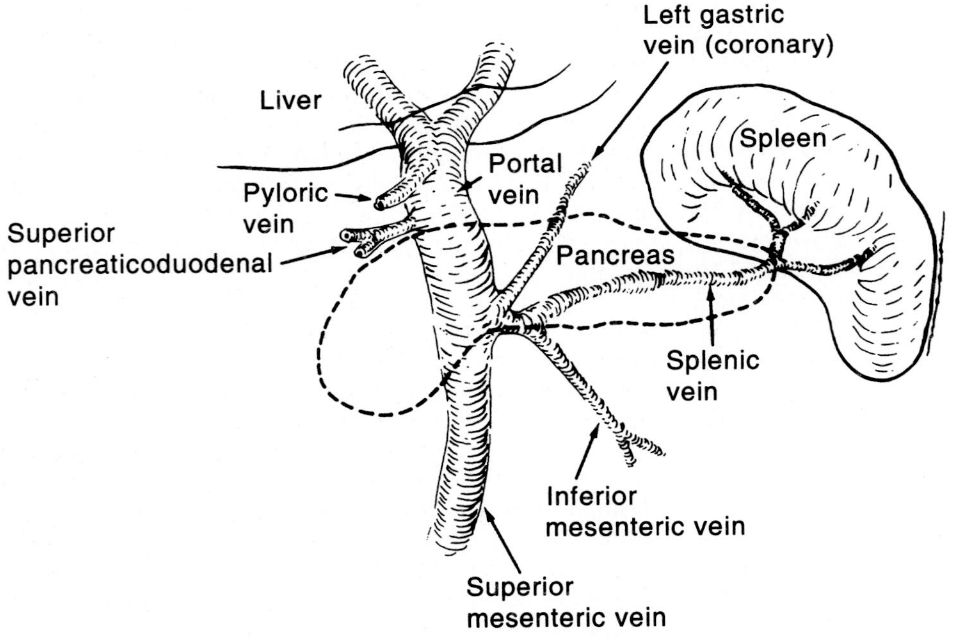

Figure 19-5 Anatomy of the portal circulation. (Reprinted with permission from Rikkers LF. Portal hypertension. In: Goldsmith HS, ed. *Practice of Surgery: General Surgery*. Vol. 3, Chap. 4. Philadelphia, PA: Harper & Row, 1981.)

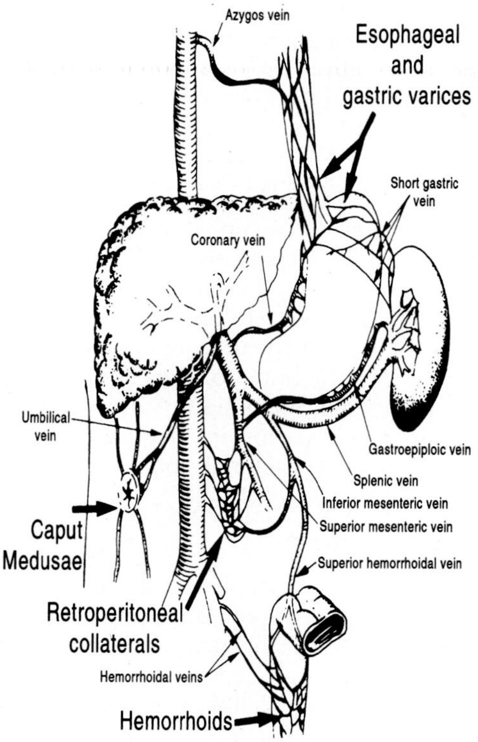

Figure 19-6 Sites of portal-systemic collateralization. (Reprinted with permission from Rikkers LF. Portal hypertension. In: Goldsmith HS, ed. *Practice of Surgery: General Surgery.* Vol. 3, Chap. 4. Philadelphia, PA: Harper & Row, 1981.)

(nephrotic syndrome, protein-losing enteropathy, malnutrition); carcinomatosis; pancreatic, chylous, or bile ascites; and end-stage renal disease. The differential diagnosis emphasizes the need for diagnostic paracentesis in the patient with newly diagnosed ascites. Studies on the fluid should include cytology, cell count and differential, amylase, triglyceride and protein levels, pH, and bacterial cultures.

In patients with portal hypertension related to cirrhosis and without complicating features, the cell count and differential of ascitic fluid usually shows a predominance of monocytes with a total neutrophil cell count of fewer than 250 cells/mL. The cytology shows nonneoplastic cells. The amylase level is less than or equal to the serum amylase level, as is the triglyceride level. Bacterial cultures are negative. The pH is usually 7.3 or greater in noninfected ascites, and the protein content is usually less than 2.5 g.

Ascites in portal hypertension can lead to substantial morbidity. Umbilical, groin, and other abdominal wall hernias can enlarge dramatically with the added pressure of ascites. The skin overlying hernias can become thinned and ulcerated. Rupture of the hernias can occur and is associated with a high mortality rate. Spontaneous bacterial peritonitis occurs in approximately 10% of cirrhotic patients with ascites. It is usually associated with an ascitic fluid white blood cell count of more than 500 cells/mL and a predominance of neutrophils. The mechanism of inoculation is speculative, but most infections are monomicrobial with enteric organisms. This disorder is associated with an exceedingly high mortality rate and requires aggressive antibiotic therapy.

The decreased circulating volume in the patient with significant ascites leads to decreased renal blood flow, increased circulating levels of aldosterone, and redistribution of renal blood flow. As a result, urinary volume and urinary sodium concentration are decreased. Ultimately, renal failure can occur. This unfortunate but common sequence is called hepatorenal syndrome, but there is no clear evidence to show that it represents anything other than profound prerenal azotemia secondary to intravascular volume depletion. Acute renal failure against a background of ascites rarely occurs spontaneously but, sadly, is usually precipitated by overzealous use of diuretics.

Treatment

Medical management effectively controls ascites in more than 90% of patients. Fluid intake is moderately restricted, and sodium intake is limited to less than 40 mEq/day. Diuresis begins with spironolactone, an aldosterone antagonist, which promotes sodium excretion. The dose is gradually increased until urinary excretion of sodium exceeds that of potassium. If further diuresis is necessary, loop or thiazide diuretics are cautiously added. When the ascitic volume severely limits respiration or mobility and rapid decompression is desired, therapeutic paracentesis is performed. Large volumes (8 to 10 L) can safely be removed in one sitting. At paracentesis, it is probably prudent to administer salt-poor albumin intravenously to replace the estimated protein content of ascites that is withdrawn.

Rarely, when medical management and paracentesis fail, more invasive treatment is required. One option is the placement of a peritoneal venous shunt. This device is a tube approximately the diameter of intravenous tubing that originates in the peritoneal cavity and runs subcutaneously to its insertion in the internal jugular vein. The peritoneal end has multiple side-hole perforations, and the tubing contains a one-way valve that precludes the reflux of blood into the tubing. When properly functioning, these devices restore circulating volume and enhance urinary output. Placement is technically simple, but peritoneal-venous shunts are associated with a number of complications (e.g., infection, occlusion of the tubing by proteinaceous debris, congestive heart failure). Variceal bleeding can also occur as a result of the increased venous pressure associated with increased circulating volume.

Portosystemic shunts (Fig. 19-7) are another means of controlling ascites by reducing portal pressure. At one time, surgical portacaval shunts were used for this purpose, but this effort was largely abandoned. Today, radiologically placed portosystemic shunts are occasionally used in the treatment of ascites. These **transjugular intrahepatic portacaval shunts (TIPS)**, although associated with less pro-

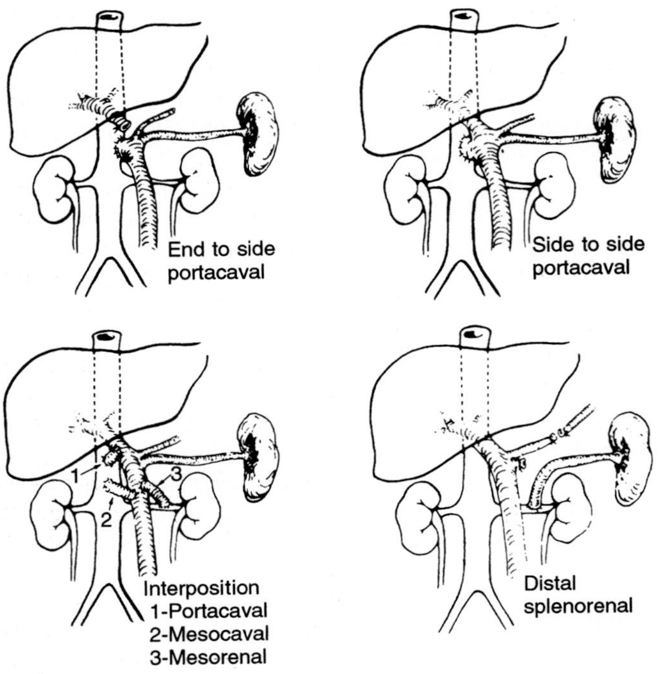

Figure 19-7 Surgical portal–systemic shunts.

cedure-related morbidity than surgical shunts, are not uniformly successful. Like surgical shunts, they often merely trade ascites for encephalopathy. Both TIPS and surgically constructed central shunts (nonselective) allow portal blood to bypass the metabolic actions of the liver. As a result, amino acid imbalances may occur and are believed to play an important role in hepatic encephalopathy (discussed below).

Hepatic Encephalopathy

Hepatic encephalopathy is a neuropsychiatric disorder that can develop in patients with severe liver disease. Clinical features include confusion, obtundation, tremor, asterixis, and fetor hepaticus (sweet, slightly feculent smell of the breath noted in advanced liver disease). The pathogenesis of encephalopathy is not understood. A number of theories have been advanced, including increased circulating levels of toxins (e.g., ammonia), the presence of false neurotransmitters (e.g., aromatic amino acids), and the concerted effect of two or more metabolic abnormalities (e.g., alkalosis, hypoxia, infection, electrolyte imbalance). Certain factors can precipitate encephalopathy. Among these are infection, gastrointestinal bleeding, constipation, dehydration, and metabolic disorders. In some cases, the ingestion of even modest amounts of dietary protein induces encephalopathy.

The diagnosis of hepatic encephalopathy is made clinically. The serum ammonia level is often elevated in encephalopathic patients, but this test lacks sufficient specificity to be diagnostic. Certain electroencephalographic patterns are seen in encephalopathy, but again, they are not diagnostic. It is important to exclude other causes of altered mental status (e.g., acute intoxication, organic brain syndrome and infection, injury or tumor in the central nervous system).

Treatment

In patients with hepatic encephalopathy, protein intake is moderately restricted. In patients who have gastrointestinal bleeding or constipation, the gut is purged. One particularly useful substance is lactulose, which can be administered by mouth, nasogastric tube, or enema. Lactulose not only acts as a cathartic but also alters the pH in the colon and inhibits bacterial production of ammonia. Intraluminal antibiotics (e.g., neomycin) decrease ammonia production by decreasing bacterial flora.

Variceal Bleeding

Although ascites and encephalopathy cause substantial morbidity in the portal hypertensive population, the complication that is clearly associated with the greatest mortality is bleeding from esophageal varices. The percentage of patients with cirrhosis who have esophageal varices is not known, but only approximately 30% of patients who have varices bleed from them. Esophageal varices are submucosal veins that become dilated and fragile in the presence of portal hypertension. As noted earlier, esophageal varices are collateral routes that drain the short gastric and coronary (left gastric) veins from the portal system into the azygous vein in the systemic venous circulation. The risk of rupture of these veins varies directly with their intraluminal pressure. However, what causes rupture of a given vein at a given time is unclear. Theories include spontaneous rupture, erosion by esophagitis, and disruption by passing food. Two aspects of therapy for variceal bleeding must be considered: cessation of the acute bleeding and prevention of recurrent bleeding.

Cessation of Acute Bleeding

The mortality rate per admission for variceal bleeding is greater than 20%. This staggering figure speaks to the need for rapid, aggressive management. The initial goal of treatment is volume resuscitation through large-bore intravenous lines to maintain tissue perfusion. As with other causes of massive hemorrhage, the volume that is lost is blood. Thus, replacement consists predominantly of blood components, particularly in variceal bleeding, because the salt and water in crystalloid solutions may later contribute to ascites formation. Although it is important to restore adequate circulating volume, it may be equally important to refrain from excessive volume replacement. Variceal pressure varies directly with central venous pressure. Thus, excessive volume replacement may lead to further bleeding. Urinary output is the best clinical indicator of circulatory perfusion. For this reason, a urinary catheter is placed early in the resuscitation effort. The hemoglobin and coagulation factors are monitored frequently to determine the adequacy of blood component therapy. Oxygen is also administered, and the hemoglobin–oxygen saturation closely monitored.

It is critical to establish the diagnosis of variceal bleeding early in the course of the disease so that therapy can be properly directed. The diagnoses of cirrhosis and portal hypertension can often be made from the history and physical examination (e.g., temporal muscle wasting, spider angiomata over the chest, ascites, splenomegaly). However, numerous studies show that as many as 50% of acute upper gastrointestinal bleeds in cirrhotic patients originate not from esophageal varices, but from such sources as peptic ulcer disease and Mallory-Weiss tears (mucosal tears at the gastroesophageal junction). Endoscopy is necessary to determine the source of bleeding. It is performed as soon as possible because the passage of even a few hours may not only prevent identification of the source of bleeding, but may also delay appropriate therapy. Gastric lavage before endoscopy is beneficial both in achieving a thorough examination and in purging blood from the gut, thus abating the subsequent development of encephalopathy from the extra protein load. Lavage is not performed with cold solutions because they can cause rapid loss of body temperature, which, among other things, can induce coagulopathy. During endoscopy, the diagnosis is made by visualizing the bleeding varix or by documenting the presence of varices and the absence of other bleeding sources.

Pharmacologic Therapy

Pharmacologic therapy for variceal hemorrhage is usually well tolerated and has no adverse effect, even if there is a nonvariceal cause of bleeding. For this reason, it is initiated before the diagnosis of variceal bleeding is confirmed. Intravenous **somatostatin** acts promptly to decrease variceal bleeding by splanchnic vasoconstriction and decrease of portal venous flow. It decreases or halts variceal bleeding in more than 50% of patients and has few clinically significant side effects. Intravenous vasopressin also acts by splanchnic vasoconstriction, but in prospective randomized trials was not as effective as somatostatin in controlling variceal hemorrhage. The vasoconstrictive effect of vasopressin is not limited to the splanchnic circulation. If given to patients with atherosclerotic disease, the coronary and peripheral vasoconstriction can cause serious complications (e.g., myocardial infarction, limb ischemia). The simultaneous infusion of nitroglycerin with vasopressin ameliorates these complications and may help to stop variceal bleeding.

Endoscopic Therapy

Endoscopic therapy is effective in approximately 80% of patients with acute variceal hemorrhage. One form of endoscopic therapy is sclerotherapy, in which small amounts of caustic solutions are injected either into or adjacent to varices to induce edema and scarring and obliterate the variceal lumen. A number of complications can occur, including additional bleeding from tearing a delicate varix, ulceration of the epithelium over the varix, perforation of the esophagus, and dissemination of the sclerosing agent to the pulmonary or systemic circulation.

To accomplish the same effect of luminal obliteration of the varix without many of the complications of sclerotherapy, banding of varices is now generally used. This treatment is similar to the banding of internal hemorrhoids, which has been successfully used for years. A hollow extension of the endoscope is placed in contact with the epithelium surrounding a varix, and suction is applied to elevate both the epithelium and the underlying varix. A very small rubber band is then used to encircle and tightly gather the varix, thus obliterating its lumen. Banding is at least as effective as sclerotherapy in the cessation of acute variceal hemorrhage, and has few of its undesirable side effects.

One limitation on both forms of endoscopic therapy is that the varices must be clearly seen for accurate and safe application. Thus, if the patient has massive active bleeding that fills the lumen of the esophagus, it may not be possible to proceed with endoscopic therapy. Another limitation of endoscopic therapy is that it is much more difficult to apply safely to gastric varices than to esophageal varices.

Luminal Tamponade

When both pharmacologic and endoscopic treatments fail to control variceal hemorrhage, luminal tamponade can be applied. The **Sengstaken-Blakemore tube** (Fig. 19-8) is one specific device available for luminal tamponade, but a number of other tubes with various modifications are available. All of these devices have a distal port to suction the luminal contents of the stomach, a large round balloon that places traction on the gastric fundus and tamponades the submucosal veins that approach the esophagus, and, above that, a cylindrical balloon to directly tamponade the esophageal varices. If the available device does not have a port proximal to the esophageal balloon to suction swallowed saliva, then a second tube is placed for this purpose. When properly applied, variceal tamponade effectively controls variceal bleeding in approximately 90% of cases. However, a number of serious complications (e.g., aspiration, asphyxiation, esophageal rupture) can occur. Thus, placement and maintenance of these tubes follows a very strict protocol. One other limitation of variceal tamponade is that it can be applied only for a relatively short period (24 to 36 hours) because of the risk of necrosing underlying tissue. Thus, a plan must be devised for further treatment when the tamponade is released.

Transjugular Intrahepatic Portacaval Shunt

TIPS can be attempted to control acute variceal hemorrhage. This procedure consists of cannulating the jugular vein and directing a semirigid wire into a large hepatic vein with subsequent puncture of the hepatic vein wall, the intervening hepatic parenchyma, and the wall of a large portal vein branch nearby. An expandable metallic stent is then used to dilate and maintain a channel be-

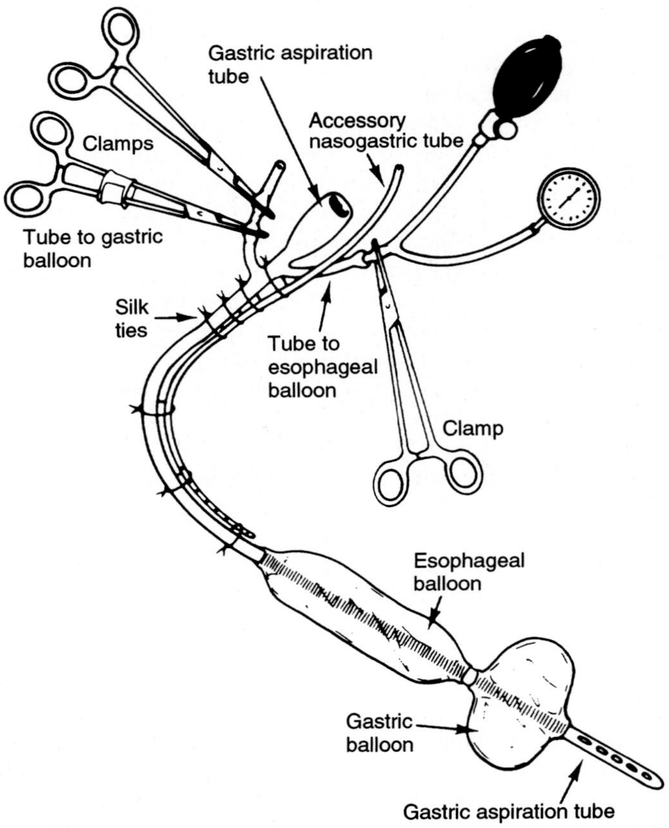

Figure 19-8 Sengstaken-Blakemore tube.

tween the portal and hepatic vein branches. This procedure is truly a portacaval shunt that is created within the liver. The diameter of the lumen of the channel is adjusted until the reduction in portal pressure is sufficient to halt the variceal bleeding. TIPS is technically accomplished in approximately 95% of patients. Except in profoundly coagulopathic patients, it is highly successful in controlling acute variceal hemorrhage.

After the acute variceal hemorrhage is controlled, attention is turned to correcting ascites, encephalopathy, and any other problems (e.g., sepsis, malnutrition). At the same time, plans are made to prevent recurrent variceal hemorrhage.

Prevention of Recurrent Variceal Hemorrhage

As noted earlier, in most patients, varices do not bleed. However, once variceal bleeding occurs, the chance of repeated bleeding approaches 70%. Therefore, therapy to prevent recurrent bleeding should be initiated following the index bleed. A number of options are available to prevent recurrent bleeding. The choice of therapy for a given patient depends on several factors. During the initial hospital stay, the patient is thoroughly evaluated to arrive at a thoughtful plan for preventing recurrent hemorrhage. A hepatitis profile is obtained as well as a history of ingestion of alcohol or exposure to other hepatotoxins (e.g., acetaminophen, nonsteroidal antiinflammatory drugs). A reliable social history is also important because the long-term success of some forms of therapy depends heavily on patient accessibility and reliability. One of the most important factors in determining future therapy is an estimation of the functional reserve of the liver. **Child's classification** (Table 19-1) uses readily available clinical information to make this estimation. The portal venous anatomy of the patient is also important because it may strongly influence the choice of definitive therapy. This anatomy is best shown by venous phase angiography (Fig. 19-9), with selective injection of the superior mesenteric and splenic arteries. At the same time that these studies are done, images are obtained of the left renal vein and inferior vena cava, which may serve as outflow tracts for shunt procedures. At the time of angiography, a hepatic vein tributary is cannulated to obtain the free and wedged hepatic vein pressures. Subtracting the former from the latter provides an estimate of the sinusoidal pressure within the liver, which is a reflection of the portal venous pressure. Angiography may also provide diagnostic information if portal or hepatic vein occlusion is identified.

Options for prevention of recurrent variceal bleeding include medical, endoscopic, radiologic, and surgical therapy. Medical therapy centers on the use of β-blockade to decrease flow to the portal vein and hence to the varices. In most centers this is used as an adjunct. The choice between endoscopic therapy, surgical shunt, and TIPS

Table 19-1 Child's Classification

Criteria	Good Risk (A)	Moderate Risk (B)	Poor Risk (C)
Serum bilirubin (mg/100 mL)	< 2.0	2.0–3.0	> 3.0
Serum albumin (mg/100 mL)	> 3.5	3.0–3.5	< 3.0
Ascites	None	Easily controlled	Not easily controlled
Encephalopathy	None	Minimal	Advanced
Nutrition	Excellent	Good	Poor

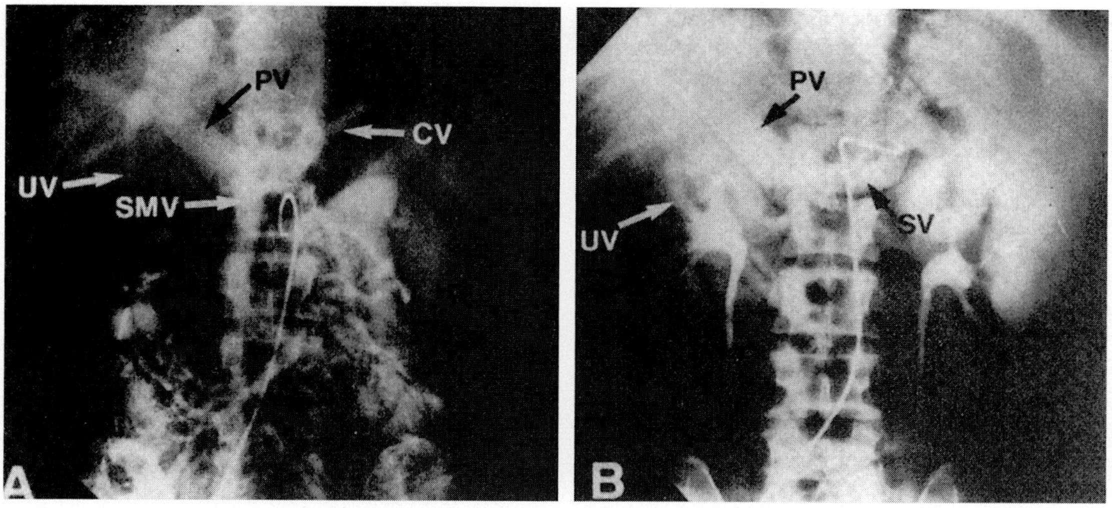

Figure 19-9 A and B, Venous phase of an angiogram showing the superior mesenteric vein (*SMV*), portal vein (*PV*), splenic vein (*SV*), common vein (*CV*), and umbilical vein (*UV*).

should take into account the functional hepatic reserve, the reliability of the patient to return for additional studies and treatment, and the degree of access the patient has to prompt medical care (i.e., the distance the patient lives from a center providing the necessary services and the ability of the patient to overcome financial obstacles to care). Endoscopic therapy is often used as primary treatment, regardless of the status of hepatic reserve, and TIPS is increasingly used as definitive therapy—either primarily or after failure of endoscopic therapy. It has been clearly established that the incidence of rebleeding is higher with endoscopic therapy than with TIPS, and the incidence of encephalopathy is greater with TIPS than endoscopic therapy. The long-term survival is approximately equal for the two. Both of these modalities require careful long-term surveillance. Surgical shunts, though clearly more invasive and associated with greater initial procedural risk, have excellent long-term patency with a low risk of recurrent bleeding and, therefore, require much less long-term followup. Surgical shunts are best applied in Child's A and B patients. The operative mortality in Child's C patients does not justify shunting when less invasive options are available. Liver transplantation (discussed below) is performed for liver failure and not for variceal bleeding, per se. However, all Child's C patients should undergo transplant evaluation.

Endoscopic Therapy

The same forms of endoscopic therapy that are available for acute bleeding (sclerotherapy and banding) can also be used on a long-term basis to prevent recurrent bleeding. The aim is to systematically eradicate all visible esophageal varices through a series of endoscopic sessions over the first few weeks. It is then necessary to periodically identify and treat newly developed variceal channels through continuing surveillance. One problem with endoscopic therapy is that eradication of esophageal varices often leads to the development of gastric varices, which are much less successfully treated endoscopically. Rebleeding rates approach 60% with endoscopic therapy, but the bleeds are generally not as severe as in the primary setting. Overall, there is about a 30% failure rate with long-term endoscopic therapy.

Transjugular Intrahepatic Portacaval Shunt

TIPS, described earlier in association with acute variceal bleeding, is also used to prevent variceal bleeding. Indeed, it is now performed much more commonly than surgical shunting. These devices are initially successful in decreasing portal pressure but they have two recurrent problems. The first is the high rate of encephalopathy (30%) that accompanies a patent TIPS. Because these procedures are radiographically constructed portacaval shunts, it is not surprising that they share this complication with their surgically created equivalents. The other problem with TIPS is a high rate of thrombosis due to intimal hyperplasia along the intrahepatic course of the metallic shunt unless it is carefully monitored with ultrasonography. Stenosis or occlusion occurs in more than 50% of patients by 1 year. The result is a substantial incidence (18% to 30%) of recurrent variceal hemorrhage. Because of this possibility, TIPS patients must be monitored every few months using Doppler ultrasound or angiography. If stenosis or occlusion develop, dilation or restenting is necessary to prevent recurrent bleeding.

Surgical Therapy

For decades, surgical shunting was the only effective means of preventing recurrent variceal hemorrhage. With the advent of endoscopic therapy and then TIPS, surgical shunting is much less commonly performed. Three forms of surgical shunts are used to prevent recurrent variceal hemorrhage. In **portosystemic (total) shunts**, large-caliber connections are made between some point in the portal circulation and a point in the systemic circulation, either by direct anastomosis or using an interposition graft. The many options (see Fig. 19-7) are hemodynamically equivalent. Portosystemic shunts very effectively prevent bleeding and control ascites. However, they divert portal flow to such a great degree that deterioration of hepatic function and hepatic encephalopathy frequently occur. **Selective shunts**, including the distal splenorenal and coronary-caval shunt, decompress varices and prevent variceal bleeding while preserving portal flow to the liver. They do so by decompressing only the gastrosplenic compartment into the systemic circulation. These shunts are as effective as portosystemic shunts at preventing variceal hemorrhage, but produce much lower rates of encephalopathy. Selective shunts have excellent long-term patency. The small-bore portacaval ("partial") shunt was designed to achieve the same goals as selective shunts, but is much more easily performed. In this operation, a small-diameter (8 to 10 mm), short (2 to 3 cm), and straight piece of polytetrafluoroethylene (PTFE) graft is sewn between the portal vein and the inferior vena cava. Partial shunts, too, have excellent long-term patency with much lower rates of encephalopathy than those seen with total shunts.

Nonshunt operations control bleeding by interrupting blood flow to the varices. One option is division and reanastomosis of the esophagus, which is usually done with an end-to-end stapling device. Another is devascularization of the stomach and lower esophagus, usually with splenectomy, to halt flow through the varices. Although nonshunt operations are successful in other parts of the world for certain disease conditions, they are rarely performed in the United States.

Prognosis

The most important indicator of long-term survival in patients who have bled from varices (regardless of the therapy chosen) is the functional reserve of the liver. Because cirrhosis, both with continued alcohol abuse and with viral hepatitis, tends to progress relentlessly, only 50% of patients who have had variceal bleeding survive for 5 years without liver transplantation.

END-STAGE LIVER DISEASE AND LIVER TRANSPLANTATION

End-stage liver disease has many recognized complications, some of which are life-threatening. Liver transplantation is now considered standard treatment for many causes of acute and chronic liver failure. However, significant risks are associated with the transplant procedure, and it is costly. Additionally, there is limited organ availability, and the procedure commits the transplant recipient to lifelong immunosuppressive therapy, with its inherent risks. Thus, physicians must exercise careful judgment to determine which patients can be treated with medical measures or less complicated surgical procedures and which ones are likely to require transplantation because of disease progression. See Chapter 24, Transplantation, for further discussion regarding liver transplantation.

Indications for Transplantation

Patients who are under consideration for liver transplantation usually have irreversible hepatic failure for which there is no suitable alternative therapy. Thus, for most patients, medical measures are tried initially to treat specific complications associated with cirrhosis and liver failure. Transplantation is considered only when these measures are not effective. Three common severe complications seen in association with end-stage liver disease are hepatic encephalopathy, intractable ascites (which may be associated with spontaneous bacterial peritonitis), and variceal hemorrhage. When these occur as isolated complicating factors in patients with otherwise well-preserved hepatic synthetic function, then attention can be directed toward correcting the isolated problem (e.g., performing a portal–systemic or peritoneal–venous shunt procedure). However, when complications occur in the patient with advanced liver disease, they serve as markers of declining hepatic functional reserve, and consideration is usually given to liver transplantation.

Liver transplantation in adults is generally performed for two major indications: chronic, progressive advanced liver disease and **fulminant hepatic failure.** Other indications (in < 10% of patients) include unresectable malignancies and inborn errors of metabolism in patients who may not have underlying cirrhosis. Table 19-2 lists contraindications to liver transplantation.

Chronic liver disease usually results from either hepatocellular injury (e.g., viral hepatitis, alcohol-induced injury) or cholestatic liver disease (e.g., primary biliary cirrhosis, sclerosing cholangitis) (discussed later). Because of the risks and expense associated with transplantation, patients are usually considered for this procedure when their 1- to 2-year survival rate is estimated at 50% or less. Although it is sometimes difficult to predict expected survival in patients with advanced liver disease, certain markers assist in this prediction. For example, in patients with chronic liver disease, clinical factors

Table 19-2 Absolute Contraindications to Liver Transplantation

Uncontrolled sepsis
HIV–positive status
Extrahepatic malignancy
Active alcohol or substance abuse
Advanced cardiac or pulmonary disease

that indicate advanced liver disease include nutritional impairment and muscle wasting, hepatic encephalopathy, difficult-to-control ascites, variceal hemorrhage, and renal insufficiency.

Laboratory parameters may be altered depending on the etiology of liver failure. When cirrhosis has a hepatocellular cause, the prothrombin time is prolonged beyond 18 to 20 seconds (international normalized ratio [INR] ≥ 2.0). A serum albumin level of less than 2.5 to 3.0 g/L is associated with diminished hepatic synthetic reserve. Patients whose cirrhosis has a cholestatic etiology may have near-normal prothrombin times and serum albumin values of 3 g/L or greater. However, elevation of the serum bilirubin above 10 mg/dL suggests advanced liver disease in this group. Laboratory parameters are only guides to hepatic functional reserve and must be considered in the context of the clinical condition of the individual patient. When patients have complications of liver disease (e.g., difficult-to-manage ascites, variceal hemorrhage, marginally controlled encephalopathy), the decision to proceed with transplantation rather than to continue observation of the patient is likely to be made.

Chronic and Progressive Advanced Liver Disease

Chronic Hepatitis C

Chronic hepatitis C infection is one of the most common indications for liver transplantation today. Hepatitis C was previously categorized under the heading non-A, non-B hepatitis, but molecular techniques allowed identification of this single-stranded RNA virus in 1989. Although it was a common cause of transfusion-associated hepatitis in the past, this risk is now less than 0.05% per unit of blood product transfused with current testing of banked blood. Many patients with chronic hepatitis C have such identifiable risk factors as previous drug use, previous transfusions, and multiple sexual partners, but approximately 50% have no definable risk factors. Its course is usually slowly progressive, and most patients have chronic infection for 10 to 20 years before complications of liver disease occur or a liver transplant is needed. Only approximately 20% of patients clear the hepatitis C virus in response to acute infection.

After liver transplantation for chronic hepatitis C, reinfection of the transplanted liver is nearly universal, but fortunately, the course of hepatocellular injury is indolent in most patients. New strategies, including antiviral therapies, are under investigation, but no effective measures to prevent allograft infection have been established. Although the short-term results of liver transplantation for hepatitis C are satisfactory in most cases, it is not known how often patients require retransplantation in long-term followup.

Chronic Hepatitis B

Chronic hepatitis B infection, unlike hepatitis C infection, shows a marked propensity to cause significant hepatocellular injury in the transplanted allograft, with a high incidence of early graft loss and death of the transplant recipient. Although at one time hepatitis B infection was an absolute contraindication to liver transplantation, many centers now use hepatitis B immunoglobulin to suppress viral expression in the posttransplant recipient. Although there is short-term success with this approach, the long-term outcome is not known.

Alcoholic Liver Disease

Transplantation for alcoholic liver disease is one of the most controversial indications for liver transplantation. With intensive pretransplant screening, including completion of an alcohol rehabilitation program and a period of supervised abstinence (usually ≥ 6 months), the risk of recidivism is less than 10% to 15%. Of those who consume alcohol after transplantation, continued alcohol use to the point of causing liver disease in the allograft is extremely rare. For reasons that are not well understood, as many as one-third of patients with a history of alcohol abuse also have serologic markers for hepatitis C infection without other known risk factors.

Autoimmune Hepatitis

Autoimmune hepatitis can usually be distinguished from other causes of chronic liver disease on the basis of immunologic and serologic testing. These patients usually have positive antinuclear or other self-directed antibodies. Initial treatment is usually with immunosuppressive medication, including corticosteroids and azathioprine. Patients in whom this treatment fails are usually good candidates for liver transplantation. Recurrent disease does not usually occur in the transplanted liver.

Hemochromatosis

Hemochromatosis is an autosomal recessive disease that causes iron overload as a result of excessive absorption from the intestinal tract. Multiple organs are affected by iron deposition, including the liver, heart, pancreas, spleen, adrenal glands, pituitary, and joints. The peak incidence of liver disease is between 40 and 60 years of age. Men show clinical manifestations and cirrhosis earlier than women, who may be protected by iron loss during menstruation and childbirth. Treatment in recognized patients is with serial phlebotomy. Withdrawal of 500 mL blood/week is often required until the excessive iron stores are depleted. Effective treatment may reverse many of the damaging effects of iron deposition. Hemochromatosis is associated with a significant risk of hepatocellular carcinoma, up to 200 times that of other patients with cirrhosis. This risk is not fully diminished by phlebotomy. Liver transplantation is effective for patients with hemochromatosis and end-stage cirrhosis, but may be complicated by the preexisting cardiomyopathy and diabetes often found in these patients. The increased absorption of iron continues after liver transplantation, necessitating careful surveillance, even in patients who undergo successful transplantation.

Wilson's Disease

Wilson's disease is a rare autosomal recessive disorder of copper metabolism. Patients have increased deposition of copper in the liver, corneas (Kayser-Fleischer rings), kidneys, brain, and other locations. Patients with Wilson's disease have decreased circulating levels of ceruloplasmin and increased urinary excretion of copper. In normal individuals, excess copper is excreted into bile, but patients with Wilson's disease appear to have diminished biliary excretion. Some patients with Wilson's disease may have acute hepatitis and fulminant hepatic failure, whereas others have chronic progressive liver disease. Patients who have chronic liver disease are initially treated with D-penicillamine, which chelates copper and increases urinary excretion. Liver transplantation is effective in patients with fulminant failure and those in whom initial medical therapy fails. After transplantation, the metabolic defect is corrected, and no further damage from excessive copper occurs.

α_1-Antitrypsin Deficiency

α_1-Antitrypsin deficiency is an autosomal dominant disorder that causes varying degrees of lung and liver damage over a patient's lifetime. The diagnosis is established by the determination of low levels of serum α_1-antitrypsin levels and confirmed with phenotypic studies. Most patients with liver disease have relatively mild pulmonary involvement, but more advanced pulmonary disease can complicate attempts at liver transplantation. There is no effective medical treatment, except for supportive measures. After liver transplantation, α_1-antitrypsin levels return to normal as the recipient takes on the phenotype of the transplanted liver.

Primary Biliary Cirrhosis

Primary biliary cirrhosis, which primarily affects middle-aged women, causes progressive bile duct destruction, probably from cytotoxic T cells. Patients often have pruritus without jaundice and usually have a positive antimitochondrial antibody finding ($\geq$ 1/40). The course of the disease may be indolent, with patients living 10 years or longer from presentation. Elevation of the serum bilirubin level is associated with disease progression and usually prompts consideration of liver transplantation.

Primary Sclerosing Cholangitis

Primary sclerosing cholangitis is an idiopathic disease that causes chronic fibrotic strictures that can involve any portion of the intrahepatic or extrahepatic biliary tree. One-half to two-thirds of patients also have inflammatory bowel disease, usually ulcerative colitis. The risk of cholangiocarcinoma is increased in patients with primary sclerosing cholangitis, and rapid progression of disease should prompt a search for malignant strictures within the biliary tree. Disease progression in patients with primary sclerosing cholangitis is more variable than in patients with primary biliary cirrhosis. When patients become jaundiced and do not have a correctable biliary stricture (usually with stenting, but occasionally with surgical bypass), then transplantation is considered. After transplantation, patients who have primary sclerosing cholangitis and ulcerative colitis require close colonic surveillance because of the increased risk of colon carcinoma.

Fulminant Hepatic Failure

Fulminant hepatic failure occurs when massive hepatocyte necrosis or severe impairment of liver function occurs. These patients do not have evidence of chronic liver disease. Liver dysfunction occurs within 8 to 12 weeks of the onset of symptoms. In these patients, hepatic encephalopathy develops and can progress to coma, brainstem herniation, and death without liver replacement. The prothrombin time is usually significantly prolonged, and reversible renal insufficiency (hepatorenal syndrome) may develop. Because these patients do not have chronic liver disease, muscle wasting and portal hypertension usually are not present. For this reason, liver transplantation is technically easier to perform than in the setting of chronic liver disease. However, because of the rapidly advancing nature of liver dysfunction in this setting, most patients die within 1 to 2 weeks of presentation without liver transplantation.

At most centers, fulminant hepatic failure is the indication for approximately 5% to 10% of liver transplantations. Common causes of fulminant hepatic failure include viral infection and hepatotoxic drugs (e.g., anesthetic drugs, acetaminophen, isoniazid). Mushroom poisoning occurs in certain areas of the United States (Pacific Northwest) and Europe, where wild mushrooms are gathered and eaten by unsuspecting individuals.

Because of the rapid progression of fulminant hepatic failure, patients require an aggressive and accelerated workup in addition to aggressive supportive measures. Patients in hepatic coma usually undergo placement of an intracerebral pressure monitor so that adequate cerebral perfusion pressures can be maintained and increases in cerebral pressures minimized. To be successful, liver transplantation must be performed before irreversible brain injury occurs. Some patients with milder forms recover without liver transplantation, but the period of observation cannot extend for too long, or it may not be possible to obtain a suitable donor liver in time to perform a successful transplant. Thus, the decision to proceed with liver transplantation requires careful judgment by the treating physicians, who must weigh the risks of death without a transplant against the potential commitment to lifelong immunosuppression in a patient who might otherwise recover without this procedure. Clinical trials with extracorporeal liver support systems are underway. These systems may prevent cerebral injury while the injured liver recovers or until a suitable donor liver is located. In the future, these systems may successfully assist patients during this critical period.

SUGGESTED READINGS

Blumgart LH, Fong Y, eds. *Surgery of the Liver and Biliary Tract.* 3rd Ed. London: WB Saunders, 2000.

Carr-Locke DL, Branch SM, Byrne WJ, et al. Technology assessment status evaluation: transvenous intrahepatic portosystemic shunt (TIPS). *Gastrointest Endosc* 1998;47:584–587.

de Franchis R, Primignani M. Natural history of portal hypertension in patients with cirrhosis. *Clin Liver Dis* 2001;5:645–663.

Garcia N Jr, Sanyal AJ. Portal hypertension. *Clin Liver Dis* 2001;5: 509–540.

Gournay J, Lake JR. Management of common problems after liver transplantation. *Adv Gastroenterol Hepatol Clin Nutr* 1996;1(2):59–72.

Hughes KS. Resection of the liver for colorectal carcinoma metastases: a multi-institutional study of indications for resection. *Surgery* 1998; 103:278–288.

Iannitti DA, Henderson JM. Portal hypertension. *Clin Liver Dis* 1997; 1:99–114.

Imperiale TF, Teran C, McCullough AJ. A meta-analysis of somatostatin versus vasopressin in the management of acute esophageal variceal hemorrhage. *Gastroenterology* 1995;109:1289–1294.

Lake JR, ed. Advances in liver transplantation. *Gastroenterol Clin North Am* 1993;22(2).

Maddrey WC, Sorrell MF, eds. *Transplantation of the Liver.* 2nd Ed. Norwalk, CT: Appleton & Lange, 1995.

Mazzaferro V, Regalia E, Doci R, et al. Liver transplantation for the treatment of small hepatocellular carcinomas in patients with cirrhosis [Comment]. *N Engl J Med* 1996;334(11):693–699.

Nagorney DM. Benign hepatic tumors: focal nodular hyperplasia and hepatocellular adenoma. *World J Surg* 1995;19:13–18.

Papatheodoridis GV, Goulis J, Leandro G, et al. Transjugular intrahepatic portosystemic shunt compared with endoscopic treatment for prevention of variceal rebleeding: a meta-analysis. *Hepatology* 1999; 30:612–622.

Sherlock S. *Diseases of the Liver and Biliary System.* 8th Ed. London: Blackwell, 1991.

Vargas HE, Gerber D, Abu-Elmagd K. Management of portal hypertension-related bleeding. *Surg Clin North Am* 1999;79:1–22.

Zervos EE, Rosemurgy AS. Management of medically refractory ascites. *Am J Surg* 2001;181:256–264.

20

GARY L. DUNNINGTON, MD ■ SUSAN KAISER, MD, PHD
ELIZABETH PERALTA, MD ■ LECIA APANTAKU, MD

Breast

OBJECTIVES

1 Categorize the risk factors for breast cancer into major and minor factors.
2 Provide the guidelines for routine screening mammography.
3 Describe the diagnostic workup and management for common benign breast conditions, including breast pain, cysts, fibroadenoma, nipple discharge, and breast abscess.
4 List the diagnostic modalities and describe their sequence in the workup of a patient with a breast mass or nipple discharge.
5 Describe the preoperative evaluation for a patient with breast cancer.
6 Provide the differential diagnosis of a breast lump in a woman in her 20s and in a woman in her 60s.
7 Describe how ductal cancer in situ differs from invasive breast cancer. Describe its role as a risk factor for invasive cancer.
8 Explain the rationale for breast conservation treatment as the preferred therapeutic option for most stage I and stage II breast cancers.
9 Describe the rationale for adjuvant therapy, radiation therapy, and hormonal therapy in the treatment of breast cancer.
10 Describe the expected survival and local recurrence rates after treatment for early breast cancer.

Familiarity with evaluation of the breast and an understanding of breast disease are critically important for primary care physicians and surgeons. This chapter focuses on the evaluation of the patient who is undergoing routine screening as well as the patient who has a breast complaint. Breast surveillance and the appropriate treatment of breast problems have become prominent aspects of health care for women, because breast cancer is common, often curable, and almost always at least treatable. It is estimated that 212,600 people in the United States (211,300 women and 1300 men) will be diagnosed with breast cancer in 2003, or 32% of all new cancers diagnosed in women. Also in 2003, 39,800 women will die of breast cancer, or 15% of all women who die of cancer. The rate of breast cancer in women has shown a slow but steady rise over the past 25 years; presently, it is estimated that one in eight women will develop breast cancer during their lifetime. The death rate has remained relatively stable over the past 70 years, with a recent trend toward decline thought to be related to earlier diagnosis and possibly to improvements in treatment.

ANATOMY

The breast is a heterogeneous structure composed of glandular, ductal, connective, and adipose tissue. It is located on the anterior chest wall, superficial to the pectoralis major muscle. The breast may extend from the clavicle superiorly to the sixth rib inferiorly, and from the midsternal line medially into the axilla laterally (Fig. 20-1). The mammary gland has approximately 15 to 20 lobes that are embedded in fibrous and adipose tissue. These lobes radiate from the central nipple area. Each lobe has an excretory duct that drains into the lactiferous sinus beneath the nipple. Cooper's ligaments are connective tissue structures that are derived from the superficial fascia of the skin that suspend the breast on the chest wall. Skin dimpling, produced by retraction of Cooper's ligaments, may be associated with underlying malignancy. The breast is a well-vascularized organ that receives its blood supply predominantly from the perforating branches of the paired internal mammary arteries and from branches of the lateral thoracic artery. The axillary, subclavian, and intercostal veins

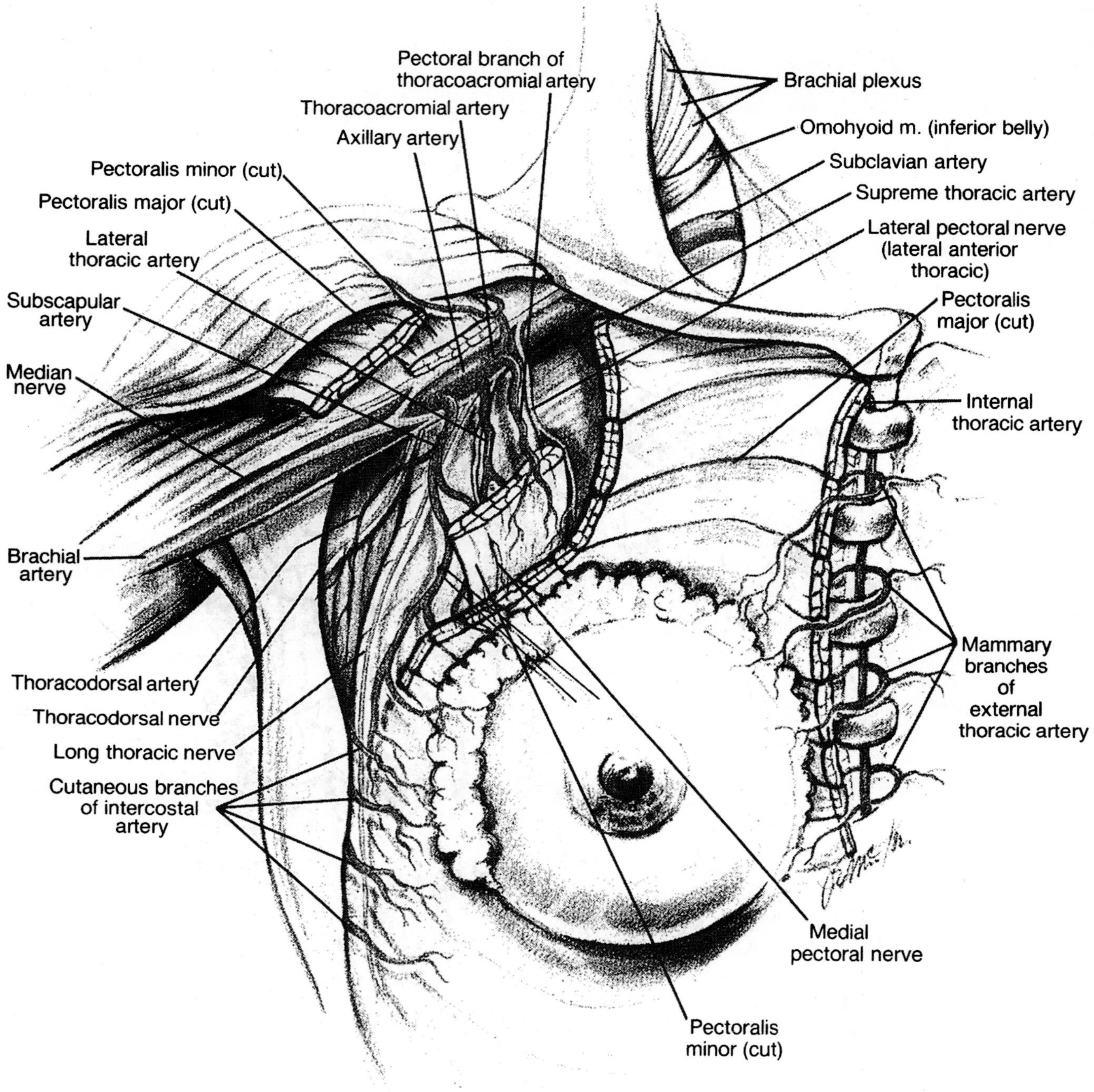

Figure 20-1 Normal breast anatomy showing vascular and neural origins.

receive venous drainage from the breast. The long thoracic, thoracodorsal, and intercostobrachial nerves are intimately associated anatomically with the breast and the axillary space. The long thoracic nerve courses vertically along the superficial surface of the serratus anterior muscle in the region of the axilla. It provides motor innervation to the serratus anterior muscle, which abducts and laterally rotates the scapula and holds it against the chest wall. The thoracodorsal nerve, which is located posteriorly in the axillary space, innervates the latissimus dorsi muscle, which adducts, extends, and medially rotates the arm. The medial pectoral nerve most commonly pierces the pectoralis minor en route to the pectoralis major while innervating both. In 15% to 20% of patients, the nerve passes lateral to the pectoralis minor en route to the pectoralis major. For this reason, it is vulnerable to injury during axillary dissection. The intercostobrachial nerves, which are the lateral cutaneous branches of the first and second intercostal nerve, course across the axillary space to provide cutaneous innervation to the inner aspect of the upper arm and the axilla. The primary route of lymphatic drainage of the breast is to the axilla (75%), with most of the rest to the internal mammary nodes (Fig. 20-2). Lymphatic drainage of the breast is thought to follow an orderly pattern, so that drainage is first to a lower level lymph node and subsequently to the higher levels. Consequently, if the lowest node is negative for malignant cells, it may safely be assumed that there is no nodal involvement at other levels. This is the rationale for sentinel lymph node biopsy in the surgical treatment of early breast cancer: the lowest

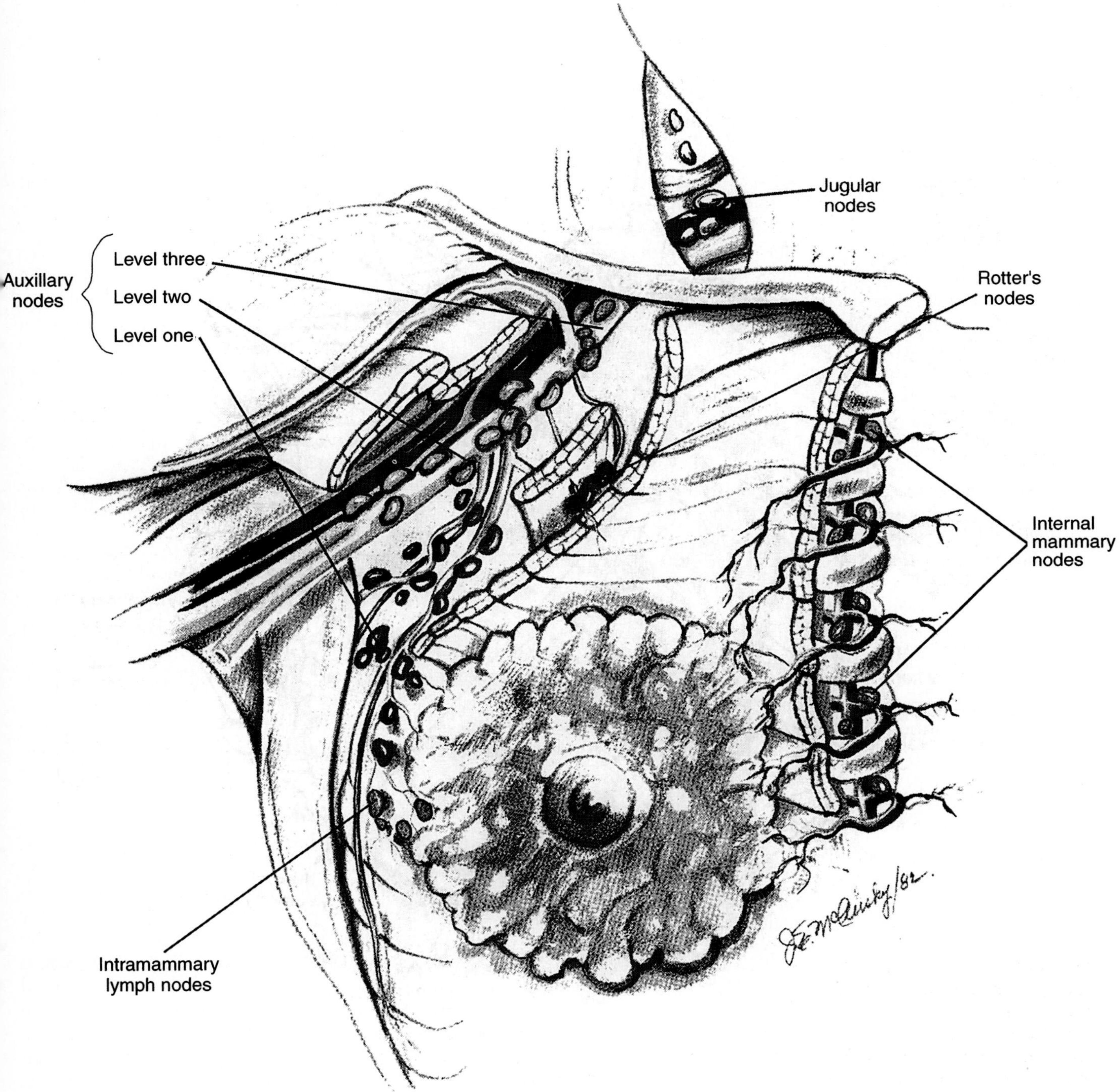

Figure 20-2 Lymphatic drainage of the breast.

node draining the cancer, usually an axillary node but occasionally an internal mammary node, is identified and biopsied. If this lymph node is negative for malignant cells, involvement of any other node is rare, and axillary dissection can be avoided.

PHYSIOLOGY

The female breast is a modified apocrine gland that undergoes considerable structural and physiologic changes during a woman's lifetime. Increased hormonal production by the ovary at puberty causes ductal budding and the initial formation of acini, which are proliferations of the terminal ducts lined with secretory cells for milk production. With each menstrual cycle, preovulatory estrogen production stimulates proliferation of the breast ductal system. After ovulation, decreased estrogen and progesterone levels cause a decrease in ductal proliferation. In pregnancy, when estrogen and progesterone levels remain relatively high, there is continued hypertrophy and budding of the ductal system, with associated acinar development. The sudden decrease in hormone levels in the postpartum period, associated with prolactin secretion from the pituitary gland, precipitates the onset of lactation. Postmenopausally, in the absence of the hormonal stimulus for cyclic proliferation of the breast ductal system, breast parenchyma is progressively lost and replaced by adipose tissue. The male breast is anatomically composed of the same heterogeneous tissue as the female breast, but it does not undergo cyclic hormonally related changes. Physiologic gynecomastia occurs in over one-half of adolescent males. For these young patients the enlarged breasts may be asymmetric and tender secondary to a physiologic excess of plasma estradiol relative to plasma testosterone. This adolescent gynecomastia usually resolves by age 20. In young girls, adolescent or juvenile hypertrophy is a postpubertal persistence of epithelial and stromal growth that can result in very large breasts. Often this occurs in the absence of any systemic hormonal imbalances. Physiologic gynecomastia is also prevalent in a significant percentage of aging men. This is manifest by either bilateral or unilateral breast enlargement often associated with breast tenderness. This gynecomastia is secondary to a relative hyperestrinism with falling plasma testosterone levels and increasing conversion of androgens to estrogens in peripheral tissues. In the absence of a palpable mass or significant symptoms, this condition does not require clinical evaluation.

CLINICAL PRESENTATION AND EVALUATION: ASSESSMENT OF BREAST CANCER RISK

A complete medical history, risk assessment, and focused physical examination should be obtained from any woman with breast complaints. Table 20-1 summarizes essential elements of the history. Risk assessment is useful primarily in women without complaints, since diagnostic and therapeutic approaches in women who do have complaints are determined by the nature of the problem rather than by the level of risk. In other words, complaints should not be disregarded because the risk is low. Most women who develop breast cancer *do not* have significant risk factors.

Table 20-1 Key Elements in the History of a Patient With a Breast Complaint

History of current problem (duration, timing, intensity)
Previous breast problems including biopsies
Results of recent mammography
Family history of breast cancer, ovarian cancer
Age at onset of menses and natural or surgical menopause
Age at first full-term pregnancy, number of pregnancies
Use of birth control pills, hormone replacement therapy
Current medications
Past medical and surgical history

Abnormalities occurring in young women, those under the age of 30, are likely to be related to benign pathologies such as fibrocystic changes, cysts, and fibroadenomas. Abnormalities in postmenopausal women, such as pain, nipple discharge, and new masses, are much more likely to be related to malignancies. Diagnostic problems most often arise in the intermediate group: women aged 30 to 50, who may have either benign or malignant pathology.

Breast cancer risk factors are statistical associations and do not define causality. A greater number of risk factors (Table 20-2) suggests greater risk, but the nature of these interactions is not well understood and awaits further study.

Hormone replacement therapy (HRT) has long been known to be associated with an increased risk of breast cancer. Recent large, well-constructed studies have also shown that the only significant benefit of HRT is in treatment of menopausal symptoms, and that it does not decrease the risk of fracture or heart disease. HRT is no longer recommended for most women.

Major risk factors for breast cancer include female sex, increasing age, family history (particularly if related to breast cancer genes), and proliferative pathology with atypia on biopsy. The older women get, the more likely they are to be diagnosed with breast cancer, but at the same time they become less likely to die from it. Risk is greater for women with first-degree relatives with bilateral premenopausal breast cancer and much greater for women with this factor and **atypical hyperplasia** themselves.

Currently, factors for which no link to breast cancer has been established include environmental pollution, breast implants, lack of exercise, smoking, abortions, antiperspirants, and underwire brassieres.

Table 20-2 Breast Cancer Risk Factors

Factor	Category	Relative Risk	Comment
Age			Increasing risk with increasing age
Alcohol consumption	Hormonal	1.5 for 2–5 drinks/day	Appears to be dose-dependent
Birth control pills	Hormonal		If current or within the past 10 years
BRCA-1 or BRCA-2	Genetic		Accounts for 5% of all cases. Lifetime risk of developing breast cancer with either of these genes is 56%–85%
Early menarche	Hormonal		Age 12 or younger
Family history of breast or ovarian cancer	Genetic	2 if one relative, 5 if two relatives	First-degree relatives (mother, sister, or daughter), and male relatives with breast cancer
Hormone replacement therapy	Hormonal	At least 2 if older than age 59	If within the past 5 years. The additional risk is greater with combination replacements than with estrogen replacement alone
Late first-term pregnancy	Hormonal		Age 30 or older
Late menopause	Hormonal		Beginning age 55 or older
Lobular carcinoma in situ (LCIS)		8–11	20% chance of developing an invasive carcinoma within 15 years, somewhere in either breast
Multiple previous biopsies			Statistical association, even if the pathology was completely benign
No term pregnancies	Hormonal		If age 30 or older
Personal history of breast cancer		4–5	Average risk 0.5%–1% per year over the next 15 years, independent of the risk of recurrence of the original breast cancer
Proliferative histology on biopsy		1.5–2 if proliferative, 4–5 if atypical hyperplasia	Does not include LCIS or ductal carcinoma in situ (DCIS)
Race			White women have slightly higher risk (but a lower death rate) than African American women. Asian, Hispanic, and Native American women have lower risk
Radiation exposure		3 if exposure > 90 rads	Previous radiation therapy for chest malignancy, repeated chest fluoroscopy, or exposure to nuclear incident
Sex			Females are at greater risk
Weight			Complex relationship between obesity and breast cancer risk is not fully understood. It does not appear to be related to dietary fat intake

Physical Examination of the Breasts

A systematic approach to the physical examination of the breasts includes both inspection and palpation. The examination begins with the patient in the sitting position. The breasts are inspected first with the arms at the patient's side, second with the arms elevated toward the ceiling, third with the patient pressing tightly at her waist to contract the pectoralis muscles, and finally with the patient leaning forward. These maneuvers are complementary in aiding the detection of dimpling of the skin, a sign of malignancy. Inspection also allows for assessment of breast symmetry, the presence of any discoloration (e.g., redness, ecchymosis), and the presence of edema. The nipples are inspected to be certain that they are everted and without rash or ulceration. With the patient still in the sitting position, both axillae are examined, with the patient's arm resting over the forearm of the examiner to relax the shoulder musculature, allowing for full assessment of axillary contents. Lymph nodes are best detected as the examiner pushes superiorly in the axilla, then moves the fingertips inferiorly against the chest wall, trapping lymph nodes between the finger and the chest wall. A careful lymph node examination also involves palpation in the supraclavicular fossae. Palpation of the breasts in the sitting position is discouraged because it often yields false-positive findings for the examiner (as well as for the patient during self-examination). The breasts should be examined with the patient supine and the arm resting comfortably above the head. This position spreads breast tissue out over the chest wall, allowing more accurate detection of abnormalities.

There are several different methods of palpating the

breast. The important element is to use a pattern that ensures that every part of the breast is examined with the pads (not the tips) of the index, long, and ring fingers, from the sternum to the axilla and from the clavicle to below the inframammary crease. Irregularities are palpated between the skin and the chest wall, not between the two hands of the examiner. Many experienced examiners find that the strip method, palpating in adjacent vertical strips, is the most thorough and reliable. Others use a "spokes of a wheel" or a spiral pattern. In addition, the precise size of the mass should be described with the use of a measuring instrument. The examiner should note whether the mass is tender or nontender, its mobility, and its texture. It is not necessary to squeeze the nipples during a breast examination because unilateral elicited discharge is almost always normal, particularly in younger women. With a history of **spontaneous nipple discharge**, the source of the discharge should be localized with systematic palpation from the outer breast to the nipple circumferentially around the areola. If discharge is identified, the color should be noted, as well as whether it is ever spontaneous, whether it is bloody, whether more than one duct orifice is involved, and whether it is bilateral. Unilateral bloody single-duct spontaneous discharge is more likely to result from an underlying malignancy, especially if it is associated with a mass in the breast.

Diagnostic Evaluation

For many years the gold standard for breast screening for normal adult women has consisted of monthly breast self-examination, yearly mammography for women aged 40 and older, and yearly breast physical examination by a health care professional. Over the last few years, the value of breast self-examination has been questioned, since it has never been shown to improve survival. Breast self-examination has been shown to dramatically increase the number of benign breast biopsies. The current recommendations from the American Cancer Society are shown in Table 20-3.

Mammography

Screening mammography includes two views of each breast: craniocaudal and mediolateral oblique, with identifiable markers placed on the nipple and any visible or palpable mass lesions (Fig. 20-3). Comparison of these two two-dimensional views allows relatively accurate localization of a feature. If necessary, other views, including magnification or compression views, may be taken. It is crucial in evaluating mammograms to compare them to previous studies, since changes over time may allow earlier identification of a lesion, or classification of an otherwise alarming abnormality as probably benign. Mammograms have a 10% false-negative rate, so a negative mammogram is not sufficient to decide that no cancer is present. New technologies such as computer-assisted detection (CAD) may assist the radiologist in detecting more subtle cancers.

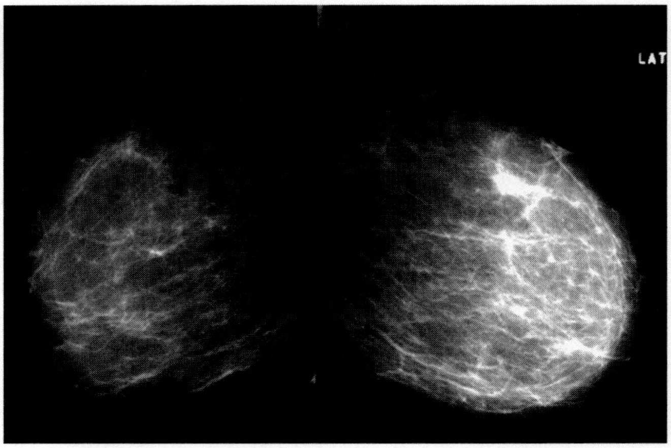

Figure 20-3 Mediolateral views of right and left breasts showing a spiculated lesion.

The x-ray dosage for a standard mammogram is about 0.2 rad (1 rad = 1 cGy = 10 mSv), although thicker breasts require higher doses. For comparison, the average person on Earth is exposed to 0.24 rad per year. A chest radiograph is about 0.01 rad. Chest computed tomography (CT) gives a breast dose of as much as 5 rad.

Masses of various types, including those too small to be palpable, are common mammographic abnormalities. Suspicious masses are those with irregular or spiculated margins; round or oval smooth masses are usually benign, although it may not be possible to tell whether they are solid or cystic. **Microcalcifications** are also common; they are considered suspicious if pleomorphic, linear, or branching, especially if they increase in number from one

Table 20-3 American Cancer Society Recommendations for Breast Cancer Detection in Asymptomatic Women

Age Group	Clinical Breast Examination	Breast Self-Examination	Mammogram
≥ 20 to 39	Every 3 years	Monthly (optional)	–
≥ 40	Yearly	Monthly (optional)	Yearly

mammogram to the next. Large round calcifications are rarely associated with malignancy.

Ultrasound (Sonogram)

Ultrasound is a completely noninvasive imaging test with no known adverse effects other than its cost. Its accuracy depends a great deal on the sophistication of the equipment and skill of the sonographer. It is most useful to characterize palpable lesions or suspicious areas found on mammogram or physical examination, especially in women under the age of 30, where the likelihood of breast cancer is low. It is not a useful routine screening test, because it is very difficult to establish that the entire breast has been interrogated. Using ultrasound, it is simple to distinguish solid masses from cysts, and simple cysts from complex cysts. Calcifications can sometimes be identified, but ultrasound is not a sensitive or reliable technique for their identification or evaluation.

Benign sonographic features of masses include sharply defined borders, central enhancement, and absence of internal echoes (characteristic of cysts). Suspicious features include poorly defined margins, heterogeneous internal echoes, "taller than wide" (caused by a lack of compressibility), and irregular internal shadowing.

Magnetic Resonance Imaging

Magnetic resonance imaging (MRI) uses radio waves in magnetic fields, after injection of gadolinium, to produce detailed images. The resolution of the images is much better when a dedicated breast coil, not available in every institution, is used.

Dense breast tissue, scar, and implants, which may make mammography less sensitive, do not interfere with MRI diagnosis. Although still in development, MRI may have a sensitivity and specificity significantly greater than that of mammography. The high cost, about 10 times as much as a mammogram, remains the major barrier for increased use. MRI is showing increasing benefit for evaluation of the high-risk patient with dense breasts on mammography as well as for local disease staging for ductal carcinoma in situ and lobular cancer. Recent technology allows MRI-directed breast biopsy when a worrisome lesion is identified.

Tissue-Sampling Techniques

The definitive diagnosis of breast lesions depends on microscopic examination, which can be divided into cytology and histology. Cytology is the description of individual cells, which can categorize them as benign or malignant but cannot identify if a malignancy is invasive. Histology describes not only the characteristics of individual cells but also their relationships to each other, that is, the architecture of the tissue.

Diagnosis of breast lesions is currently performed most commonly in the physician's office or the radiology suite. This approach is preferred over biopsy in the operating room, since a needle diagnosis of cancer usually allows definitive treatment to be accomplished with only a single trip to the operating room. Current breast biopsy options include:

Fine-needle aspiration cytology (FNAC): Using a needle and syringe, cells are obtained from a mass lesion, smeared on a slide, fixed, stained, and examined under a microscope. The lesion can be located by palpation or with mammographic or sonographic guidance.

Core-needle biopsy: Using a special large needle under local anesthesia, small thin cores of tissue are obtained and set in formalin for microscopic examination. As with FNAC, the lesion can be located by palpation or with mammographic or sonographic guidance, using a biplanar or stereolactic approach to localize the lesion.

Open biopsy: Through a skin incision, all (excisional biopsy) or part (incisional biopsy) of a lesion is removed and sent for microscopic examination. If the lesion is not palpable, mammography or ultrasound can be used to locate it and a wire can be placed through it percutaneously. This wire is left in place to guide the surgeon to the lesion in the operating room (needle-directed breast biopsy).

Evaluation of the Patient With a Breast Mass

The evaluation of a patient presenting with a "breast mass" depends on patient age and physical findings. If the examination reveals areas of increased density typical of fibrocystic changes and no discrete breast mass, the patient should be reevaluated in 3 months, particularly if premenopausal, to evaluate for cyclical changes. If there is a question as to whether the physical findings indicate areas of breast thickening or a breast mass, a workup is clearly indicated. In the patient less than 30 to 40 years of age, the workup should begin with ultrasound; in the patient greater than 40 years, the workup should include mammography with or without ultrasound. Clearly, all patients felt to have a certain discrete mass on breast exam require tissue diagnosis. Figure 20-4 presents an algorithm for evaluation of a palpable mass.

BENIGN CONDITIONS OF THE BREAST

Breast Pain

Mild, cyclic bilateral breast tenderness and swelling is a common experience a few days preceding the menses and rarely prompts medical consultation. Although it is unusual for the presence of breast cancer to be signaled by pain, persistent or unilateral pain and tenderness can be a cause of alarm. A thorough clinical evaluation and appropriate diagnostic workup should be performed. Musculoskeletal causes and angina should be considered, and breast imaging such as mammogram and ultrasound

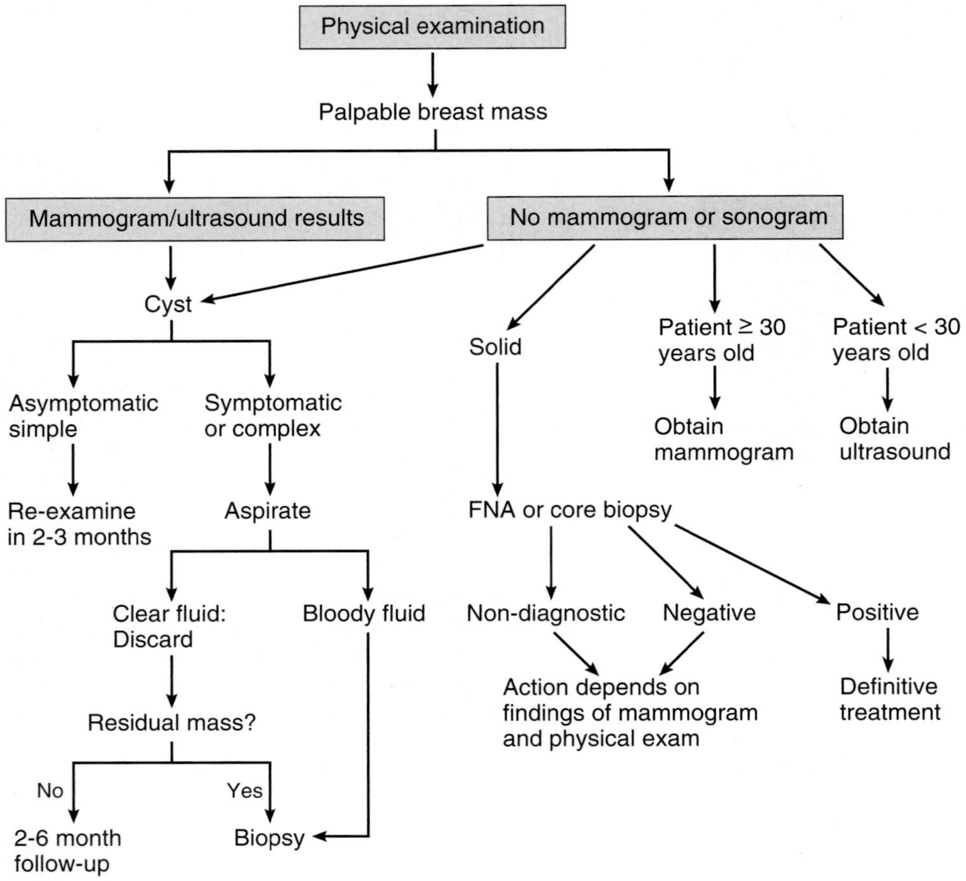

Figure 20-4 Algorithm for evaluation of a palpable mass.

should be used to rule out a malignancy. In the absence of any physical or radiologic abnormality, reassurance and a followup examination in a few months often provide adequate relief.

Hormonal stimulation of glandular breast tissue is thought to be the underlying cause of breast pain, or mastalgia. Discontinuing hormone replacement therapy in postmenopausal women with breast pain is recommended. Other therapeutic measures include use of a compressive elastic style of bra (sport or minimizer bra), decreasing caffeine consumption, nonsteroidal antiinflammatory analgesics, and evening primrose oil capsules. Danazol, an androgen analogue, is often effective in relieving breast pain and tenderness, but it should only be used after failure of the previous measures because of its adverse effects, including deepening of the voice and hirsutism.

Fibroadenoma

Fibroadenoma is a very common benign tumor of the breast. It usually occurs in young women (late teens to early 30s), although it may develop at any age. Typically, the fibroadenoma is 1 to 3 cm in size and is palpated as a freely movable, discrete, firm, rounded mass in the breast. Histologically, fibroadenomas are composed of fibrous stromal tissue and tissue clefts lined with normal epithelium. **Fine-needle aspiration** or **core biopsy** can establish the diagnosis. Fibroadenomas resemble normal mammary lobules in that they show lactation in pregnancy and involution in menopause, an example of the ANDI (aberrancies of normal development and involution) concept that supports observation rather than excision.

For young women with a typical clinical presentation, an ultrasound consistent with fibroadenoma, and cytologic or histologic diagnosis of fibroadenoma, excision is not required if the fibroadenoma is small (< 2.5 cm). In this group, 6-month followup for 18 months is important to establish stability of the lesion. Approximately 50% of fibroadenomas in younger women involute within 5 years. Hormonal stimulation during pregnancy may cause rapid growth of a fibroadenoma and require its excision. Giant fibroadenoma is an uncommon benign tumor in adolescent girls. Core-needle biopsy should be performed prior to excision to distinguish the relatively rare phyllodes tumor, a usually benign (90%) tumor of the stromal elements requiring wide margins of resection to prevent local recurrence.

Breast Cyst

A cyst is the most common cause of breast mass in women in their fourth and fifth decades of life. Cysts may be soli-

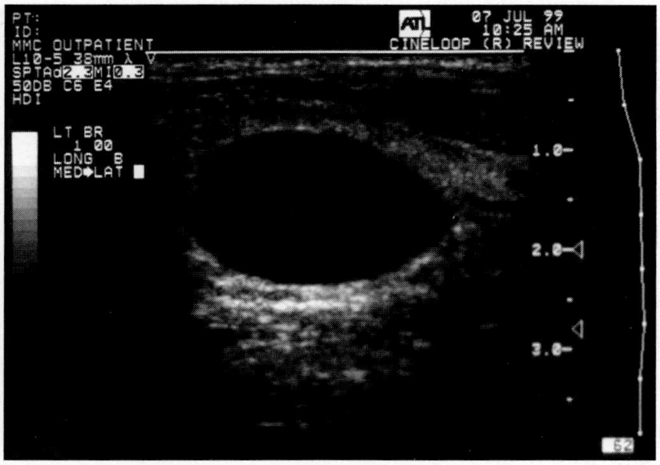

Figure 20-5 Ultrasound of a simple cyst.

tary or multiple and present as firm, mobile, slightly tender masses, often with less well-defined borders compared to fibroadenomas. Unlike fibroadenomas, the size and degree of tenderness of a cyst typically fluctuates with the menstrual cycle. Screening mammography will frequently detect nonpalpable cysts. Ultrasonography is very useful in demonstrating a simple cyst as a well-demarcated, hypoechoic mass with posterior enhancement of transmission (Fig. 20-5). Such an appearance is diagnostic and does not require biopsy. Aspiration may be performed on large, symptomatic cysts. The resulting fluid may be straw-colored or greenish, and cytologic analysis is unnecessary.

The ultrasound appearance of complex cysts shows internal echoes or an associated solid component. Mammography and core-needle biopsy are warranted in this setting.

Nipple Discharge

The most common cause of nipple discharge is duct ectasia, a nonneoplastic condition characterized by multiple dilated ducts in the subareolar space. The nipple discharge may be clear, milky, or green-brown. The discharge should be applied to occult blood test paper, and further evaluation should be performed when blood is present. Persistent, spontaneous discharge from a single duct and bloody discharge are considered pathologic. The incidence of malignancy is 10% to 15% in unilateral, bloody nipple discharge. The great majority of cases are caused by intraductal papilloma, a benign local proliferation of ductal epithelial cells that typically presents in women in their fourth or fifth decade of life.

Systematic palpation around the nipple–areolar complex can frequently identify the discharging duct. Mammography is important to evaluate for malignancy. Ductography is seldom helpful because it does not alter the subsequent management. In the absence of clinical or radiologic evidence of malignancy, duct excision through a circumareolar incision allows definitive histologic diagnosis and eliminates the discharge with a cosmetically acceptable result.

Breast Abscess and Mastitis

Presence of an exquisitely tender, fluctuant mass indicates abscess formation. Ultrasound is helpful to demonstrate drainable fluid collections. Repeated aspiration combined with antibiotics may allow resolution of the abscess without open drainage. In nonlactating women, especially smokers, recurrent breast abscesses may occur with chronic inflammation and fistula formation between the skin and the duct. Treatment includes antibiotics with coverage of anaerobic organisms followed by excision of the subareolar ducts including the fistula tract.

Inflammatory cancer occasionally mimics breast abscess. Biopsy of any mass associated with an abscess should be performed at the time of drainage.

Mastitis presents with pain and erythema of the breast, most commonly in lactating women. The causative organisms in this setting are usually staphylococci or streptococci. Appropriate antibiotics such as dicloxacillin or clindamycin should bring prompt relief. Breast-feeding may continue on the unaffected breast, while use of a breast pump is helpful to reduce congestion of the infected breast.

BREAST CANCER

Approximately one of every eight women will have breast cancer in her lifetime. It is the most frequently diagnosed nonskin cancer, and the second leading cause of cancer death in women. Although incidence rates have been increasing, the rate of increase has slowed in the past decade. Approximately 25% of new cancers are in situ. The rise in the detection of ductal carcinoma in situ is a result of the increased use of screening mammography, which detects breast cancers before they are palpable.

The earliest sign of a breast cancer is usually an abnormality on a mammogram. As breast cancers grow, they can produce a palpable mass that is often hard and irregular. Other signs may include thickening, swelling, skin irritation, or dimpling. Nipple changes due to breast cancer can include scaliness and dryness, ulceration, retraction, or discharge.

In most cases of breast cancer, the cause is unknown, but many risk factors such as hormonal and dietary factors have been identified. About 10% of cancers are related to genetic factors. Approximately 1% of breast cancers occur in men. They are usually diagnosed and treated in the same way as breast cancer in women.

Histologic Types of Breast Cancer

Lobular carcinoma in situ (LCIS) is considered a marker for the increased risk of developing invasive ductal or lobular carcinoma in either breast in the future. It is often

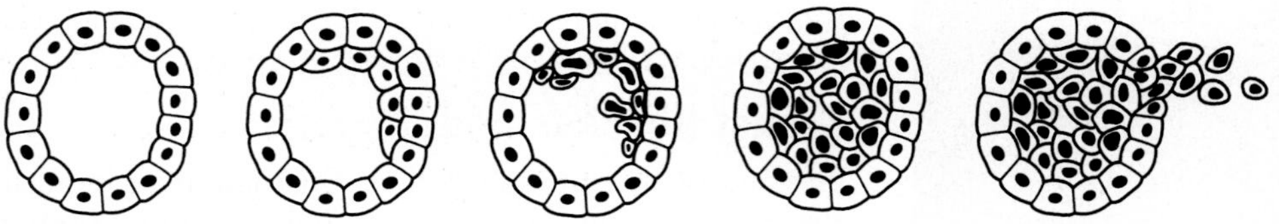

Figure 20-6 The evolution from normal duct to invasive cancer. (Adapted with permission from Love SM. *Dr. Susan Love's Breast Book.* Reading, MA: Addison-Wesley Longman, 1990;192. Copyright 1990, 1991 by Susan M. Love, MD. Reprinted by permission of Addison-Wesley Longman, Inc.)

identified incidentally with excision of other breast pathology.

Ductal carcinoma in situ (DCIS) is a preinvasive form of ductal cancer. If not treated adequately, invasive cancer may develop in 30% to 50% of patients over 10 years (Fig. 20-6). The typical appearance of DCIS on mammography is microcalcifications; there is rarely a mass on physical examination or mammography. The histologic types of DCIS include solid, cribriform, micropapillary, and comedo-type. DCIS can be classified on the basis of nuclear grades 1, 2, and 3, with grade 1 being the most favorable. Patients with comedo-type necrosis and/or high-grade lesions have an increased risk of recurrence and of the lesion developing into invasive cancer.

Infiltrating ductal carcinoma constitutes approximately 90% of invasive breast cancers. It produces the characteristic firm, irregular mass on physical examination. These masses are characteristically more well defined mammographically and histologically than infiltrating lobular cancers.

Infiltrating lobular carcinoma makes up approximately 10% of breast cancers and is often difficult to detect mammographically and on physical examination because of its indistinct borders. It is characterized by a higher incidence of multicentricity in the same breast and by its presence in the contralateral breast.

Tubular carcinoma, a very well-differentiated form of ductal carcinoma, constitutes approximately 1% to 2% of breast cancers. It is so named because it forms small tubules, randomly arranged, each lined by a single uniform row of cells. This subtype tends to occur in women who are slightly younger than the average patient with breast cancer. The prognosis is better than with other infiltrating ductal carcinomas.

Medullary carcinoma, another variant of infiltrating ductal cancer, is characterized by extensive tumor invasion by small lymphocytes and is slightly less well differentiated than tubular carcinoma. It constitutes approximately 5% of breast carcinomas. At diagnosis, it tends to be rapidly growing and large, and it is often associated with DCIS. It less commonly metastasizes to regional lymph nodes and has a better prognosis than the typical infiltrating ductal carcinoma.

Colloid or mucinous carcinoma is also a variant of infiltrating ductal cancer and accounts for approximately 2% to 3% of breast carcinomas. It is characterized histologically by clumps and strands of epithelial cells in pools of mucoid material. It grows slowly and occurs more often in older women. The pure type has a relatively good prognosis.

True papillary carcinoma accounts for approximately 1% of breast carcinomas. These tumors can be difficult to distinguish histologically from intraductal papilloma, a benign lesion. They tend to be quite small, and even when they metastasize to regional nodes, they have a better prognosis than ductal carcinomas because of their slower rate of growth.

Inflammatory carcinoma accounts for 3% of all breast cancers and presents with skin edema (peau d'orange) and erythema. The skin edema is secondary to dermal lymphatics congested with malignant cells that are generally ductal in origin. Inflammatory carcinoma of the breast has a poor prognosis, with approximately 25% of patients alive 5 years later. Malignancies that rarely occur in the breast include sarcomas, lymphomas, and leukemia.

Paget's disease of the nipple is a cutaneous nipple abnormality, which may be moist and exudative, dry and scaly, erosive, or just a thickened area. The patient may note itching, burning, or sticking pain in the nipple. As time passes, the lesion spreads out from the duct orifice. Histologically, the dermis is infiltrated by Paget's cells, which are of ductal origin, large and pale, with large nuclei, prominent nucleoli, and abundant cytoplasm. Paget's disease of the nipple is seen in approximately 3% of breast cancers and is usually, but not always, associated with an underlying malignancy, which is palpable in half of cases. It may originate in DCIS or in an invasive cancer.

Paget's disease of the nipple is often misdiagnosed as a simple dermatologic eruption and treated with ointments and creams for prolonged periods, during which time the cancer progresses. If a lesion is clinically suspicious for Paget's disease, a nipple biopsy should be done.

Staging

The treatment for breast cancer depends on the likelihood of local recurrence and distant spread. The most common areas of breast cancer metastasis are bone, lung, liver, and brain. The risk for distant spread is related to tumor size and lymph node involvement with cancer. The tumor,

Table 20-4 TNM Staging System for Breast Cancer

Primary Tumor (T)

Tis	Carcinoma in situ
T1	Tumor ≤2 cm
T2	Tumor > 2 cm, ≤5 cm
T3	Tumor > 5 cm
T4	Tumor any size with extension to chest wall or skin

Regional Lymph Nodes (N)

NO	No lymph node metastasis
N1	Metastasis in one to three axillary lymph nodes
N2	Metastasis in four to nine axillary lymph nodes
N3	Metastasis in 10 or more axillary lymph nodes

Distant Metastasis (M)

MO	No distant metastasis
M1	Distant metastasis

Stage Grouping

0	Tis	NO	MO
I	T1	NO	MO
IIA	TO	N1	MO
	T1	N1	MO
	T2	NO	MO
IIB	T2	N1	MO
	T3	NO	MO
IIIA	TO	N2	MO
	T1	N2	MO
	T2	N2	MO
	T3	N1	MO
	T3	N2	MO
IIIB	T4	NO	MO
	T4	N1	MO
	T4	N2	MO
IIIC	Any T	N3	MO
IV	Any T	Any N	M1

node, metastasis (TNM) status defines the patient's stage of disease (Table 20-4).

Besides TNM status, other factors are taken into account when planning therapy for breast cancer. These include the estrogen receptor status, the histopathologic grade of the tumor, and the mitotic index. Her-2-neu, an oncogene produced by some tumors, predicts a poorer prognosis as well as the likelihood of a response to Herceptin, a monoclonal antibody, in the event of a relapse to standard therapy.

When the patient's risk for metastatic disease is low (tumor size < 5 cm and no palpable lymphadenopathy), only chest radiograph and complete blood count are necessary prior to surgery. Patients with more advanced disease should have chest and abdominal CT scans as well as bone scans before surgical treatment.

Treatment of Breast Cancer

Breast cancer treatment is best viewed as a multidisciplinary effort involving breast imagers, breast and plastic surgeons, medical and radiation oncologists, pathologists, gynecologists, oncology nurses, social workers, and psychiatrists. The treatment of breast cancer concerns both local treatment (surgery and radiation) and adjuvant treatment (chemotherapy and hormone therapy) designed to decrease systemic recurrence.

Surgery

Lumpectomy, wide excision, and partial mastectomy refer to the excision of a malignancy with a margin of microscopically normal tissue on all sides. Lumpectomy may be used in the treatment of ductal carcinoma in situ and invasive carcinoma and is usually followed by breast irradiation.

Simple, or total, mastectomy removes the entire breast with the pectoralis major fascia. Modified radical mastectomy is simple mastectomy with axillary dissection. Radical mastectomy, in which the breast, both pectoralis muscles, axillary contents, and the overlying skin are removed, was developed by Halsted at a time when no other treatments were available. It causes disfigurement and upper extremity dysfunction and is no longer used except in unusual circumstances (e.g., invasion of the pectoralis muscles).

Axillary treatment has evolved over the past 10 years from routine dissection to a more selective approach. Axillary dissection removes the level I and level II lymph nodes, including the nodes in the axillary fat pad (level I), below the pectoralis major muscle and behind the pectoralis minor muscles (level II). Axillary dissection is indicated in the presence of lymph node metastases. In a clinically negative axilla, sentinel lymph node biopsy employs injection of a radioactive colloid and/or blue dye to identify the first lymph node that receives drainage from the breast. Typically, only one or two nodes will pick up the marker. These nodes may be removed with a smaller incision and less risk of disruption of the lymphatic drainage of the arm. Staging of the regional nodes is then based upon the histopathologic analysis of the sentinel node.

The option of breast reconstruction should be discussed with all patients and can be performed immediately after mastectomy or may be delayed. The breast mound may be reconstructed using prosthetic implants or autologous tissue obtained from rectus abdominus or latissimus dorsi musculocutaneous flaps.

Choosing a Surgical Option

The choice of surgical option should balance the extent of disease with the morbidity of treatment. Noninvasive disease (DCIS) does not require axillary staging. Lumpectomy is usually feasible in tumors under 4 cm, depending on the size of the breast. A recurrence rate of 30% for lumpectomy alone usually mandates postoperative radiation, which is delivered in daily fractions over a 6-week period. Occasionally, lumpectomy alone without radiation is adequate treatment with very small, low-grade tumors with wide margins of excision, particularly in the elderly.

Involvement of the nipple, as in Paget's disease, requires excision of the nipple–areolar complex by lumpectomy or mastectomy. Dermal lymphatic involvement, diffuse or multiple tumors, unwillingness or inability to undergo radiation therapy, and the expectation of a cosmetically unacceptable result are contradictions to lumpectomy.

It is important for a patient to understand that there is no statistically significant difference in cure (survival) or chance of recurrence between breast-conserving therapy and mastectomy. Local recurrence after lumpectomy is treated with mastectomy, but survival is determined by systemic recurrence.

Prophylactic (bilateral simple) mastectomy is an option for patients at a very high risk of breast cancer. This group includes those with a combination of high-risk lesions on biopsy (atypical ductal hyperplasia, LCIS) and a strong family history. Patients who carry one of the breast cancer genes (**BRCA-1**, BRCA-2) are also offered the option. This procedure reduces the risk of breast cancer by 90%, compared to 49% in chemoprevention with tamoxifen.

Chemotherapy

The use of adjuvant chemotherapy has increased remarkably over the last several years. The most common regimen currently used includes cyclophosphamide, doxorubicin, and 5-fluorouracil given over 9 to 10 weeks at 3-week intervals. Another regimen used with increasing frequency is a course of doxorubicin and cyclophosphamide followed by a course of a taxane. Indications for chemotherapy include premenopausal and postmenopausal patients with node-positive disease or tumors greater than 1 cm. With increasing age, hormonal therapy alone may be utilized, particularly for node-negative disease greater than 1 cm. More recently, the addition of a novel class of drugs, the taxanes, has shown improved disease-free and overall survival rates.

Hormonal Therapy

Tamoxifen is used to treat estrogen-receptor–positive (ER-positive) tumors, particularly in postmenopausal women, and it may have some benefit for ER-negative tumors in postmenopausal women. Its role in premenopausal women is less well established, but it is often used in this setting after chemotherapy. In addition to decreasing recurrence, tamoxifen decreases the incidence of contralateral breast cancer by approximately 40%. No benefit is shown for continuing tamoxifen longer than 5 years. Newer aromatase inhibitors are being used with increasing frequency as an alternative to tamoxifen. The aromatase inhibitors as a class of drugs have been shown to decrease circulating estrogen levels by approximately 90% in postmenopausal women. Anastrazole is one of the first to be compared with tamoxifen in a clinical trial. It may be superior to tamoxifen in prolonging disease-free survival. It also appears to cause fewer hot flashes, but may be associated with a greater incidence of osteoporosis than tamoxifen.

Treatment for Recurrent and Metastatic Breast Cancer

Local tumor recurrence in the breast after breast conservation (lumpectomy, axillary dissection, and radiation) is treated with mastectomy. If radiation was never given, a small recurrence is treated with lumpectomy and radiation. Local recurrence after mastectomy is treated with surgical excision, if possible, and radiation to the chest wall. Early recurrences are treated with systemic chemotherapy. Local recurrence has a good prognosis in the absence of concomitant systemic recurrence.

Metastatic disease is treated with chemotherapy. Brain metastases, which are often multiple, are treated with radiation. Bony metastases are treated with radiation and surgical fixation if there is a high risk of fracture. For pain reduction, biphosphonates and ^{89}Sr are undergoing trials. Second-generation aromatase inhibitors (anastrozole, letrozole) are also used for recurrent and metastatic breast cancer.

Complications of Breast Cancer Treatment

Complications of Surgery

Complications of surgery for breast cancer are similar to those for other surgical procedures and include wound infection, seroma, and hematoma formation. In addition, a poor cosmetic result and a local recurrence of 5% to 12% can occur after breast-conserving therapy. Modified radical mastectomy can lead to flap necrosis and a local recurrence rate of 5% to 10%. Axillary lymph node dissection can cause **lymphedema** and decreased range of motion in the shoulder. Rarely, injury to the long thoracic nerve or to the thoracodorsal nerve causes "winged scapula" and latissimus dorsi paralysis, respectively. The intercostobrachial nerve is sometimes divided as it passes through the axillary fat pad and may result in loss of sensation to the skin of the inner upper arm. These complications are, for the most part, avoided with sentinel node biopsy.

After axillary dissection, blood should not be drawn and blood pressure cuffs should not be placed on the ipsilateral arm. Infections should be avoided and treated promptly in an effort to prevent permanent lymphedema.

Complications of Chemotherapy, Hormonal Therapy, and Radiation

Common side effects of chemotherapy are nausea, vomiting, leukopenia, thrombocytopenia, and alopecia. Less common adverse effects include cardiotoxicity from doxorubicin, sepsis, and hemorrhagic cystitis. The development of recombinant erythropoietin and **granulocyte colony-stimulating factor** has made it possible to maintain hematocrit and neutrophil counts at acceptable levels, decreasing the likelihood of nadir sepsis and allowing more aggressive treatment.

Common side effects of tamoxifen are hot flashes, fluid retention, vaginitis, and thrombocytopenia. Though less common, serious side effects are endometrial carcinoma, vascular thrombosis, and pulmonary embolism.

A common side effect early after radiation treatment is breast edema with altered sensation. Chronic changes progress to fibrosis and hyperpigmentation. Rare complications are pneumonitis and bone necrosis. Radiation oncologists use tangential fields to minimize the radiation dose to all but breast tissue.

Prognosis

The most important prognostic factors for breast cancer are related to stage of disease (Table 20-5). Axillary lymph node status is the single most important factor in determining disease-free and overall survival, followed by tumor size and ER-receptor status. Other possible prognostic factors such as growth factors and proteases are being investigated. The risk of developing a second primary breast cancer is approximately 1% per year for the first 15 years. The risk of recurrence, while never reaching 0%, decreases over time.

Table 20-5 Five-Year Relative Survival Rates for Patients With Treated Breast Cancer by Stage

Stage	Survival Rate (%)
I	96
II	82
III	53
IV	18

Rates adjusted for deaths from other causes.

Followup

Followup for breast cancer patients should include bilateral mammogram 6 months after completion of radiation therapy following lumpectomy and yearly thereafter. After modified radical mastectomy, contralateral breast mammogram should be performed annually. Physical examination should be every 3 to 6 months for 3 years and then annually. Other studies to detect metastasis are not cost-effective and should be performed only when indicated by symptoms or physical findings.

SUGGESTED READINGS

Cox C, Salud C, Harrinton M. The role of selective sentinel lymph node dissection in breast cancer. *Surg Clin North Am* 2000;80(6):1759–1777.

Fisher B, Costantino J, et al. Tamoxifen for prevention of breast cancer: report of the National Surgical Adjuvant Breast and Bowel Project P-1 Study. *J Natl Cancer Inst* 2003;90:1371–1388.

Hughes LE, Mansel RE, Webster DJT. *Benign Disorders and Diseases of the Breast.* 2nd Ed. Philadelphia, PA: WB Saunders, 2000.

Morrow M, Wong S, Venta L. The evaluation of breast masses in women younger than forty years of age. *Surgery* 1998;124(4):634–641.

Singletary SE. Revisions of the breast cancer staging system: the sixth edition of the American Joint Committee on Cancer Staging Manual. *Breast Diseases: A Year Book Quarterly* 2002;13(2):114–119.

21

Surgical Endocrinology

■ **THYROID GLAND**
Nicholas P.W. Coe, MD
■ **PARATHYROID GLANDS**
Karen R. Borman, MD, Nicholas P.W. Coe, MD
■ **ADRENAL GLANDS**
Roshni Rao, MD, Richard B. Wait, MD, PhD
■ **MULTIPLE ENDOCRINE NEOPLASIA SYNDROMES**
Karen R. Borman, MD

OBJECTIVES

Thyroid Gland

1. Discuss the evaluation and differential diagnosis of a patient with a thyroid nodule.
2. List the different types of carcinoma of the thyroid gland and their cell type of origin; discuss the appropriate therapeutic strategy for each.
3. Understand the major risk factors for carcinoma of the thyroid gland and the prognostic variables that dictate therapy.
4. Describe the symptoms of a patient with hyperthyroidism; discuss the differential diagnosis and treatment options.

Parathyroid Glands

1. Understand the role of the parathyroid glands in the physiology of calcium homeostasis.
2. List the causes, symptoms, and signs of hypercalcemia.
3. Know the difference between primary, secondary, and tertiary hyperparathyroidism.
4. Discuss the evaluation and differential diagnosis of a patient with hypercalcemia.
5. Understand the management of acute and severe hypercalcemia.
6. Describe the indications for surgery for hyperparathyroidism.
7. Describe the complications of parathyroid surgery.

Adrenal Glands

1. Describe the clinical features of Cushing's syndrome and discuss how lesions in the pituitary, adrenal cortex, and extra-adrenal sites are distinguished diagnostically.
2. Discuss the medical and surgical management of Cushing's syndrome in patients with an adrenal adenoma, with a pituitary adenoma causing adrenal hyperplasia, and with an adrenocorticotropic hormone (ACTH)-producing neoplasm.
3. Describe the pathology, clinical features, laboratory findings, workup, and management of a patient with primary aldosteronism.
4. Discuss adrenal cortical carcinoma, including its presentation, signs and symptoms, diagnostic workup, and management.
5. Discuss pheochromocytoma, including its associated signs and symptoms, appropriate diagnostic workup, and treatment.
6. Discuss the management and evaluation of an incidentally discovered adrenal mass.
7. Discuss the causes of adrenal insufficiency in the surgical setting as well as the associated clinical and laboratory findings.

Multiple Endocrine Neoplasia Syndromes

1. Describe the multiple endocrine neoplasia syndromes and their surgical treatment.

THYROID GLAND

ANATOMY

The thyroid gland forms two lobes in the neck, anterior to the larynx. The lobes are connected by the thyroid isthmus at approximately the second tracheal ring (Fig. 21-1). It is the first endocrine gland to appear during embryonic development, at approximately 24 days after conception. It begins as a thickening on the floor of the pharynx at the site of the foramen cecum on the adult tongue. This endodermal thickening grows caudally, as the thyroglossal duct, into the neck, passing ventral to the embryonal hyoid bone and thyroid cartilage. The duct disappears by the 50th day of gestation, but may persist anywhere along its migratory pathway as the pyramidal lobe of the thyroid (in 50% of adults) or as a thyroglossal duct cyst. In addition, the ultimobranchial body that stems from the fourth pharyngeal pouch epithelium contributes to the thyroid. This body is the origin of the C cells.

The adult thyroid gland weighs 15 to 25 g and is supplied by the superior (the first branch of the external carotid artery) and inferior (a branch of the thyrocervical trunk that arises from the subclavian artery) thyroid arteries (Fig. 21-2). Venous drainage occurs through the superior, middle, and inferior thyroid veins. The thyroid gland lies anterior to the trachea. It is covered anteriorly by the skin and platysma muscle and anterolaterally by the sternocleidomastoid, sternohyoid, and sternothyroid muscles. The parathyroid glands (discussed later) are posterior to the thyroid gland.

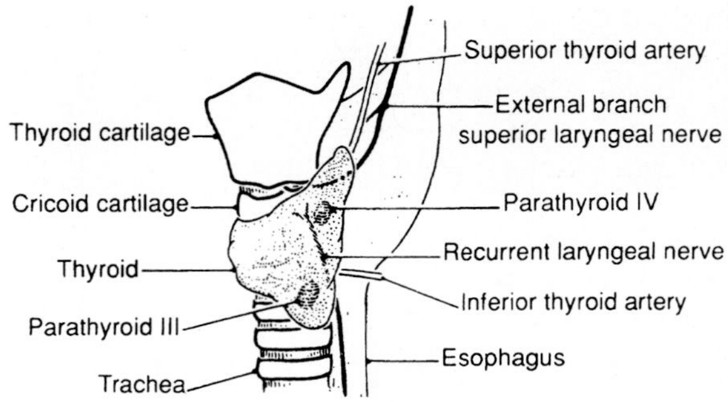

Figure 21-2 The adult thyroid gland.

PHYSIOLOGY

The thyroid gland has two distinct groups of hormone-producing cells. **Follicular cells** produce, store, and release **thyroxine (T_4)** and **triiodothyronine (T_3)**, major regulators of the basal metabolic rate. **Parafollicular cells,** or C cells, secrete calcitonin, a hormone that has a minor role in maintaining calcium homeostasis.

Follicular cells efficiently capture iodide from the circulation, which appears to be the rate-limiting step in thyroid hormone synthesis. Thyroid cells concentrate **iodine** to levels 30 times that found in normal tissues. The iodide (I^-) is then oxidized to I^+ or to iodine (I^0). This reaction is catalyzed by the membrane-bound enzyme thyroid peroxidase (TPO). This reaction, called organification, occurs on the apical membranes of the follicular cells, which form the boundary of an extracellular storage space called the **follicle. Thyroglobulin** is a large (molecular weight [MW] = 660 kDa) glycoprotein that is synthesized by the follicular cells and then secreted into the follicle. The tyrosine residues of thyroglobulin are iodinated by the I^0 or I^+ species, forming monoiodotyrosine (MIT) and diiodotyrosine (DIT), which then couple to form the iodothyronines T_3 (MIT + DIT) and T_4 (DIT + DIT). This iodinated thyroglobulin is the storage form of the thyroid hormones that are kept in the follicle (Fig. 21-3). When **thyroid-stimulating hormone** (TSH, or thyrotropin) stim-

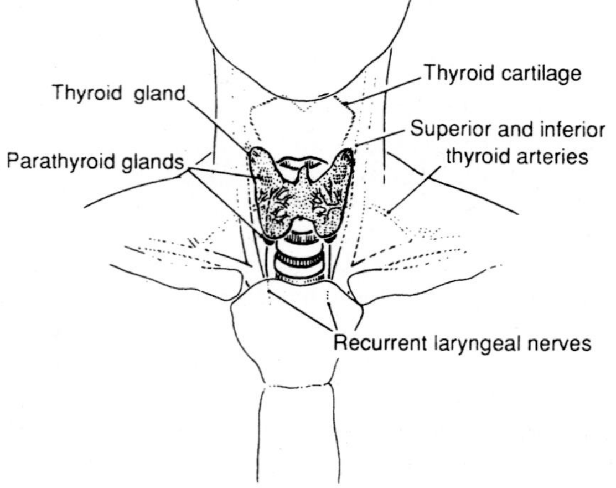

Figure 21-1 The thyroid gland.

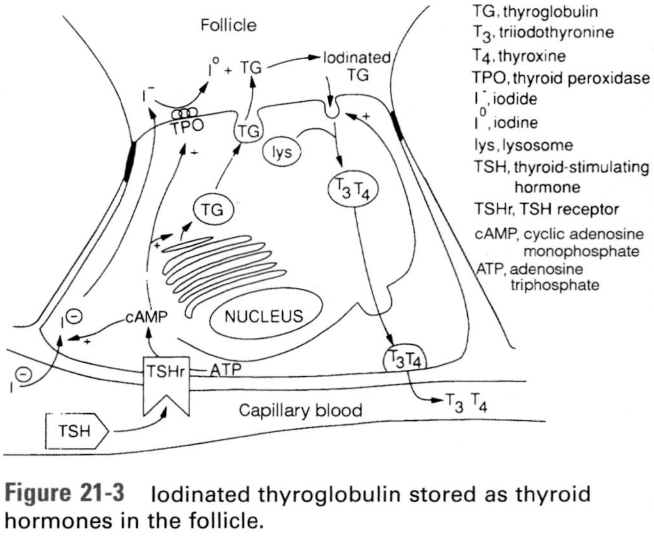

Figure 21-3 Iodinated thyroglobulin stored as thyroid hormones in the follicle.

ulates the thyroid gland to release active hormone, the iodinated thyroglobulin from the follicle is taken into the follicular cell by endocytosis. There, it is hydrolyzed to T_3 and T_4, which are then released into the circulation. The thyroglobulin itself is not released except under pathologic conditions. T_3 and T_4 are the active forms of circulating hormone. Most (80%) of the circulating hormone is T_4, but T_3, which is generated by the peripheral conversion of T_4 to T_3, is the most active form of thyroid hormone. This reaction can also produce reverse T_3 (rT_3), an inactive form of the hormone.

Follicular cell function is controlled by the anterior pituitary–derived TSH, which stimulates the thyroid to release T_3 and T_4. TSH also stimulates the cell to increase the means of producing thyroid hormones, which includes increasing both thyroglobulin synthesis and iodide transport efficiency. TSH production, in turn, is controlled by two mechanisms. Thyrotropin-releasing hormone (TRH), which is secreted by the hypothalamus into the hypothalamic–pituitary portal venous system, increases TSH release. If excessive concentrations of T_3 and T_4 are present, however, a negative feedback system shuts off the secretion of TSH and probably TRH (Fig. 21-4).

The other hormone-producing cells in the thyroid, the parafollicular cells or C cells, are derived from the neural crest cells of the ultimobranchial body. When these cells are stimulated by high serum calcium levels, they secrete the hormone calcitonin, which inhibits osteoclast activity, thus decreasing the calcium level. Calcitonin secretion, which is also affected by serum estrogen and vitamin D levels, does not normally play a major role in regulating serum calcium levels. Its function probably is to protect the skeleton from excessive scavenging during times of high calcium demand (e.g., growth, pregnancy, lactation). The absence of calcitonin production (e.g., after total thyroidectomy) appears to have no demonstrable negative physiologic effect.

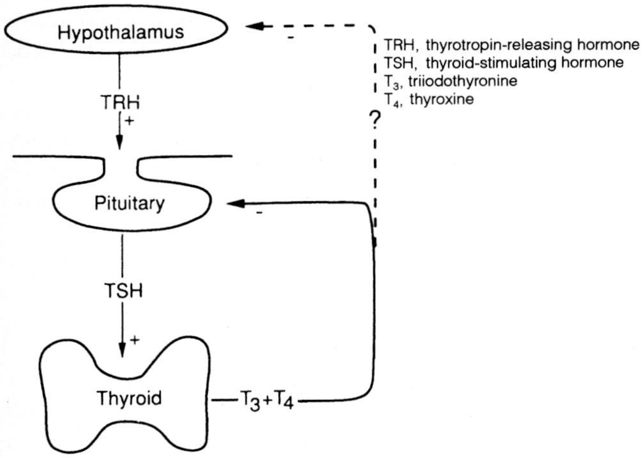

Figure 21-4 The hypothalamus–pituitary–thyroid axis.

PATHOPHYSIOLOGY

Thyroid Nodule

Palpable thyroid nodules occur in 4% of the population of the United States: Half are solitary and half are multinodular. The frequency of undetected nodules is unknown, but autopsy studies suggest that the true incidence is much higher. At autopsy, 50% of thyroid glands contain one or more nodules, and 12% have a solitary nodule. Thyroid nodules are a common presentation of a potentially curable cancer.

Clinical Presentation and Evaluation

In evaluating a patient with a thyroid nodule, a thorough history and physical examination should be performed. Although thyroid cancer is more common in women, a solitary lesion in a man is significantly more likely to be malignant than a comparable nodule in a woman. Although the initial evaluation is the same, a heightened index of suspicion should be maintained in a man with a thyroid nodule. Certain factors, such as the duration of the presence of a nodule, and local symptoms, such as pain, pressure, or hoarseness, may suggest local invasiveness and should be assessed. The patient should be asked about symptoms of toxicity because toxic adenomas can present as a solitary palpable thyroid nodule. A family history of multiple endocrine neoplasia (MEN) syndrome should be investigated.

A history of childhood radiation is significant because radiation exposure increases the risk of thyroid cancer, which is often multicentric. Beginning at a dose of as low as 200 rad, the risk rises as the dose increases to 2000 rad. A dose of radiation greater than 2000 rad usually causes actual destruction of the thyroid tissue. Patients may have radiation exposure as the result of treatment of an enlarged thymus in infancy or treatment for ringworm, acne, tubercular lymphadenopathy (therapies popular between 1930 and 1955), capillary hemangioma, or keloid scars (still used occasionally today). Patients who lived in the Ukraine or the Gomel region of Belorussia at the time of the Chernobyl incident (1986) are also at significant risk.

Although the primary concern in patients with a thyroid nodule is to confirm or exclude carcinoma, many patients have symptoms from benign disease. Multinodular goiters, especially those that extend retrosternally, and occasionally thyroids associated with Hashimoto's thyroiditis, may grow to great size and cause symptoms of compression with a feeling of choking and difficulty breathing or swallowing. These patients may present for thyroidectomy to relieve their symptoms.

The physical examination should include careful palpation of the remainder of the thyroid gland and regional lymph nodes. Symptoms of compression in patients whose goiter is retrosternal may be confirmed by eliciting a Pemberton's sign. Raising the arms above the head, as while brushing the hair, may cause venous compression at the thoracic inlet, with engorgement of the head and neck and a feeling of strangulation. Indirect laryngoscopy is indicated when there is hoarseness or when the signs and symptoms suggest malignancy. The simplest baseline laboratory study is a TSH test. A low level suggests thyrotoxicosis, and a high level suggests underactivity (e.g., associated with Hashimoto's thyroiditis). Thyroid function is measured whenever the TSH is abnormal. These tests are available at some institutions as "thyroid function tests" and generally include TSH and T_4 and sometimes T_3. Other combinations of these and other tests may be offered. In general, it is better practice to order tests that are appropriate for the clinical setting rather than ordering broad panels of tests. For example, in a patient with Graves' disease, a T_4, T_3, TSH, thyroxine-binding globulin (TBG), and thyroid-stimulating antibody (TSab) tests should be ordered. This combination would be inappropriate for a patient without toxic symptoms or signs where a TSH alone may be sufficient.

Serum calcium levels are measured in patients who have a history of radiation exposure (which may also cause parathyroid adenoma) or a family history of MEN syndrome. Patients who are related to someone who has MEN-2 syndrome should also have urinary catecholamines and catecholamine metabolites screened for functional **pheochromocytoma.** Medullary carcinoma is the only thyroid cancer that reliably expresses a tumor marker that is measurable in the serum (calcitonin). Serum thyroglobulin levels may be elevated in follicular or papillary carcinomas, but not reliably so. Thyroglobulin levels may also be elevated in benign diseases.

Fine-needle aspiration cytology (FNA) is extremely accurate and is the single most important study in evaluating a thyroid mass. Only 3% of patients with a benign diagnosis on FNA have thyroid cancer, and 85% of nodules identified as malignant on FNA are cancers at resection. FNA has decreased unnecessary operative procedures in patients with benign nodules and increased the probability that surgery will be performed only on patients with malignant nodules. The major difficulty remains in patients whose FNA diagnosis is indeterminate, usually those with follicular neoplasms. Follicular adenomas are often difficult to distinguish from follicular carcinomas because the distinction rests on architectural characteristics, such as capsular and vascular invasion, which are not detectable by cytology. In these cases, surgical resection is necessary to obtain a diagnosis.

Ultrasound examination of the neck may be used to supplement physical examination to determine whether a nodule is cystic or solid, whether additional nodules or nodes exist, and the exact size of the nodule (Fig. 21-5). Multiple nodules, usually benign, are difficult to evaluate with percutaneous FNA and may require surgical resection for diagnosis. If a solitary thyroid nodule is cystic, it is aspirated with a fine needle. If the fluid obtained is cytologically benign and the mass disappears, the nodule is considered resolved, and no further evaluation or treatment is necessary. Recurrent cystic nodules are reaspirated and reevaluated cytologically as necessary. Most cystic masses resolve after a single needle aspiration. The presence of a residual mass after complete aspiration of a thyroid cyst may warrant surgical resection, particularly if the cytologic findings are suspicious. A thyroid nodule that is solid on ultrasound also requires aspiration or biopsy for diagnosis.

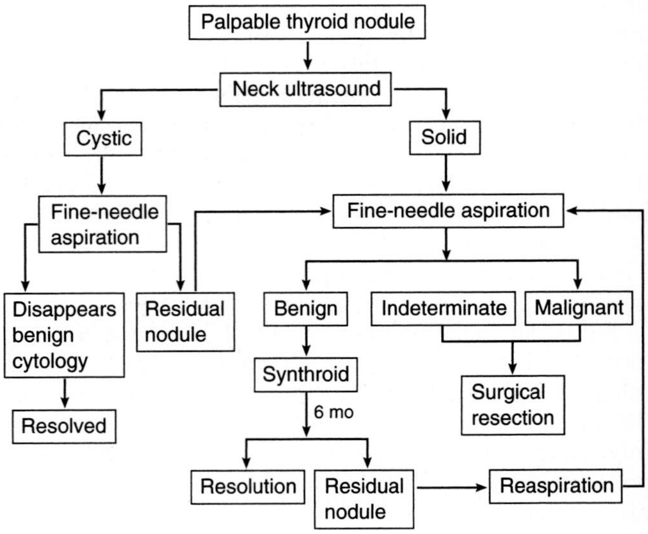

Figure 21-5 Ultrasound examination of the neck can determine whether a nodule is cystic or solid, whether additional nodules or nodes exist, and the exact size of the nodule. Follicular neoplasms are commonly intermediate on aspiration.

Treatment

Patients with solid nodules that are diagnosed as benign on FNA may be offered the option of being followed for a period of 3 to 6 months while being treated with oral thyroid hormone to suppress TSH stimulation of tumor growth. The decrease in TSH should be to the midnormal or low-normal range and should be carefully monitored to ensure the adequacy of suppression. Suppression to very low levels was used in the past but this is associated with an increased risk of osteoporosis and new onset atrial fibrillation and is no longer recommended. If the nodule remains the same size, it is reaspirated. If it shrinks, suppression therapy is continued. If it enlarges on suppressive therapy, it has a higher risk of being a cancer and must be excised.

Surgical exploration in a patient with a thyroid nodule is undertaken with a working diagnosis of cancer. The initial procedure is thyroid lobectomy and isthmectomy to remove the ipsilateral lobe of the thyroid gland as well as the isthmus (see Fig. 21-6). Simple nodulectomy incompletely removes the tumor and should not be performed. Lobectomy allows the pathologist to assess the relation between the nodule and its surrounding thyroid tissue to determine whether it is malignant. If the pathologist can-

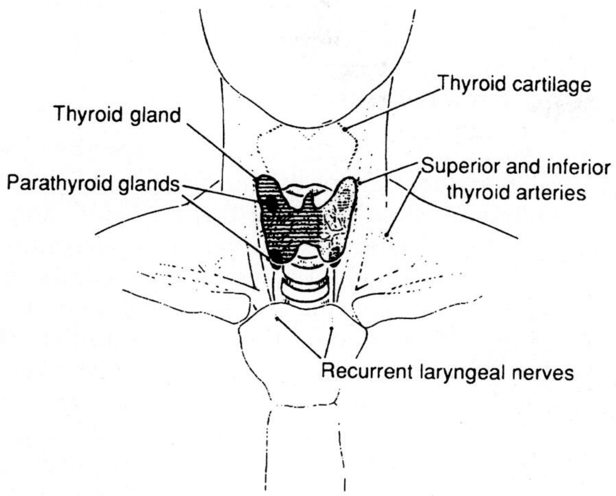

Figure 21-6 Thyroid lobectomy and isthmectomy.

not provide a definitive diagnosis on frozen-section analysis, especially in the case of follicular neoplasms, no further surgery is undertaken at that time. Definitive therapy is dictated by the permanent pathologic analysis and may require completion thyroidectomy in a few days. If frozen-section analysis of the specimen shows cancer, further resection (total thyroidectomy) is performed if it is indicated according to the criteria in Table 21-1. In patients with symptomatic thyroid enlargement, the extent of thyroidectomy is dictated by the disease. Lobectomy may be sufficient, or subtotal or total thyroidectomy may be necessary to remove all diseased tissue. Surgical resection should be definitive if possible because reoperation poses much greater risk to the nerves and parathyroids.

In performing lobectomy or total thyroidectomy, great care is taken to preserve the parathyroid glands and their blood supply. Occasionally, autografting of a parathyroid into the sternocleidomastoid muscle is necessary if the glandular blood supply is injured during the procedure. Preservation of the recurrent laryngeal nerve and the external branch of the superior laryngeal nerve is also essential. Injury to the recurrent laryngeal nerve causes paralysis of the ipsilateral vocal cord, which is immobile in the paramedian position. The other cord may not be opposable, leaving the patient with a weak, breathy voice. Bilateral injury causes total loss of speech and airway control and requires tracheostomy. Injury to the external branch of the superior nerve results in loss of voice quality. Transient hypoparathyroidism or neurapraxia of the nerves is more common than permanent injury, and it usually resolves without sequelae. Hemorrhage, always a risk with any surgical procedure, is uncommon.

Hyperthyroidism

Hyperthyroidism is a syndrome that is caused by excessive secretion of thyroid hormone. The most common cause is **Graves' disease**, or diffuse toxic **goiter.** Less commonly, hyperthyroidism is caused by one (**toxic adenoma**) or more (**toxic multinodular goiter**) hyperfunctioning nodules. Less common causes include thyrotoxicosis factitia, a condition that is caused by the ingestion of excessive amounts of exogenous thyroid hormone, and struma (synonymous with goiter) ovarii, a condition in which the hyperactive thyroid tissue is found in an ovarian teratoma or dermoid.

The lifetime risk of hyperthyroidism is approximately

Table 21-1 Common Problems at Presentation of Thyroid Malignancy and Their Management

Diagnosis	Incidence (%)	Age (Yr)	Size	Extrathyroidal Invasion	Lymph Nodes	Surgical Therapy[a,b]
Well-differentiated	70–80	< 45	< 2 cm	None	±	Thyroid lobectomy and isthmusectomy or total thyroidectomy; removes only abnormal nodes
Papillary		> 45	> 1 cm	Often	±	Total thyroidectomy
Follicular	10–20	Any	Any	−	−	Total thyroidectomy
		Any	Any	+	−	Total thyroidectomy
Medullary	7	Any	Any	±	±	Total thyroidectomy and median lymph node dissection
Anaplastic	3	Any	Any	±	±	Nonsurgical therapy

[a] Thyroid replacement (thyroid-stimulating hormone) is recommended for patients with well-differentiated thyroid cancer after surgery.
[b] Radioactive iodine (^{131}I) is recommended for all patients with well-differentiated thyroid cancer and extrathyroidal disease that demonstrate uptake on a postsurgical^{131} scan.

5% for women and 1% for men. Graves' disease occurs predominantly in young women (8:1 ratio). The yearly rate of occurrence for women 20 to 30 years of age is 59: 100,000. For women older than 60 years of age, it is 38: 100,000. The incidence of toxic adenoma is lower and less well defined. However, between 10% and 30% of patients with hyperthyroidism may have toxic adenomas, and approximately 75% of these have a single toxic adenoma.

Graves' Disease

Clinical Presentation and Evaluation

Graves' disease (Robert J. Graves, Irish physician, 1797–1853) is a syndrome of diffuse goiter with hyperthyroidism (the most common component), exophthalmos, tachycardia, and tremor. Heat intolerance and weight loss are also common.

The signs and symptoms (Table 21-2) are those of a hypermetabolic state resulting from excessive production of thyroid hormone. The ophthalmologic effects of Graves' disease cover a continuum from a stare with lid lag, to proptosis, to deformity of the periorbital tissues with optic nerve involvement and complete loss of vision.

Serum TSH levels in thyrotoxicosis can determine whether the hyperthyroidism is pituitary-dependent or independent. In thyroid causes of hyperthyroidism, serum TSH levels are decreased, whereas in pituitary causes, they are increased. Total T_3 and T_4 levels are measured, along with the amount of TBG, because elevated T_4 levels may reflect increased serum TBG (e.g., in pregnancy). Alternatively, free T_3 and T_4 estimations are not affected by altered TBG levels. A low level of TSH in the presence of high thyroid hormone levels establishes thyroid-dependent hyperthyroidism, the most common situation.

The hyperthyroidism associated with Graves' disease is caused by a circulating immunoglobulin G, called TSAb, that is directed against the TSH receptors on the follicular cells of the thyroid. This antibody stimulates the thyroid to generate and secrete thyroid hormone, but the sensitivity to the negative feedback system that controls normal thyroid function is lost. Thus, TSAb causes excessive production of T_3 and T_4 and progressive hyperthyroidism. The pathogenesis of the exophthalmos and pretibial myxedema of Graves' disease is not well understood.

Treatment

The three possible treatments for Graves' hyperthyroidism are: (1) medical blockade of the hormone and its effects, (2) radioiodine ablation of active thyroid tissue, and (3) surgical resection. Iodide, administered as potassium iodide or as Lugol's solution (5% iodine plus potassium iodide), temporarily inhibits the release of thyroid hormone from the gland. The reason for this counterintuitive effect (the Wolff-Chaikoff effect) is not fully understood. As plasma iodide levels rise, increasing amounts are organified until a critical point is reached. After the critical point, the binding of iodide to tyrosine residues decreases dramatically. The synthesis of an unknown inhibitory iodine-containing compound within the thyroid during exposure to excess iodine has been postulated. The effect is short-lived (1 to 2 weeks).

Propranolol and other beta-blockers ameliorate some of the peripheral effects of excess thyroid hormone. These drugs decrease the peripheral conversion of T_4 to T_3 rather than block beta activity. Both iodide and propranolol may have a role in the short-term management or preoperative preparation of patients with hyperthyroidism, but do not provide definitive therapy.

Thionamides (e.g., propylthiouracil [PTU], methimazole [Tapazole]) interfere with the synthesis of thyroid hormones in the gland by inhibiting iodide organification and iodotyrosine coupling. They also reduce the rate of peripheral conversion of T_4 to T_3. Approximately one-third of patients who tolerate thionamide therapy remain in remission after 6 to 12 months of treatment with PTU; however, a significant percentage (5% to 10%) have adverse reactions to the drug (Table 21-3).

The other two-thirds of patients need more definitive treatment with either surgery or radioiodine. The isotope of choice for the radioablation of hyperactive thyroid tissue is ^{131}I. A dose of 80 $\mu Ci/g$ estimated thyroid tissue is effective for most patients and has a low incidence of inducing early hypothyroidism. A second and even a third dose may

Table 21-2 Symptoms and Signs of Hyperthyroidism

Central Nervous System	Cardiovascular and Respiratory Systems	Other Systems
Nervousness	Tachycardia	Lid lag
Restlessness	Palpitations	Proptosis or exophthalmos
Emotional lability	Arrhythmias	Ophthalmopathy
Fast speech	Dyspnea	Increased sweating
Fine tremor		Fatigue
		Weakness
		Hair loss
		Leg swelling
		Pretibial myxedema

Table 21-3 Complications of Treatment in Graves' Hyperthyroidism

Treatment	Complication	Frequency (%)
Subtotal thyroidectomy	Hypothyroidism	20
Total or subtotal	Recurrent hyperthyroidism	< 5
thyroidectomy	Superior laryngeal nerve injury	< 1
Radioiodine ablation	Recurrent laryngeal nerve injury	< 1
Thionamides	Hypoparathyroidism	< 2
	Hypothyroidism	20
	Early	50
	Late	15–20
	Delayed control requiring:	5
	Second radioiodine treatment	60–70
	Third radioiodine treatment	5–10
	Recurrent/persistent hyperthyroidism	0.02
	Intolerance of medication including:	
	Cholestasis	
	Arthralgia	
	Headache	
	Neuritis	
	Dependent edema	
	Reversible granulocytopenia	

be necessary if the patient has hyperthyroidism after 6 months (see Table 21-3). Over a period of 5 to 10 years, however, hypothyroidism occurs in 50% to 70% of these patients. Radioiodine ablation is safe and effective, and long-term followup of these patients suggests that radiation exposure does not appear to cause secondary thyroid cancer. This result probably occurs because the **radioactive iodine** is taken up so avidly by thyroid cells that the cellular radiation dose completely destroys the cells rather than simply altering their DNA. Subsequent neck exploration in these patients shows minimal, if any, residual thyroid tissue. Therapy with radioactive iodine does not appear to cause injury to the parathyroids, agranulocytosis, or any other radiation-induced phenomena. External beam radiotherapy plays no role in the treatment of hyperthyroidism.

Subtotal (Fig. 21-7) or total **thyroidectomy** (discussed under the medullary cancer section below) can also be used to treat Graves' hyperthyroidism. These procedures provide rapid control of the disease and eliminate exposure to radioactivity. Some studies show total thyroidectomy to be superior to subtotal thyroidectomy because it avoids the possibility of recurrent thyrotoxicosis. Although earlier reports suggested a higher incidence of injury to the nerves or parathyroids with total thyroidectomy, recent data document the safety of the procedure in experienced hands. Surgery may be chosen as the definitive therapy for patients who are pregnant or wish to become pregnant within a year of therapy, cannot comply with antithyroid medications or followup because of mental or emotional incapacity, are allergic to iodine, or refuse antithyroid drugs or radioiodine ablation. However, most clinicians favor radioiodine ablation over surgery.

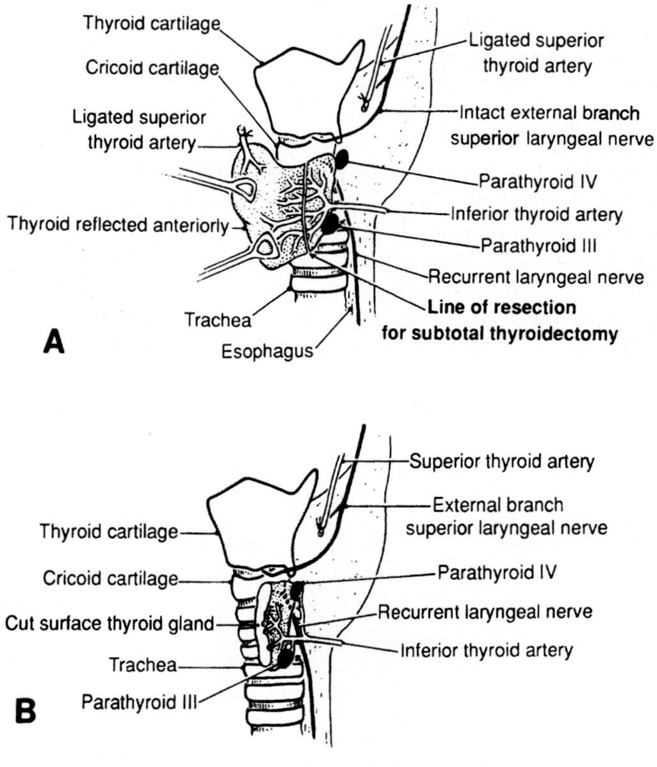

Figure 21-7 **A**, Anteromedial reflection of the thyroid gland. **B**, Anatomy after bilateral subtotal thyroid lobectomy for Graves' disease.

None of the antithyroid therapies significantly affect the exophthalmos or pretibial myxedema that is associated with Graves' disease. These manifestations may respond to local or systemic cortisol treatment, and external beam radiation therapy is occasionally used for severe ophthalmopathy. However, stabilization and regression of these signs and symptoms are reported most consistently after total thyroidectomy. This effect is thought to occur by lessening the generalized autoimmune response by removing all thyroid tissue.

Toxic Adenoma

Toxic adenoma is a solitary tumor of the thyroid gland that produces excessive amounts of thyroid hormone and causes clinically overt hyperthyroidism. Malignancy in a toxic nodule is rare. The hyperthyroidism is similar to that seen in Graves' disease. However, patients do not have associated ophthalmopathy or pretibial myxedema because toxic adenoma is not an autoimmune phenomenon such as Graves' disease.

Clinical Presentation and Evaluation

Serum thyroid hormone levels show high T_3 and T_4 and suppressed TSH, consistent with an autonomous thyroid source for the excessive thyroid hormone production. The differentiation between hyperthyroidism caused by Graves' disease and that caused by toxic adenoma depends on the characteristics of the thyroid on physical examination and scan. In patients with Graves' disease, the thyroid is diffusely enlarged. In patients with toxic adenoma, it is normal or small, with a palpable nodule that is "hot," or functional, on thyroid scan.

Treatment

The initial treatment is similar to that for Graves' disease, but definitive treatment depends more on surgery because resolution after treatment with PTU or methimazole is rare. After preoperative preparation, usually with propranolol or one of the thionamides, the lobe with the "hot" nodule is excised by thyroid lobectomy and isthmectomy (Fig. 21-6). Surgery is also considered optimal therapy for a toxic multinodular goiter (**Plummer's disease**). Total or subtotal thyroidectomy is indicated, especially if the goiter is large and associated with symptoms such as compression. In general, radioactive iodine ablation is not considered appropriate therapy for toxic adenoma or Plummer's disease. Although the overactive thyroid elements can be ablated, recurrence is more common than with Graves' disease because of the intrinsic autonomy of the thyroid tissue.

Thyroid Carcinoma

The annual incidence of **thyroid carcinoma** is 36 to 60 cases per 1 million people. The death rate is approximately nine per 1 million people. It is twice as common in women as in men, occurring primarily in those 25 to 65 years of age. Thyroid cancers can arise from any of the cells that make up the gland. Follicular cells give rise to well-differentiated thyroid cancers (papillary and follicular varieties). Parafollicular cells give rise to medullary carcinoma, and lymphoid cells give rise to lymphoma. Hürthle cell or oxyphil cell tumors are a variant of follicular neoplasms and arise from follicular cells. When analyzed by electron microscopy and immunohistochemistry, anaplastic tumors appear to arise from follicular cells, although they have dedifferentiated to the point that they are no longer recognizable as such by light microscopy.

General Principles of Treatment

Surgery is the therapy of choice for localized thyroid cancer, unless the tumor is an anaplastic carcinoma or a lymphoma (see below). The type of surgical resection used for more favorable forms of thyroid cancer, papillary or follicular lesions, is dictated by the extent of disease and the aggressiveness of the tumor (Table 21-1; see Figs. 21-6 and 21-8). The prognosis for papillary and follicular tumors is generally good, and the disease seldom shortens life expectancy. The survival benefit demonstrated by some studies and the ease of long-term followup when no thyroid tissue remains in the neck justify the risk of complications (e.g., recurrent laryngeal nerve injury, hypoparathyroidism) posed by total thyroidectomy. These risks are minimal if the surgeon is experienced.

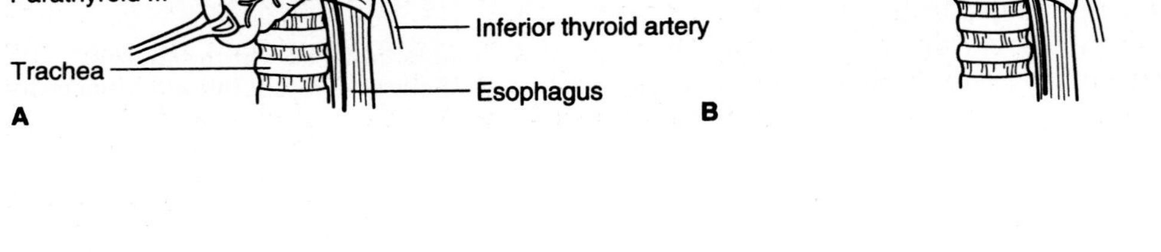

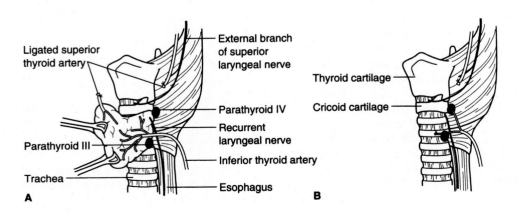

Figure 21-8 **A,** Anteromedial reflection of the thyroid gland. **B,** Anatomy after total thyroidectomy.

Papillary Carcinoma

Papillary carcinoma is the most common thyroid malignancy in the United States, occurring in approximately 70% to 80% of cases.

Clinical Presentation and Evaluation

Tumors with a mix of papillary and follicular features are classified with the papillary cancers because they have similar biologic behavior. Papillary carcinomas are characterized by concentric layers of calcium (psammoma bodies) found in the stalk formations that give this cancer its name. Because papillary cancers grow slowly, most patients with these tumors have an excellent prognosis. Poor prognosis is associated with male sex, age older than 50 years, a primary tumor larger than 4 cm, less–well-differentiated cells, and locally invasive or distant metastatic disease. Metastases are primarily to regional lymph nodes, although this finding is not associated with a significantly worse prognosis, particularly in young women.

Treatment

Lesions in patients with a good prognosis are treated by thyroid lobectomy and isthmectomy (see Fig. 21-6) or total thyroidectomy (see Fig. 21-8A, *B*). All patients with lesions that show evidence of a poor prognosis should undergo total thyroidectomy.

The extent of surgery, either lobectomy or total thyroidectomy, has been hotly debated in the endocrine literature. Several risk stratification systems assess *a*ge, *m*etastatic disease, *e*xtent of disease, and tumor *s*ize (AMES; Lahey Clinic) or *a*ge, histologic grade, *e*xtent of disease, and tumor *s*ize (AGES; Mayo Clinic) as prognostic factors. Other classifications of risk assess similar factors. Previously, patients who had lesions smaller than 3 cm were considered to have a good prognosis. Current data suggest, however, that optimal therapy should include total thyroidectomy and postoperative radioiodine ablation of residual or metastatic disease for any lesion larger than 1 cm. On the basis of these data, virtually all patients should undergo total thyroidectomy; stratification into risk groups is necessary only for prognostic calculations, not to dictate the choice of operation. Removal of obviously involved lymph nodes is generally advocated, but random sampling plays little role in planning therapy and has no place in the treatment of thyroid cancer. All of these patients will receive thyroid hormone replacement, but because thyroid cancer cells are to some degree TSH-dependent, TSH should be suppressed to midnormal or low levels by adjusting the hormone replacement dosage to avoid the potential trophic effect of this hormone on cancer cells.

Distant metastases are usually to the lungs and bones. Excision of all thyroid tissue in the neck facilitates scanning for metastases and treatment of those lesions with radioiodine if they are identified. Scanning and radioactive iodine therapy are not possible if thyroid tissue remains in the neck because the isotope is preferentially taken up by this tissue. Although thyroid cancers are often thought of as "cold," this designation is in reference to normal thyroid tissue. Well-differentiated thyroid cancer metastases often take up radioiodine and can be imaged in areas, such as lung, that do not. Pulmonary metastases more commonly take up iodine and may be cured with aggressive treatment with radioiodine, but bony metastases may need additional treatment with external beam radiation therapy. Although small trials of doxorubicin and cisplatin have been undertaken, there is no well-documented, effective chemotherapy for well-differentiated thyroid cancer.

Follicular Carcinoma

Follicular carcinoma occurs less commonly than papillary carcinoma, accounting for 10% to 20% of cases, except in iodine-deficient areas of the world.

Clinical Presentation and Evaluation

Follicular carcinomas have a monotonous, relatively uniform appearance of microfollicles, without the more complex papillations seen in papillary carcinoma. They closely resemble follicular adenomas on cytologic and frozen-section examination. On permanent section, they are distinguished from adenomas by the presence of capsular and vascular invasion. Follicular cancers also grow slowly, and the prognosis is good for patients with small, minimally invasive tumors. Larger or more invasive tumors have a poorer prognosis. Poor prognostic indicators include age greater than 45 years, local invasion to contiguous neck structures, and distant metastases.

Treatment

Papillary and follicular carcinomas are considered well-differentiated cancers. Treatment for both is similar (including operative options). Metastases are usually hematogenously disseminated to lung and bone. These lesions may concentrate iodine and be amenable to radioiodine therapy after the thyroid gland is removed.

Medullary Carcinoma

Medullary thyroid carcinoma (MTC) constitutes approximately 7% of all thyroid cancers. Of patients with this cell type, 20% have a genetically transmitted, autosomal dominant inheritance pattern associated with either familial medullary carcinoma or MEN type 2A or 2B (discussed later).

Clinical Presentation and Evaluation

In patients with familial medullary cancer or MEN-2, the tumor is always present in both thyroid lobes. The sporadic variant of MTC usually occurs unilaterally. Patients with MTC have a worse prognosis than patients with well-differentiated papillary or follicular carcinoma; only 50% of patients survive 10 years. Medullary cancer is demonstrated by plasma screening that shows elevated calcitonin levels or by screening with a calcium and pentagastrin infusion test that shows elevated calcitonin.

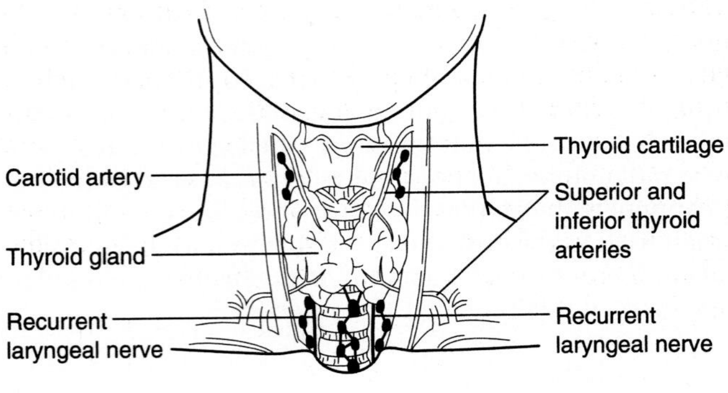

Figure 21-9 Removal of the cervical lymph nodes medial to both carotid arteries to treat medullary cancer, which requires a total thyroidectomy and central lymph node dissection.

Treatment

Medullary cancer without obvious lymph node metastases requires total thyroidectomy and central lymph node dissection (removal of the cervical lymph nodes medial to both recurrent laryngeal nerves and carotid arteries [Fig. 21-9]). Its tendency to have early lymph channel and bloodborne metastasis and its worse overall prognosis warrant an aggressive approach. Modified radical lymph node dissection is performed if there is lymph node involvement.

Anaplastic Carcinoma

Anaplastic carcinoma of the thyroid gland is an extremely aggressive neoplasm. It arises from the follicular cells, but is nearly totally dedifferentiated. Surgical resection does not appear to improve the outcome because it provides only palliative airway relief. The prognosis is dismal. Chemotherapy and external beam radiation therapy are equally ineffective. Patients are considered to have Stage IV disease at presentation, and few survive longer than 2 years.

Lymphoma

Lymphoma can present as a thyroid mass lesion and is treated similarly to lymphomas that present in other sites. To distinguish a lymphoma from florid **Hashimoto's thyroiditis**, a core-needle or open biopsy may be necessary.

■ PARATHYROID GLANDS

ANATOMY AND MORPHOLOGY

The **parathyroid glands** are yellow-brown, ovoid, soft, and mobile and have attached fatty tissue. Ninety percent of adults have four glands. Each gland normally weighs 30 to 50 mg and measures about 5 mm in its greatest dimension. As parathyroid glands pathologically enlarge, they become darker brown and firmer and are surrounded by less fat. The superior parathyroid glands develop from the fourth branchial pouches, while the inferior parathyroid glands and thymus gland develop from the third branchial pouches and migrate caudad together. Parathyroid blood supply is usually from multiple branches of the inferior thyroid arteries. Venous drainage is to the internal jugular, subclavian, and innominate veins. The superior glands are most commonly posterior and lateral to the recurrent laryngeal nerve and superior to the inferior thyroid artery, and they are often just beneath the thyroid capsule. The inferior glands are typically anterior and medial to the recurrent laryngeal nerve in the space between the inferior thyroid pole and the superior aspect of the cervical thymus. Inferior glands are often beneath either the thyroid capsule or the thymic capsule. Although the superior parathyroid glands are more consistent in their location, any of the parathyroid glands can be ectopically positioned along the path of their descent from the pharynx, within the thyroid gland, posterior in the neck, or even in the mediastinum (see Fig. 21-2).

PHYSIOLOGY AND PATHOPHYSIOLOGY

The parathyroid glands synthesize and secrete **parathyroid hormone** (PTH). This hormone, along with the interdependent factors of vitamin D, renal calcium excretion, bone turnover, and intestinal calcium absorption, regulates calcium homeostasis. Calcium is a vital cation that plays a key role in cardiac and neuromuscular conduction, catalyzes numerous cellular processes, and serves as an essential skeletal component. Magnesium and calcitonin are among the secondary factors in the maintenance of calcium homeostasis.

PTH is an 84-amino-acid peptide secreted only by the parathyroid glands. It is closely related to serum calcium levels through a very sensitive, rapid, inverse feedback loop. Hypocalcemia stimulates and hypercalcemia inhibits PTH secretion. Plasma PTH is rapidly cleaved into active N-terminal and inactive C-terminal fragments. The N-terminal fragment half-life is about 3 minutes compared to about 18 hours for the C-terminal fragment. The N-terminal portion is metabolized in the liver while C-terminal metabolites are excreted in the urine. PTH directly increases calcium resorption in the proximal convoluted renal tubule and increases phosphate clearance. PTH secretion is not influenced by serum phosphate levels. PTH directly mobilizes calcium from bone that is in equilibrium with the extracellular fluid (rapid phase) and by osteoclast activation and bone reabsorption (slow phase). PTH indirectly increases gastrointestinal absorption of calcium by stimulating vitamin D production.

Vitamin D is a fat-soluble vitamin that is formed when skin is exposed to sunlight (Fig. 21-10). Cholecalciferol (vitamin D_3) undergoes 25-hydroxylation in the liver, generating 25-OH-vitamin D_3, followed by hydroxylation in the kidney by 1α-hydroxylase to the most active form, 1,25-dihydroxy-vitamin D_3. Vitamin D directly enhances gas-

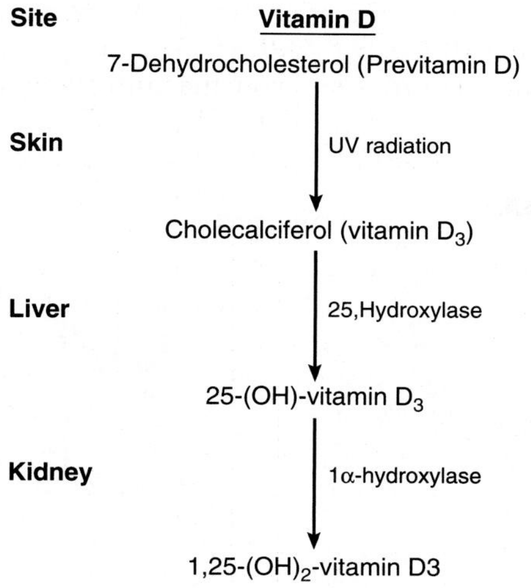

Figure 21-10 Vitamin D synthesis.

trointestinal (GI) tract calcium absorption. Low vitamin D levels increase PTH secretion and thereby increase 1α-hydroxylase activity.

Serum magnesium usually fluctuates with serum calcium in an inverse relationship with PTH. However, severe hypomagnesemia paradoxically inhibits PTH secretion. Calcitonin is produced in the parafollicular, or C, cells of the thyroid. High-dose calcitonin inhibits osteoclastic bone reabsorption. The precise physiologic role of calcitonin in maintaining calcium homeostasis is unknown. Elevated calcitonin levels (e.g., medullary thyroid carcinoma) or decreased levels (e.g., after total thyroidectomy) do not significantly affect serum calcium levels. Calcitonin is thought to be important at times of calcium stress such as puberty, pregnancy, or lactation.

Primary Hyperparathyroidism

In **primary hyperparathyroidism**, the tight inverse relationship between PTH and serum calcium is disturbed, and PTH is elevated with respect to the serum calcium, even though the serum calcium may remain within the normal range. Serum phosphate is often low and renal function is normal. Three distinct lesions can cause primary hyperparathyroidism: **parathyroid adenoma** (85%), **parathyroid hyperplasia** (15%), or parathyroid carcinoma (< 1%). PTH secretion is increased and the homeostatic set point for calcium is presumably reset at a higher value with all three. Excess PTH secretion leads to increased GI absorption of calcium, increased urinary calcium excretion, and bone loss. Adenoma, or uniglandular disease, refers to a single enlarged gland and is a benign process. The abnormal gland, though enlarged, is rarely palpable preoperatively. Typical adenomas measure 1 to 2 cm in size and weigh 500 to 1500 mg. With progressively earlier diagnosis of primary hyperparathyroidism, adenoma sizes and weights are decreasing. Hyperplasia, or multiglandular disease, is diagnosed when multiple glands are grossly abnormal. Hyperplasia is also a benign process that affects all glands, although gland enlargement may be asymmetric. Primary parathyroid hyperplasia most commonly is sporadic but may be inherited, either alone or as part of a multiple endocrine neoplasia syndrome. The distinction between adenoma and hyperplasia is becoming more blurred as newer operative strategies depend less on the gross appearances of the parathyroid glands.

Secondary and Tertiary Hyperparathyroidism

Secondary hyperparathyroidism most often occurs in patients with renal failure. Impaired glomerular filtration causes phosphate retention and decreased serum calcium levels. With fewer functioning nephrons, the amount of 1α-hydroxylase available to hydroxylate 25-OH-vitamin D decreases. Lower 1,25-dihydroxy-vitamin D levels lead to less GI absorption of calcium and further hypocalcemia. These changes stimulate excess PTH secretion by all parathyroid tissue in an attempt to restore calcium and phosphorus homeostasis. Continued nephron loss leads to chronic overstimulation of PTH secretion, elevated PTH levels, and parathyroid hyperplasia plus hyperphosphatemia (Fig. 21-11). The multiple abnormalities in calcium, phosphate, and vitamin D metabolism have extremely deleterious effects on bone mineralization and may lead to soft tissue calcium deposition with subsequent tissue destruction (e.g., tendon rupture, skin necrosis). Secondary hyperparathyroidism can also occur because of low vitamin D levels related to nutritional deficiencies or lack of sun exposure.

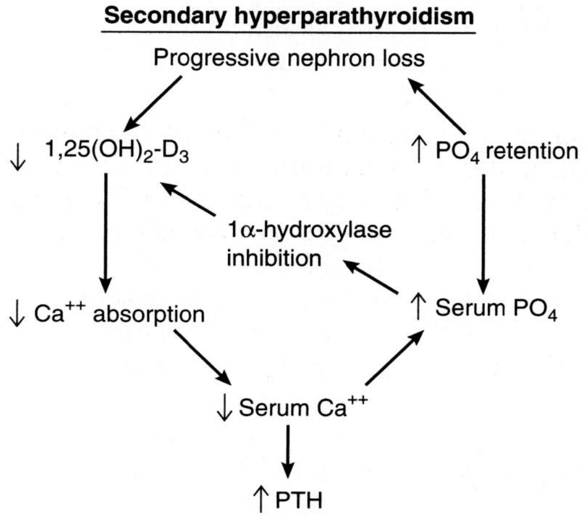

Figure 21-11 In secondary hyperparathyroidism, progressive nephron loss leads to phosphate retention, decreased calcium absorption, inhibition of 1α-hydroxylase, and decreased activation of vitamin D. These factors lead to decreased serum calcium and increased secretion of parathyroid hormone. PTH, parathyroid hormone.

In **tertiary hyperparathyroidism**, one or more of the chronically stimulated, hyperplastic glands of a patient with secondary hyperparathyroidism becomes an autonomous producer of PTH. Even with successful renal transplantation and correction of serum levels of phosphate and calcium, PTH levels remain elevated. Tertiary hyperparathyroidism behaves in most ways like primary hyperparathyroidism, although multiglandular disease is more common than in primary hyperparathyroidism.

Clinical Presentation and Evaluation

A patient with primary hyperparathyroidism classically presents with some or all of the complaints suggested in the mnemonic, "stones, bones, groans, moans, and psych overtones." Formerly the most common presentations involved urolithiasis (stones) or bone diseases including bone resorption with cyst (osteitis cystica) and brown tumor formation (bones). Less commonly seen were abdominal pain from peptic ulcers or pancreatitis (moans), diffuse joint and muscle pains, fatigue and lethargy (groans), and neuropsychiatric abnormalities including depression or worsening psychosis (psych overtones).

Currently, most patients are minimally, if at all, symptomatic and are found when unrelated laboratory testing reveals them to be hypercalcemic. Once repeat testing confirms hypercalcemia, the clinical challenge is to develop a differential diagnosis. A directed history may uncover the classic complaints, but more commonly discloses poorly defined constitutional or neuropsychiatric symptoms such as a decreased sense of well-being or behavioral changes. Medications, both prescription (e.g., diuretics) and nonprescription (e.g., calcium supplements), should be documented. Family history may suggest inherited hypercalcemia syndromes. History and physical examination should also seek evidence of occult malignancy.

The most common cause of outpatient hypercalcemia is primary hyperparathyroidism, and the most frequent source of inpatient hypercalcemia is malignancy, either via paraneoplastic syndrome or bony metastases. Further workup after excluding drug-induced hypercalcemia begins with simultaneous serum calcium and PTH levels. Modern PTH assays detect the whole PTH peptide by double antibody techniques and are known as "intact" assays (Fig. 21-12). Table 21-4 lists diseases associated with hypercalcemia arranged into those associated with or without elevated PTH. Elevated PTH occurs only with primary hyperparathyroidism, familial hypercalcemic hypocalciuria (FHH, also called familial benign hypercalcemia), or vitamin D deficiency. Urinary calcium and serum vitamin D levels can help differentiate among the causes of increased PTH. A calcium:creatinine clearance ratio of less than 0.05 indicates FHH, and the family history may be confirmatory.

Obtaining a serum parathyroid hormone–related peptide (PTHrP) level might be useful when occult malignancy is a concern (Table 21-4). PTHrP, encoded on chromosome 12 and expressed by almost all cells, may represent a primitive precursor to PTH, which is encoded on chromosome 11 and expressed only by parathyroid cells. The role of PTHrP in calcium metabolism is unknown. PTHrP may help maintain calcium homeostasis during pregnancy, since PTHrP, unlike PTH, crosses the placenta. All forms of PTHrP described thus far are longer peptides than PTH but have the same initial 34 N-terminal amino acids as PTH. PTHrP does not cross-react with intact PTH assays. Tumors of epithelial origin may secrete PTHrP and cause hypercalcemia as a paraneoplastic syndrome. The most common primary malignancy producing PTHrP is bronchial squamous cell carcinoma; others include breast, renal, and ovarian cancers. Bone destruction by primary cancers (e.g., multiple myeloma) or lytic bony metastases causes hypercalcemia without elevation of PTHrP. Vitamin D analogues are secreted by some tumors (e.g., lymphoma) and can produce hypercalcemia without PTH or PTHrP elevations. Increased activation of 25-OH-vitamin D by macrophages in granulomatous lesions (e.g., sarcoidosis) can lead to hypercalcemia without increased PTH or PTHrP. Lithium appears to interfere with the calcium-PTH feedback loop; a history of bipolar disorder or a therapeutic lithium level should point to this possibility.

Secondary hyperparathyroidism is present to some degree in most end-stage renal disease patients. Intact PTH levels are often elevated, calcium is usually normal, and phosphate and creatinine are increased. PTH fragments and their metabolites, especially C-terminal fragments, have prolonged half-lives and elevated levels in chronic renal failure, while vitamin D is often low. Typical manifestations of disease are bone pain, soft tissue calcifications, and pruritus.

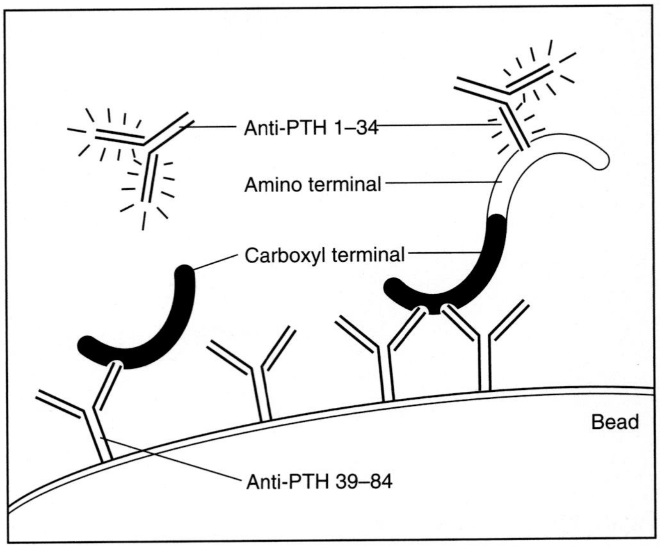

Figure 21-12 Intact parathyroid hormone (PTH) assay. An antibody recognizing PTH 39–84 binds carboxyl fragments in the midpoint and C-terminus of the molecule. A second antibody recognizes the amino terminal region of PTH (1–34).

Table 21-4 Differential Diagnosis of Hypercalcemia

Diagnosis	PTH	PTHrP
Primary hyperparathyroidism	High	Low
Tertiary hyperparathyroidism	High	Low
Familial hypercalcemic hypocalciuria	High, normal, or low	Low
Lithium therapy	High or normal	Low
Paraneoplastic syndrome (humoral hypercalcemia of malignancy)	Low	High
Osteolytic metastases	Low	Low
Multiple myeloma	Low	Low
Drug-induced hypercalcemia	Low	Low
Granulomatous disease	Low	Low
Hypervitaminosis D	Low	Low
Milk-alkali syndrome	Low	Low
Nonparathryoid endocrine disease	Low	Low
Immobilization	Low	Low
Idiopathic	Low	Low

PTH, parathyroid hormone; PTHrP, parathyroid hormone–related peptide.

Treatment

Medical

Acute, severe hypercalcemia is managed by large volume infusion of saline to restore intravascular volume and to initiate a saline diuresis, which in turn triggers calciuresis. Loop diuretics are used adjunctively. Drugs may be added to decrease bone turnover (e.g., bisphosphonates, calcitonin). Acute dialysis is rarely required. Treatment directed at any underlying malignancy or other precipitating condition is added where appropriate (e.g., steroids for sarcoidosis).

Currently, there is no definitive medical treatment for primary or tertiary hyperparathyroidism. Bisphosphonates (e.g., Fosamax) and selective estrogen receptor modulators (e.g., Evista) can help to slow and sometimes even prevent bone loss. However, these drugs are relatively ineffective in primary and tertiary hyperparathyroidism and are generally reserved for patients who are prohibitive operative risks. For end-stage renal disease patients, improved techniques of dialysis, better vitamin D supplements, and effective oral phosphate binders have markedly improved the medical control of secondary hyperparathyroidism and decreased the incidence of significant bony disease.

Surgical

For patients with overt symptoms or signs of primary hyperparathyroidism (e.g., urolithiasis), operation is clearly indicated. In the absence of major, life-limiting comorbidities, patients with metabolic derangements due to primary hyperparathyroidism (e.g., hypercalciuria, decreased bone density) are also best served by surgery. If operation is deferred, serial evaluations for progressive organ dysfunction are appropriate and require a cooperative, compliant patient. Operative indications for patients with no or minimal symptoms are somewhat less clear. Outcomes data are confounded by the difficulty in distinguishing between the constitutional symptoms of primary hyperparathyroidism and the aches and pains of daily life and aging. Newer, less invasive techniques of parathyroid exploration offer a simpler, low morbidity procedure with few risks, short convalescence, and reduced costs. When compared to the inconvenience and cost of observation with serial metabolic evaluations and the inherent risks of prolonged hyperparathyroidism, surgery is being recommended increasingly by endocrinologists and surgeons for even minimally symptomatic patients.

For end-stage renal disease patients, renal transplantation remains the most effective long-term treatment of both their renal disease and their secondary hyperparathyroidism. Parathyroidectomy is sometimes indicated for ongoing bone loss, soft tissue calcifications, or severe pruritus, particularly for patients who are not transplant candidates. Parathyroidectomy is occasionally indicated for patients on lithium who develop hypercalcemia and who cannot be managed with alternative medications such as Divalproex.

Operative Strategies

Classic exploration for sporadic primary hyperparathyroidism includes visualization of all cervical glands, characterization of the disease by the surgeon based upon gross morphology as uniglandular (adenoma) or multiglandular (hyperplasia), and resection of sufficient parathyroid tissue to restore long-term eucalcemia while preventing hypoparathyroidism.

Single-gland resection is performed for adenoma and

subtotal (three and one-half gland) resection for hyperplasia. Special considerations, such as total parathyroidectomy with forearm autotransplantation and cryopreservation of excised tissue, may apply in familial disease states (see multiple endocrine neoplasia). Classic bilateral exploration is most often performed under general anesthesia.

Two-directed, also known as "minimally invasive" or "targeted," operative strategies have been developed for sporadic primary hyperparathyroidism: intraoperative PTH (ioPTH) assay monitoring and radioguidance. Both approaches require that an abnormal parathyroid gland be identified preoperatively to guide the surgeon to the appropriate side of the neck. Such preoperative localization is usually done by sestamibi radionuclide scanning, and a nonlocalizing scan precludes radioguided operation. Other imaging modalities (e.g., cervical ultrasonography) may lateralize an abnormal parathyroid gland and support an ioPTH-based approach. Both of the directed operations can be performed under cervical block anesthesia combined with conscious sedation or under general anesthesia.

With the *radioguided strategy*, the patient is injected with sestamibi about 2 hours prior to the start of neck exploration. The incision is placed over the point of maximal radioactivity as detected by a handheld gamma probe. Dissection follows the radioactivity signal to expose abnormal parathyroid tissue, which is excised. Radioactivity should equalize throughout the neck after adenoma removal, and the adenoma should have a radioactivity count at least 20% above the neck background count. Failure to meet these radioactivity criteria mandates full neck exploration.

For the *ioPTH-directed strategy*, a peripheral blood-sampling device is inserted before neck exploration and a baseline sample drawn for ioPTH assay, which is an intact PTH assay modified to shorten the turnaround time to 20 minutes. It can be performed on portable equipment stationed adjacent to the operating room. A limited incision is made to expose the preoperatively localized abnormal parathyroid gland, which is then excised. Serial blood samples for ioPTH are drawn at 5-minute intervals after excision. A decrease of ioPTH level of greater than 50% from baseline and into the normal range at the 10-minute sample indicates resection of sufficient parathyroid tissue to restore long-term eucalcemia. Failure of the ioPTH level to drop appropriately leads to continued neck exploration.

Directed parathyroidectomy normally allows patients to be discharged either the same day or on the first postoperative day. Minimal analgesics are required and convalescence is typically brief. Patients are sometimes discharged on calcium supplements to be weaned as outpatients; this is primarily determined by surgeon preference and patient access to urgent health care.

Since secondary hyperparathyroidism is by definition a multiglandular hyperplasia, at least subtotal parathyroidectomy (three and one-half gland) should be performed. Total parathyroidectomy with forearm autotransplantation is preferred by some surgeons, although published results are similar for both procedures. More recently, some surgeons have chosen to omit forearm autotransplantation after total parathyroidectomy since patients may have residual rests of cervical parathyroid tissue that are sufficient to support calcium homeostasis. Cervical thymectomy is typically performed with operations for secondary hyperparathyroidism, since the inferior parathyroid glands and many parathyroid cell rests are adjacent to or within the cervical thymus.

Operations for tertiary hyperparathyroidism are guided by the intraoperative findings, most often multiglandular disease leading to either total parathyroidectomy with forearm autotransplant or subtotal parathyroidectomy. There is little experience with directed operative approaches to tertiary disease.

Minimally invasive, endoscopic approaches to parathyroid exploration are being investigated but currently offer little, if any, advantage over the available directed strategies.

Complications

The most serious complication of parathyroidectomy, recurrent laryngeal nerve injury, should be extremely rare. Persistent hypercalcemia because of failure to identify the adenoma or all hyperplastic glands occurs in 1% to 5% of patients in most large series. Transient, early postoperative hypoparathyroidism sometimes occurs because of suppression of the remaining normal parathyroid tissue by the hyperfunctioning gland(s). Patients with established bone disease appear to be at increased risk for early hypoparathyroidism. Persistent hypoparathyroidism should be rare ($<$ 1%). In addition to monitoring calcium postoperatively, phosphate levels should also be measured. Preoperative hypophosphatemia should be corrected by successful operation. In the "hungry bone" syndrome, phosphate is taken up by the bone with calcium and the phosphate will remain low. These patients will require larger doses of supplemental calcium until the condition resolves spontaneously.

Reoperative Surgery

In the event of persistent or recurrent hypercalcemia, the patient should be restudied to ensure that the diagnosis of hyperparathyroidism is secure. Radionuclide and anatomic imaging studies are performed. When conventional imaging is unrevealing, transfemoral selective venous sampling in the neck and mediastinum may be necessary to localize the source of the excess PTH. Ironically, most persistent hyperplastic tissue is found in the neck. Cervical reoperation carries substantially greater risk of recurrent nerve injury and permanent hypoparathyroidism than primary operation. Mediastinal abnormal parathyroid glands can sometimes be ablated by angioembolization or removed thoracoscopically.

■ ADRENAL GLANDS

ANATOMY

The adrenal (or suprarenal) glands are small (approximately 3 to 5 g each), yellow, triangular-shaped paired glands located behind the peritoneum of the posterior abdominal wall, closely associated with the upper poles of the kidneys (Fig. 21-13). The right adrenal gland lies posterior to the liver and posterior and lateral to the inferior vena cava. The left adrenal gland is lateral to the aorta and just behind the superior border of the pancreatic tail.

It is critical for the surgeon to be familiar with the vasculature of the adrenal glands. There are usually three small adrenal arteries delivering blood to each adrenal gland, simply named the superior, middle, and inferior adrenal arteries, and originating from the inferior phrenic arteries, aorta, and the renal arteries, respectively. The adrenal veins are remarkably consistent in their location and drainage, but differ by side. The right adrenal vein is 2 to 5 mm long, takes off from the anterior aspect of the adrenal gland, and drains into the posterolateral aspect of the vena cava. The left adrenal vein arises from the lower portion of the gland and travels inferiorly to drain into the left renal vein.

The adrenal gland can be divided into two primary areas based on embryologic development of the tissue types: the cortex, which is derived from the mesoderm, and the medulla, which arises from neural crest cells. The cortex has three layers, the outer zona glomerulosa, the middle zona fasciculata, and the inner zona reticularis. The medulla is the only endocrine organ whose activity is controlled entirely by nervous impulses. The innervation of the adrenal medulla is unusual in that there are no postganglionic cells. Preganglionic fibers from the sympathetic nervous system end directly on the medullary cells.

PHYSIOLOGY: ADRENAL CORTEX

Each zone of the adrenal cortex produces its own distinct hormones, which reflect the compartmental steroid synthetic pathways. All of these hormones are ultimately derived from cholesterol, which is converted to Δ-pregnenolone. The latter serves as the precursor for the glucocorticoids, mineralocorticoids, and androgenic steroids produced by the cortical cells (Table 21-5).

The *zona glomerulosa* produces and secretes mineralocorticoids, the most predominant of which is aldosterone. Aldosterone has a short half-life of only 15 minutes and is metabolized in the liver. Aldosterone secretion is primarily regulated by the rennin–angiotensin system in a negative feedback fashion, and is also influenced by plasma potassium concentration. In response to a decrease in renal blood flow, the juxtaglomerular cells within the kidney produce renin, which cleaves angiotensinogen into angiotensin I, which is then converted by angiotensin-converting enzyme (ACE) in the lung into angiotensin II. Angiotensin II directly stimulates aldosterone release from the zona glomerulosa cells, which, in turn, increase the exchange of sodium for potassium and hydrogen ions in the distal nephron. Thus, aldosterone increases sodium reabsorption in the kidney while promoting potassium wasting. It therefore has a significant effect on the body's electrolyte composition and fluid volume as well as blood pressure.

The *zona fasciculata*, regulated by circulating adrenocorticotropic hormone (ACTH) produced by the pituitary, secretes the glucocorticoid *cortisol*. Cortisol is involved in the intermediate metabolism of carbohydrates, proteins, and lipids. It increases the blood glucose levels by decreasing insulin uptake and stimulating hepatic gluconeogenesis. Cortisol also slows amino acid uptake and peripheral protein synthesis, and increases peripheral lipolysis.

Normal individuals produce 10 to 30 mg of cortisol

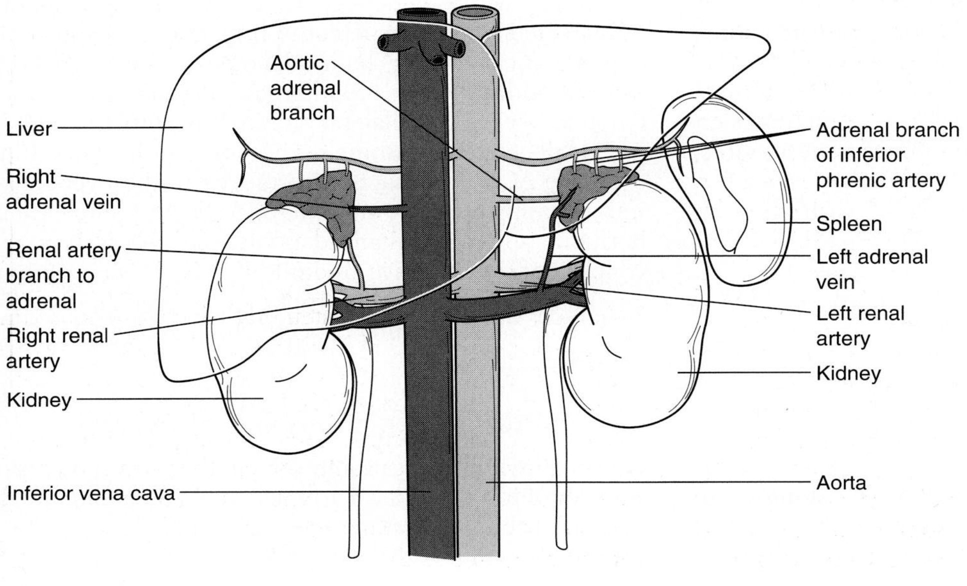

Figure 21-13 Anatomy of the adrenal glands showing their relations to adjacent structures and their blood supply.

Table 21-5 Correlation of Adrenal Zones With Disease Syndromes and Abnormal Adrenal Function

Adrenal Zone	Hormone Produced	Normal Function	Hypersecretory Syndrome	Symptoms	Pearls
Zona glomerulosa	Aldosterone	Electrolyte metabolism	Conn's syndrome	Hypokalemia	Insuppressible hyperaldosteronism and suppressed plasma renin
				Hypertension	
				Muscle weakness	
Zona fasciculata	Cortisone	Protein and carbohydrate metabolism	Cushing's syndrome or disease	Buffalo hump	Exclude exogenous intake of glucocorticoids
	Hydrocortisone			Violaceous striae	
				Moon facies	
				Truncal obesity	
				Hypertension	
Zona reticularis	Progesterone	Sexual differentiation	Adrenogenital syndrome	Virilism/feminization	Presents in early childhood
	Androgen			Hyponatremia	
	Estrogen			Hypertension	
Medulla	Epinephrine	Sympathetic response	Pheochromocytoma	Episodic hypertension	10% are: Malignant, Bilateral, Familial, Extrarenal
	Norepinephrine			Headache	
				Sweating	
				Palpitations	

daily in a diurnal rhythm. Cortisol has a half-life of approximately 90 minutes and is metabolized primarily by the liver. The natural byproducts of cortisol metabolism can be measured in the urine as *17-hydroxycorticosteroids*. Prolonged effects of high levels of cortisol include induction of a catabolic state, proximal muscle wasting, truncal obesity, insulin-resistant diabetes, impaired wound healing, and immunosuppression.

The cells of the *zona reticularis* respond to ACTH by converting pregnenolone to 17-hydroxypregnenolone, which is then converted to dehydroepiandrosterone (DHEA), the major sex steroid produced by the adrenal glands. DHEA is converted by local tissues into testosterone. Adrenal production of sex hormones is responsible, in part, for the development of male secondary sexual features. Abnormal production can cause virilization in women.

PATHOPHYSIOLOGY

Hyperadrenocorticism (Cushing's Syndrome and Cushing's Disease)

Cushing first described the syndrome now known to be associated with hypercortisolism in 1932. **Cushing's syndrome** refers to the many signs and symptoms associated with hypercortisolism, no matter what the cause. The most common cause of the syndrome is exogenous administration of corticosteroids. **Cushing's disease,** on the other hand, refers to a specific cause of Cushing's syndrome — an ACTH-producing pituitary adenoma, which produces bilateral adrenal cortical hyperplasia and is responsible for approximately 70% of cases of endogenous Cushing's syndrome.

Cushing's syndrome of adrenal origin can be classified as either ACTH independent or ACTH dependent. ACTH-independent hypercortisolism may be caused by adrenocortical tumors, both adenomas (10% to 25% of patients with Cushing's syndrome), adrenal cortical carcinomas (8%), or bilateral adrenal hyperplasia (1%). ACTH-dependent Cushing's syndrome can be caused by excessive ACTH production secondary to the hypothalamus releasing excessive amounts of corticotropin-releasing hormone (CRH); pituitary adenomas (Cushing's disease), which produce excessive amounts of ACTH; or extrapituitary ACTH-producing tumors (such as bronchial carcinoids and small-cell lung cancer, which are found in 5% to 10% of cases).

Clinical Presentation of Cushing's Syndrome

Cushing's syndrome is usually seen in the third and fourth decades of life and has a 4:1 female:male preponderance. The classic clinical features include central obesity (90%), hypertension (80%), diabetes (80%), weakness (80%), purple striae (70%), hirsutism (70%), and moon face (60%). A number of other symptoms can be seen, including depression, mental changes, osteoporosis, kidney stones, polyuria, fungal skin infections, poor wound healing, menstrual disturbances, and acne. In patients with Cushing's syndrome due to ectopic ACTH and pituitary tumors, melanotropins (melanocyte-stimulating hormones, or MSHs) are also secreted, leading to increased skin pigmentation.

Diagnosis of Cushing's Syndrome

In patients with suspected Cushing's syndrome, a complete history and physical examination looking for the previously mentioned symptoms is critical. The initial screening should involve the measurement of glucocorticoid hormones or their breakdown products. A 24-hour urinary excretion of free cortisol and 17-hydroxycorticosteroid reveals elevated levels. In addition, the plasma cortisol level is generally elevated. The diurnal variation in glucocorticoid secretion (high levels in the morning, declining during the day, with lowest levels in the evening) and the ability of the adrenal gland to increase cortisol secretion in response to ACTH stimulation are either lost or blunted. Mild hyperglycemia, glycosuria, hypokalemia, and elevated carbon dioxide content are inconsistent findings in Cushing's syndrome.

The overnight low-dose **dexamethasone suppression test** is used to confirm the presence of Cushing's syndrome and to discriminate between Cushing's syndrome and Cushing's disease. Humans produce about 30 mg of cortisol a day. One milligram of dexamethasone, given orally, will suppress ACTH secretion and decrease adrenal cortisol production. Normal subjects will have fasting cortisol levels less than 3 to 5 μg/dL (or will decrease their level by 50%) the morning after the dose is given. Patients with Cushing's syndrome will not be suppressed below 12 μg/dL, because this low dose of dexamethasone will not suppress cortisol production from autonomous adrenocortical tumors or adrenals that are being stimulated by nonpituitary sources of ACTH. If the plasma cortisol level is not suppressed by this dose of dexamethasone, the patient has Cushing's syndrome (Fig. 21-14). The next step is to determine the etiology of the autonomous hypersecretion.

Plasma ACTH measurement by immunometric assay is a direct method to determine hypersecretion. Very low levels of ACTH indicate hyperadrenocorticism due to primary adrenal causes such as adenoma, nodular hyperplasia, or carcinoma. Very high levels of ACTH are diagnostic for a pituitary adenoma or ectopic ACTH secretion. To distinguish between these two etiologies, a high-dose dexamethasone test is used. A dose of 8 mg of dexamethasone is given over 24 hours, and plasma cortisol levels are then determined. Patients with pituitary adenomas should have plasma cortisol levels that are lower by at least 50%. Patients with ectopic ACTH production will not be suppressed by even this high dose of dexamethasone and will continue to have very high levels of ACTH. Patients suspected of having pituitary adenomas should have a magnetic resonance imaging (MRI) study of the pituitary, and

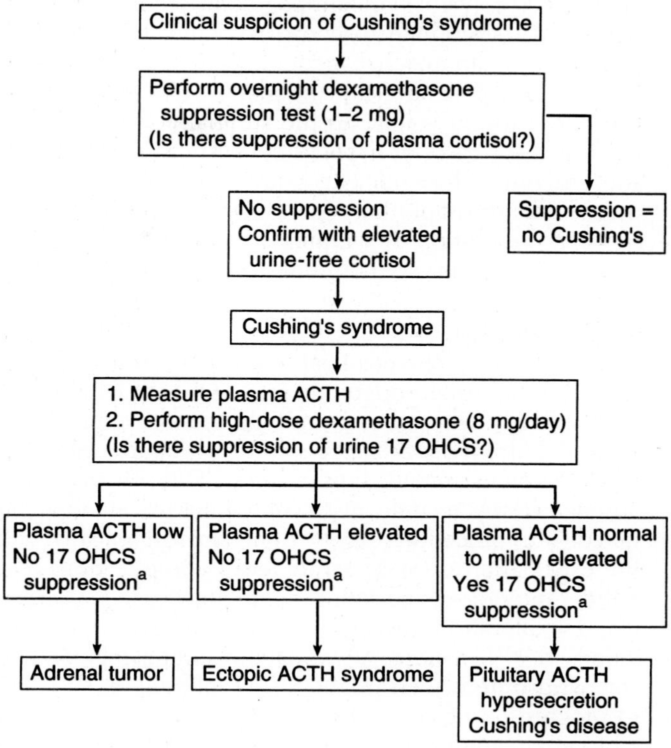

Figure 21-14 Algorithm for management of a patient whose symptoms suggest Cushing's syndrome. ACTH, adrenocorticotropic hormone. [a]Refers to whether dexamethasone suppresses 17-hydroxycorticosteroid levels in the urine.

if no tumor is located, inferior petrosal sinus sampling for ACTH should be considered. Patients suspected of having ectopic ACTH production should have a computed tomography (CT) scan of the chest, since bronchial carcinoids and lung cancers are the most common cause.

CT and MRI are helpful in identifying adrenal lesions. The initial radiologic study used to localize adrenal pathology in these patients should be an abdominal CT scan or MRI with thin cuts through areas of the adrenal glands. These high-resolution studies have a sensitivity rate of 95%. An autonomous adenoma usually appears as a unilateral mass 2 cm or larger, with a normal or atrophic contralateral gland. A unilateral mass larger than 4 to 6 cm is suspicious for a carcinoma. Bilateral adrenal enlargement suggests adrenal hyperplasia. Although not often indicated, adrenal photoscanning or scintigraphy with radiolabeled cholesterol (NP-59) is useful in localizing adrenal tumors and evaluating their functional status. Adenomas and hyperplasia will take up NP-59, while carcinomas rarely do. Angiography or other invasive testing is not often indicated.

Treatment: Cushing's Disease

Medical Therapy

Cushing's disease can be temporarily controlled with the use of agents that inhibit steroid biosynthesis such as metyrapone, ketoconazole, or aminoglutethemide. Nearly all patients will eventually develop a tolerance to these medications. This approach is generally reserved for patients who are very poor surgical candidates. A DDT derivative, **mitotane**, which is toxic to the adrenal cortex, has been used in some cases of hyperadrenocorticism with modest success, although its side effects are serious and quite common. Radiation of pituitary adenomas can also be effective; however, resolution of symptoms may take up to a year, and recurrence is very common.

Surgical Therapy

The treatment of choice in patients with Cushing's disease caused by a pituitary adenoma is transphenoidal microadenomectomy, which has an initial cure rate approaching 95%. Recurrent disease necessitating a second exploration produces a cure rate of approximately 50%. Bilateral total adrenalectomy is indicated when pituitary therapy has failed. This procedure may be done laparoscopically, with the expectation of significantly fewer complications than either anterior or posterior open approaches. Adrenal gland exploration reveals pathologic changes in these glands in 90% of cases. After bilateral adrenalectomy, **Nelson syndrome** is seen in about 20% of patients. It is due to progression of an ACTH-secreting pituitary adenoma. This enlargement can cause hyperpigmentation, headaches, exophthalmos, and visual field loss.

Primary Adrenal Cushing's Syndrome

Adrenal Adenoma

Solitary adenomas are the cause of primary adrenal hypercortisolism in 80% to 90% of patients. As a result of the hypersecretion of cortisol and inhibition of ACTH, the remaining adrenal tissue on the ipsilateral side and the contralateral adrenal tissue becomes significantly atrophic, functioning poorly until the adenoma or gland containing the adenoma is removed. The treatment of choice is therefore unilateral adrenalectomy, although some surgeons are now advocating removal of the diseased portion of the gland only (partial adrenalectomy). The procedure is best accomplished through a laparoscopic approach, which results in earlier discharge, less pain, and fewer wound infections than the open posterior approach. All of these patients should receive perioperative doses of steroids, and because the remaining adrenal tissue stays poorly functional for many months, patients should be maintained on maintenance doses of prednisone (5 mg q AM and 2.5 mg q PM) or hydrocortisone until normal adrenal function has returned as determined by normalization of results on the **ACTH stimulation test**. This may take as long as 12 to 18 months.

Primary Adrenal Hyperplasia

Primary adrenal hyperplasia of either the primary pigmented nodular (PPNAD) form or the macronodular (PPNAD) form may occur in a small percentage of patients. Treatment of these patients usually requires total bilateral adrenalectomy, which then necessitates lifelong steroid replacement therapy.

Primary Aldosteronism

Primary aldosteronism (Conn's syndrome) was first described by Jerome Conn in 1955. Patients with primary aldosteronism produce excess aldosterone from a solitary adenoma, diffuse hyperplasia, or nodular (adenomatous) hyperplasia of the adrenal cortex. Adrenal cortical carcinoma is the cause in less than 1% of cases. The syndrome is twice as common in women as in men, and most commonly occurs between the fourth and sixth decades of life. Although it is not a common cause of hypertension, it is becoming increasingly recognized, and now is estimated to be present in up to 20% of all patients presenting to a hypertension treatment center. The syndrome may account for as much as 50% of those patients with hypertension and concomitant hypokalemia.

Clinical Presentation

Excess aldosterone increases total body sodium, decreases potassium levels, and increases extracellular volume, which results in metabolic alkalosis and hypertension. Hypomagnesemia, tetany, and periodic paralysis may also be seen. The classic biochemical findings include persistently elevated plasma and urinary aldosterone levels and decreased plasma renin activity that cannot be stimulated to rise. Aldosterone is normally secreted in response to a reduced effective blood volume and renal blood flow, sodium depletion (or restriction), or potassium loading. It stimulates absorption of sodium at the distal convoluted and cortical collecting tubules. Sodium is reabsorbed at the expense of hydrogen and potassium ions.

Diagnosis

Primary hyperaldosteronism is defined as inappropriate hypersecretion of aldosterone in the absence of activation of the renin–angiotensin system. It is most commonly diagnosed by the presence of the triad of hypertension, hypokalemia, and high aldosterone levels concomitant with low plasma renin activity. Although most studies report that 80% to 90% of these individuals manifest hypokalemia, other investigations report that as many as half may not show evidence of significant hypokalemia unless given a sodium load. Of these patients, 55% to 60% have an adrenal adenoma, while 35% to 45% have bilateral hyperplasia. Rarely, an adrenal cortical adenoma can be a part of MEN type I syndrome or familial Conn's syndrome. Bilateral adenomas have also been described, as have nonfunctional adenomas (incidentalomas) in the presence of bilateral hyperplasia. The vast majority of adenomas are unilateral, are 1 to 2 cm in diameter, and have a classic chrome yellow color when sectioned.

Secondary hyperaldosteronism is a normal homeostatic

response to volume or salt depletion. It is associated with elevated plasma renin activity and elevated or high normal aldosterone levels. It can be seen in association with cirrhosis, nephrotic syndrome, and congestive heart failure.

The diagnostic goal when confronted by a patient with suspected Conn's syndrome should be to determine whether primary hyperaldosteronism is present. In those patients with confirmed hyperaldosteronism, the goal is then to differentiate between adrenal adenomas, which can be treated surgically, and bilateral hyperplasia, which should be treated pharmacologically. Initial screening of patients with hypertension and hypokalemia, sustained hypertension refractory to medication, or very severe hypertension or hypertension in young patients should include an upright plasma aldosterone concentration (PAC) and a plasma renin activity (PRA). A PAC of greater than 20 with a PAC:PRA ratio of greater than 30 is 90% sensitive for the presence of primary hyperaldosteronism.

A sodium-loading test is used to distinguish between primary and secondary hyperaldosteronism. In this test, 200 mEq/day of sodium is given for 3 to 4 days, and then plasma and 24-hour urine collections are measured for aldosterone, potassium, and plasma renin activity. If plasma and urinary aldosterone levels are increased and plasma renin activity is suppressed, primary hyperaldosteronism is confirmed. Because this test is very sensitive to the effects of extrinsic medications, antihypertensive sympathetic inhibitors (e.g., clonidine, alpha-methyldopa) should be discontinued for 1 week, diuretics for 4 weeks, and spironolactone for 6 weeks prior to the study.

One aid in distinguishing between the causes of primary hyperaldosteronism is the upright postural stimulation test. Aldosterone levels are measured after 4 hours of upright posture. In patients with an aldosteronoma, the rennin–angiotensin system is nearly completely suppressed, so that postural stimulation will not increase plasma aldosterone levels. Some patients may even have a decrease in their aldosterone levels after postural stimulation. Patients with bilateral adrenal hyperplasia (idiopathic aldosteronism) will have an increase in their plasma aldosterone after postural stimulation. This response is theoretically caused by increased sensitivity of diffusely hyperplastic adrenocortical tissue to small increases in angiotensin II that are induced by upright posture.

Further differentiation between adrenal adenoma and idiopathic hyperaldosteronism can be achieved with CT or MRI. These studies will identify adenomas as small as 0.5 cm in over 80% of patients. If CT scan reveals a unilateral adenoma in a patient under 40 years of age, this may be assumed to be the cause of the hyperaldosteronism. If the CT scan is not diagnostic, shows bilateral enlarged adrenals, or shows an adenoma in a patient greater than 40 years of age, it is now recommended by many that a selected venous sampling for aldosterone levels be performed. This test is the most precise method of localizing an adenoma. Aldosterone and cortisol levels are obtained from the adrenal veins and the lower inferior vena cava. Cortisol levels are obtained to normalize for dilution. Aldosterone:cortisol ratios that are four to five times higher on one side than the other are indicative of unilateral disease and indicate surgical treatment by adrenalectomy. Selective venous sampling is increasingly being used because of the occasional finding of nonfunctional adenomas (incidentaloma) in the presence of bilateral hyperplasia, especially as a patient's age increases.

Treatment

Patients with unilateral aldosteronomas should have their potassium levels normalized with potassium and spironolactone, if indicated, prior to surgical intervention. Laparoscopic unilateral adrenalectomy is then the treatment of choice. In 70% of patients whose adenomas are removed, blood pressure becomes normal. The remainder will require modest antihypertensive therapy. Patients with hyperaldosteronism that cannot be localized to one adrenal gland are managed with spironolactone and symptomatic treatment. In most of these patients, bilateral adrenal hyperplasia (diffuse disease) is the cause of the hyperaldosteronism, and bilateral adrenalectomy is not recommended.

Adrenal Cortical Carcinoma

Adrenal cortical carcinomas (ACCs) are rare tumors — the incidence is estimated to be one case per 1.7 million people. These tumors can occur at any age, but demonstrate a peak incidence in the fourth and fifth decades. They also show a slight left-sided and female preponderance. Bilateral tumors are seen in 5% of cases, and 50% to 70% of patients develop symptoms related to hypersecretion of hormones — primarily Cushing's syndrome.

Most ACCs are large (mean diameter of 12 cm), encapsulated, and friable and have extensive central necrosis and hemorrhage. It is often difficult to differentiate large benign adrenal neoplasms from malignant lesions purely on the basis of cellular characteristics. Venous or capsular invasion and distant metastases are the most reliable signs of malignancy. However, tumor necrosis, intratumoral hemorrhage, marked nuclear and cellular pleomorphism, and the presence of many mitotic figures per high-power field all strongly support the diagnosis of ACC.

Clinical Presentation

Over 50% of patients present with Cushing's syndrome, 15% present with virilizing, feminizing, and purely aldosterone-secreting carcinomas, and 10% have tumors that are found to secrete hormones only by biochemical studies. An abdominal mass is a common finding. Nearly half of patients will have metastatic disease (to lungs, liver, etc.) at the time of diagnosis. Symptoms from metastases — weight loss, weakness, fever, or bone pain — are also frequently seen. Children are more likely to have tumors that produce excess androgens. Women with virilizing tumors may exhibit hirsutism, temporal balding, increased muscle mass, and amenorrhea. Boys may present with precocious puberty. Men with virilizing tumors will typically present with gynecomastia, testicular atrophy, impotence, or decreased libido.

Diagnosis

CT scan is the imaging modality of choice for adrenal lesions. Features on abdominal CT that suggest that an adrenal mass is a carcinoma include irregular margins or borders, heterogeneity, evidence of central necrosis, stippled calcifications (15% to 30% of cases), regional adenopathy, invasion of adjacent structures, and the presence of metastases to the liver or other visceral structures. ACCs may be large enough to show anatomic distortions or abnormalities on a plain abdominal radiograph, an excretory urogram (intravenous pyelogram), or an adrenal ultrasound.

ACCs have a predilection for extension through the adrenal vein into either the renal vein (left-sided neoplasms) or the inferior vena cava (right-sided neoplasms). MRI can be helpful in delineating extension. Adrenal angiography and venography are rarely indicated in the workup of adrenal cortical carcinoma.

Treatment

The treatment of choice for adrenal carcinoma is surgical excision with removal of all visible tumors. Resection is possible in 80% of cases; however, survival after complete resection is only about 55% at 5 years. In presentations with early disease, adrenalectomy and excision of involved regional lymph nodes may be all that is necessary. If there is presence of local invasion or visceral metastases, ipsilateral nephrectomy and resection of contiguous structures or hepatic metastases is indicated. Postoperatively, corticosteroid replacement is usually necessary because of atrophy of the contralateral gland secondary to the suppression of ACTH secretion caused by hypersecretion of cortisol by the tumor.

Chemotherapy is indicated in patients who have metastatic or unresectable tumors. Mitotane (ortho-para-DDD) is the most common agent. Multiagent regimens that may include cisplatin, suramin (polysulfonated naphthylurea), VP-16, gossypol (spermatotoxin), 5-fluorouracil, and doxorubicin have also been used, with little or no improvement over ortho-para-DDD alone. ACC is relatively resistant to radiation therapy; however, the adrenal bed is generally treated with radiation postoperatively. The role of radiation remains controversial. Repeat resection for locally recurrent adrenal carcinoma may be beneficial.

The overall prognosis of ACC is poor. Median survival is 15 months. Five-year survival is between 42% and 62% after resection. As better imaging modalities allow these tumors to be diagnosed at earlier stages, this poor prognosis may improve.

Incidentally Discovered Adrenal Mass

With increasing use of CT scanning of the abdomen, MRI, and ultrasound, incidentally discovered adrenal masses (incidentalomas) are becoming more commonly reported. Adrenal tumors are usually diagnosed on the basis of clinical symptoms. The incidentally discovered mass is typically asymptomatic, however, and therefore presents a unique challenge for the managing physician. The prevalence of **adrenal incidentaloma** has been estimated to be 2.3% at autopsy and between 0.6% and 5% when upper abdominal CT scans are evaluated. Approximately 33% of incidentally discovered adrenal masses are benign cortical adenomas, 22% are metastases to the adrenal gland, 3% are adrenal cysts, 1.7% are adrenal cortical carcinomas, and between 1% and 5% are pheochromocytomas. The risk of malignancy over time for masses defined as benign has been estimated to be one per 1000, although up to 25% of these lesions may increase in size over time. The risk of carcinoma increases markedly in lesions greater than 6 cm, and the risk of lesions becoming hyperfunctional over time (estimated to be 1.7%) increases in lesions greater than 4 cm.

The diagnostic approach to the adrenal incidentaloma should be focused first on determining the functional status of the tumor, and second on determining if the lesion is or has significant risk of being malignant.

Diagnosis

The initial step in determining the potential seriousness of an adrenal incidentaloma is to establish whether it is hormonally active. This may prove to be difficult because basal hormonal measurements in most patients with incidentalomas are normal. The biochemical evaluation should therefore be directed by a careful history and physical examination, which should include an evaluation for symptoms or signs related to possible metastatic disease, and/or symptoms consistent with hormone-secreting tumors. A recent National Institutes of Health consensus conference held on the management of the "clinically inapparent adrenal mass" concluded that the evaluation of all patients should include a 1 mg dexamethasone suppression test and a measurement of plasma-free metanephrines. It was also their recommendation that patients with hypertension should have serum potassium, plasma aldosterone, and plasma renin activity measured to determine the aldosterone:plasma renin ratio. All functional tumors should undergo surgical excision.

The existence of "subclinical" Cushing's syndrome in patients with incidentaloma has been a subject of increasing concern. This entity is characterized as mild autonomous cortisol hyperproduction in the absence of any specific clinical signs of Cushing's syndrome, and has been found to be associated with decreased insulin sensitivity with abnormal glucose tolerance, and slight-to-moderate increases in blood pressure. Studies have also demonstrated that these patients have an increased cardiovascular risk profile as compared with normal individuals. Whether these patients should be treated by adrenalectomy is still debated.

The most common cancers involving the adrenal

glands are metastatic. Lung, breast, and colon cancers are the most common primary cancers to metastasize to the adrenals. This is probably the most common setting in which fine-needle aspiration biopsy (FNAB) is performed to evaluate a solid mass of the adrenal gland. Prior to FNAB, biochemical studies to rule out pheochromocytoma and aldosteronoma should be performed to prevent catecholamine crisis and death. Purely cystic adrenal lesions can also be evaluated by FNAB: If clear fluid is aspirated, the lesion is benign and the lesion can be followed.

Treatment

All hyperfunctional adrenal tumors should be removed regardless of size. If there is no evidence of adrenocortical or medullary hyperfunction, loss of diurnal rhythm, and suspicion for malignancy on CT scan or MRI, and if the adrenal mass is smaller than 3 to 4 cm, the patient can be followed with two or more abdominal CT scans at least 6 months apart and repeated endocrine followup for 4 years. If there is no evidence of enlargement of the adrenal mass or development of hyperfunction during that time, it is reasonable to follow the patient thereafter and to monitor for any changes. Adrenal masses larger than 6 cm should surgically be excised because of the high likelihood of malignancy. Although a laparoscopic approach is recommended for most patients with adrenal masses, those with large tumors (> 6 cm) may require open surgery to provide the optimal oncologic resection. Many surgeons have adopted the approach that all lesions greater than 4 cm should be treated surgically, although this approach is not universally accepted. Treatment of tumors between 3 and 6 cm remains controversial. It is in this group that more data will be needed to determine the best approach for treatment. Patients in this group with subclinical Cushing's syndrome may benefit from surgical treatment.

Tumors of the Adrenal Medulla: Pheochromocytoma

Pheochromocytomas have an incidence among hypertensive patients of 0.1% to 2%. They are found in 0.1% of autopsies and constitute about 5% of adrenal tumors found incidentally on CT scans. These tumors arise from chromaffin tissue and secrete excess catecholamines. Episodic hypertension is the hallmark in these patients as a result of vasoconstriction from alpha-adrenergic stimulation and increased cardiac output from beta-adrenergic stimulation. Of these tumors, 85% to 90% arise from the adrenal medulla, with the right being more commonly affected than the left. They may also arise from extra-adrenal sites (**paraganglionoma**) of chromaffin tissue in the peripheral autonomic nervous system. These sites may be anywhere from the base of the skull to the pelvis, but are most often found in a para-aortic position. Approximately 10% of these tumors are malignant, 10% are bilateral, 10% are found in children, 10% are familial, and 10% are extra-adrenal (rule of 10s).

Clinical Presentation

The classic triad of pheochromocytomas involves episodic hypertension associated with palpitations, headache, and sweating. These symptoms are a direct result of the effects of sustained or paroxysmal secretion of norepinephrine and/or epinephrine. Patients may also experience a sense of impending doom, significant anxiety, weight loss, and constipation. Physical signs of an attack may include pallor, flushing, and sweating. Most attacks are short-lived, lasting 15 minutes or less, and can be precipitated by trauma (including invasive medical procedures), physical activity, exertion, changes in position, alcohol intake, micturition, smoking, or labor in pregnant patients.

The hallmark manifestation of these tumors, hypertension, can occur in one of three patterns: episodic, sustained, or widely fluctuating superimposed on sustained hypertension. Of these patients, 50% have sustained hypertension, while some patients may exhibit only mild clinical symptoms, making the diagnosis difficult. Pheochromocytoma typically presents as a sporadic tumor, but may also be found as a part of the MEN type 2 syndrome. Pheochromocytomas are also associated with many familial disorders, including **von Recklinghausen's disease, von Hippel-Lindau disease**, and **Sturge-Weber syndrome**.

Diagnosis

Patients suspected of harboring a pheochromocytoma or functional paraganglionoma should be screened by measuring plasma-free metanephrine and normetanephrine levels. This test is highly sensitive and in many institutions has recently replaced the traditional screening method of measuring levels of catecholamines and their metabolites (metanephrine, normetanephrine, and vanillylmandelic [VMA]) in the urine, although urine screening may still be necessary in selected patients because of the incidence of false-positive results obtained in measuring plasma-free metanephrine and normetanephrine. Catecholamine levels do not correlate with tumor size. Multiple medications (i.e., tricyclic antidepressants, benzodiazepines, amphetamines, labetalol) interfere with these levels and should be discontinued prior to testing. The measurement of serum epinephrine and norepinephrine has a sensitivity of only 75%, but may lead to the diagnosis in rare cases in which transient rises in plasma catecholamines during paroxysmal attacks are the sole finding.

Of pheochromocytomas, 98% are located in the abdominal cavity. Other locations include the bladder and the organ of Zuckerkandl—an area of chromaffin tissue inferior to the take-off of the inferior mesenteric artery and anterior to the aorta. Most pheochromocytomas of the adrenal glands secrete both norepinephrine and epinephrine. To convert norepinephrine to epinephrine, phenylethanolamine-N-methyltransferase (PNMT) must be induced. Extraadrenal tumors do not have a high enough cortisol level around them to induce this enzyme, and thus usually only secrete norepinephrine. Plasma normetanephrine levels are elevated in 97% of patients with adrenal pheochromocytoma and in 100% of patients with extraadrenal pheochromocytomas. A plasma metanephrine/normetanephrine ratio of less than 0.2 is indicative of an extraadrenal tumor.

Localization

CT scan has been the first-line imaging study used for localization of a possible pheochromocytoma. MRI is equally as sensitive in identifying adrenal tumors, but has an advantage in that the T2 weighted image of a pheochromocytoma has a brightness three times that of liver, thus making the lesion "light up." Finally, ^{131}I-metaiodobenzylguanidine (MIBG) is selectively taken up by the chromaffin tissue in pheochromocytomas, and thus scintigraphy helps to localize these lesions. This test is primarily used to locate occult tumors or paraganglionomas.

Treatment

Once the diagnosis of pheochromocytoma is confirmed, surgical excision is the standard of care. However, it is critical that the patient be appropriately prepared for surgery. The first step is the administration of the alpha-adrenergic blocking agent phenoxybenzamine in a daily dose sufficient to control blood pressure. Dosing typically starts at a dose of 10 mg two to three times daily. The dose should be increased until the signs of excess catecholamine release have disappeared and the patient develops mild postural hypotension. In addition, adequate circulating blood volume should be maintained by having the patient drink plenty of fluids. Once the patient has achieved adequate alpha-blockade, patients who demonstrate tachycardia or arrhythmias may require treatment with a beta-blocker. It is critical to initiate beta-blockade therapy only after adequate alpha-blockade has been achieved. Patients with pheochromocytoma have severe peripheral vasoconstriction, increased systemic vascular resistance, and increased cardiac afterload. To maintain perfusion, patients compensate by increasing heart rate and stroke volume. Therefore, if a beta-blocker is initially given, the mechanisms by which the patient has compensated for the severe vasoconstriction are removed, and cardiovascular collapse may occur.

Surgical excision can be performed via an open approach through the midline or a transverse abdominal approach. Adrenalectomy can also be performed laparoscopically through either a flank, retroperitoneal, or transabdominal approach. The laparoscopic approach has been associated with a shorter hospital stay and a lower postoperative morbidity rate. Patients undergoing adrenalectomy for pheochromocytoma may become hypotensive after ligation of the adrenal vein or removal of the gland because of profound vasodilation (especially if the patient has not been adequately hydrated during the preoperative period). Intravenous fluids and pressor support may be needed during the initial postresection period.

Treatment Complications

The morbidity and complications associated with adrenalectomy are typically a consequence of the underlying adrenal pathology. For example, among patients who are undergoing adrenalectomy for Cushing's syndrome, the increased susceptibility to infection, deep venous thrombosis, poor wound healing, and mild glucose intolerance are primarily consequences of hypercortisolism.

Intraoperative complications include hypertension and hemorrhage secondary to inadvertent injury to the adrenal vein or vena cava, especially during right adrenalectomy. Hemorrhage can be avoided by using meticulous surgical technique. The surgeon should secure control of the venous drainage of the adrenal gland and divide the adrenal vein before manipulating any tumors. The risk of significant changes in blood pressure during adrenalectomy for pheochromocytoma is minimized with adequate preoperative preparation that includes volume replacement and adrenergic blockade. Intraoperative hypertension, usually associated with manipulation of the pheochromocytoma, is managed with nitroprusside.

Perhaps the most important postoperative complication of adrenalectomy is the onset of occult **adrenal insufficiency** or Addisonian crisis as a result of inadequate glucocorticoid replacement. Patients who undergo unilateral adrenalectomy for an adrenal cause of Cushing's syndrome are treated with hydrocortisone perioperatively, because the contralateral adrenal gland is assumed to be suppressed until proven otherwise. Patients who undergo bilateral adrenalectomy for Cushing's disease (adrenal hyperplasia) or bilateral pheochromocytomas require lifelong glucocorticoid replacement. Patients who undergo unilateral adrenalectomy for primary hyperaldosteronism, pheochromocytoma, or a nonfunctional adrenal tumor (e.g., adrenal cyst, myelolipoma) do not need cortisol replacement unless they were receiving steroid therapy prior to surgery.

Treatment of patients with corticosteroids is relatively common, and thus consideration must be given to treating these patients during the perioperative period. In these patients, ACTH secretion is inhibited and native adrenal cortisol release is likewise impaired, even after relatively short courses of steroid therapy. These patients cannot respond normally to the stress of surgery by increasing their secretion of cortisol and will have relative **adrenal insufficiency** in the perioperative period unless adequate replacement is given. Postural hypotension or dizziness, nausea, vomiting, abdominal pain, weakness, fatigability, hyperkalemia, and hyponatremia are common symptoms and signs of adrenal insufficiency. The patient may not have all of these findings, but the presence of any one of them in a patient in the correct clinical setting must raise the index of suspicion. When adrenal insufficiency is suspected in an unstable patient, it is appropriate to draw blood to measure cortisol and then immediately to give the patient parenteral steroids (100 to 200 mg hydrocortisone IV).

Care of patients after adrenalectomy who require long-term cortisol replacement should include careful followup to ensure the intact function of the patient's hypothalamic–pituitary–adrenal (HPA) axis before weaning them from steroids. The standard method is to establish that the patient has adequate adrenal reserve (i.e., demonstrate the ability of the remaining adrenal gland to respond appropriately to ACTH). This can be accomplished by using an ACTH stimulation test, which involves administering 250 mg of synthetic ACTH by IV bolus or IM injection after a baseline plasma cortisol level has been drawn. Plasma cortisol is then measured at 30 and 60 minutes. The test is performed before 9:00 AM. If the baseline cortisol level is 20 mg/dL or greater and increases more than 7 mg/dL, then the HPA axis is normal. If the cortisol level is less than 20 mg/dL and increases less than 7 mg/dL, then the HPA axis is abnormal. Until the HPA axis is normal, the patient requires some steroid replacement therapy.

■ MULTIPLE ENDOCRINE NEOPLASIA SYNDROMES

Familial endocrine tumor syndromes, inherited as autosomal dominant conditions, are divided into three types: **MEN-1, MEN-2A,** and **MEN-2B.** Another autosomal dominant condition, **familial medullary thyroid carcinoma (FMTC),** is also inherited, but it is associated only with **medullary thyroid carcinoma** and no other endocrine abnormalities.

MULTIPLE ENDOCRINE NEOPLASIA TYPE 1

MEN-1 is an inherited endocrine disorder that combines parathyroid hyperplasia with other endocrine neoplasms, usually pancreatic islet cell and anterior pituitary tumors. Many other endocrine and nonendocrine tumors occur, but less commonly. Carcinoid tumors and lipomas are the most frequent (Table 21-6).

Multiple Endocrine Neoplasia Type 1 Genetics and Screening

MEN-1 is an autosomal dominant disorder with a high degree of penetrance but variable expressivity (i.e., 50% of the offspring will have the syndrome, but each child may not express all component diseases). The causative gene in MEN-1 is a tumor suppressor gene located on the long arm of chromosome 11 that encodes the protein **menin**. Inactivating germline mutations can occur across a wide region of the gene. The heterogeneity of mutations complicates genetic screening for MEN-1. Specific mutations as detected by the MEN-1 germline mutation test have been localized for 80% of MEN-1 kindreds. More complex testing may allow carrier identification when the MEN-1 germline mutation test is negative. Genetic test results are useful for MEN-1 patient counseling but, unlike MEN-2, do not mandate therapeutic interventions. Periodic biochemical screening is required for MEN-1 carriers and for patients in whom DNA-based tests are not possible.

Biochemical screening should begin during the second or third decade of life. Concomitant history and physical examination should seek evidence for MEN-1 component diseases. Screening of MEN-1 carriers is performed annually. When DNA tests are not feasible or informative, individuals at 50% risk (i.e., first-degree relatives of known MEN-1 patients) should be screened every 3 years. Screening includes tests for the common lesions of MEN-1 (calcium, prolactin, fasting glucose and insulin, gastrin). Other tests are added based upon individual patient evaluation and family history. Patients from MEN-1 kindreds with known mutations who have negative genetic testing do not require further genetic or biochemical screening.

Calcium and PTH levels should be measured in all patients newly presenting with islet cell tumors, since the absence of hyperparathyroidism virtually excludes MEN-1.

Multiple Endocrine Neoplasia Type 1 Parathyroid Disease

Primary hyperparathyroidism is the most common endocrine disorder in MEN-1, occurring in over 90% of cases, but represents only about 3% of all cases of primary hyperparathyroidism. The mean age of onset is 25 years, much

Table 21-6 Multiple Endocrine Neoplasia Type I: Gland Involvement

Glands and Sites Involved	Type of Disease	Estimated Penetrance by Age 40 (%)
Parathyroid	Hyperplasia	90
Pancreas	Islet cell tumors	70
Pituitary	Adenoma	35
Adrenal	Adenoma or carcinoma	25
Enterochromaffin system	Carcinoid tumor	15
Soft tissue	Lipoma	30
	Facial angiofibroma	85
	Collagenoma	70

younger than for sporadic primary hyperparathyroidism. The clinical manifestations are similar for MEN-1 and for sporadic disease, including asymptomatic hypercalcemia, constitutional and neuropsychiatric complaints (weakness, fatigue, irritability, depression), urinary tract findings (urolithiasis, hypercalciuria), abdominal pain (peptic ulcer disease, pancreatitis), and bone disease (decreased bone density, bone pain, fractures). As for sporadic disease, MEN-1 hyperparathyroidism is diagnosed by serum calcium and PTH levels. Assessment of metabolic disease (e.g., hypercalciuria, osteoporosis) may guide therapeutic recommendations for minimally symptomatic patients.

Hyperparathyroidism in MEN-1 affects all parathyroid glands, although the hyperplasia may be asymmetric. The neoplastic genetic stimulus is not eliminated by parathyroidectomy, so recurrence rates are much higher for MEN-1 hyperparathyroidism (> 50% at 10 years) than for sporadic disease (< 5%). Because recurrence is common, the timing of operation is controversial, especially for patients with few symptoms and limited metabolic disease. MEN-1 patients with hypercalcemia and hypergastrinemia should undergo parathyroidectomy first for optimal control of gastrin secretion.

Since MEN-1 hyperparathyroidism is inevitably multiglandular, a bilateral neck exploration is performed; preoperative localizing studies (e.g., sestamibi radionuclide scan) are unnecessary before initial operation. Either total (four gland) parathyroidectomy with forearm autotransplant or subtotal (three and one-half gland) parathyroidectomy is appropriate. The cervical thymus should always be removed because supernumerary glands can occur and are usually within the thymus. Parathyroid tissue can be cryopreserved for forearm reimplantation in the rare patient who is permanently hypoparathyroid postoperatively.

Multiple Endocrine Neoplasia Type 1 Islet Cell Disease

Neuroendocrine tumors of the small bowel and pancreas (islet cell tumors) are found at autopsy in 80% of MEN-1 patients, but are less often diagnosed during life. Tumors are considered functional when they secrete ectopic hormones and generate a clinical syndrome. Functional islet tumors most often secrete gastrin or insulin, and less commonly glucagon, vasoactive intestinal peptide (VIP), somatostatin, and growth hormone–releasing factor (GRF). The most common islet cell neoplasm in MEN-1 secretes pancreatic polypeptide (PP) and is nonfunctional, while gastrinoma is the most frequent functional tumor. Islet cell tumors may be malignant, and there is a direct correlation between tumor size and the rate of metastases. The clinical presentations of MEN-1 patients with islet cell tumors are similar to those of patients with islet neoplasms but without MEN. Symptoms of hormonal excess do not often appear before age 40 and malignant lesions are very rare before age 30.

Clinical Presentation and Evaluation

Gastrinomas are present in 40% of MEN-1 patients, and 25% of gastrinoma patients have MEN-1. Gastrinomas cause the Zollinger-Ellison syndrome in which hypergastrinemia leads to hypersecretion of gastric acid manifested by severe peptic ulcer disease, secretory diarrhea, and esophagitis. Fasting serum gastrin levels greater than 100 pg/mL and basal acid output greater than 15 mEq/hr while a patient is off all antisecretory medications are diagnostic of Zollinger-Ellison syndrome. The secretin stimulation test may be helpful in equivocal cases. Gastrin level increases of greater than 200 pg/mL after intravenous secretin injection occur only with Zollinger-Ellison syndrome (see Chapter 14, Stomach and Duodenum, for further discussion of Zollinger-Ellison syndrome).

Patients with insulinoma have neuroglycopenic symptoms when fasting, ranging from drowsiness to seizures and coma. Many patients gain weight, as they try to minimize symptoms by eating frequently. Insulinoma is diagnosed by a supervised fast. The triad of neuroglycopenic symptoms, serum glucose less than 45 mg/dL, and serum insulin greater than 5 μU/mL occurring within 72 hours is diagnostic of insulinoma. Blood C-peptide and proinsulin levels are elevated with insulinoma and are combined with urinary sulfonylurea testing to exclude factitious hypoglycemia.

Tumors other than gastrinoma and insulinoma occur more rarely. Glucagonoma is associated with hyperglycemia, cachexia, and anemia plus necrolytic migratory erythema, a red, scaling, pruritic, migratory rash. Elevated plasma glucagon levels are diagnostic. VIPoma patients have profuse watery diarrhea, severe hypokalemia, and hypochlorhydria. The diagnosis is excluded by stool volume less than 700 mL/day and is confirmed by elevated plasma VIP levels. Somatostatinoma is manifested by cholelithiasis, hyperglycemia, weight loss, and steatorrhea plus elevated blood somatostatin levels. Tumors secreting predominantly GRF present as acromegaly, but less than 5% of acromegaly cases are caused by GRFomas. Plasma GRF levels are elevated. Nonfunctional islet cell tumors may produce PP, which does not cause a clinical syndrome. Blood PP levels are also elevated with many functional islet tumors.

Once the biochemical diagnosis of an islet cell tumor is secure, the tumor must be localized. Tumors that produce insulin, glucagon, VIP, and somatostatin are generally found within the pancreas. The proximal pancreas and the duodenal wall are the most common sites for gastrinomas. There is no ideal localizing test. CT scan and endoscopic ultrasound are the most helpful preoperative studies. Other options include MRI, octreotide radionuclide scan, and angiography. Octreotide uptake depends upon the tumor density of type 2 somatostatin receptors. Tumors may be detected directly during arteriography as a vascular blush. Tumors may also be indirectly localized to a region of the pancreas by provocative angiography during which secretin (for gastrinoma) or calcium (for insulinoma or gastrinoma) is injected selectively into regional arteries while hepatic venous hormone output is measured. Regional localization can also be done using portal venous branch sampling, but this test is seldom done due to the morbidity of transhepatic portal system catheterization. Some patients with clear biochemical evidence of an islet cell neoplasm still have no tumor identified preoperatively. Endoscopy with duodenal transillumination and pancreatic ultrasonography may aid tumor identification intraoperatively.

Treatment

Therapeutic goals for patients with MEN-1 or sporadic islet cell tumors include controlling symptoms of hormonal excess and extirpating malignancy. Excess hormone secretion and its effects are fairly well controlled by medications, except for insulinoma. Multiple islet tumors are common with MEN-1 and may be synchronous, metachronous, or both. Most insulinomas are benign, but the majority of gastrinomas are malignant. At least 60% of the remaining islet neoplasms are malignant, except for GRFoma, of which 30% are cancers. Initial staging discloses liver metastases in at least half of patients with malignant islet tumors except insulinomas, which present with hepatic metastases in less than 5% of cases. Both primary and metastatic islet cell cancers grow more slowly than most other gastrointestinal malignancies.

Surgery is appropriate for virtually all insulinomas, since most are benign and since medications poorly control life-threatening symptoms. Surgery is indicated to resect most other islet tumors without known metastases. Primary surgery is usually indicated for sporadic gastrinomas, but is more controversial in MEN-1. MEN-1 gastrinomas are usually multiple, malignant, and often located where resection requires pancreaticoduodenectomy. Long-term eugastrinemia is uncommon postoperatively. Proton pump inhibitors effectively control gastric acid secretion. Surgery for hyperparathyroidism facilitates the management of Zollinger-Ellison syndrome, and parathyroidectomy should precede operation for gastrinoma in hypercalcemic patients. Resection of limited hepatic metastases from any islet tumor may be curative, and hepatic transplantation is occasionally performed. Debulking of primary or metastatic lesions may palliate disabling symptoms of hormonal excess.

Multiple Endocrine Neoplasia Type 1 Pituitary Disease

Clinical Presentation and Evaluation

Nearly all pituitary tumors in MEN-1 patients secrete prolactin, producing irregular menses, galactorrhea, infertility, and impotence. Rarely, pituitary tumors secrete other hormones, including ACTH, growth hormone, and TSH. These tumors are associated with Cushing's disease, acromegaly, and hyperthyroidism, respectively. The diagnosis of each hormonal syndrome is based on recognizing clinical signs and symptoms and obtaining elevated hormone levels. MRI or CT scan of the sella and visual field examination are obtained. About two-thirds of tumors are microadenomas (< 1 cm). Bitemporal hemianopsia can occur when large tumors compress the optic chiasm.

Hypercortisolism in MEN-1 patients has multiple potential origins, including pituitary adenoma, ectopic ACTH from carcinoid or islet cell tumor, or adrenal cortical tumor. Treatment depends upon determining the precise cause and may require multiple, complex diagnostic studies such as dexamethasone suppression testing and petrosal sinus sampling. Biochemical assessment is combined with imaging of the pituitary, adrenals, and, if ectopic ACTH is suspected, the chest and pancreas.

Treatment

Prolactinomas can usually be controlled with bromocriptine. Refractory or large tumors may require resection via the transphenoidal route or craniotomy. Occasionally, external beam radiotherapy is chosen as the primary treatment. Patients with hypercortisolism should have the primary tumor resected. Drug therapy or bilateral adrenalectomy may be indicated in rare cases.

Multiple Endocrine Neoplasia Type 1 Secondary Tumors

Less common tumors associated with MEN-1 include carcinoids, lipomas, thyroid or adrenal adenomas, and, rarely, adrenal cortical carcinoma (see Table 21-6). Carcinoid tumors are malignant and should be resected. Thyroid and adrenal adenomas require no treatment unless hyperfunctional. Adrenal cancers and symptomatic lipomas are excised.

MULTIPLE ENDOCRINE NEOPLASIA TYPE 2A, TYPE 2B, AND FAMILIAL MEDULLARY THYROID CARCINOMA

The MEN-2A, MEN-2B, and FMTC syndromes are inherited endocrine disorders, all of which include medullary thyroid cancer (MTC) as the primary component (Table 21-7). In MEN-2A, MTC occurs with adrenal pheochromocytoma and primary hyperparathyroidism. Both pheochromocytoma and MTC are present in MEN-2B, but hyperparathyroidism is absent and is replaced by a characteristic phenotype. MEN-2A patients outnumber MEN-2B patients by 3:1. FMTC patients have MTC as their only inherited endocrine disorder. MTC arises from the parafollicular or C cells of the thyroid. Hereditary MTC is multifocal, bilateral, and associated with C-cell hyperplasia. C cells secrete calcitonin. Basal and stimulated calcitonin levels are obtained preoperatively and followed sequentially postoperatively by a tumor marker. Lymphatic and distant metastatic patterns are similar for hereditary and sporadic MTC.

Table 21-7 Multiple Endocrine Neoplasia Type 2A, Multiple Endocrine Neoplasia Type 2B, and Familial Medullary Thyroid Carcinoma: Genetic Abnormalities and Associated Diseases

Endocrine Syndrome	Chromosome	Gene	Clinical Expression	Percentage Who Have Trait
MEN-2A	10	RET	MTC	100
			Pheochromocytoma	50
			Parathyroid hyperplasia	25
MEN-2B	10	RET	MTC	100
			Phenotype	100
			Pheochromocytoma	50
FMTC	10	RET	MTC	100

FMTC, familial medullary thyroid carcinoma; MEN, multiple endocrine neoplasia; MTC, medullary thyroid carcinoma; RET, a transmembrane protein kinase receptor.

Multiple Endocrine Neoplasia Type 2/ Familial Medullary Thyroid Carcinoma Genetics and Screening

MEN-2A, MEN-2B, and FMTC are autosomal dominant disorders, and MTC is expressed during life in virtually all gene carriers. About 20% of all MTC is hereditary. The responsible gene is located in the pericentromeric region of chromosome 10 and is known as the **RET proto-oncogene**. RET mutations enhance cellular growth. MEN-2/FMTC mutations affect a limited number of codons, so that genetic testing is simpler and more reliable than for MEN-1. Genetic screening has largely replaced calcitonin screening. RET DNA analysis utilizes lymphocytes extracted from a peripheral blood sample, may be performed soon after birth, and is performed once in a lifetime. Patients at risk but with negative RET testing do not require further screening. Positive RET results lead to thyroidectomy and further evaluation. At least 10% of apparently "sporadic" cases of MTC and of pheochromocytoma will prove to be due to MEN-2/FMTC. RET testing should be done on all "sporadic" MTC and pheochromocytoma patients.

Multiple Endocrine Neoplasia Type 2A

MEN-2A deaths are due to MTC. Reliable genetic screening now allows early identification of MEN-2A within known kindreds. RET-positive patients should undergo total thyroidectomy before age 6 to prevent MTC. Even in patients this young, C-cell hyperplasia or early MTC is often present. When the diagnosis or operation is delayed, cervical lymphadenectomy may also be appropriate. Patients with palpable tumors have very high recurrence rates and often die of disease, despite total thyroidectomy and extensive lymph node dissections. Distant metastases are to lung, liver, and bone. Survival rates after thyroidectomy in MEN-2A currently are intermediate between FMTC and MEN-2B, but could approach 100% using genetic screening. Management of persistent or recurrent postoperative hypercalcitonemia is controversial.

Nearly 50% of MEN-2A patients will develop pheochromocytomas. The tumors are almost always in the adrenal glands and are very rarely malignant. Symptoms, if present, are similar to those for sporadic pheochromocytoma. The biochemical diagnosis is made by measuring plasma or urinary catecholamines. Tumors detected only by screening often produce lesser amounts of catecholamines. Tumor localization is primarily by CT scan. MIBG radionuclide scan or MRI is sometimes helpful. Bilateral adrenalectomy is performed when bilateral adrenal imaging abnormalities are present. When the disease appears unilateral, treatment is controversial, ranging from unilateral adrenalectomy with close followup to bilateral resection. The 50% risk of contralateral tumor development must be balanced against the lifelong risk of Addisonian crisis. Laparoscopic adrenalectomy is often feasible for these less hormonally active, small tumors. Screening for pheochromocytoma should precede all operations for MTC, and, when screening is positive, adrenalectomy should precede thyroidectomy.

Nearly 25% of MEN-2A patients will develop primary hyperparathyroidism, though less severe than that in MEN-1 patients and at a later age. The disease always affects all four glands, although hyperplasia may be asymmetric. Symptoms are similar to those in patients with sporadic disease. Diagnosis is made using blood calcium and PTH levels. Either total parathyroidectomy (four glands) with forearm autotransplantation or subtotal resection (three and one-half glands) is appropriate. Resected parathyroid tissue can be cryopreserved for later reimplantation if permanent hypoparathyroidism develops. If abnormal parathyroid glands are encountered during thyroidectomy for MTC, at least subtotal parathyroidectomy is appropriate, even for normocalcemic patients. Screening for pheochromocytoma should precede parathyroid operations, and, when screening is positive, adrenalectomy should precede parathyroidectomy.

MEN-2A is sometimes associated with Hirschsprung's disease and with cutaneous lichen amyloidosis.

Multiple Endocrine Neoplasia Type 2B

Patients with MEN-2B have a characteristic phenotype with features evident soon after birth. They include marfanoid habitus, prognathism, puffy lips, bumpy tongue, and hyperflexible joints. Corneal nerve hypertrophy is seen on slit lamp examination. RET testing is confirmatory. Among the MEN/FMTC syndromes, MTC is most aggressive in MEN-2B, with distant metastases reported as early as the first year of life. RET-positive patients should undergo thyroidectomy and central neck lymphadenectomy before age 6 months.

The presentation, diagnosis, and management of pheochromocytoma in MEN-2B patients are identical to those of MEN-2A. Hyperparathyroidism is absent in MEN-2B. Ganglioneuromas occur at multiple sites in MEN-2B patients, and in the colon can lead to severe constipation and megacolon.

Familial Medullary Thyroid Carcinoma

MTC is least virulent in FMTC, and patient survival exceeds that for MEN-2A, MEN-2B, and sporadic MTC. The age of onset of MTC is later in FMTC kindreds than in MEN-2A or MEN-2B kindreds. In small kindreds, distinguishing MEN-2A from FMTC may be difficult, since MTC is the first manifestation of both syndromes. FMTC patients should therefore undergo thyroidectomy in early childhood, similar to MEN-2A patients. Definitive diagnosis of FMTC is made using RET testing plus rigorous kindred criteria that includes longitudinal observation of multiple kindred members. Equivocal cases should be classified as MEN-2A so that potentially curative thyroidectomy is not delayed and so that pheochromocytoma is not missed. By definition, FMTC has no other associated familial endocrinopathies.

SUGGESTED READINGS

Thyroid Gland
Thyroid Nodule

Hegedus, L. The thyroid nodule. *N Engl J Med* 2004;351:1764.

Hermus, RA, Huysman DA. Drug therapy: treatment of benign nodular thyroid disease. *N Engl J Med* 1998;338:1438.

Hyperthyroidism

Ginsberg, J. Diagnosis and management of Graves' disease. *Can Med Assoc J* 2003;168:575.

Soh Y, Duh QY. Diagnosis and management of hot nodules (Plummer's disease). *Probl Gen Surg* 1997;14:165.

Winsa B, Rastad J, Larrson E, et al. Total thyroidectomy in therapy-resistant Graves' disease. *Surgery* 1994;116:1068.

Thyroid Carcinoma

Hay ID, Grant CS, et al. Unilateral total lobectomy: is it sufficient surgical treatment for patients with AMES low risk papillary thyroid carcinoma? *Surgery* 1998;124:958–4966.

Mazzaferri EL, Kloos RT. Current approaches to primary therapy for papillary and follicular thyroid cancer. *J Clin Endocrinol Metab* 2001;86:1447.

Mazzaferri EL, Sissy JM. Long-term impact of initial surgical and medical therapy on papillary and follicular cancer. *Am J Med* 1994;97:418.

Schlumberger MJ. Papillary and follicular thyroid carcinoma. *N Engl J Med* 1998;338;297.

Singer P, Cooper DS, Daniels GH, et al. Treatment guidelines for patients with thyroid nodules and well differentiated thyroid cancer. *Arch Intern Med* 1996;156:2165.

Parathyroid Glands

Bilizekian JP, Silverberg SJ. Asymptomatic primary hyperparathyroidism. *N Engl J Med* 2004;350:1746.

Chan FKW, Koberle LMC, Thys-Jacobs S, et al. Differential diagnosis, causes, and management of hypercalcemia. *Curr Probl Surg* 1997;34:445.

Clark OH. Editorial: how should patients with primary hyperparathyroidism be treated? *J Clin Endocrinol Metab* 2003;88:3011.

Eigelberger MS, Clark OH. Surgical approach to primary hyperparathyroidism. *Endocrinol Metab Clin North Am* 2000;29:479.

Adrenal Glands

Endocrinol Metab Clin North Am. 2000;29. Entire issue devoted to incidentalomas.

Findling JW, Doppman JL. Biochemical and radiologic diagnosis of Cushing's syndrome. *Endocrinol Metab Clin North Am* 1994;23:511–537.

Halpin VJ, Norton JA. Adrenal insufficiency. In: Wilmore DW, et al., eds. ACS care of the surgical patient. *Sci Am* 1997.

NIH state-of-the-science statement on management of the clinically inapparent adrenal mass ("incidentaloma"). *NIH Consens State Sci Statements* 2002 Feb 4–6;19(2):1–25.

Scott HW. *Surgery of the Adrenal Glands.* Philadelphia, PA: JB Lippincott, 1990.

Terzolo M, Pia A, Ali A, et al. Adrenal incidentaloma: a new cause of the metabolic syndrome. *J Clin Endocrinol Metab* 2002;170(3):1043.

Multiple Endocrine Neoplasia Syndromes

Brandi ML, Gagel RF, Angeli A, et al. Consensus: guidelines for diagnosis and therapy of MEN Type 1 and Type 2. *J Clin Endocrinol Metab* 2001;86:5658–5671.

Chi DD, Moley JF. Medullary thyroid carcinoma. *Surg Oncol Clin North Am* 1998;7:681–706.

Phay JE, Moley JF, Lairmore TC. Multiple endocrine neoplasia. *Semin Surg Onc* 2000;18:324–332.

22

JAMES C. HEBERT, MD ■ KENNITH H. SARTORELLI, MD

Spleen

OBJECTIVES

1. Discuss the anatomy and functions of the spleen.
2. Discuss the workup and management of a patient with splenic injury.
3. Discuss the role of splenectomy in hematologic abnormalities.
4. Distinguish between splenomegaly and hypersplenism, and discuss their causes.
5. Discuss the consequences of splenectomy and the potential methods to reduce the associated risks.

To many of the ancients, the spleen was an enigma. At one time, functions such as laughter and swiftness were attributed to the spleen. We now realize that the spleen, the largest mass of lymphoid tissue in the body, plays a key role in maintaining the integrity of an individual's immune and hematologic status.

ANATOMY

The spleen develops from the dorsal mesogastrium and is present by the sixth week of gestation. The spleen resides in the left upper quadrant of the abdomen, which is bounded by the diaphragm superiorly and the lower thoracic cage anterolaterally. The spleen is intimately associated with the pancreas, stomach, left kidney, colon, and diaphragm by a series of suspensory ligaments (Fig. 22-1). The ligaments of the spleen are also derived from the dorsal mesogastrium. The splenorenal, gastrosplenic, splenocolic, and splenophrenic ligaments provide direct fixation of the spleen to the left upper quadrant. The short gastric vessels run through the gastrosplenic ligament. The splenic vessels and the tail of the pancreas traverse the splenorenal ligament. Laxity of the splenic ligaments may cause excessive mobility of the spleen, allowing it access to the lower quadrants of the abdomen (wandering spleen). This condition is treated with splenopexy to the left upper abdomen. The spleen is encased in a capsule that becomes thin and fibrotic by adulthood. Traction on the spleen or its supporting ligaments by blunt or operative trauma may cause bleeding from capsular avulsion. A normal spleen weighs between 75 and 150 g and is the size of the patient's fist.

The spleen is an extremely vascular organ that receives approximately 5% of the cardiac output. The organ has a dual arterial blood supply. The splenic artery provides the primary inflow, with additional contributions from the short gastric arteries (Fig. 22-2). The splenic artery is a branch of the celiac artery and courses along the superior border of the pancreas, dividing into two or more branches before ultimately entering the spleen at its hilum. There are usually four to six short gastric arteries derived from the left gastroepiploic artery. Vexing bleeding from the short gastric vessels can be encountered during splenectomy or operations on the stomach (e.g., fundoplication).

Venous drainage of the spleen occurs through the splenic and short gastric veins. The course of the splenic vein parallels that of the splenic artery. The splenic vein joins the superior mesenteric vein to form the portal vein.

A variety of developmental disorders affect the spleen. The most common developmental anomaly is the presence of **accessory spleens** in addition to a normal spleen. Accessory spleens are found in 10% to 30% of the population and are believed to result from failure of separate splenic masses in the dorsal mesogastrium to fuse. These splenic buds are then carried to various locations by the migration of the splenic ligaments. The most common sites for accessory spleens, in order of decreasing frequency, are the splenic hilum, splenocolic ligament, gastrocolic ligament, splenorenal ligament, and omentum (Fig. 22-3). Failure to recognize accessory spleens may

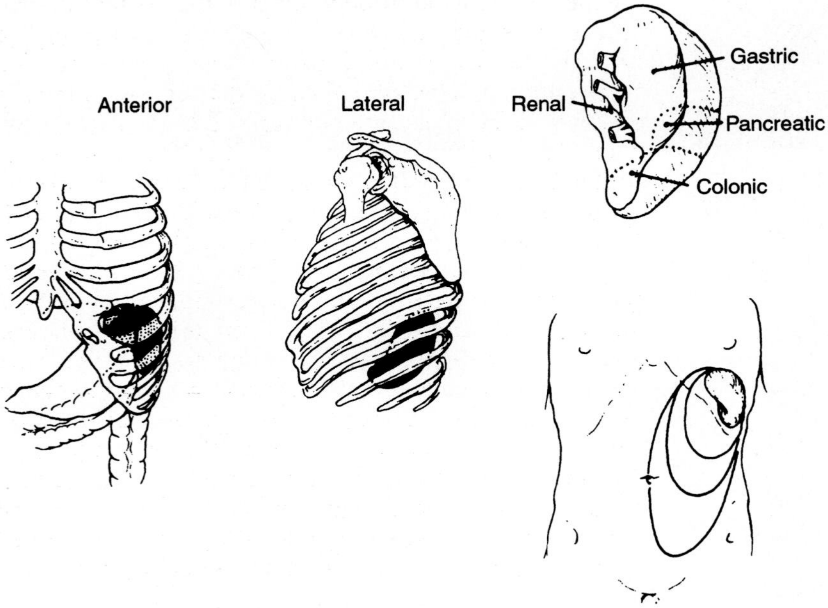

Figure 22-1 Normal external relations of the spleen.

lead to relapse of various hematologic disorders after splenectomy.

Polysplenia is the presence of multiple small spleens, with no normal spleen. Polysplenia is associated with multiple anomalies, including severe cardiac defects, situs inversus, and biliary atresia. Absence of the spleen (asplenia), a lethal condition, is also associated with severe cardiac anomalies and situs inversus. Splenogonadal fusion is a rare disorder of development, in which splenic tissue is found in the scrotum, often attached to the testicle.

PHYSIOLOGY

The spleen has several distinct functions, including hematopoiesis, blood filtering, and immune modulation. The function of the spleen is intimately related to its microstructure. Central to its microstructure is its microcirculation (Fig. 22-4). A trabecular meshwork of fibrous tissue joins the fibroelastic capsule to the hilum of the spleen and surrounds the entering blood vessels. Blood enters the

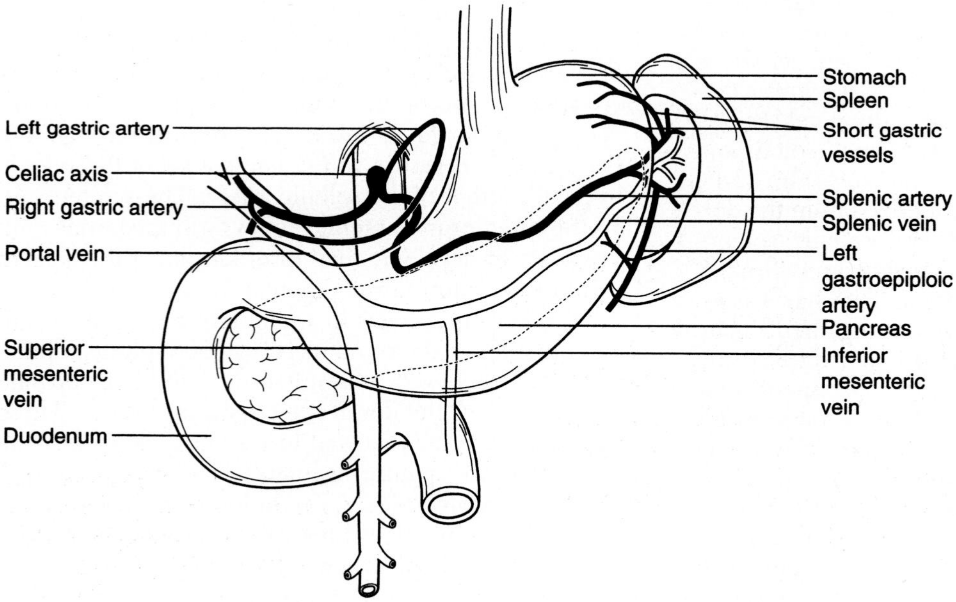

Figure 22-2 Blood supply to the spleen.

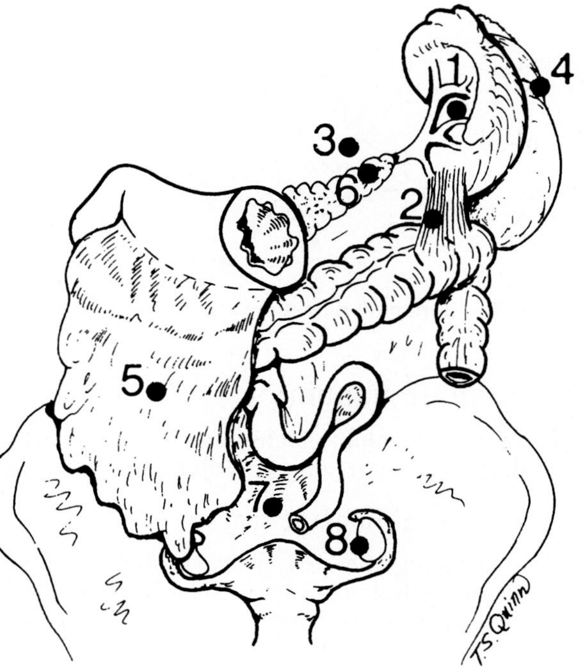

Figure 22-3 Normal internal relations of the spleen (stomach removed) and location of accessory spleens. **1,** Splenic hilum. **2,** Splenocolic ligament. **3,** Gastrocolic ligament. **4,** Splenorenal ligament. **5,** Greater omentum. **6,** Tail of the pancreas. **7,** Mesentery. **8,** Gonadal.

splenic parenchyma through central arteries that branch off the trabecular arteries. These central arteries course through the **white pulp,** where they are surrounded by periarterial lymphatic sheaths that consist primarily of T-lymphocytes and macrophages that can process soluble antigens. Some blood flows into the surrounding lymphatic follicles, where B-lymphocytes can proliferate in germinal centers. Mature antibody-producing cells (plasma cells) are found here. Blood that leaves the white pulp flows into a marginal zone, where it is directed either back to the white pulp or through terminal arterioles into the **splenic cords of Billroth** in the **red pulp** (open circulation). In the reticular network of the cords, which have no endothelial cells, blood percolates slowly and comes into contact with numerous macrophages before they enter the endothelial-lined sinuses. The red pulp is the site of removal of antibody-sensitized cells and particulate material. In some pathologic conditions, blood is shunted from the marginal zone directly into the sinuses (closed circulation), bypassing much of the critical filtering function.

The spleen is a site of fetal extramedullary hematopoiesis, but this activity usually ceases by birth in normal humans.

In its capacity as a blood filter, the spleen culls abnormal and aged erythrocytes, granulocytes, and platelets from the nearly 350 L/day of blood that passes through it. As red blood cells near the end of their lives, they lose membrane integrity as a result of declining adenosine triphosphate levels. As a result, they are marked for destruction. Abnormal and senescent red blood cells cannot de-

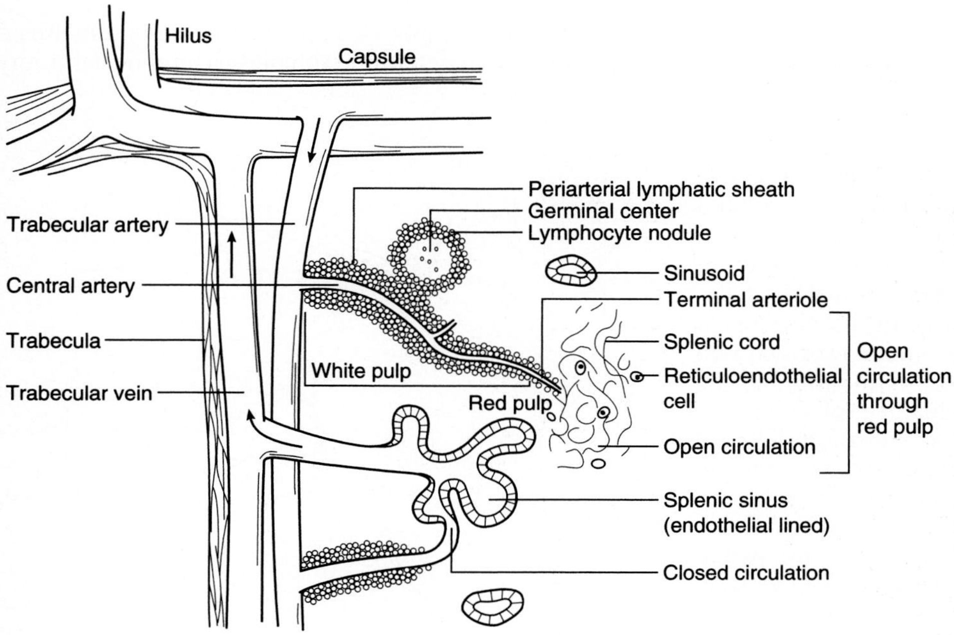

Figure 22-4 Microanatomy of the spleen, with its functional components, showing both open and closed circulations.

form appropriately to enter the splenic sinuses through the fenestrations in the endothelium. Therefore, they are removed in the red pulp. In addition, as red blood cells deform to enter the splenic sinuses as they leave the red pulp, cellular inclusions are pinched off from the cells. This "pitting" function removes nuclear remnants, such as **Howell-Jolly bodies,** from red blood cells. It also removes other red blood cell inclusions, such as **Heinz bodies** (denatured hemoglobin) and **Pappenheimer bodies** (iron inclusions).

The role of the spleen in the sequestration and destruction of granulocytes and platelets under normal circumstances is not well understood. Normally, one-third of the body's platelets are stored in the spleen. Abnormal splenic processing of platelets occurs in several disease processes and causes marked thrombocytopenia. Splenectomy is usually followed by thrombocytosis.

The spleen plays an important role in the immune system and is part of the reticuloendothelial system. It also provides both nonspecific and specific immune responses. A nonspecific response has two arms: (1) clearance of opsonized particles and bacteria by fixed splenic macrophages and (2) opsonin production. **Opsonins** that are produced by the spleen include properdin, tuftsin, and fibronectin. Properdin activates the alternative pathway of the complement system. Tuftsin facilitates macrophage phagocytosis. The specific immune response of the spleen includes antigen processing and antibody production by splenic lymphocytes that are present in the white pulp. The spleen is the body's largest producer of immunoglobulin M (IgM), and splenectomy causes a marked decrease in IgM and opsonin production. Because of its mass and its position in the circulation, the spleen probably plays a major role in modulating the systemic cytokine response to infection. However, little is understood about this role.

GENERAL DIAGNOSTIC CONSIDERATIONS

Physical Examination

A normal spleen is difficult to palpate because of its size and position. The long axis of the spleen is located behind and parallel to the 10th rib in the midaxillary line. A normal adult spleen is approximately 12 cm long and 7 cm wide. Splenic palpation and percussion are used to determine the size of the spleen. The edge of an enlarged spleen may be palpated at the costal margin and may extend into the left iliac fossa. Rarely, it crosses the midline into the right iliac fossa (see Fig. 22-1). An enlarged spleen usually is not tender. Therefore, discomfort on palpation alerts the clinician to the possibility of an infective process, splenic infarction, or splenic trauma. Palpation of the spleen is accomplished either bimanually (Fig. 22-5) or with Middleton's method (Fig. 22-6). Table 22-1 shows the pathologic conditions that are associated with the need for splenectomy. Percussion of the spleen causes an area of splenic dullness in the left upper quadrant. Feces in the colon or fluid in the stomach may falsely suggest splenomegaly.

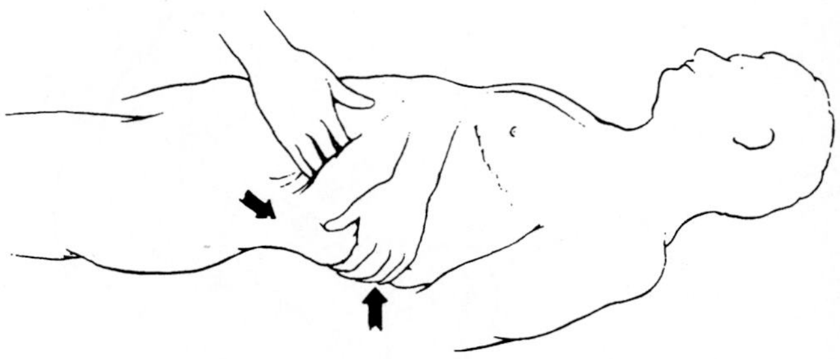

Figure 22-5 Bimanual palpation of the spleen.

Radiographic Imaging

A variety of radiographic techniques are available to aid in the diagnosis and treatment of disorders of the spleen.

Plain Abdominal Roentgenogram

Abdominal radiographs may yield information that suggests splenomegaly as a result of displacement of the colon or stomach, an elevated left diaphragm, or a large splenic shadow (Fig. 22-7). Left-sided rib fractures may suggest splenic trauma.

Ultrasound

Ultrasound is a useful tool to evaluate splenomegaly and to show splenic cysts or abscesses (Fig. 22-8). Abdominal ultrasound is rapidly gaining acceptance as a means to evaluate patients with traumatic injury (see discussion in the abdominal trauma section of Chapter XX, Trauma). Gas within the intestinal tract may interfere with visualization of the spleen and other structures.

Computed Tomography

Computed tomography (CT) scan is the most useful imaging technique to determine splenic size and detect injury

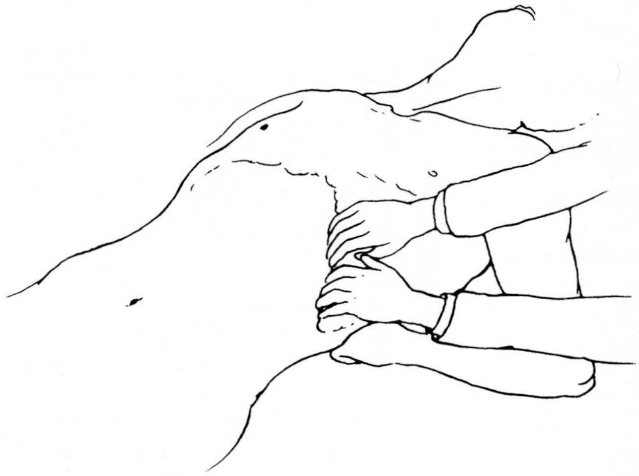

Figure 22-6 Palpation of the spleen with Middleton's method.

Table 22-1	Indications for Splenectomy

Splenic rupture (repair of the spleen is preferred in certain patients)
- Trauma
- Spontaneous
- Iatrogenic injury

Hematologic disorders
- Hematolytic anemias
- Hereditary spherocytosis
- Hereditary elliptocytosis
- Thalassemia minor and major (rare)
- Autoimmune hemolytic anemia not responsive to steroid therapy
- Thrombocytopenia
- Idiopathic thrombocytopenic purpura
- Immunologic thrombocytopenia associated with chronic lymphocytic leukemia or systemic lupus erythematosis
- Thrombotic thrombocytopenic purpura (rarely)

Hypersplenism associated with other diseases
- Inflammation
- Infiltrative diseases
- Congestion

Leukemia and lymphoma

Other diseases
- Splenic abscess (often associated with drug abuse or AIDS)
- Primary and metastatic tumors
- Splenic cysts
- Splenic artery aneurysm

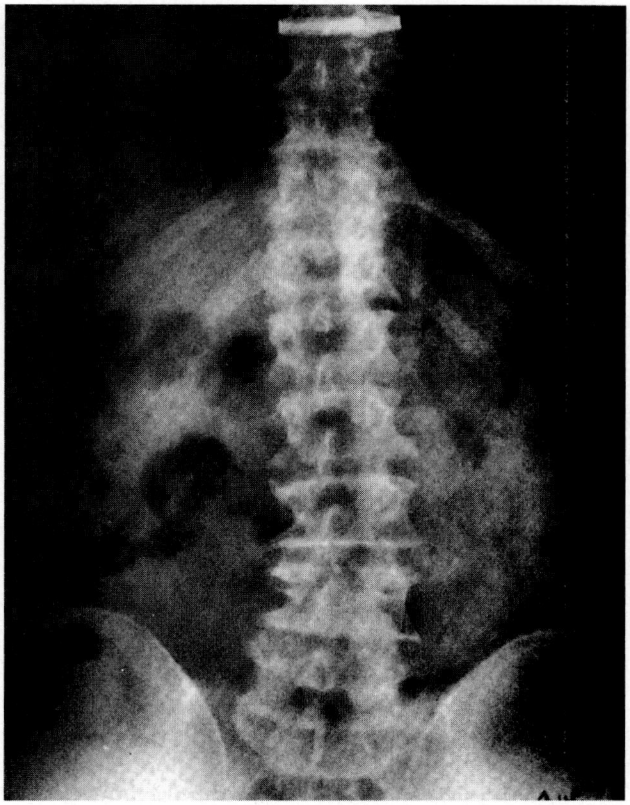

Figure 22-7 Plain film of the abdomen showing an enlarged spleen (radiopaque shadow in the left upper quadrant).

(Fig. 22-9). CT scans also provide useful information about other potential disease processes or injuries in adjacent organs. Splenic cysts and abscesses are clearly shown by CT scans, and percutaneous drainage can be performed under CT guidance. CT scans are useful to follow splenic injuries and to obtain information about the patency of splenic vessels.

Radionuclide Scans

Colloid suspensions of technetium are taken up by the reticuloendothelial system and give information about splenic size and function. Radionuclide scans are useful to look for missed accessory spleens after unsuccessful splenectomy to control hematologic disorders. They are used infrequently today.

Angiography

Angiography is useful in showing splenic vein thrombosis and aids in planning portal venous decompressive procedures. Angiography is also helpful in showing splenic tumors. Splenic artery embolization may be a useful adjunct to control bleeding before laparoscopic splenectomy. Partial splenic embolization is used to control hypersplenism in children with portal hypertension and to control bleeding in splenic injuries.

Surgical Disorders of the Spleen

The spleen is subject to a variety of disorders that may require surgical intervention (see Table 22-1). Trauma is the most common reason for splenectomy. Alternatives to splenectomy (e.g., partial splenectomy, embolization, image-guided percutaneous drainage procedures) are often used successfully.

Splenic Trauma

The spleen is the most commonly injured organ after blunt abdominal trauma and the second most commonly injured organ after penetrating abdominal trauma. Traditionally, injuries to the spleen were treated with prompt splenectomy. The recognition of the entity of **overwhelming postsplenectomy infection,** coupled with a better understanding of the immunologic function of the spleen, led to attempts at splenic preservation when feasible.

Clinical Presentation and Evaluation

Three general mechanisms of splenic injury occur: penetrating, blunt compressive, and blunt deceleration. The extent of penetrating injuries depends on the device used to create the injury (firearm versus knife). Penetrating trauma, particularly with firearms, often involves the

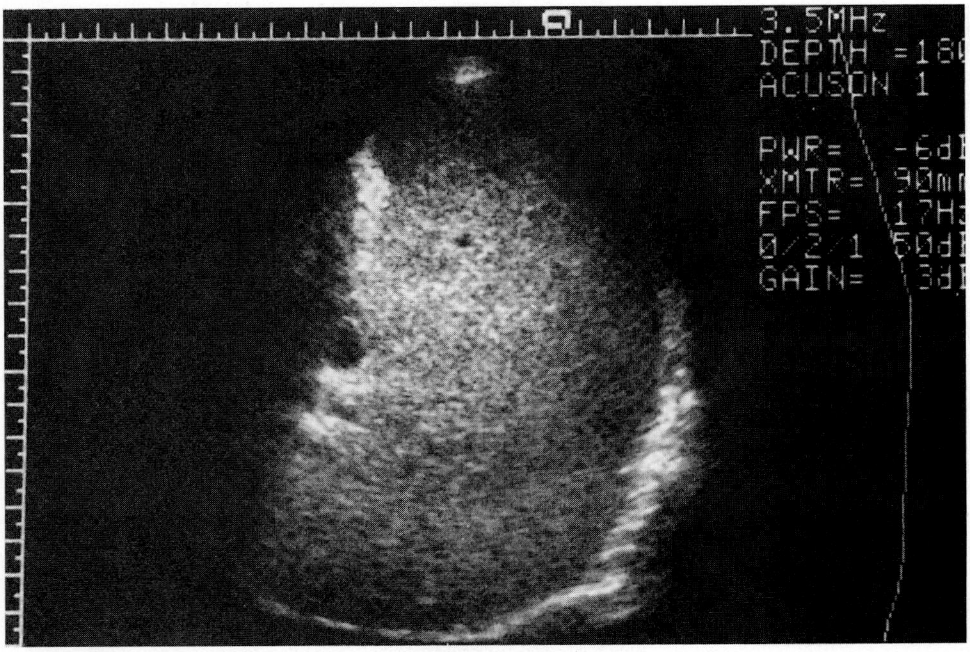

Figure 22-8 Ultrasound of the left upper quadrant showing an enlarged spleen. In this case, splenomegaly is secondary to myelofibrosis.

splenic vasculature as well as adjacent organs. Because of the fixation of the spleen afforded by the splenic ligaments, the spleen is prone to blunt compressive injuries as well as capsular avulsion from rapid decelerations. In adults, the ribs may provide some protection to the spleen. However, rib fractures are present in 20% of spleen injuries, and the rib fragments may contribute to the spleen injury. The compliant thoracic cage of children provides little protection to the spleen from blunt forces. A scale of severity for splenic injuries was devised by the American Association for the Surgery of Trauma (Table 22-2). All patients should be resuscitated according to the guidelines of the Advanced Trauma Life Support Course of the American College of Surgeons.

In evaluating patients for splenic injury, the physician should look for signs and symptoms of local peritoneal irritation and acute hemorrhage. Signs of peritoneal irritation include left upper quadrant tenderness to palpation, pain at the top of the left shoulder (**Kehr's sign**), and percussion dullness of the left flank (**Ballance's sign**). When evaluating patients with penetrating trauma, it must be remembered that the diaphragm and underlying spleen may ascend as high as the fourth intercostal space during inspiration. Any penetrating injury from the level of the

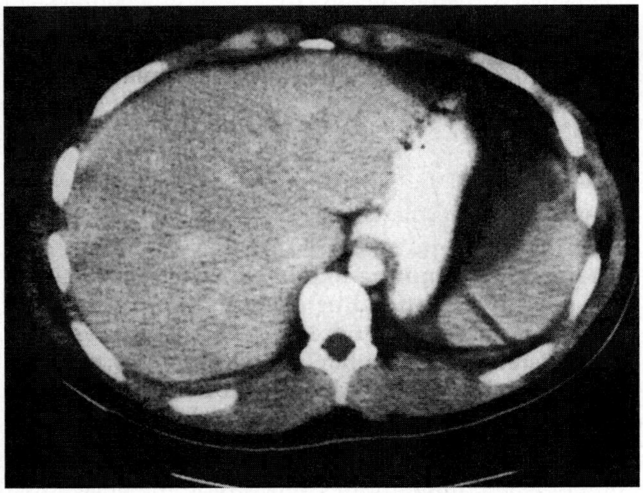

Figure 22-9 Computed tomography scan of the abdomen showing a subcapsular hematoma of the spleen.

Table 22-2 Grades of Splenic Injury

Grade	Description
I	Hematoma: Subcapsular < 10% surface area Laceration: < 1 cm deep
II	Hematoma: Subcapsular 10%–50% surface area Parenchymal < 5 cm diameter Laceration: 1–3 cm deep, not involving trabecular vessels
III	Hematoma: Subcapsular > 50% surface area Parenchymal > 5 cm diameter Any expanding or ruptured Laceration: > 3 cm deep or involving trabecular vessels
IV	Laceration: Segmental vessels involved with devascularization < 50%
V	Completely shattered spleen or hilar vascular injury with devascularization

nipples down may traverse the peritoneal cavity, and patients with signs of intraperitoneal hemorrhage should undergo prompt celiotomy.

The evaluation of patients with blunt abdominal trauma is complicated by the high incidence of concomitant neurologic and orthopedic injuries. Isolated splenic injury occurs in only 30% of patients. Hemodynamically unstable patients who have signs of blunt abdominal trauma require prompt celiotomy. Stable patients who have signs of abdominal injury and those whose neurologic status is impaired require evaluation with CT scan, ultrasound, or diagnostic peritoneal lavage. If splenic injury is present, several treatment options exist.

Treatment

Splenectomy is performed if the spleen is extensively injured (grade V) or if the patient is profoundly unstable. In stable patients, attempts at splenic preservation with splenorrhaphy or nonoperative management are undertaken.

Splenorrhaphy is operative repair of the spleen. If at least 50% of the splenic volume is preserved, the immune function of the spleen should remain intact. Techniques of splenorrhaphy include debridement of devitalized tissue followed by compression with microcrystalline collagen, pledgeted suture repair, and the creation of polyglycolic acid mesh slings to provide hemostatic compression. Splenorrhaphy is abandoned if the patient has persistent hypotension or extensive additional intraabdominal injuries.

Splenic autotransplantation by placing splenic fragments in the omentum or peritoneal cavity should be avoided. This procedure does not preserve splenic function and may lead to a high risk of bowel obstruction, requiring further surgery that is associated with troublesome bloody adhesions.

Nonoperative management of splenic injuries is the treatment of choice in hemodynamically stable children. It is also gaining acceptance in adults. For nonoperative therapy to be successful, the patient must be hemodynamically stable, with an isolated splenic injury, usually grades I through III by CT scan. Protocols must be followed. Treatment is undertaken in a very controlled environment by a surgical team experienced in the management of splenic trauma. Protocols vary from institution to institution. Usually, the patient is given bed rest initially in an intensive care unit, and serial physical examinations are performed and hematocrits checked. If the patient shows any signs of shock or has evidence of continued bleeding, then celiotomy is undertaken. Patients who remain hemodynamically stable are followed closely, usually for approximately 1 week in the hospital and then for 6 to 12 weeks of restricted activity. CT or ultrasound is usually obtained to check for splenic healing before the patient is allowed to return to full activity. Nonoperative therapy is successful in more than 85% of children and 70% of adults. Concerns about nonoperative therapy include delayed splenic rupture, risk of transfusions, and missed associated injuries. Although these concerns are real, they are not borne out by experience.

Disorders of Splenic Function

Disorders of the spleen are classified as either functional or anatomic. Functional disorders are considered in terms of too little function (**hyposplenism** and **asplenia**) or excess function (**hypersplenism**). Congenital asplenia or hyposplenism is extremely rare. Splenectomy is the most common reason for the asplenic state, although other conditions (e.g., sickle cell anemia) may lead to a functional asplenic state. The size of the spleen is not related to its hematologic function. Splenomegaly (anatomic enlargement of the spleen) is caused by a variety of conditions (Table 22-3) and should not be confused with hypersplenism (excess function of the spleen). Hypersplenism is characterized by **cytopenia** (anemia, leukopenia, and

Table 22-3 Classification of Splenomegaly (Based on Degree of Enlargement)

Light	Moderate	Great
Chronic passive congestion	Rickets	Chronic myelocytic leukemia
Acute malaria	Hepatitis	Myelofibrosis
Typhoid fever	Hepatic cirrhosis	Gaucher's disease
Subacute bacterial endocarditis	Lymphoma (leukemia)	Neimann-Pick disease
Acute and subacute infection	Infectious mononucleosis	Thalassemia major
Systemic lupus erythematosus	Pernicious anemia	Chronic malaria
Thalassemia minor	Abscesses, infarcts	Leishmaniasis
	Amyloidosis	Splenic vein thrombosis
		Leukemic reticuloendotheliosis (hairy-cell leukemia)

thrombocytopenia, alone or in combination) and normal or hyperplastic cellular precursors in the bone marrow. Cytopenia results from increased sequestration of the cells in the spleen, increased destruction of cells by the spleen, or production of antibody in the spleen, leading to increased sequestration and destruction of cells. Hyposplenism also occurs with normal or enlarged spleens (multiple myeloma, sickle cell anemia).

There are three hematologic disorders of splenic function for which splenectomy may be helpful: **hemolytic anemia, immune thrombocytopenic purpura** (ITP), and cytopenia associated with splenomegaly from other diseases (secondary hypersplenism).

Hemolytic Anemia

Splenectomy may aid in the management of hereditary hemolytic anemias and some cases of acquired immune hemolytic anemias. Hereditary hemolytic anemias are classified into three broad areas: membrane structural abnormalities, metabolic abnormalities, and **hemoglobinopathies** (Table 22-4).

Hereditary spherocytosis, an autosomal dominant trait, is characterized by abnormally shaped, rigid red cells as a result of a deficiency in spectrin, a membrane component that is essential for deformability. These rigid erythrocytes cannot pass into the splenic sinuses and become sequestered in the red pulp. Splenectomy is usually indicated because it allows red cells to survive and hematocrit to reach near-normal values postoperatively. An intraoperative search for an accessory spleen is also performed. The severity of the disease is related to the amount of spectrin produced, and the disease runs in families. Occasionally, the disease is so severe that young children require splenectomy. Splenectomy is deferred if possible, however, until the patient is at least 5 years old because the risk of overwhelming postsplenectomy sepsis is much higher in young children.

Other types of membrane structural abnormalities are less common, but may require splenectomy. A cholecystectomy is performed at the time of splenectomy for hemolytic anemia because pigment gallstones are quite common.

Hemolytic anemias caused by metabolic abnormalities (e.g., pyruvate kinase deficiency, glucose-6-phosphate dehydrogenase [G6PD] deficiency) are not responsive to splenectomy. In G6PD deficiency, the erythrocyte membrane is injured by certain oxidizing drugs, which should be discontinued.

Hemoglobinopathies, which are abnormalities in hemoglobin structure, can lead to red cell deformity and subsequent hemolytic anemia. Sickle cell disease is an autosomal recessive disease. The homozygous state is more

Table 22-4 Hereditary Hemolytic Anemias

Type	Inheritance	Defect	Usefulness of Splenectomy
Abnormal membrane structure			
Spherocytosis	Autosomal dominant	Deficiency in spectrin (membrane component essential for deformability) Rigid erythrocytes cannot pass through splenic vasculature and are sequestered, leading to progressive splenomegaly	Usually
Elliptocytosis	Autosomal dominant	Decreased levels of spectrin; relatively mild in most cases	Rarely
Pyropoikilocytosis	Autosomal recessive	Rare variant of spherocytosis	Usually
Xerocytosis		Water loss leading to increased concentration of hemoglobin	Rarely
Hydrocytosis		Abnormality in erythrocyte Na^+/K^+ transport	Often
Metabolic abnormalities			
Pyruvate kinase deficiency	Autosomal recessive	Decreased ATP generation leads to membrane destruction	Rarely
Glucose-6-phosphate dehydrogenase deficiency	Sex-linked recessive	Pentose phosphate shunt is blocked and membrane is injured by oxidation injury from certain drugs (e.g., sulfamethoxazole, ASA, phenacetin, nitrofurantoin)	Never
Hemoglobinopathies			
Sickle cell	Autosomal recessive (homozygous more severe)	Valine substitute for glutamic acid at position 6 of β-chain of HbA; rigid, sickle-shaped cells at low O_2	Rarely
Thalassemias	Many varieties	Deficits in the synthesis of one or more subunits of Hb	Rarely

ATP, adenosine triphosphate; ASA, aminosalicylic acid; Hb, hemoglobin.

severe than the heterozygous state. In sickle hemoglobin, valine is substituted for glutamic acid at position six of the beta chain of hemoglobin A. This substitution causes a conformational change in structure that leads to the formation of a rigid sickle-shaped red cell at low oxygen saturations. In addition to hemolytic anemia, sickle cells cause an increase in blood viscosity that leads to stasis and subsequent thrombocytosis. Ischemia occurs as a result and leads to fibrosis in a variety of organs. Most patients with homozygous sickle cell anemia are functionally asplenic because of repeated splenic infarcts and fibrosis. Occasionally, splenectomy is useful in the treatment of patients with splenomegaly in hemolytic crisis. This treatment is usually useful early in the disease.

Thalassemias are characterized by deficits in the synthesis of one or more subunits of hemoglobin. There are many varied types. In thalassemia major (homozygous β-thalassemia), splenectomy is beneficial in reducing the requirements for transfusion, the physical discomfort from massive splenomegaly, and the potential for rupture. In thalassemia minor (heterozygous β-thalassemia), splenectomy can decrease the need for transfusion and the problems associated with iron overload. In general, patients who have thalassemia and undergo splenectomy are at the highest risk for overwhelming postsplenectomy infection. For this reason, alternatives to total splenectomy (e.g., splenic embolization, partial splenectomy) are successful in these patients.

Acquired autoimmune hemolytic anemias are caused by exposure to chemicals, drugs, infectious agents, inflammatory processes, or malignancies. In many cases, a cause is not readily identified. Red blood cells from patients with autoimmune hemolytic anemias are coated with immunoglobulin, complement, or both, which results in a positive direct Coombs' test. Coombs'-negative hemolytic anemia is usually secondary to drugs, toxins, or infectious agents, and is best treated by removing the responsible agent. Patients with Coombs'-positive hemolytic anemia should receive corticosteroid therapy and treatment for any underlying disorders. Splenectomy is indicated when steroids are ineffective, when high doses are required, and when toxic side effects develop during steroid treatment. Splenic sequestration studies and red cell survival may help to select patients who will respond to splenectomy. Further, anemias associated with warm reactive antibodies (usually IgG) do not include complement activation. They are associated with splenic sequestration and usually respond to splenectomy. Hemolytic anemias associated with cold reactive antibodies (usually IgM) are characterized by complement binding and agglutination. Hemolysis occurs in peripheral locations in response to cool environmental temperatures. Splenectomy is usually not helpful in these cases.

Thrombocytopenia

Thrombocytopenia has a variety of causes (Table 22-5). Splenectomy is appropriate only in idiopathic, immune-mediated thrombocytopenias (those in which a cause cannot be found). These platelet disorders are usually characterized by the coexistence of a low platelet count, a normal or increased number of megakaryocytes in the bone marrow, and the absence of other hematologic disorders or splenomegaly. The medication history is important, particularly the history of drugs that interfere with platelet function (e.g., aspirin) or other therapeutic agents that are known to cause thrombocytopenia.

Table 22-5 Classification of Thrombocytopenia

- Decreased production
  - Hypoproliferation (toxic agents, sepsis, radiation, myelofibrosis, tumor involvement of marrow)
  - Ineffective platelet production (megaloblastic anemia, Guglielmo's syndrome)
- Splenic sequestration (congestive splenomegaly, myeloid metaplasia, lymphoma, Gaucher's disease)
- Dilutional loss (after massive transfusion)
- Abnormal destruction
  - Consumption (disseminated intravascular coagulation)
  - Immune mechanisms
  - Splenectomy sometimes indicated (idiopathic thrombocytopenic purpura, chronic lymphocytic leukemia, systemic lupus erythematosus)
  - Splenectomy not indicated (drug-induced thromboc topenia, neonatal thrombocytopenia, posttransfusion purpura)

Patients with thrombocytopenia often have multiple petechiae (pinpoint lesions that result from breakage of small capillaries or increased permeability of the arterioles, capillaries, or venules). Petechiae occur in areas of the body that encounter pressure and are characteristic of thrombocytopenia. Purpura causes a confluence of petechiae. Ecchymoses are extensive purpuric lesions that indicate that blood has spread along fascial planes. Ecchymoses are more suggestive of a coagulation disorder than of thrombocytopenia.

If the platelet count is low and coagulation disorders were ruled out by appropriate laboratory tests, then all medications should be discontinued. Antiplatelet antibodies should be measured because they are elevated in 85% of patients with immune cytopenic purpura. The bone marrow is evaluated to determine the number of megakaryocytes. In disorders of platelet destruction (e.g., ITP), the bone marrow shows either normal or increased numbers of megakaryocytes.

Immune Thrombocytopenic Purpura. Acute ITP usually occurs after an acute viral infection. It has an excellent prognosis in children younger than 16 years of age. Approximately 80% of these patients have a complete, permanent, spontaneous recovery without therapy. Chronic ITP is primarily a disease of young adults. It affects women more often than men. Patients are best treated initially with a course of corticosteroid therapy. If patients do not respond with an elevated platelet count, splenectomy is performed.

In patients who respond to steroid therapy, splenectomy is recommended if thrombocytopenia occurs after steroids are tapered. Patients who initially respond to steroid therapy fare better after splenectomy than those who do not respond to steroids. Patients who have any sign of intracranial bleeding during steroid therapy require emergency splenectomy. Of patients who undergo splenectomy, 75% to 85% respond permanently and require no further therapy. If platelet counts are less than 20,000, platelets should be available for transfusion. Transfusion of platelets is performed after the spleen is removed because transfused platelets are rapidly destroyed in the spleen. For patients who do not respond or who relapse after splenectomy and who do not improve with corticosteroids, treatment with vincristine and γ-globulin shows some success.

Thrombotic Thrombocytopenic Purpura. Thrombotic thrombocytopenic purpura is a disease of the arteries or capillaries. It is characterized by thrombotic episodes and low platelet counts. The constellation of clinical features in virtually all cases consists of fever, purpura, hemolytic anemia, neurologic manifestations, and signs of renal disease. Plasma pheresis, a therapy aimed at removing plasma-derived factors that cause platelet aggregation, is usually successful, either alone or in combination with antiplatelet therapy, whole-blood exchange transfusions, and steroids. Splenectomy is arguably indicated if these measures fail.

HIV-Associated Thrombocytopenia. Infection with HIV may lead to HIV-associated thrombocytopenia. HIV-positive patients and those with AIDS and symptomatic HIV-associated thrombocytopenia that is resistant to medical therapy appear to benefit from splenectomy. Sustained resolution of thrombocytopenia is seen in 60% to 80% of these patients. Splenectomy is performed without an undue increase in morbidity and mortality rates. Splenectomy does not appear to accelerate the conversion rate to AIDS in HIV-positive patients.

Hypersplenism Associated With Other Diseases

A number of clinical syndromes are characterized by destruction of various formed elements of the blood. The cardinal features include splenomegaly; some reduction in the number of circulating blood cells affecting granulocytes, erythrocytes, or platelets in any combination; a compensatory proliferative response in the bone marrow; and the potential for correction of these hematologic abnormalities by splenectomy. Both infiltrative and congestive forms of splenomegaly are associated with hypersplenism (Table 22-6). In patients with splenomegaly, sequestration of both red cells and platelets occurs. Red cell transit time through the spleen increases proportionately with splenomegaly. Platelet survival is not usually affected; however, platelet sequestration by the enlarged spleen is increased. For this reason, thrombocytopenia is usually apparent before anemia in patients with hypersplenism associated with splenomegaly.

Table 22-6 Diseases Associated With Hypersplenism

Infiltrative disease of the spleen
- Benign conditions (Gaucher's disease, Niemann-Pick disease, amyloidosis, extramedullary hematopoiesis)
- Neoplastic conditions (leukemias, lymphoma, Hodgkin's disease, primary tumors, metastatic tumors, myeloid metaplasia)

Congestive disease of the spleen
- Portal hypertension
- Splenic vein thrombosis

Miscellaneous diseases
- Felty's syndrome (rheumatoid arthritis, splenomegaly, neutropenia)
- Sarcoidosis
- Porphyria erythropoietica

Hypersplenism is suggested by splenomegaly. Peripheral blood smears may show pancytopenia, isolated thrombocytopenia, anemia, or leukopenia. Most cases of hypersplenism, however, show pancytopenia. The bone marrow is usually hyperplastic. In myelofibrosis, a bone marrow examination shows increased deposition of collagen. The diagnostic approach is dictated by the accompanying features (e.g., hematologic findings, lymphadenopathy, portal hypertension, liver dysfunction, systemic infection). For a variety of reasons, splenectomy is indicated for patients with splenomegaly and hypersplenism. Splenectomy is indicated for hypersplenism if the platelet count is less than 50,000, with evidence of bleeding; if the neutrophil count is less than 2000, with or without frequent intercurrent infections; or if the patient has anemia requiring blood transfusion. In myelofibrosis with myeloid metaplasia as well as other cases of extramedullary hematopoiesis, splenectomy is indicated only when the clinical evidence suggests that the compensatory hematopoietic function of the enlarged spleen is outweighed by accelerated sequestration and destruction of red cells.

In most cases of secondary hypersplenism, splenectomy does not completely alleviate the cytopenia. Postoperatively, however, a dramatic increase in the number of platelets may occur and may be associated with thrombosis and thromboembolism, particularly in myelofibrosis. Close postoperative monitoring of platelets is essential.

Congestive Splenomegaly. Hypersplenism associated with **congestive splenomegaly** as a result of liver failure and the vascular consequences of portal hypertension requires treatment of the hypertension rather than splenectomy. Splenectomy is contraindicated as a primary treatment in this setting because it eliminates the possibility of performing a selective splenorenal shunt procedure, which is a more appropriate treatment for portal hypertension. In this setting, splenectomy may also lead to portal vein thrombosis and complicate potential liver transplantation.

Infiltrative Splenomegaly. In benign cases of **infiltrative splenomegaly** (e.g., Gaucher's disease, an autosomal recessive disorder that causes abnormal accumulation of glucocerebrosides in the reticuloendothelial cells), partial splenectomy and splenic embolization are used instead of splenectomy to treat hypersplenism and abdominal discomfort caused by massive splenomegaly.

Felty's Syndrome. Some patients with rheumatoid arthritis have leg ulcers or other chronic infections, with associated splenomegaly and neutropenia. In these patients, circulating antibodies against neutrophils are found. Splenectomy is controversial because the response is unpredictable. Splenectomy is usually performed for **Felty's syndrome** when severe recurrent infections or intractable leg ulcers occur.

Hematologic Malignancies

Splenectomy is not indicated for acute leukemia. For patients with chronic leukemia, splenectomy is indicated for some cases of hypersplenism and for symptoms associated with massive splenomegaly.

Leukemic reticuloendotheliosis (hairy cell leukemia) is an indolent, progressive form of chronic leukemia. Ongoing hepatomegaly and splenomegaly occur as the disease progresses and the leukemic cells infiltrate the spleen and liver. In the recent past, splenectomy was believed to be an important therapeutic intervention early in the treatment of hairy cell leukemia. Recently, α-interferon and 21-deoxycoformycin were introduced as first-line treatments. Splenectomy is now reserved primarily for palliating cytopenias and symptoms of splenomegaly.

Splenectomy as part of a staging laparotomy to match treatment with extent of disease is now rarely performed for Hodgkin's disease because of improvements in imaging technologies and changes to more systemic forms of therapy (see the discussion of Hodgkin's lymphoma in Chapter 25, Surgical Oncology). Splenectomy for non-Hodgkin's lymphoma is rarely indicated except in patients with massive splenic enlargement that causes local pressure on the abdominal viscera, or symptomatic hypersplenism (see the discussion of non-Hodgkin's lymphoma in Chapter 25, Surgical Oncology).

Further Technical Considerations for Splenic Surgery

Splenectomy may be accomplished by traditional open means or by minimally invasive techniques. Open splenectomy is performed with either a midline incision or a left subcostal incision (Kehr's incision). The keys to safe splenectomy are mobilization of the spleen and control of the splenic vasculature. Complete mobilization of the spleen is mandatory for partial splenectomy and to evaluate and repair splenic injuries. It is important not to take the short gastric vessels too close to the stomach to avoid injury of the gastric wall. Care is also taken to avoid injuring the tail of the pancreas at the splenic hilum. Splenectomy for hematologic disease is not complete until a thorough search for accessory spleens is made. Drains are not routinely left after splenectomy.

Increasingly, laparoscopic splenectomy is performed successfully for splenectomy necessitated by ITP, hereditary spherocytosis, and HIV-related thrombocytopenia. The principles for laparoscopic splenectomy are the same as those for open splenectomy. However, it is necessary to morselize the spleen in special bags that are removed through the small incisions. Occasionally, surgeons make a larger lower abdominal incision to remove very large spleens in fragments.

Consequences and Complications of Splenectomy

Hematologic Changes

In a normal patient, after the spleen is removed, the white blood cell count increases by an average of 50% over baseline. In some cases, the number of neutrophils increases to 15,000 to 20,000 mm^3 in the initial postoperative period. The white blood cell count usually returns to normal within 5 to 7 days. Elevation beyond this period suggests infection.

The peripheral smear of a patient who underwent splenectomy routinely shows Howell-Jolly bodies, Pappenheimer bodies, and pitted red cells on phase microscopy. Some red blood cells may show abnormal morphology. The absence of these findings after splenectomy for hematologic disease suggests that an accessory spleen was missed. A radionuclide spleen scan may be useful for identifying retained splenic elements.

The platelet count increases by 30% between 2 and 10 days after splenectomy and usually returns to normal within 2 weeks. **Thrombocytosis** (platelet count > $400{,}000/mm^3$) occurs in as many as 50% of patients. Theoretically, this increase predisposes the patient to thrombotic complications (e.g., pulmonary embolism). However, little evidence supports a correlation between absolute platelet count and thrombosis. Most thromboses and pulmonary emboli occur in patients who have myeloproliferative disorders. Postoperative therapy with platelet inhibitors (e.g., aspirin, dipyridamole) is justified in patients who have myeloproliferative disease and platelet counts greater than $400{,}000/mm^3$ and in all other patients after splenectomy if the platelet count is greater than $750{,}000/mm^3$. Treatment continues until the platelet count returns to normal. Anticoagulation with heparin or warfarin therapy is not beneficial and should be avoided.

Immune Consequences

The risk of postsplenectomy sepsis varies with the age of the patient and the reason for splenectomy. In otherwise normal children, the potential risk is approximately 2% to 4%. In adults, it is approximately 1% to 2%. Patients who undergo splenectomy for hematologic disorders are at the highest risk. The overall incidence of postsplenectomy sepsis is 40 times that of the general population, and these patients are at risk for fatal sepsis at any time after splenectomy.

Overwhelming infections are usually caused by encapsulated organisms. *Streptococcus pneumoniae* (pneumococcus) is the most common agent (75%), followed in decreasing frequency by *Haemophilus influenzae, Neisseria meningitidis*, beta-hemolytic streptococcus, *Staphylococcus aureus, Escherichia coli,* and *Pseudomonas.* Viral infections, most commonly herpes zoster, may be severe in splenectomized patients. Some parasitic infections (babesiosis, malaria) also overwhelm the splenectomized host.

Overwhelming infections with encapsulated bacteria (e.g., pneumococcus) are insidious in onset, often mimicking a cold or flu. Within a few hours, patients may become septic, and death may ensue rapidly (24 to 28 hours) despite vigorous antibiotic therapy. Adrenal infarction causing adrenal insufficiency is often associated with these infections (Waterhouse-Friderichsen's syndrome).

Polyvalent pneumococcal polysaccharide vaccines are given after total splenectomy or conservative splenic operation for trauma. Patients with splenic trauma who are managed nonoperatively are also vaccinated. Neither the surgeon nor the patient should consider this vaccine full protection against overwhelming postsplenectomy sepsis. Both clinical and experimental evidence suggests that splenectomized patients may not respond well to pneumococcal polysaccharide antigens. Children who are younger than 2 years of age also do not become effectively immunized. In addition, pneumococcal types that are not contained in the vaccine (or other bacteria) may cause overwhelming sepsis. Patients who undergo elective splenectomy should be immunized well in advance of surgery. The exact timing for immunization is unknown, but longer than 1 week before surgery is probably sufficient. After splenectomy, it is wise to wait until the patient is nutritionally intact and recovers from other injuries before administering the vaccination. Vaccinations against *H. influenzae* type B and *N. meningitidis* are available and should be considered for asplenic patients. Conjugate vaccines are now available and recommended for children; however, their efficacy after splenectomy is not clearly defined.

Long-term antibiotic prophylaxis with oral penicillin is a reasonable approach in immunologically compromised patients (e.g., renal transplant recipients), those receiving chemotherapy, and children younger than 6 years of age who undergo splenectomy. This approach does not provide definite prophylaxis for a number of reasons, including lack of compliance, inconvenience, and bacterial resistance.

People who undergo splenectomy should carry identification that explains their medical condition. They should also be instructed to contact their physician at the first sign of any minor infection (e.g., cold, sore throat). Antibiotics should be prescribed and the patient followed closely.

Anatomic Complications After Splenectomy

Morbidity and mortality rates after splenectomy are relatively low. Older patients and those with severe underlying conditions have the highest morbidity and mortality rates.

Atelectasis is the most common problem after splenectomy. It is usually caused by reduced respiratory excursion secondary to high abdominal incisions and irritation of the diaphragm. Atelectasis usually resolves within 2 to 3 days if it is properly treated. Improperly treated, atelectasis can progress to pneumonia. Pleural effusions may be associated with atelectasis, but are more often associated with a subphrenic abscess. Subphrenic fluid may collect in the space left by the spleen. This situation occurs secondary to bleeding, inflammation, or leak of pancreatic fluid as a result of injury to the tail of the pancreas. Abscesses are more likely to occur if the gastrointestinal tract is opened. The placement of prophylactic drains increases the risk of subphrenic abscess. These drains are rarely used unless a pancreatic injury is identified. Subphrenic abscesses are usually apparent within 5 to 10 days after surgery. Signs include fever, pain, pleural effusion, prolonged atelectasis, pneumonia, and prolonged leukocytosis. Ultrasonography and CT scanning are useful for identifying abscesses. Once identified, they are promptly drained, either percutaneously with image guidance or operatively.

Injury to the pancreas occurs in 1% to 3% of patients who undergo splenectomy. It may be clinically unrecognized and cause mild hyperamylasemia or may cause clinical pancreatitis, pancreatic fistula, or pancreatic pseudocysts. Serum amylase or lipase determination on the second to fourth day after surgery may help to identify the pancreatic injury. Symptoms and signs (nausea and vomiting, abdominal distension, abdominal pain and pulmonary complications, such as those seen with a subphrenic abscess) usually develop within 4 to 5 days after splenectomy.

Likewise, injury to the stomach may occur while the short gastric vessels are being divided. This injury may lead to the development of a subphrenic abscess or gastrocutaneous fistula. Some surgeons advocate nasogastric decompression for 2 to 3 days after splenectomy to avoid gastric distension and prevent complications. Care is taken to reinforce the gastric wall, where the short gastric vessels have been clipped or ligated in close proximity to the gastric wall, to prevent problems.

Bleeding at splenectomy usually occurs when it is performed for massive splenomegaly (because of the friability of dilated veins).

Persistent hemorrhage after splenectomy occurs in less than 1% of cases. It usually occurs in patients who undergo splenectomy for thrombocytopenia, especially those in whom the platelet count does not respond to splenectomy. Reoperation to gain hemostasis is considered if bleeding continues after coagulation abnormalities are corrected or if hemodynamic instability occurs.

SUGGESTED READINGS

Altamura M, Caradonna L, Amati L, et al. Splenectomy and sepsis: the role of the spleen in immune-mediated bacterial clearance. *Immunopharmacol Immunotoxicol* 2001;23(2):153–161.

Chadburn, A. The spleen: anatomy and anatomical function. *Semin Hematol* 2000;37(Suppl):13–21.

Coon, WW. Surgical aspects of splenic disease and lymphoma. *Curr Probl Surg* 1998;35(7):543–646.

Fixler, J, Styles L. Sickle cell disease. *Pediatr Clin North Am* 2002;49(6): 1193–1210.

Hansen, K, Singer, DB. Asplenic-hyposplenic overwhelming sepsis: postsplenectomy sepsis revisited. *Pediatr Dev Pathol* 2001;4(2): 105–121.

Katkhouda,N, Mavor, E. Laparoscopic splenectomy. *Surg Clin North Am* 2000;80(4):1285–1297.

Lo L, Singer, ST. Thalassemia: current approach to an old disease. *Pediatr Clin North Am* 2002;49(6):1165–1191.

Peitzman AB, Ford HR, Harbrecht BG, et al. Injury to the spleen. *Curr Probl Surg* 2001;38(12):932–1008.

Stasi R, Provan D. Management of immune thrombocytopenic purpura in adults. *Mayo Clin Proc* 2004;79(4):504–522.

Tse WT, Lux SE. Red blood cell membrane disorders. *Br J Haematol* 1999;104(1):2–13.

23

JAMES F. MCKINSEY, MD ■ PETER F. LAWRENCE, MD
BRUCE L. GEWERTZ, MD

Diseases of the Vascular System

OBJECTIVES

Arterial Disease: Atherosclerosis, Aneurysms, Peripheral Arterial Occlusive Disease, and Cerebrovascular Insufficiency

1. Describe five risk factors for the development of atherosclerosis.
2. List three specific sites that have a predilection for atherosclerotic plaque, and explain why this predilection exists.
3. List at least two clinical sequelae of atherosclerosis and three ways to retard the atherosclerotic process.
4. List the common sites and relative incidence of arterial aneurysms.
5. List the symptoms, signs, differential diagnosis, and diagnostic and management plans for a patient with a rupturing abdominal aortic aneurysm.
6. Discuss the risk factors, indications, and contraindications for repair in patients with nonruptured abdominal aortic aneurysms.
7. Compare the presentation, complications (i.e., frequency of dissection, rupture, thrombosis, and embolization), and treatment of thoracic, abdominal, femoral, and popliteal aneurysms.
8. Define and discuss the prevention of the common complications of aneurysm surgery.
9. Describe the pathophysiology of intermittent claudication, and differentiate this symptom from leg pain from other causes.
10. Describe the diagnostic approach and medical management of arterial occlusive disease of the upper and lower extremities.
11. Describe the treatment options available for chronic occlusive disease of the distal aorta and iliac arteries, superficial femoral and popliteal arteries, and tibial and peroneal arteries.
12. List the criteria to help differentiate among venous, arterial, diabetic, and infectious leg ulcers.
13. List four indications for amputation, and discuss the methods used to select the amputation site.
14. Describe the clinical manifestations, diagnostic workup, and surgical indications for chronic renal artery occlusion.
15. Describe the natural history and causes of acute arterial occlusion, and differentiate between embolic and thrombotic occlusion.
16. List six signs and symptoms of acute arterial occlusion, and outline its management (e.g., indications for medical versus surgical treatment).
17. Define and differentiate among the following:
    - **A** Amaurosis fugax
    - **B** Transient ischemic attacks
    - **C** Cerebrovascular accident (stroke)
18. Outline the diagnostic methods and the management of a patient with asymptomatic carotid artery disease.

19 List the differential diagnoses and outline a management and treatment plan for patients with transient ischemic attacks and stroke due to carotid disease.

20 Differentiate between hemispheric and vertebrobasilar symptoms.

Venous Disease: Superficial Vein Thrombosis, Deep Vein Thrombosis, Pulmonary Embolus, Chronic Venous Insufficiency, and Varicose Veins

1 Identify the usual initial anatomic location of deep vein thrombosis, and discuss the clinical factors that lead to an increased incidence of this problem.

2 Identify the noninvasive testing procedures used to diagnose deep vein thrombosis and venous valvular incompetence.

3 Outline the differential diagnosis of acute edema associated with leg pain.

4 Describe five modalities to prevent the development of venous thrombosis in surgical patients.

5 Describe the methods used to administer anticoagulant and thrombolytic agents. Discuss how the adequacy of therapy is evaluated, and describe the contraindications to therapy.

6 Describe the clinical syndrome of pulmonary embolus, and identify the order of priorities in diagnosing and caring for an acutely ill patient with life-threatening pulmonary embolus.

7 List the indications for surgical intervention in venous thrombosis and pulmonary embolus.

8 Describe the management of a patient with varicose veins and chronic venous insufficiency.

9 Outline the diagnostic, nonoperative, and operative management of venous ulcers.

Vascular Trauma

1 List the indications for arteriography in a patient with a possible arterial injury to the extremities.

2 In a patient with recent trauma, outline the physical findings, diagnostic plan, and treatment for suspected arterial injury.

Vasospastic and Lymphatic Disorders

1 List five underlying diseases or disorders associated with vasospastic changes in the extremities, and discuss their diagnosis and treatment.

2 Describe the anatomic mechanisms that cause thoracic outlet compression syndrome, and discuss the appropriate diagnostic studies and treatment.

3 Define lymphedema praecox, lymphedema tarda, primary lymphedema, and secondary lymphedema.

4 Explain the pathophysiology of lymphedema and discuss its treatment.

ARTERIAL DISEASE

Anatomy

The three layers of the arterial wall are the intima, media, and adventitia (Fig. 23-1). The internal elastic lamina separates the intima from the media, and the external elastic lamina separates the media from the adventitia. The endothelium, which is derived from hemangioblasts, lines the inner aspect of the intima and has a collective mass that is greater than that of the liver. The endothelial layer was previously believed to be an inert interface between blood and the arterial wall, but it is now known that the endothelial cells are highly active metabolically. The endothelium functions as an antithrombotic surface that expresses protein C, protein S, antithrombin 3, and nitric oxide, and aids in the regulation of vascular tone by both vasodilation and vasoconstriction. The myogenic tone of the blood vessels is further modified by the production of endothelium-derived relaxing factor and prostacyclins, which contribute to arterial vasodilation. Conversely, platelet-derived growth factor and angiotensin II trigger arterial vasoconstriction.

The media is the thickest layer of the arterial wall. It is composed chiefly of smooth muscle cells, along with a connective tissue matrix that includes elastin, collagen, and proteoglycans. The strength of the media is derived from collagen. Its elasticity is provided by elastin. The smooth muscle cells and surrounding matrix are organized into discrete circular bundles, or lamellae. Larger vessels, which have more than 28 lamellar units, have vasovasorum that penetrate the adventitia to perfuse the media. Arteries that have fewer than 28 lamellar units are oxygenated directly from the blood within the vessel. The adventitia is the outermost layer. It extends beyond the external elastic lamina and is composed of loose connective tissue, fibroblasts, capillaries, and neural fibers. The adventitia provides little strength to the artery. It is the site of vessel nutrition and neural innervation and is important in containing hemorrhage after trauma or aneurysmal rupture.

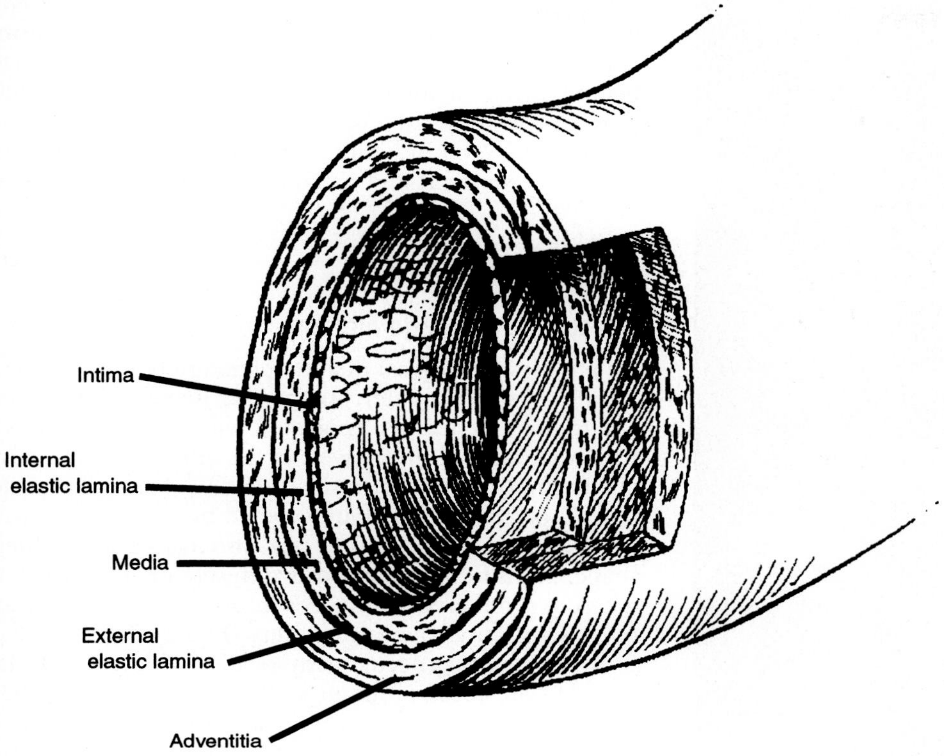

Figure 23-1 Layers of the arterial wall.

Atherosclerosis

The most common cause of arterial stenosis and occlusion is **atherosclerosis,** a degenerative disease that is characterized by endothelial cell dysfunction, inflammatory cell adhesion and infiltration, and the accumulation of cellular and matrix elements, leading to the formation of fibrocellular plaques. In the end stages of the disease, advanced plaques impede blood flow and lead to the well-known ischemic syndromes of angina pectoris, intermittent **claudication** of the arms or legs, and renovascular hypertension. More sudden events (e.g., myocardial infarction, stroke, atheroembolism) may be caused by unstable plaques, which may rupture the fibrous cap into the lumen, hemorrhage in the substance of the plaque, and ultimately cause acute occlusion or **embolism.**

Risk factors for the development of atherosclerosis include cigarette smoking, hypertension, abnormalities in cholesterol metabolism (elevated levels of low-density lipoprotein and depressed levels of high-density lipoprotein), diabetes mellitus, obesity, coagulation disorders, and regions of turbulence within the arterial circulation; the Framingham Study has shown the additive effect of multiple risk factors. The first signs of atherosclerosis may appear as early as childhood or adolescence. They are manifested by lipid- and macrophage-laden fatty streaks that form on the endothelial surface. These lesions progress to fibrous plaques that are usually located at areas of flow disturbance. Fibrous plaques generally consist of lipid-laden macrophages encapsulated by collagen and elastin. As the fibrous plaque matures, regions within the plaque become necrotic and eventually rupture, leading to plaque ulceration. Within these complex plaques, regions of microcalcification develop that can progress to significant calcium deposits. Although atherosclerosis is usually considered a systemic disease, plaques tend to localize in specific regions. The most common sites of atherosclerotic plaques are within the coronary arteries, the carotid bifurcation, the proximal iliac arteries, and the adductor canal region of the arteries of the legs. Regions of arterial bifurcation are most predisposed to the development of atherosclerotic plaques because of turbulence at the flow divider that results in regions of low shear stress and flow stagnation (Fig. 23-2). This stasis allows greater contact time between the atherogenic factors in the blood (e.g., lipids) and the vessel wall. It appears that smoking is a greater risk factor for peripheral atherosclerosis (incidence nine times that of the normal population) than for coronary atherosclerosis (incidence four times that of the normal population).

The common sequelae of atherosclerosis are: (1) myocardial infarction or angina pectoris as a result of coronary atherosclerosis; (2) **transient ischemic attack (TIA)** or stroke as a result of carotid bifurcation atherosclerosis; and (3) lower extremity ischemia that causes intermittent claudication, difficulty in walking, **rest pain,** or gangrene. Less common clinical presentations are renal hypoperfusion due to renal artery stenosis and small bowel ischemia due to mesenteric stenosis or occlusion. The symptoms of arterial stenosis are caused by either gradual progressive occlu-

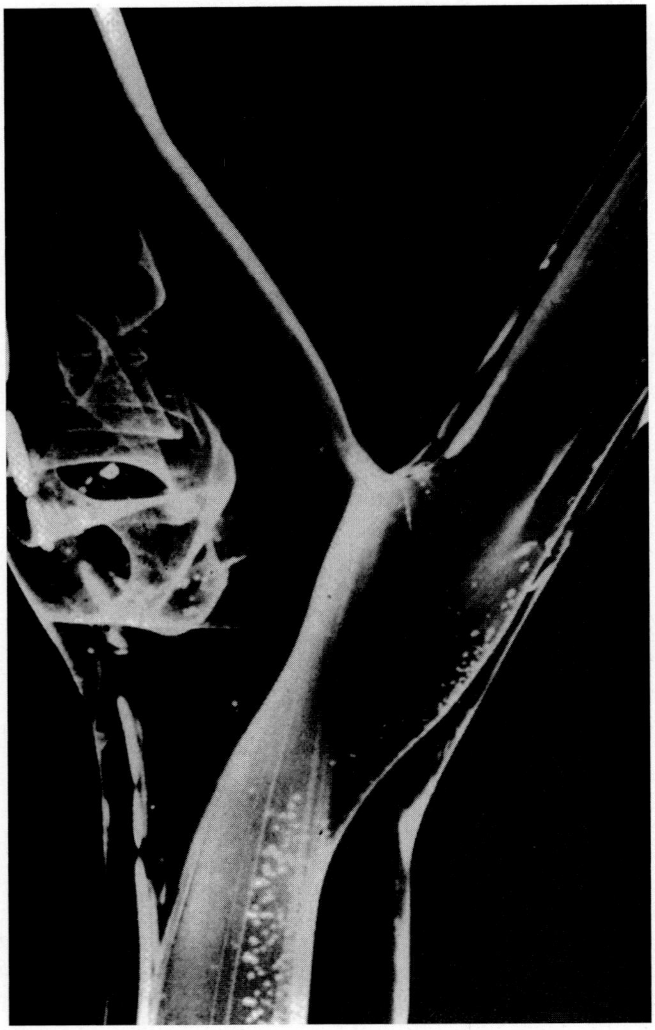

Figure 23-2 Glass model of the carotid bifurcation. Hydrogen gas bubbles show the streamlining of flow fields at the carotid flow divider and the complex counterrotating helical pattern at the arterial wall opposite the flow divider. (Reprinted with permission from Zarins CK, Glagov S. Arterial wall pathology in atherosclerosis. In Rutherford RB, ed. *Vascular Surgery.* 4th Ed. Vol. 1. Philadelphia, PA: WB Saunders, 1996:214.)

sion from an enlarging plaque that limits distal perfusion or a sudden **thrombosis** of the artery at a region of stenosis. Sudden arterial occlusion does not allow for the development of collateral arterial channels, but gradual stenosis of the artery allows for the development of arterial collaterals to maintain distal perfusion. The result is either sudden ischemia or more gradual-onset chronic ischemia. Plaque ulcerations often become a nidus for thrombus formation or platelet deposition. Distal embolization of this material may produce an acute occlusive event and sudden onset of symptoms.

Atherosclerosis is a progressive event. The best way to retard its progression is to modify the atherosclerotic risk factors. Programs that use a combination of risk factor modifiers such as beta-blockers, statins, angiotensin-converting enzyme (ACE) inhibitors, and nutrition have been shown to dramatically reduce the incidence of cardiovascular events. Exercise has a protective effect by increasing the level of high-density lipoproteins, which enhance the transport and metabolism of other lipids.

Aneurysms

Anatomy and Epidemiology

An **aneurysm** is a focal dilation of an artery to more than 1.5 its normal diameter. Aneurysms may be either true aneurysms (generally associated with atherosclerosis), which include all three layers of the arterial wall, or false aneurysms (**pseudoaneurysms**), which occur secondary to trauma or infection and are covered by only a thickened fibrous capsule. Aneurysms are also classified by their shape. A fusiform aneurysm is diffusely dilated, whereas a saccular aneurysm is an eccentric outpouching of an otherwise normal-appearing artery (Fig. 23-3).

Aneurysms may occur in any location within the arterial tree, but are most common in the infrarenal aorta, iliac arteries, and popliteal arteries (Table 23-1). It is estimated that 2% to 3% of men older than 70 years of age have an aortic aneurysm, but patients with high-risk factors may have an incidence of up to 10%. Aneurysmal formation is a systemic and familial disease. A patient with one popliteal aneurysm has a 60% chance of having an aneurysm in the contralateral popliteal artery and a 50% chance of harboring an abdominal aortic aneurysm (AAA). Approximately 20% of patients with AAAs have a first-degree relative with the same disease.

Pathophysiology

Approximately 90% of all aneurysms are associated with atherosclerosis. Atherosclerosis probably impairs the diffusion of nutrients and allows for metalloproteinase-mediated arterial wall degeneration. Recent studies have demonstrated increased levels of matrix-metalloproteinase (MMP)-2 and MMP-9 in early AAA, and abundance of MMP-9 levels in patients with larger AAA. The poorly developed vasovasorum of the infrarenal aorta likely contributes to this effect, explaining the predilection of aneurysm formation in this location. Less common causes of aneurysm formation include connective tissue disease (Marfan's syndrome, Ehlers-Danlos syndrome), infection (mycotic aneurysm), cystic medial degeneration, disruption of anastomotic connections (anastomotic pseudoaneurysm), and trauma (traumatic pseudoaneurysm) (Table 23-2).

The most serious complication of aneurysms is their propensity for enlargement and rupture. The growth rate of aneurysms is unpredictable. Although most AAAs enlarge at an average rate of approximately 0.3 cm/year, the range of expansion rates is wide; some aneurysms double

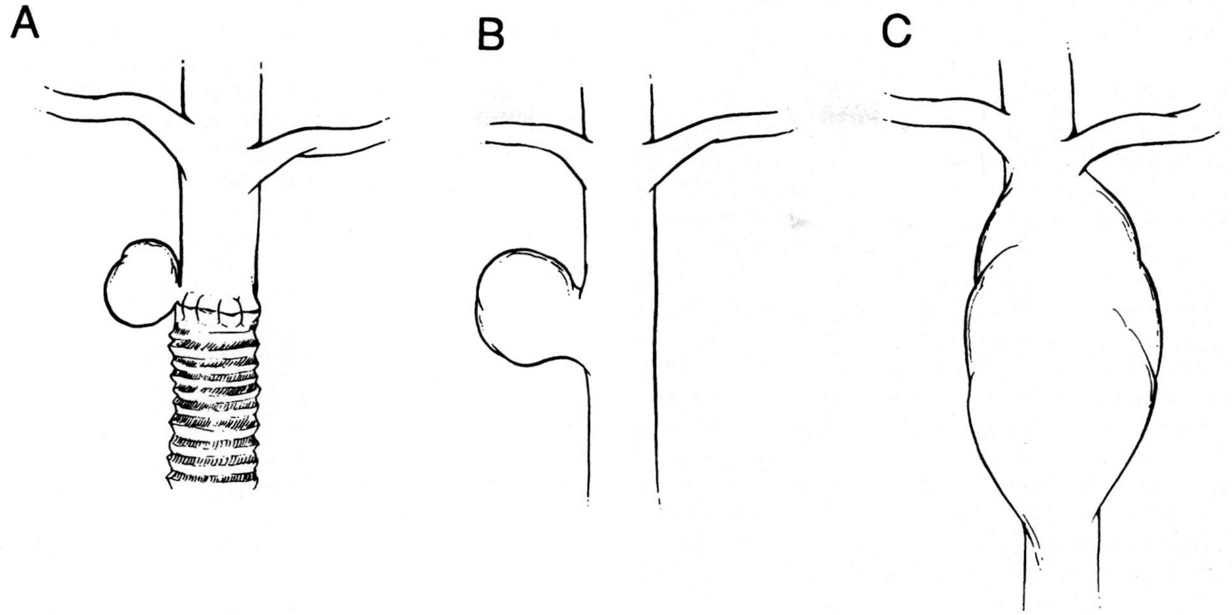

Figure 23-3 Classification of aneurysms. **A,** Pseudoaneurysm. **B,** Saccular atherosclerotic aneurysm. **C,** Fusiform atherosclerotic aneurysm.

in size over a few months. The size of an aneurysm is critically important because the risk of rupture is diameter-dependent. According to a modification of the law of Laplace, the larger and thinner an aneurysm grows, the higher its tangential wall stress *(J)*:

$$J = P \times r/t,$$

where P = intraluminal pressure, r = aneurysm radius, and t = wall thickness.

The slow flow within the aneurysmal portion of the artery can also lead to thrombus formation along the wall,

Table 23-1 Localization and Incidence of Abdominal Aneurysms

Location of Aneurysm	Incidence
Abdominal aortic artery	1.5%–3.0%
Common iliac artery	20%–40% present with AAA 0.03% isolated, without AAA
Splenic artery	0.8% 60% of all splanchnic artery aneurysms
Renal artery	0.1%
Hepatic artery	0.1%
Superior mesenteric artery	0.07%
Celiac axis	0.05%

AAA, abdominal aortic artery.

Table 23-2 Etiology of Aneurysmal Disease

- Congenital
  - Idiopathic
  - Tuberous sclerosis
  - Turner's syndrome
  - Poststenotic dilation
- Inherited abnormalities of connective tissue
  - Marfan's syndrome
  - Ehlers-Danlos syndrome
  - Cystic medial necrosis
- Dissection
- Infections
  - Mycotic
  - Posttraumatic
  - Infection of existing aneurysm
- Inflammatory
- Aneurysms associated with pregnancy
  - Splenic artery
  - Mesenteric vessels
  - Renal artery
- Aneurysms associated with arteritis
  - Takayasu's disease
  - Giant cell arteritis
  - Polyarteritis nodosa
  - Systemic lupus erythematosus
- Pseudoaneurysm
- Nonspecific aortic aneurysms: "atherosclerotic"

which may either embolize (peripheral aneurysms) or stimulate MMPs and aneurysm growth.

Clinical Presentation and Evaluation

Aneurysms are usually discovered as asymptomatic pulsatile masses on routine physical examination or during diagnostic tests for other conditions. Approximately 20% of aneurysms cause symptoms, including localized pain or tenderness, thrombosis or distal embolization that causes peripheral ischemia, and rupture (Fig. 23-4). The clinical presentation reflects the location of the aneurysm. Abdominal and thoracoabdominal aortic aneurysms tend to be discovered during routine examination or, if ruptured, as a clinical catastrophe that causes acute back pain, hypotension, and hemodynamic collapse. Popliteal and femoral aneurysms rarely rupture, but laminated thrombus along the wall can dislodge and embolize into the arteries of the calf and foot, causing acute arterial ischemia. Carotid artery aneurysms may cause either asymptomatic pulsatile neck masses or cerebrovascular ischemia, including TIAs or stroke.

The diagnosis of aortic and peripheral artery aneurysms may be made during a careful physical examination. If an aneurysm is suspected, the patient should undergo diagnostic evaluations. The best screening tool for aortic and peripheral aneurysms is ultrasonography. A well-performed ultrasound assesses the size and general location of the aneurysm with more than 95% accuracy. If the diagnosis of AAA is established, the patient should undergo computed tomography (CT) scanning to evaluate the full extent of the aneurysm and better assess the need for intervention. In the past, most AAAs were further evaluated with invasive contrast angiography. Because of improvements in the performance and interpretation of CT scans, however, many patients proceed to operation without angiography if they are relatively free of atherosclerotic arterial occlusive disease. Routine angiography is still advised for peripheral artery aneurysms to plan the arterial reconstruction.

Treatment

The natural history of AAAs is to enlarge and rupture. Patients with AAAs have a greatly decreased life expectancy compared with age-matched controls. Aneurysm rupture is expected to cause as many as 60% of deaths. The risk of rupture is directly related to the diameter of the aneurysm; most clinical studies show that a 4-cm AAA has an annual risk of rupture of less than 5% (5-year risk of rupture is 25%), but the annual rate increases to 15% when the AAA reaches 6 cm (Fig. 23-5). Two recent studies, the United Kingdom

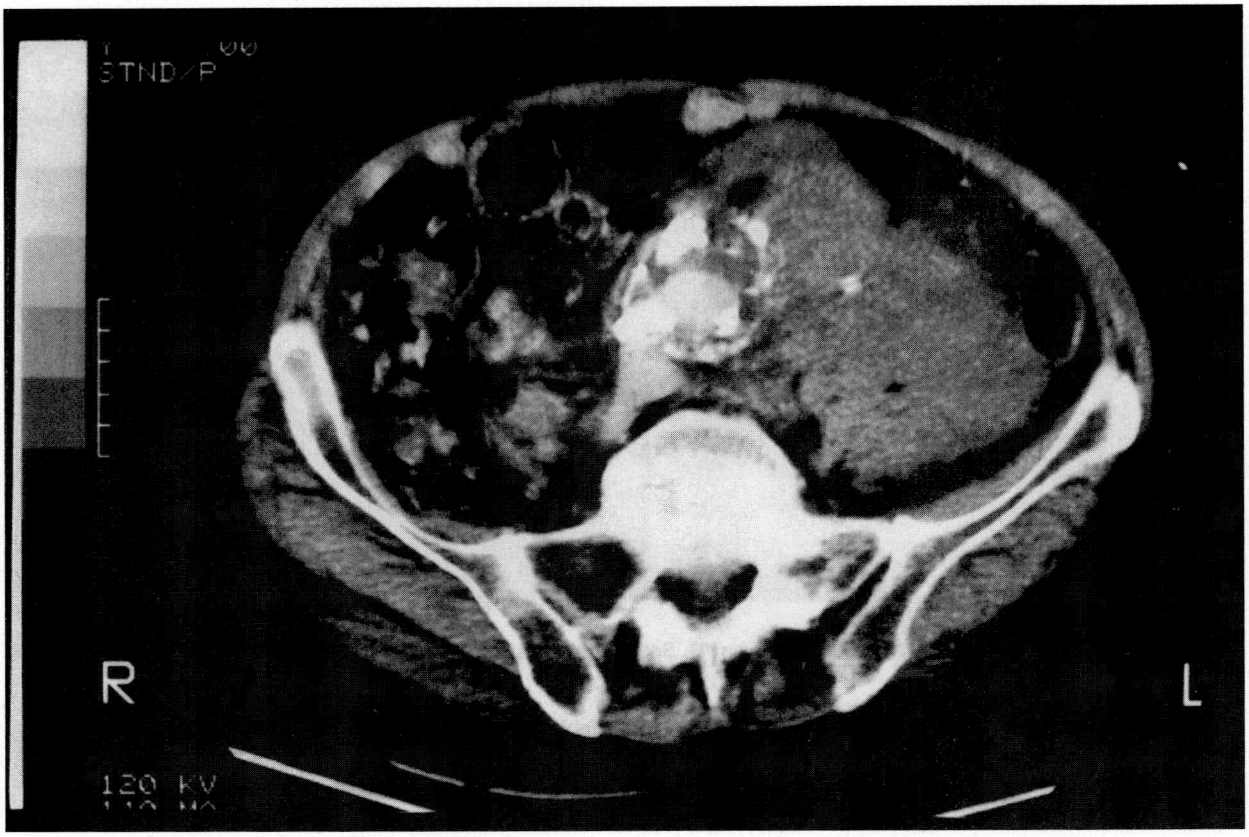

Figure 23-4 Computed tomography scan of a calcific abdominal aortic aneurysm with a contained rupture into the left retroperitoneum.

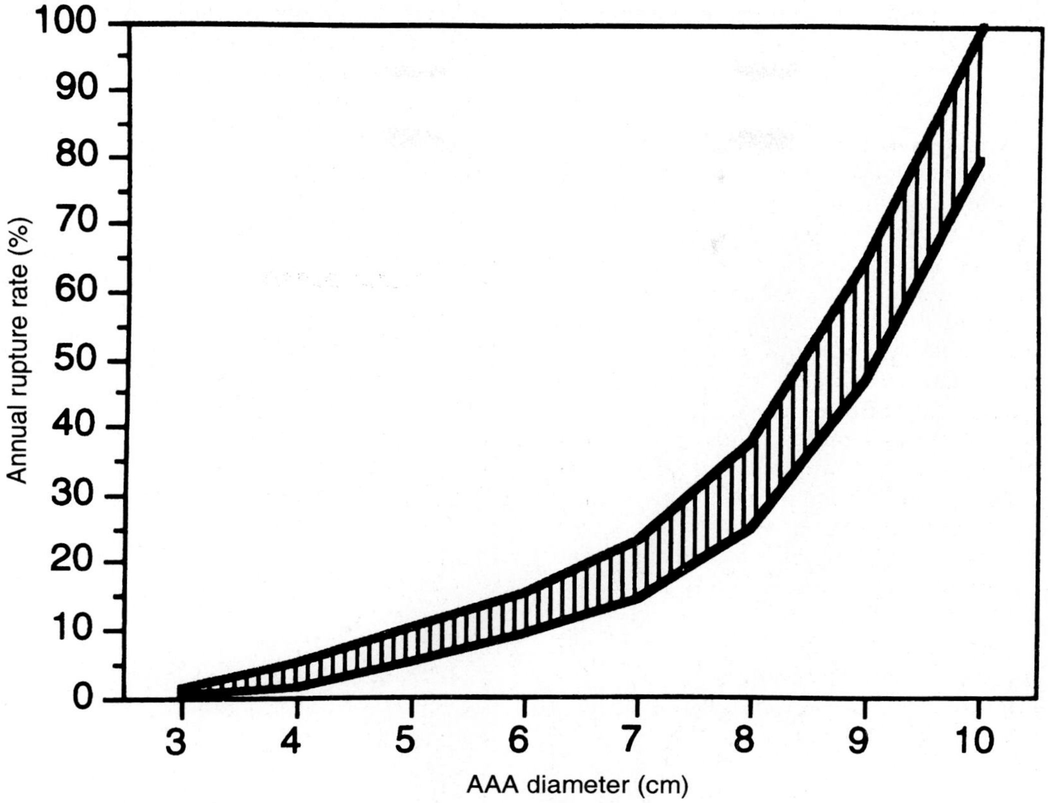

Figure 23-5 The annual risk of aneurysm rupture according to size. AAA, abdominal aortic artery. (Reprinted with permission from Sampson LN, Cronenwett JL. Abdominal aortic aneurysm. *Probl Gen Surg* 1995;2:385–417.)

Small Aneurysm Trial and the VA Cooperative Small Aneurysm study, demonstrated that "all cause" mortality was equivalent in patients with asymptomatic AAAs between 4 cm to 5.5 cm. This would indicate that patients may be followed by surveillance with asymptomatic AAAs less than 5.5 cm. However, other studies have noted that women have a fourfold increased risk of rupture in aneurysms greater than 5 cm, probably due to the smaller size of the native aorta. Patients with serious risk factors (e.g., coronary artery disease, renal insufficiency, pulmonary disease) are managed more conservatively. Nonetheless, most clinicians recommend repair whenever the anticipated risk of rupture exceeds the risk of surgery. This occurs in patients with an AAA greater than 5.5 cm or one that is tender on exam. The conventional elective surgical treatment of AAAs is usually accomplished with an abdominal incision. The normal proximal aorta and distal arteries are dissected and isolated. After heparinization, the aorta is clamped and the aneurysm incised. A prosthetic graft is sewn in place and covered with the residual aneurysm sac (Fig. 23-6). Aneurysms that involve the iliac arteries or the more proximal portions of the abdominal or thoracic aorta are technically more challenging, but good results are consistently reported in modern series. The operative mortality for elective repair of an infrarenal AA is less than 5% in good-risk patients. The evolution of sophisticated catheter techniques and devices led to the development of the endovascular graft as an alternative to traditional operative AAA repair. The procedure involves placing prosthetic grafts with wire supports and attachment sites through the femoral or iliac arteries into the infrarenal aorta and iliac arteries (Fig. 23-7). The first aortic stent grafts were originally designed for repair of an aneurysm of the aorta without iliac involvement; however, they did not afford long-term success mainly due to leaks at the distal aortic attachment site. This has led to endovascular grafts that bridge the infrarenal aorta to both iliac arteries. Endovascular repair of abdominal aortic aneurysms is associated with decreased blood loss, a shortened hospital stay, and a more rapid return to normal activity. The disadvantages of endovascular repair include the need for an intensive followup requiring annual abdominal CT scans, an increased rate of secondary interventions to correct problems with the fixation of the aortic graft, leakage of blood into the aortic aneurysm sac, and increased renal dysfunction secondary to the contrast agents used for visualization of the graft and the aorta during implantation. Recent studies have shown decreased short-term mortality with endovascular repair compared to conventional open aortic repair, but long-term data are still required.

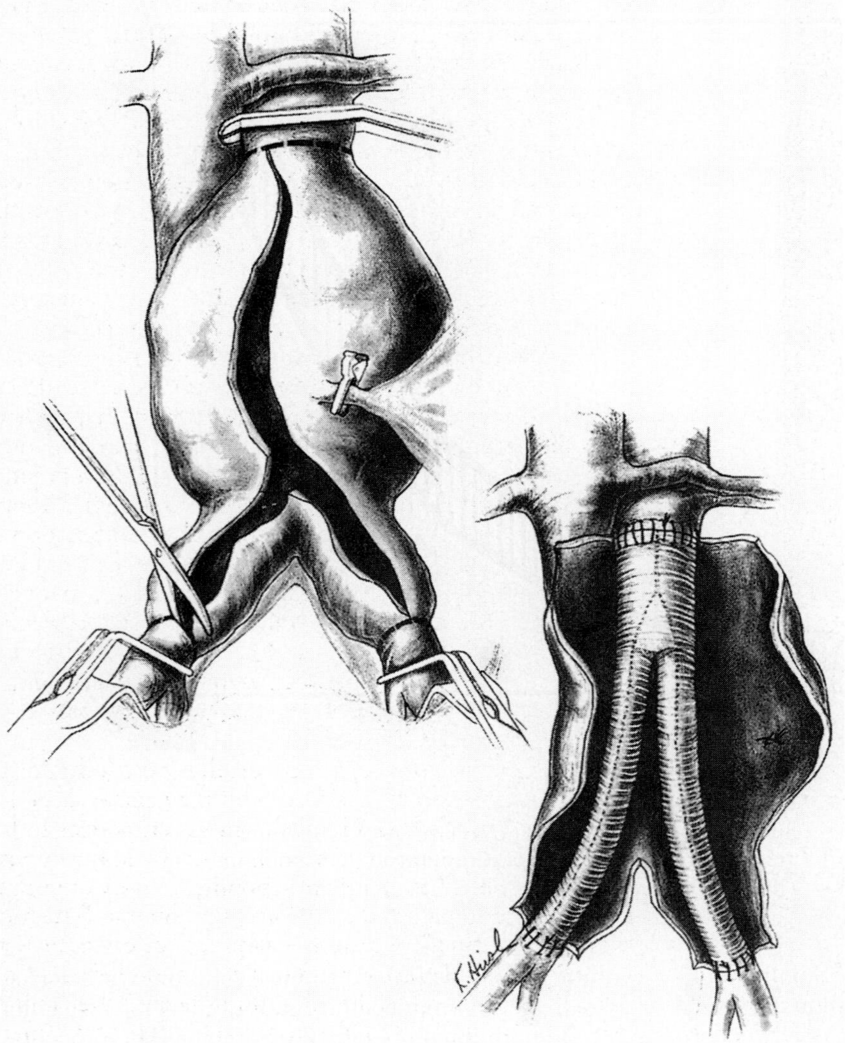

Figure 23-6 Repair of an abdominal aortic aneurysm and a bilateral iliac artery aneurysm with an aortoiliac bypass graft. (Reprinted with permission from Zarins CK, Gewertz BL. Aneurysms. In: *Atlas of Vascular Surgery.* New York, NY: Churchill Livingstone, 1989:51.)

Patients who have rupture of an aneurysm have a dismal prognosis unless they are immediately treated. Patients who present with a pulsatile abdominal mass, hypotension, and back or flank pain must be taken to the operating room for repair. They should be carefully resuscitated with fluid and blood products while being prepared for operation. Current practice is a technique of "restricted resuscitation" of volume, titrated to a systolic blood pressure, to maintain it between 70 and 80 mm Hg with maintenance of mental status. This technique strives to minimize ongoing blood loss through the aortic defect. Even in the best of hands, the survival rate for operations for AAA rupture is less than 50%, and many survivors have major complications, including renal dysfunction, myocardial infarction, extremity amputation, and cerebrovascular accident. Endografts are being increasingly used to repair ruptured AAAs.

Popliteal aneurysms are generally repaired if they exceed 2 cm in diameter, if there is evidence of thrombus formation in the aneurysm wall, or following distal embolization. As stated earlier, preoperative angiography is essential for planning the reconstruction and, occasionally, for delivering thrombolytic (clot busting) therapy to recanalize thrombosed distal vessels. In contrast to AAA repair, popliteal aneurysm repair is best accomplished with open surgery. The preferred conduit is saphenous vein graft, because of its superior patency record for below-the-knee revascularization, although prosthetic graft may be used for short segment popliteal aneurysms.

Complications

Immediate complications after elective repair of aortic aneurysms include myocardial infarction (3% to 16%), renal failure (3% to 12%), colonic ischemia (2%), distal emboli, and hemorrhage. Long-term complications include aortic graft infection, graft thrombosis, and pseudoaneurysm formation. Aortic graft infection can occur 5 to 7 years later as a pseudoaneurysm, because of the breakdown of the graft-to-artery anastomosis. Gradual disruption of the proximal or

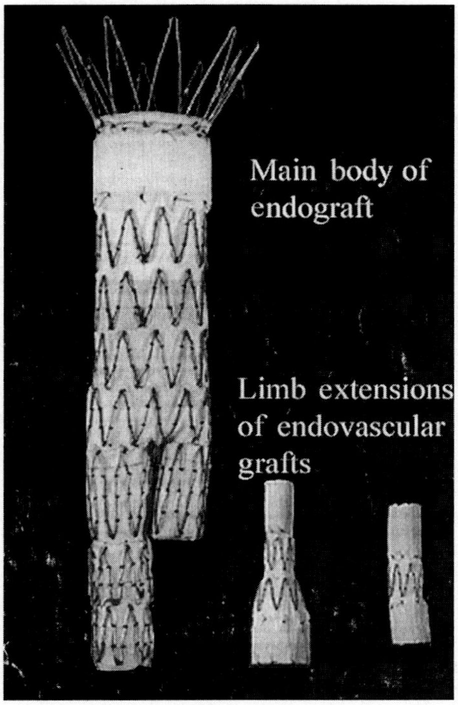

Figure 23-7 Example of an endovascular aortic stent graft (Zenith; Cook, Inc., Bloomingdale, Indiana.) There is a main body of the graft that is implanted in the aorta just below the renal arteries and then limb extensions that are intussuscepted into the gates for extension into the iliac arteries. The diameter of the distal aspect of the extension limbs comes in multiple sizes to allow for treatment of different-sized iliac arteries.

distal anastomotic suture lines, unassociated with infection, may cause anastomotic pseudoaneurysms to form. They are usually amenable to repair with interposition grafting.

After aortic repair, colonic ischemia can result from the disruption of pelvic arterial collateral flow, ligation of the inferior mesenteric artery, or perioperative hypotension. The patient with postoperative colonic ischemia will have colonic emptying, guaiac-positive diarrhea, or abdominal pain. Patients who have diarrhea immediately postoperatively, with or without blood, should undergo sigmoidoscopy to further evaluate the viability of the sigmoid colon and rectum. If the colon is frankly infarcted, then the affected colonic portion should be resected and a colostomy performed. However, if the colon appears dusky, but without frank necrosis, then the patient is treated with blood pressure support, broad-spectrum antibiotics, and frequent repeat sigmoidoscopy to follow the ischemic recovery.

Endoleak is a complication associated with the endovascular repair of aortic and iliac aneurysms. An endoleak represents leakage of blood into the aneurysm sac. Endoleaks are classified as types I to IV. A type I endoleak represents an attachment site leak at either the proximal or distal attachment site. This is associated with a high rate of expansion and rupture and should be repaired with either placement of an additional graft or stent or replacement of the endovascular graft with an open repair. A type II endoleak represents persistent flow into and out of the aneurysm sac from lumbar or inferior mesenteric arteries. Generally, type II endoleaks are not treated unless there is expansion of the aneurysm sac or symptoms. Type III endoleaks occur from a modular disconnection between components of the stent graft or a tear in the fabric of the graft. They should be repaired when identified. A type IV endoleak is due to leakage of blood through the graft and generally will resolve once the anticoagulation therapy is reversed at the conclusion of the surgical procedure.

Graft infection, with or without a fistula between the aorta and duodenum (**aortoenteric fistula**), is a devastating long-term complication with a mortality rate that exceeds 50%. It should be suspected in any patient with an aortic graft who has chronic infection, sepsis, abdominal pain, or gastrointestinal bleeding. The diagnosis is often difficult to establish, but may be confirmed with a combination of CT or white blood cell scanning, blood cultures, endoscopy, and surgical exploration. Some patients are managed with antibiotics and in situ graft replacement (replacing the graft with a new graft at the same site), but most undergo graft excision with duodenal repair and either autogenous replacement or extraanatomic bypass to restore extremity perfusion.

Popliteal artery aneurysms classically cause either distal emboli or thrombosis. Distal emboli may cause "blue toe syndrome," in which a mural thrombus embolizes to the digital vessels of the foot, resulting in localized thrombosis and gangrene. Thrombosis of a popliteal artery aneurysm has a poor prognosis and a 50% amputation rate. The morbidity rate is high because the popliteal artery aneurysm generally thromboses only after it has showered multiple emboli to the lower extremity, thrombosing the outflow vessels. This sequence has prompted the use of preoperative thrombolytic therapy to lyse the obstructed outflow vessels before arterial reconstruction.

Aortic Dissection

Aortic dissection results from a tear in the intima, with extension of a pulsatile blood column traveling through the media of the thoracic and abdominal aorta. These lesions classically begin in the thoracic aorta (Stanford type A involves the ascending thoracic aorta and type B is limited to the descending aorta), but the dissection can extend into the abdominal aorta and compromise the arterial blood supply to the mesenteric circulation, renal circulation, spinal cord, or distal extremities. Complications from an ascending aortic dissection are related to either retrograde or antegrade propagation of the dissection. With retrograde dissection toward the aortic valve, the origins of the coronary arteries can be obstructed, resulting in acute myocardial ischemia. The dissection can also extend into the aortic valve leaflets and result in acute aortic valve insufficiency. The most devastating complication is proximal extension of the dissection into the aortic root and free rupture into the pericardial sac, which results in cardiac tamponade. Dissection can also extend into the brachiocephalic vessels and cause stroke. The diagnosis of an aortic dissection is confirmed by transesophageal echocardiography, CT scan, or angiography. Acute management of aortic dissection is directed at lowering the blood pressure and heart rate to decrease the stress on the arterial wall. Acute intervention is reserved for dissections that involve the ascending aorta or those that begin in the descending thoracic aorta and occlude the mesenteric, renal, or iliac vessels and result in sudden ischemia. Enlargement of a chronic dissection with aneurysm formation is the main indication for elective repair.

Peripheral Arterial Occlusive Disease

Occlusion or stenosis of the arteries of the lower extremities is usually called peripheral arterial disease (PAD). Common sites that are predisposed to the development of atherosclerotic plaques include the iliac, superficial femoral, and tibial arteries. Specific symptoms are dictated by the number and severity of occlusions, the degree of collateralization, and the patient's tolerance to limitations in walking distance. Stenosis or occlusion of the aorta and iliac arteries (aortoiliac occlusive disease) is more common in adults between 40 and 60 years of age. The predilection to aortoiliac disease is increased by cigarette smoking, hypertension, and hyperlipidemia. Disease confined below the inguinal ligament is known as femoropopliteal occlusive disease. The most common pattern of occlusion is disease of the distal superficial femoral artery within the adductor (Hunter's) canal. Femoropopliteal occlusive disease may be asymptomatic unless a patient participates in extensive exercise, due to collateralization from the profunda femoris artery. Involvement of the arteries below the popliteal trifurcation is called tibial occlusive disease or simply distal disease. Tibial occlusive disease is common in patients with diabetes, end-stage renal failure, and advanced age.

Physiology

Large atherosclerotic plaques occlude the arterial lumen, impede blood flow, and diminish blood pressure distal to the stenosis. The loss of pressure (for steady flow of a Newtonian liquid) is described by Poiseuille's law:

$$\Delta P = 8Q\,L\,\eta/\pi\, r_i^4,$$

where ΔP = change in pressure, Q = volume of blood flow, L = arterial length, η = density, and r = arterial radius. As noted, the loss in pressure is directly proportional to the volume of blood flow and the arterial length, but inversely proportional to the fourth power of the radius. A decrease in radius has the most profound effect on ΔP. In general, ΔP is small until the reduction in diameter is approximately 50% (75% reduction in cross-sectional area), when it increases exponentially with greater narrowing.

The enlargement of an atherosclerotic plaque is the leading cause of development of symptoms of peripheral vascular arterial occlusive disease. Studies have shown that the vessel initially adapts to the atherosclerotic plaque and enlarges its overall diameter. Once maximal enlargement is attained, this compensation is exhausted, and the luminal area is progressively decreased by the atherosclerotic process (Fig. 23-8). Other potential causes of arterial occlusive disease are Buerger's disease (thromboarteritis obliterans) and cystic adventitial disease. Although it is much less common, extraluminal compression of the arterial system can occur as a result of compression of the artery by aberrant muscular bands (e.g., popliteal artery entrapment syndrome and cervical rib).

Clinical Presentation

Ischemia of the lower extremity can cause intermittent claudication, ischemic rest pain, skin ulceration, and gangrene. The degree of ischemia determines the type or extent of presentation. Claudication, from the Latin *claudatio* (to limp), is characterized by reproducible pain in a major muscle group that is precipitated by exercise and relieved by rest. The joints and foot are generally spared, because they have little muscle mass. Although these patients maintain adequate arterial perfusion at rest, arterial occlusions prevent the augmentation of blood flow that is necessary to meet the metabolic demands of active mus-

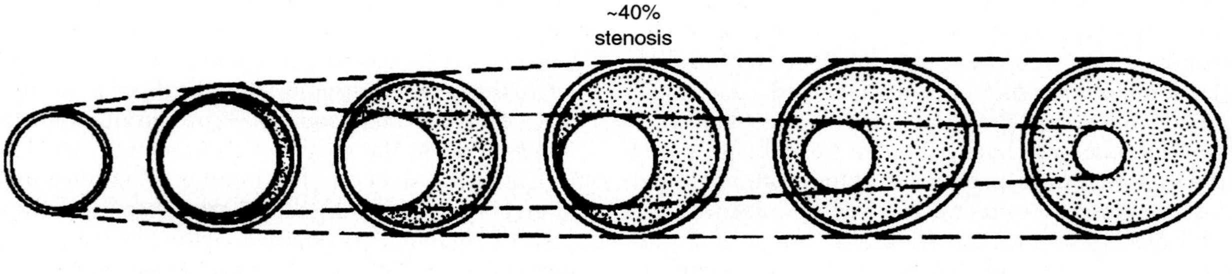

Figure 23-8 Proposed arterial adaptation to enlarging atherosclerotic plaques. Initially, the artery enlarges to maintain the luminal diameter despite the enlarging plaque. After the plaques create a stenosis of more than 40%, the artery can no longer adapt, and a luminal stenosis develops. (Reprinted with permission from Glagov S, Weisenberg E, Zarins CK, et al. Compensatory enlargement of human atherosclerotic coronary arteries. *N Engl J Med* 1987;316:1371.)

cles during exercise. The result is conversion to anaerobic metabolism and local metabolic acidosis. The muscle groups that are affected by claudication are always distal to the level of arterial obstruction. Hence, aortoiliac occlusion classically causes Leriche syndrome (defined by impotence, absence of femoral pulses, lower extremity claudication, and muscle wasting of the buttocks). Occlusion of the superficial femoral artery causes calf, but not thigh, claudication, since the thigh blood supply comes from the profunda femoris artery.

The natural history of untreated claudication is generally benign. In the Framingham study, the risk of major amputation was only 5% within 5 years if claudication was treated conservatively. With cessation of cigarette smoking and an organized exercise program, as many as 50% of patients with claudication improve and their symptoms completely resolve. The most common cause of death in patients with claudication is a cardiac or cerebral event.

Ischemic rest pain indicates more advanced peripheral ischemia, just as rest angina is a more advanced form of exertional angina. Most commonly, patients have pain in the toes and metatarsal heads while lying down at night. Temporary relief is achieved by dangling the legs over the side of the bed or standing and walking around the room. By making the feet more dependent, gravitational hydrostatic pressure increases venous pressure, slows capillary flow, and temporarily enhances oxygen delivery. Rest pain is caused by nerve ischemia of tissues that are most sensitive to hypoxia. Nocturnal cramps in the calf muscle, unassociated with impairment of blood flow, can usually be distinguished from true rest pain by the location of the pain (calf versus distal foot) and the absence of advanced ischemic changes in the skin.

Ulceration of the skin of the toes, heel, or dorsum of the foot can occur as a result of arterial insufficiency. Even minor trauma (e.g., friction from an ill-fitting shoe), incorrect nail care, or a small break in the skin can lead to chronic, progressive ulceration as a result of insufficient arterial perfusion. Ulcerations usually cause pain, except in patients with diabetes, who often have associated peripheral neuropathy. Ischemic ulcers may have a punched-out appearance and a pale or necrotic base. By comparison, venous ulcerations usually occur at the level of the medial or lateral malleolus ("gaiter zone"). They are usually associated with venous pooling and red blood cell extravasation that leads to an orange–brown skin discoloration secondary to hemosiderin deposition. The ulcers are located at the level of the medial and lateral malleoli because of the presence of perforating veins that connect the superficial and deep venous systems at the level of the ankle. Venous ulcerations may have a granulating base and are usually associated with significant edema and/or scarring of the subcutaneous tissue (lipodermatosclerosis). Treatment of venous stasis ulcerations is generally conservative (discussed later).

Diabetic ulcerations are painless and are located on the plantar or lateral aspect of the foot. They are a direct result of the neuropathy of diabetes. Because of the injury to the autonomic, motor, and sensory nerves, the skin becomes dry and the foot can become deformed (Charcot's foot) and asensate. The changes associated with diabetes are worsened by the arterial occlusive process that usually accompanies diabetes.

The outlook for patients with rest pain is far worse than that for patients with claudication. If untreated, nearly 50% of patients with rest pain need amputation for intractable pain or gangrene within a short period.

Dry and wet gangrene are differentiated clinically. Dry gangrene is mummification of the digits of the foot without associated purulent drainage or cellulitis. Wet gangrene is gangrene associated with ongoing infection. The severely ischemic foot is an excellent nidus for the colonization and growth of bacteria and is generally malodorous, with copious purulent drainage. The outlook is ominous, with potential sepsis and immediate limb loss, unless the necrotic tissue is removed and the limb is revascularized.

Physical Examination

Routine evaluation of patients with peripheral vascular disease (PVD) includes a thorough physical examination and noninvasive vascular testing. A search for coexisting vascular disease by auscultation for cervical **bruits,** precordial gallops or murmurs, and pulsatile masses or bruits in the abdomen is mandatory. Examination of the lower extremity includes inspection, palpation, and auscultation. Inspection of the legs and feet in a patient with PVD may show loss of hair on the distal aspect of the leg, muscle atrophy, color changes in the leg, and ulcers or gangrene. Patients with severe PVD often have Buerger's sign (dependent rubor). With dependency of the foot, pooling of oxygenated blood in the maximally dilated arteriolar bed distal to an arterial occlusion causes the foot to appear ruborous (red). When the extremity is elevated, hydrostatic pressure decreases, allowing drainage of pooled blood, and the foot becomes white (pallor). Palpation should include investigation of the presence and character of the arterial pulsations at the groin (femoral artery), at the popliteal fossa (popliteal artery), at the dorsum of the foot (dorsalis pedis artery), and posterior to the medial malleolus (posterior tibial artery). All questionable pulses should be confirmed by Doppler ultrasound. Patients who do not have palpable pulses should be examined with continuous-wave Doppler ultrasound. The Doppler probe emits 2- to 10-MHz ultrasonic waves that are reflected by flowing red blood cells and detected by a receiving crystal. The frequency shift between the transmitting and the receiving crystals is proportional to the velocity of the moving particles and provides a qualitative assessment of the degree of stenosis. Normally, a triphasic waveform is seen, representing the forward flow of systole, reversal of the arterial velocity waveform against the relatively high-resistance vascular bed, and resumption of forward flow during diastole. If proximal stenosis is present, the pulse volume from cardiac contraction loses kinetic energy crossing the area of stenosis and does not have enough energy to recoil against the vascular outflow bed. As a result, the Doppler signal becomes biphasic. With further progression of proximal arterial stenosis, the waveform becomes more blunt and widened, and it eventually becomes monophasic (Fig. 23-9).

In addition to this qualitative assessment of disease, the systolic pressure within the arteries of the foot can be determined. A blood pressure cuff is inflated in the calf and then slowly deflated while the Doppler signal is monitored. The pressure at which a signal reappears is the systolic pressure within the artery. The pressure is normalized for all patients by dividing the ankle pressure by the systolic blood pressure in the arm and calculating the **ankle-brachial index** (ABI). In general, an ABI less than 0.8 is consistent with claudication, whereas an ABI less than 0.4 is usually associated with rest pain or tissue loss.

Advances in ultrasound technology have led to better anatomic correlation with arterial duplex scanning. Duplex scanners provide visualization of blood flow within the artery in two dimensions and calculate the velocity of flowing blood. In regions of significant stenosis, high-velocity jets are seen as blood travels through the narrow lumen.

Patients with severe lifestyle-limiting claudication, rest pain, or gangrene should undergo diagnostic magnetic resonance arteriography (MRA) or contrast arteriography. Arteriography is performed with a percutaneous femoral artery puncture, advancement of a wire and catheter into the abdominal aorta, and injection of radiopaque contrast agent for visualization of the distal arterial tree. Complications of these tests, including idiosyncratic dye reactions, contrast agent nephropathy, and puncture site hemorrhage, are infrequent, but mandate careful patient selection. MRA is increasingly being used to evaluate blood flow in small vessels, although it currently overestimates the degrees of some stenoses.

Differential Diagnosis

Intermittent claudication can be differentiated from musculoskeletal or neurogenic pain by a careful history, physical examination, and noninvasive vascular evaluation. Neurogenic lower extremity pain is usually not located in major muscle groups and is rarely precipitated by exercise. Straight-leg raised lifts and findings of sensory examinations may be abnormal. Musculoskeletal pain is often present at rest. Pain secondary to spinal stenosis is relieved by bending forward while walking. It often radiates down the limb and is not relieved immediately (< 5 minutes) by resting. If the clinical assessment is confusing, patients should be walked on a treadmill. Claudicators will drop their ABI when symptoms occur, while other causes of leg pain will not.

Diagnostic Angiograms in Vascular Disorders

Angiography has been traditionally considered to be the "road map for the surgeon." However, the development over the past 10 to 15 years of endovascular therapy for PAD, including the rise of minimally invasive balloon angioplasty stents and thrombolysis, has led to the angiogram playing a more important role in intervention. "Diagnostic" angiography is increasingly being replaced by duplex ultrasonography to identify peripheral arterial stenoses and occlusions. Magnetic resonance angiography and CT angiography have been replacing intraarterial angiography for diagnosis. Consequently, intraarterial angiography is used as the initial step in the treatment of PAD prior to placement of arterial balloons and stents.

The most commonly used technique for angiography involves puncture of a peripheral artery, with passage of an intravascular catheter for selective injection of arteries (Seldinger technique) (Fig. 23-10). A needle and then a guidewire are percutaneously inserted into the femoral artery and advanced into the aorta under X-ray guidance. A catheter is then inserted over the wire into the aorta. After removal of the wire, liquid contrast is injected into the catheter. This contrast mixes with the blood and is radiopaque. Wherever the blood travels so does the contrast and regions of enlargement (aneurysms) or narrowing (stenosis) are visualized. The femoral artery is often used; axillary and brachial arteries are also used.

The principal complications of angiography include

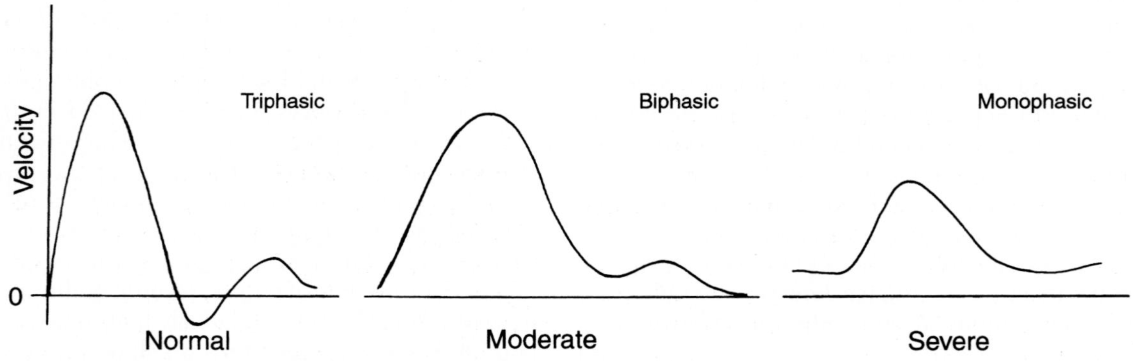

Figure 23-9 A Doppler ultrasound instrument provides an analog display of blood flow velocity (waveform). With progressive occlusion, the waveform changes from triphasic to biphasic to monophasic.

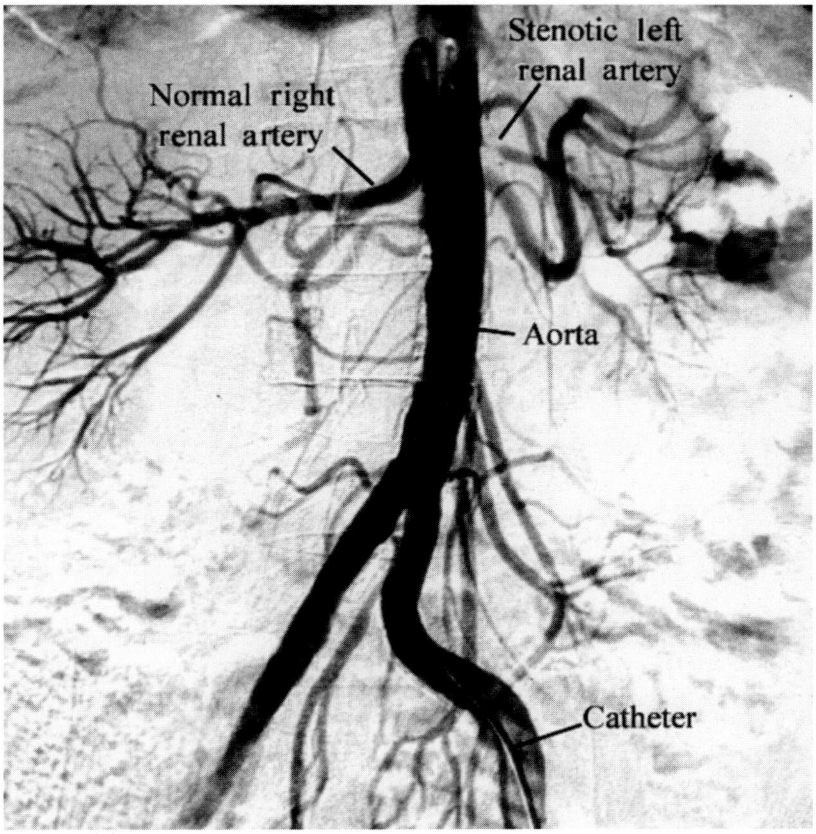

Figure 23-10 Example of an angiogram of the abdominal aorta. A proximal left renal artery stenosis is visualized.

bleeding around the puncture site, thrombosis at the puncture site from an intimal flap caused by passage of the catheter, formation of a pseudoaneurysm, hypersensitivity reaction to the iodinated dye, and contrast-related renal toxicity, especially in diabetic patients. Bleeding may be immediate or delayed and may cause a pseudoaneurysm later. The initial presentation of local bleeding includes paresthesias in the involved limb because of compression of adjacent nerves. Thrombosis usually occurs within 6 hours of arterial puncture, but may occur days later. Pseudoaneurysms secondary to catheter trauma may be thrombosed by duplex-directed compression, especially in patients who are not undergoing anticoagulation therapy. If compression therapy is not successful, then surgical exposure, with closure of the puncture site and repair of the injured intima, is appropriate.

In patients with known hypersensitivity to iodinated contrast material, steroids and antihistamines can be administered before the procedure to decrease the incidence and severity of reactions. All patients should be questioned carefully about previous allergic reactions before angiography or venography is performed. Hydration before and after angiography is important in all patients, particularly those with renal insufficiency. Judicious use of diuretic also decreases nephrotoxicity

Treatment

Medical

As many as 50% of patients with intermittent claudication obtain significant relief with cessation of smoking and a regimented exercise program. Treatment with cilostazol (Pletal) is often helpful, although the extent of improvement ranges from 30% to 50%. Some patients with painless ischemic ulcers respond to conservative local therapy while they are followed closely for progression or the development of gangrene. Since atherosclerosis is a generalized disease, all PVD patients should be treated with beta-blockers, statins, and ACE inhibitors to reduce the rate of progression of atherosclerosis.

Endovascular Treatment of PAD. Since the first reported success of balloon dilation of coronary vessels in 1979, the technique of percutaneous transluminal angioplasty (PTA) has been used to treat short segment stenosis of peripheral arteries (Fig. 23-11*A* and *B*). PTA entails the passage of a thin wire (0.014 to 0.035 inch) through the region of stenosis or occlusion from a remote percutaneous puncture site. A balloon catheter is then passed over the wire and inflated in the region of narrowing, thereby dilating the vessel and increasing the luminal diameter. This

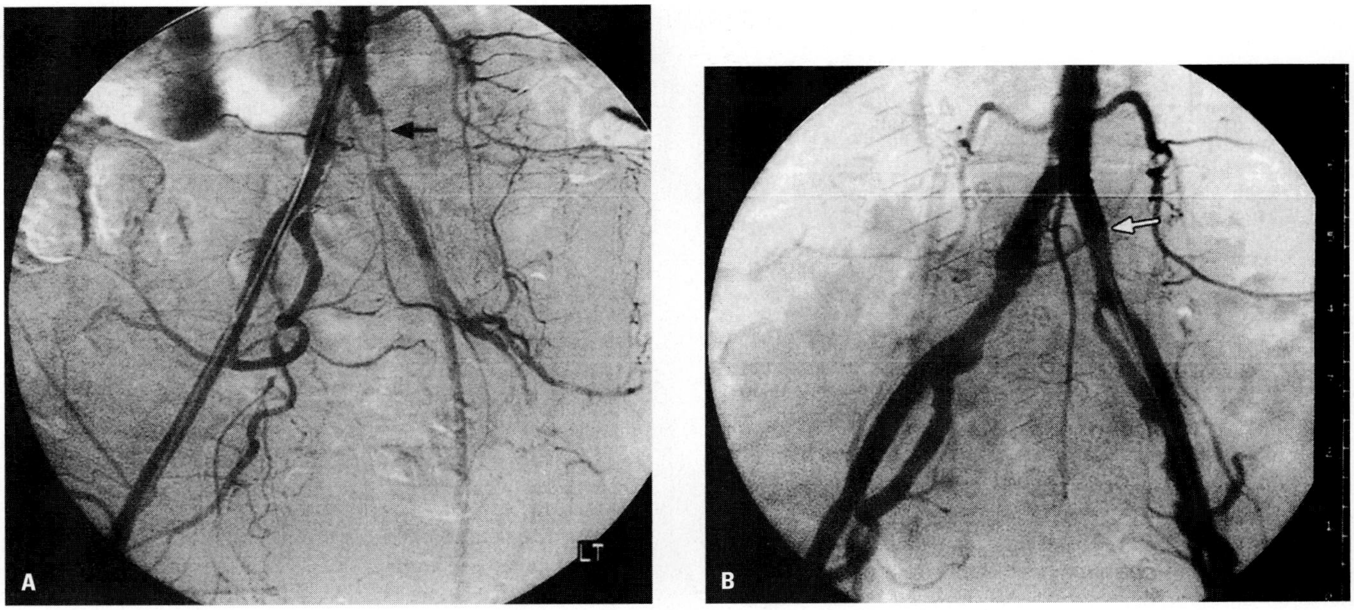

Figure 23-11 **A,** Angiogram showing a short segment occlusion of the proximal left common iliac artery (*solid arrow*). **B,** Successful percutaneous balloon angioplasty of the iliac lesion (*open arrow*).

has been expanded to include long-segment stenosis and even occlusion in the last 10 years. Subintimal dissection of an occluded artery can also be performed to create a new channel that can angioplastied to allow flow through the wall of the vessel without a surgical bypass. PTA can be complicated by both acute vessel occlusion and restenosis. The incidence of interval restenosis has been reported to be between 20% and 50% in most arterial beds at 1 year. Acute vessel occlusion is best ascribed to elastic recoil, vasospasm, plaque rupture, and dissection. Introduction of percutaneous transluminal coronary angioplasty (PTCA) combined with stenting of the coronary vessels has resulted in decreased acute occlusion, decreased overall rate of re-intervention, and decreased angiographic incidence of restensosis when compared to PTCA alone.

Experience in percutaneous intervention on noncoronary vascular lesions has shown similar results. Table 23-3 summarizes studies in both renal and iliac arterial sites. The renal vessels have demonstrated between 11% and 26% angiographic restenosis at more than 6 months; iliac vessels demonstrate 68% to 93% primary patency at 1 year by clinical exam and noninvasive testing. Unlike data in PTCA/stent studies, the peripheral stent studies have less rigorous angiographic followup, relying more on noninvasive studies and clinical endpoints, therefore increasing the potential for underreporting of asymptomatic restenosis (reduction of lumen diameter $\geq$ 50%).

Angioplasty of the infrapopliteal and tibial vessels is reserved for patients who are poor surgical risks or who only need to heal a traumatic foot ulcer, because only 40% to 50% of these vessels remain patent after 1 year. Carotid angioplasty and stenting has recently been proposed for treatment of carotid atherosclerosis and will be compared with carotid surgery in future clinical trials.

Stents have improved the technical result of angioplasty and reduced the incidence of acute vessel occlusion; however, studies demonstrate the potential for later reduction of luminal diameter associated with stent placement. The complication of luminal diameter reduction from 6 months to 1 year postprocedure is best explained by development of neointimal hyperplasia. This has been described as an inflammatory mediated process resulting in prolonged cellular proliferation, monocytic invasion, and ultimately smooth muscle cell migration and collagen deposition. Restenosis due to in-stent intimal hyperplasia continues to limit the long-term efficacy of minimally invasive interventions. Multiple adjunct procedures are being used to decrease the incidence of restenosis, including treating the stents with a coating of antimyoproliferative agents, brachytherapy, and synthetic coverings. These techniques are still being evaluated for long-term success.

Surgical

Endarterectomy. Endarterectomy (excision of the diseased arterial wall, including the endothelium, the occluding plaque, and a portion of the media) is the standard operative treatment for carotid bifurcation atherosclerosis. Endarterectomy has more limited usefulness in the treatment of lower extremity occlusive diseases because lower extremity atherosclerotic disease is often extensive, with no discrete starting or ending points. Few patients with aortoiliac disease are candidates for aortoiliac endarterectomy,

Table 23-3 Success of Percutaneous Angioplasty

Iliac Artery

	n	Initial Success	2-Year Patency
Vorwerk et al.	121	97%	88%
Strecker et al.	116	100%	95%
Henry et al.	184	99%	91%
Martin et al.	140	97%	71%

Renal Angioplasty/Stent

	n	Initial Failure	Complications	Patency
Losinno, 1993	256	5%	7.6%	86% (102 months)
Bonelli, 1995	396	20%	8%	83% (43 months)
Blum, 1997	74	0%	4%	89% (24 months)

but many surgeons use local endarterectomy of the common femoral artery and profunda femoral arteries to improve outflow for an aortofemoral bypass graft.

Bypass Procedures. Bypass procedures are the principal operative treatment for PAD. Aortoiliac occlusive disease is usually treated with aortobifemoral bypass. With a combination of abdominal and groin incisions, a prosthetic graft is sutured to the infrarenal aorta and tunneled through the retroperitoneum to both femoral arteries (Fig. 23-12). In cases of concomitant superficial artery occlusion, the profunda femoris artery is the primary outflow bed. Aortofemoral bypass grafting is a durable procedure with a 5-year patency rate of greater than 90%. Aortofemoral bypass graft limb occlusion is usually caused by the progression of distal outflow disease, which limits blood flow through the graft, causing stasis and thrombosis.

If the patient is a prohibitive surgical risk for an intraabdominal procedure or has had multiple intraabdominal procedures or infections (hostile abdomen), extraanatomic bypasses are considered. Extraanatomic bypasses include axillary artery–femoral artery bypass grafts and femoral artery–femoral artery bypass grafts. These grafts are tunneled in the subcutaneous tissue. In critically ill patients, this procedure may be performed with local anesthesia and intravenous sedation. The patency rates for extraanatomic bypasses are lower than those for aortofemoral bypass grafts, especially in the presence of superficial femoral artery occlusion. Occlusions can also occur secondary to the longer length of the bypass graft. Graft compression or kinking also may occur within the subcutaneous tunnels.

In patients with rest pain and occluded superficial femoral arteries with proximal profunda femoral artery stenoses, opening the stenoses (profundaplasty) can assist by increasing perfusion through the collaterals. However, if the ischemia has progressed to tissue loss or gangrene, it is unlikely that the profundaplasty alone can adequately increase arterial inflow into the leg to heal the ulcerative lesions. In this case, arterial bypass is performed.

Patients who have femoropopliteal occlusive disease are best treated with bypass of the occluded segment. Duplex arterial imaging or diagnostic arteriography is used to ensure that the patient has adequate arterial inflow into the femoral arteries as well as to identify the distal target vessel—usually the popliteal or tibial artery. Bypass to the popliteal artery above the knee is performed with either the patient's own veins (autologous vein) or a polytetrafluoroethylene graft with equivalent initial results. In contrast, prosthetic bypasses to arteries below the knee function more poorly. These distal bypass procedures are best accomplished with autologous vein (Table 23-4). Saphenous vein bypass grafts can be reversed so that the venous valves are in the same direction as arterial flow. The disadvantages of this orientation are the need for complete removal of the vein from its nutrient bed as well as a potential size mismatch between the proximal aspect of the saphenous vein and the small distal artery. Alternatively, in situ bypasses can be performed in which the saphenous vein is left in its normal anatomic position and the vein valves are disrupted with a valvulotome. This approach allows a better size match between the artery and the vein. Disadvantages of in situ bypass include endothelial injury during passage of the valvulotome and the possibility of missing a valve cusp (retained valve). Arteries (e.g., radial, subscapular) can occasionally be used for bypass to small vessels in the leg or foot.

Postoperative duplex graft surveillance of saphenous vein bypass grafts is effective in identifying regions of anastomotic and graft stenosis that, if uncorrected, could lead to graft failure. The combination of duplex graft surveillance and surgical reintervention with repair of stenotic lesions, which occurs in 20% of grafts, results in higher

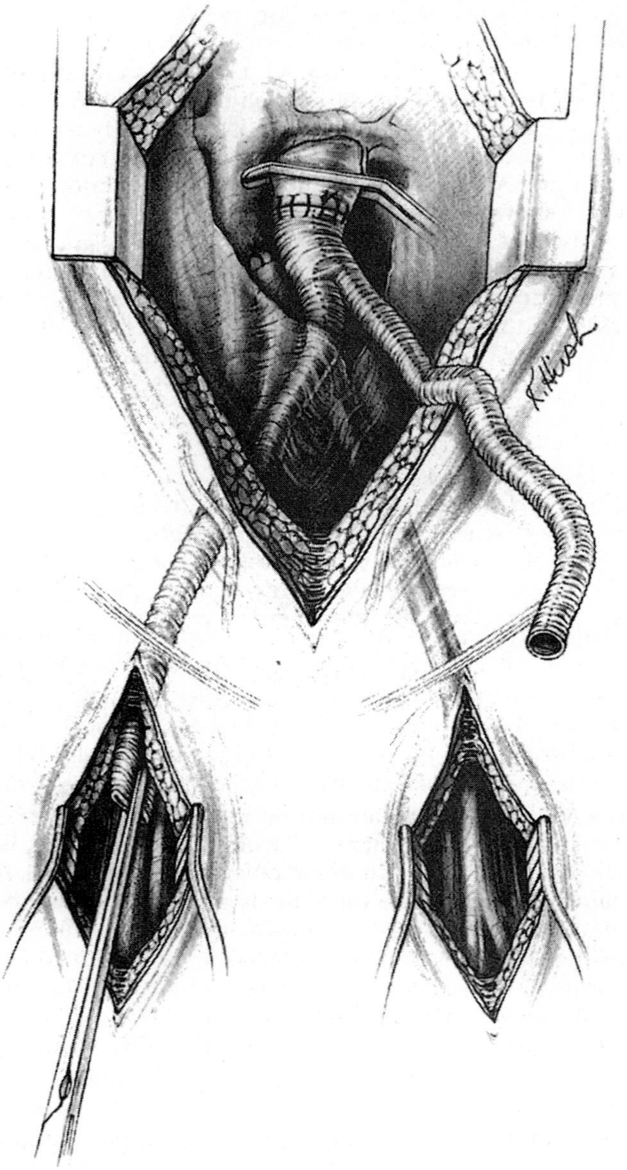

Figure 23-12 Aortobifemoral bypass graft showing the creation of the retroperitoneal tunnels to the groins. (Reprinted with permission from Zarins CK, Gewertz BL. Aneurysms. In: *Atlas of Vascular Surgery.* New York, NY: Churchill Livingstone, 1989:125.)

long-term patency of the saphenous vein bypass graft. The assisted patency rates of these vein grafts approach 90%. In contrast, if a stenosis of a saphenous vein graft is allowed to progress to occlusion and then is revised, the patency rate at 2 years is only 30%.

Immediate complications of arterial bypass graft procedures are often caused by technical problems (e.g., postoperative bleeding from the anastomotic site, graft thrombosis, hematoma in the graft tunnel, lymphatic leakage that results in a lymphocele). Because many patients with peripheral arterial occlusive disease have concomitant coronary artery disease, renal insufficiency, or pulmonary obstructive disease, postoperative complications are always a concern.

Aortoduodenal fistula is one of the most devastating complications of aortofemoral bypass grafting. If it is not properly covered, the aortic graft anastomosis can erode into the third portion of the duodenum and contaminate the aortic graft with duodenal contents. In this circumstance, the arterial anastomosis is weakened, and massive bleeding can occur into the bowel. A long-term problem associated with arterial bypass graft procedures is progressive arterial occlusive disease of the outflow vessels that results in graft thrombosis. Graft infection and pseudoaneurysm formation can also occur, and do so more frequently when prosthetic graft is used.

Amputation. Amputation may be the only option in patients with severe rest pain or gangrene who are not candidates for revascularization or who do not have a suitable target vessel for a distal bypass. Partial foot amputation, with removal of areas of gangrene, may be required to augment a successful distal bypass. An amputation is virtually never performed for venous disease without coexisting arterial insufficiency. In general, the more distal the amputation is, the better is the rehabilitation potential. Distal amputations include toe, transmetatarsal, and Syme's (ankle) amputations. If arterial inflow is inadequate and an arterial bypass cannot be performed, then a below-the-knee (BKA) or above-the-knee (AKA) amputation may be required.

It is important to choose the appropriate site for amputation to ensure adequate wound healing. If there is an occluded and unreconstructable superficial femoral artery and if there are no distal vessels below the knee, a BKA amputation is often the lowest level that will heal. If the perfusion pressure is greater than 50 mm Hg at the popliteal artery and the ABI is greater than 0.6, then healing is expected in more than 70% of cases. It is important to attempt to preserve the knee joint, because significantly more energy is required to ambulate with an AKA prosthesis.

AKA amputation is required when profound ischemia and gangrene extend to the knee. At this higher amputation level, healing is likely, even in advanced ischemia. AKA amputation is also indicated in patients who are bedridden or a high surgical risk because of other medical conditions.

Chronic Intestinal Ischemia

Pathophysiology

The visceral arterial supply includes the celiac axis, superior mesenteric artery, and inferior mesenteric artery. If one of the major visceral vessels becomes stenotic or occluded, the gastroduodenal artery and marginal artery can supply significant collateral flow (Fig. 23-13). After occlu-

Table 23-4 Outcomes of Infrainguinal Arterial Bypasses

Graft Type	2-Year Patency (%) Primary/Secondary	4-Year Patency (%) Primary/Secondary
Above-knee femoropopliteal, PTFE	75	60
Above-knee femoropopliteal, vein	80	70
Below-knee femoropopliteal, PTFE	60	40
Below-knee femoropopliteal, vein	75–80/90	70–75/80
Femoral-tibial bypass, PTFE	30	20
Femoral-tibial bypass, vein	70–75/80–90	60–70/75–80

PTFE, polytetrafluoroethylene.

sion of two of the three major arterial pathways to the visceral organs, patients often have visceral ischemic symptoms.

Clinical Presentation

The clinical manifestations of chronically decreased blood supply to the intestine (chronic intestinal ischemia) include postprandial abdominal pain and weight loss. Postprandial pain usually occurs 1/2 to 1 hour after meals and ranges from a persistent epigastric ache to severe, disabling, cramping pain. Other symptoms include early satiety and abdominal bloating. Many patients have a fear of food because of postprandial pain and limit their oral intake. This factor accounts for the significant weight loss seen in many patients. Associated comorbid atherosclerotic symptoms are often present (e.g., coronary artery disease, claudication, cerebrovascular accident). The malnutrition associated with chronic visceral ischemia suggests a differential diagnosis that includes disseminated carcinomatosis and primary visceral malignancies.

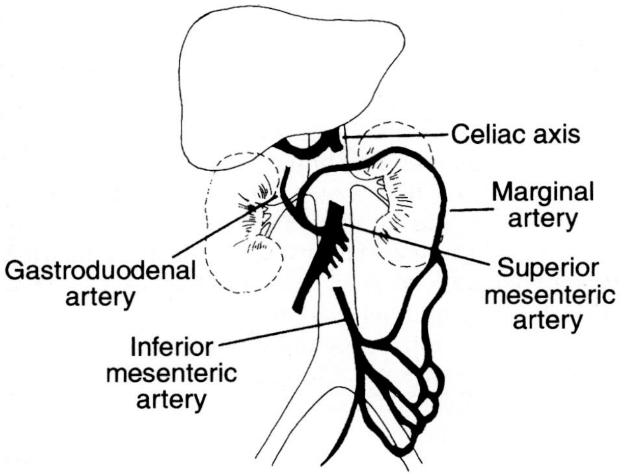

Figure 23-13 The intestinal circulation is characterized by three main vessels: the celiac axis, superior mesenteric artery, and inferior mesenteric artery. Collaterals connect these vessels so that chronic occlusion of one vessel is well compensated.

Diagnosis

Many patients see a surgeon only *after* an extensive gastrointestinal workup. The diagnosis is based on an accurate history and physical examination as well as noninvasive duplex ultrasound studies and mesenteric angiography of the visceral vessels. The noninvasive duplex scan assesses the flow within the visceral vessels as well as the presence of a proximal arterial stenosis. The limitation of the duplex scan is its inability to evaluate the visceral vessels if a significant amount of bowel gas is present. To confirm the diagnosis, arteriograms are used to show hemodynamically significant lesions of at least two of the three major visceral vessels and evidence of collateral flow circumventing the stenotic mesenteric vessel. Evaluation of the proximal superior mesenteric artery and celiac axis is made by a lateral arteriogram, which demonstrates the origin of these vessels, which have anterior positioning off the aorta.

Treatment

Mesenteric revascularization should be considered in patients who have a history that is consistent with mesenteric ischemia as well as angiographic evidence of significant arterial occlusive disease of the visceral vessels. In these cases, mesenteric revascularization usually provides symptomatic improvement and prevents catastrophic mesenteric infarction.

Proximal mesenteric artery balloon angioplasty is being used more frequently, but because of the acute angle of the origin of the visceral vessel, requires a great level of expertise to place the balloon and stents in the superior mesenteric artery.

Surgical revascularization options include endarterectomy of the proximal visceral vessels or bypass with vein or synthetic conduits. Most patients have symptomatic improvement with revascularization of a single mesenteric vessel. However, many experienced surgeons routinely revascularize at least two of the visceral vessels to maximize the durability of the repair.

Renal Artery Stenosis

Renal artery stenosis is the most common cause of surgically correctable hypertension. Stenoses can result from atherosclerosis, fibromuscular dysplasia, or posttraumatic subintimal dissections. Although renovascular hypertension accounts for approximately 5% of the total incidence of hypertension, this mechanism is responsible for a disproportionate fraction of hypertension in children and young women and for new-onset hypertension in the elderly. Renovascular hypertension is often refractory to medical management, and patients usually require multiple antihypertensive medications to partially control their hypertension. In addition, progressive renal failure due to reduced perfusion may mandate revascularization to avoid dialysis. Other causes of surgically correctable hypertension include pheochromocytoma, aldosterone-secreting tumors, and descending thoracic aortic coarctation.

Anatomy

Atherosclerotic renal artery lesions usually occur in the proximal to middle portion of the renal artery and often represent an extension of an aortic plaque into the renal artery ostium. In contrast, fibromuscular dysplasia most commonly involves the middle to distal portion of the renal artery, with sparing of the proximal aspect of the renal artery (Fig. 23-14). **Fibromuscular dysplasia** is a hyperplastic, fibrosing process of the intima, media, or adventitia. It is three times more common in women than in men, and it usually occurs in the second to fourth decade. Bilateral involvement is seen in as many as 50% of cases.

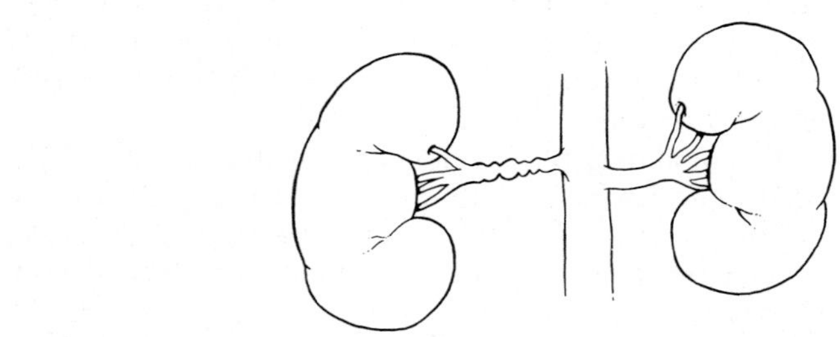

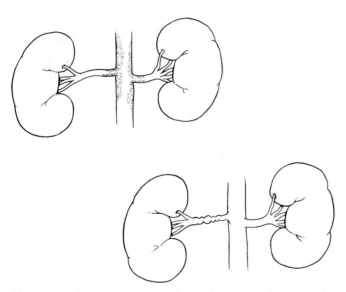

Figure 23-14 **A,** Stenotic lesions of the renal artery cause hypoperfusion of the kidney and activation of the renin–angiotensin system. As a result, significant hypertension occurs. Atherosclerotic lesions usually involve the origin to the middle portion of the renal artery. **B,** Fibromuscular hyperplasia involves the middle to the distal portion of the renal artery.

Pathophysiology

Critical stenosis of the renal artery causes decreased blood pressure and flow to the kidney as well as decreased glomerular filtration. This change stimulates the renal juxtaglomerular apparatus to produce renin, which catalyzes the conversion of angiotensinogen to angiotensin I. Angiotensin-converting enzyme then converts angiotensin I to angiotensin II, a potent vasoconstrictor. Angiotensin II also stimulates the production of aldosterone, causing sodium retention and increased plasma volume. This combination of vasoconstriction and sodium retention causes a hypertensive state.

Physical Examination

Most untreated patients have profound diastolic hypertension with diastolic pressures occasionally exceeding 120 mm Hg. An epigastric or flank bruit may be noted on auscultation of the abdomen and suggests turbulent flow within the renal artery.

Diagnosis

Renal duplex scan, renal perfusion scan, renal function studies, and intravenous urography (IVP) are used as screening studies to separate patients with renal vascular hypertension from the general hypertensive population. The high incidence of false-negative results limits reliance on these studies. Urograms may contribute to the diagnosis of renal ischemia by showing: (1) a decrease in renal size secondary to hypoperfusion; (2) ureteral notching as a result of compression by collateral blood vessels; and (3) a delayed nephrogram with hyperconcentration of contrast. More important, urography may exclude other primary renal parenchymal pathology.

A functional test for renovascular hypertension is the captopril challenge test. Captopril, an angiotensin II–converting enzyme inhibitor, prevents the conversion of angiotensin I to angiotensin II. Because of the blockage of synthesis of angiotensin II, more renin is produced and plasma renin levels are elevated after captopril administration. A positive captopril test also leads to a decrease in the glomerular filtration rate because of the blockage of the effect of angiotensin II on the efferent arteriole of the renal glomeruli. There was early enthusiasm for renal vein renin samplings as an accurate diagnostic test for renal vascular hypertension. Unfortunately, in patients with bilateral renal artery stenosis, the ratio may be 1, with both renal arteries producing higher levels of renin.

Renal duplex ultrasonography can assess the flow velocity profile in both renal arteries as well as the juxtarenal aorta. A significant difference in renal artery velocities (renal artery:aorta ratio $>$ 3.5:1) suggests the presence of a hemodynamically significant renal artery stenosis. The duplex scan can also determine the renal parenchymal size to determine whether one of the kidneys is atrophying as a result of ischemia. The sensitivity and specificity of renal artery duplex ultrasonography for detecting significant renal artery stenosis is greater than 90%.

The definitive diagnosis of renal artery stenosis is confirmed by angiography. Renal arteriography not only detects renal artery stenoses but also assists in determining kidney size by evaluating the postinjection nephrogram.

Treatment

Antihypertensive medications are usually ineffective in controlling renovascular hypertension. However, angiotensin II–converting enzyme inhibitors are avoided in cases of bilateral renal artery stenosis because these drugs decrease the glomerular filtration rate and may cause renal failure.

In patients with severe hypertension and hemodynamically significant renal artery stenosis, some form of renal revascularization should be considered. Fibromuscular dysplasia responds exceptionally well to percutaneous transluminal balloon angioplasty in all age groups. Current experience with fibromuscular disease in pediatric patients and young adults suggests that more than 95% of patients are cured or significantly improved with renal artery angioplasty. Atherosclerotic lesions of the proximal renal artery are less responsive to angioplasty because the renal artery plaque is usually an extension of an aortic plaque. These lesions are more likely to return to their original degree of stenosis. The use of a metallic stent after angioplasty provides better results in these cases. The risk of surgical intervention for failure of endovascular repair of renal artery stenosis is the same as for primary surgical procedures, so many vascular specialists recommend endovascular repair as the initial method of treatment for renal artery stenosis, with reservation of open surgical bypass for those patients that fail endovascular intervention.

Surgical treatment for renal vascular hypertension is performed in patients who have recurrent stenosis after angioplasty. It is also performed when lesions are not correctable with angioplasty. Surgical interventions include endarterectomy of the atherosclerotic lesions and bypass to the renal artery from the aorta, the hepatic arteries, or the splenic arteries.

Acute Arterial Occlusion

Clinical Presentation

Acute occlusion of an extremity or visceral vessel can cause limb, intestinal, or life-threatening ischemia. Etiologies of acute arterial occlusion include in situ thrombosis of preexisting atherosclerotic occlusive disease, arterial emboli, vascular trauma (either penetrating or blunt), and thrombosis of a preexisting arterial aneurysm. Patients with preexisting arterial occlusive disease may have a history of claudication or intestinal angina before arterial thrombosis occurs and acute symptoms of ischemia develop. These patients may already have a moderate collateral bed and therefore may have less acute symptoms. In contrast, patients with arterial emboli, vascular trauma, or thrombosis of a preexisting aneurysm are asymptomatic before the arterial occlusion occurs and may have more profound ischemic symptoms.

The great majority (80%) of arterial emboli originate in the left side of the heart. Thrombi form in the left atrium in patients with atrial fibrillation and in akinetic or hypokinetic regions of previous myocardial infarction. These thrombi can dislodge and embolize to the peripheral circulation. Nonthrombotic emboli can also occur from atherosclerotic lesions of the aorta and aortic valve. Mural thrombi within thoracic, abdominal aortic, and popliteal aneurysms can also cause distal embolization.

The most common site of embolic occlusion is the femoral artery. Other common sites are the axillary, popliteal, and iliac arteries; the aortic bifurcation; and the mesenteric vessels.

The classic presentation of limb-threatening acute arterial occlusion includes the "six *P*s": *p*allor, *p*ain, *p*aresthesia, *p*aralysis, *p*ulselessness, and *p*oikilothermia (change in temperature). These changes are limited to the area distal to the region of acute arterial occlusion. For example, with femoral artery occlusion, the ischemic changes (one or more of the six *P*s) occur in the distal thigh, calf, or foot.

Acute mesenteric ischemia results from arterial occlusion (embolus or thrombosis), mesenteric venous occlusion, or nonocclusive mesenteric ischemia (especially vasospasm). Embolization to the superior mesenteric artery accounts for approximately 50% of all cases of acute mesenteric ischemia; 25% of cases occur secondary to thrombosis of a preexisting atherosclerotic lesion. Most superior mesenteric artery emboli lodge just distal to the origin of the middle colic artery, approximately 3 to 10 cm from the origin of the superior mesenteric artery (Fig. 23-15). Nonocclusive mesenteric ischemia accounts for an additional 25% of cases of acute mesenteric ischemia. The

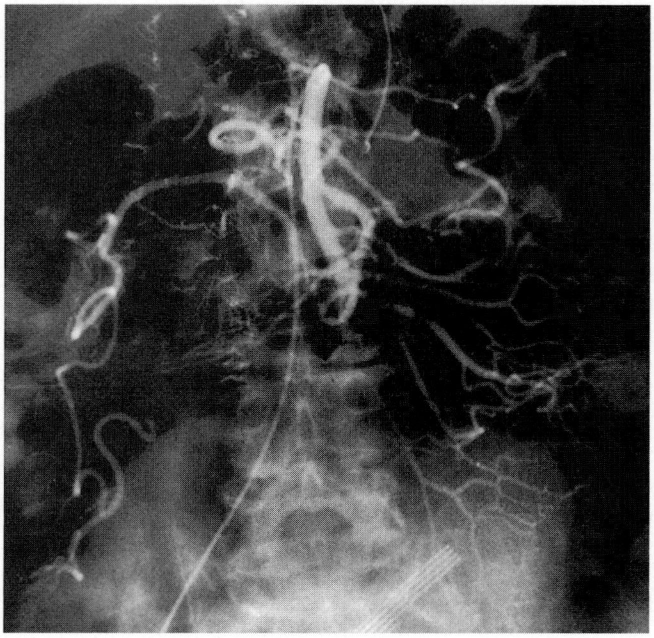

Figure 23-15 Acute embolus of the proximal superior mesenteric artery (*solid arrow*).

etiology of nonocclusive mesenteric ischemia is multifactorial, but usually involves moderate to severe mesenteric atherosclerotic lesions in association with a low cardiac output state or the administration of vasoconstricting medications or digitalis.

Treatment

Patients with acute arterial occlusion require rapid evaluation and diagnosis to prevent limb-, bowel-, or life-threatening ischemia. Anticoagulation with intravenous heparin is administered to prevent further propagation of the thrombus. Contraindications to anticoagulation include a history of gastrointestinal bleeding, a new neurologic deficit, head injury, ongoing sites of active bleeding, and antibodies to heparin. Aggressive fluid resuscitation and correction of ongoing systemic acidosis should be performed. Patients who are in critical condition may require inotropic support. Dextran and mannitol offer advantages as part of the treatment of acute arterial occlusion. Dextran enhances the electronegativity of the red blood cells and the vessel wall and leads to a decrease in the propagation of thrombus. Dextran and mannitol function as an oncotic load to draw free water back into the bloodstream and hemodilute the blood. Interventions should not be significantly delayed to allow for correction of the acidosis because the ongoing ischemia is the primary contributor to the acid–base disturbance.

In cases of limb-threatening ischemia, immediate surgical thrombectomy or embolectomy is performed. Preoperative arteriogrphy may be of benefit in patients who have a history of arterial occlusive disease. In patients with sudden acute ischemia, arteriograms should be avoided and immediate surgical revascularization performed, based on physical examination and the level at which the pulse is absent.

The surgical approach is directed toward rapidly reperfusing the threatened extremity or organ. This reperfusion can be accomplished by embolectomy, endarterectomy, or surgical bypass. The results of revascularization are variable and depend on the extent of the occlusive disease and the duration of ischemia. In embolic occlusion, embolectomy is performed through peripheral vessels with specialized balloon-tipped catheters. Careful, complete thrombectomy is performed both proximally and distally. Distal thrombectomy is essential because nearly one-third of patients with arterial occlusions have additional thrombus past the point of occlusion. Pathologic evaluation should be performed of all emboli, especially in the absence of atrial fibrillation, to ensure that the embolus is not of tumor (e.g., myxomatous) origin. If the embolus is of thrombotic origin, its shape may give a good indication of its origin.

After extremity or organ revascularization, the reperfused organ is examined to determine the extent of tissue damage and the potential for edema. If there was lengthy lower extremity ischemia (> 4 hours), fasciotomy is often required to decompress the muscular compartments and prevent compression of the arteries, nerves, and veins (i.e., compartment syndrome). Unfortunately, the mortality rate from acute arterial occlusion is relatively high. This high rate is related to the advanced age of the patient population as well as to comorbid factors (e.g., myocardial disease). In the case of embolic arterial occlusion, postoperative anticoagulation should be considered because as many as one-third of patients have recurrent embolus or thrombosis without anticoagulation within 30 days.

In patients who have acute arterial ischemia without signs of profound ischemia to either the limb or the intestine, thrombolytic therapy can be considered. The goal of thrombolysis is to reperfuse the limb gradually, causing fewer systemic effects and a lower probability of compartment syndrome than a surgical approach. This approach requires arterial cannulation of the area proximal to the area of occlusion and administration of a thrombolytic agent (urokinase or tissue plasminogen activator). However, if there are signs of critical ischemia, thrombolytic therapy is aborted and surgical revascularization is performed emergently.

Cerebrovascular Insufficiency

Cerebrovascular insufficiency can result from arterial occlusive, ulcerative, or aneurysmal disease of the carotid or vertebral arteries. The most devastating complication of cerebral vascular insufficiency is stroke. Stroke is the third leading cause of death in North America and the leading cause of long-term disability. Each year, more than 500,000 new strokes and 200,000 stroke-related deaths occur. The medical cost of managing patients after stroke is estimated at $15 billion to $20 billion per year.

Strokes are caused by infarction or hemorrhage within the cerebral hemispheres. Approximately 75% of cerebral infarctions are caused by embolism from atherosclerotic plaques in the carotid arteries of the neck. Although medical management, including antihypertensive, hypocholesterolemic, and antiplatelet agents, may help to prevent carotid atheroembolism, the most effective strategy is angioplasty or removal of the plaque through carotid endarterectomy (CEA).

Anatomy

Blood reaches the brain through the paired carotid and vertebral arteries. The right and left carotid arteries originate from the innominate artery and the aortic arch, respectively. The vertebral arteries arise from the proximal portions of the subclavian arteries. The common carotid arteries in the midneck bifurcate into the external carotid arteries (which supply the muscles of the face) and the internal carotid arteries. The internal carotid arteries have no branches in the neck, but they enter the petrous portion of the skull and give rise to the ophthalmic artery of the eye and the anterior and middle cerebral arteries that serve the cerebral cortex. The paired vertebral arteries form a single blood vessel within the brainstem (basilar artery) and then give rise to the posterior cerebral arteries and the arteries of the cerebellum. The arteries of the anterior and posterior circulation are part of a rich collateral network of vessels (circle of Willis) that is composed of the P1 segments of the posterior cerebral arteries, the posterior communicating arteries, the A1 segments of the anterior cerebral arteries, and the anterior communicating artery. Theoretically, an intact circle of Willis allows cerebral perfusion to be maintained in the face of occlusion or stenosis of one or more of the main branches. Unfortunately, this collateral network is complete in less than 25% of people.

Physiology

Approximately 15% of the cardiac output is directed to maintain cerebral perfusion. The resting total cerebral blood flow is 100 mL/min/100 g brain matter, with as much as 50 to 60 mL/min/100 g directed to the more cellular gray matter and 20 mL/min/100 g to the less cellular white matter. Cerebral ischemia can result once the total perfusion is less than 18 mL/min/100 g brain matter. Cerebral infarction can occur after the cerebral perfusion decreases to less than 8 mL/min/100 g.

A number of mechanisms maintain cerebral blood flow in the face of systemic hypotension or fixed lesions in the named arteries. Baroreceptors located at the carotid sinus sample and regulate blood pressure and heart rate. Further, cerebral vessels dilate in response to decreased perfusion pressure (autoregulation). This change is probably mediated by local receptors in the vascular smooth muscle and by autoregulatory autocoids (e.g., nitric oxide).

Pathophysiology

Although cerebral ischemia occasionally results from systemically induced decreased blood flow, atheroembolism is by far the most common cause of cerebral infarction. Cerebral embolism may originate from any source between the left atrium and cerebral arteries, including the atrial appendage, left ventricle, aortic valve, aortic arch, carotid bifurcation, and carotid siphon. The most common source is an atherosclerotic lesion at the carotid bifurcation. Experimental models show that the carotid bifurcation contains areas of low and oscillatory shear stress. This finding may account for the transfer of circulating cellular elements to predisposed segments of the arterial wall and the development of occlusive plaques. Like any lesion in the body, most plaques are eventually covered with a fibrous cap, or scar, and separated from the circulation. Occasionally, however, the fibrous cap is disrupted, allowing embolism of exposed plaque elements or laminated thrombus. Less common causes of carotid arterial occlusive disease include fibromuscular dysplasia, Takayasu arteritis, arterial dissection, and trauma.

Hypoperfusion can cause neurologic deficits in the watershed areas between the perfused territories of the main cerebral arteries, where collateral flow is marginal. Sudden thrombosis of the carotid artery can cause massive cerebral infarction or may be asymptomatic if there is adequate collateral circulation from the contralateral carotid artery and the basilar artery (silent occlusion).

Clinical Presentation and Evaluation

Symptoms of cerebral vascular insufficiency are classified according to the location of the deficit, its duration, and the presence of cerebral infarction. These symptoms can be either transient or permanent. **Amaurosis fugax** (fleeting blindness) is a transient monocular blindness that is caused by emboli to the ipsilateral ophthalmic artery. Classically, amaurosis fugax is described as a curtain of blindness being pulled down from superior to inferior and involving the eye ipsilateral to the carotid lesion. TIAs are short-lived, often repetitive changes in mentation, vision, or sensorimotor function that are completely reversed within 24 hours. Most TIAs last seconds to minutes before they resolve completely. Because TIAs often involve the middle cerebral artery distribution, patients often have contralateral arm, leg, and facial weakness. A stroke-in-evolution is a rapid progressive worsening of a neurologic deficit. A cerebral infarction, or **cerebrovascular accident,** is a permanent neurologic deficit, or stroke. Cerebral CT scan or MRI of a patient who had a stroke shows a region of nonviable cerebral tissue. Atherosclerotic carotid artery disease is not the only etiology of these clinical presentations. TIAs are also caused by migraines, seizure disorders, brain tumors, intracranial aneurysms, and arteriovenous malformations.

The severity of the neurologic deficit is determined by the volume and location of the ischemic area of the brain. The most commonly involved area is the perfused territory of the middle cerebral artery (parietal lobe), which is the main outflow vessel of the carotid artery. Hypoperfusion of the middle cerebral artery causes contralateral hemiparesis or hemiplegia and, occasionally, paralysis of the contralateral lower part of the face (central seventh nerve paralysis). Difficulty with speech (aphasia) is noted if the dominant hemisphere is involved. The left hemisphere is dominant in nearly all right-handed people and most left-handed people.

Patients with ischemia of the brain tissue that is supplied by the anterior cerebral artery have contralateral monoplegia that is usually more severe in the lower extremity. Posterior cerebral artery ischemia may result from carotid artery occlusive disease, but is also related to obstruction of both vertebral arteries or the basilar artery. Dizziness or syncope may be accompanied by visual field defects, palsy of the ipsilateral third cranial nerve, and contralateral sensory losses.

Diagnosis of Cerebrovascular Disease

As with most syndromes of vascular insufficiency, the diagnosis is usually suggested by the history alone. A carefully elicited history may also localize the neuroanatomic deficit and the offending arterial lesion. Physical examination should include a thorough neurologic examination as well as a search for evidence of arterial occlusive disease in other vascular beds. The classic finding in a patient with carotid stenosis is a cervical bruit (high-frequency systolic murmur) heard during auscultation with a stethoscope placed at the angle of the jaw. Unfortunately, there is little correlation between the degree of stenosis and the pitch, duration, or intensity of the bruit. A minimal stenosis can produce a loud bruit, but a near-total occlusion may not produce a bruit at all. A bruit can also be produced from other cervical blood vessels or transmitted from the aortic valve. Because of the close proximity of the carotid artery to the ear, some patients actually note a buzzing or heartbeat in their ear referred from the carotid stenosis. During ophthalmologic examination, small, yellow refractile particles (Hollenhorst plaques) may be seen at the branch point of the retinal vessels. These plaques are cholesterol emboli from a carotid artery, aortic arch, or aortic valve plaque. Fisher plugs are due to platelet emboli and are not refractile.

Noninvasive tests can characterize the extent of carotid artery stenosis without the use of arteriography. Candidates for noninvasive testing include patients with cerebrovascular symptoms, those with cervical bruit, and, in some cases, those who are undergoing major vascular procedures (e.g., coronary artery bypass grafting). Noninvasive, yet direct, evaluation of the extracranial and carotid arterial vessels is obtained with Doppler ultrasound. The nature of the plaque (soft, calcific, or ulcerated) and its precise location (common versus external versus internal carotid artery) can be determined with both carotid arterial systems. The accuracy of imaging is enhanced by combining B-mode ultrasound with Doppler-derived assessments of blood flow velocity (duplex scan). A limitation of duplex scanning is the inability to assess the intracranial circulation and the origins of the common carotid arteries from the aortic arch. Occasionally, visualization of the bifurcation is impaired by calcification of the vessels. In more than 90% of patients with carotid bifurcation plaque, no further diagnostic test is needed to institute therapy.

The definitive study of the extracranial carotid arterial system is arteriography. Arterial injections offer the clearest definition of carotid plaques and potential ulcerations (Fig. 23-16). Arteriography is indicated in patients who have a potential aortic arch or intracranial lesion, those with uncertain symptoms, and those in whom the carotid stenosis cannot be clearly visualized on duplex ultrasonography. Complications are rare, but can be devastating. They include cerebrovascular accident (approximately 0.5% of cases).

Recent improvements in cerebral MRI and magnetic resonance angiography have led to increased application in patients with carotid occlusive disease. MRI is useful for evaluation of the brain for infarction, tumor, arteriovenous malformation, and hemorrhage. Magnetic resonance angiography provides detailed visualization of the carotid arterial system without requiring arterial puncture and injection (Fig. 23-17).

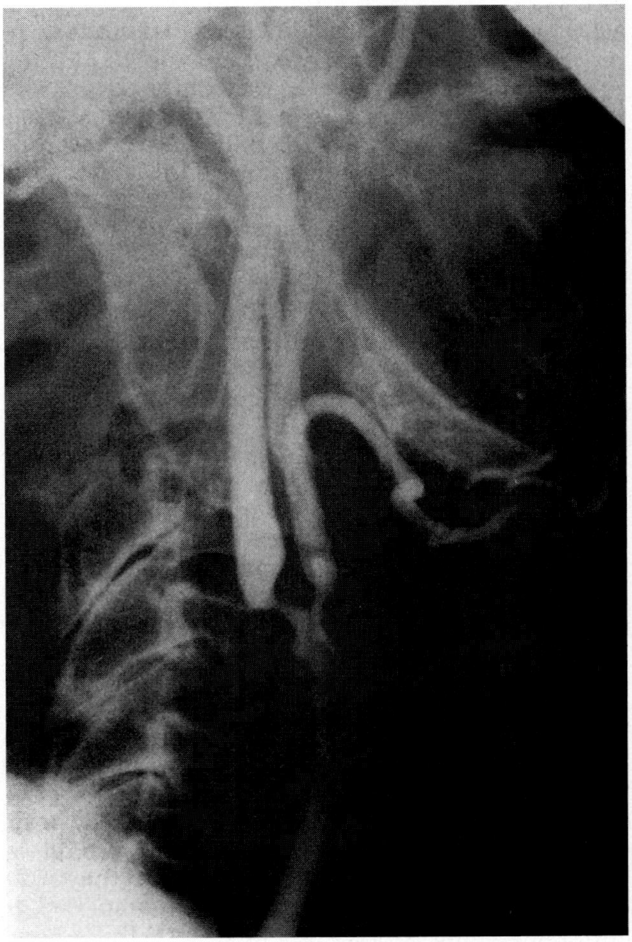

Figure 23-16 Angiogram of an internal carotid stenosis showing an ulcerative and stenotic atherosclerotic lesion at the carotid bifurcation in a patient who has transient ischemic attacks.

Treatment

Medical therapy for cerebrovascular disease is directed at the control of risk factors (e.g., hypertension, hyperlipoproteinemia) and anticoagulation or administration of antiplatelet drugs (e.g., aspirin, clopidogrel, or Coumadin). Anticoagulation and antiplatelet therapy are most commonly used in patients with ulcerative nonstenotic lesions or severe intracranial disease because surgical therapy would not change the natural history of the disease process. A prospective randomized study (North American Symptomatic Carotid Endarterectomy Trial [NASCET]) evaluated the treatment of patients with 50% to 70% and more than 70% internal carotid artery stenosis and cerebrovascular symptoms in the distribution of the affected carotid artery. After 2 years of followup, researchers found that in symptomatic patients who had more than 70% ipsilateral stenosis and were managed with antiplatelet therapy alone, the risk of cerebrovascular accident or death was approximately 26% compared with 9% in patients who were

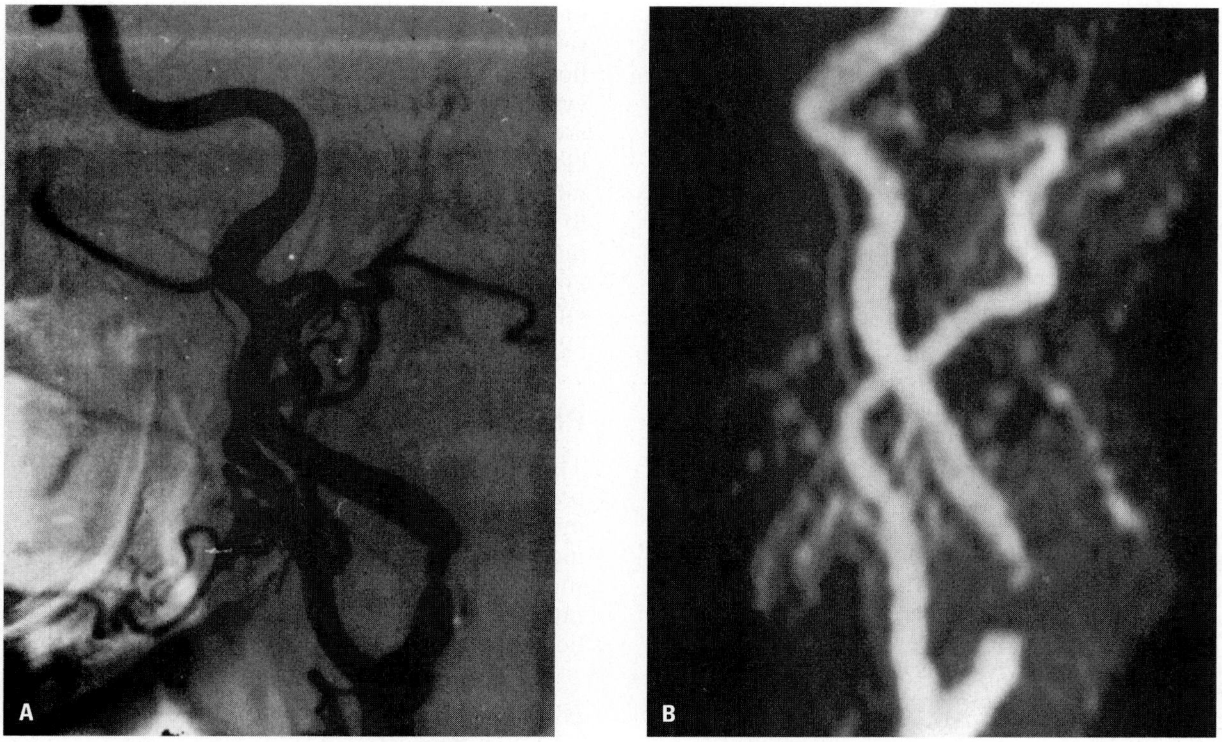

Figure 23-17 **A,** A conventional cerebral angiogram. **B,** A magnetic resonance angiogram in the same patient.

treated with CEA. The risk in patients with 50% to 69% stenosis was also reduced with CEA. Asymptomatic patients with documented 60% or greater carotid stenosis were studied (Asymptomatic Carotid Atherosclerosis Study [ACAS]). The risk of stroke in the medically managed group was calculated at 11% in 5 years. CEA reduced the risk to 5%. These findings firmly established the role of CEA in the prevention of stroke in patients with significant carotid stenosis.

In experienced hands, the morbidity and mortality rates for CEA are less than 2%. Recurrent lesions may occur in as many as 10% of endarterectomized arteries, so long-term followup with serial ultrasonography is advised. Restenosis within 2 years usually represents intimal hyperplasia, whereas late recurrence is usually a manifestation of recurrent atherosclerosis.

Carotid angioplasty with placement of a metallic stent has been evaluated and is being used with increasing frequency to treat both symptomatic and asymptomatic carotid stenosis. There appear to be nearly equivalent stroke rates associated with either CEA or carotid stenting, but there may be a decreased risk of myocardial infarction with carotid stenting. This procedure allows percutaneous treatment of carotid stenosis without the risk of surgical intervention. The long-term results of carotid stenting are still pending but appear promising. A clinical trial, CREST, will compare CEA with carotid angioplasty/stent and determine subgroups in which each treatment is preferable.

Vertebral Basilar Disease

The classic syndrome of vertebral basilar insufficiency is subclavian steal syndrome, which is associated with subclavian or innominate artery occlusive disease. Symptoms occur when an occlusive lesion that is located proximal to the origin of the vertebral vessel decreases perfusion pressure in the subclavian artery. The vertebral artery then functions as a collateral pathway to the arm circulation. During arm exercise, vascular resistance in the arm decreases, and flow is reversed in the vertebral artery. As a result, basilar arterial blood flow and perfusion pressure are decreased (Fig. 23-18). Symptoms of posterior cerebral and cerebellar ischemia are common and include lightheadedness, syncope, and nausea correlated with arm exercise. Supraclavicular bruits are often detected, and blood pressure in the ipsilateral brachial artery is usually reduced by at least 40 mm Hg. Because of the increased length of the left subclavian artery relative to the right, there is a three to four times increased incidence of left subclavian stenosis and subclavian steal syndrome.

In patients with associated carotid artery disease, CEA alone may relieve the symptoms of vertebral basilar insufficiency by increasing collateral flow to the posterior cere-

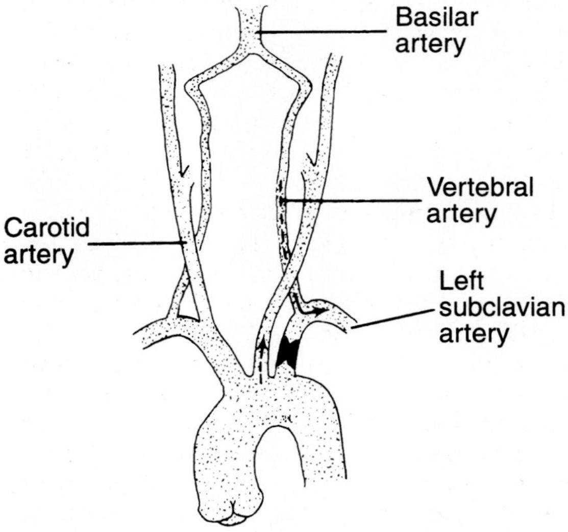

Figure 23-18 Subclavian steal syndrome. Proximal occlusion of the left subclavian artery causes retrograde flow of blood through the left vertebral artery, "stealing" blood from the basilar circulation and causing transient dizziness and syncope with arm exercise.

bral artery and cerebellum. However, in most symptomatic patients with subclavian steal syndrome, the most commonly performed procedures are carotid–subclavian bypass and reimplantation of the subclavian artery into the proximal common carotid artery. These procedures restore normal blood flow to the subclavian artery and allow antegrade perfusion of the vertebral artery.

VENOUS DISEASE

Venous disease is one of the most common medical conditions affecting adults. Approximately 40% of adults have some form of venous disease, including varicose veins, **postthrombotic syndrome**, venous ulcers, and spider veins or telangiectasias.

Anatomy

The venous system is divided into peripheral and central systems. The central venous system includes the inferior and superior vena cava, iliac veins, and subclavian veins. The peripheral venous system includes the upper and lower extremity venous systems as well as the venous drainage of the head and neck region. The extremity veins are further classified as either superficial or deep. The superficial system of the lower extremity is composed of the greater and lesser saphenous veins and their tributaries. The deep venous system is composed of the large veins that travel with the major named arteries of the extremity. The common femoral, superficial femoral, and profunda femoral veins parallel the arteries of the same names. The anterior tibial, posterior tibial, and peroneal veins are almost always paired, so that the calf has six primary deep veins in contrast to three primary arteries. Unidirectional flow back to the heart is maintained by a series of bicuspid vein valves. These vein valves prevent reflux of blood back toward the lower extremity during standing. The superficial and deep venous systems communicate through perforating veins that direct blood from the superficial system to the deep system. Incompetency of the valves and perforating veins as a result of scarring or distension allows retrograde flow from the deep system into the superficial system and can cause varicosities, chronic venous insufficiency, and venous ulcerations.

Physiology

The muscular compartments of the calf are critically important in the venous circulation. Muscular contraction increases pressure within the compartments, thereby forcing blood back to the heart. Unlike the deep veins, the superficial veins are not surrounded by muscular compartments and therefore are not emptied by muscular contraction.

Pathology

In 1856, Virchow identified a triad of risk factors for deep vein thrombosis. It included stasis, venous endothelial injury, and hypercoagulable states. Other risk factors include pregnancy, the use of oral contraceptives, a history of deep vein thrombosis, surgical procedures, sepsis, and obesity. Bony and soft tissue trauma to the legs is a common cause of endothelial injury. Stasis and venous distension may also injure the venous endothelium. The pathophysiology of venous disease is generally caused by obstruction of the venous system, venous valvular insufficiency, or elements of both.

Superficial Vein Thrombosis

Thrombosis of a superficial vein causes swelling, erythema, and tenderness along its course. Patients who have superficial thromboses are managed with nonsteroidal antiinflammatory agents and warm compresses. They do not require bed rest.

Deep Vein Thrombosis

Approximately 500,000 patients per year have deep vein thrombosis (DVT). If pulmonary thromboembolism occurs, in-hospital mortality rates are 10%.

Clinical Presentation

As many as 50% of episodes of hospital-acquired DVT are asymptomatic. The remaining patients have local pain secondary to inflammation and edema. DVT of the left iliac venous system is four times more common than that of the right iliac venous system because of the potential for compression of the left iliac vein by the aortic bifurcation.

Unfortunately, in a small percentage of patients, the first symptom of DVT is pulmonary embolism.

Diagnosis

Physical examination of a patient with a lower-extremity DVT may show unilateral extremity swelling or pain. Calf pain precipitated by dorsal flexion of the foot (Homan's sign) is present in fewer than 50% of cases. Because the accuracy of diagnosis based on clinical and physical examination alone is only 50%, more objective diagnostic studies are needed to confirm the presence of DVT before treatment. In addition to DVT, the differential diagnosis of acute edema and leg pain includes congestive heart failure, trauma, ruptured plantaris tendon, acute or chronic arterial insufficiency, infection, lymphangitis, lumbosacral strain, sciatica, muscle hematoma, and renal failure.

The accuracy of duplex ultrasound is greater than 95% in diagnosing DVT because it can characterize venous blood flow and visualize the venous thrombus. A Doppler ultrasound can document the loss of the normal augmentation of venous flow with distal compression and the variation of venous flow with respiration. Normally, lower extremity venous flow decreases with inspiration as a result of increased intraabdominal pressure. The accuracy of duplex scanning is decreased in the tibial veins because of the occasional difficulty encountered when visualizing these small veins within the muscular compartments. In unusual cases, CT scans of the abdomen and pelvis, with intravenous contrast material, may aid in the diagnosis of pelvic and vena caval thrombosis. If the results of noninvasive diagnostic tests are not definitive, venography is performed.

Prophylaxis

Deep vein thrombosis with a potential for pulmonary embolus is a significant risk for patients undergoing major surgery. Preoperative prophylaxis has an impact in reducing DVT. Prophylactic measures include mechanical therapy (intermittent segmental compression device, early ambulation, and passive range of motion) and pharmacologic therapy (subcutaneous heparin, dextran, aspirin, or Coumadin).

Treatment

The goals of treatment include decreasing the risk of pulmonary embolus and preventing further propagation of the venous thrombus. Primary therapy includes anticoagulation with subcutaneous low–molecular-weight or intravenous heparin and elevation of the extremity. After the patient is adequately anticoagulated with heparin, long-term anticoagulation is begun with sodium warfarin (Coumadin). Coumadin therapy is monitored to maintain a therapeutic prothrombin time and international normalized ratio (INR). Sodium warfarin inhibits the vitamin K–dependent factors for both the procoagulant factors (II, VII, IX, X) and the anticoagulant factors (protein C and protein S). Because the half-lives of protein C and protein S are less than those of the procoagulant factors, for a short time after the initiation of Coumadin therapy, the patient may become hypercoagulable. Coumadin skin necrosis is a catastrophic complication of this rare hypercoagulable state. It can cause significant loss of skin, especially skin overlying poorly vascularized regions (i.e., adipose tissue). For this reason, heparin anticoagulation is maintained during the beginning of Coumadin therapy. Contraindications to anticoagulation therapy include bleeding diathesis, gastrointestinal ulceration, recent stroke, cerebral arteriovenous malformations, recent surgery, hematologic disorders (e.g., hemophilia), and bone marrow suppression as a result of chemotherapy.

Anticoagulation therapy prevents further propagation of the thrombus, but does not actually dissolve or lyse the existing thrombus. Fibrinolysis occurs gradually, through the endogenous plasminogen system, or may be stimulated by the administration of exogenous urokinase or tissue plasminogen activator (TPA). Definite indications for thrombolytic therapy include subclavian vein thrombosis, acute renal vein thrombosis, and acute superior vena cava occlusion by the thrombus. Its application is also being investigated for routine use in lower-extremity DVT. It is uncertain whether venous valvular function can be preserved with successful thrombolytic therapy. Surgical thrombectomy is usually reserved for cases of limb-threatening ischemia. Even in complete iliofemoral thrombosis with massive edema (phlegmasia cerulea dolens or phlegmasia alba dolens), venous thrombectomy has limited usefulness because more than 50% of thromboses recur. Thrombolysis is the preferred treatment.

Pulmonary Embolism

Pulmonary embolism results from the migration of venous clots to the pulmonary arteries. Clots may originate in any large vein, especially those that arise from the iliac, femoral, and large pelvic veins.

Clinical Presentation

Patients with pulmonary embolism may have no specific clinical findings or may have massive cardiovascular collapse. The classic clinical presentation (Table 23-5) includes pleuritic chest pain, dyspnea, tachypnea, tachycardia, cough, and hemoptysis. Right-sided heart strain is seen

Table 23-5 Clinical Presentations of Pulmonary Embolus

Pleuritic chest pain (70%)
Dyspnea and tachypnea (80%)
Tachycardia (45%)
Hemoptysis (25%–30%)
Associated findings
Cough and rales
Right heart failure

on electrocardiogram. Patients with hypercoagulable conditions are predisposed to DVT and pulmonary embolism.

Diagnosis

Chest radiography is rarely diagnostic for pulmonary embolus. A pleural effusion is present in as many as one-third of patients with pulmonary embolus. The classic wedge-shaped region of atelectasis from a pulmonary embolus (Westermark sign) is rarely noted. Chest radiography is most useful for ruling out other potential pulmonary pathology. The definitive diagnosis of pulmonary embolism is made by CT scan of the chest, ventilation–perfusion lung scan, or pulmonary angiogram. A wedge-shaped or lobar defect seen on perfusion scan without a ventilation deficit indicates a high probability of pulmonary embolism. Chest CT scan often shows both the thrombus in the pulmonary artery and the infarcted lung parenchyma. Pulmonary angiogram has a specificity and a sensitivity of greater than 98%, but it is an invasive procedure.

Evaluation for hypercoagulability with measures of protein C, protein S, antithrombin 3, factor V Leiden, and anticardiolipin antibodies should be performed in patients with spontaneous DVT.

Treatment

The primary therapy for pulmonary embolism is anticoagulation, in an attempt to prevent further pulmonary emboli. If the patient is hemodynamically unstable, inotropic support may be required. If the patient remains stable but is compromised as a result of the pulmonary embolus, thrombolytic therapy is considered. There is no direct correlation between clot size, cardiopulmonary dynamics, and other risk factors and survival in patients with acute embolism. Multiple small emboli cause cardiovascular collapse as often as massive emboli.

If a patient with lower-extremity or pelvic venous thrombus has a contraindication to anticoagulation or has a pulmonary embolism while anticoagulated (failure of anticoagulation), a mechanical filter device can be placed in the inferior vena cava. This device traps emboli before they reach the pulmonary artery. Vena caval filters are permanent or removable and can be placed with a percutaneous catheter. Percutaneous pulmonary embolectomy suction devices aid in the removal of large clots from the pulmonary artery. If the patient becomes profoundly hypotensive and hypoxic despite intubation and vasopressor support, pulmonary artery embolectomy (Trendelenburg operation) may be considered. Unfortunately, direct surgical removal of the embolus is associated with a mortality rate of more than 80%.

Varicose Veins

Incidence

Venous disease, including varicose veins, spider veins, and postthrombotic limbs with edema and ulcers, is among the most common diseases in the United States. It is estimated that more than 40% of the adult population has varicose veins and that 6% of adults will develop a venous ulcer during their lifetime. In addition, the recurrence of venous ulcers is high, and most patients live for long periods with open ulcers, punctuated with periods of healing. Consequently, venous problems are not only extremely common but also important to the health care system.

Anatomy

Knowledge of venous anatomy is critical to understanding venous disease. The superficial, perforating, and deep systems interconnect, with blood flowing from the superficial to the deep system, and with valves preventing reflux from proximal to distal and from the deep to the superficial systems. Since 85% to 90% of the venous return is in the deep system, establishing its presence and patency is a key to treatment, and removal of the superficial veins has little consequence on blood flow physiology as long as the deep system is patent.

Primary Varicose Veins

Superficial veins often are not associated with other perforating or deep venous involvement, and therefore are considered "primary." The most common cause of primary varicose veins is incompetence of the saphenofemoral valve at the junction of the saphenous vein with the femoral vein in the inguinal region. Incompetence of the valve results in proximal vein dilation and progressive incompetence of distal veins. Eventually, the dilated vein results in valve incompetence of the entire saphenous vein as well as branch veins. The visible portion of the incompetent veins is usually in the calf, where they are closer to the skin. In spite of proximal incompetence, many patients request treatment only when the calf veins become visible.

Symptoms

Superficial varicose veins cause symptoms of heaviness and fatigue after prolonged standing, night cramps, and occasionally superficial thrombophlebitis or hemorrhage from superficial veins.

Diagnosis

Although physical examination is helpful in establishing the presence of varicose veins, the critical determinant of the approach to treatment is the competency of the saphenofemoral junction valve, which often cannot be determined by physical examination. Duplex ultrasound is the best diagnostic test for valve incompetence and should be used in all patients with symptoms. If the saphenous vein is not assessed for competency, then an incompetent saphenous vein may be left in place, leading to recurrence. Venography visualizes the leg veins well, but is rarely needed and may cause phlebitis. Plethysmography assesses reflux in the superficial and deep system, but has little role in primary varicose veins.

Treatment

The treatment of primary varicose veins has changed dramatically in the past 10 years, and, like many areas of surgery, has become less invasive.

1 "Stripping" of the saphenous vein. The saphenous vein may be removed by a technique of stripping, where the vein is exposed at each end and then removed by passing a disposable or metal catheter up the vein from the ankle or knee. A suture is tied around the vein at the saphenofemoral junction and the vein is then removed or "stripped." This technique is being used less frequently, since it is associated with a slightly longer patient recovery with more postoperative pain than minimally invasive approaches.
2 Saphenous ligation. Ligating the saphenous vein flush with the femoral vein in the fossa ovalis can eliminate the saphenous reflux. Although this technique eliminates reflux, there are often other connecting veins that maintain the patency and reflux, resulting in a higher rate of recurrence. Therefore, this technique is currently not favored by most surgeons.
3 Radiofrequency ablation or laser closure of the saphenous vein. This technique is the least invasive and is performed by accessing the saphenous vein below the knee with a needle, using ultrasound guidance. A wire is then passed into the vein, followed by a sheath and then a radiofrequency or laser catheter. After the catheter has been passed up to the saphenofemoral junction, the catheter is used to heat the vein. The heat contracts collagen and thromboses the vein, leading to closure.
4 Branch vein excision by stab phlebectomy. The branches of the saphenous vein can be removed with small incisions that allow the vein to be visualized and removed with small instruments or clamps. The resulting scars are very small and nearly invisible.

Secondary Varicose Veins and Venous Ulcers

Varicose veins in these patients reflect an underlying venous disease state, such as postthrombotic from DVT or proximal obstruction due to tumor compression.

Clinical Presentation

The leg is typically swollen and pigmented in the "gaiter" zone of the ankle. The pigmentation is a reflection of chronic venous hypertension, which is worsened in the standing position. The term "lipodermatosclerosis" refers to the end stage of venous hypertension, when the chronic venous hypertension leads to fibrosis of the tissue around the ankle and pigmentation, due to leakage of red blood cells into the tissue.

Diagnosis

The duplex ultrasound remains the best diagnostic test for secondary varicose veins and venous ulcers, although plethysmography or intravenous pressure catheters can also measure high venous pressure, which coexists with valve incompetence. The most important role of duplex scanning, though, is to identify the incompetent perforating veins and to mark their position so that they can be ligated.

Treatment

The initial treatment is nonsurgical. Eliminating swelling of the ankle, by using compression hose, can reduce or prevent pigmentation and fibrosis. Unfortunately, compliance is poor in many patients, since they do not see the immediate benefit of the support hose and dislike the cost of the hose and the discomfort associated with wearing the hose. If the fibrosis and pigmentation persist, there is a high likelihood of developing a venous ulcer, characterized by its location in the medial ankle, depth above the fascia, and association with pigmented, fibrotic skin. Venous ulcers will heal with compression wraps, but also may require removal of incompetent superficial veins and ligation of the perforating veins that enter under the ulcer and cause the ulcer. A "Linton" procedure refers to the open surgical technique of ligating perforating veins. It is associated with a high incidence of wound complications and is currently rarely used. Subfascial endoscopic perforator surgery (SEPS) ligates the same veins using a closed laparoscopic technique, with small incisions in normal tissue above the lipodermatosclerosis. Radiofrequency ablation is now being used to close perforator as well as incompetent saphenous veins.

Chronic Venous Insufficiency

Chronic venous insufficiency is a direct result of local venous hypertension. Causes of venous hypertension include deep venous valvular incompetence, venous obstruction as a result of intrinsic or extrinsic compression, and reflux from perforating veins.

Clinical Presentation

The clinical manifestations of chronic venous insufficiency are chronically swollen legs, hyperpigmentation, and venous stasis ulceration.

Diagnosis

Physical examination shows an orange–brown skin discoloration at the level of the ankle with hemosiderin deposition, lower extremity edema, superficial varicosities, and/or ulceration. Venous stasis ulceration usually occurs at the medial and lateral malleoli of the ankle. These chronic changes in the lower extremity occur as a result of venous hypertension and are usually postthrombotic, but may also be caused by congenital primary deep valvular incompetence.

Noninvasive vascular laboratory evaluation includes venous duplex ultrasonography, which allows visualization of venous flow as well as reflux through incompetent deep and perforator venous valves. Likewise, a duplex scan can directly visualize a deep vein chronic occlusion or note the inability of the vein to be compressed secondary to the mass of the venous thrombus. If the noninvasive duplex scan is not diagnostic, magnetic resonance or contrast venography may be necessary.

Treatment

The initial management of lower extremity edema with potential ulceration of chronic venous insufficiency is the use of gradient compression stockings. In patients with venous ulceration, meticulous wound care is required to prevent infection during healing. A medicated, tightly applied dressing of three or four layers (Unna's boot or Profore) may be required. If the wound does not heal, but the edema is controlled, split-thickness skin grafting may accomplish wound healing. Stripping/removal of the refluxing superficial veins, as well as surgical interruption of perforating veins, may be necessary to heal venous ulcers (SEPS procedure).

ARTERIOVENOUS MALFORMATIONS

Arteriovenous malformations result from abnormal embryologic development of the maturing vascular spaces, producing pathologic arteriovenous connections that involve small and medium-sized vessels. There is an equal male:female ratio, and the lower extremities are involved two to three times as often as the upper extremities. Although lesions are present at birth, most become clinically significant only in the second and third decade as they gradually enlarge. On palpation, a vibration, or **thrill,** is often noted over the level of the arteriovenous connection. In larger arteriovenous malformations, skin ulceration and bleeding are troublesome complications. Rarely, congenital arteriovenous fistulae produce cardiac enlargement and heart failure as a result of increased blood flow to the right side of the heart.

The management of symptomatic, localized congenital arteriovenous malformations is surgical excision. However, the treatment of large or diffuse lesions can be extremely difficult and is associated with a high recurrence rate. An alternative to surgery is percutaneous intraarterial or intravenous sclerosis of the main feeding artery and outflow veins to decrease the amount of blood that is shunted from the arterioles to the venules.

Acquired arteriovenous fistulae are abnormal communications between the arteries and veins, but they usually result from iatrogenic injuries (arterial catheterizations) or penetrating trauma (gunshot or knife wounds). These fistulae are often associated with a false aneurysm and involve large vessels (common femoral artery–common femoral vein fistula). A palpable thrill or bruit may be present. Venous hypertension and venous stasis changes occur with long-standing arteriovenous fistulae.

All acquired traumatic arteriovenous fistulae should be repaired to prevent the development of complications (e.g., cardiac failure, local pain, aneurysmal formation, limb length discrepancy in children, chronic venous hypertension). Direct compression of postcatheterization arteriovenous fistulae is often effective, especially if anticoagulants are not used. Operative intervention requires complete dissection and separation of the involved vessels and appropriate vascular repair. To exclude some arteriovenous communications nonoperatively, coated metallic stents are also used.

VASCULAR TRAUMA

Blood vessels are injured directly by penetrating trauma (e.g., stab wounds, gunshot wounds), blunt trauma (especially fractures of the long bones), and during treatment of other structures adjacent to blood vessels. In high-speed collisions involving motor vehicles or aircraft, vessels may be partially or totally disrupted by the shearing stress of sudden acceleration and deceleration. Patients with arterial injuries may have obvious signs (e.g., external hemorrhage, absence of distal pulses), but the signs of vascular injury are often subtle. Hemorrhage may be occult and confined to soft tissue or body cavities. Other findings that indicate vascular injury include acute arteriovenous fistulae (associated with to-and-fro murmurs or palpable thrills), neurologic deficits and paresthesias (as a result of nerve compression by adjacent hematomas), or organ-specific deficits that reflect obstruction of the main arterial supply (e.g., cerebral infarction with carotid artery injuries). Injury to the endothelial surface (intimal flaps) may not cause thrombosis for hours or days and therefore cannot be diagnosed by physical examination until the complication occurs. A common misconception is that a patient who has an arterial injury must have a reduced or absent distal pulse. This finding only occurs if the injury is hemodynamically significant.

Immediate diagnosis and treatment of arterial injuries is indicated to avoid excessive blood loss and to restore extremity or organ blood flow. If the diagnosis is missed on initial evaluation, late complications may be much more difficult to treat. These late complications include pseudoaneurysms, gradual enlargement of small lacerations in vessels, high-volume arteriovenous fistulae with venous insufficiency and high-output cardiac failure, and delayed thrombosis from untreated intimal flaps or dissections.

The poor reliability of physical diagnosis in accurately assessing the location and extent of vascular injury mandates investigation when penetrating trauma occurs near blood vessels, even if no overt signs of injury are present. If the patient has a viable extremity with an ABI of 1.0, then limb-threatening arterial injury is unlikely and the vessels that are near the region of trauma can be further evaluated by noninvasive duplex studies. If the extremity is ischemic, then angiography is indicated, unless the delay puts the limb or organ at significant risk. Because of the tremendous concussive energy of high-velocity missiles, extensive damage can result, even from near-misses. Specific types of blunt trauma (especially dislocation of the knees and elbows) are so often associated with arterial contusions and intimal disruption that duplex ultrasonography or arteriography is prudent, even if no symptoms are present.

Although the consequences of venous injury are not as severe as those of arterial trauma, venous laceration must be considered in any patient who has evidence of excessive blood loss and no arterial lesion on angiography. Magnetic resonance venography can usually confirm and localize the injury. Venous injury also predisposes the patient to the development of deep venous thrombosis.

Immediate vascular repair may be as simple as ligation or lateral suture of the injured vessel. In some cases, bypass grafts are needed, with resection of the vessel. In these cases, it is preferable to use an autologous vein from an uninjured extremity, because this conduit has a high patency rate and a low infection rate, even in the face of contamination. Repair of a concomitant major venous injury in an extremity results in a higher patency rate for the arterial repair.

VASOSPASTIC DISORDERS AND LYMPHATIC DISORDERS

Raynaud's Syndrome

Episodic digital vasospasm involving the hands and feet was first described by Maurice Raynaud in 1862. Raynaud's syndrome is cold- or emotion-induced episodic digital ischemia. As many as 90% of patients are female, and 50% have an associated autoimmune disease (e.g., scleroderma, lupus erythematosus, rheumatoid arthritis, Sjögren's syndrome). Some appear to have a work-related syndrome caused by the use of vibratory machinery. Unilateral Raynaud's syndrome is more common in men and is often associated with proximal arterial disease of the large vessels (e.g., subclavian stenosis, occlusion).

The clinical aspects may vary, but the classic Raynaud's attack has three distinct phenomena (white, blue, red syndrome). Exposure to cold initially causes profound vasospasm and blanching of the digits (white). After 15 minutes, cyanosis is evident, presumably from venous filling with delayed venous emptying (blue). Later, the digits and hands become hyperemic as vasospasm lessens and flow to the digits is restored (red).

The diagnosis of Raynaud's syndrome is made from the history and physical examination. Coexistent symptoms of connective tissue disorders are often elicited. Laboratory tests (e.g., sedimentation rate, complement assay, antinuclear antibody assay) often confirm the immunologic disorders associated with the syndrome. It is important to document all pulses by physical examination and Doppler auscultation.

Treatment consists of discontinuing any medications that cause reduced cardiac output or vasospasm and that are associated with Raynaud's syndrome (e.g., ergotamines, oral contraceptives, beta-blockers). Other pharmacologic agents, especially alpha- and calcium channel–blocking agents, are used to decrease the tendency toward vasospasm. Sympathetic blocks with xylocaine and sympathectomy are occasionally used, although sympathectomy is not an effective treatment, since sympathetic fibers regenerate over time. Revascularization of an ischemic extremity may markedly improve the symptoms in patients with arterial occlusive disease.

Thoracic Outlet Syndrome

Symptoms that mimic a vasospastic disorder may occur in thoracic outlet syndrome (TOS). This syndrome is often seen in young and middle-aged women. Symptoms are caused by compression or irritation of the brachial plexus and, to a much lesser extent, the subclavian artery, as they pass through the thoracic outlet and the costoclavicular space.

Anatomic causes of the syndrome include an elongated transverse process of the seventh cervical vertebra; a fully developed cervical rib; congenital bands in the outlet related to the cervical rib, middle scalene muscle, or anterior scalene muscle; and a narrowed costoclavicular space, often because of a previously fractured rib or clavicle, with callus formation.

Paresthesias of the arm and hand reflect neurologic compression and are much more common than arterial symptoms. When arterial symptoms occur, they include coldness of the hand and arm, pallor, and muscle fatigue. In rare cases, stenosis of the subclavian artery causes an aneurysm and/or emboli to the hand. Subclavian vein thrombosis may also occur.

Evaluation of these patients involves a detailed history and a thorough physical examination to document localized scalene muscle tenderness and radicular phenomena. Adson's test (disappearance of the radial pulse on abduction and external rotation of the shoulder), said to be indicative of thoracic outlet syndrome in the early literature, is now considered relatively nonspecific. Cervical spine radiographs are obtained to identify cervical ribs or bands. Nerve conduction velocity across the outlet and local anesthetic injection of the anterior scalene muscle are used to determine the etiology of symptoms. Angiography is recommended only if arterial occlusion or embolization is suspected.

After the diagnosis is confirmed, nonsurgical treatments, including physical therapy and Botox injection of the anterior scalene muscle, are attempted in patients with neurogenic TOS. If symptoms persist, surgical decompression of the outlet may be warranted. The most commonly used procedure is resection of the first thoracic rib, removal of any cervical ribs, and division of the anterior scalene muscle. Patients with vasculogenic TOS (artery or vein) require immediate thrombolysis of clot, followed by surgical repair of the affected artery or vein.

Lymphatic Disorders

The lymphatic system serves a number of functions, including drainage of proteins and extracellular fluid that are lost from the capillary circulation and removal of bacteria and foreign materials. Lymphedema occurs when lymph transport and transcapillary fluid exchange are impaired. In these situations, the production of lymph continues at a constant rate, but drainage is inadequate, and protein-rich fluid accumulates in the limb. The high osmolality of the lymphatic fluid attracts even greater amounts of extracellular fluid.

Primary lymphedema is classified as congenital lymphedema (present at birth and rare), lymphedema praecox (starting early in life, usually at 10 to 15 years of age), and lymphedema tarda (starting after 35 years of age). The lymphangiographic appearance further divides primary lymphedema into hyperplasia (numerous large, dilated lymphatic vessels are present; usually associated with lymphedema tarda) and hypoplasia (lymphatics are few in number and small in caliber; usually associated with lymphedema praecox). Acquired lymphedema occurs after recurrent infection, radiation, surgical excision, or neoplastic invasion of regional lymph nodes.

Patients with lymphedema usually have diffuse painless enlargement of the extremities. With time, the soft "pitting" edema becomes "woody" as progressive fibrosis of the connective tissue occurs.

Treatment includes both medical and surgical management, neither of which can cure the process. The use of high-pressure (40 to 50 mm Hg) support hosiery, avoidance of prolonged standing, lymphatic massage, sequential compression devices, and meticulous foot care to minimize lymphangitis are the primary medical therapies. Lymphangitis is treated aggressively with antibiotics, elevation, and bed rest. Patients with recurrent infection are candidates for continuing antibiotic therapy. Patients with long-standing acquired lymphedema are at a small increased risk of lymphosarcoma and should be examined frequently.

Surgical intervention is considered only if medical management fails. Surgical approaches fall into two categories: reconstruction of the lymphatic drainage (lymphangioplasty) and excision of varying amounts of subcutaneous tissue and skin. Unfortunately, the results of surgery are often disappointing and should be reserved for patients with extensive edema who have failed medical therapy.

SUGGESTED READINGS

Atherosclerosis

Zierler RE. Haemodynamics for the vascular surgeon. In: Moore W, ed. *Vascular Surgery: A Comprehensive Review*. Philadelphia, PA: Elsevier, 2005.

Aneurysm

Cao P, Verzini F, Parlani G, et al. Clinical effect of abdominal aortic endografting: 7-year concurrent comparison with open repair. *J Vasc Surg* 2004;40(5):841–848.

Arterial Occlusive Disease

Dormandy JA, Rutherford RB. Management of peripheral arterial disease (PAD). TASC Working Group: TransAtlantic Inter-Society. *J Vasc Surg* 2000;31(1Pt2):S1–S296.

Cerebrovascular Insufficiency

Lepore MR, Stanbergh 3rd WC, Salartash K, et al. Influence of NASCET/ACAS trial eligibility on outcome after carotid endarterectomy. *J Vasc Surg* 2001;34(4):58–86.

Mayo SW, Eldrup-Jorgensen J, Lucas FL, et al. Carotid endarterectomy after NASCET and ACAS: a statewide study. *J Vasc Surg* 1998;28(6):1017–1023.

Jordan WD, Alcocer F, Wirthlin DJ, et al. High-risk carotid endarterectomy: challenging carotid stent protocols. *J Vasc Surg* 2002;35(1):16–22.

Venous Disease

Callan MJ. Epidemiology of varicose veins. *Br J Surg* 1994;81:167–173.

Merchant RT, DePalma RG, Kabnick LS. Endovascular obliteration of saphenous reflux: a multicenter study. *J Vasc Surg* 2002;35:1190–1196.

24

OSCAR H. GRANDAS, MD ■ HILARY SANFEY, MD
MITCHELL H. GOLDMAN, MD

Transplantation

OBJECTIVES

1 List the organs and tissues that are currently being transplanted, and give the statistics for graft survival for organs from living related and cadaver donors.
2 List the criteria used to establish death for the purpose of organ and tissue donation.
3 Given a potential donor, list the acceptable and exclusionary criteria for the donation of each organ and tissue.
4 Describe the methods of organ preservation during the interval from recovery to transplantation for the kidney, liver, pancreas, heart, and lung. List the acceptable intervals for preservation.
5 Define autograft, isograft, allograft, xenograft, orthotopic graft, and heterotopic graft.
6 List the current forms of immunosuppression for transplantation, and describe their mechanisms of action and specific side effects.
7 Distinguish among hyperacute accelerated acute, acute, and chronic rejection in terms of pathophysiology, interval from transplant, histology, and prognosis.

The concept of tissue replacement, or transplantation, is based on the idea that patients who have end-stage disease of critical organs can be kept alive beyond the useful life of these organs and tissues. Until the middle of the 20th century, the failure of any organ that is essential to life was uniformly fatal. However, technologies to sustain life despite transient organ failure were slowly developed. Two examples are early dialysis for acute renal failure and the refinement of respirators for respiratory insufficiency. The experimental techniques of organ and tissue transfer were attempted in humans, mostly in the form of kidney transplantation and skin grafting. Early attempts at kidney transplantation failed because the understanding of immunology did not evolve as rapidly as the surgical techniques for organ replacement. Now, because of improved understanding of immunology and of organ and tissue preservation, end-stage failure of several organs essential to life no longer dooms the patient. In addition, tissues that are not vital to life (e.g., cornea, bone, skin, dura) can be transplanted, improving the quality of many lives.

ORGAN AND TISSUE DONATION

Organs and tissues for transplantation come from either cadaver donors or living donors. Even though grafts from living related donors have the advantages of increased graft survival, ready availability, and immediate graft function, cadaver donors are the major source of graft tissues. Kidney, segmental pancreas, segmental liver, lung, small bowel, and bone marrow grafts can be taken from living donors. All other organs and tissues are procured from cadavers. The total number of organ donors has increased by 78% from 7092 in 1992 to 12,607 in 2001. This rise consists of a 154% increase in living donors (2572 in 1992, 6526 in 2001) and a 35% increase in deceased donors (4520 in 1992, 6081 in 2001). Recently, there has been an acceptance of the concept of "emotionally" related or voluntary unrelated living donation of kidneys. Spouses, distant relatives, friends, and even strangers who have expressed an interest in donation without remuneration are being accepted as donors in an attempt to alleviate the shortage of donors for the growing waiting list. The resulting graft survival of these living unrelated donations is intermediate between that of related and deceased donor transplants.

The recognition of a potential cadaver donor is the initial step in organ donation. Solid organs can be transplanted if they remain perfused in situ until the time of retrieval. Therefore, any patient who has normal cardiac function and has been pronounced dead using **brain**

death criteria is a potential donor. To increase the supply of noncardiac organs, the use of donors whose hearts are no longer beating has gained increased attention, especially when the donor organs can be rapidly cooled in situ after cardiac function ceases.

The diagnosis of **brain death** must be made before organ recovery is performed. The clinical neurologic examination remains the standard for the determination of brain death. The primary physician or a neurologic specialist usually makes this diagnosis. The President's Commission for the Study of Ethical Problems in Medicine and Biochemical and Behavioral Research defined brain death and endorsed criteria that are used as guidelines. These guidelines are separated into clinical criteria and confirmatory objective studies. Clinical criteria indicate that the individual is totally unresponsive to stimuli (Table 24-1). Clinical situations that mimic complete unresponsiveness (e.g., barbiturate or opiate overdose, profound hypothermia) must be excluded or corrected. Confirmatory studies support the diagnosis of brain death, but this diagnosis may be made by clinical criteria only. Evaluation of the potential donor requires serial observations over a period of 6 to 24 hours. During this time, referral by the primary hospital staff to the organ procurement organization is initiated.

Eligible donors are previously healthy people who have irreversible central nervous system injury as a result of trauma, cerebrovascular accident, central nervous system tumors, or cerebral anoxia. Contraindications to donation include most chronic medical problems, malignancy other than primary brain tumors, cardiac arrest that causes prolonged warm ischemia of organs, uncontrolled infection, and HIV infection. Additionally, a relative contraindication to donation is preexisting hypertensive cardiovascular disease. Utilization of organs from donors with positive viral serology poses a threat of viral transmission and subsequent disease. Transplantation of livers and kidneys from hepatitis B core (HBc) Ab+ and hepatitis C virus (HCV) Ab+ donors into recipients with appropriate serologic and viral profiles poses minimal risk of posttransplantation morbidity and mortality from viral transmission or disease. The federal Centers for Disease Control also advise against using individuals as donors whose history or behavior makes them high risk for having transmissible disease. Individuals who indulge in risky sexual behavior, who use intravenous drugs, or who have been recently incarcerated in correctional institutions are considered high risk for harboring transmissible disease. Expanded criteria for kidney donors are those older than 60 years of age and with a history of hypertension, cerebrovascular accident as a cause of death, and a final preprocurement creatinine level of greater than 1.5 mg/dL.

For specific organs and tissues, age is a relative contraindication to donation. Acute or chronic diseases that affect certain organs may exclude them from consideration. A history of hepatic disease excludes liver donation. A history of hepatitis B excludes most organ and tissue donation, but organs may be used in selected cases where the recipient has antibody protection. Preexisting renal disease excludes kidney donation, and diabetes mellitus precludes pancreatic donation. Cardiac trauma, coronary artery disease, pneumonia, and advanced age exclude cardiac and heart–lung donation. Donors who are older than 35 to 40 years of age may require coronary catheterization to rule out significant cardiac disease. Pulmonary trauma, pneumonia, and respiratory compromise preclude lung donation. Bronchoscopy may be required to rule out infection. Minimal hypertension may not be a contraindication to kidney donation, although severe hypertension is an absolute contraindication to cardiac or renal donation. Laboratory studies and biopsy are useful to determine the acceptability of donor organs (Table 24-2).

Table 24-1 Criteria to Determine Cessation of Brain Function

Clinical Signs	Confirmatory Tests
Absence of spontaneous respirations	Sustained apnea when disconnecting respirator
Absence of pupillary light reflex	
Absence of corneal reflex	Electroencephalogram
Absence of oculocephalic or oculovestibular reflex	Radionuclide brain scan
	Cerebral angiography
Unresponsiveness to stimuli	Transcranial Doppler ultrasonography
Known cause for condition	
Duration of condition over time	
Known irreversibility	

Table 24-2 Laboratory Studies Used to Determine Acceptability of Organs for Transplantation

Laboratory Study	Evaluated Organ
Cardiac catheterization, echocardiogram	Heart, heart-lung
Electrocardiogram	Heart, heart-lung
Chest radiograph	Heart, lung, heart-lung
Creatinine phosphokinase with MB bands	Heart, heart-lung
Bronchoscopy	Lung
BUN, creatinine	Kidney
Glucose	Pancreas
Liver function tests	Liver
Blood, urine, sputum culture	All
Hepatitis screen	All
Serologic test for syphilis	All
HIV	All
Blood group	All

BUN, blood urea nitrogen.

Consent for organ or tissue donation is obtained through a signed donor card, the appropriate driver's license designation (usually a consent sticker), a consent statement, or a will. The U.S. system of organ donation relies on obtaining written consent for donation from next of kin. If a medical examiner is involved, permission may also be required from both the medical examiner and the legal guardian. Public education efforts emphasize the fact that the optimal situation for organ donation occurs when the family has previously discussed and agreed on organ donation.

Donor Management

After the donor is declared brain dead, treatment is directed toward optimizing organ function. Ventilation is maintained with a mechanical respirator, and arterial blood gases are monitored. Because many patients who have closed head injuries are purposefully dehydrated to decrease cerebral edema, vigorous rehydration may be necessary. If vigorous hydration with crystalloid or colloid is inadequate to maintain end organ perfusion, a vasopressor (dopamine or dobutamine) is used. Vasoconstrictors are avoided because of their vasospastic effect on the renal and splanchnic beds. Donors who have massive diuresis because of diabetes insipidus may require vasopressin. Although oliguria is often corrected with hydration, diuretics (e.g., furosemide, mannitol) may help to initiate and maintain urinary output. Monitoring of cardiac and pulmonary function is imperative when a heart, heart–lung, or lung donation is considered. Bone, skin, dura, fascia, and cornea donors do not need a functioning cardiovascular system, and the corresponding tissue can be procured as many as 12 to 24 hours after the cessation of cardiac and respiratory function.

Organ Preservation

Effective preservation of whole organs after recovery enhances the success of cadaveric transplantation by providing time for distant transplant centers to retrieve the needed organs, perform precise tissue typing and crossmatching between donor and recipient, prepare the recipient, and work with national and international organ-sharing programs. The most critical steps in the preservation of solid organs are rapid organ cooling and sterile storage in a cold environment (Table 24-3).

The kidney, heart, lung, liver, and pancreas are routinely flushed in situ with a cold solution to stop metabolism rapidly. Usually, hyperosmotic (325 to 420 mOsm/L) or hyperkalemic solutions are used. In some situations, a colloid is added. The organs are subsequently removed, individually packaged in sterile containers, and placed in ice. Hypothermic (7°C to 10°C) continuous pulsatile machine perfusion with a colloid solution is used to extend renal preservation time. Pulsatile machine preservation is sometimes administered with an apparatus that includes a pulsatile pump, a membrane oxygenator, and tubing connected to the renal artery. The colloid solution is continuously recirculated. Cryopreservation with cryoprotec-

Table 24-3 Preservation Methods and Useful Durations

Organ	Preservation Method	Typical Solution	Useful Duration
Kidney	Ice slush	Hyperosmotic Hyperkalemic	24–96 hr
	Hypothermic pulsatile perfusion	Colloid solution	96 hr
Heart	Ice slush	Crystalloid with cardioplegia	6 hr
Liver	Ice slush	Hyperosmotic Hyperkalemic	12–24 hr
Pancreas	Ice slush	Hyperosmotic Hyperkalemic	24 hr 24 hr
Heart-lung	Ice slush	Crystalloid with/without cardioplegia	3–6 hr
Lung	Ice slush	Pulmonoplegia	6–10 hr
Small bowel	Ice slush	Hyperosmotic	Hours
Eyes			
Scleral grafts	Freezing	With/without glycerin	Several months
Cornea	Refrigeration Cryopreservation	Storage media	3–14 days Several months
Skin	Cryopreservation Lyophilization	Glycerin, DMSO	Indefinitely
Skeletal tissue	Cryopreservation Lyophilization	Glycerin, DMSO	Indefinitely

DMSO, dimethyl sulfoxide.

tants (e.g., glycerin, dimethyl sulfoxide) and **lyophilization** (freeze-drying) are useful in preserving skin, skeletal, and scleral tissues. Nutrient media and normothermic or hypothermic preservation are used with cornea, skin, cartilage, and bone.

Organ and Tissue Allocation

After organs and tissues are recovered from the cadaver donor, a national allocation system is used to distribute these lifesaving and health-restoring resources appropriately. Organ allocation is regulated through a contract from the federal government by the **United Network for Organ Sharing (UNOS)** in Richmond, Virginia. UNOS is the national headquarters for the listing of patients who need an organ for transplantation (Table 24-4). All organs that are recovered from donors are registered with UNOS. As organs become available, the computer listing process matches the patients on the waiting list and the organs. All organs are usually matched according to ABO compatibility. In addition, kidneys and kidney–pancreas combinations are distributed according to human leukocyte antigen (HLA) match and waiting time. Hearts, livers, and lungs are primarily shared on the basis of ABO match. However, the seriousness of the recipient's condition, distance from the donor center, size match, and waiting time are used to determine which ABO-matched recipient has priority. The national program allows sharing of these scarce resources equitably while balancing medical and ethical issues. The numerous committees of UNOS, which represent all aspects of organ donation, procurement, and transplantation, oversee this process. UNOS attempts to increase donation and to ensure that organs are distributed fairly, with the best possible results.

Tissues and cornea are distributed through appropriate local and national banking systems. The allocation of musculoskeletal tissue is different because several tissues can be banked for long periods. Therefore, tissue allocation is managed through well-organized tissue banks that have a variety of tissues "on the shelf." Centers that perform tissue transplantation can obtain the necessary tissues as specific needs arise. There is no national computer system similar to UNOS for tissue allocation. However, standards for tissue procurement, processing, storage, and distribution have been established by the American Association of Tissue Banks and the Food and Drug Administration. Distribution of corneal grafts is based on local waiting lists. For bone marrow, there is a national computer network of living donors that allows volunteers to donate perfectly matched bone marrow to those in need.

IMMUNOLOGY

Transplantation involves a surgical procedure that transfers tissue from one site to another in the same individual or between different individuals. An **autograft** is tissue that is transplanted from one site of the body to another in the same individual (e.g., skin graft removed from the leg and placed on a wound elsewhere). An **isograft** is tissue that is transferred between genetically identical individuals (e.g., renal transplant between monozygotic twins). An **allograft** is tissue that is transplanted between genetically dissimilar individuals of the same species (e.g., cadaver donor renal transplant). A **xenograft** is tissue that is transferred between individuals of different species (e.g., porcine skin grafted onto a human burn victim). An **orthotopic graft** (orthograft) involves placement of an organ in the normal anatomic position. An orthotopic graft usually necessitates removal of the native organ (e.g., cardiac transplantation). A **heterotopic graft** involves placement of an organ at a site different from the normal anatomic position (e.g., renal transplantation).

The success of a graft depends on the degree of genetic similarity between the organ and the host, on the ischemia reperfusion injury induced by the cold storage, and on the effectiveness of the immunosuppressive means used to alter host response. In vitro testing can identify favorable donor–recipient genetic combinations. In addition, the discovery of new immunosuppressive agents has led to better graft survival, fewer and less severe episodes of rejection, and less risk of infection. The result is an improved outlook for patients who require transplantation.

Immune competence in humans is based primarily on

Table 24-4 Number of Patients on UNOS Waiting Lists by Organ Needed and ABO Blood Group, August 1, 2003

Organ	O	A	B	AB	Total
Kidney	30,790	26,414	13,273	2,379	58,305
Heart	2092	1187	359	69	3707
Heart-lung	96	61	22		183
Liver	8897	6329	2031	483	17,740
Lung	1902	1447	421		3926
Pancreas	702	508	178	34	1,422
Total	45,892	26,414	13,273	2379	87,958

UNOS, United Network of Organ Sharing.

preformed humoral antibody responses. The presence of an incompatible ABO blood group or a preformed complement-dependent antibody directed toward the donor tissue is usually a contraindication to transplantation. Antibodies may be present at birth (e.g., ABO blood group antibodies), or they may be acquired. Successful transplantation requires ABO blood group compatibility for organs that express ABO antigens (e.g., kidney, heart). If ABO blood group–directed antibodies are present in the blood that is perfusing an organ that contains one or more of these antigens, antibody-mediated killing of the endothelium occurs. The result is thrombosis and organ necrosis, as seen in **hyperacute rejection.** Acquired antibodies directed against **human leukocyte antigens** (HLA system) may form in response to blood transfusions, pregnancy, or previously transplanted organs. These antibodies are complement-dependent and are cytotoxic to tissue that has similar surface antigens. The pretransplantation **crossmatch** test is the final immunologic screening step, and it determines the presence of preformed antibodies. Recipient serum must be tested for the presence of these antibodies with a microcytotoxicity test that uses donor lymphocytes as target antigens. If recipient antibodies are present, lymphocyte killing takes place, with a resultant positive crossmatch. A more sensitive technique is the flow cytometry crossmatch, which can detect very low levels of circulating antibodies. Positive flow cytometry crossmatches have been associated with a higher rate of early acute rejection. If certain organs are transplanted in the presence of a positive crossmatch, circulating anti-HLA antibodies attach to the endothelium of the donor organ. If complement is present, these antibodies destroy the organ. Circulating preformed antibodies may be neutralized and removed with the use of plasmapheresis and infusion of IV immunoglobulin G (IgG). In renal transplantation, preformed alloantibodies against HLA antigens are identified using the same technique against a panel of known cells containing most of the known HLA specificities. Panel reactive antibodies (PRAs) are identified periodically in the patients awaiting transplants, and the information is used to determine which patients are highly reactive and which recipients are more likely to react against a donor with similar specificities.

The genetic loci for both humoral and cellular immune responses are located on the short arm of the sixth chromosome. These loci are responsible for two classes of histocompatibility molecules. Class I antigens are single-chain glycoproteins and are cataloged as HLA, B, or C. These antigens are present on all nucleated cells and are inherited in an autosomal codominant fashion. The subloci are genetically transferred as haplotypes on a single segment of chromosome. Thus, a recipient shares one of two haplotypes with each parent. According to Mendelian genetics, a recipient has a 25% chance of sharing two haplotypes, a 50% chance of sharing one haplotype, and a 25% chance of not sharing a haplotype with a sibling. Unrelated individuals randomly share similar antigens. Class I antigens play an important role in the antigen-recognition phase of cellular immunity. They are detected by a serologic evaluation that uses lymphocytes and a known panel of antisera in a complement-dependent microcytotoxicity test. In living related donor kidney transplants, these antigens have a very strong correlation with graft success.

Class II antigens are glycoproteins that have two polymeric chains, each with a common subunit. These antigens are present on B-lymphocytes, dendritic cells, activated **T cells,** endothelial cells, and monocytes. Several series are found within this HLA locus, including the HLA-D locus and the HLA-Dr, Dq, and Dp loci. The antigens form the cellular arm of the immune response and are defined by the mixed lymphocyte culture (MLC) test. The MLC is a strong predictor of success in living related renal transplants. Because this test takes 5 to 7 days to perform, it is not useful in cadaver transplants, especially cardiac, liver, and pancreatic transplants. The HLA-Dr locus correlates with the D locus and can be evaluated serologically. In renal transplants, the graft success rate is approximately 20% higher with Dr-matched cadaver donors compared with Dr-unmatched donors. Heart, liver, and lung transplants require cadaver donors, and preservation time is significantly shorter than in renal transplantation. For these reasons, ABO matching and crossmatching are the most common tests performed before transplantation. In some cases, even crossmatching is disregarded when an emergency transplant is performed. However, retrospective studies have shown that the correlation between matching and graft survival persists in these organ transplants as well. Bone, skin, dura, and other cryopreserved or lyophilized tissues usually do not require typing and crossmatching before transplantation because their immunogenic activity is very weak after preservation. Better results are reported with corneal transplants after HLA matching.

Immunologic Events After Transplantation

Rejection or acceptance of a transplanted organ is an inherited characteristic. Transplantation tolerance is defined as immune unresponsiveness to graft alloantigens in the absence of ongoing therapy, but not to other (third-party) antigens. The functional characteristics of tolerance are lack of demonstrable immune reactivity to donor graft alloantigens, presence of immune reactivity to other alloantigens, and absence of generalized immunosuppression for graft maintenance.

Rejection is an immunologic attempt to destroy foreign tissue after transplantation. It is a complex and incompletely understood event. Four types of clinically identified rejection occur. The forms of allograft rejection are classified according to the time of occurrence and the immune mechanism involved.

Hyperacute Rejection

Hyperacute rejection occurs soon (minutes to several hours) after graft implantation. The organ becomes flaccid, cyanotic, and, in the case of the kidney, anuric. Histologically, polymorphonuclear leukocytes are packed in the pericapillary area, and endothelial necrosis with vascular thrombosis occurs. Hyperacute rejection is associated with preformed antibodies directed toward either ABO blood group or HLA antigens. It rarely occurs today because of the practice of crossmatching and blood group matching (Table 24-5).

Accelerated Acute Rejection

Accelerated acute rejection occurs during the first several days after transplantation. In the kidney, it is characterized by oliguria and may be accompanied by disseminated intravascular coagulation, thrombocytopenia, and hemolysis. The organ becomes swollen, tender, and congested. Histologically, extensive arteriolar necrosis and perivasculitis are present. Monocyte/macrophage infiltration of renal allografts has been shown to adversely affect graft survival. Intense CD4 deposition in the glomerular basement membrane and peritubular capillaries can be found by immunofluorescence staining. This type of rejection is believed to represent a second set of anamnestic (relating to the medical history of the patient) responses that are mediated by both antibodies and lymphocytes. Usually, the antibody crossmatch is negative, but may become positive after rejection occurs. A preformed antibody may be present at a low or undetectable level that produces a negative pretransplant crossmatch. This type of rejection is rare, and there is no effective treatment.

Acute Rejection

Even with the use of modern immunosuppressive therapy, **acute rejection** occurs in as many as 20% to 30% of cadaver donor transplants. It may even occur in well-matched living related donor transplants. This type of rejection causes organ failure. Microscopically, T-lymphocyte infiltration occurs into vascular and interstitial spaces. Organs that have severe acute rejection show evidence of endotheliitis and T-lymphocyte infiltration. Biopsy samples from patients with acute rejection that are indistinguishable on conventional histologic analysis reveal extensive differences in gene expression, which are associated with differences in immunologic and cellular features and clinical course. The presence of dense clusters of B cells may be strongly associated with severe graft rejection, suggesting a pivotal role of infiltrating B cells in acute rejection. In the kidney, glomeruli are often spared relative to other regions. In the heart, the infiltrate is usually pericapillary and is associated with interstitial edema and myonecrosis. In the liver, the infiltrate is often seen in the area of the vascular triad. In the lung, bronchiolitis occurs. Acute rejection is treated with increased doses of immunosuppression. If it is reversed, the patient has an excellent chance of retaining the graft. Repeated acute rejection may ultimately shorten the graft half-life.

Chronic Rejection

Chronic rejection is a slow, progressive immunologic process that occurs over a period of months to years. It is

Table 24-5 Rejection: General Pathology

Rejection Type	Time	Pathology	Treatment	Prognosis
Hyperacute	Immediately to hours after transplant	Swollen, edematous organ Antibody-mediated vascular thrombosis and necrosis Polymorphonuclear infiltrates	Usually prevented by crossmatching and blood group matching	Poor
Accelerated	2–5 days	Swollen, edematous organ Arterial necrosis Vasculitis Lymphocyte infiltration	No effective treatment	Poor
Acute	7–10 days; may recur during subsequent years	Mononuclear cell infiltration into vascular and interstitial spaces Endotheliitis, bronchiolar inflammation (lung) Myocyte injury (heart) Bile duct injury (liver)	Increased immunosuppression or change to different regimen	80%–90% reversal
Chronic	Years	Obliterative vasculopathy Myocardial fibrosis and coronary obliteration (heart) Progressive bile duct loss (liver) Bronchiectasis, pleural thickening (lung)	No effective treatment At best, prevention of acute deterioration	Relentless deterioration

characterized by vascular intimal hyperplasia, lymphocytic infiltration, and atrophy and fibrosis of renal, cardiac, or hepatic tissue. Chronic rejection is mediated by both immune and nonimmune mechanisms through poorly understood mechanisms. The healing process after repeated episodes of acute rejection, chronic graft injury by a delayed type of hypersensitivity response, chronic ischemia, antibody formation, calcineurin-inhibitor toxicity, and enhanced transforming growth factor (TGF)-β production have been proposed as alternative stimuli for the development of chronic allograft dysfunction.

Immunosuppressive Drug Therapy

All recipients of allografts require immunosuppressive therapy. The sole exception is a patient who receives a transplanted organ from an identical twin (isograft). Because of their lack of lymphatic drainage, the eyes are an immune-privileged site. Thus, matching and systemic immunosuppression are rarely required for corneal transplants. However, when rejection occurs, topical steroids are used. The role of immunosuppression is twofold: (1) to provide maintenance suppression of the immune system to prevent rejection and (2) to treat episodes of rejection if the recipient "breaks through" the maintenance program. Immunosuppressive agents are classified as biologic or pharmacologic. They are the main components of immunosuppressive programs. Other immunosuppressive modalities (e.g., radiation therapy, plasmapheresis, thoracic duct drainage) are of historic interest only in solid-organ transplantation.

Immunosuppressive agents are always used in combination (Table 24-6), because no single agent or technique provides adequate therapy. For this reason, agents are often chosen to modulate the immune system at various times after transplantation and to complement each other by suppressing the immune system at different levels or by different mechanisms. Multimodal therapy reduces the toxicity and side effects of individual drugs by enabling lower doses of each while still maintaining an adequate level of immunosuppression. Some agents prevent the recognition of antigens. Others depress cellular clonal expansion. Some agents affect cellular cytotoxicity during an episode of rejection, and others prevent the formation or release of cytokine (Table 24-7). All agents reduce the recipient's resistance to infection and increase the recipient's susceptibility to both routine and opportunistic organisms (e.g., fungi, viruses, parasites, protozoa). These agents also reduce the recipient's ability to provide immunosurveillance against tumors. As a result, transplant recipients have a 10-fold to a 100-fold increase in the incidence of tumors, especially lymphomas and skin cancers.

Table 24-6 Clinically Available Immunosuppressive Agents and Techniques in Organ Transplantation

Pharmacologic	Biologic
Azathioprine	Polyclonal sera
Cyclophosphamide	Monoclonal sera
Cyclosporine	Daclizumab
Tacrolimus	Basiliximab
Sirolimus	
Steroids	
Mycophenolate mofetil	

Pharmacologic Agents

Pharmacologic agents can be classified as corticosteroids, calcineurin inhibitors, inhibitors of nucleotide metabolism, inhibitors of the protein TOR (target of rapamycin), or lymphocyte-trafficking modulators.

The most commonly used immunosuppressive agents are corticosteroids (prednisone, methylprednisolone). These compounds are used to provide maintenance immunosuppression and, in higher doses, to treat rejection. Their mechanism of action is poorly understood, but steroids are lympholytic and inhibit the release of interleukin-1 from macrophages. Prednisone is the most common steroid preparation used in transplantation. Initial doses start at 1 to 2 mg/kg, tapering to 0.1 to 0.25 mg/kg 1 year after transplant. The complications of steroid use are variable and include dyspepsia, cataracts, osteonecrosis, Cushing's syndrome, acne, capillary fragility, and glucose intolerance. There are some protocols in effect that eliminate steroids after a period of posttransplant therapy.

Cyclosporine (Sandimmune, Neoral, Gengraf) is an undecapeptide that blocks the secretion of interleukin-2, a T-cell growth factor. It prevents the proliferation and maturation of cytotoxic T cells that cause graft rejection. This drug is a potent immunosuppressant and is used for maintenance therapy in combination with other agents. It is not effective in the treatment of rejection. Complications include dose-dependent nephrotoxicity, hyperlipidemia, hyperuricemia, hepatotoxicity, hyperkalemia, hypertension, gingival hyperplasia, tremors, and breast fibroadenomas. Whole blood levels of cyclosporine are routinely monitored to ensure maximal therapeutic benefit and minimize complications. Since cyclosporine is metabolized in the liver by the cytochrome P_{450} system, liver disease and drugs that interact with or are metabolized competitively by that system should be monitored closely for effects on cyclosporine levels and toxicity as well as for their own toxicities. Examples of such drugs are barbiturates, phenytoin, imidazole antifungals, macrolide antibiotics, and rifampin.

Tacrolimus (Prograf) is a macrolide antibiotic. Its mechanism of action is similar to that of cyclosporine (inhibiting the production of interleukin-2 and other cytokines). It is more potent than cyclosporine, and it suppresses both B- and T-cell activity. It is used for maintenance immunosuppression in combination with steroids and azathioprine (or mycophenolate mofetil). Tacrolimus

Table 24-7 Drugs Used for Immunosuppression

Name	Use	Mechanism of Action	Side Effects
Corticosteroids (prednisone, Medrol)	Maintenance, rejection therapy	Lympholysis, inhibition of IL-1 release	Cushing's syndrome, dyspepsia, osteonecrosis, cancer
Azathioprine (Imuran)	Maintenance	Inhibition of nucleic acid synthesis	Bone marrow depression, venoocclusive hepatic disease, arthralgia, pancreatitis, red cell aplasia, cancer
Cyclosporine (Sandimmune, Neoral, Gengraf)	Maintenance	[tbInhibition of secretion and formation of IL-2 (by inhibiting calcineurin)	Nephrotoxicity, hypertension, hyperkalemia, hepatotoxicity, hirsutism, gingival hyperplasia, tremors, breast fibroadenomas, cancer
Tacrolimus (FK-506 [Prograf])	Maintenance, treatment of refractory rejection	Inhibition of production of IL-2	Nephrotoxicity, glucose intolerance, neurotoxicity, cancer
Mycophenolate mofetil (CellCept)	Maintenance	Inhibition of inosine monophosphate dehydrogenase	Gastrointestinal intolerance, neutropenia
Sirolimus	Maintenance	Inhibitor TOR	Neutropenia, dyslipidemia, impaired wound healing
OKT3 (monoclonal antibody)	Treatment of rejection	Depletion of T cells, modulation of CDS receptor from surface of T cells	Fever, chills, pulmonary edema, cerebritis, lymphoproliferative disorders
Polyclonal antilymphocyte preparations	Induction therapy Treatment of rejection	Depletion of lymphocytes	Anaphylaxis, fever, leukopenia, thrombocytopenia, lymphoproliferative disorders, cytokine-release syndrome
Daclizumab, basiliximab	Induction therapy	Block IL-2 receptor	Minimal

IL, interleukin; TOR, target of rapamycin.

is effective in the treatment of refractory rejection. Its side effects include dose-dependent nephrotoxicity, glucose intolerance, infections, and a higher incidence of lymphoproliferative disorders. As with cyclosporine, drug monitoring is essential and P_{450} interacting drugs should be carefully scrutinized.

Azathioprine (Imuran) is an antimetabolite. It is metabolized to its active form, 6-mercaptopurine, by the liver. It acts principally to inhibit the synthesis of nucleic acid. Therefore, it is a relatively nonspecific agent, and it affects all replicating cells of the body. Its major side effect is bone marrow depression manifested by leukopenia and thrombocytopenia. These effects are dose-dependent. Other side effects include veno-occlusive hepatic disease, arthralgias, pancreatitis, and red cell aplasia. It is used for baseline immunosuppression but never to treat rejection directly. It is always used with other immunosuppressants. Recently, it has been supplanted by mycophenolate mofetil.

Mycophenolate mofetil (CellCept) was approved for clinical transplantation in 1995. Its mechanism of action differs from that of the other compounds; it is a noncompetitive, reversible inhibitor of inosine monophosphate dehydrogenase (the enzyme necessary to convert inosine monophosphate to guanosine monophosphate) and is a specific T- and **B-cell** antimetabolite. Because only lymphocytes require the de novo synthesis of guanosine monophosphate, mycophenolate mofetil profoundly inhibits T- and B-cell function. This drug is used in combination with steroids and cyclosporine or tacrolimus for maintenance therapy. Its use for chronic rejection is under review. The compound is particularly effective in transplant populations that are at high risk for rejection (e.g., African Americans, children, previously transplanted patients). Its major side effect is gastrointestinal intolerance manifested as diarrhea and abdominal discomfort.

Sirolimus or rapamycin (Rapamune) is a macrolide antifungal that interferes with the intracellular signaling pathways of the IL-2–dependent clonal expansion of activated T lymphocytes. Like the calcineurin inhibitors, it binds to a cytoplasm-binding protein (FKBP). The ligand engages a protein, target of rapamycin (TOR), a key regulatory kinase, which, once inhibited, reduces cytokine-dependent cellular proliferation. Sirolimus is approved as an adjunctive agent in combination with prednisone and calcineurin inhibitors. Some trials have been designed to test sirolimus as a primary agent with low-dose or calcineurin inhibitor avoidance regimens.

Biologic Agents

Biologic agents are either polyclonal or monoclonal sera that are prepared by immunizing an animal (e.g., horse, rabbit, mouse, and rat) with human lymphocytes or thymocytes. The polyclonal sera antithymocyte globulin (Thymoglobulin) and antilymphocyte globulin (ATGAM) are beneficial when used as induction therapy during the first 1 or 2 weeks of therapy for solid-organ transplant recipients or to treat acute cellular rejection. These preparations are usually given intravenously and are never used for maintenance therapy. Monoclonal antibodies have been prepared against various cell-surface receptors on the T cell and are directed against specific T-cell subsets, not against the entire T- or B-cell population. One of these antibodies, OKT3, is directed against the CD3 receptor on the T cell and is used for prophylactic induction therapy as well as for treatment of acute cellular rejection. The humanized anti-TAC (anti-CD25) monoclonal antibody preparations, daclizumab (Zenapax) and basiliximab (Simulect), block the IL-2 receptor, which is upregulated only in activated T cells. Both of these agents have a half-life greater than 7 days. When used as induction therapy, these agents complement the effect of calcineurin inhibitors. Biologic agents are often used in place of calcineurin inhibitors early after renal transplantation when there is acute tubular necrosis to obviate the nephrotoxic effects of the calcineurin inhibitors.

Blood transfusions, either donor-specific or random, are still believed to provide protection against rejection. Premeditated donor blood transfusion is occasionally carried out in living donor transplantation. The mechanism is still poorly understood, but may be related to the formation of blocking antibodies. These antibodies cover up recognition antigens on the donor cells and prevent them from being recognized as nonself. There is, however, a 15% risk of allosensitization to both the specific donor and to other random donors as well. Infusion of donor bone marrow into the recipient of a solid organ is a similar manipulation of the immune system that may encourage donor-specific immunomodulation and prevent rejection.

New Immunosuppressive Drugs

Several compounds are currently under development. Some modify currently used immunosuppressants, minimizing their side effects or improving their pharmacologic characteristics; others have a novel mechanism of action.

Everolimus (SDZ-RAD) is a derivative of sirolimus with improved oral bioavailability. ERL80A is an enteric-coated form of mycophenolate sodium that may produce fewer gastrointestinal side effects than mycophenolate mofetil. FTY720 is a novel compound that alters lymphocyte trafficking. It reduces the number of T and B cells in the peripheral blood while increasing their number in the lymph nodes, resulting in decreased allograft infiltration. FK-778 is a malononitrilamide, which is an analog of the active metabolite of leflunomide, which inhibits proliferation of T and B cells. HuM291 is a humanized form of OKT3 that may have less first-dose cytokine release. Anti-CD3 immunotoxin is a conjugate of a murine anti-CD3 monoclonal antibody with mutant diphtheria toxin; it promotes allograft tolerance in nonhuman primates. Campath-1H (Alemtuzumab), a humanized anti-CD52 monoclonal antibody that depletes T and B lymphocytes, natural killer cells, and some monocytes and macrophages, has been tested in renal transplantation in humans in combination with cyclosporine monotherapy with good results. CTLA4-Ig, a fusion protein, blocks CD28-mediated costimulatory signals and prolongs graft survival or introduces long-term graft acceptance in several animal models.

END-STAGE RENAL DISEASE AND KIDNEY TRANSPLANTATION

Dialysis

Treatment of end-stage renal failure often involves long-term hemodialysis or peritoneal dialysis to maintain life. Because of the availability of maintenance dialysis, kidney transplantation is usually a nonemergency procedure that allows tissue typing and matching, long-term survival without transplant, and survival after transplant rejection. The principle of dialysis is simple: on one side of the semipermeable membrane is the extracellular fluid of the patient; on the other side of the membrane is the material that is to be discarded. Products of normal metabolism that are not excreted by the failed kidney accumulate in the extracellular fluid, pass through the semipermeable membrane to the dialysate solution, and are discarded. Hemodialysis requires connection of the patient's vascular space to a dialysis machine. In acute situations, large cannulae are inserted into the venous circulation through the femoral, jugular, or subclavian veins. For long-term hemodialysis, permanent access to the circulation is achieved by the creation of an autologous arteriovenous fistula, connecting an artery to a vein in an easily accessible and reusable area (e.g., radial artery and cephalic vein just above the anteromedial elbow joint). A vascular bridging conduit of polytetrafluoroethylene (PTFE) graft may be placed in a subcutaneous tunnel, with one end sewn to an artery and the other to a vein to provide a large-caliber shunt for hemodialysis. In peritoneal dialysis, access to the peritoneal membrane requires a transabdominal indwelling catheter that is used for infusion and drainage of dialysate fluid. Most procedures to place hemodialysis and peritoneal catheters are performed under local anesthesia.

Patients on dialysis who await a transplant for 2 years have a three times greater chance of losing their new kidneys than do those who wait less than 6 months. Those on dialysis the longest often are sicker at the time of the transplantation and thus will not do as well as those who are on dialysis for a short time. There is 22% mortality in the first year of dialysis and 60% mortality in 5 years. For patients on dialysis, the longer the wait, the more complications they develop. Most patients who undergo kidney transplantation have to wait up to 3 years for donor organs. It has been shown that even after waiting 3 years, patients live an average of 10 years longer if they undergo transplantation. Renal transplantation is associated with a significantly improved survival compared with hemodialysis in patients with end-stage renal disease caused by type 1 diabetes mellitus. This seems to be a result of a reduced incidence of cardiovascular complications after renal transplantation compared to those remaining on dialysis.

Indications for Transplant

A patient who has end-stage renal failure from any cause may be a candidate for transplant, regardless of the type or duration of dialysis support required. The acceptable age range for kidney recipients is 1 to 70 years, although infants and patients who are older than 70 years of age can be successfully transplanted. The patient should be currently free of infections and free of cancer for at least 5 years. Patients with localized cancers (e.g., skin cancer) may undergo transplantation after successful excision of the lesion. Other chronic disease processes should be minor, self-limited, or under control (e.g., a patient with known coronary artery disease should be optimally treated and show cardiovascular stability before undergoing renal transplantation).

Transplant Procedure

Kidney transplantation is nearly always a heterotopic allograft, placed in the extraperitoneal iliac fossa (Fig. 24-1). The renal artery and vein are sewn to a corresponding iliac vessel, and the ureter is implanted in the urinary bladder. Technical variations are common and include intraabdominal graft placement in infants and small children as well as donor-to-recipient ureter-to-ureter anastomosis instead of donor-ureter-to-recipient-bladder ureteroneocystostomy.

Treatment of the renal transplant recipient involves methods used for any operative procedure as well as those specific to the patient. Ambulation, diet, and medication orders are much the same as for patients who undergo operations such as herniorrhaphy or appendectomy. Early

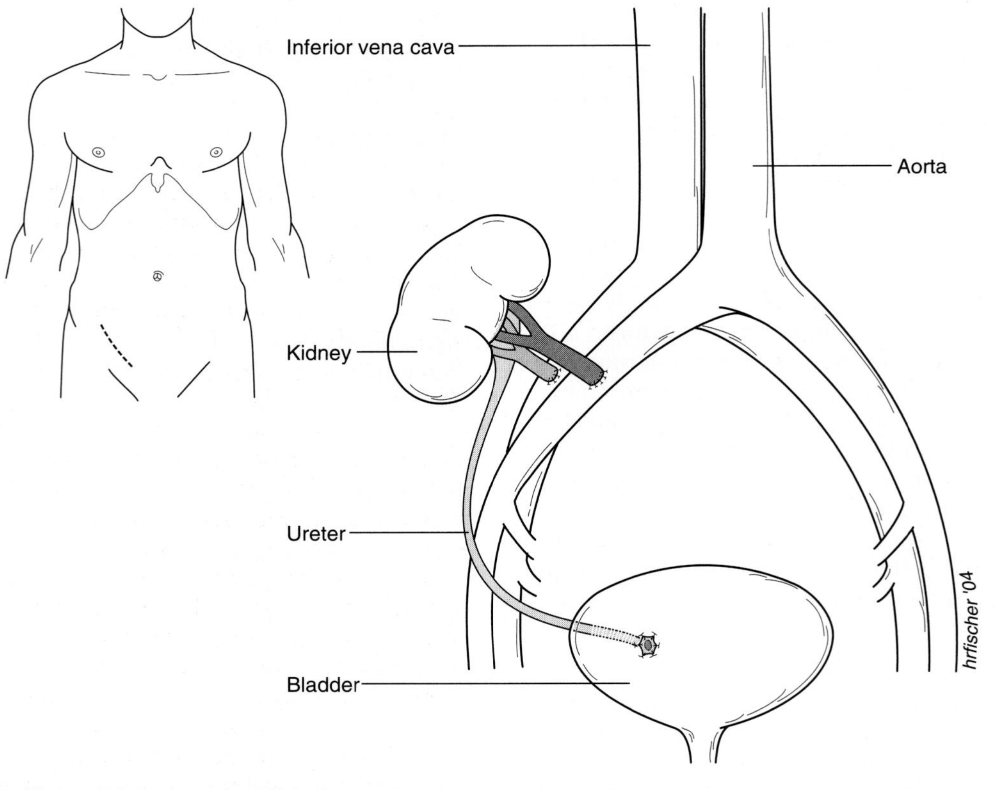

Figure 24-1 A heterotopic human renal allograft in the right extraperitoneal iliac fossa. The renal artery and vein anastomoses are end to side, respectively, to the common iliac artery and vein. A tunneled ureteroneocystostomy allows normal micturition.

postgraft care involves hourly monitoring of vital signs and urine output. Immunosuppression for renal transplantation varies from center to center. Signs and symptoms of acute rejection include increasing serum creatinine, proteinuria, hypertension, fever, decreasing urine output, and, occasionally, low-grade abdominal pain. Acute rejection is treated by modulation of the immune response to prevent graft loss while allowing for suitable host defense mechanisms to lessen the intensity of severe, acute infection. Usually, intravenous methyl-prednisolone, OKT3, or antithymocyte globulin therapy is given for several days. Acute rejection is usually reversible.

Complications

Renal complications after renal transplantation are described in Table 24-8. Nonrenal early complications include infections and cardiovascular events (e.g., postoperative myocardial infarction, cerebrovascular accident, deep vein thrombosis). Kidney transplant recipients are usually treated prophylactically for ulcer disease with an H_2 receptor blocker. Infections are the most common complications (see Fig. 24-2 for timing of infections in relation to transplantation). They may be common (e.g., pneumococcal pneumonia) or unusual (e.g., necrotizing fasciitis from a rare fungus). Organisms that cause clinical infection in the immunosuppressed host include cytomegalovirus (CMV), common bacteria, fungi, and protozoa such as *Pneumocystis carinii*. CMV infection is one of the most common infections in all transplants. It is manifested by fever, malaise, weakness, gastrointestinal bleeding, esophagitis, ophthalmitis, and cerebritis. The disease results from the infection of a seronegative recipient by a positive donor or from reactivation of the recipient endogenous viral load by excessive immunosuppression, especially in the context of biologic agents. Prophylactic therapy with acyclovir or one of the newer antiviral agents is common.

Table 24-8 Complications of Renal Transplantation

Type	Early	Late
Renal	Massive diuresis	Ureteric stenosis
	Ureter anastomotic leak	Vascular anastomotic stenosis (aneurysm)
	Hemorrhage	
	Lymphocele	Recurrent primary renal disease
	Rejection	
	Rupture	Neoplasia
	Thrombosis	
Nonrenal	Infection	Infection
	Myocardial infarction	Progressive atherosclerotic vascular disorders, hypertension
	Steroid-induced acne	
	Peptic ulcer disease	Hepatic disease
	Thromboembolic disorders	Cushing's syndrome
		Diabetes mellitus
		Aseptic joint necrosis
		Cataract
		Posttransplant lymphoproliferative disorder

Prognosis

The results of kidney transplantation have improved since 1975. Functional graft survival rates of 80% to 88% for cadaveric kidneys and 95% for living related donor organs at 1 year are now common (Table 24-9). In addition, patient survival now exceeds 95% at 1 year. Rates of infection-related deaths have fallen drastically. These improvements are the result of better selection of patients with end-stage renal failure and recognition of the limits of antirejection therapy. Overuse of immunosuppressive therapy does not result in better graft survival and is detrimental to patient survival. The loss of a renal allograft requires a return to dialysis, but second and subsequent renal allografts are often performed successfully.

Although complications occur, kidney transplantation is the model of solid-organ replacement therapy. In the United States, more than 14,000 patients undergo this procedure annually.

PANCREAS AND ISLET CELL TRANSPLANTATION

Indications

Pancreatic transplantation is the only form of treatment of type I diabetes mellitus that establishes a long-term, insulin-independent, normoglycemic state. To achieve this end, either whole-organ, segmental, or islet cell transplantation is offered to patients who have this disease. As of October 2000, over 16,000 pancreas transplants had been reported to the International Pancreas Transplant Registry (IPTR). These include over 11,000 performed in the United States and over 4000 from outside the United States. The majority of all transplant cases per year were Simultaneous Pancreas Kidney, with Pancreas After Kidney increasing significantly over time to more than 10% per year and Pancreas Transplant Alone to about 5% per year. Although successful whole-organ or islet-cell-only transplantation affords the patient normoglycemia, the effect of pancreatic transplantation on the chronic complications of diabetes mellitus is less clear. However, peripheral neuropathy may improve, and diabetic retinopathy may stabilize. In patients who undergo simultaneous kidney–pancreas transplants, the kidney may be protected because glomerular and mesangial changes (signs of early diabetic damage) are absent from the kidney after simultaneous kidney–pancreas transplantation. Unfortunately,

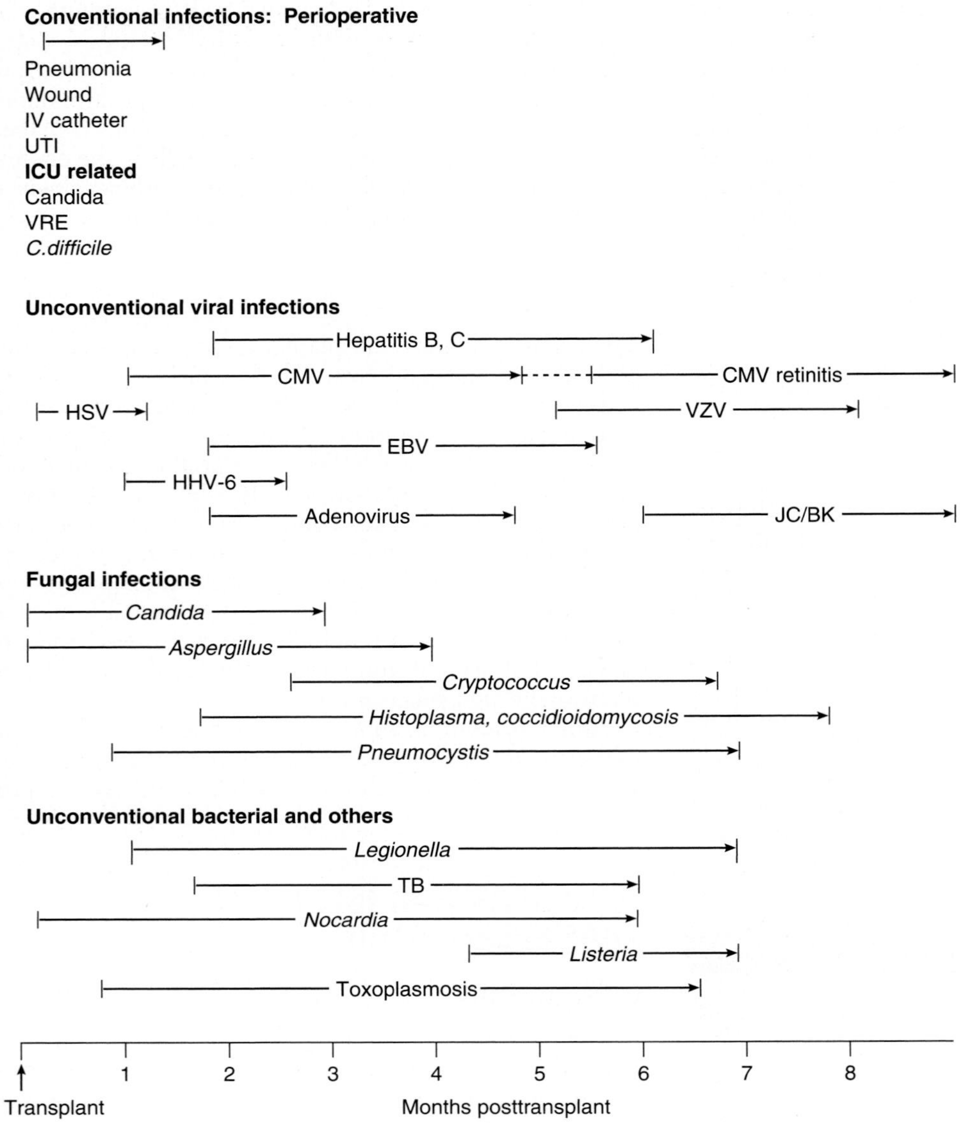

Figure 24-2 Timing of infections in relation to transplantation.

the effects of pancreatic transplantation on the main causes of morbidity and mortality in diabetic patients (e.g., vascular disease, infection) are missing. The last 2 decades of work in this field showed that patients who have diabetes and functioning pancreatic grafts could enjoy perfect metabolic control and the freedom from dietary restrictions.

Whole-Organ Pancreas Transplantation

In the past, a variety of techniques were used for this operation. Today, the procedure is mostly standardized.

Procedure

The donor pancreas and duodenal C-loop are transplanted together in the pelvis of the recipient (Fig. 24-3**A** and **B**). The operation is performed intraperitoneally. The arterial supply of the pancreas, including the splenic and superior mesenteric arteries, is reconstructed using a donor iliac artery Y-graft, which is anastomosed to the recipient iliac artery. The pancreatic venous drainage (donor portal vein) is attached to the recipient iliac vein. The donor duodenal C-loop is used to drain the donor pancreatic exocrine secretions. Since 1995, many centers have switched from bladder to enteric drainage of the exocrine secretions in simultaneous kidney–pancreas transplantation (SKPT). Enteric exocrine drainage may be performed with either systemic (systemic-enteric; S-E) or portal (portal-enteric; P-E) venous delivery of insulin. Although controversy exists regarding the optimal surgical technique, excellent survival rates are achieved with all three techniques. P-E drainage is not associated with a higher risk of pancreas thrombosis or with a lower incidence of acute rejection. Enteric drainage is not associated with a higher risk of

Table 24-9 Graft and Patient Survival at 3 Months, 1 Year, 3 Years, 5 Years, and 10 Years (%)

		Follow-up Period				
Organ and Survival Type		**3 Months**	**1 Year**	**3 Years**	**5 Years**	**10 Years**
Kidney: Deceased donor	Graft survival	93.5%	88.4%	78.5%	63.3%	36.4%
	Patient survival	97.3%	94.0%	88.4%	79.9%	59.4%
Kidney: Living donor	Graft survival	96.8%	94.4%	88.3%	76.5%	55.5%
	Patient survival	99.0%	97.7%	94.7%	89.7%	79.4%
Pancreas alone	Graft survival	87.4%	81.2%	57.1%	32.4%	16.2%
	Patient survival	100.0%	98.6%	86.0%	77.8%	68.2%
Pancreas after kidney	Graft survival	86.5%	78.3%	60.2%	45.5%	16.4%
	Patient survival	97.9%	95.5%	89.3%	77.3%	64.7%
Kidney-pancreas	Kidney graft survival	97.0%	95.1%	89.8%	83.9%	64.0%
	Pancreas graft survival	97.0%	94.9%	89.8%	84.3%	63.3%
	Patient survival	97.1%	95.1%	89.2%	82.6%	60.8%
Liver: Deceased donor	Graft survival	85.8%	80.2%	71.4%	63.5%	45.1%
	Patient survival	91.1%	86.4%	79.5%	72.4%	59.4%
Liver: Living donor	Graft survival	83.0%	76.3%	72.4%	73.0%	42.7%
	Patient survival	91.0%	85.2%	80.2%	85.6%	85.2%
Intestine	Graft survival	78.3%	67.2%	44.9%	19.7%	0.0%
	Patient survival	92.3%	84.6%	72.9%	48.6%	50.0%
Heart	Graft survival	89.0%	84.4%	77.5%	68.1%	46.4%
	Patient survival	89.5%	85.1%	78.6%	69.8%	50.0%
Lung	Graft survival	87.3%	76.2%	57.5%	40.5%	17.5%
	Patient survival	88.2%	77.4%	59.3%	42.5%	22.7%
Heart-lung	Graft survival	73.9%	60.1%	41.8%	46.9%	28.1%
	Patient survival	73.4%	59.6%	44.8%	48.6%	29.7%
Kidney-liver	Kidney graft survival	84.5%	78.3%	70.4%	54.5%	55.4%
	Liver graft survival	84.7%	79.2%	72.2%	58.8%	56.4%
	Patient survival	85.0%	79.6%	75.2%	61.5%	61.0%

Source: OPTN/SRTR data as of August 1, 2002.
URREA; UNOS. 2002 Annual Report of the U.S. Organ Procurement and Transplantation Network and the Scientific Registry of Transplant Recipients: Transplant Data 1992–2001 [Internet]. Rockville, MD: HHS/HRSA/OSP/DOT; 2003 [modified 2003 Feb. 18; cited YYYY MMM D] Available from: http://www.ustransplant.org/annual.html.
Multi-organ transplants are excluded except where specified. Living donor transplants excluded unless explicitly listed. Heterotopic heart and liver transplants excluded.
Survival is calculated for transplants during 1999–2000 for 3 months and 1 year; 1997–1998 for 3 years; 1995–1996 for 5 years; and 1990–1991 for 10 years.
Graft survival follows individual transplants until graft failure. Patient survival follows patients from first transplant of this type until death.

infection. Pancreas graft function and readmissions are similar, regardless of surgical technique.

Complications

The postoperative course of combined whole-organ pancreatic–kidney transplantation is more complicated than that of kidney transplantation alone. More episodes of rejection occur, and they require more immunosuppression. Subsequently, the patients have more infectious complications and longer hospital stays. The frequency of vascular complications is similar to that of renal transplant patients, but urinary complications (e.g., infection, leakage, minor bleeding) are greater in pancreas transplant patients if the anastomosis is performed to the bladder. Pancreas-alone transplants have similar complications, including anastomotic leak, vascular thrombosis, and urinary complications, but rejection episodes are more difficult to monitor.

Prognosis

The success rates for whole-organ pancreas transplantation approach those for other solid-organ transplantations. Some series report patient survival rates of 95% and graft survival rates of more than 80%. These rates are comparable to those for renal transplantation. Patients who undergo successful pancreatic transplants report an increased sense of well-being and better overall rehabilitation.

Islet Cell Transplantation

Islet cell transplantation offers the potential for long-lasting strict glucose control. Recent strides have been made by increasing the number of viable islets from a donor pancreas with the use of new, gentler digesting agents. Techniques to culture or freeze the islets may eventually provide an islet banking and distribution system for elective

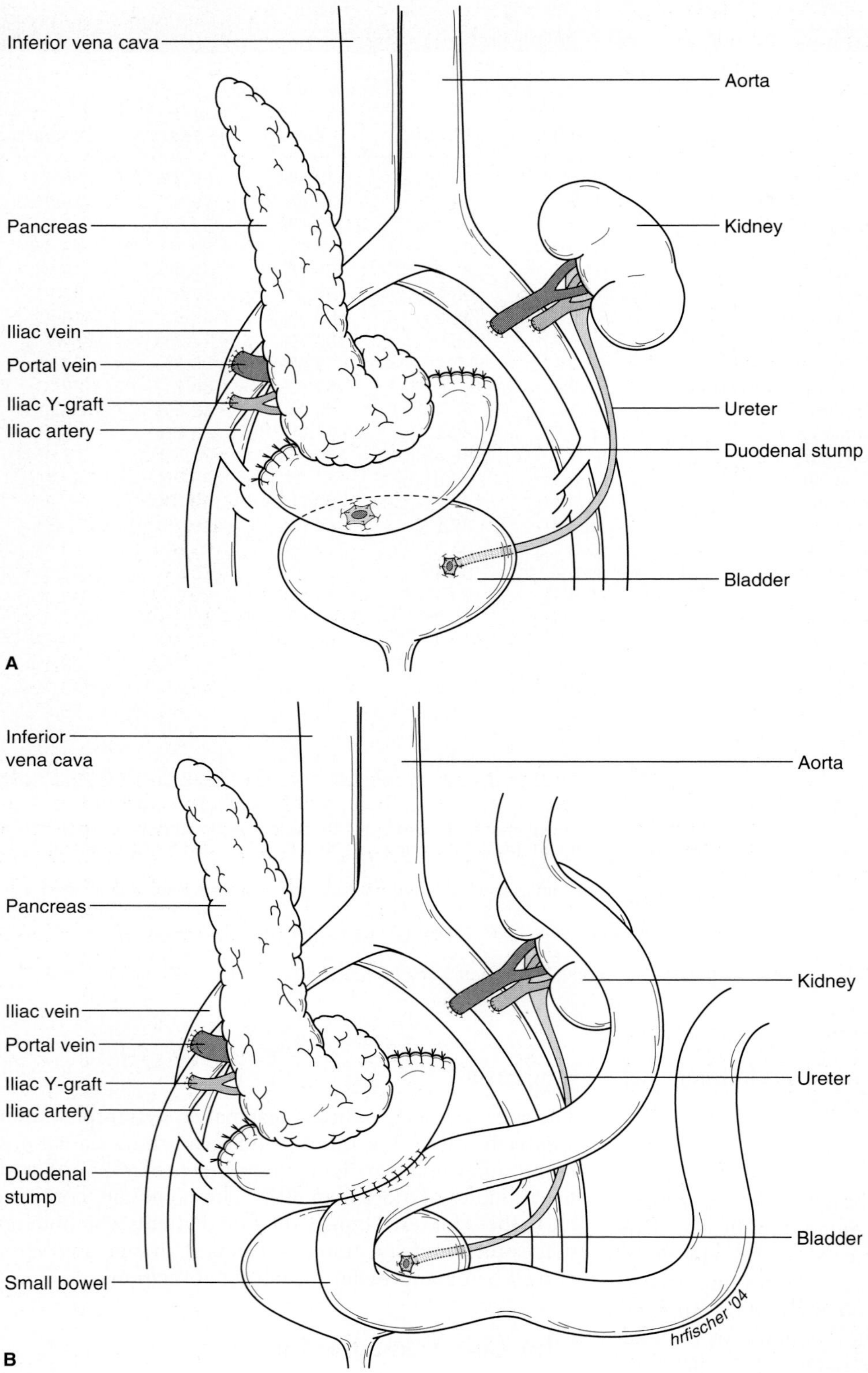

Figure 24-3 Pancreatic transplants using bladder (**A**) or enteric (**B**) drainage.

transplantation. The proper delivery system for islets is still debatable. Current options include injection into the portal vein, placement under the renal capsule, and encapsulation into immuno-isolated chambers. The increased rejection rate, the need for large numbers of islets, and the small number of donors relative to the large potential recipient pool have held back the widespread implementation of islet cell transplantation. The initiative sponsored by the Immune Tolerance Network (ITN) and the National Institutes of Health has announced preliminary results from its 36-patient multicenter clinical trial of the Edmonton Protocol for islet transplantation (portal vein injection and steroid-free immunosuppression). An early analysis confirms that the treatment for type 1 diabetes pioneered in Edmonton, Canada, can be successfully replicated at other clinical sites. Of the 15 patients able to complete their transplants, 12 (80%) are currently insulin-free, in some cases for up to 1 year. Six graft failures were reported following initial transplant. The rate of insulin independence is 52%. Differences in success rates between individual clinical centers were noted, which underscore the challenges that lie ahead in the widespread adoption of the technique.

LIVER TRANSPLANTATION

Indications

Liver transplantation is indicated in patients with irreversible, progressive liver disease who have failed medical therapy. To be considered a candidate for liver transplantation, a patient should have no evidence of malignancy other than small incidental hepatocellular tumors and should be free of infection and active substance abuse at the time of transplantation. The best results are obtained if transplantation is carried out before the onset of terminal events associated with end-stage liver failure. Table 24-10 lists diseases that are treated by liver transplantation, and Table 24-11 lists the indications for proceeding to transplantation. Cirrhosis secondary to infection with hepatitis C is now the most common indication for liver transplantation in the United States. Waiting times before transplantation may be 1 year or longer, depending on the availability of organs and the condition of the recipient. Patients with cirrhosis are prioritized on the waiting list according to their MELD score (Model for End-Stage Liver Disease). The MELD score is calculated using the patient's serum bilirubin, international normalized ratio (INR), and creatinine. Patients with acute or fulminant liver failure receive priority on the liver waiting list. Liver donor/recipients are matched by blood group only and a crossmatch is not required.

Procedure

There are a number of possible techniques for liver transplantation. The classic orthotopic liver transplantation uses the whole liver from a cadaver donor. After completion of the native hepatectomy, the new liver is implanted by anastomosing the suprahepatic vena cava of the donor liver to the remaining suprahepatic vena cava of the recipient and then performing an infrahepatic vena caval anastomosis (Fig. 24-4). The donor hepatic artery is sewn to the recipient artery, and the donor portal vein is sewn to the recipient portal vein. Biliary drainage is commonly achieved by duct-to-duct anastomosis in the adult and by

Table 24-10 Diseases Treated With Liver Transplantation

Benefit	Diseases
Proven	End-stage liver failure from: Cirrhosis: postnecrotic resulting from hepatitis C, autoimmune hepatitis, cryptogenic cirrhosis, alcoholic cirrhosis Primary biliary cirrhosis Primary sclerosing cholangitis Metabolic disease with and without cirrhosis: Wilson's disease, α_1-antitrypsin disease, primary hemochromatosis, and others Congenital biliary atresia (children) Congenital hepatic fibrosis
Possible	Acute liver failure, resulting from fulminant or acute toxic liver damage Budd-Chiari syndrome Cirrhosis, resulting from hepatitis B virus Certain rare primary hepatic tumors: fibrolamellar hepatocellular carcinoma, epithelioid hemangioendothelioma, endocrine tumors
Questionable	Alcoholic hepatitis
Not indicated	Metastatic cancer

Table 24-11 Indications for Liver Transplantation

Progressive end-stage liver failure secondary to chronic disease

- Gastrointestinal hemorrhage associated with coagulopathy and esophageal varices
- Progressive encephalopathy
- Progressive malnutrition and muscle wasting
- Symptomatic progression of liver deterioration (e.g., pruritus, bony fractures, malaise)
- Recurrent infections, especially spontaneous bacterial peritonitis, pneumonia, septicemia, or intrahepatic abscess seen with progressive biliary strictures
- Intractable ascites

Acute liver failure

- Encephalopathy progressing to stage III or IV coma (semicomatose or comatose, requiring mechanical ventilation)
- Progressive coagulopathy with gastrointestinal bleeding

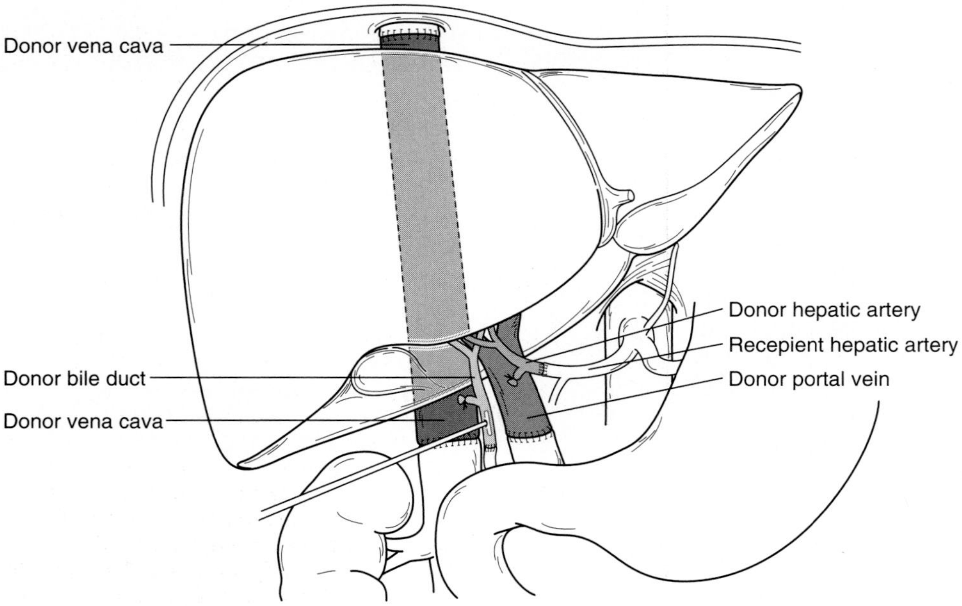

Figure 24-4 An orthotopic human hepatic allograft. End-to-end vascular anastomoses connect the donor and recipient hepatic artery, portal vein, and vena cava both suprahepatically and infrahepatically. The most commonly used common bile duct-to-duct anastomosis is shown.

Roux-en-Y choledochojejunostomy in the child. A modification of the classic technique outlined above, "the piggyback operation," allows the liver to be dissected off the vena cava without division of the cava. This method is associated with improved intraoperative hemodynamic stability and a reduced incidence of posttransplant renal insufficiency. One requirement for hepatic transplantation is size match between the donor and recipient livers. This match is particularly difficult to obtain in a timely manner in small children. This problem led to the introduction of reduced-size livers, usually the left lobe or lateral segment. The resulting segment of liver, its blood supply, and the bile duct are reimplanted into the recipient. The success rate with this procedure is equivalent to that of whole-liver grafts, and it is even used for adult recipients. In fact, split livers are used to provide transplants to two recipients. In recent years, the demand for liver transplantation has exceeded the supply of cadaveric organs, leading to the introduction of living donor liver transplantation in adults as well as children. In adults, the right lobe of the liver is removed from a living donor and transplanted into the recipient (Fig. 24-5). In children, the smaller left lobe is usually removed from the donor.

Complications

Complications of liver transplantation may be categorized as immunologic, technical, infective, drug related, systemic, or related to poor graft function (Table 24-12). Acute rejection may occur, but it is usually less common and milder than that seen in kidney transplantation. Chronic rejection may be an indication for retransplantation. Primary nonfunction is a condition in which the transplanted liver fails to function and is an indication for emergency retransplantation. Various degrees of graft dysfunction may occur and may usually be managed supportively. Untreated hepatic artery thrombosis occurring in the first week of transplantation is a devastating complication and is also an indication for urgent retransplantation. Unlike the native liver, the transplanted liver is almost totally dependent on blood supply from the hepatic artery in order to maintain the integrity of the biliary tree. Hepatic artery ischemia may therefore lead to biliary strictures. Cardiac, respiratory, and renal complications may occur after any major surgery, and liver transplantation is no exception. Late complications of liver transplantation include recurrent disease, chronic rejection, and toxicity from immunosuppressive drug therapy.

Prognosis

Patient and graft survival rates in liver transplantation approach 85% at 1 year for patients who are operated on before the terminal phase of their disease. In patients who are hospitalized in the intensive care unit at the time of transplantation, survival statistics for both the operation and the postoperative period are poor. Many patients, particularly those transplanted for viral hepatitis, are at risk of developing recurrent disease.

HEART, HEART–LUNG, AND LUNG TRANSPLANTATION

Heart Transplantation

Indications

The indication for heart transplantation is end-stage cardiac disease not amenable to other medical or surgical

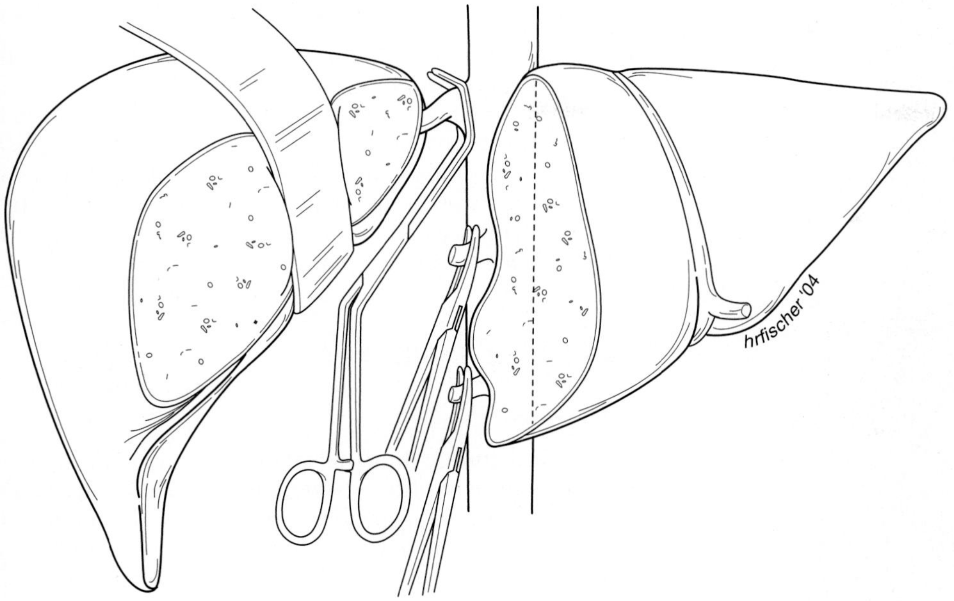

Figure 24-5 Living donor right hepatectomy. The right hepatic duct, hepatic artery, and right portal vein are divided after division of the liver. The clamp is on the right hepatic vein.

therapy. Patients who have N.Y. Heart Classification symptoms on optimal medical therapy whose prognosis for survival is less than 50% at 1 year are also suitable candidates. Age, up to 65 years, is not a contraindication. Oxygen consumption at maximal exercise, a peak VO_2 of less than 10 mL/kg/min, has been used as an objective criterion for candidacy for transplantation. The patient must be free of infection and neoplasm and have full potential for rehabilitation. Specific indications for heart transplantation include idiopathic cardiomyopathy, viral cardiomyopathy, ischemic cardiac disease, postpartum cardiomyopathy, terminal cardiac valvular disease, and hypertensive cardiomyopathy. Many patients are maintained on ventricular assist devices as a bridge to transplantation. Severe pulmonary hypertension with a fixed pulmonary vascular resistance of six Wood's units at rest (normal = 1.16 to 3) is a contraindication to heart transplantation, and heart–lung transplantation should be considered. Cardiac transplantation is most often performed in adults because many congenital cardiac defects can be corrected surgically. However, neonatal and pediatric cardiac transplantation is also performed successfully.

Table 24-12 Postoperative Complications of Liver Transplantation

Immunologic	Acute rejection
	Chronic rejection
Technical	Bleeding
	Hepatic artery thrombosis
	Portal vein thrombosis
	Biliary leak/stricture/sludge
Graft function	Primary nonfunction
	Graft dysfunction
Infection	Bacterial
	Fungal
	Viral
Systemic	Cardiac failure
	Respiratory failure
	Renal failure
Drug related	Nephrotoxicity
	Hypertension
Recurrent disease	Viral hepatitis
	Primary biliary cirrhosis/ autoimmune hepatitis

Procedure

The ideal cardiac preservation time is under 6 hours. Thus, donor and recipient surgeries are scheduled to coincide. Since the number of donors is far exceeded by the number of potential recipients, and cold time is an important consideration, hearts are distributed through the UNOS computer system to the sickest patients. These patients, who usually require mechanical or medical support in the intensive care unit, are in a hospital that is close enough to the donor hospital to enable implantation within the prescribed cold ischemia limits.

The usual cardiac transplant is a size-matched, ABO-matched orthotopic allograft. Tissue typing is usually not done preoperatively. The recipient heart is removed, and the donor heart is sewn into place by attaching the left and right atria of the donor heart to the left and right atria of the recipient. The pulmonary artery and aortic anastomoses are completed (Fig. 24-6). The heart is resuscitated and allowed to take over support of the recipient.

Some centers use heterotopic grafts. These grafts allow the recipient's heart to remain as a safety net if the donor heart is rejected. In heterotopic grafts, the donor heart is

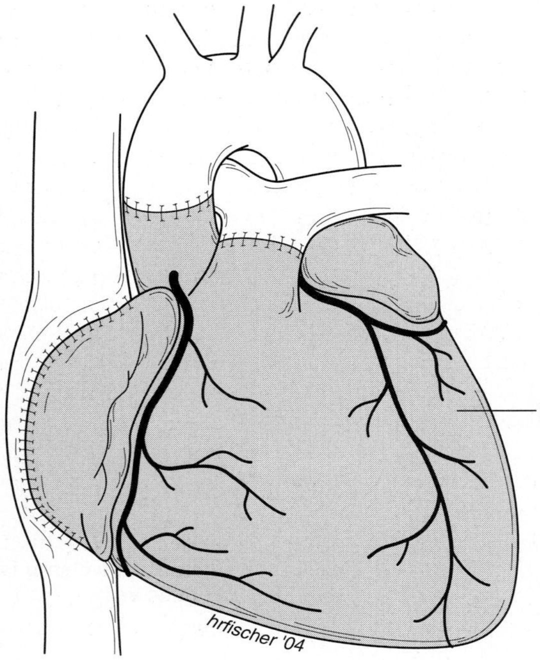

Figure 24-6 An orthotopic human cardiac allograft. The left and right atria of the graft are sutured to the posterior-most atrial walls, which remain intact in the recipient. End-to-end anastomoses of the pulmonary artery and aorta are completed before the transplanted heart is resuscitated and cardiopulmonary bypass support is terminated.

placed alongside the recipient heart, and the donor and recipient atria and aorta are anastomosed. A graft is used to connect the donor pulmonary artery to the recipient pulmonary artery.

Complications

The complications of cardiac transplantation are largely infection and rejection, with ensuing progressive cardiac failure. Early postoperative problems, in addition to infection, include respiratory, renal, and cerebrovascular complications. Late problems are limited to chronic allograft rejection and the long-term effects of immunosuppressive therapy, including calcineurin-inhibitor–induced nephropathy. Accelerated coronary artery disease occurs in some patients and may be related to chronic rejection. Retransplantation and percutaneous transluminal angioplasty are performed for this problem.

Prognosis

Newer immunosuppressive agents (e.g., cyclosporine) and the serial use of endomyocardial biopsy to diagnose rejection have improved the outcome of cardiac transplantation. The current 1-year graft and patient survival rate is 80% or higher, and the 5-year rate is 60% to 70%.

Heart–Lung Transplantation

Heart–lung transplantation is performed when severe pulmonary hypertension accompanies cardiac disease. It is also performed for congenital heart disease. In addition to the complications of cardiac transplantation, complications of heart–lung transplantation include restrictive fibrosis of the lung. Acute and chronic rejection of the lung may be manifested by bronchiolitis. The 1-year survival rate for heart–lung transplant recipients is 63%.

Lung Transplantation

Indications

Single- and double-lung transplantations are performed for patients with α_1-antitrypsin deficiency disease, interstitial pulmonary fibrosis, primary pulmonary hypertension, cystic fibrosis, and emphysema. Single- or double-lung transplantation can provide total pulmonary function to patients with end-stage pulmonary disease without suppuration and concomitant cardiac failure. An FEV_1 of less than 25%, $PaCO_2$ of greater than 55 TORR, or an elevated pulmonary artery pressure in the presence of deteriorating clinical function are good indicators of the need for pulmonary transplantation. Lung cancer is a contraindication to lung transplantation. Recipients must be free of infection and are usually younger than 65 years of age. The donor and the recipient must be of equivalent height and weight.

Complications

Rejection is the most common complication. It is diagnosed by the appearance of infiltrates on chest radiograph and is confirmed with transbronchial or transthoracic needle biopsy and bronchioalveolar lavage. Breakdown of the bronchial anastomosis is a dreaded complication that occurs in 5% of transplants. For this reason, the dose of steroids is kept as low as possible to enhance healing. In lung transplantation, acute and chronic rejection of the lung may be manifested by bronchiolitis. Obliterative bronchiolitis is the primary manifestation of chronic rejection.

Procedure

The surgery is performed through a posterolateral thoracotomy for single-lung transplants and through a transverse thoracotomy for double-lung transplants. The donor pulmonary veins are sewn to a left atrial recipient cuff after the sleeve bronchial anastomosis is performed. Finally, the pulmonary arteries are anastomosed.

Prognosis

Patient survival rates for lung transplantation are 77% at 1 year and 42% at 5 years.

INTESTINAL TRANSPLANTATION

Indications

Short-gut syndrome, the prime indication for small intestinal transplantation, has an incidence of two to three per 1 million population. The syndrome is the result of many intestinal disorders, including intestinal strangulation or infarction from midgut volvulus, obstruction, or internal hernias; trauma; and vascular accidents of the mesenteric vessels. Other associated diseases include Crohn's disease, low-grade tumors, and necrotizing enterocolitis. Candidates for transplantation must depend on parenteral nutrition. Some transplant centers perform cluster-graft transplantation, including liver, pancreas, and small bowel, after upper abdominal exenteration.

Procedure

The donor bowel may come from a living relative or from a cadaver. A segment of small bowel at least 100 to 150 cm long is necessary to provide an adequate absorptive surface. The allograft may be heterotopic or orthotopic. It is preferable to provide for venous drainage into the recipient's portal system. The ends of the bowel may be anastomosed to the recipient's remaining bowel or brought up to the abdominal wall as an ostomy. The latter approach allows easy observation and biopsy to monitor rejection or ischemia.

Complications

Complications include rejection, graft-versus-host disease, and sepsis from the translocation of bacteria through the bowel mucosal barriers.

Prognosis

The results of small-bowel transplantation are tenuous. The procedure is considered experimental and is performed only at centers that have specific protocols. Graft survival is typically less than 3 years, and in many cases, less than 1 year.

TRANSPLANTATION OF OTHER ORGANS AND TISSUES

Occasionally, allografts of parathyroid tissue, bone, and skin are successful. The use of cyclosporine and matching for bone marrow transplantation added to the success of these procedures. Allografts of skin, bone, fascia, dura, endocrine organs, corneas, and blood vessels are used clinically in a variety of situations or are being studied in several centers. Most of the musculoskeletal tissues that are used for transplantation are either lyophilized, fresh frozen, or fresh grafts. Lyophilized bone is used to replace deficits that are created surgically, to fill spaces, and to aid in posttraumatic reconstruction. Lyophilization significantly reduces the immunogenicity of the tissue while leaving a matrix for bony regrowth (osteotransduction) or promoting new bone growth (osteoinduction). Either particles or larger pieces of bone are used. Allograft fascia and whole joints are also used in reconstructive orthopedic surgery. When available, cryopreserved human allograft valves are used for aortic valve replacement. These valves do not require postoperative anticoagulation. They seem to be repopulated with recipient endothelial cells early after implantation. Allograft veins and arteries are used in peripheral vascular surgery when no autogenous veins are available for limb salvage. The results are significantly poorer than with autogenous material. Although graft patency may be improved with full immunosuppression, the risk of complications of the immunosuppressants must be weighed against the need for the allograft vessel.

SUGGESTED READINGS

Auchincloss H Jr. In search of the elusive Holy Grail: the mechanisms and prospects for achieving clinical transplantation tolerance. *Am J Transplant* 2001 May;1(1):6–12.

Bonnefoy-Berard N, Revillard JP. Mechanisms of immunosuppression induced by antithymocyte globulins and OKT3. *J Heart Lung Transplant* 1996;15:435–442.

Cecka M, Terasaki P. The UNOS renal transplant registry. *Clin Transplants* 2002:1–20.

Gordon RD, Todo S, Tzakis AG, et al. Liver transplantation under cyclosporine: a decade of experience. *Transplant Proc* 1995;23:1393–1396.

Halloran PF. Aspects of allograft rejection: part IV. Evaluation of new pharmacologic agents for prevention of allograft rejection. *Transplant Rev* 1995;9:138–146.

Mihalov ML, Gattuso P, Abraham K, et al. Incidence of post-transplant malignancy among 674 solid-organ-transplant recipients at a single center. *Clin Transplant* 1996;10:248–255.

Shapiro AM, Lakey JR, Ryan EA, et al. Islet transplantation in seven patients with type 1 diabetes mellitus using a glucocorticoid-free immunosuppressive regimen. *N Engl J Med* 2000; 343(4):230–238.

Sutherland DER, Gruessner RWG, Gores PF. Pancreas and islet transplantation: an update. *Transplant Rev* 1994;8:185–206.

Snydman DR. Epidemiology of infections after solid-organ transplantation. *Clin Infect Dis* 2001;33:Suppl 1, S5–S8.

Trulock EP, Edwards LB, Taylor DO, et al. The Registry of the International Society for Heart and Lung Transplantation: twentieth official adult lung and heart-lung transplant report—2003. *J Heart Lung Transplant* 2003;22(6):625–635.

Wiesner RH, McDiarmid SV, Kamath PS, et al. MELD and PELD: application of survival models to liver allocation. *Liver Transplant* 2001 Jul;7:567–580.

Williams KA, Coster DJ. Clinical and experimental aspects of corneal transplantation. *Transplant Rev* 1993;7:44–64.

Wood RFM, Pockley AG. Small bowel transplantation. *Transplant Rev* 1994;8:64–72.

25

NICHOLAS P. LANG, MD ■ MICHAEL STONE, MD
CHRIS DE GARA, MD ■ JAMES WARNEKE, MD

Surgical Oncology: Malignant Diseases of the Skin, the Lymphatics, and Soft Tissue

OBJECTIVES

Malignant Diseases of the Skin

1. Describe the etiologies and incidences of basal and squamous cell carcinomas.
2. Discuss the clinical characteristics, treatment methods, and prognoses for basal and squamous cell carcinomas.
3. List the predisposing factors for and the four categories of melanoma.
4. List four signs and symptoms of a malignant melanoma.
5. Outline the steps to confirm a diagnosis and determine the extent of malignant melanoma.
6. On the basis of the extent of a malignant melanoma, describe the recurrence potential and prognosis.
7. Outline the local, regional, and systemic therapies for malignant melanoma.

Malignant Diseases of the Lymphatics and Soft Tissue

1. List the signs and symptoms of Hodgkin's lymphoma and non-Hodgkin's lymphoma.
2. Describe the workup for a patient suspected to have lymphoma.
3. Describe the role of the surgeon in the staging of Hodgkin's lymphoma and non-Hodgkin's lymphoma.
4. List the clinical features of a sarcoma in the trunk or abdomen and in the extremity.
5. Describe the considerations in the evaluation of sarcoma, including the techniques of biopsy, and studies to identify the extent (stage) of the disease.
6. Discuss the treatment of sarcomas, including surgery, radiation therapy, and chemotherapy.

Table 25-1	Characteristics of Malignant Skin Lesions
Change in pigmentation (darker or lighter)	
Rapid growth	
Bleeding	
Crusting	
Pain, itching, or other discomfort	
Loss of skin appendages, hair follicles, etc.	
Regional lymphadenopathy	
Serous exudate	
Raised borders	
Central ulceration	

MALIGNANT DISEASES OF THE SKIN

Nearly every individual has nine to 15 freckles, moles, or other aberrations of the skin. Although the most common malignant tumor in the United States is skin cancer, it is impractical to remove every lesion from every individual. Fortunately, the vast majority of lesions are benign, and many lesions are of only cosmetic importance. Many patients, however, raise questions about the malignant potential of skin lesions and whether removal is necessary. For this reason, every physician should be aware of the characteristics of malignant skin lesions so that appropriate therapy can be instituted in a timely fashion. Table 25-1 lists the characteristics that should arouse suspicion for malignancy. They should be committed to memory.

BASAL CELL AND SQUAMOUS CELL CARCINOMA

Incidence and Etiology

In the United States, the increase in the number of participants in outdoor activities and the preoccupation with maintaining an attractive appearance with a suntan are accompanied by a rise in the number of cases of skin cancer. Unfortunately, just as the link between cigarette smoking and carcinoma of the lung is firmly established, there is clear evidence that one etiology of skin cancer is chronic exposure to sunlight.

Approximately 40% of all new cancers in humans are skin cancers. The vast majority of these are either **squamous cell carcinoma** (SCC) or **basal cell carcinoma** (BCC). Approximately 1 million new cases of nonmelanoma skin cancers are diagnosed annually, compared with 55,100 cases of **melanoma.** These figures show an increase of 15% to 20% over the incidence reported only a decade earlier by the National Cancer Institute. Of the two most common lesions, BCC accounts for 70% of cases and SCC for 25%. Fortunately, the cure rate for these nonmelanoma neoplasms is as high as 97% with current therapeutic modalities. However, approximately 2340 people die annually from nonmelanoma skin cancers. The skin is the most easily accessible portion of the body for diagnostic observation, and early diagnosis of skin malignancies facilitates treatment and cure. For these reasons, the physician must recognize these tumors and their potentially premalignant precursors early and institute prompt therapy. Although skin cancers may remain curable as they increase in size, the cosmetic and functional deformity that results from the excision of a large tumor makes reconstruction of the defect a formidable challenge (Figs. 25-1 to 25-5). Further, although BCCs rarely metastasize, SCCs, especially those that are poorly differentiated, clearly have metastatic potential.

Tumor incidence increases with age. Most patients are older than 65 years of age at the time of diagnosis. There is a 3:1 predominance of these tumors in men, possibly because of employment patterns that require greater sun exposure.

A variety of etiologic factors are implicated in the development of BCC and SCC. The most common factor is solar radiation, especially ultraviolet B light in the spectrum of 290 to 320 nm. For this reason, physicians who practice in sunny climates tend to see more patients with BCC and SCC. The cumulative effect of solar radiation causes irreversible epidermal damage. These tumors are

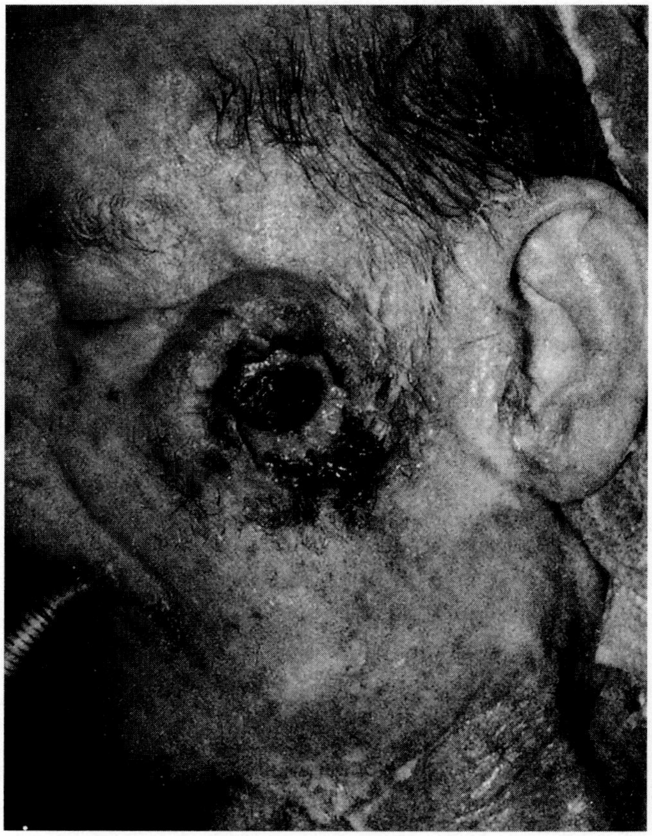

Figure 25-1 Large, neglected squamous cell carcinoma of the left cheek of a man who is approximately 79 years old. The tumor extends nearly to the periosteum of the zygomatic bone.

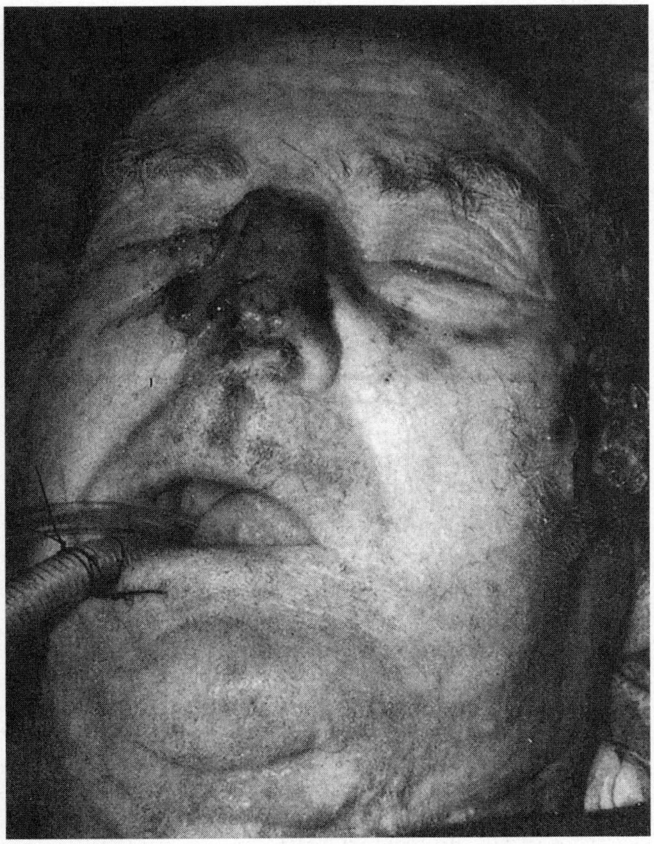

Figure 25-2 Synchronous squamous cell carcinoma of the nose in the patient shown in Figure 25-1. The tumor is eroding through the entire nasal skin and portions of the cartilage.

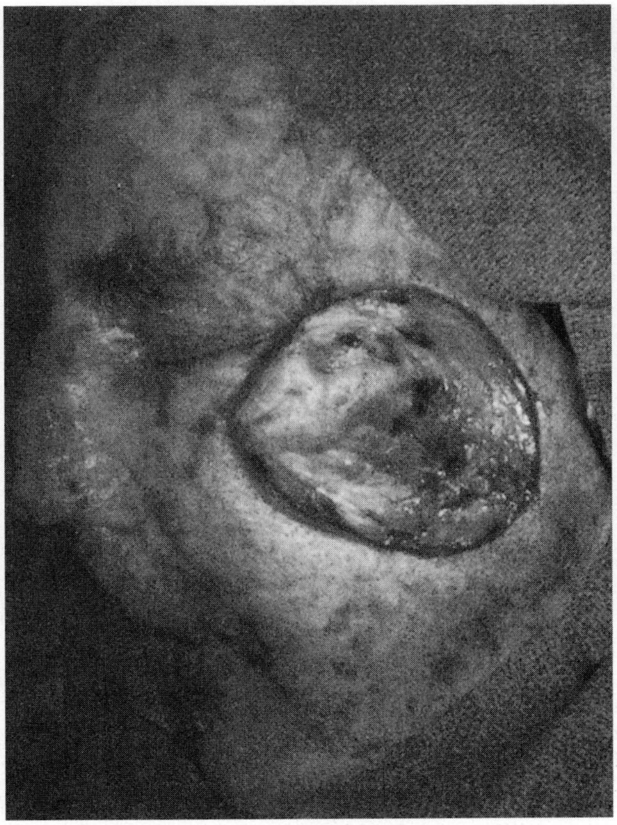

Figure 25-3 After the tumor is excised, portions of the zygoma are seen near the lateral aspect of the eye.

often seen in association with other skin changes caused by solar radiation, including wrinkling, telangiectasis (dilated blood vessels), actinic keratosis (erythematous, gritty-surfaced lesions), and solar elastosis (yellow papules). Given this relation to sun exposure, it is not surprising that approximately 80% to 90% of tumors are found in the head and neck area and on the back of the hands.

Chemical exposure is a second factor implicated in the development of skin cancer. The first finding of a specific cause for cancer is credited to Pott in 1775. Pott showed the relation between soot and carcinoma of the scrotum in chimney sweeps. Other examples include arsenic, paraffin oil, creosote, pitch, fuel oil, coal, and psoralens, plus ultraviolet A photochemotherapy. Cigarette smoking is also associated with SCC of the lip, mouth, and nonmucosal skin.

Another cause of skin cancer is chronic burn scars, where SCC can arise. Marjolin first described this process of malignant ulceration in burn scars (**Marjolin's ulcers**) in 1828. Carcinomas that develop in burn scars are aggressive and can be rapidly lethal. Epidermoid carcinoma also develops within chronically draining skin sinuses and fistulae (e.g., at the site of a chronic osteomyelitis infection, chronic pilonidal sinus). These tumors also tend to be highly malignant. Finally, virus infections may play a role in the development of some skin cancers. For example, human papilloma virus is seen in SCC of the genital area.

Genetic and ethnic factors, as reflected in skin complexion, play an important predisposing role in the development of SCC and BCC. Fair-skinned Caucasians with light hair and eye color are at greater risk than those with darker pigmentation. Because these tumors are unusual in black patients, melanin may afford protection against the damage caused by solar radiation. Another example of genetic influence is **xeroderma pigmentosum,** which is a rare, genetically transmitted disease that is characterized by faulty DNA repair of ultraviolet damage. Patients who have this abnormality eventually have numerous cutaneous neoplasms (Fig. 25-6). Albinism, epidermodysplasia verruciformis, and basal cell nevus syndrome are other genetically determined skin diseases that are associated directly with an increased risk of cutaneous SCC.

The frequency of skin cancer is increased in patients who are immunosuppressed for organ transplantation. Because the kidney is the most commonly transplanted organ, kidney transplant patients make up the majority of the at-risk group. However, patients who undergo heart transplantation have a higher incidence of premalignant and malignant nonmelanoma skin cancers than the nonimmunosuppressed population. In general, patients who

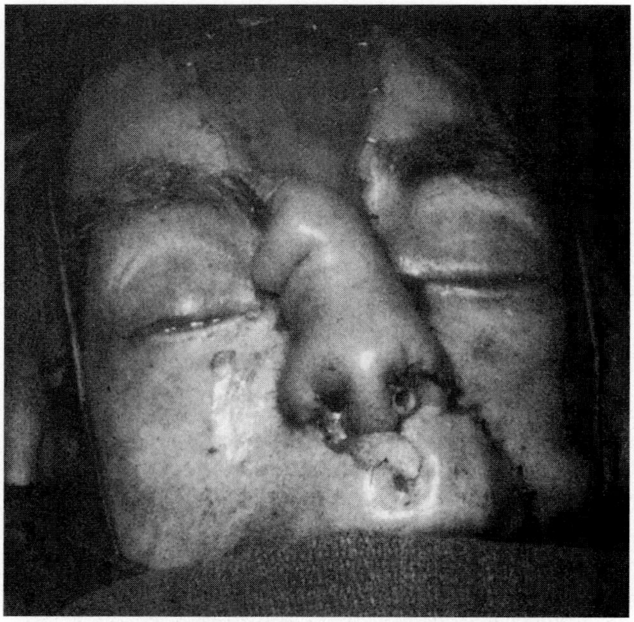

Figure 25-4 The nasal skin and portions of the nasal cartilage were removed. The nose was reconstructed with a forehead flap and a left nasolabial flap. The resulting forehead defect was covered with a split-thickness skin graft. The cheek defect was also repaired with a skin graft.

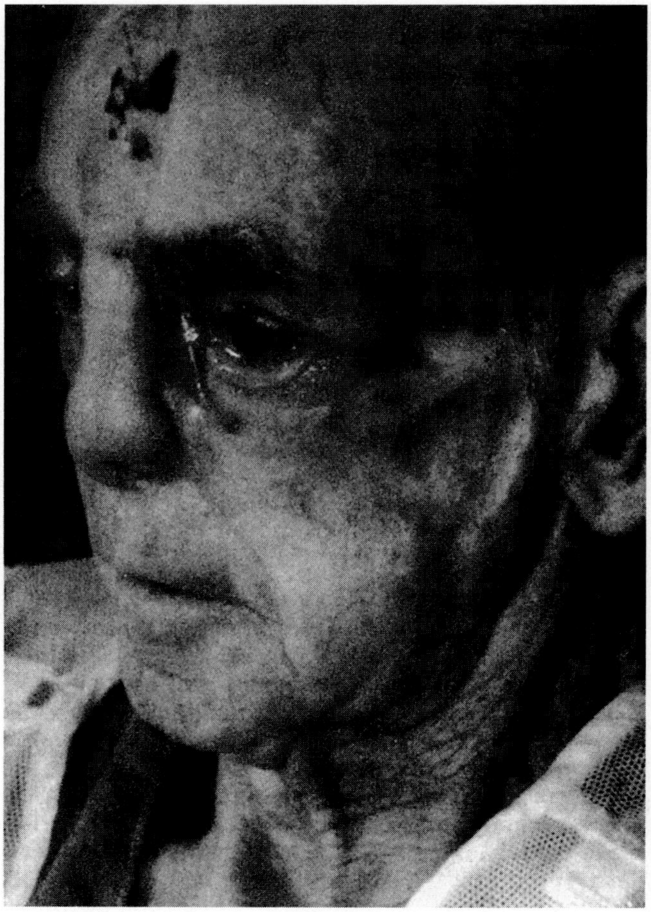

Figure 25-5 The patient's appearance approximately 1 month after completion of the reconstruction.

undergo heart transplantation are older, receive more immunosuppressive treatment, and have the shortest interval from transplantation to the development of the first lesion. Skin cancers in transplant patients are more virulent. The local growth rate and the metastatic rate are both increased.

Although less common today, radiation is another physical agent that is responsible for the development of malignant skin tumors, usually SCC. This phenomenon is particularly true for dentists and physicians who use x-ray equipment without appropriate protection and in patients who receive radiation treatment for benign skin conditions (e.g., acne).

Basal Cell Carcinoma

Clinical and Histopathologic Characteristics

BCC arises from the basal layer of germinating cells of the skin epithelium or from epithelial appendages (e.g., hair follicles, sebaceous glands). Usually, these lesions grow slowly and are nonaggressive. However, if the tumor is left untreated, it destroys normal tissue, including cartilage, in its growth path. These tumors also spread microscopically a significant distance beyond the visible lesion. Although a number of descriptive forms were proposed based on appearance, only three major varieties are discussed here.

Nodular BCC typically begins as a smooth, dome-shaped, round, waxy, or pearly papule (Fig. 25-7). The lesion may take as long as 1 year to double in size. It may have telangiectases on the surface that bleed readily when traumatized. As the tumor enlarges, the center tends to undergo necrosis, forming an ulcer with the potential to invade into deep structures (rodent ulcer) (Fig. 25-8) including the skull, orbit, or brain.

Pigmented BCC is similar to the nodular form, except that it contains melanocytes that impart a dark brown or blue-black color. Understandably, it may be confused with melanoma.

Morphealike or **fibrosing BCC** is an indurated, yellow plaque with ill-defined borders. The overlying skin remains intact for a long time. The skin looks shiny and taut because the tumor causes an intense fibroblastic response that gives it a scarlike appearance (Fig. 25-9). This variety is less common than the nodular form and is more often initially overlooked. The margins of this form of BCC are very difficult to identify because the tumor cells invade normal tissue well beyond the visible margins.

Histologically, BCC consists of masses of darkly stained

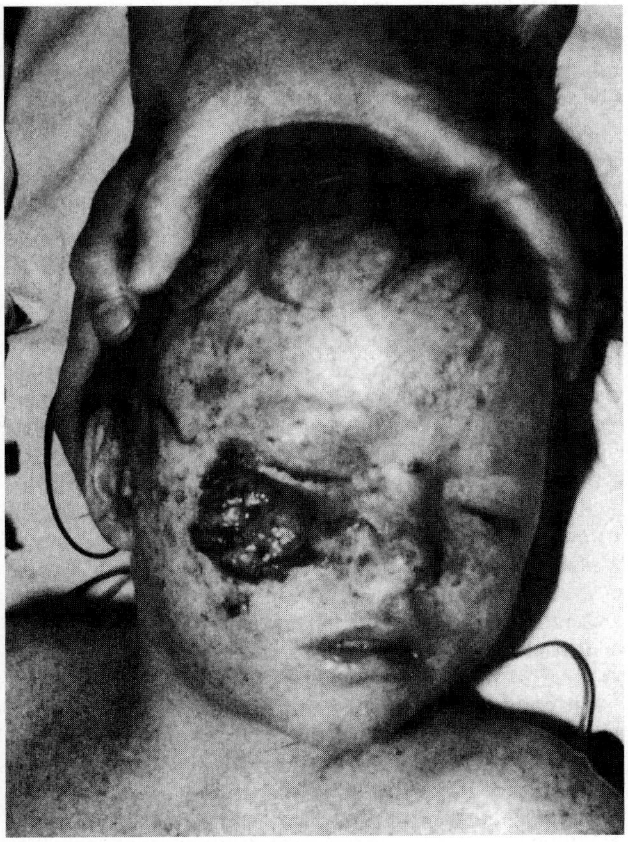

Figure 25-6 Large squamous cell carcinoma on the right cheek of a 4-year-old child with xeroderma pigmentosum.

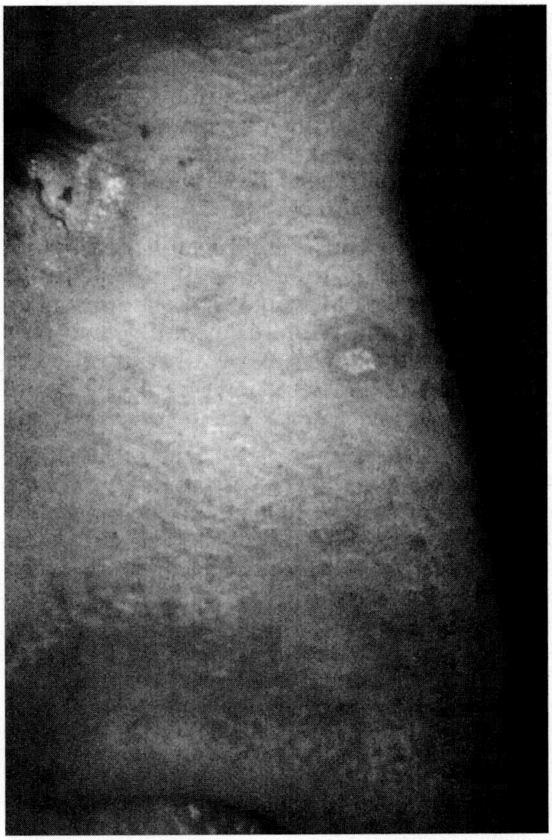

Figure 25-7 Small, early basal cell carcinoma on the lateral bridge of the nose of a woman who is approximately 50 years old. The lesion was elliptically excised, with clear margins.

cells that extend downward from the basal layer of epithelium and into the dermis and subcutaneous tissue. The tumor rarely shows rapid early growth. It causes no pain or discomfort and the patient may defer seeking medical attention until the lesion is well advanced. Alternatively, the patient may first seek care because of troublesome bleeding from the tumor when it is traumatized (e.g., by shaving).

Treatment

Effective therapy for both BCC and SCC centers on two major principles: recognition of the lesion and complete removal or destruction of the tumor. For small ($\leq$ 0.5 cm) typical BCC (translucent, pearly, raised edges and telangiectasia), many dermatologists recommend cryotherapy (freezing the tumor) or electrodesiccation and curettage (using a sharp spoonlike instrument with electrocautery to remove the bulk of the tumor). Both of these treatments take several weeks to heal. The disadvantage of both of these modalities is that complete tumor excision is not guaranteed because tissue surrounding the tumor is destroyed and is not examined microscopically for tumor cells. Most surgeons recommend excision for the management of BCC. To ensure complete tumor removal, a 1-cm margin of normal tissue is included in the resected specimen. A minimum margin of 0.5 cm is included for a lesion that is located near a critical anatomic feature (e.g., eyelid). With a morphealike, or fibrosing, tumor, a pathologically negative margin is required; however, a 1.5-cm margin is suggested. For these difficult locations or histologies, Mohs micrographic surgical technique may be used. This method is usually performed by a dermatologist and consists of the following steps: (1) at the time of removal, the specimen is carefully labeled to show its orientation (e.g., superior margin, anterior); (2) a diagram is drawn of the position of the specimen in relation to the surrounding structures; (3) frozen sections are carefully examined to determine proximity of the tumor to the resection margin; (4) if the margins are clear of tumor, the surgical wound is closed primarily, skin is grafted, or a flap is turned to provide coverage; (5) if there is uncertainty about the margin of the specimen, additional tissue is sent for frozen-section examination; (6) if the wound is large, it is covered with a sterile dressing until the results are obtained, at which point a graft or flap is applied. Closure is postponed to prevent the harvest of an insufficient graft or flap if additional resection is necessary.

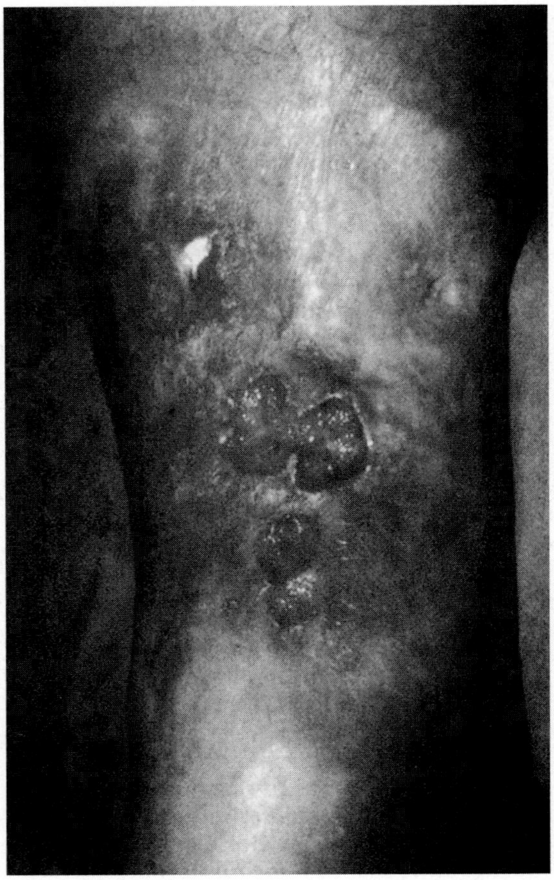

Figure 25-8 Recurrent basal cell carcinoma on the leg of a 63-year-old man. These ulcers form as the lesion penetrates more deeply, outstrips its blood supply, and undergoes central necrosis.

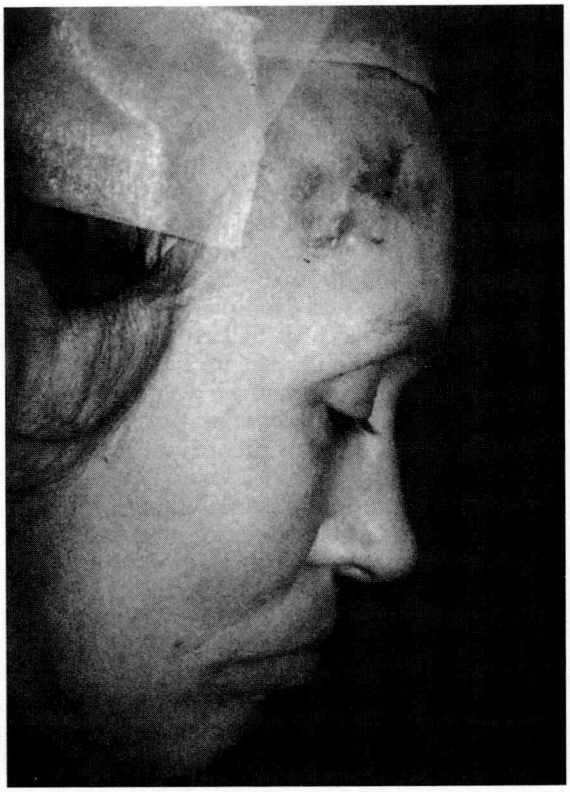

Figure 25-9 Large morphea-type basal cell carcinoma of the forehead. The fibrous tissue reaction causes a scarlike appearance.

Another modality useful in patients with many superficial BCCs is treatment with topical therapy using 5-fluorouracil (5-FU). The treatment requires application of a lotion or cream once or twice per day for approximately 1 month. The dosage is adjusted (1%, 2%, or 5% 5-FU concentration) to achieve moderate erythema. The discomfort of this erythema causes some patients to discontinue treatment.

Prognosis

With adequate surgical excision, approximately 95% of patients are cured. Tumor cells left at the margins usually cause recurrence at the site of tumor removal. However, 20% of patients who have a single BCC have a second lesion within 1 year. Of patients who have multiple tumors, 40% have an additional BCC within 1 year. Some patients experience a field change within the skin that increases their susceptibility to the further development of BCC tumors. Therefore, long-term skin surveillance at 6-month to 1-year intervals is imperative after tumor resection in all patients with BCC.

Squamous Cell Carcinoma

Clinical and Histopathologic Characteristics

SCC differs from BCC in a number of ways, the most important of which is the potential of SCC for metastatic spread. Usually, the lesions reach considerable size before metastases occur. While size is important, another predictor of spread is the grade of the SCC. Grade I has less than 25% undifferentiated cells, while grade IV has greater than 75%. The higher the number of undifferentiated cells is, the worse the prognosis is. Approximately 75% of SCC tumors occur in the head and neck. The lower lip is the most common site. The tumor may arise de novo or from an area with preexisting skin damage, burn scars, chronic ulcers, osteomyelitic sinuses, or chronic granulomas. SCC is also seen in scars from chronic discoid lupus erythematosus. For any chronic nonhealing ulcer of the leg that is increasing in size and is not responding as expected to appropriate therapy, biopsy should be performed in four quadrants to rule out SCC. Bowen's disease, a skin condition that is characterized by chronic scaling and occasionally by a crusted, purple, or erythematous raised lesion, is carcinoma in situ that has not yet broken through the epidermal–dermal junction. Over time, this lesion may become frankly invasive SCC.

It is not clear how often metastatic spread occurs from SCC, although, considering all SCC tumors, the rate of metastasis is probably low (approximately 1% to 2%). However, tumors that arise as a result of thermal injury, draining osteomyelitic sinuses, chronic ulcers, and Bowen's disease tend to metastasize more often than tumors that arise in sun-damaged skin. Tumors that arise either de novo or in sun-damaged skin and penetrate 8 mm or more from the surface are more likely to metastasize.

Clinically, the tumor arises as an erythematous firm papule on normal or sun-damaged skin. It grows relatively slowly and is, at first, difficult to distinguish from a hyperkeratotic lesion. As the tumor enlarges, it forms a nodule, with central ulceration surrounded by firm induration. Beneath the area of ulceration is a white or yellow necrotic base. When this base is removed, a craterlike defect remains (Fig. 25-10). It does not have the pearly, raised margins of BCC tumors (see Fig. 25-7). SCC tumors often have crusts or scabs as a result of repetitive trauma, bleeding, or leakage of the serous exudate (Fig. 25-11). As with BCC lesions, SCC lesions may enlarge and erode through adjacent tissue, causing considerable destruction (Fig. 25-12).

Microscopically, the tumors are irregular nests of epidermal cells that infiltrate the dermis to varying depths and show varying degrees of differentiation. The more differentiated the tumor is, the greater is the number of epithelial pearls (keratinous material) seen in the depths of the tumor.

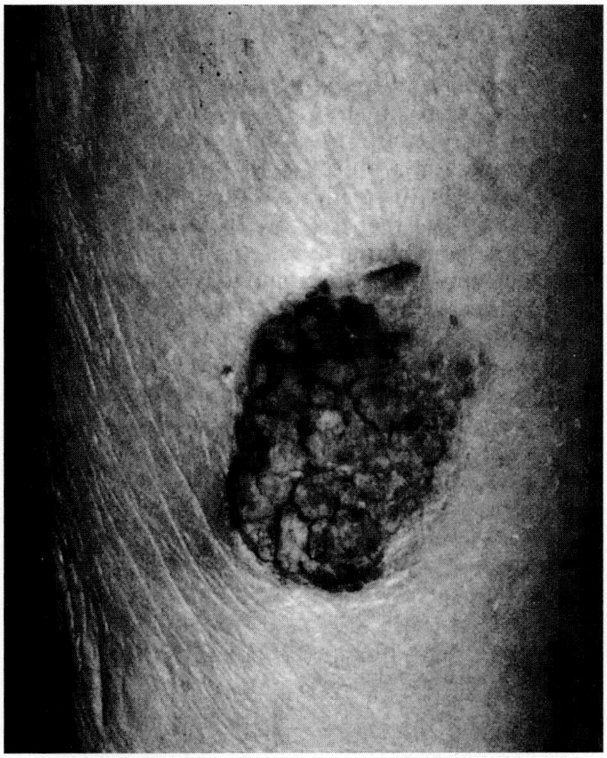

Figure 25-11 Large squamous cell carcinoma of the leg covered by a crust of congealed serous fluid and blood. When the crust is removed, the underlying lesion bleeds considerably.

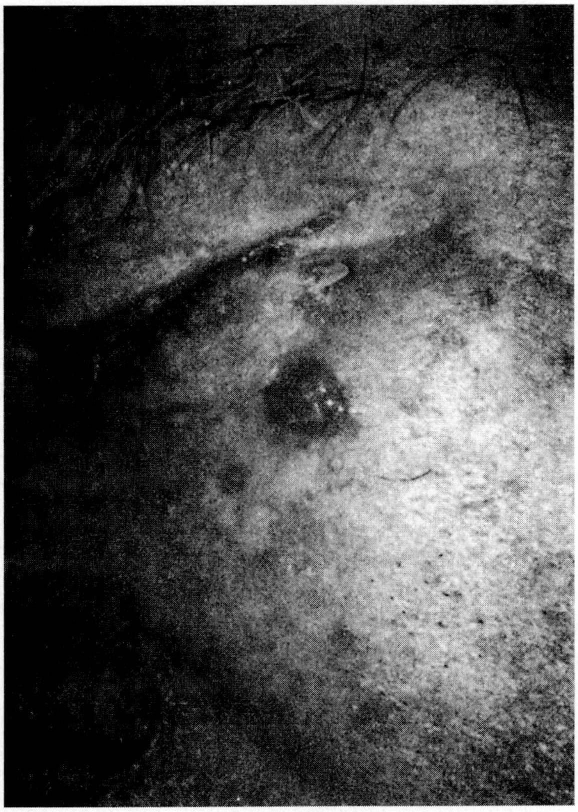

Figure 25-10 Ulcerlike appearance of a small squamous cell carcinoma of the cheek of a 56-year-old man.

Treatment

The considerations for the treatment of SCC lesions are essentially the same as those for BCC lesions. The standard margin of resection is 1 cm, and the same criteria apply for skin grafting and flap coverage. A major difference is the occasional need for lymph node dissection, with excision of the primary lesion.

Sentinel node biopsy should be considered for poorly differentiated or large cancers. For details of the technique, see the treatment subsection of the melanoma section below.

Prognosis

As with BCC, the prognosis for small lesions is excellent, with a cure rate of 95%. In larger lesions that penetrate the subcutaneous tissue, the risk of nodal metastasis increases substantially. After lymph node involvement occurs, the prognosis is poor. Two-thirds of patients with SCC that has penetrated into the subcutaneous tissue may die. Nearly all patients with lymph node involvement eventually die of their disease. Followup in patients with excised SCC lesions should be as rigorous as in patients with BCC. The

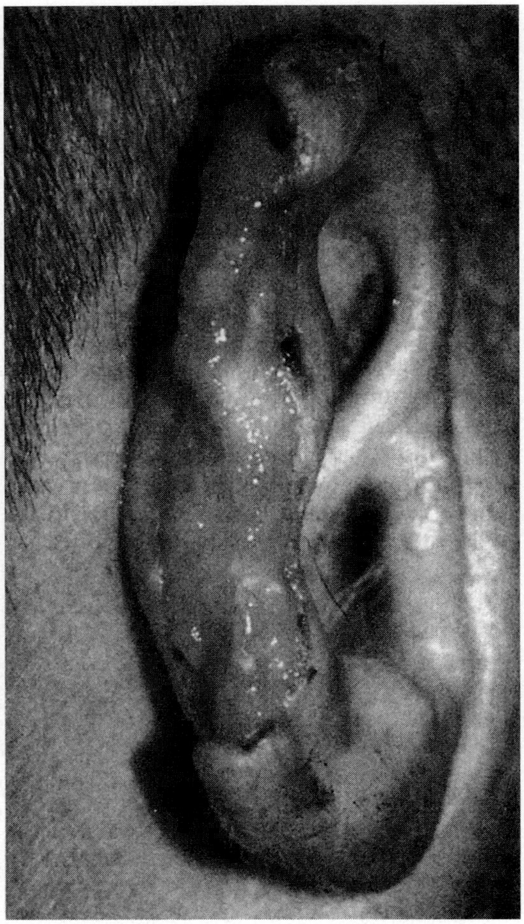

Figure 25-12 Posterior aspect of an ear eroded by squamous cell carcinoma that extends into the ear cartilage. This patient came to the emergency room after a dog bit his ear. Careful examination of the lesion raised the index of suspicion for a skin malignancy. A frozen-section biopsy confirmed the lesion as squamous cell carcinoma.

patient is examined every 6 months for local recurrence, evidence of regional nodal metastasis, or new lesions.

MELANOMA

Incidence and Etiology

The frequency of melanoma is increasing. Although it is much less common than BCC or SCC, it is the cause of 77% of deaths from skin cancer. The risk factors for melanoma are easily identified, even by the layperson. Consequently, early detection is a reasonable goal that should result in improved cure rates. To ensure maximum benefit to the patient, the physician should assist the patient with early diagnosis, correct staging, and treatment.

In 2004, melanoma accounted for approximately 10% of all cancer cases in the United States (approximately 55,100 cases) and approximately 1.4% of cancer deaths. It represents only 5% of cutaneous neoplastic growth, but its malignant potential is more aptly represented by the fact that melanoma causes 78% of deaths from skin cancer. The age variation progresses from 0.4 cases per 100,000 people who are 10 to 19 years old to 35 cases per 100,000 people who are older than 80 years old. In addition, the incidence of this disease continues to increase with the current lifetime risk of developing melanoma, at one in 81 for women and one in 57 for men. This increase does not appear to be the result of more complete reporting or an alteration in the pathologic criteria for diagnostic inclusion.

Several studies in Australia, New Zealand, and the United States show an increased incidence of melanoma near the equator. Melanomas occur with increased incidence on the lower legs in women and on the trunk in men. These data suggest that exposure to sunlight has a role in the etiology of melanoma, but they do not explain the occurrence of melanoma in areas of the body that have minimal exposure to sunlight.

The incidence of melanoma is influenced by skin pigment, with the lowest rates (0.8 per 100,000 population) occurring among blacks. On the other hand, incidence rates among the Celtic population in Australia and New Zealand are the highest in the world (40 per 100,000). In the United States, the incidence varies from 15 per 100,000 among males in Los Angeles to 5.3 per 100,000 among females in New Orleans.

Approximately one-fourth of cutaneous melanomas occur in the head and neck area. Of these, 88% occur outside the protected area (hair-bearing scalp). This suggests, but does not prove, a solar etiology for melanoma in this area. The fact that melanoma is more common among white-collar than blue-collar workers and that melanoma can occur on mucus membranes both suggest sun exposure is not the sole cause of melanoma. The site distribution of malignant melanoma in blacks is strikingly different from that in whites. In Uganda, approximately 70% of melanomas are found on the plantar surface, compared with 6% in whites. Likewise, 8% of melanomas in Uganda occur in the nasopharynx, an extremely rare site in the white population. All of these factors seem to influence the development of melanoma, but no single explanation is satisfactory for all locations and frequencies of melanoma.

The etiology of melanoma is not known. However, 50% to 60% of melanomas arise from or near benign nevi. The triggering event for malignant transformation is not known. Benign nevi are extremely common, and very few become malignant. The one exception is **congenital giant hairy nevus** (bathing trunk nevus), which undergoes malignant transformation to melanoma in 10% to 30% of untreated lesions.

Familial malignant melanomas account for 8% to 12% of all melanomas. As many as 44% of patients who have multiple primary melanomas have a family history of this tumor. Familial melanomas tend to occur at a younger age than sporadic tumors. Of patients who have a melanoma, 3% to 5% have a second primary melanoma. In these patients, the risk is calculated at 900 times that of the population at large.

A third recognized risk factor for hereditary melanoma is **familial atypical mole and melanoma syndrome (FAM-M)**, previously called dysplastic nevus syndrome. Hereditary melanoma and FAM-M represent an autosomal dominant gene with high penetrance. These lesions are associated with genetic alterations in chromosomes 1p, 6q, 7, and 9 and are implicated in the pathogenesis of familial melanoma. A tumor suppressor gene in chromosome 9p21 is probably involved in familial melanoma as well as sporadic melanoma. Several kindreds with familial melanoma have large premalignant nevi, predominantly over the shoulders, upper chest, and back. Genetic predisposition to malignant melanoma is also associated with the hereditary syndrome xeroderma pigmentosum.

Embryology of Melanocytes

Melanocytes are derived from neural crest tissue. During early gestation, the cells migrate to the skin, uveal tract, meninges, and ectodermal mucosa. Melanocytes reside in the skin (in the basement layer of the epidermis) and elaborate melanin pigment under a variety of stimuli.

The number of melanocytes per unit area of skin surface does not correlate with the propensity for melanoma to develop. The density of melanocytes in Caucasians and African Americans is approximately the same for any skin site. Differences in skin pigmentation are determined by the melanosome-pigment package that is passed out of the melanocyte, by way of its dendritic processes, and phagocytized by surrounding keratinocytes. These cells then migrate up to the epidermis, where they cause the phenotypic patterns and degrees of skin coloration observed in people.

Clinical and Histopathologic Characteristics

A convenient guide for the recognition of melanoma is the ABCD rule. A refers to Asymmetry: One-half of the mole does not match the other half. B is for Border: The edges are ragged, irregular, or blurred. C refers to Color: There is variation in the color with differing shades of brown or black, or there may be patches of red, white, or blue. D is for Diameter: The lesion is larger than 6 millimeters (the size of a pencil eraser) or is growing larger since the last evaluation.

Excluding ocular lesions, as many as 11 types of melanoma are described. For this discussion, melanoma is classified as **lentigo maligna melanoma, superficial spreading melanoma, nodular melanoma,** and **acral lentiginous melanoma.** Melanoma has two distinct growth patterns. The horizontal, or lateral, growth phase results in increasing lesion size, but less risk of distant spread while the deep, or vertical, growth phase is more dangerous because of increased likelihood of invasion and metastatic spread. The radial growth phase is characterized by abnormal melanocytes that extend centrifugally in the epidermis, with minimal invasion of the papillary dermis. In superficial spreading melanoma, these large epithelioid cells occur in nests and as an intradermal component at least three rete pegs away from the area of invasion. These cells have relatively uniform nuclei, with an abundance of dusky cytoplasm. The vertical growth phase consists of malignant cells that invade the dermis for variable distances. Cells may vary in appearance from one cluster to another. Lymphocytes are common around these invading cells.

Lentigo maligna melanoma (Hutchinson's freckle) is a type of melanoma that is characterized by a long period of development and by its tendency to occur on the sun-exposed areas of the face, head, and neck of older people. It usually begins as a circumscribed macular patch of mottled pigmentation, showing shades of dark brown, tan, or black. The median age at diagnosis is approximately 70 years. This type of melanoma constitutes 10% to 15% of cutaneous melanomas and is the most benign cutaneous melanoma (Fig. 25-13). It commonly occurs in areas that

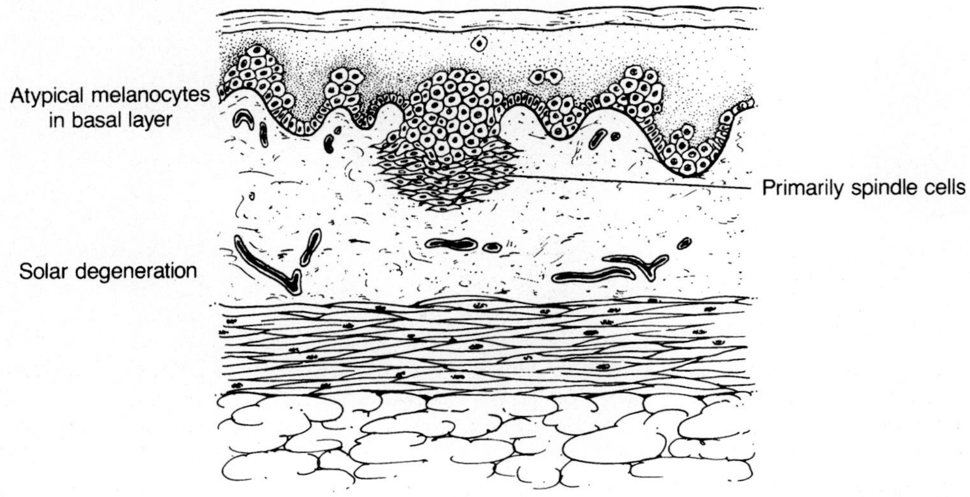

Figure 25-13 Lentigo maligna melanoma.

are heavily exposed to the sun. Women are affected more often than men. The lesions are large, flat, and tan or brown. As the vertical growth phase begins to develop, the lesions become focally elevated. The basic tan-brown pattern of the radial growth phase persists during this period. The elevation is either lighter or darker than the surrounding radial growth phase. The rarity of rose and pink colors in the radial growth phase distinguishes lentigo maligna melanoma from superficial spreading melanoma.

Superficial spreading melanoma accounts for approximately 70% of all cutaneous melanomas. It is intermediate in malignancy and affects the sexes equally. The legs are most commonly affected in women, and the back is most commonly affected in men. The peak incidence of superficial spreading melanoma occurs in the fifth decade (Fig. 25-14). This tumor has both radial and vertical growth phases. The radial growth phase is characterized by melanoma cells within the epidermis and papillary dermis and by a host response of inflammatory cells, fibroblasts, and the formation of new blood vessels. The radial growth phase of superficial spreading melanoma is more obviously elevated than the radial growth phase of lentigo maligna melanoma. The vertical growth phase of superficial spreading melanoma seems to develop more rapidly than that in lentigo maligna melanoma and is heralded by the appearance of a palpable nodule. Early superficial spreading melanoma lesions are a haphazard combination of colors (usually tan, brown, blue, and black). Many lesions also have areas of rose and pink. The common characteristics of variation in color, marginal notching, and loss of skin creases distinguish this lesion from the more common intradermal junctional nevus. More advanced lesions have palpable nodularity, which indicates the development of a vertical growth phase. Satellite nodules also may surround them. Some of these tumors have pale areas that represent areas of spontaneous regression.

Nodular melanoma is the most malignant type, involving almost exclusively a vertical growth phase. It accounts for approximately 12% of all cutaneous melanomas. Nodular melanoma occurs twice as often in men as in women (Fig. 25-15). The host cellular response is usually less than that seen with other types of melanoma. Clinically, these lesions develop quickly and have a palpable nodular component in their earliest stages. Nodular melanoma is blue-black. The variability in color and margins that is seen with superficial spreading melanoma is rare in the nodular type.

Acral lentiginous melanoma occurs on the palms and soles and in subungual sites. This melanoma has some of the growth characteristics of both superficial spreading and nodular melanoma. The exact prognostic significance of these different characteristics has not been determined in a large series. Acral lentiginous melanoma (Fig. 25-16), however, seems to have a worse prognosis than superficial spreading melanoma, but it is not as severe as nodular melanoma. This melanoma has both a radial and a vertical growth phase. In the subungual location, the radial growth phase may simply be a streak in the nail associated with irregular tan-brown staining of the nail bed.

In addition to the types listed earlier, melanoma may arise in the eye; in a giant hairy nevus; in the oral, vaginal, and anal mucous membranes; in a blue nevus; or in a visceral organ. Ocular melanoma is unusual because a high proportion of those that spread metastasize to the liver. Melanoma occasionally occurs as a metastatic lesion without a demonstrable primary site.

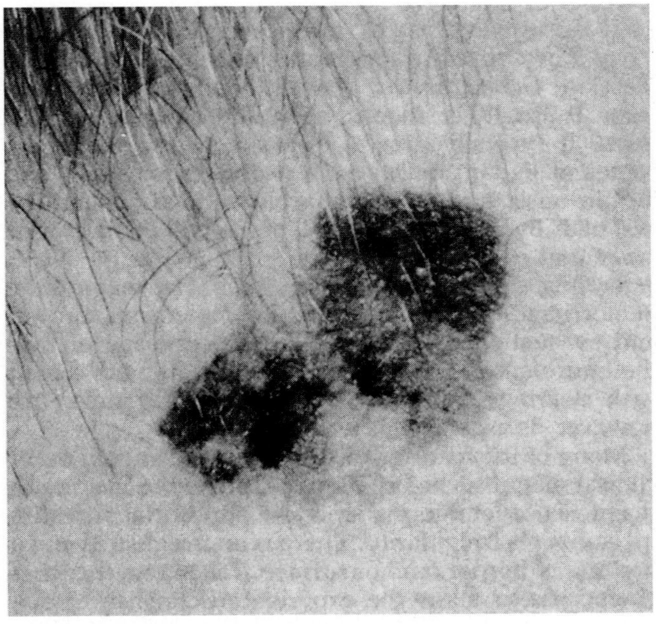

Figure 25-14 Superficial spreading melanoma.

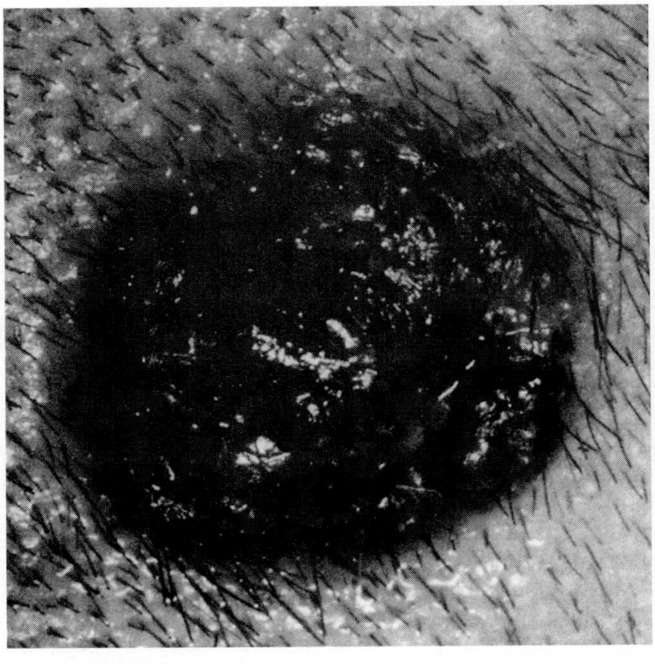

Figure 25-15 Nodular melanoma.

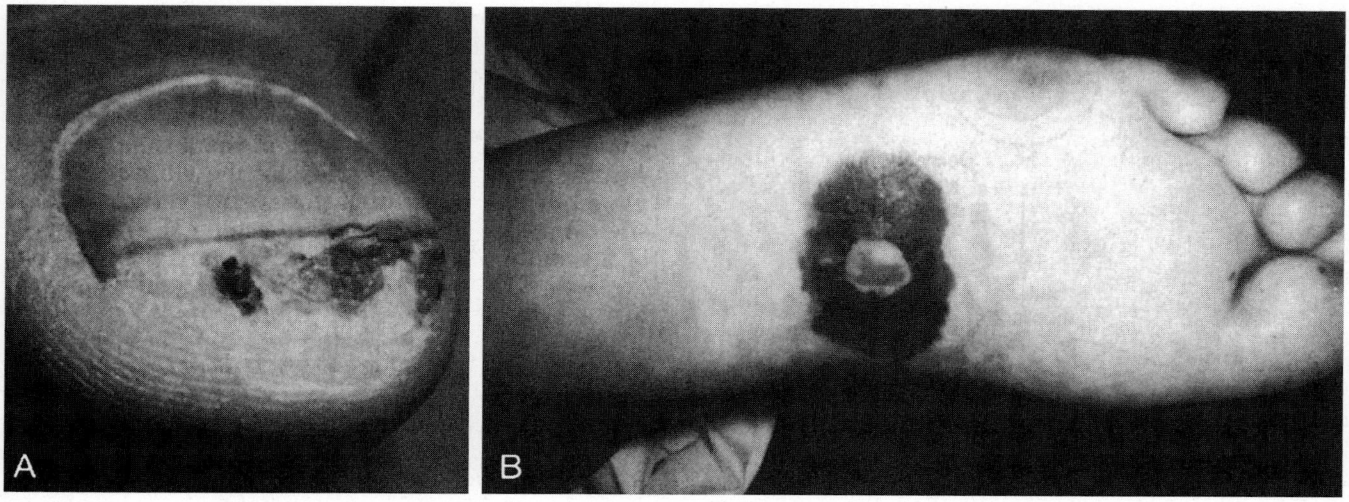

Figure 25-16 **A** and **B**, Acral lentiginous melanoma.

Diagnosis

Lesions that are occasionally confused with cutaneous melanoma are **junctional nevi, compound nevi, intradermal nevi, blue nevi, BCCs, seborrheic keratoses, dermatofibromas,** and subungual hemorrhage. These entities can often be differentiated clinically by a dermatologist using dermatoscopy. Characteristics that help with the differentiation of these lesions from melanoma are listed here. Junctional nevi usually appear during the early years of life and are particularly apparent during adolescence. They vary in size from a few millimeters to several centimeters. They are light to dark brown, with a flat, smooth surface and irregular edges. Compound nevi are usually brown or black, with a raised nodular surface that often contains hair. They are usually smaller than 1 cm and occur in all age groups. Intradermal nevi can be very large, although they are usually less than 1 cm in diameter. Their color varies from light to dark brown, and they may have a raised warty or smooth surface. The presence of coarse hairs distinguishes them from other nevi. Blue nevi are smooth blue-black lesions that are smaller than 1 cm, with well-defined, regular margins. They usually occur on the face, the dorsum of the feet and hands, and the buttocks. They are rarely associated with malignant melanoma. BCCs are most common in middle-aged people. A pigmented BCC tumor is usually blue-black, with raised edges and capillary neovascularity. Initially, the lesion is smooth, but it can become ulcerated. Seborrheic keratoses are occasionally black. They are usually 1 cm or larger and typically appear as raised and warty, with a greasy consistency. They appear to be stuck onto the skin. Dermatofibromas are occasionally dark brown. They are usually smooth, slightly raised, and without hairs. They typically grow very slowly and never become malignant. A malignant version of this tumor, dermatofibrosarcoma protuberans, also occurs as a slow-growing tumor that may rarely be pigmented. Subungual hemorrhage is usually sudden in onset and is sharply defined beneath the nail bed. By comparison, subungual melanoma has a gradual onset and has poorly demarcated streaks that extend along the axis of the nail. The diagnosis of hemorrhage is confirmed by puncturing the nail and evacuating the blood. In time, the entire subungual hemorrhage migrates distally, and the nail bed clears. Subungual melanoma, however, is a persistent lesion. However, if there is any question about a lesion, histologic examination provides the necessary confirmatory evidence.

Many of the features of cutaneous melanoma permit clinical diagnosis before biopsy. The key to making the diagnoses of lentigo maligna and superficial spreading melanoma is irregularity (e.g., color, border, and surface). Taken together, these characteristics allow the experienced clinician to diagnose most melanomas. Patients, however, have many other types of pigmented lesions that require diagnosis. Although it is possible to be quite certain about some pigmented lesions, many others require biopsy for histologic examination before therapy can be planned. Nodular melanoma does not have the border variability seen in lentigo maligna and superficial spreading melanoma. However, it does have the variability of color and does cause a raised nodule. Its color, thickness, and rapid growth permit easy clinical diagnosis.

Accurate microstaging is very important in the management of melanoma. The person who performs the biopsy must provide the pathologist with adequate and satisfactory material to make the diagnosis and determine the stage, which is based on maximum tumor thickness. If possible, a biopsy includes complete excision of the lesion, with a small margin of normal tissue, so that the pathologist can accurately stage the lesion. If this procedure is not practical because of size or location, the second choice is to perform an incisional biopsy. To help the pathologist stage the lesion correctly, the specimen must include the thickest portion of the lesion. Because shave biopsies provide no information on depth of the tumor, this method should not be used when dealing with melanoma.

Excisional Biopsy

Excisional biopsy is preferred when possible because the entire lesion is available for step-section histopathologic analysis to determine the depth of penetration. This information is critical for further management. Before local anesthesia is initiated, the physician outlines an ellipse around the lesion with 2- to 4-mm margins. The long axis of the ellipse is placed to permit easy therapeutic reexcision of the site. In general, the long axis of the ellipse is directed toward the node-bearing area. In addition, the physician confirms that the planned defect can be closed easily without undue tension. After the ellipse is outlined, field block local anesthesia is administered with a single injection at either end of the ellipse, infiltrating into normal tissue rather than into the tumor. Full-thickness skin and subcutaneous tissue are excised as part of the biopsy. After the bleeding points are controlled, the skin is reapproximated with alternating simple and vertical mattress stitches to give a smooth, straight closure (Fig. 25-17). If the size or location of the primary site prevents excisional biopsy, then an incisional biopsy is performed.

Incisional Biopsy

The prognosis is not compromised by the use of incisional biopsy as long as definitive therapy is initiated promptly.

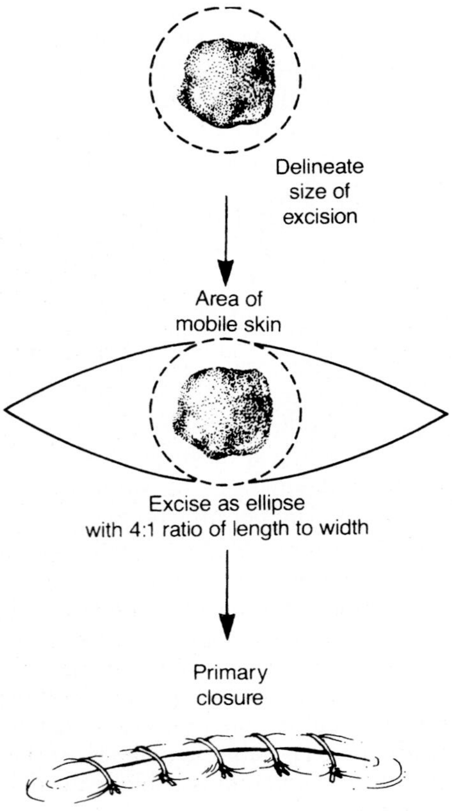

Figure 25-17 Scalpel excision with primary closure is used for smaller lesions.

Selection of the biopsy site is critical because of the effect of tumor thickness on prognosis. An incisional biopsy must include some of the thickest part of the pigmented lesion to allow correct microstaging. The placement of the incisional biopsy should not compromise definitive surgical therapy. Incision planning and anesthesia administration should be as outlined above for an excisional biopsy. Where possible, the normal skin involved in the biopsy site is used to close the biopsy site.

Staging

In the last 20 years, a better understanding of the growth and development of primary melanoma lesions has allowed surgeons to design treatment tailored to the characteristics of the primary lesion and to predict outcome on the basis of these characteristics. The features of the tumor that seem most important in determining prognosis are thickness, ulceration, nodal metastases, and distant metastases. Two systems are used to determine tumor depth of invasion (microstaging) of malignant melanomas. The **Clark system** for primary melanoma is based on the histologic level of invasion of the tumor. Level I lesions are confined to the epidermis, level II lesions invade the papillary layer of the dermis, level III lesions reach the junction of the papillary and reticular layers, level IV lesions invade the reticular dermis, and level V lesions invade the subcutaneous fat. Survival is best for level I lesions and worst for level V lesions. A disadvantage of this system is that different pathologists may interpret the levels of invasion variably.

The disadvantage of the Clark microstaging system is addressed by the **Breslow system,** which uses an ocular micrometer to measure the thickness of the tumor in millimeters at the deepest point of its vertical growth. Thicker tumors have a worse prognosis (see Table 25-2). The Breslow system allows more objective evaluation and easier comparison among pathologists.

The TNM (tumor, node, metastasis) system combines information from the Breslow system, whether the lesion is ulcerated, and information about the status of lymph nodes and distant metastases to provide a comprehensive staging system (Table 25-2).

Malignant melanoma can spread through both the lymphatic and blood routes. Lymphatic spread can present clinically as in-transit metastases or as enlarged nodes. In-transit metastases occur when melanoma cells are trapped between the primary tumor and regional lymph nodes and produce a region of subcutaneous metastases more than 3 cm from the primary site. Mechanical blockage of afferent lymph drainage by either metastatic disease or lymph node dissection is believed to be the cause of these in-transit metastases. Distant metastasis from melanoma may occur in any tissue, with skin, subcutaneous tissue, and distant lymphatic sites being most common. Lung, brain, liver, and bone are less frequent sites. Evaluation of large numbers of patients has led to the recognition that within the group with distant metastatic disease, those with spread to skin, subcuta-

Table 25-2 TNM Classification: AJCC–UICC Melanoma Staging System

Stage	TNM	Criteria	5-yr Survival
IA	T1a	Primary melanoma < 1.0 mm thick without ulceration and Clark's level II/III	91%–99%
IB	T1b	Primary melanoma < 1.0 mm thick with ulceration or Clark's level IV/V	90%–92%
	T2a	Primary melanoma 1.01–2.0 mm thick without ulceration	88%–90%
IIA	T2b	Primary melanoma 1.01–2.00 mm thick with ulceration	76%–79%
	T3a	Primary melanoma 2.01–4.0 mm thick without ulceration	78%–80%
IIB	T3b	Primary melanoma 2.01–4.0 mm thick with ulceration	62%–65%
	T4a	Primary melanoma > 4.0 mm thick without ulceration	65%–70%
IIC	T4b	Primary melanoma > 4.0 mm thick with ulceration	43%–47%
IIIA	N1a	1 node with micrometastasis only	65%–73%
	N2a	2–3 nodes with micrometastasis only	58%–69%
IIIB	N1a	1 node, with micrometastasis only with ulceration of the primary lesion	49%–57%
	N2a	2–3 nodes with micrometastasis only with ulceration of the primary lesion	43%–55%
	N1b	1 node, with macrometastasis	54%–64%
	N2b	2–3 nodes, with macrometastasis	41%–52%
IIIC	N1b	1 node, with macrometastasis with ulceration of the primary lesion	25%–34%
	N2b	2–3 nodes with macrometastasis, with ulceration of the primary lesion	20%–28%
	N3	4 or more metastatic notes, or matted nodes, or in-transit/satellite metastasis	24%–29%
IV	M1a	Metastasis to skin or subcutaneous tissue	16%–22%
	M1b	Metastasis to lung	4%–10%
	M1c	Metastasis to other visceral sites	8%–10%

AJCC, American Joint Committee on Cancer Staging; UICC,
Used with permission of the American Society of Clinical Oncology. The original source for this material is Balch CM, Buzaid AC, Soong SJ, et al. Final version of the American Joint Committee on Cancer staging system for cutaneous melanoma. *J Clin Oncol* 2001;19:3635–3648.

neous tissue, or lymphatic sites fare better than those with spread to lung or to all other visceral sites (Table 25-2).

Treatment

The two questions about local therapy concern the proper width of excision and the proper depth of excision. Current recommendations (based on prospective randomized trials) are 1-cm radial margins of resection for melanomas less than 1 mm thick and 2-cm margins of excision (when possible) for intermediate-thickness melanomas (1 to 4 mm). In general, excision sites should be closed primarily and skin grafts avoided. Skin grafts may be necessary for distal extremity lesions. In most cases, the excision extends through the subcutaneous tissue to the level of the underlying fascia. Excision of the fascia with the lesion does little to prevent the spread of melanoma.

There is general agreement that if regional lymph nodes are abnormal on physical examination (clinical stage III), regional node dissection is performed. There is also agreement that if these nodes are not palpable and the primary lesion is less than or equal to 1 mm thick (clinical stage I), regional node dissection is not indicated because the incidence of metastatic disease from these lesions is extremely low. Sentinel node biopsy, described below, directs the management of regional lymph nodes in other cases of stage I and stage II melanoma. This method allows the surgeon to selectively biopsy the draining node basin and manage the patient based on the biopsy result.

The development of intraoperative lymphatic mapping for early-stage melanoma began as a technique to permit identification of the draining lymphatics from melanomas with ambiguous drainage such as those occurring in the midback. Surgeons quickly recognized this method could also identify the first node (sentinel node) reached by the tumor cells escaping from the primary site of the melanoma. By examining the sentinel node, a decision could be made to leave the node basin intact (sentinel node negative) or to remove the nodes because the sentinel node was positive. This approach uses a dye (isosulfan blue), a radiolabeled material (often ^{99m}Tc sulfur colloid), or a combination of the two injected intradermally around the site of the melanoma or on either side of the biopsy scar. The best results occur when the vital blue dye and lymphoscintigraphy methods are combined. An incision is made over the regional lymph basin. The blue-stained sentinel node is identified and examined with a hand-held gamma counter. If the counts are elevated, the node is removed and submitted for histologic examination and immunohistochemical studies. If the sentinel node is negative, there is a 99% chance that the remaining lymph nodes are not involved with metastatic melanoma, as shown by long-term followup. If the sentinel node is positive, then a complete node dissection is required because the probability of finding other positive lymph nodes is significant. Recent reports indicate the sensitivity and predictive value of this method can be improved by the use of immunohistochemistry methods that identify proteins unique to melanoma cells and by the use of reverse transcriptase-polymerase chain reaction to identify genes unique to melanoma cells. While these methods increase the sensitivity of melanocyte detection, the routine use of reverse transcriptase-polymerase chain reaction in staging melanoma is still under evaluation to determine its utility and predictive value.

Interferon-α appears to be a beneficial adjuvant therapy for melanoma patients with node metastases based on three randomized trials. However, there was overall survival benefit in only two of the trials. Treatment with interferon has significant side effects that limit the drugs used in some patients.

The management of distant disease is rarely curative and is determined primarily by its location and symptoms. Metastatic disease to the brain is usually treated with either radiation therapy alone or with a combination of surgical removal and whole-brain radiation. Pulmonary nodules, if few in number, may be resected, but this practice is not generally followed. While these patients may undergo chemotherapy, there is not currently a standard treatment. Enrollment in a clinical trial may be the best approach. Distant spread to an extremity that involves in-transit metastases may be managed by regional limb perfusion with a chemotherapeutic agent (e.g., L-phenylalanine mustard) and hyperthermia. This treatment is beneficial only if the disease is confined to that extremity and there are no data indicating that it prolongs patient life. Regardless of the protocol, the response rate is low (20%), even when partial and complete responses are combined. No effective chemotherapy is available for either primary or metastatic melanoma. Most patients who have recurrent metastatic melanoma are treated according to a protocol so that data collection can continue and treatment be improved.

Immunotherapy as an adjuvant to surgical treatment remains an important but incompletely achieved goal. Trials underway are testing a variety of vaccines, dosages, and routes of administration. Access to these agents in most cases requires participation in a clinical trial.

Radiation is rarely used as the single treatment for melanoma. However, it is used to treat metastatic disease (e.g., whole-brain radiation after brain metastasis). New fractionation methods, with higher single doses given less often, increased the response rate from 35% to 75%.

Prognosis

To improve our understanding of melanoma behavior, Balch et al. analyzed 17,600 patients that had staging information and outcome data available. In stages I and II (disease limited to the primary site), both the Clark and Breslow systems of microstaging allow patients to be subdivided into different risk categories for recurrent disease and eventual death (see Table 25-2). In general, the risk of recurrence after excision of a primary melanoma is extremely low if the melanoma is less than or equal to 1 mm thick. On the other hand, if the melanoma is greater than 4 mm, the probability of both recurrence and death is extremely high. Overall, the 5-year survival rate for patients with stage I disease is 92%. For patients with stage II disease, 5-year survival varies from 79% for the thinnest lesion (T3) without ulceration to 45% for the thickest lesion (T4) with ulceration. While Balch et al. found thickness and ulceration were the most important factors, patient age, gender, and site of the tumor were also predictors of recurrence in localized melanoma.

In stage III (disease spread to the draining lymph nodes), the presence of metastatic disease in the regional lymph nodes is an ominous prognostic sign. The clear finding that melanoma has spread beyond the primary site decreases the 5-year disease-free survival rate to between 24% and 70%. The prognosis worsens as the number of involved lymph nodes increases.

In stage IV (disease spread to distant sites), patients survive an average of 6 months, with less than 10% living 5 years. Patients who have only skin and lymph node metastases fare better (median survival of 14 months) than those with visceral metastases (median survival of 4 months).

MALIGNANT DISEASES OF THE LYMPHATICS AND SOFT TISSUE

HODGKIN'S LYMPHOMA AND NON-HODGKIN'S LYMPHOMA

Lymphomas are malignancies that arise in the lymphoid tissues of the body. Collections of lymphoid cells occur in the lymph nodes, the white pulp of the spleen, Waldeyer's ring, the thymus gland, and lymphoid aggregates in the submucosa of the respiratory and gastrointestinal tracts (**Peyer's patches**). The two major subgroups of malignant lymphoma are **Hodgkin's lymphoma** (13%) and **non-Hodgkin's lymphoma** (87%). Lymphomas are classified based on immunohistopathologic standards (Table 25-3). Lymphomas originate from **B cells, T cells,** histiocytes, or other lymphoid cells.

Hodgkin's Lymphoma

Incidence and Etiology

The incidence of Hodgkin's lymphoma follows a bimodal curve, with peaks in young adulthood (late 20s) and in older adults (mid 70s). The average age of a patient with Hodgkin's lymphoma is 32 years. The incidence in the

Table 25-3 Lymphoid Neoplasms Recognized by the International Lymphoma Study Group

B-cell neoplasms

I. Precursor B-cell neoplasm: precursor B-lymphoblastic leukemia/lymphoma
II. Peripheral B-cell neoplasms
  1. B-cell chronic lymphocytic leukemia, prolymphocytic leukemia or small lymphocytic lymphoma
  2. Lymphoplasmacytoid lymphoma or immunocytoma
  3. Mantle cell lymphoma
  4. Follicle center lymphoma, follicular
     Provisional cytologic grades: I (small cell), II (mixed small and large cell), III (large cell)
     Provisional subtype: diffuse, predominantly small cell type
  5. Marginal zone B-cell lymphoma
     Extranodal (MALT-type with or without monocytoid B cells)
     Provisional subtype: nodal (with or without monocytoid B cells)
  6. Provisional entity: splenic marginal zone lymphoma (with or without villous lymphocytes)
  7. Hairy cell leukemia
  8. Plasmacytoma or plasma cell myeloma
  9. Diffuse large B-cell lymphoma[a]
     Subtype: primary mediastinal (thymic) B-cell lymphoma
  10. Burkitt's lymphoma
  11. Provisional entity: high-grade B-cell lymphoma, Burkitt-like[a]

T-cell and putative NK-cell neoplasms

I. Precursor T-cell neoplasm: precursor T-lymphoblastic lymphoma or leukemia
II. Peripheral T-cell and NK-cell neoplasms
  1. T-cell chronic lymphocytic leukemia or prolymphocytic leukemia
  2. Large granular lymphocyte leukemia
     T-cell type
     NK-cell type
  3. Mycosis fungoides or Sezary syndrome
  4. Peripheral T-cell lymphomas, unspecified[a]
     Provisional cytologic categories: medium cell, mixed medium and large cell, large cell, or lymphoepithelioid cell
     Provisional subtype: hepatosplenic $\gamma\delta$ T-cell lymphoma
     Provisional subtype: subcutaneous panniculitic T-cell lymphoma
  5. Angioimmunoblastic T-cell lymphoma
  6. Angiocentric lymphoma
  7. Intestinal T-cell lymphoma (with or without associated enteropathy)
  8. Adult T-cell lymphoma or leukemia
  9. Anaplastic large cell lymphoma, $CD30^+$, T- and null-cell types
  10. Provisional entity: anaplastic large-cell lymphoma, Hodgkin's-like

Hodgkin's lymphoma

I. Lymphocyte predominance
II. Nodular sclerosis
III. Mixed cellularity
IV. Lymphocyte depletion
V. Provisional entity: lymphocyte-rich classical Hodgkin's lymphoma

[a] These categories probably include more than one disease entity.
MALT, mucosa-associated lymphoid tissue; NK, natural killer.
Adapted with permission from Harris NL, Jaffe ES, Stein H, et al. A revised European-American classification of lymphoid neoplasms: a proposal from the International Lymphoma Study Group. *Blood* 1994;84(5):1361–1392. Copyright American Society of Hematology, used with permission.

United States has declined significantly since the 1980s and was estimated to be 7880 cases in 2004.

The etiology of Hodgkin's lymphoma is unknown. Various theories are postulated, including infectious causes (e.g., Epstein-Barr virus). The cellular origin of Hodgkin's lymphoma is also uncertain, although it may involve the monocyte–macrophage cell line.

Clinical Presentation and Evaluation

Hodgkin's lymphoma usually causes asymptomatic cervical lymphadenopathy (60% to 80%). Supradiaphragmatic disease occurs initially in 90% of young adults who have Hodgkin's lymphoma. In older adults, however, the likelihood of subdiaphragmatic disease is 25%. Systemic symptoms (fever, night sweats, and loss of more than 10% of body weight) indicate a worse prognosis. Hodgkin's lymphoma may be localized or disseminated. Patients also may have signs and symptoms because of the mass effect of mediastinal or retroperitoneal disease.

All patients must undergo a thorough evaluation, including a complete physical examination. Particular attention is paid to the peripheral lymph node regions. A chest radiograph is also needed. The next step is excisional biopsy of an enlarged, abnormal lymph node. If multiple sites are enlarged, biopsy is performed on cervical rather than axillary or inguinal nodes, since these sites are more likely to show reactive changes and therefore be nondiagnostic. After the histologic diagnosis is made, a bone marrow biopsy is obtained. Finally, the liver, spleen, and retroperitoneal nodes are evaluated with computed tomography (CT) scan.

In the past, staging laparotomy was an important part of the pretreatment evaluation of a patient with Hodgkin's disease. Staging laparotomy includes splenectomy and biopsy of the splenic hilar, celiac, porta hepatis, mesenteric, paraaortic, and iliac nodes. Bilateral wedge and needle biopsies of the liver are also performed. In an attempt to maintain fertility after radiation treatment in premenopausal women, the ovaries are positioned in a retrouterine site and sutured to presacral fascia (oophoropexy).

Now, staging laparotomy rarely plays a role in the evaluation of patients with Hodgkin's disease. Its use is limited to patients with minimal stage disease. The issue for the physician is differentiating patients who may have limited disease treatable by radiation from those who have more extensive disease and need chemotherapy. Over the last few decades, the need for staging laparotomy has decreased as imaging studies have permitted greater accuracy in staging, and treatment patterns have changed with greater use of chemotherapy. For example, staging laparotomy is not necessary in patients who have a large mediastinal mass and in older patients who have mixed or lymphocyte-depleted histology. These patients require systemic therapy, and laparotomy does not alter the course of treatment.

Staging

The Revised European-American Classification of Lymphoid Neoplasms/World Health Organization (REAL/WHO) classification system groups Hodgkin's lymphoma histologically into five categories: nodular lymphocyte predominate, lymphocyte rich, nodular sclerosis, mixed cellularity, and lymphocyte depleted. Nodular sclerosis is the most common histologic type (relative frequency of 70%). Histologically, Hodgkin's lymphoma appears as a tumor with a large reactive background of lymphocytes, eosinophils, and plasma cells, with a few malignant mononuclear cells and multinuclear giant cells (Reed-Sternberg cells). The Reed-Sternberg cell has a classic "owl eye" appearance (Fig. 25-18). This cell must be present for the diagnosis of Hodgkin's lymphoma to be made. Reed-Sternberg cells are also present in other disorders, including mononucleosis and other inflammatory conditions, and with phenytoin (Dilantin) therapy.

The Cotswolds classification is used to stage Hodgkin's lymphoma (Table 25-4). This classification identifies patients as stage A (asymptomatic) or stage B (fevers, night sweats, and weight loss). Stage classification is based on the involvement of single, multiple, or disseminated sites of one or more extralymphatic organs.

Treatment

The treatment of Hodgkin's lymphoma is determined by staging. Radiation therapy plays a role in the treatment of early-stage disease (stages I and II). When used, radiation is administered in doses of 30 Gy to 40 Gy to areas of known involvement and to neighboring nodal basins that are likely to represent the next area of spread. Chemotherapy, with or without radiation therapy, is recommended for advanced disease.

Chemotherapy significantly alters the prognosis of patients with Hodgkin's lymphoma, with cure achieved in 80% of cases. Two common regimens are nitrogen mustard, vincristine, procarbazine, and prednisone (MOPP); and doxorubicin (adriamycin), bleomycin, vinblastine, and dacarbazine (ABVD).

Prognosis

The prognosis for patients with Hodgkin's lymphoma is excellent. Risk factors include the stage of disease at the time of treatment and the histology. The lymphocyte-predominant group appears to have the best prognosis, followed by the nodular-sclerosis group. With adequate staging and therapy, 80% of patients are cured. The risk of a second tumor after treatment (thought to be secondary to the treatment) continues to increase with time. The risk of leukemia reaches a plateau of approximately 3% at 10 years.

Non-Hodgkin's Lymphoma

Non-Hodgkin's lymphomas are a diverse group that represent a large spectrum of malignancies. Their histology, immunology, and clinical characteristics are heterogeneous.

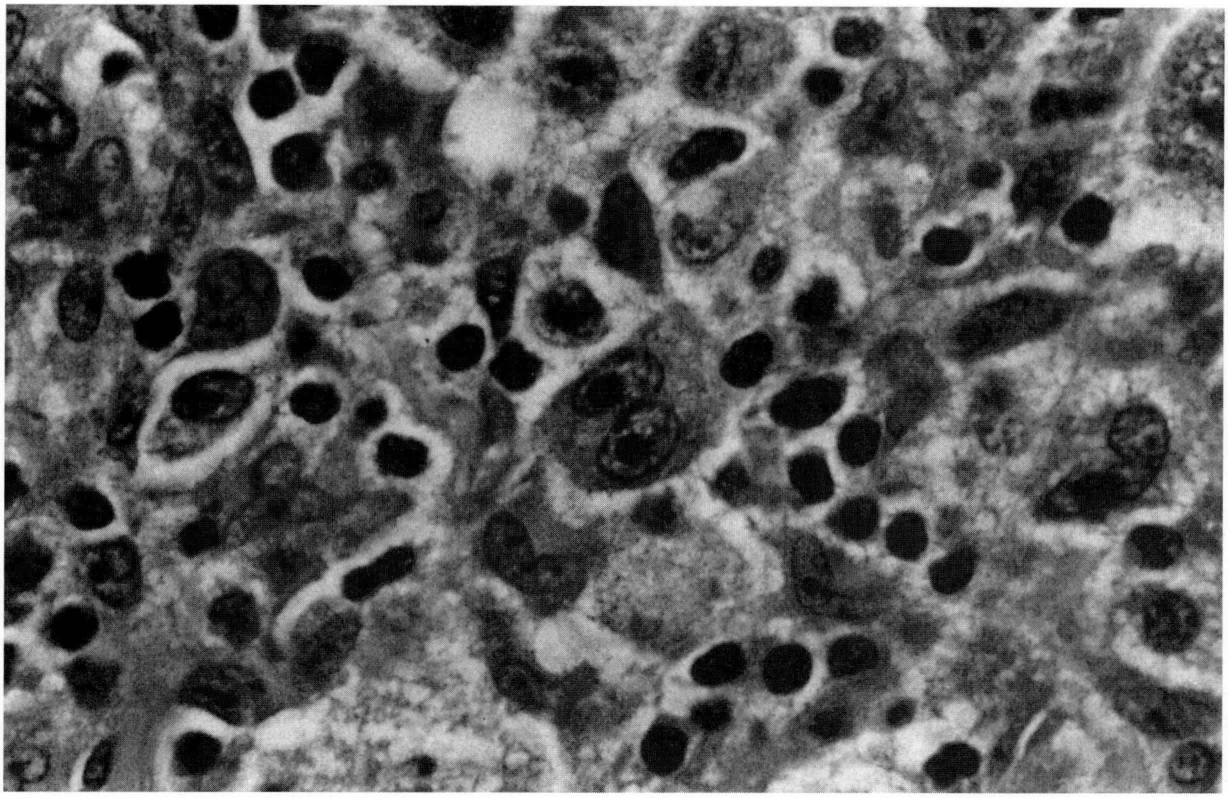

Figure 25-18 Hodgkin's lymphoma, mixed cellularity subtype. A classic, diagnostic bilobulated Reed-Sternberg cell is surrounded by a variety of cell types, including malignant Hodgkin's cells and benign small lymphocytes and histiocytes (hematoxylin and eosin × 1000). (Courtesy of Dr. Rogers Griffith, Department of Pathology, Rhode Island Hospital, Providence, Rhode Island.)

Incidence and Etiology

Since 1970, the incidence of non-Hodgkin's lymphoma has nearly doubled. In 2004, approximately 54,370 new cases were expected to be diagnosed. Non-Hodgkin's lymphoma appears to be associated with HIV, although the increased incidence is not entirely explained by the rise in the number of cases of AIDS.

As with Hodgkin's lymphoma, the etiology of most types of non-Hodgkin's lymphoma is unclear. The incidence appears to increase in association with immunosuppression. Patients with AIDS and those who undergo organ transplantation are at increased risk for this disorder. Viruses can cause specific lymphomas. Epstein-Barr virus infection is associated with Burkitt's lymphoma, and human T-cell lymphoma virus-1 is associated with a T-cell lymphoma that is found in the Caribbean Islands.

Clinical Presentation and Evaluation

Most patients with non-Hodgkin's lymphoma are asymptomatic at presentation, although 20% have systemic symptoms (fever, night sweats, or weight loss). Patients may have enlarged lymph nodes, with gastrointestinal symptoms that include nausea, vomiting, and bleeding. Unlike Hodgkin's lymphoma, non-Hodgkin's lymphoma tends to be disseminated. Patients may have symptoms secondary to the extent of spread. Some dramatic presentations include superior vena cava syndrome, acute spinal cord compression, mucosal-associated lymphatic tissue (MALT) lymphomas, and meningeal involvement. MALT represents lymphomas that occur outside the lymph nodes (gastrointestinal tract, thyroid, breast, or skin).

The evaluation of patients with non-Hodgkin's lymphoma begins with a complete history and physical examination. Next, diagnostic studies are performed, including complete blood count, liver function tests, chest radiograph, and CT scan of the chest, abdomen, and pelvis. Bone marrow biopsy is then performed. Patients with intermediate-grade non-Hodgkin's lymphoma with bone marrow involvement and those with high-grade non-Hodgkin's lymphoma may require lumbar puncture because central nervous system involvement is increased in these groups. Staging laparotomy is usually not indicated because these patients tend to have disseminated disease, in contrast to those with Hodgkin's lymphoma, who tend to have localized disease that progresses by involvement of contiguous node basins.

Table 25-4 Cotswolds Staging for Hodgkin's Lymphoma

Stage	Findings
I	Involvement of a single lymph node region or lymphoid structure (e.g., spleen, thymus, Waldeyer's ring) or a single extralymphatic organ or site
II	Involvement of two or more lymph node regions on the same side of the diaphragm (hilar nodes, when involved on both sides, constitute stage II disease); localized contiguous involvement of only one extralymphatic organ or site and lymph node region on the same side of the diaphragm (IIE). The number of anatomic regions involved should be indicated by a subscript (e.g., II_3)
III	Involvement of lymph node regions on both sides of the diaphragm (III), which may be accompanied by involvement of the spleen (III_S), of or by localized contiguous involvement of only one extralymphatic organ site (III_E), or both (III_{SE})
III_1	With or without involvement of splenic, hilar, celiac, or portal nodes
III_2	With involvement of para-aortic, iliac, and mesenteric nodes
IV	Diffuse or disseminated involvement of one or more extralymphatic organs or tissues, with or without associated lymph node involvement (involved organs should be identified by a symbol)
Designations Applicable to any Disease Stage	
A	No symptoms
B	Fever (temperature > 38°C), drenching night sweats, unexplained weight loss > 10% of body weight within past 6 months
X	Bulky disease (a widening of the mediastinum by more than one-third of the presence of a nodal mass with a maximal dimension > 10 cm)
E	Involvement of a single extranodal site that is contiguous or proximal to the known nodal site
CS	Clinical stage
PS	Pathologic stage (as determined by laparotomy)

Used with permission of the American Society of Clinical Oncology. The original source for this material is Lister T, Crowther D, Sutcliff S, et al. Report of a committee convened to discuss the evaluation and staging of patients with Hodgkin's disease: Cotswolds meeting. *J Clin Oncol* 1989;7:1630.

Classification and Staging

Many histologic classification systems are used for non-Hodgkin's lymphoma. These include the Rappaport and the Working Formulation systems as well as the REAL/WHO (Table 25-3). The latter system incorporates morphology, immunophenotype, and genetic characteristics to give a comprehensive list of diseases with distinct clinical characteristics. The stage is determined with the Ann Arbor system, although this system is somewhat limited because non-Hodgkin's lymphoma tends to occur in disseminated form. In 1993, the International Non-Hodgkin's Lymphoma Prognostic Factors Project devised a new classification system (Table 25-5) that groups patients based on risk of relapse. This system is used in conjunction with staging information to determine the optimal patient treatment plan.

Treatment

The treatment of non-Hodgkin's lymphoma is variable, depending on the histologic subtype, the stage, and the risk of relapse. Surgery, radiation therapy, and chemotherapy are the treatment options. The primary role of surgery is for diagnosis, although it is sometimes an important aspect of treatment. Localized gastric and small-bowel non-Hodgkin's lymphoma may be effectively treated with resection (see Chapter 14, Stomach and Duodenum, and Chapter 15, Small Intestine and Appendix). Surgery may also be indicated to treat complications (perforation, obstruction) of the disease or those associated with treatment (perforation). Radiation therapy is useful in localized non-Hodgkin's lymphoma, although this presentation is unusual. Radiation therapy is also used for complications related to mass effect (e.g., superior vena cava obstruction, spinal cord compression).

Non-Hodgkin's lymphoma tumors are primarily treated with chemotherapy. A variety of agents and treatment protocols are used. The response to chemotherapy and the duration of remission are related to tumor grade and stage.

Prognosis

To determine the prognosis, tumor grade and stage are considered. Low-grade tumors tend to follow an indolent course, and if left untreated, patients often survive 5 years or longer. On the other hand, high-grade tumors may progress rapidly if they are not treated and may result in death. These high-grade tumors respond well to chemotherapy. Factors that affect responsiveness in patients with high- and intermediate-grade tumors have been defined. The prognosis is poor in patients who are older than 60 years of age, have systemic symptoms (fever, night sweats, weight loss), and have bulky disease, and in those who have extranodal disease and bone marrow or gastrointestinal involvement.

SARCOMA

Soft Tissue Sarcoma

Adult soft tissue sarcomas are rare tumors derived from embryonic mesoderm. Unlike more common solid tumors, such as breast, lung, and colorectal cancer, they are not derived from epithelial tissues. Less than 1% of all cancers are sarcomas. Of sarcomas, 66% occur in the extremity, 20% on the trunk, and 13% in the retroperitoneum. There are over 50 subtypes, the most common

Table 25-5 International Non-Hodgkin's Lymphoma Prognostic Factors Project

Category	Risk Factors[a] (n)	Complete Response Rate (%)	2-yr Survival (%)	5-yr Survival (%)
Low risk	≤ 1	87	84	73
Low-intermediate risk	2	67	66	50
High-intermediate risk	3	55	54	43
High risk	4 or 5	44	34	26

[a] Risk factors include age (≥60 yr), stage (I/II versus III/IV), extranodal sites (≤1 or > 1), performance status (Eastern Cooperative Oncology Group ≤1 versus 2), and lactic dehydrogenase level (normal versus abnormal).

Adapted with permission from The International Non-Hodgkin's Lymphoma Prognostic Factors Project. A predictive model for aggressive non-Hodgkin's lymphoma. *N Engl J Med* 1993;329:987–994.

being malignant fibrous histiocytoma (24%), leiomyosarcoma (21%), and liposarcoma (19%) (Fig. 25-19). As with other malignancies, the stage of the tumor determines patient outcome, and, somewhat peculiar to sarcoma, stage is largely determined by grade. Sarcoma is particularly prone to local recurrence if incompletely excised in the first instance. The complex nature and rarity of the tumor means that it is best managed by a multidisciplinary team of oncologists (surgical, radiation, and medical), supported by a dedicated sarcoma pathologist.

Incidence and Etiology

In the United States in 2004, 8680 new cases of sarcoma were reported, with 3660 deaths from sarcoma estimated.

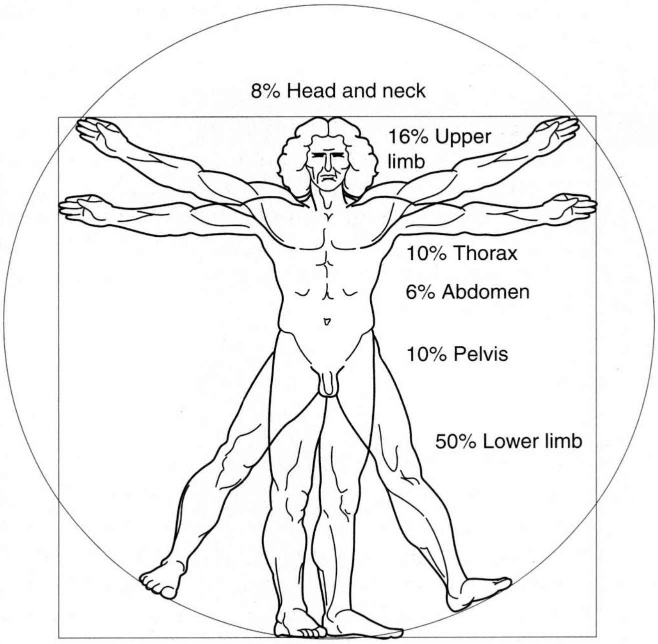

Figure 25-19 Site distribution of adult soft tissue sarcoma.

In Alberta, Canada (population 3 million), in 2003, there were 80 new sarcomas, in contrast to 1600 new breast cancers, 1100 new colorectal cancers, and 1400 new lung cancers. Patients with sarcoma may present with a history of trauma to the area; however, a causal relationship has never been established. It is more likely that injury calls attention to the preexisting tumor. Risk factors that have been associated with sarcoma occurrence include occupational exposure, radiation, chronic lymphedema, and both germ-line and somatic mutations in oncogenes and tumor suppressor genes.

A variety of chemical agents and carcinogens have been linked to the development of sarcoma. Asbestos (hydrated silicate) is associated with the development of pleural mesothelioma. The phenoxyacetic acid herbicides (lawn pesticides) and their byproducts, dioxin and Agent Orange, have been associated with increased incidence of sarcomas, most notably in soldiers who fought in the Vietnam War. The manufacture of polyvinyl chloride (PVC) has been associated with the development of the particularly aggressive sarcoma hepatic angiosarcoma.

There is an eightfold to 50-fold increase in incidence of sarcoma reported in patients treated with radiation for carcinoma of breast, cervix, ovary, testes, and lymphatic system. To be diagnosed as a radiation-associated sarcoma, the lesion must be in the radiated field, be of different histology to the tumor originally treated with radiation, and develop after a latency period of at least 3 years.

Lymphangiosarcoma can occur in chronic lymphedema. Angiosarcoma in the context of lymphedema from a radical axillary dissection for a carcinoma of the breast is known as Stewart-Treves syndrome.

Gene rearrangements have been found in Ewing's sarcoma, clear-cell sarcoma, myxoid liposarcoma, alveolar rhabdomyosarcoma, desmoplastic small round-cell tumors, and synovial sarcoma. Oncogenes implicated so far include MDM2, N-myc, c-erB2, and ras oncogenes.

Germ-line mutations in the tumor suppressor gene p53 cause the Li-Fraumeni syndrome and increase the risk of rhabdomyosarcoma as well as early-onset breast carcinoma and other neoplasms. Germ-line mutations in the neurofibromatosis type l gene *NF1* produce Von Recklinghausen syndrome and increase the incidence of neurofibrosarcoma (10%). Gardner's syndrome (a subset of familial polyposis patients) is associated with an increased incidence of desmoid tumors (aggressive fibromatosis). The familial polyposis syndromes are due to a mutation in the *APC* gene. In addition, somatic mutations in the p53 tumor suppressor gene have been reported in 30% to 60% of soft tissue sarcomas. Mutations or deletions in the Rb gene can lead to the development of retinoblastoma.

Clinical Presentation and Evaluation

Soft tissue sarcomas arise from a variety of cell types and are difficult to diagnose, with expert pathologists disagreeing on 24% to 40% of individual cases (Table 25-6). Using panels of immunohistochemical stains, a pathologist can more accurately identify the more common histologic types (Fig. 25-20). Tumor grade (Table 25-7) also provides important prognostic information.

In addition to histologic subtype, sarcomas can be divided into those with limited metastatic potential and those with significant metastatic potential (Table 25-8). Lymph node metastases are not a common feature of sarcoma, occurring in less than 5% of tumors, except specific histologic subtypes such as epithelioid sarcoma, rhabdomyosarcoma, clear cell sarcoma, and angiosarcoma. As with other cancers, sarcoma is staged according to the American Joint Committee on Cancer (AJCC) staging criteria (Table 25-9). The stage assigned depends on tumor grade, tumor size, and the presence of metastases and nodes.

Patient outcome is influenced by tumor size, with smaller lesions (≤ 5 cm [T1 lesions]) having a better prognosis. Tumor grade also influences outcome, with higher-grade lesions being more likely to spread or to recur. In addition, T staging is further divided into tumors that are above (a) or below (b) the superficial fascia. This staging system not only has major prognostic significance, but also guides the multidisciplinary sarcoma team in patient management.

The overall clinical behavior of most sarcomas is similar and is determined by anatomic location, grade, and size of tumor. The metastatic tumor spread is hematogenous, the primary site being the lung; however, in advanced disease, subcutaneous metastases are not uncommon. For intra- and retroperitoneal disease, liver metastases and eventual sarcomatosis (extensive sarcoma tumor nodules within the peritoneal cavity) are common in the terminal phases of the disease.

Sarcoma is predominantly a surgical disease. The goal is to resect the tumor with at least a 2-cm margin of normal tissue surrounding the tumor. Where the ability to achieve a 2-cm margin is in doubt, owing to close proximity of vital structures (e.g., major nerves or arteries), adjuvant (in addition to, but after surgery) or neoadjuvant (in addition to, but before surgery) radiotherapy is employed. This strategy not only improves the limb-sparing rate (fewer amputations), but also improves local control. Administering neoadjuvant radiotherapy for retroperitoneal tumors can be problematic given the limited tissue tolerances of certain organs (e.g., liver, 2000 rads). When margins are positive or very close (< 2 mm), the local recurrence rate approaches 100%.

Sarcoma is notable in that approximately one-third of patients are asymptomatic at the time of presentation. As a consequence, some of these tumors may grow extremely large (20 to 30 cm). Sarcoma tends not to invade other structures, but rather to have a pushing type of growth. In addition, these tumors tend not to compress luminal structures such as the gut or vessels. The presence of significant neurovascular or gastrointestinal compressive or obstructive symptoms implies locally advanced disease. Addi-

Table 25-6 Histologic Classification of Soft Tissue Tumors

Tumor Type	Benign	Intermediate	Malignant
Fibrous	Nodular fasciitis	Aggressive fibromatosis	Fibrosarcoma
Fibrohistiocytic	Xanthoma	Atypical fibroxanthoma	Fibrous histiocytoma
Lipomatous	Lipoma	Atypical lipoma	Liposarcoma
Smooth muscle	Leiomyoma	Hemangioendothelioma	Leiomyosarcoma
Gastrointestinal stromal	GIST		GIST
Skeletal muscle	Rhabdomyoma		Rhabdomyosarcoma
Tumors of blood and lymph vessels	Hemangioma/ lymphangioma		Angiosarcoma/ hemangiopericytoma
Peripheral nerve sheath	Schwannoma		
Neuroectodermal	Ganglioneuroma		Ewing's sarcoma

GIST, gastrointestinal stromal tumor.

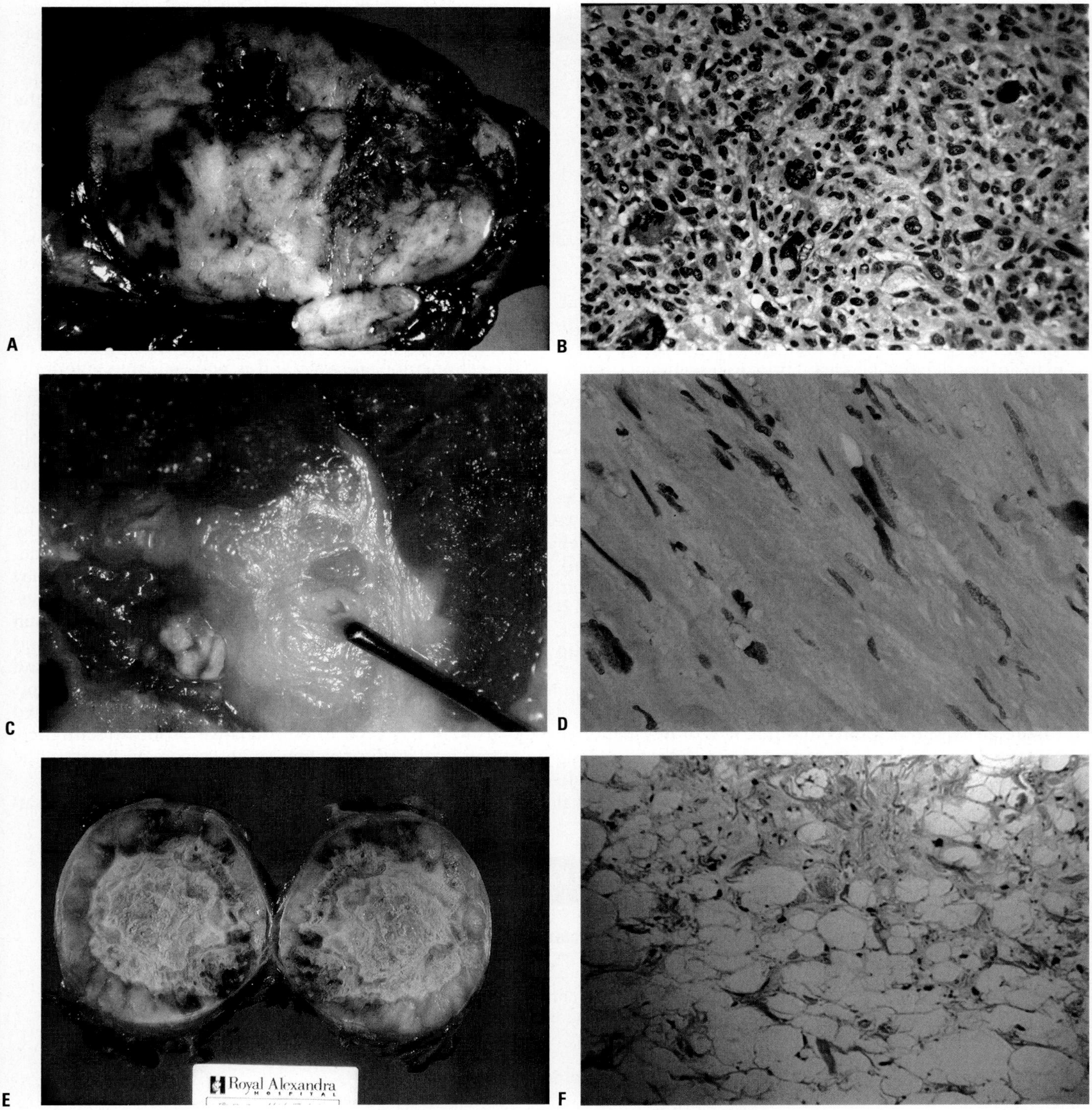

Figure 25-20 Common sarcoma histology types.

tional worrisome clinical features are a history of a rapid growth of tumors and the presence of lymphadenopathy.

Treatment

When a patient presents with a clinically suspicious mass, appropriate imaging and staging studies are carried out to determine the extent of local disease and whether there is any metastatic disease (see Fig. 25-21). Next, a core biopsy is undertaken, and if this yields inadequate tissue for diagnosis, then an open biopsy is performed in the axial plane that would be used for excision of the lesion. Resection with adequate margins of normal tissue will be suffi-

Table 25-7 Histologic Grading of Sarcoma

Parameter	Low (G1)	Intermediate (G2)	High (G3)
Cellularity	+	++	+++
Differentiation	+++	++	+
Pleomorphism	+	++	+++
Mitotic rate	+	++	+++
Necrosis	–	+	++
Hemorrhage	–	–	++

cient for the management of small (≤ 5 cm), superficial, well-differentiated lesions. All other tumors require multidisciplinary management, with many of the components of treatment decided by a team prior to resectional surgery.

Superficial

Superficial extremity sarcomas are defined by the AJCC staging system as those superficial to the deep fascia. Figure 25-22 shows an example of a young woman with type 1 neurofibromatosis in whom a single neurofibroma degenerated into a neurofibrosarcoma. Figure 25-22*B* shows neovascularization of the skin overlying the tumor as well as café-au-lait spots visible on the anterior abdominal wall. Wide resection, including 2-cm margins of skin and subcutaneous tissue plus the deep fascia, was performed, followed by rotation flap and skin graft of the resultant defect. The lesion was low grade and did not require any adjuvant chemotherapy or radiotherapy.

Deep

Figure 25-23 shows a sarcoma in a 56-year-old man who presented with a 3-month history of a rapidly expanding mass involving the adductor compartment of the thigh. The skin overlying the lesion was hot to the touch. Radical external beam radiotherapy (6500 rads over 6 weeks) was administered to arrest the rapid growth and to assist in achieving negative surgical margins. Surgery was performed 6 weeks following completion of radiotherapy. Owing to the proximity of neurovascular bundles to the tumor, the ability to achieve a wide resection was not possible. To preserve the limb, a "marginal" resection (close or narrow margins) was obtained. Owing to the high grade and aggressive nature of this lesion, the patient received 6 cycles of adriamycin-based chemotherapy postoperatively. While the use of chemotherapy in this situation is common, the benefit to the patient remains difficult to prove.

Retroperitoneal Sarcoma

Figure 25-24 demonstrates a large right retroperitoneal liposarcoma, which has pushed the right kidney out from the retroperitoneal space and is now palpable anteriorly. Two components of the tumor are visible: the darker area more consistent with simple fat laterally, and a more solid central component compressing the aorta. A thoracoabdominal incision is necessary to completely excise this tumor. An on-block resection is required involving not only resecting the tumor, but also the right kidney and adrenal gland and right colon. For large lesions high in the left retroperitoneum, the spleen, portions of the stomach, diaphragm, pancreas, and duodenal jejunal flexion may also need to be resected to completely remove the tumors. The ability to achieve a wide resection margin with such large tumors within the peritoneum or retroperitoneum is impossible owing to vital structures. Liposarcomas respond poorly to adjuvant or neoadjuvant chemoradiotherapy. Given the size and location of the tumor, it is anticipated that there is a 60% to 80% chance of local recurrence, and ultimately the development of sarcomatosis within the peritoneal cavity.

Figure 25-25A shows a CT scan of a large pelvic sar-

Table 25-8 Metastatic Potential of Various Sarcoma Histologies

Low Metastatic Potential	Intermediate Metastatic Potential	High Metastatic Potential
Desmoid tumor	Myxoid liposarcoma	Alveolar soft part sarcoma
Atypical lipomatous tumor	Myxoid malignant fibrous histiocytoma	Angiosarcoma
Dermatofibrosarcoma protuberans	Extraskeletal chondrosarcoma	Clear cell sarcoma ("melanoma of soft parts")
Hemangiopericytoma		Epithelioid sarcoma
		Extraskeletal Ewing's sarcoma
		Extraskeletal osteosarcoma
		Malignant fibrous histiocytoma
		Liposarcoma (pleomorphic and dedifferentiated)
		Leiomyosarcoma
		Neurogenic sarcoma (malignant schwannoma)
		Rhabdomyosarcoma
		Synovial sarcoma

Table 25-9 American Joint Committee on Cancer Staging Criteria for Soft Tissue Sarcomas

Primary tumor (T)

TX Primary tumor cannot be assessed
T0 No evidence of primary tumor
T1 Tumor ≤5 cm in greatest dimension
  T1a Tumor above superficial fascia
  T1b Tumor invading or deep to superficial fascia
T2 Tumor > 5 cm in greatest dimension
  T2a Tumor above superficial fascia
  T2b Tumor invading or deep to superficial fascia

Regional lymph nodes (N)

NX Regional lymph nodes cannot be assessed
N0 No regional lymph node metastasis
N1* Regional lymph node metastasis
  *Note: Presence of positive nodes (N1) is considered stage IV.

Distant metastasis (M)

MX Presence of distant metastasis cannot be assessed
M0 No distant metastasis
M1 Distant metastasis

Histopathologic grade (G)

GX Grade cannot be assessed
G1 Well differentiated
G2 Moderately differentiated
G3 Poorly differentiated
G4 Poorly differentiated or undifferentiated (four-tiered system only)

Stage grouping

Stage I	T1a, 1b, 2a, 2b	N0	M0	G1–G2	G1
Stage II	T1a, 1b, 2a	N0	M0	G3–G4	G2–G3
Stage III	T2b	N0	M0	G3–G4	G2–G3
Stage IV	Any T	N1	M0	Any G	Any G
	Any T	Any N	M1	Any G	Any G

There are two columns for grade to reflect two different grading systems: one ranges from G1 to G4, the other from G1 to G3. Adapted with permission from Green FL, Page DL, Fleming ID, et al., eds. *AJCC Cancer Staging Manual.* 6th Ed. New York, NY: Springer-Verlag, 2002: 193–197.

coma. The rectum, prostate, urethra, and bladder are intimately related to this 12-cm tumor, and, as a consequence, an anterior and posterior total pelvic exenteration (i.e., removal of the tumor, rectum, and bladder with permanent colostomy and ileoconduit) was necessary to completely resect this tumor. Figure 25-25*B* is the postresection CT scan, showing loops of small bowel filling the space left by the pelvic organs and tumor.

Management of Local Recurrence

Even in the presence of local recurrence, soft tissue sarcoma remains primarily a surgical disease. Typically, these sarcomas will recur within 2 years (80%) of the original tumor presentation. Confirmation of the diagnosis of local recurrence can usually be made on **fine-needle aspiration biopsy** (FNAB) cytology. Imaging studies (CT and/or magnetic resonance imaging [MRI]) are required to delineate the extent of local recurrence and determine further resectability. Additional imaging studies are carried out (CT thorax) to restage the patient for metastatic disease. Local excision of local recurrence is always attempted; however, the need to obtain wide margins is of less paramount importance. The outcome of patients who develop local recurrence is poorer than that of those who do not, and further local recurrence and subsequent development of metastatic disease is heavily dependent on the adequacy of the original surgery, grade of the original tumor, and subsequent recurrences. Dedifferentiation from low to high grade is uncommon, but may occur in liposarcoma. If not previously administered, radiotherapy may be of value in controlling further local recurrence or making unresectable local recurrence resectable.

Management of Distant Disease

Isolated lung metastases can be treated with thoracotomy and metastasectomy. Generally, however, metastatic disease implies an inability to cure the patient, who will be offered palliative therapy. Response rates to chemotherapy are poor: 20% to 40% partial response and rare complete

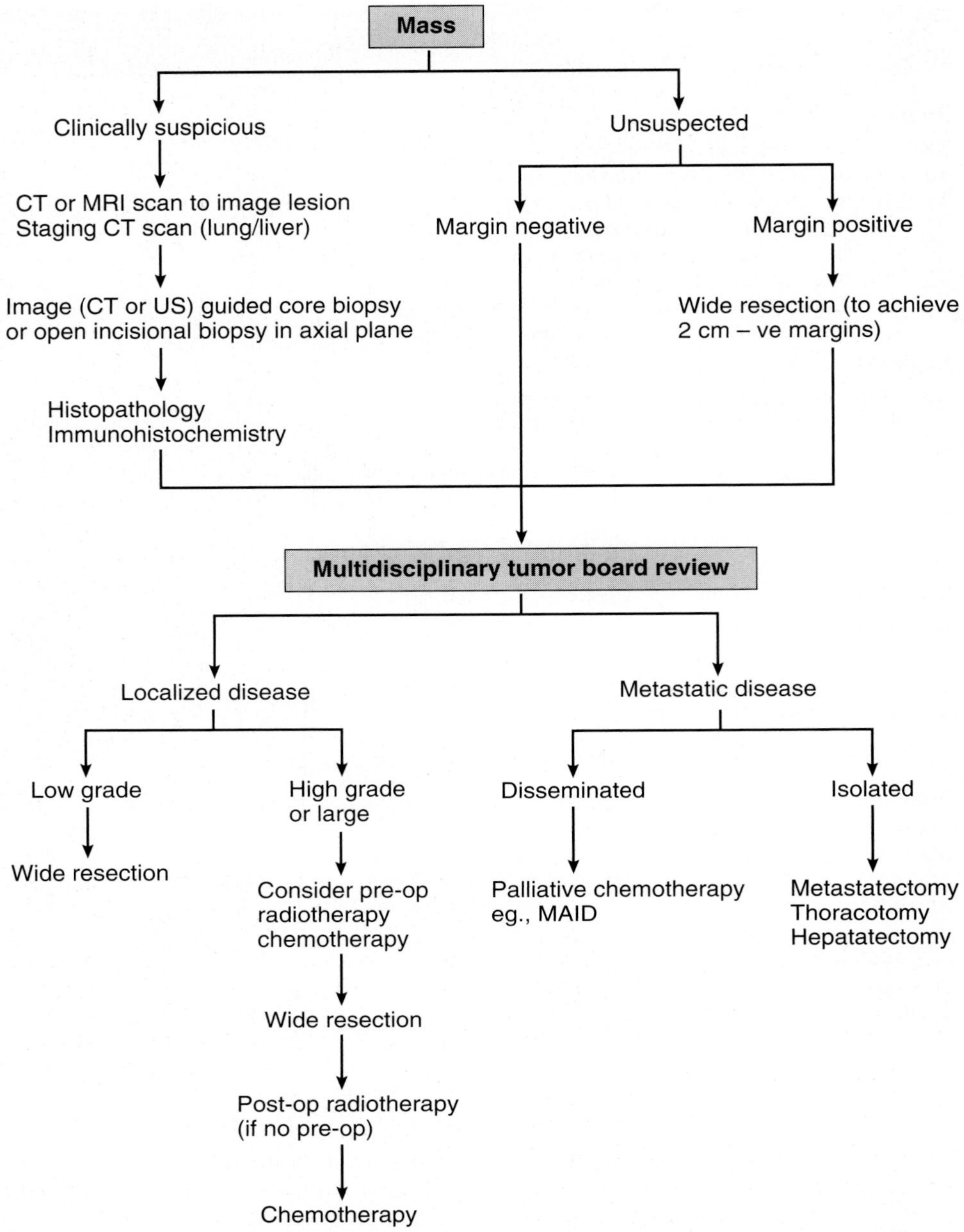

Figure 25-21 Management algorithm for adult soft tissue sarcoma.

response. Currently, MAID (mesna, doxorubicin, ifosfamide, and dacarbazine) is often administered every 4 weeks for 4 months prior to reassessing the patient with CT scanning. Occasionally, long-term survival can be achieved, but generally metastatic sarcoma patients will die of their disease in 12 to 18 months.

Prognosis

Overall, patient outcome is 50%; 5-year survival ranges from 90% for superficial low-grade tumors to 20% for advanced (metastatic disease, large, deep, or high-grade local) disease. In addition, resection margin involvement is an unfavorable survival factor (Table 25-10). No blood tests are of value in the followup of soft tissue sarcoma. For patients with superficial low-grade sarcomas excised for cure, clinical examination every 6 months (for the first 2 years), then yearly, is adequate followup. For deep-extremity or retroperitoneal sarcomas, imaging with CT or MRI will detect local recurrence. Because these tumors have a risk of metastasizing, a CT of the thorax is commonly used, beginning every 6 months for 2 years, followed by yearly exams. However, data from the National Cancer Institute suggest that chest radiography is adequate.

A 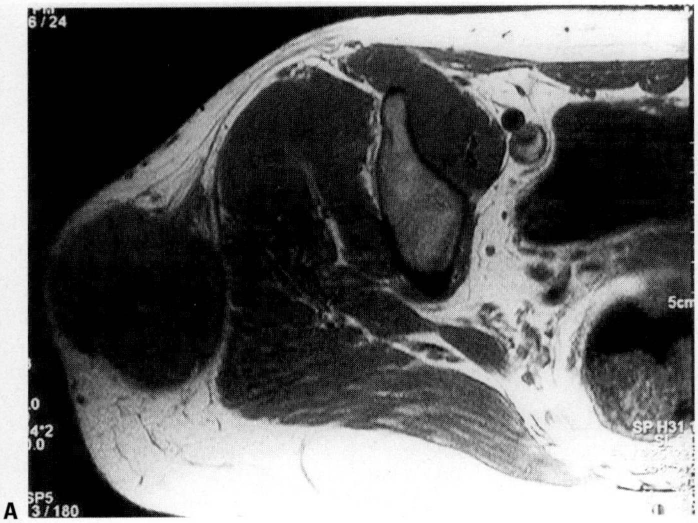

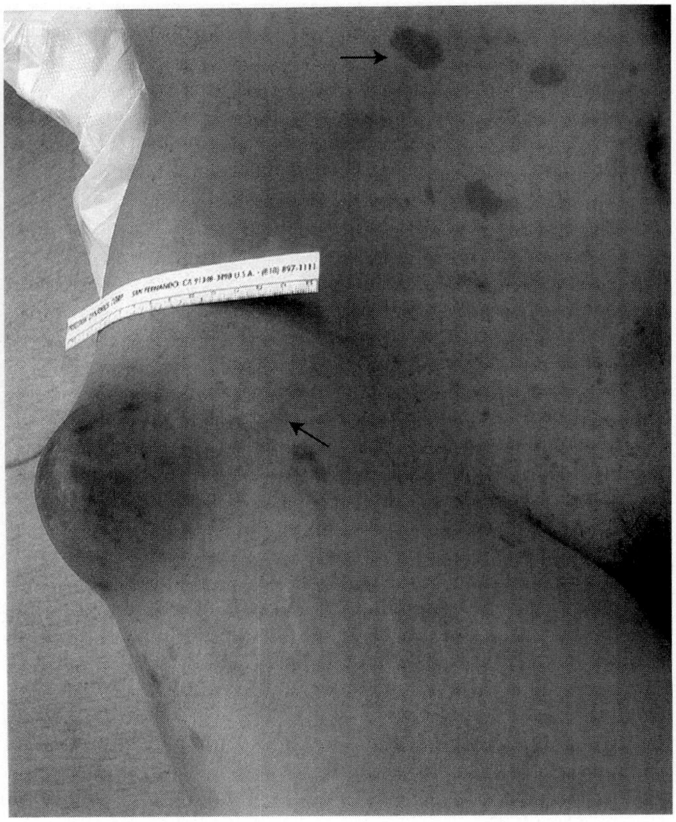

B

Figure 25-22 Neurofibrosarcoma in a patient with type 1 neurofibromatosis (G1T2N0M0). **A**, Magnetic resonance image. **B**, Clinical view. Lower arrow shows area of neovascularization; upper arrow shows café-au-lait spot.

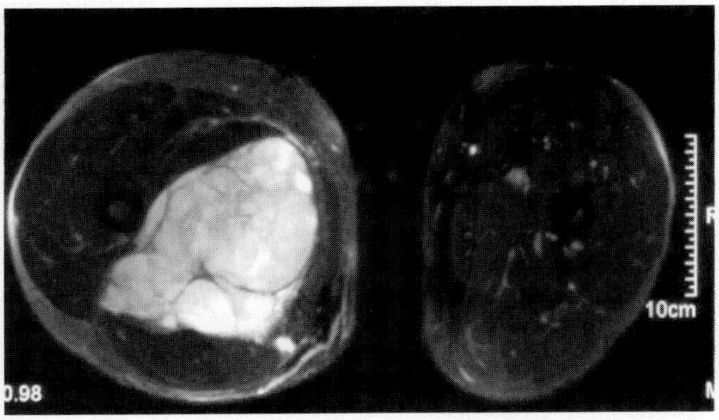

Figure 25-23 Sarcoma of the thigh (G3T2N0M0).

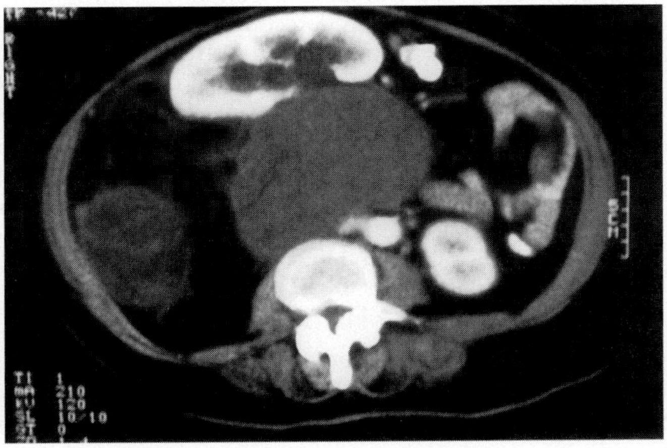

Figure 25-24 Retroperitoneal liposarcoma.

Specific Sarcomas and Sarcomalike Lesions

Gastrointestinal Stromal Tumor

Gastrointestinal stromal tumor represents a subgroup of sarcoma of gastrointestinal neural origin (see Fig. 25-26). These tumors are unique in that they have a specific genetic makeup and may express CD34 (hematopoietic progenitor cell antigen) and CD117 (C-kit protein, a membrane receptor with a tyrosine kinase component) with antigens. In the past, this tumor had a poor prognosis; however, the recent development of targeted chemotherapy in the form of tyrosine kinase inhibitor (imatinib mesylate) has shown impressive results in reversing and stabilizing metastatic disease. Treatment remains resection of the tumor with negative margins, and clinical trials are ongoing to determine the long-term results of tyrosine kinase inhibitors in metastatic as well as in the adjuvant setting.

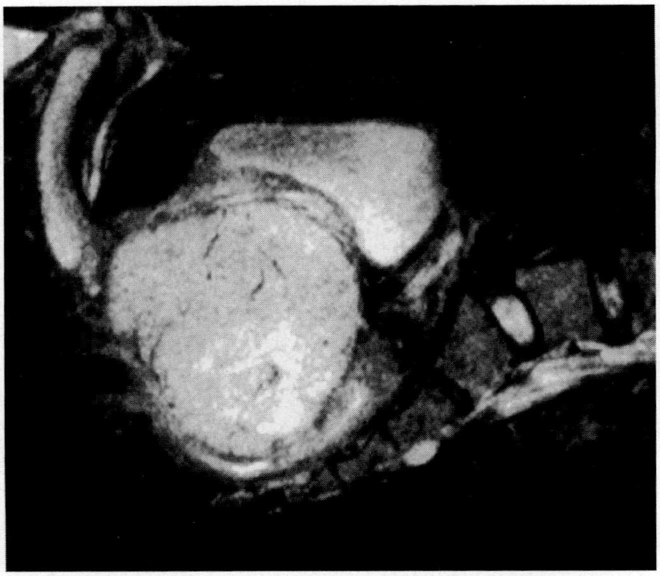

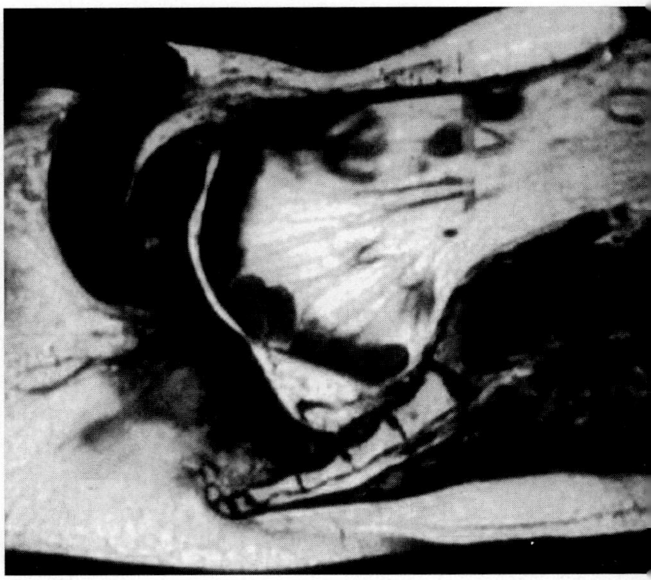

A B

Figure 25-25 Pelvic sarcoma. **A,** Preoperative scan. **B,** Postoperative scan.

Dermatofibrosarcoma Protuberans

This unusual skin and subcutaneous lesion has limited, if any, metastatic potential (less than 5%). However, if completely excised with positive margins, local recurrence is guaranteed. These lesions typically have a long-time course and may recur over a 25-year time period. The local recurrence potential is easy to underestimate, but with wide resection margins and appropriate reconstruction, a cure can be assured. Figure 25-27 shows the obvious nodularity of this subcutaneous lesion in the suprapubic area. A wide resection was taken incorporating the rectus abdominus muscle, which was subsequently reconstructed with mesh. It was possible to achieve closure of the resultant defect by advancing the abdominal wall flap to achieve an incision similar to those used for an abdominoplasty "tummy tuck."

Desmoid (Aggressive Fibromatosis)

Desmoid represents an intermediate grade malignancy of fibrous tissue. An example of the CT appearance of this lesion is seen in Figure 25-28. Typically, these lesions have a propensity for local recurrence and infiltration within muscle and soft tissue. Treatment consists of a wide resection. When this is not possible, radiotherapy may provide a reasonable chance of reducing the risk of local recurrence. More recently, evidence has emerged that these tumors may respond to nonsteroidal antiinflammatory drugs, tamoxifen, or some combination of these agents. Response to these agents is typically slow, but continues for months or years. For advanced or recurrent lesions, radiation and chemotherapy are also important treatment modalities.

Table 25-10 Prognostic Factors for Soft Tissue Sarcomas

	Prognosis	
Factor	**Favorable**	**Unfavorable**
Grade	Low	High
Size	< 5 cm	> 5 cm
Primary site	Superficial	Deep
Surgical margin	Clear	Involved

Kaposi's Sarcoma

In the past, Kaposi's sarcoma (KS) was largely limited to elderly Jewish men of Mediterranean descent and to peo-

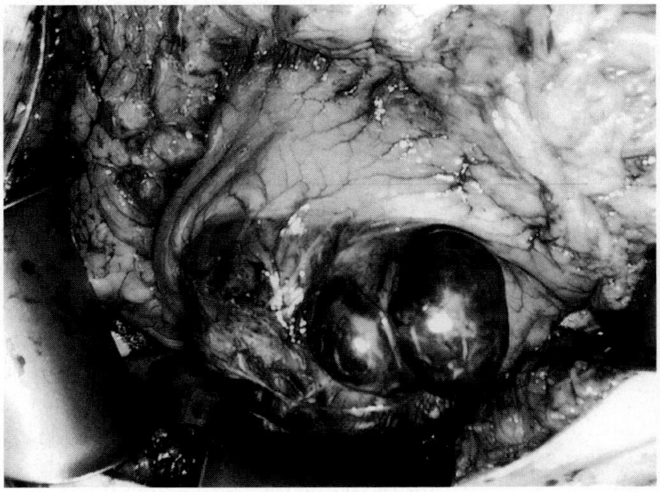

Figure 25-26 Gastrointestinal stromal tumor of the stomach (GIST).

A B C

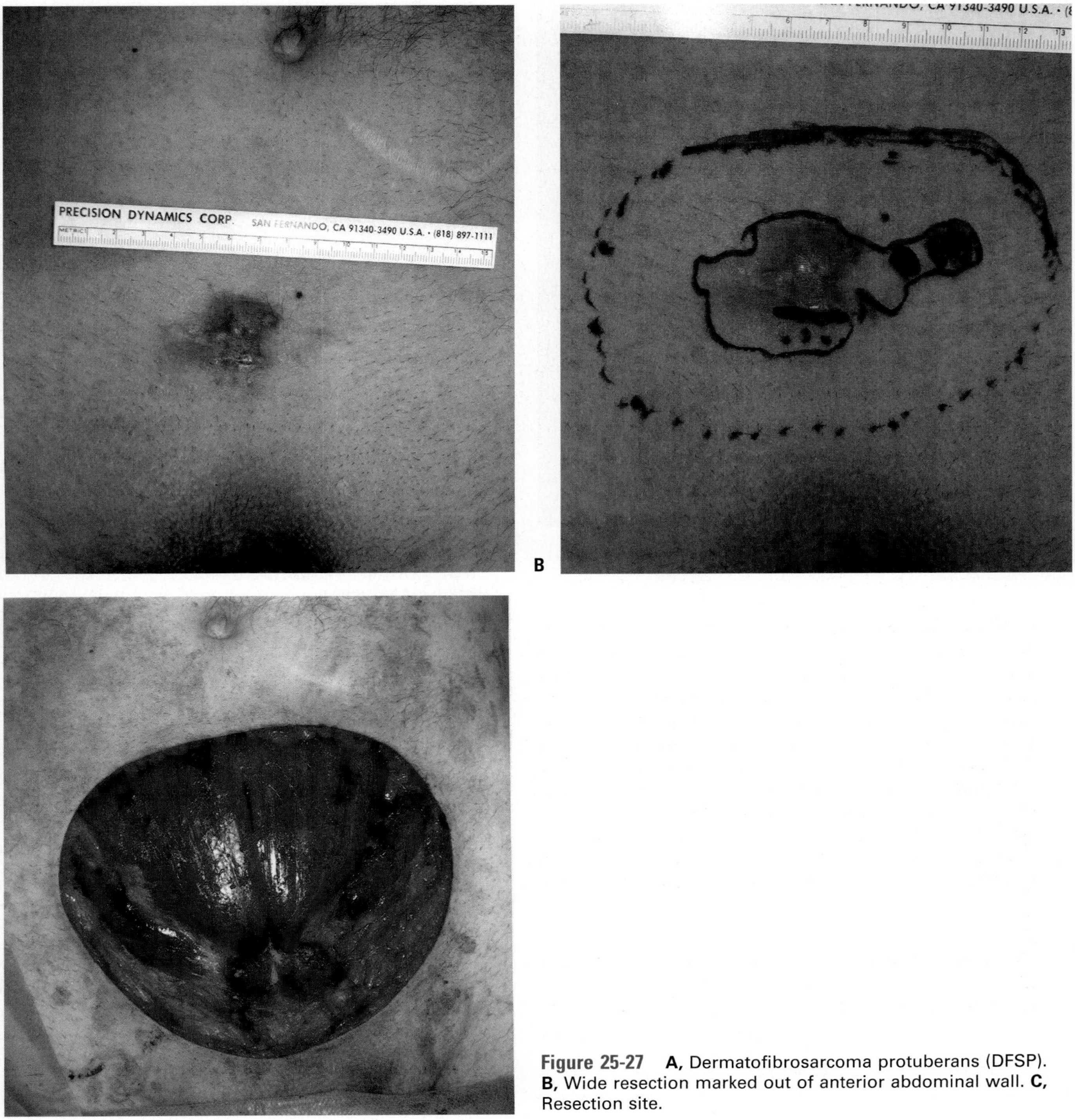

Figure 25-27 **A,** Dermatofibrosarcoma protuberans (DFSP). **B,** Wide resection marked out of anterior abdominal wall. **C,** Resection site.

ple from sub-Saharan Africa. With the AIDS epidemic, the incidence of Kaposi's sarcoma has increased. There are now four subtypes of KS based on epidemiologic variations: classic KS, African endemic KS, iatrogenic KS, and epidemic, AIDS-associated KS. Kaposi's sarcoma is the most common neoplastic complication of AIDS. Homosexual and bisexual men are much more likely to have Kaposi's sarcoma than others with AIDS. This finding suggests a sexually transmitted etiology in this patient population, and the agent appears to be human herpesvirus 8. Iatrogenic KS occurs in patients immunosuppressed by drug therapy. These lesions may regress if the immunotherapy can be stopped.

Kaposi's sarcoma lesions initially appear as flat, blue

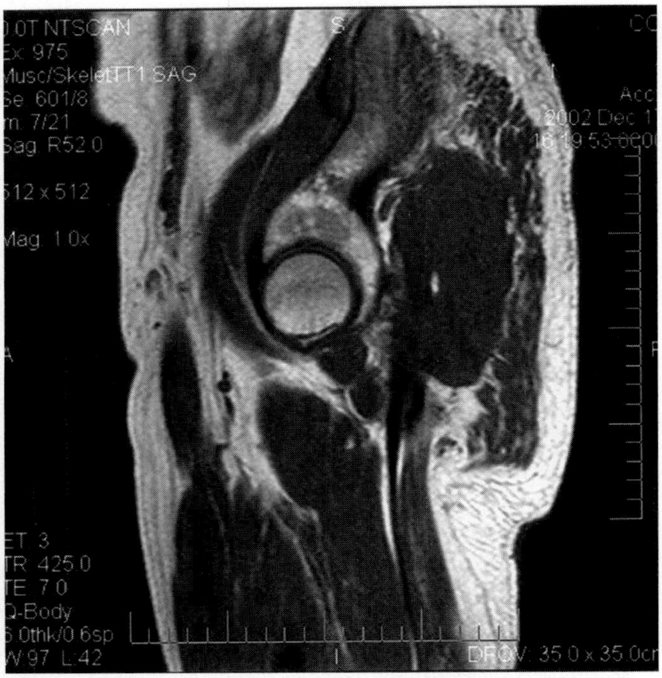

Figure 25-28 Aggressive fibromatosis of the buttock.

patches that resemble a hematoma. Later, they become raised, rubbery nodules. Non-AIDS Kaposi's sarcoma is typically found on the lower extremities. AIDS-related Kaposi's sarcoma often begins in the perioral mucosa. The palate is the most common site. AIDS-related Kaposi's sarcoma is often multifocal, with rapid spread to the lymph nodes. It often involves the gastrointestinal tract. Biopsy shows endothelial cells, with fibroblasts, spindle cells, and increased capillary growth. These malignancies are considered angiosarcomas.

Surgical excision or local radiation is effective for small, localized lesions. Agents such as vinblastine, bleomycin, and doxorubicin produce responses in more advanced cases. Patients with AIDS-related Kaposi's sarcoma have a far worse prognosis because of immunodeficiency, the presence of opportunistic infection, and the inability to use conventional multidrug regimens. Local radiation shrinks these lesions and provides palliation. Treatment includes single-drug regimens with vinblastine or VP-16.

SUGGESTED READINGS

Malignant Diseases of the Skin

Armstrong BK, English DR. Cutaneous malignant melanoma. In: Schottenfeld D, Fraumeni JF, eds. *Cancer Epidemiology and Prevention*. 2nd Ed. New York, NY: Oxford University Press, 1996: 1282–1312.

Balch CM, Buzaid AC, Soong SJ, et al. Final version of the American Joint Committee on Cancer staging system for cutaneous melanoma. *J Clin Oncol* 2001;19:3635–3648.

Balch CM, Houghton AN, Milton GW, et al. *Cutaneous Melanoma*. Philadelphia, PA: JB Lippincott, 1992.

Balch CM, Houghton AN, Peters L. Cutaneous melanoma. In: DeVita VT, Hellman S, Rosenberg SA, eds. *Cancer: Principles and Practice of Oncology*. 4th Ed. Philadelphia, PA: JB Lippincott, 1993: 1499–1542.

Fleming ID, Cooper JS, Henson DE, et al. *American Joint Committee on Cancer Staging Manual*. 5th Ed. Philadelphia, PA: Lippincott-Raven, 1997.

Greene FL, Page DL, Fleming ID, et al. *AJCC Cancer Staging Manual*. 6th Ed. New York, NY. Springer-Verlag, 2002.

Jemal A, Tiwari RC, Murray T, et al. Cancer statistics, 2004. *CA: Cancer J Clin* 2004;54(1):8–29.

Leffell DJ, Carucci JA. Management of skin cancer. In: DeVita VT, Hellman S, Rosenberg SA, eds. *Cancer: Principles and Practice of Oncology*. 6th Ed. Philadelphia, PA: Lippincott Williams & Wilkins, 2001:1976–2002.

Lotze MT, Dallal RM, Kirkwood JM, et al. Cutaneous melanoma. In: DeVita VT, Hellman S, Rosenberg SA, eds. *Cancer: Principles and Practice of Oncology*. 6th Ed. Philadelphia, PA: Lippincott Williams & Wilkins, 2001:2012–2069.

Patterson JAK, Geronemus RG. Cancers of the skin. In: DeVita VT, Hellman S, Rosenberg SA, eds. *Cancer: Principles and Practice of Oncology*. 4th Ed. Philadelphia, PA: Lippincott, 1993:1612–1650.

Sober AJ. Diagnosis and management of skin cancer. *Cancer* 1983;51: 2448–2452.

Malignant Diseases of the Lymphatics and Soft Tissue

Armitage JO, Mauch PM, Harris NL, et al. Non-Hodgkin's lymphomas. In: DeVita VT, Hellman S, Rosenberg SA, eds. *Cancer: Principles and Practice of Oncology*. 6th Ed. Philadelphia, PA: Lippincott Williams & Wilkins, 2001:2256–2315.

Brennan MF, Alektiar KM, Maki RG. Soft tissue sarcoma. In: DeVita VT, Hellman S, Rosenberg SA, eds. *Cancer: Principles and Practice of Oncology*. 6th Ed. Philadelphia, PA: Lippincott Williams & Wilkins, 2001:1841–1890.

Brennan MF, Casper ES, Harrison LB, et al. The role of multimodality therapy in soft tissue sarcoma. *Ann Surg* 1991;214(3):328–338.

Diehl V, Mauch PM, Harris NL. Hodgkin's disease. In: DeVita VT, Hellman S, Rosenberg SA, eds. *Cancer: Principles and Practice of Oncology*. 6th Ed. Philadelphia, PA: Lippincott Williams & Wilkins, 2001:2339–2388.

Hartge P, Devesa S, Fraumeni J Jr. Hodgkin's and non-Hodgkin's lymphomas. Cancer Surveys 19/20. Trends in Cancer Incidence and Mortality, 1994.

Lawrence W Jr. Operative management of soft tissue sarcomas: impact of anatomic site. *Semin Surg Oncol* 1994;10:340–346.

Mazanet R, Antman KH. Adjuvant therapy for sarcomas. *Semin Oncol* 1991;18(6):603–612.

26

RICHARD M. BELL, MD

Surgical Procedures, Techniques, and Skills

THE OPERATING ROOM

The surgical theater can be an uncomfortable place for the novice. The intensity of the environment and the regulations that govern the maintenance of a sterile field add to the awkwardness and anxiety. Fortunately, the code of conduct is straightforward and easily learned. The operating room is the arena where the student physician can actually see and touch the pathology. Surgeons use this opportunity to demonstrate how surgical therapy affects the disease process, to demonstrate living human anatomy, and to discuss normal and pathologic physiology.

Attire

Knowledge of the surgical environment and the meticulous practice of **asepsis** and **sterile technique** are required. Infectious complications increase hospital stay, patient discomfort, costs, and the risk of death and disfigurement. For the student, participation in the care of the surgical patient and admission to the surgical suite are privileges.

Proper design of facilities and regulations for attire and conduct in the surgical suite are important factors in preventing the transportation of microorganisms into the operating room. To minimize the transportation of virulent hospital pathogens directly into the surgical arena, street clothes are never worn within restricted areas of the surgical suite, and operating room attire should not be worn outside of the operating area. All persons who enter restricted areas are required to wear clean surgical apparel, including hats, scrub clothes, shoe covers, and face masks. Each item of surgical garb is designed to protect the patient from contamination from hair, fomites (objects, such as clothing, that might harbor a disease agent), and microorganisms in the air.

The hat, or hood, covers and contains all hair. It fits snugly, and elastic or drawstrings secure the edges. Personnel with long hair can wear hoods that tie under the chin.

Scrub clothes are made of a closely woven fabric that is flame resistant, lint-free, cool, and comfortable. A large variety of scrub suits are available. They should fit closely, and shirts and drawstrings should be tucked into the pants.

All persons who enter the restricted areas of the surgical suite wear shoe covers. They are changed between operative procedures and are never worn outside the operating area.

High-filtration-efficiency disposable masks are worn at all times in the operating room. These masks are tied securely to cover the mouth and nose entirely. To prevent cross-infection, masks are handled only by the strings. They are never lowered to hang loosely around the neck. Masks are changed frequently and promptly discarded after use.

Protective glasses or face shields are worn to prevent inoculation of the eyes with body fluids or irritant solutions.

Scrubbed team members also wear sterile gowns and gloves. Most institutions use water-repellent disposable gowns. Although the entire gown is sterilized, neither the back nor any area below the waist or above the chest is considered sterile after the gown is donned. The cuffs are made of stockinette to fit the wrist tightly. Sterile gloves cover the wrists.

Scrubbing

Sterilization of the skin is not possible. However, every effort is made to reduce the bacterial count and minimize the possibility of microbial contamination. The surgical scrub is a process of mechanical scrubbing with a chemical antiseptic solution. General preparations for the surgical scrub include ensuring that the fingernails are short and unpolished, removing all hand jewelry, cleaning under each fingernail, and performing a short prescrub of the hands and arms.

The details of the surgical scrub vary among institutions and with the soaps or solutions used. Students are generally given an orientation to the procedures used in the operating room early in the clerkship and the specifics of the institution's policy are explained. The following anatomic pattern of scrubbing is suggested: the fingernails, the four surfaces of each finger, the dorsal surface of the hand, the palmar surface of the hand, and the area over the wrists and up the arm, ending 2 inches above the elbow (Fig. 26-1). Because the hands are in most direct contact with the sterile field, all steps of the scrub procedure begin with the hands and end at the elbows. After the scrub, the hands and forearms are held higher than the elbows. In this way, contaminated water can roll off at the elbow and not run down the arms to contaminate the hands (Fig. 26-2). The hands and arms are also held away from the body.

To dry the hands, a folded sterile towel is grasped with one hand. The towel is allowed to unfold without touching any sterile object. One arm is dried by holding the towel in the opposite hand. Drying is begun at the fingers and hand. The arm is then rotated, and the towel is drawn up to the elbow. The used portion is never brought back into the dry area. The towel is then reversed, and the opposite hand and arm are dried with the unused part of the towel. The towel is discarded in the appropriate container.

Gowning and Gloving

A person who is gowning unassisted picks up the gown, taking care to touch only the inner surface. The gown is held by the inside and allowed to unfold, with the inside of the gown toward the body. With the hands at shoulder level, the arms are inserted into the sleeves. The arms remain extended, and the circulating nurse assists by pulling the gown over the shoulders and tying it in the back.

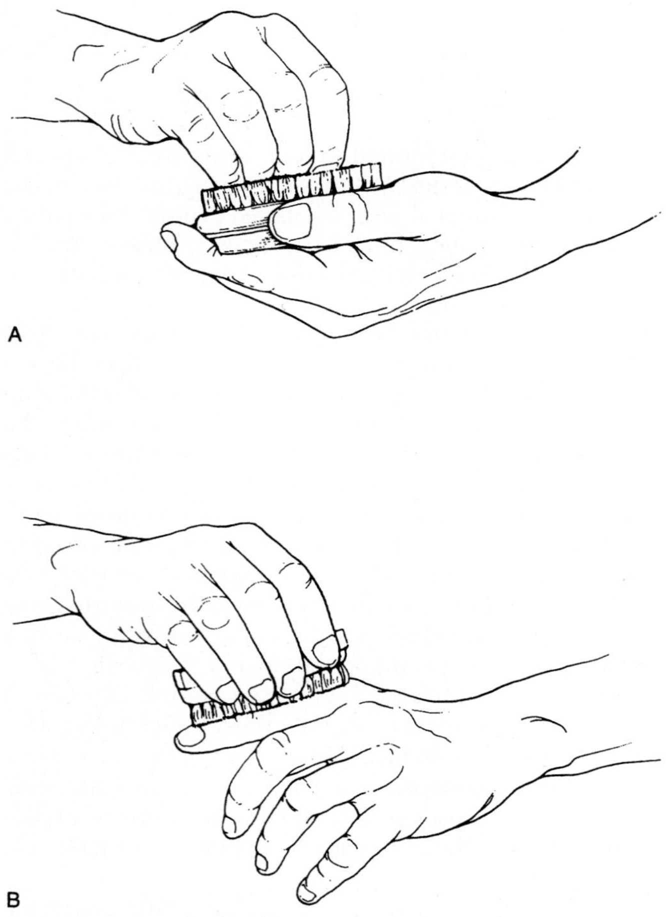

Figure 26-1 **A,** Use of a bristle brush to scrub the fingernails. **B,** The anatomic pattern of scrubbing. Four surfaces of each finger are scrubbed.

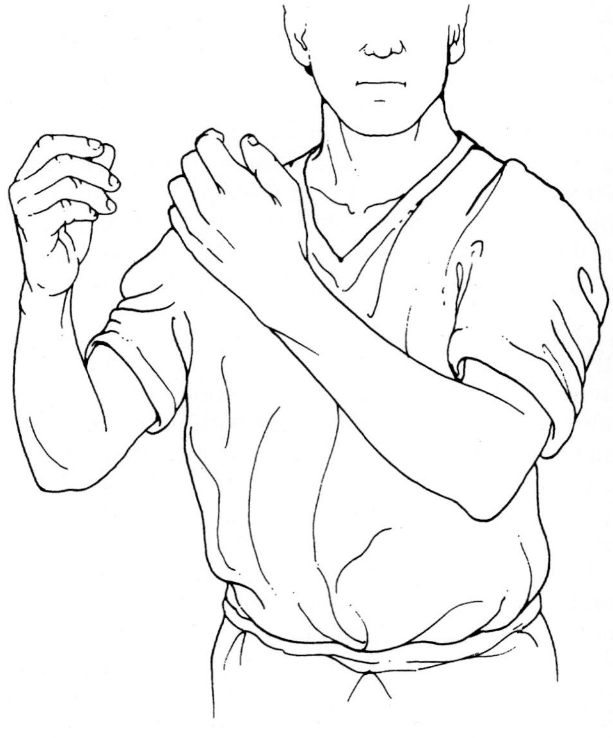

Figure 26-2 The arms and forearms are held away from the body and higher than the elbows.

If a **closed-gloving technique** is used (gowning and gloving without assistance), the hands are advanced to the edge of the cuff, but not through it (Fig. 26-3A). With this method, the gloves are handled through the fabric of the gown sleeves. The hands are pushed through the cuff openings as the gloves are pulled on. With this technique, the glove is placed palm down onto the pronated forearm of the matching hand, with the fingers of the glove pointing toward the elbow and the glove cuff on the gown wristlet (Fig. 26-3*B*). The glove is held securely by the hand on which it is placed. The other hand is used to stretch the cuff over the sleeve opening to cover the gown wristlet (Fig. 26-3*C*). The cuff is drawn back onto the wrist, and the fingers are adjusted (Fig. 26-3*D*). The gloved hand is used to position the other glove on the opposite sleeve in the same fashion (Fig. 26-3*E*).

If an **open-gloving technique** is used, the hands are advanced completely through the cuffs of the gown (Fig. 26-4). The left glove is removed from the package by placing the fingers of the right hand on the folded-back cuff, touching only the inner surface of the glove. The left hand is inserted into the glove, but the cuff is not turned up. The right glove is taken from the package by slipping the gloved left fingers under the inverted cuff and pulling the glove into the right hand. The cuffs are pulled over the gown wristlet by rotating the arm slightly.

If the **scrub nurse** assists with gowning and gloving, the nurse holds the gown open with the inner side toward the person who is gowning. The arms are inserted into the gown. The circulating nurse reaches inside the gown, grasps the sleeve seam, pulls the gown on, and ties the back closure. After the gown is on, the scrub

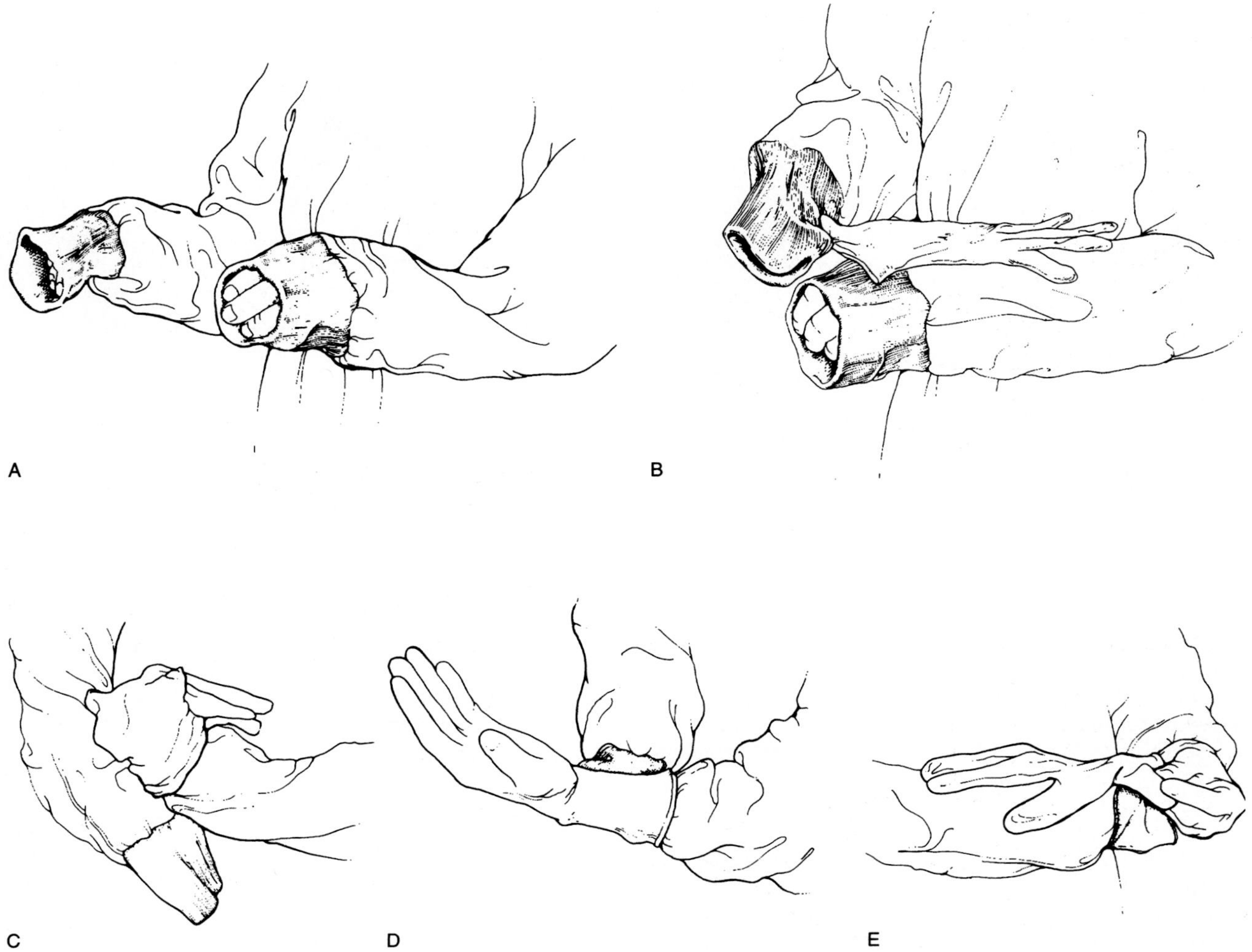

Figure 26-3 The closed-gloving technique. **A,** The hands are advanced to the edge of the cuff, but not through the cuff. **B,** The glove is placed down on the forearm, with the fingers pointed toward the elbow. **C,** The other hand stretches the glove over the gown wristlet (through the gown fabric). **D,** The cuff is drawn back onto the wrist. **E,** The gloved hand is used to pull on the remaining glove in the same way.

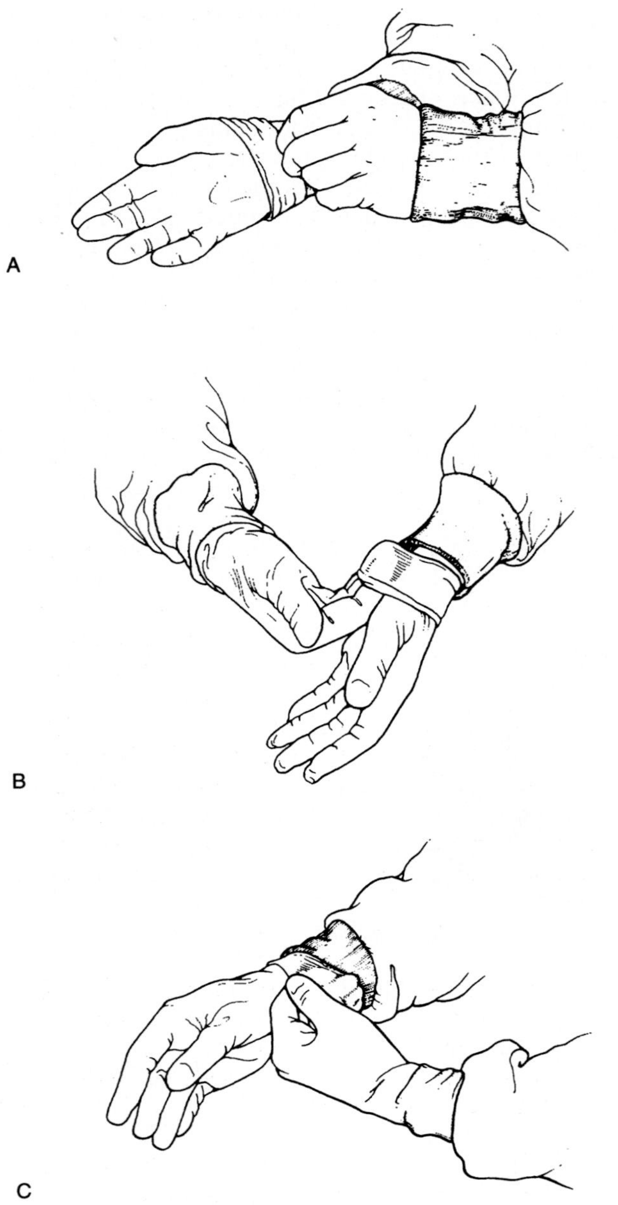

Figure 26-4 The open-gloving technique. **A,** The left ungloved hand pulls on the right glove, touching only the inner surface. **B,** The gloved fingers of the right hand are inserted under the cuff, and the glove is pulled onto the left hand. **C,** The glove cuffs are pulled over the gown wristlets.

nurse holds the gloves open, and the hands are slipped into them.

After gloving, the assisted gowning continues. The exterior ties in the front of the gown are untied. The tie that is attached to the back of the gown is handed to another person who is gowned and gloved. The other tie is held securely, and the person turns in the opposite direction to close the back panel of the gown. The tie is retrieved and tied securely at the side.

A glove that becomes contaminated is changed immediately. If a question about contamination arises, it is best to change gloves or both gown and gloves. The hand with the contaminated glove is extended to the circulating nurse, who grasps the outside of the glove cuff and pulls it off inside out. Surgical personnel should not attempt to remove a glove unassisted because the other hand may become contaminated. The sleeve wristlet is pulled down over the hand when the glove is removed because the new glove could be contaminated by the gown sleeve. If possible, another sterile team member assists with the regloving. If this assistance is not possible, the person steps aside and applies the new glove with the open-gloving technique.

To remove the gown and gloves properly, the gown is removed first by pulling it down from the shoulders and turning the sleeves inside out while the arms are pulled from the sleeves. The gloves are removed by turning them inside out, and the hands are protected by not touching the outer, soiled surface of the gloves (Fig. 26-5). As a

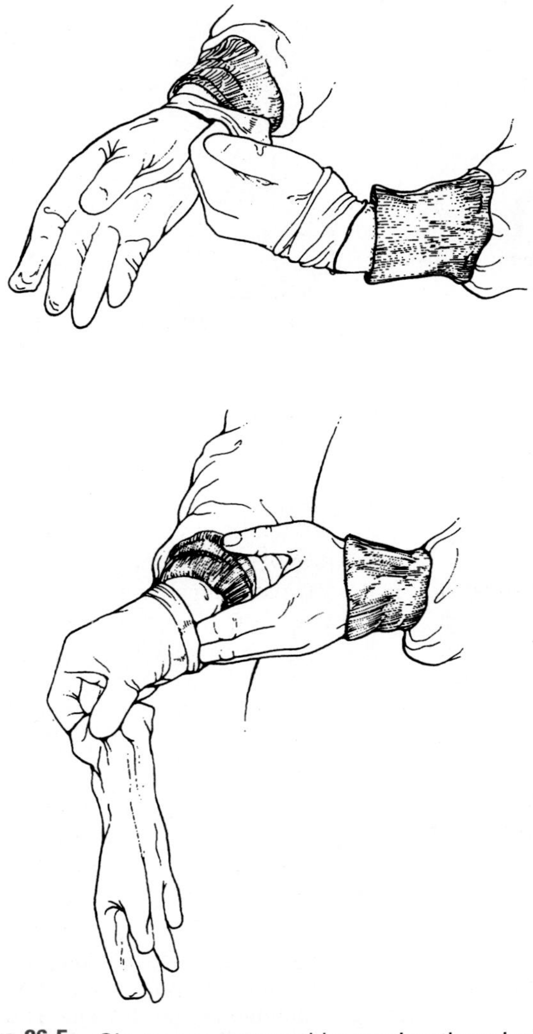

Figure 26-5 Gloves are removed by turning them inside out without touching the soiled part with the hands.

matter of courtesy and to contain contaminants, the gown and gloves are discarded in the receptacles provided.

Some procedures that are associated with large concentrations of bacteria pose additional risk of infection. These procedures are known as dirty, contaminated, or septic. Special practices may be necessary to confine potentially infectious material (e.g., intraabdominal sepsis, empyema, gross fecal contamination, perirectal abscesses). Personnel should remove the gown, gloves, shoe covers, hat, and mask before leaving the operating room.

PRINCIPLES OF ASEPSIS AND STERILE TECHNIQUE

A simple definition of asepsis is the absence of any infectious agents. However, the term is also used broadly to describe a wide variety of procedures that reduce the incidence of infection in patients and hospital personnel. These practices include sterilization of goods and supplies, disinfection of the hospital environment, **antisepsis** of animate objects, and environmental control of the operating room.

Sterilization is the process that kills all forms of living matter, including bacteria, viruses, yeast, and mold. Special equipment for this process uses **moist heat, dry heat,** or **ethylene oxide gas**.

Moist heat destroys all forms of microbial life, including spores, through denaturation and coagulation of intracellular protein. The essential factors are temperature, time, and pressure. A temperature of 250°F, a time exposure of 15 to 30 minutes, and a pressure of 15 to 17 pounds per square inch are required to kill all microorganisms. Other variables are the size, contents, and packaging methods of the materials to be sterilized.

A high-speed instrument sterilizer, the autoclave (flash sterilizer), is used for moist-heat sterilization in the operating room. The autoclave functions rapidly at a high temperature and increased pressure. To sterilize unwrapped instruments, the requirements are 270°F, 27 pounds of pressure, and minimum exposure time of 3 minutes.

Dry-heat sterilization is used only for articles that cannot tolerate the corrosive action of steam or for products that cannot be penetrated by steam or gas (e.g., petroleum products, powders, glassware, delicate instruments). In the absence of moisture, higher temperature and longer exposure times are required: 340°F for 1 hour, 280°F for 3 hours, and 250°F for 6 hours.

Sterilization with ethylene oxide gas kills bacteria by reacting with the chemical components of the cell protein. This type of sterilization is particularly useful for items that cannot withstand moisture or high heat (e.g., lensed instruments, air-powered instruments, glassware, paper or rubber products). This type of sterilization depends on gas concentration, temperature, humidity, and exposure time.

A biologic control test provides assurance of sterilization. Process monitors (e.g., heat-sensitive tape) indicate exposure to sterilization conditions, but do not ensure sterility. Packaged items are marked with a sterilization date. The time that a sterile package may be kept in storage without compromising its sterility is its shelf life. Shelf life depends on the conditions of storage, the packaging materials, the seal of the package, and the integrity of the package. Any package that is outdated, exposed to moisture, dropped on the floor, or punctured is considered contaminated.

The hospital environment is disinfected with chemical agents that destroy pathogenic bacteria on inanimate surfaces. The operating room and all furniture (e.g., operating table, instrument tables, lights) are cleaned with chemical disinfectants after each operation.

Antisepsis is the use of chemical agents to destroy bacteria on animate surfaces. Before an operative procedure is begun, personnel perform the surgical scrub on the hands and arms with antiseptic soaps. The patient's skin is also carefully prepared to create an area with reduced levels of bacteria.

Environmental control of the surgical suite is essential to minimize contamination and provide maximum protection for the patient. These factors include maintaining greater air pressure in the room than in the hallway so that air is forced out of the surgical area. Additional measures include restricting traffic, controlling the room temperature (68°F to 72°F), controlling the humidity (50%), and maintaining an air change rate of 18 to 25 times per hour.

A variety of measures and controls are used to maintain an environment that is as sterile and free of bacteria as possible. The integrity of this environment depends on strict adherence by all personnel to sterile technique. To minimize the risk of infection, attention to the following principles of sterile technique is essential:

1. Only sterile items are used within a sterile field. The sterility of these items is ensured by proper packaging, sterilization, and handling.
2. Parts of a gown that are considered sterile are the sleeves and the front from the waist to the shoulder level.
3. Tables are sterile only at table level (top). The edges and sides below table level are not sterile.
4. The edges of anything that encloses sterile contents (e.g., packaging) are not sterile.
5. Persons who are sterile touch only items that are sterile. Persons who are not sterile touch only items that are not sterile.
6. Sterile persons stay within the sterile area. Persons who are not sterile avoid entering the sterile area.
7. Sterile persons avoid leaning over an area that is not sterile. Persons who are not sterile avoid reaching over a sterile area.
8. Sterile persons minimize contact with an area that is not sterile.
9. A sterile field is created immediately before use.
10. Sterile areas are continuously kept in view.
11. If the integrity of the microbial barriers is destroyed, contamination occurs.
12. Microorganisms are kept to a minimum.

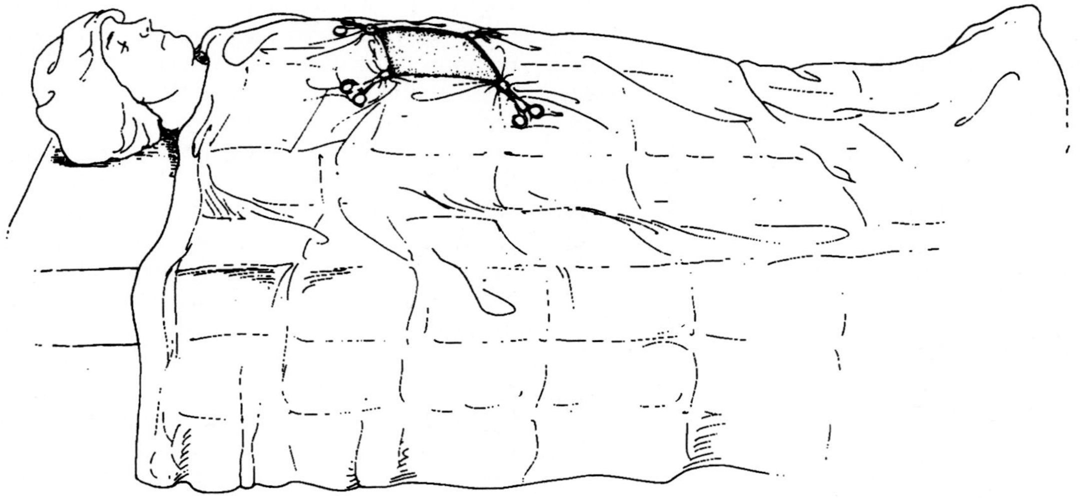

Figure 26-6 The incision site is exposed, yet isolated.

A sterile field is created by the placement of sterile sheets and towels in a specific position to maintain the sterility of the operative surfaces. The patient and the operating table are covered with drapes so that the site of incision is exposed, yet isolated (Fig. 26-6). Objects that are draped include instrument tables, basins, the Mayo stand, and trays. Sterile team members function within this limited area and handle only sterile items. All members of the operating team constantly safeguard the sterility of the operative field.

Surgical Preparation

A wide area of skin around the operative incision is meticulously prepared by shaving and scrubbing. Shaving is performed just before the procedure and ideally outside the operative theater. Skin preparation cleanses the operative site of transient and resident microorganisms, dirt, and skin oil.

Skin preparation is usually carried out from a separate table (prep table). After the patient is positioned on the operating table, one member of the surgical team prepares the patient's skin with antiseptic solution. Sterile gloves are worn. The incision line is scrubbed first, and the team member works outward, toward the periphery of the field (Fig. 26-7). Theoretically, the incision line is the cleanest area. The number of organisms increases with increasing distance from the incision site. After the lateral limits of the operative field are reached, the sponge is discarded. The process is repeated with a new sponge. The sponge is never brought from the outside of the field to repeat the scrub of the central incision area. Areas that are likely to contain large numbers of bacteria (e.g., perineum, groin, axilla) are washed last. Cleansing is done vigorously, with particular attention given to difficult areas (e.g., umbilicus). Cotton-tipped applicators may be used in the umbilical area. Towels are used to absorb excess solution and prevent the solution from pooling under the patient.

The procedure for applying antiseptic solution to various parts of the body may vary, depending on the site and the surgeon's preference. Painting of the operative area with antiseptic solution follows the same principles as the scrub (i.e., from the center toward the periphery). After the skin is prepared, the patient is ready for draping.

Draping involves covering the patient and the surrounding areas with a sterile barrier to create a sterile area. Drapes are fluid resistant, antistatic, abrasive-free, lint-free, and flexible enough to fit contours. The following standard principles for draping are followed:

1. Place drapes on a dry area.
2. Handle the drapes as little as possible. Avoid shaking them because air currents carry contaminants.
3. Make a cuff over the gloved hand to protect the hand from contacting an area that is not sterile.
4. Never reach across the table to drape the opposite side; instead, go around the table.
5. Hold the drape high enough to avoid touching areas that are not sterile.
6. After a drape is placed, do not adjust it. If a drape is placed incorrectly, discard it.
7. Unfold the drape toward the feet first.
8. Place the folded edge toward the incision to provide a smooth outline of the field. Prevent instruments or sponges from falling between the layers.
9. Any part of the drape below waist level or table level is considered contaminated and should not be handled.
10. Towel clips that are fastened through the drapes have contaminated points. Remove them only if necessary, and discard them.
11. If a hole is found after a drape is placed, cover that area with another barrier.

Draping procedures may vary from one hospital to another; however, standardized methods of application are followed.

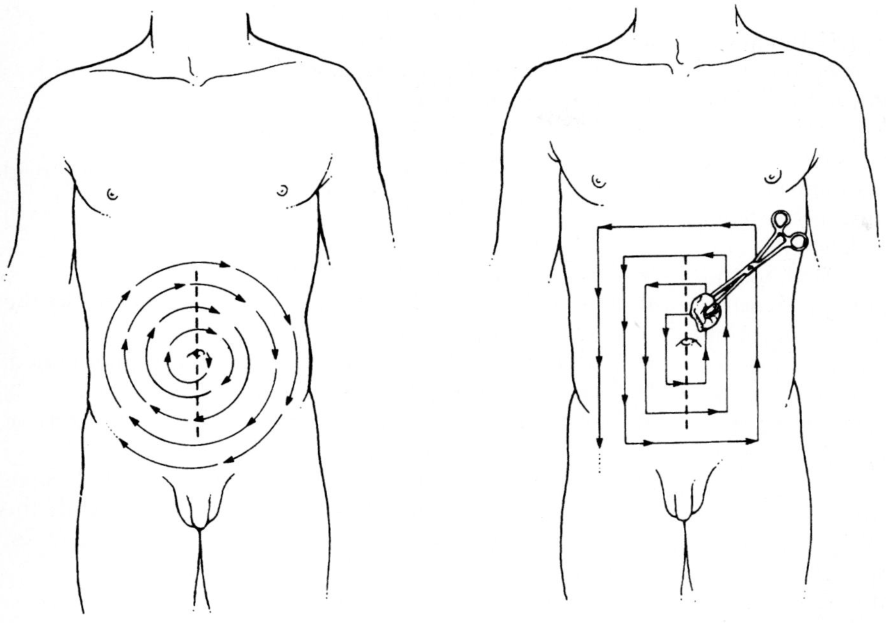

Figure 26-7 Preparation of the operative site. Movement is from the center toward the periphery.

ASSISTING IN THE OPERATING ROOM

A student is often asked to assist during an operative procedure. Assisting can produce a spectrum of emotional responses that varies from elation to fear and trepidation. Usually, undergraduates are asked to hold retractors or provide other measures to gain exposure for the operating surgeon. The assistant is often excluded from the field of view and asked to maintain an uncomfortable position while pulling on a retractor with strength that has long been spent. In addition, the assistant may feel ill, exhausted, or worried, and may anticipate a barrage of questions about regional anatomy, physiology, or surgical technique. Most surgeons respond positively to students who show an interest and some evidence of independent study about the patient or the operation. Because most surgical procedures are elective, students usually have time to become familiar with the basic operative steps.

The following checklist may help the student prepare for the role of assistant or observer in the operating room. A well-prepared student is more likely to have a positive experience and to make a contribution to the team's effort.

- What procedure is planned?
- What is the regional anatomy?
- What are the normal physiology and the pathophysiology of the organ?
- What are the surgical and nonsurgical treatment options?
- What is the effect of the procedure on the pathophysiology?
- What are the potential complications?

In most cases, the operative plan is clear (e.g., cholecystectomy for cholelithiasis). A review of the regional anatomy is always beneficial. The blood supply to the organs involved, the lymphatic drainage, and the proximity to other vital structures (e.g., relation of the common bile duct to the portal vein or hepatic artery) are important. A surgical atlas may be the best reference for anatomic detail because this type of text approaches the subject from a surgeon's perspective.

Most surgeons assume that students can describe the normal physiology of the organ or organ systems involved. An understanding of the abnormal, or pathophysiologic, process is the goal of most undergraduate clerkships.

Most problems have more than one surgical approach in addition to nonsurgical approaches (e.g., treatment for breast cancer, approach to the solitary thyroid nodule). Knowledge of how the surgical procedure reverses or changes the pathophysiologic process enhances the student's understanding of the operating room experience.

Every surgical procedure carries a risk of complication. Some complications are related to the technical aspects of the procedure (e.g., anastomotic leak or stenosis, pseudoaneurysm, common duct injury during laparoscopic cholecystectomy). Others involve physiologic or anatomic alterations caused by surgery (e.g., marginal ulcers at the site of gastrojejunostomy, dumping syndrome, afferent loop syndrome). Many surgical atlases list the common complications of each procedure. The risks of anesthesia, pulmonary compromise, atelectasis, thrombophlebitis, and wound infection are complications of many procedures.

Functioning as a good assistant can be as demanding as serving as the primary surgeon. Assisting effectively is learned behavior that requires experience and knowledge of the procedure. A good assistant anticipates the steps in the procedure and helps, rather than competes with, the operating surgeon. Keeping the field dry, anticipating the cutting of sutures, and providing adequate exposure are within the capabilities of even the novice in the operating room. Most surgeons recognize that the undergraduate student is in unfamiliar territory, and senior members of the team usually provide instruction on how to help. The assistant pays attention to the procedure and avoids distractions. For example, conversation should be limited to the case. Care is taken not to lean on the patient inadvertently while standing at the operative table because nerve damage or interference with ventilation could occur.

The surgical technician passes the requested instruments. A student who attempts to retrieve or replace instruments on the Mayo stand may disrupt the organization and flow of the operation. Many surgical technicians consider the Mayo stand hallowed ground, and trespassers are often chastised. The ability to provide the requested instruments, ties, or suture material quickly is hampered by extra hands or disorganized instruments.

The operative field is kept as tidy as possible. To contain contamination, simplify the accounting of sponges, and provide a rough estimate of blood loss, sponges that are used during the procedure are dropped into the container that is provided. Searching for a misplaced sponge tries everyone's patience. (See Table 26-1 for a list of hemostatic agents and their uses.)

The members of the surgical team remain in the room until the patient leaves or the surgeon grants permission to leave. The student should remain available to assist with application of the dressing, transfer of the patient to the stretcher, or other tasks.

Proper positioning of the patient for the operation is determined by the surgeon. The following principles are considered:

- Proper maintenance of respiration
- Unimpaired circulation
- Protection of muscles and nerves from pressure
- Accessibility and exposure of the operative field
- Uninterrupted administration of anesthetic agents
- Accessibility for administration of intravenous fluids
- Comfort and safety of the patient

The following important safety measures are observed when a patient is transferred or positioned:

- The table is securely locked in position.
- The patient's head is protected from movement by the anesthesiologist.
- Uninterrupted flow of intravenous fluids is maintained.
- Care is taken not to hyperextend the arms.
- Slow, gentle movement is used to avoid circulatory or respiratory compromise.
- The placement of pressure on nerves is avoided. Steps include ensuring that the legs are not crossed while the patient is in the supine position and placing pillows or rolls under the chest if the patient is prone.
- Nothing is allowed to obstruct tubing.

Operating tables are divided into three or more hinged sections that are flexed or extended to obtain the desired position. This procedure is often called "breaking" the table. The joints of the table are called "breaks." The operative table can be placed in a number of positions, including Trendelenburg (head down) and reverse Trendelenburg (head up). The table can also be rotated laterally, fixed, raised, or lowered. Special equipment and table attachments (e.g., safety belts, arm straps, arm boards, braces, supports, stirrups, bandage rolls) are used to stabilize the patient on the table. Although the circulating nurse assumes the major responsibility for positioning the patient, the safety of the patient during the operative procedure is a responsibility that is shared by every member of the surgical team.

Table 26-1 Hemostatic Agents and Their Uses

Hemostatic Agents	Content	Uses
Thrombin	Human or bovine thrombin	Liver, spleen, spine, neurosurgery
Fibrin sealants	Human fibrinogen Human factor XIII Human thrombin Bovine aprotinin (with various methods to inactivate blood-borne viruses)	Liver, spleen, spine, neurosurgery
Gelatin foams/sheets	Gelatin	Liver, spleen, and generally any oozing surface
Cellulose sheets	Oxidized regenerated cellulose	Liver, spleen, vascular
Avitine flour	Microfibrillar collagen	Liver, spleen, vascular, neurosurgery, spine

CLASSIFICATION OF OPERATIVE WOUNDS

Operative wounds are classified, according to the risk of contamination or infection, as clean, clean-contaminated, contaminated, or dirty. This classification allows prediction of the risk of subsequent wound infection and allows comparison of the techniques of different surgical teams.

In clean wounds, the gastrointestinal, respiratory, or urinary tract is not entered. In addition, inflammation is not present, and no break in technique occurs. The risk of infection is negligible.

In clean-contaminated wounds, the gastrointestinal, respiratory, or urinary tract is entered without significant spillage or break in operative technique. The risk of infection is minimal.

Contaminated wounds involve gross spillage of the contents of the gastrointestinal or urinary tract or a major break in operative technique. This category includes fresh traumatic wounds because of the potential for contamination. The risk of infection approaches 5%.

A wound is considered dirty if pus or a perforated viscus is encountered. Old traumatic wounds with necrotic tissue, wounds that require the excision of a foreign body, or wounds that have gross fecal contamination are also considered dirty. Because the infection rate is high if these wounds are closed primarily, they are often left open.

The prevention of wound infection in the surgical patient requires the following steps:

- Control of endogenous infection
- Strict adherence to sterile technique
- Careful operative technique and wound closure
- Reduction of exogenous or environmental sources of contamination
- Thorough, prompt cleansing and debridement of traumatic wounds
- Prevention of intraoperative wound contamination
- Use of prophylactic antibiotics in selected patients
- Adherence to sterile technique for dressing changes
- Documentation of wound infection statistics

Wound infections lead to prolonged hospitalization, significant patient discomfort, incisional hernias, and unsightly scars. Adherence to the principles described in this chapter minimizes the morbidity associated with wound infection.

A SHORT ATLAS OF COMMON SURGICAL PROCEDURES

This section describes some common surgical procedures. In this section, the numbered procedure immediately following an illustration refers to that illustration. See a complete surgical atlas for more details.

Appendectomy

Indications

Acute appendicitis
Incidental finding (usually performed after another planned procedure)

Differential Diagnosis

Gastroenteritis
Mesenteric adenitis
Pelvic inflammatory disease
Ovarian accident
  Ruptured cyst
  Torsion
  Mittelschmerz
Ectopic pregnancy
Meckel's diverticulum
Inflammatory bowel disease

Procedure

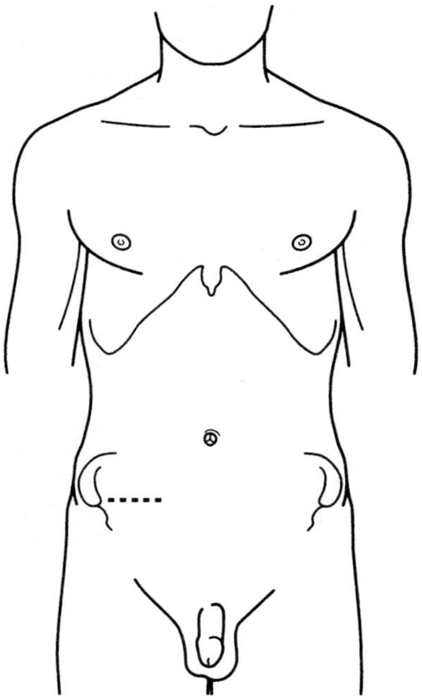

1 A transverse or oblique incision is made, usually over McBurney's point (a point between 11/2 and 2 inches superomedial to the anterior superior spine of the ilium, on a straight line joining that process and the umbilicus, where pressure elicits tenderness in acute appendicitis).

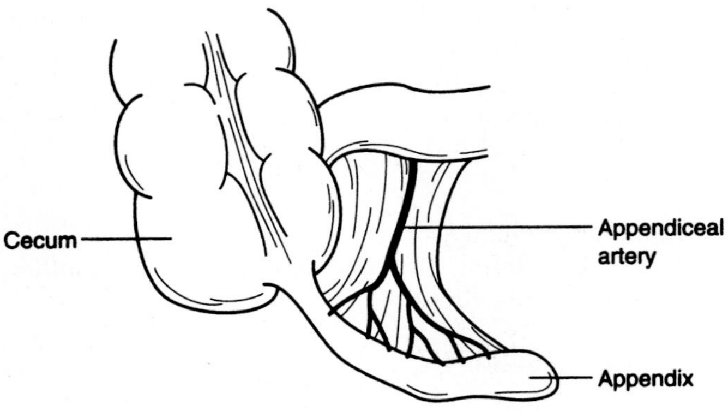

2 The cecum is mobilized into the surgical incision.

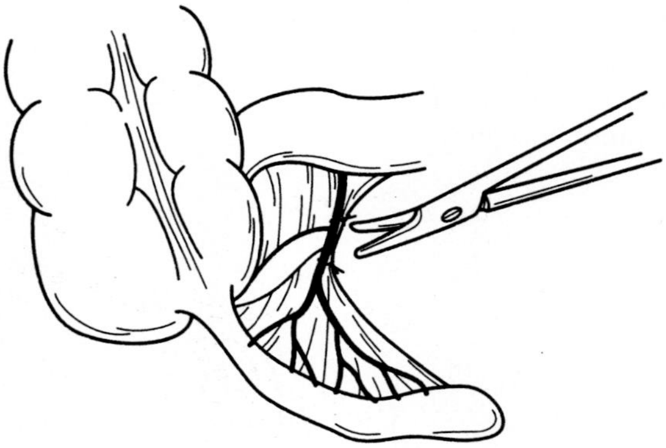

3 The mesoappendix, which contains the appendiceal artery, is divided, and the vessels are ligated.

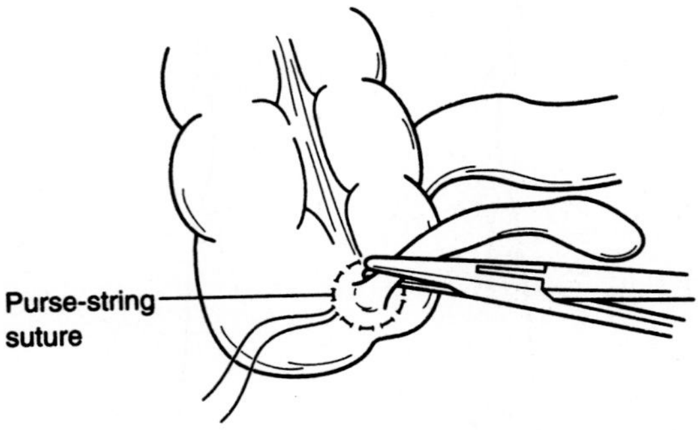

4 A purse-string suture is placed in the cecum near the base of the appendix.

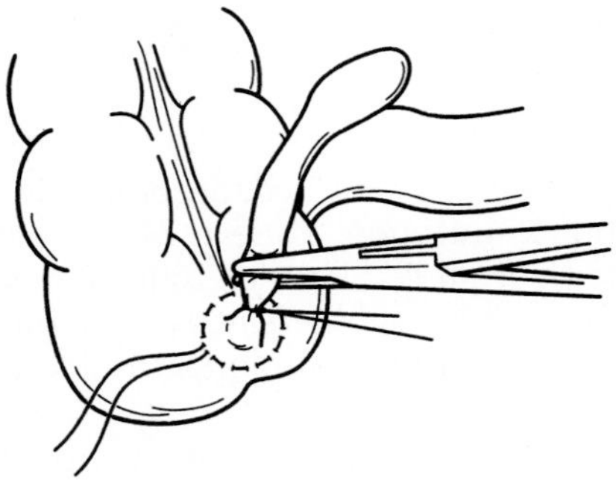

5 The base of the appendix is crushed and tied.

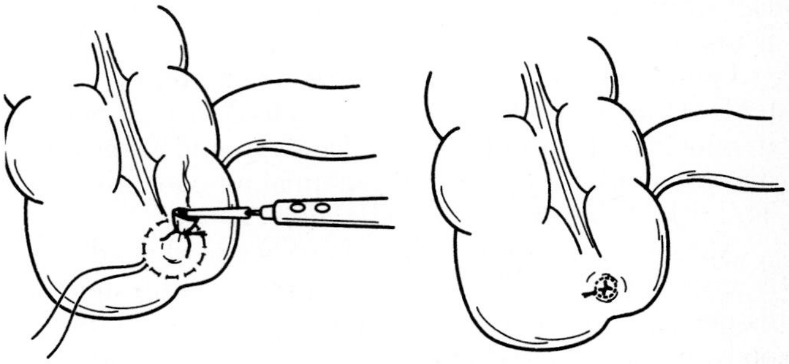

6 The mucosa of the appendiceal stump is cauterized to prevent bacterial spillage and mucocele formation. The stump is inverted, and the purse-string suture is tied securely.

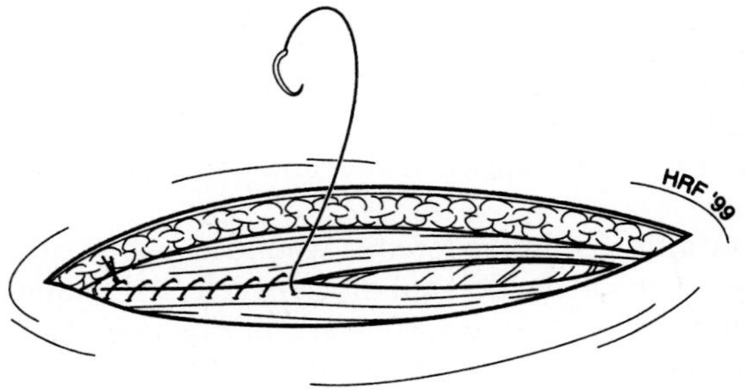

7 The cecum is returned to its normal position in the celomic cavity, and the wound is irrigated and closed in layers. The skin may be left open if the appendix is perforated.

Complications

Wound infection
Pelvic abscess
Enterocutaneous fistula
Pylephlebitis
Appendiceal perforation

Laparoscopic Appendectomy

Procedure

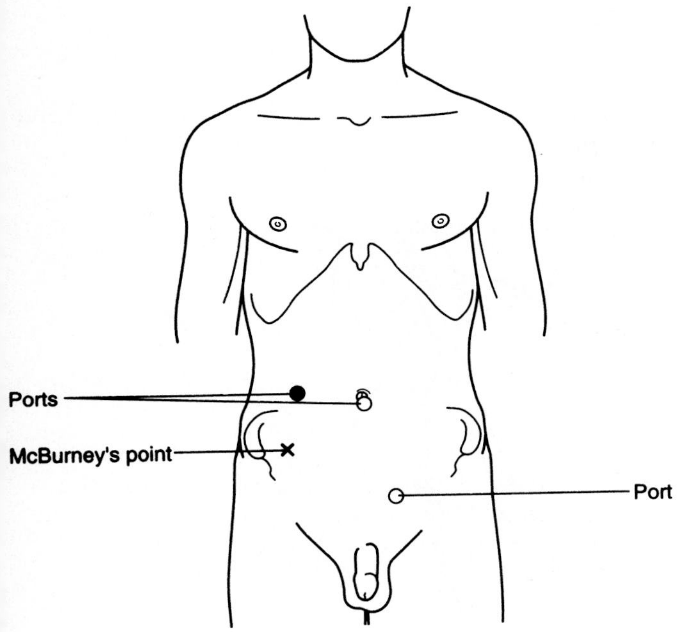

1 Ports are placed for the camera and operative tools.

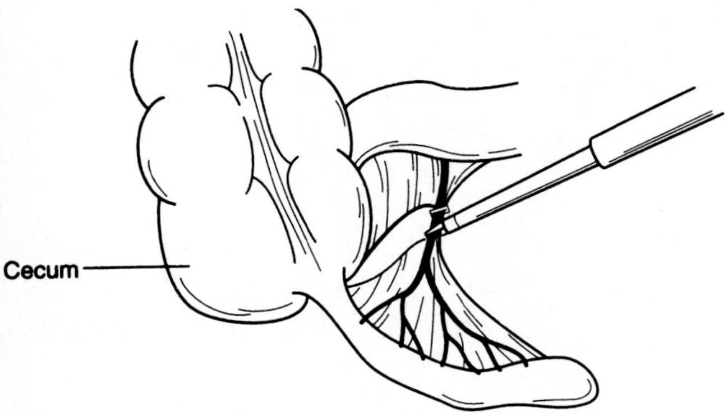

2 The cecum is mobilized, and the appendiceal vessels are clipped and divided.

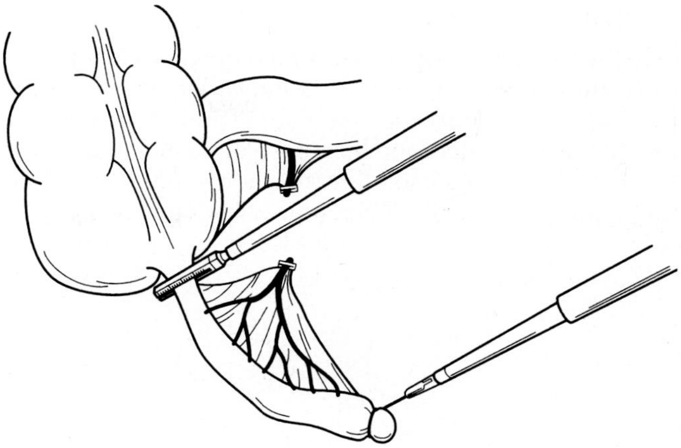

3 A stapling device is used to transect the appendix. The appendiceal stump is cauterized.

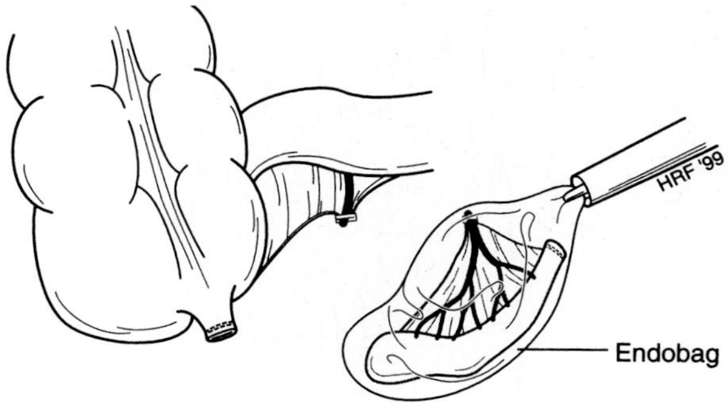

4 The appendix is placed in a plastic bag and removed. The ports are withdrawn.

Cholecystectomy

Indications

Acute or chronic cholecystitis
Cholelithiasis
Choledocholithiasis

Differential Diagnosis

Peptic ulcer disease
Pancreatitis
Gastroenteritis
Acute appendicitis
Right lower lobe pneumonia

Procedure

Whether the procedure is performed open or laparoscopically, the approach to removing the gallbladder from the liver bed is the same: the cystic artery and cystic duct are identified and ligated, and then the gallbladder is dissected from the liver. The major difference is that different instruments are used, and in open cholecystectomy the incision is larger and requires closure in layers.

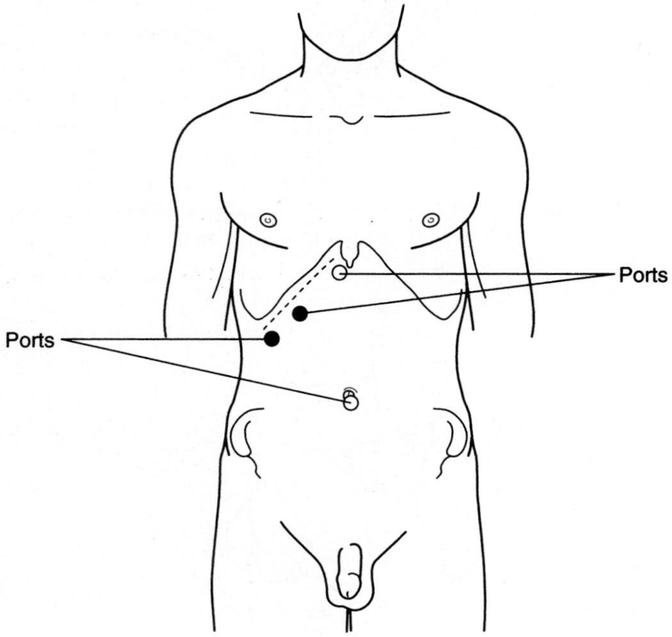

1 For the laparoscopic approach, operative and camera ports are placed.

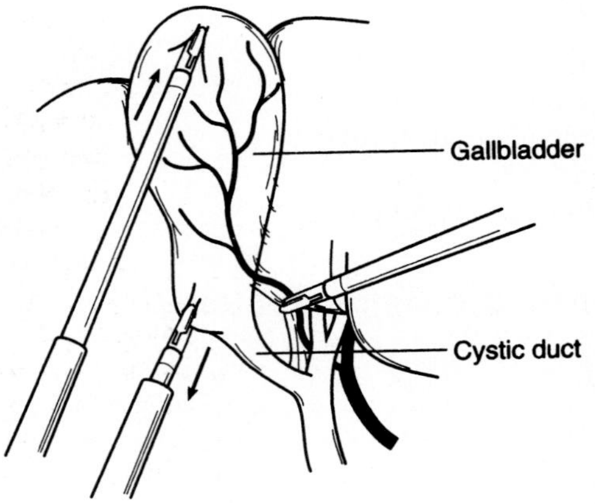

2 Dissection is performed to isolate the cystic duct and artery.

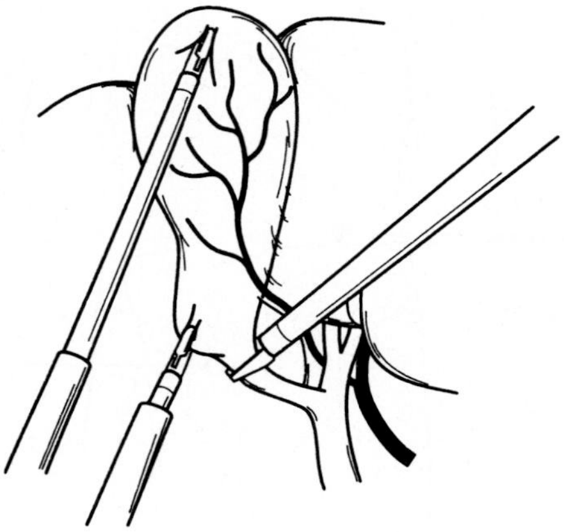

3 The cystic duct is clipped or tied proximally to prevent the migration of stones into the common duct.

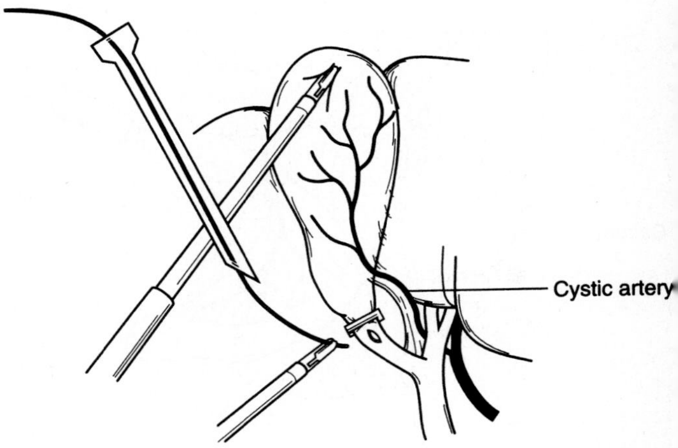

4 A cholangiogram is performed.

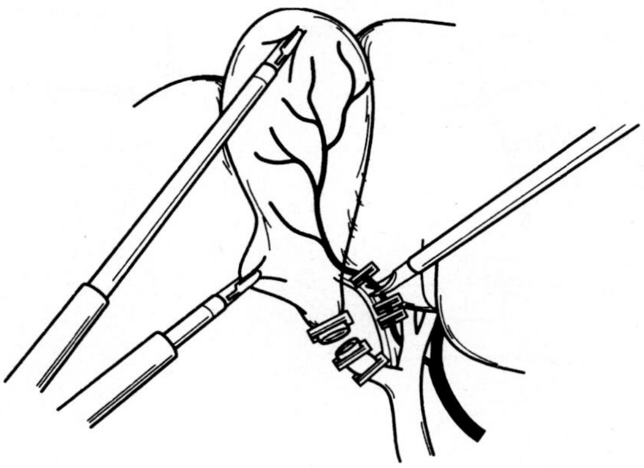

5 The cystic artery and cystic duct are tied or clipped and divided.

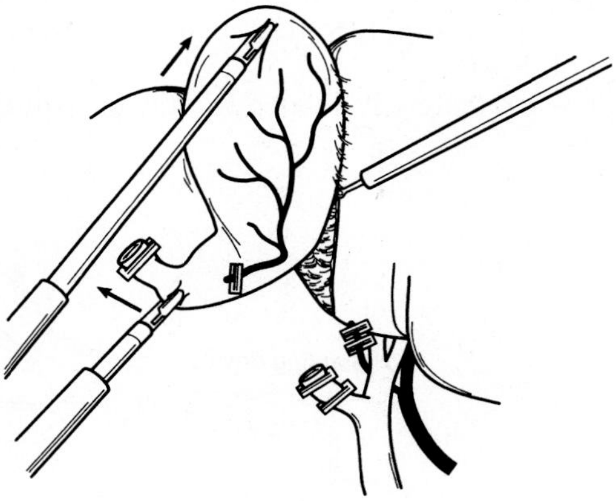

A

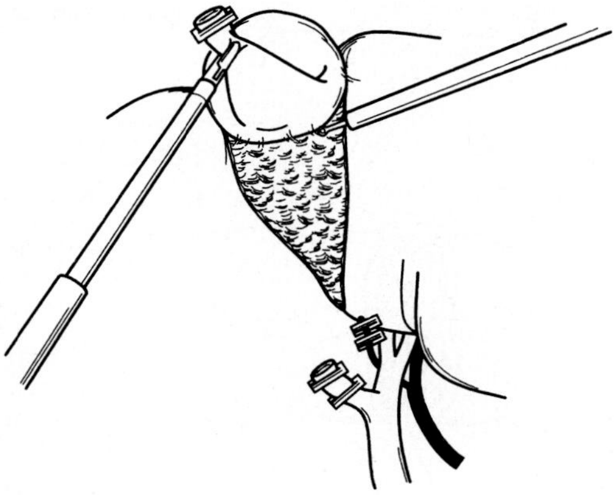

B

6 A, B. The gallbladder is removed from the liver bed with blunt, sharp, or electrocautery dissection.

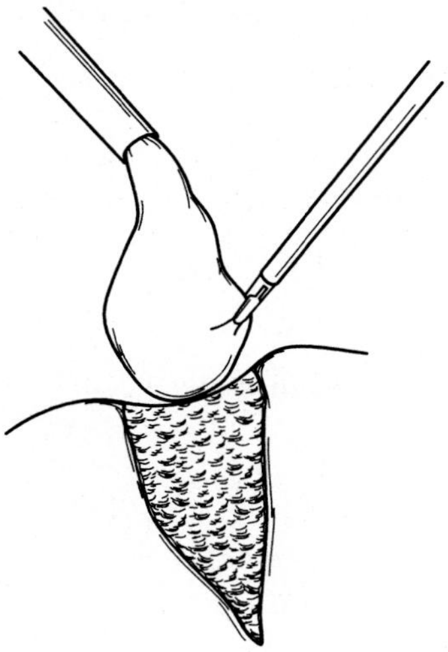

7 The gallbladder is removed through a large port.

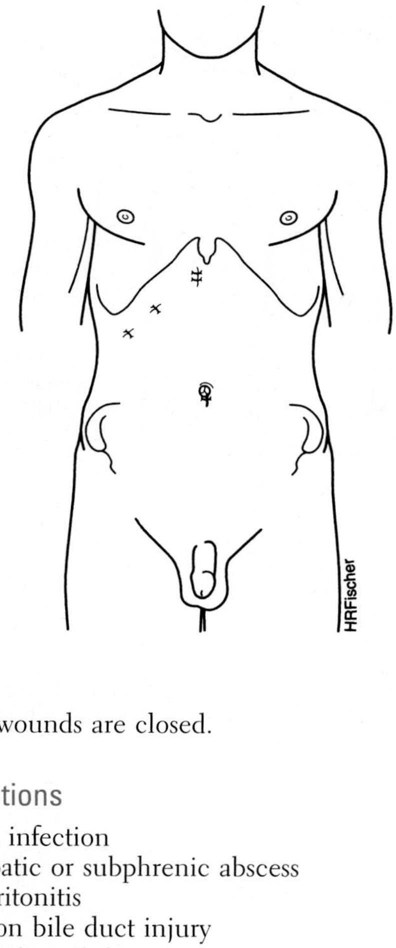

8 The wounds are closed.

Complications

Wound infection
Subhepatic or subphrenic abscess
Bile peritonitis
Common bile duct injury
Hollow viscus injury
Postoperative hemorrhage
Retained common duct stone
Pancreatitis (postoperative)

Colectomy/Small Bowel Resection

Indications

- Malignancy
- Diverticular disease
  - Hemorrhage
  - Perforation
  - Stricture
  - Obstruction
- Inflammatory bowel disease
- Trauma
- Volvulus

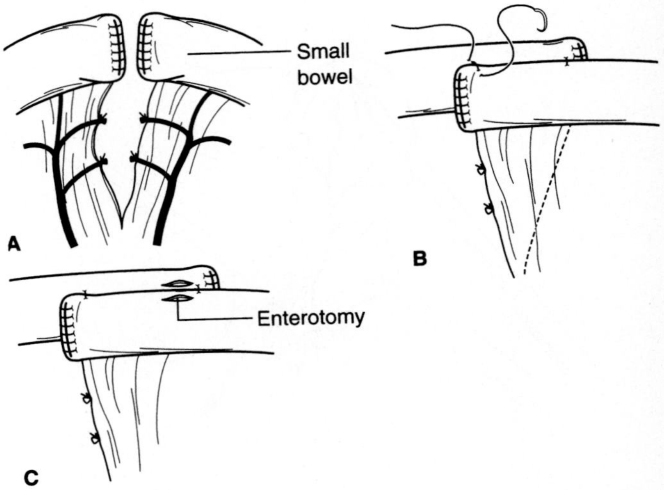

Procedure

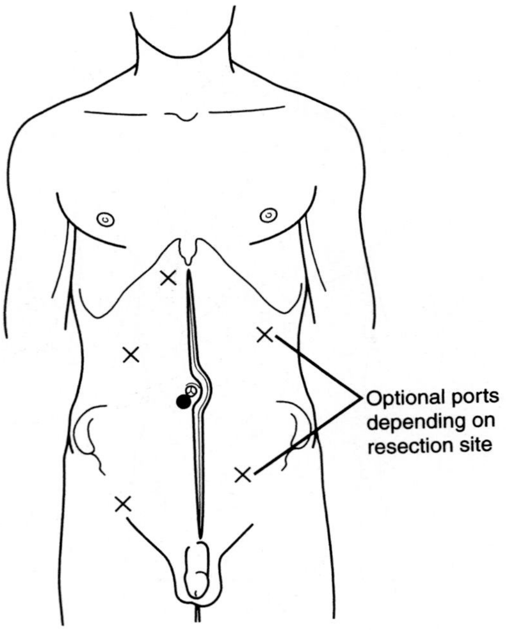

1 The colon/small bowel is approached through a midline incision or laparoscopically through the ports indicated.

2 The segment of the colon/small bowel to be resected is mobilized. Additional mobilization may be required to perform an anastomosis without tension. The blood supply to the resected segment is isolated and divided.

3 The mesentery is divided sharply or with electrocautery.

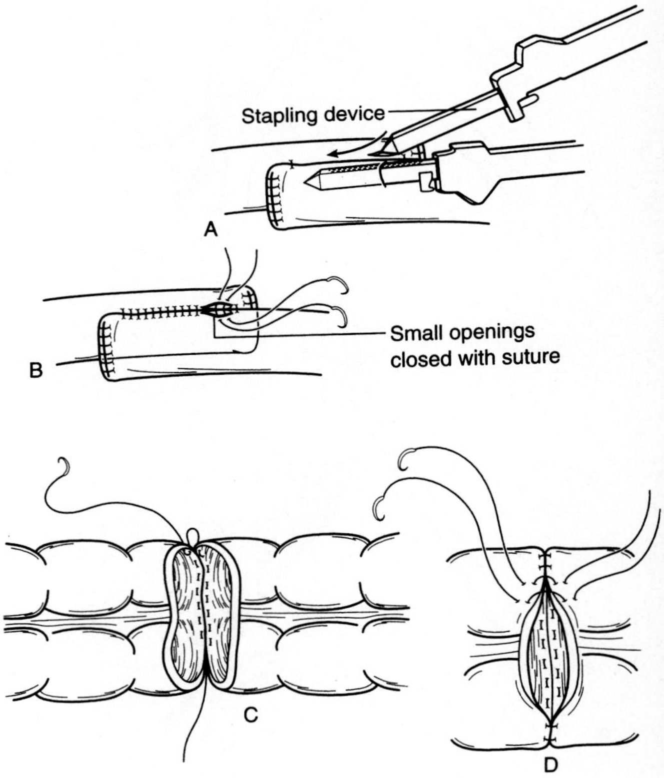

4 Reapproximation is performed by stapling (A) or sewing (B, C, D).

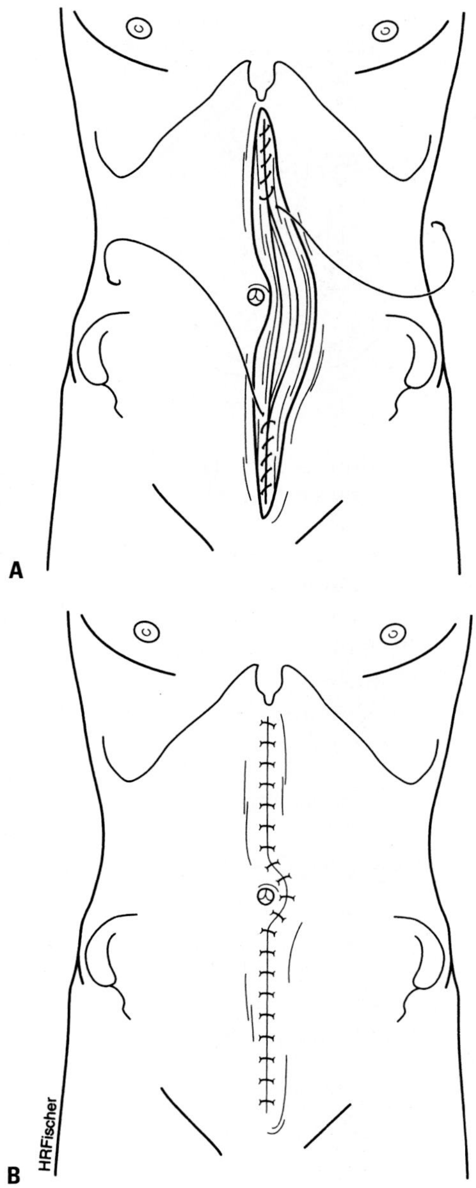

5 A, B. The incision is closed according to the surgeon's preference.

Complications

Wound infection
Pelvic abscess
Anastomotic leak
Enterocutaneous fistula
Anastomotic stricture
Recurrent disease

Splenectomy

Indications

Trauma or spontaneous rupture
Spherocytosis, pyropoikilocytosis
Immune thrombocytopenic purpura
Cytopenia with splenomegaly
Leukemia or lymphoma
Splenic abscess
Splenic cyst
Splenic aneurysm
Metastatic disease

Procedure

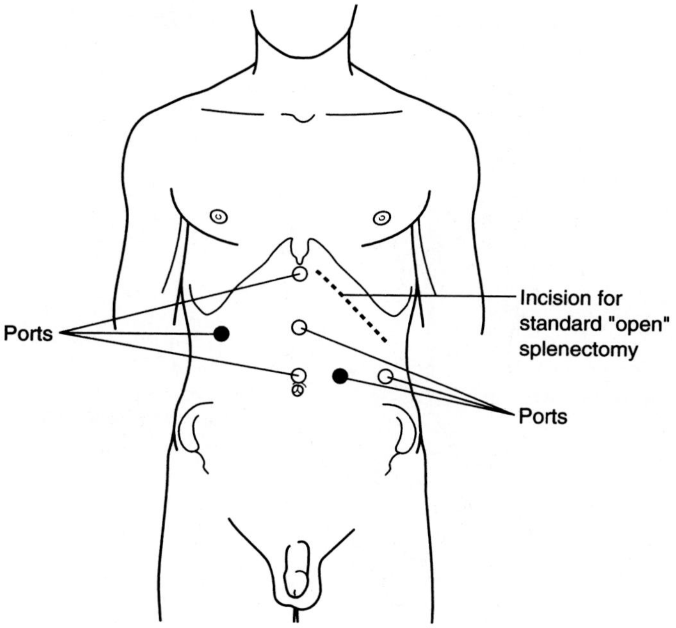

1 The celomic cavity is entered through a left subcostal incision or a midline incision, or ports are placed for a laparoscopic approach.

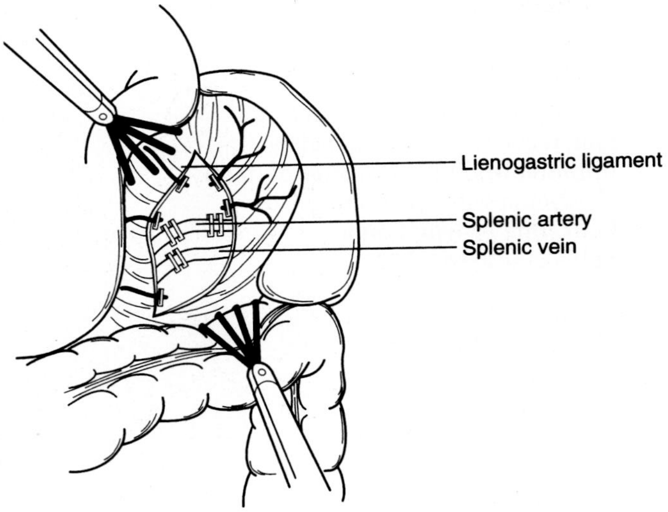

2 The lesser sac is entered by dividing the short gastric vessels in the lienogastric ligament between clips or ties.

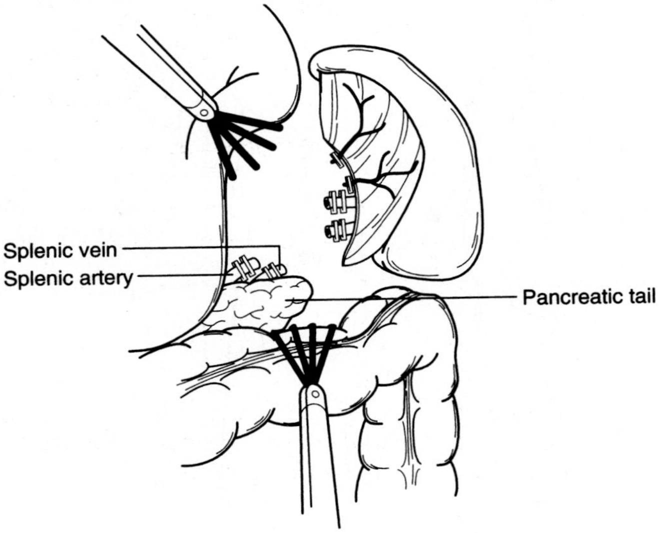

3 The splenic artery and vein may be ligated near the superior border of the pancreatic tail.

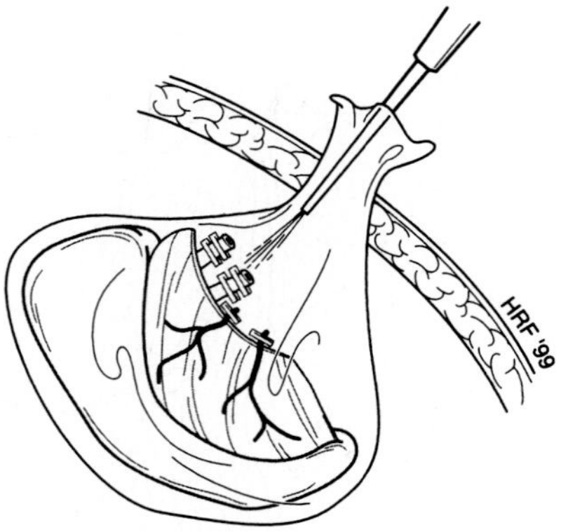

4 If the procedure is done laparoscopically, it may be necessary to purée the spleen in a bag to facilitate removal.

5 The abdomen is closed in layers according to the surgeon's preference.

Complications

Subphrenic abscess
Postoperative hemorrhage
Gastric wall necrosis
Thrombocytosis
Overwhelming postsplenectomy sepsis syndrome

Surgical Procedures on the Breast

Biopsy

Indications

Breast mass
Mammographic abnormality

Procedure

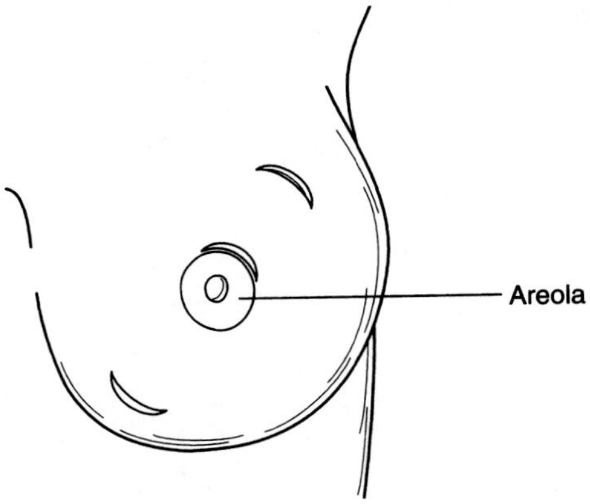

1 Biopsy is performed under general or local anesthesia. A circumareolar or skin-line incision is made.

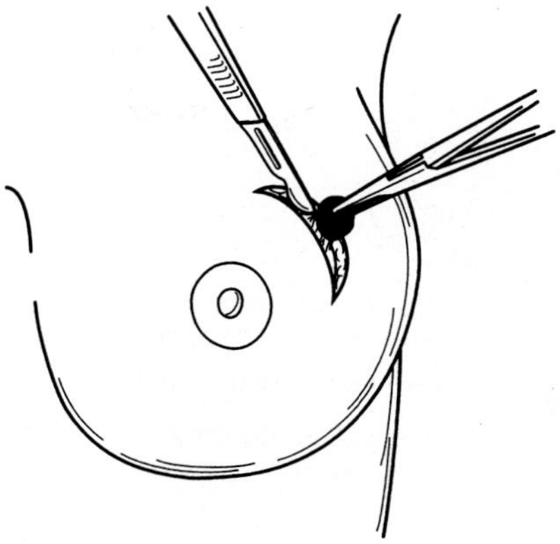

2 The mass may be grasped with a clamp and excised sharply with gentle traction.

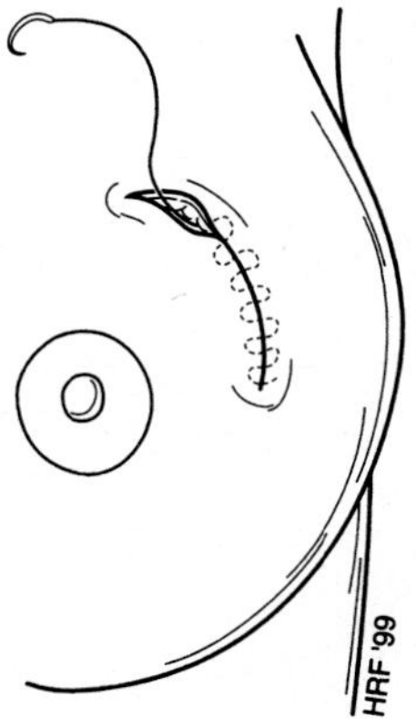

3 After hemostasis is achieved, the incision is closed with a subcuticular stitch.

Complications

Wound infection
Breast hematoma

Mastectomy

Indications

Malignant disease
High-risk histopathology

Procedure

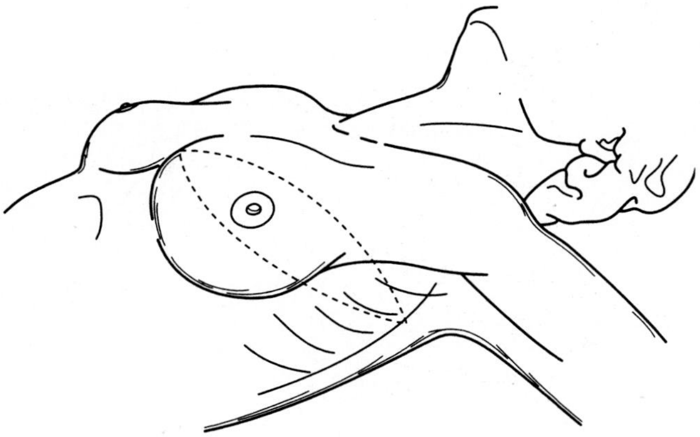

1 A transverse incision is usually used.

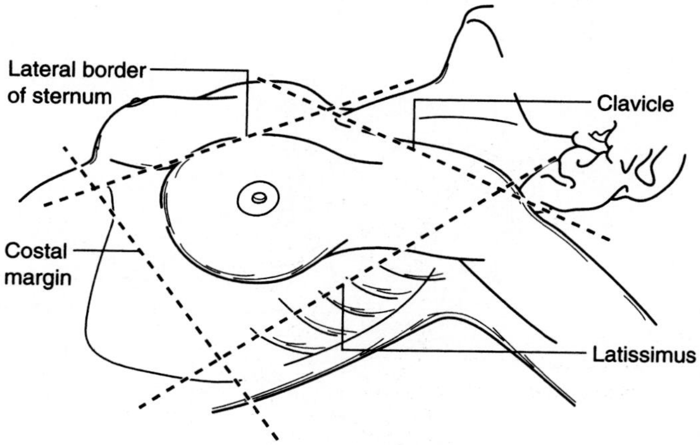

2 The limits of the dissection include the clavicle superiorly, the latissimus dorsi posteriorly, the sternum medially, and the sixth rib inferiorly.

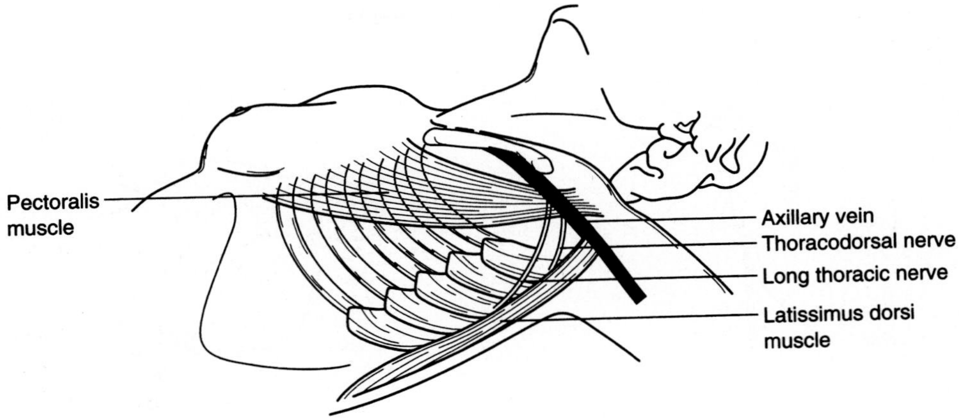

3 Axillary dissection preserves the long thoracic and thoracodorsal nerves. The axillary vein is cleaned of node-bearing from its inferior surface.

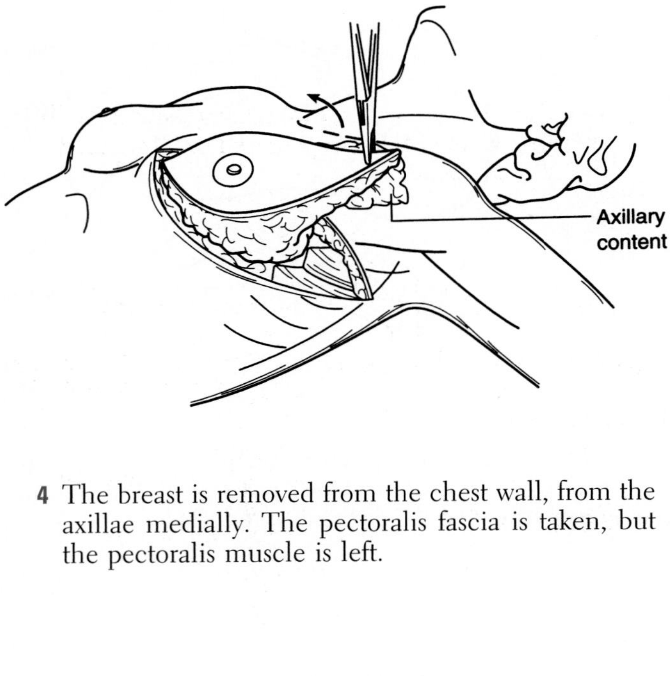

4 The breast is removed from the chest wall, from the axillae medially. The pectoralis fascia is taken, but the pectoralis muscle is left.

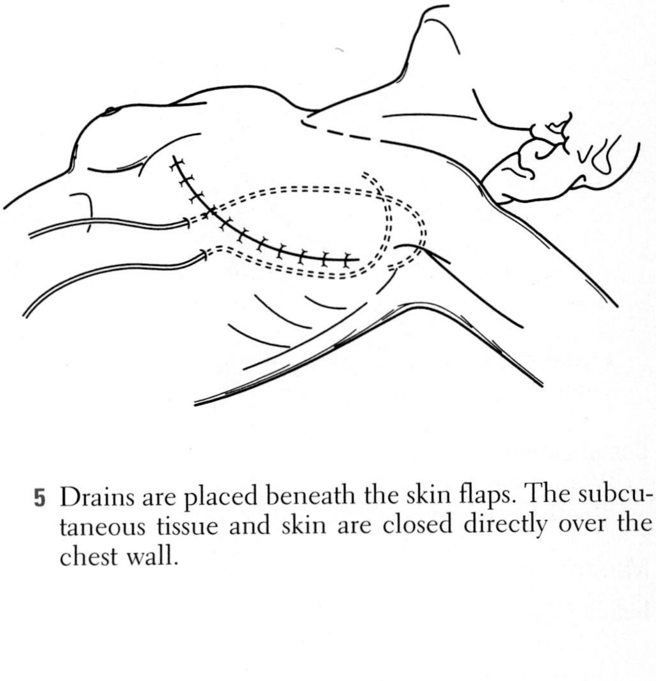

5 Drains are placed beneath the skin flaps. The subcutaneous tissue and skin are closed directly over the chest wall.

Complications

Hematoma or seroma
Flap necrosis
Axillary vein injury
Long thoracic nerve injury
Thoracodorsal nerve injury
Intercostal brachial nerve injury
Lymphedema or lymphadenitis
Recurrent disease

Partial Mastectomy (Breast Preservation)

Procedure

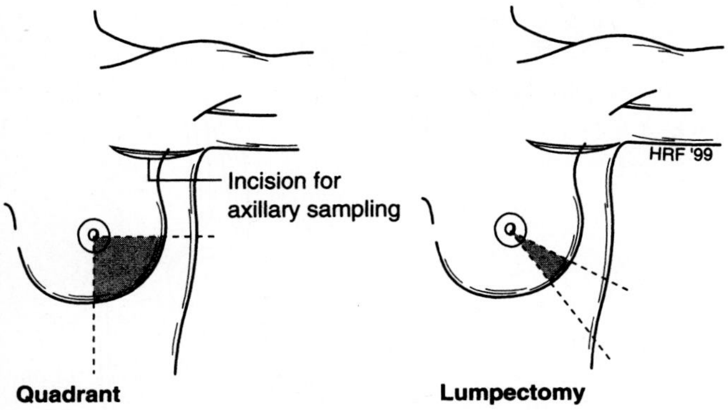

1 Breast conservation preserves the breast mound.
2 A sampling of axillary lymph nodes is usually performed with these procedures.
3 If a sentinel node is to be removed, the patient will have had an injection of a radioactive material into the breast. This tracer can be located with the use of a handheld probe. The surgeon may also inject a vital dye just before the operation to facilitate visual identification of the axillary node.

Vascular Procedures

Abdominal Aortic Aneurysm

Indications

Aneurysm larger than 5 cm
Rupture or leak
- Back pain
- Syncope
- Shock

Procedure

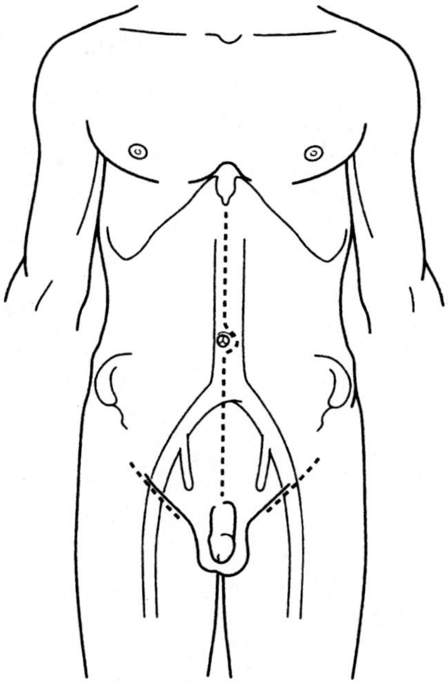

1 The aorta is approached through a generous midline incision. Both groins are prepared to allow access to the femoral vessels.

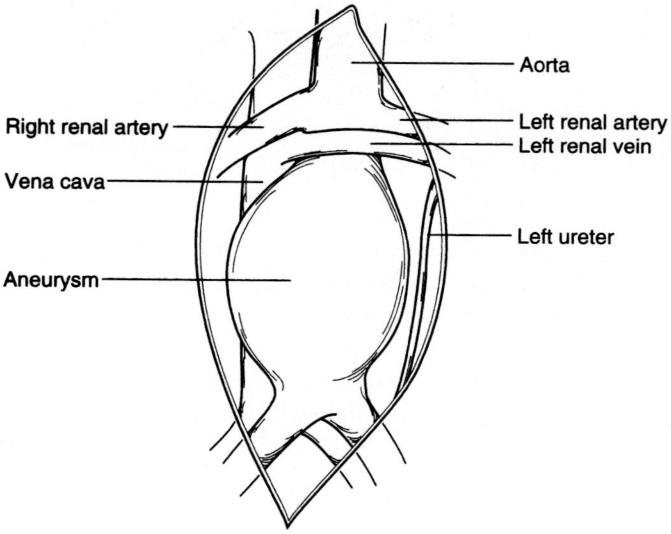

2 The small bowel is mobilized to the right side to expose the aorta. If rupture occurs, the aorta may be approached directly through the mesentery of the bowel.

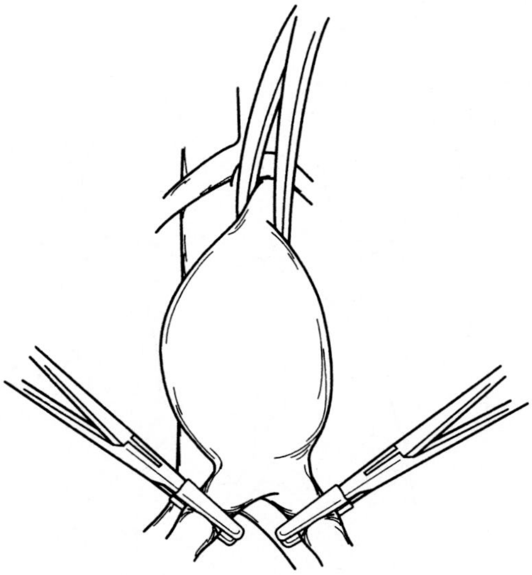

3 Proximal control of the aorta is gained either above or below the renal arteries, depending on the clinical situation. Distal control is gained below the aneurysm.

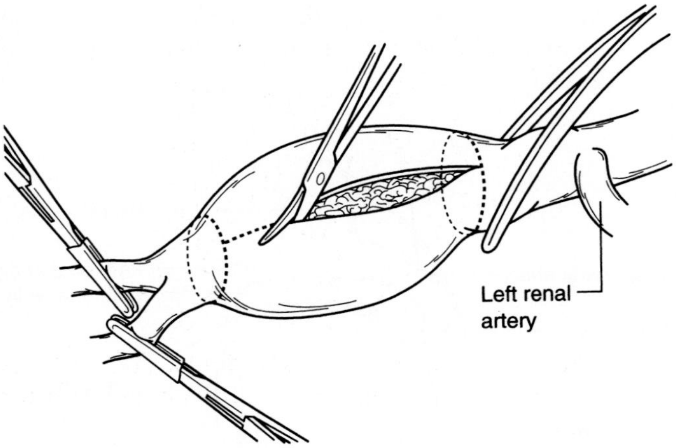

4 The aneurysm is opened after the aorta is cross-clamped, preferably below the renal arteries.

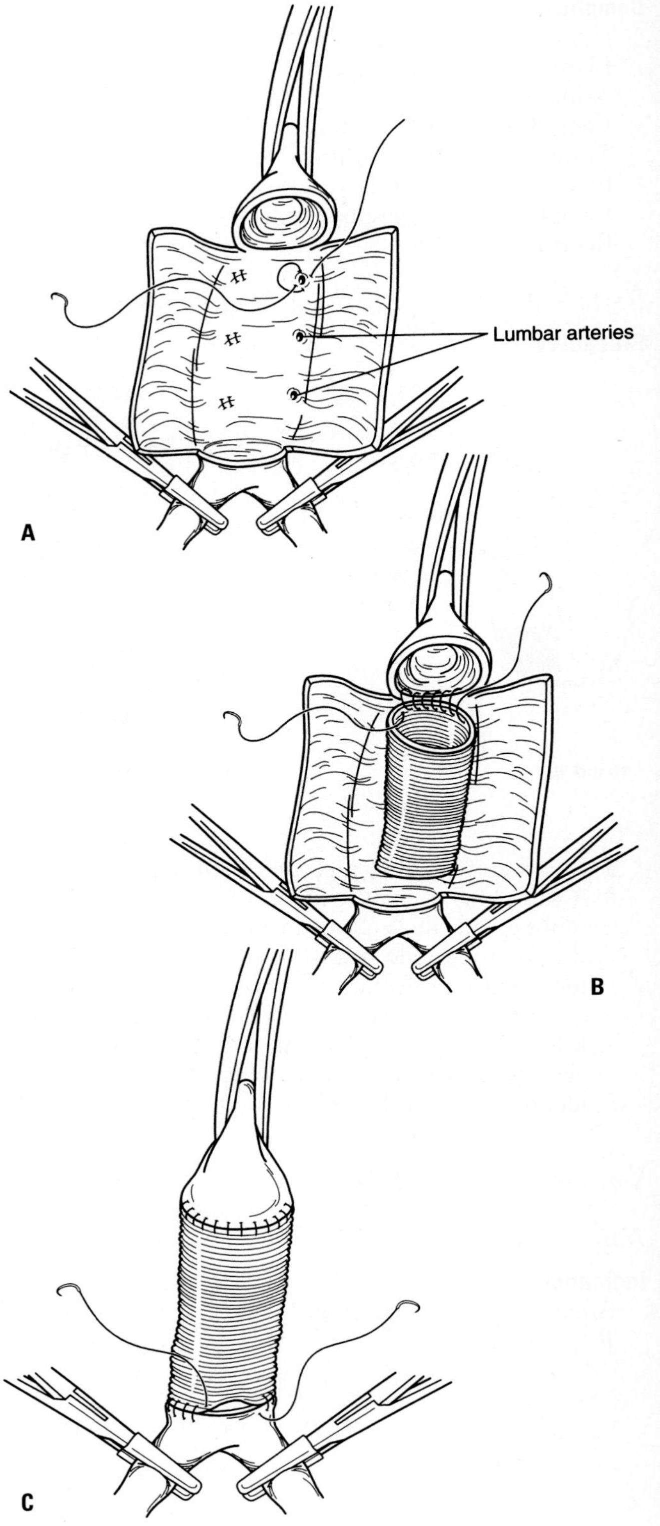

5 A, B, C. A prosthetic graft is sewn into place. The graft may be either tubular or bifurcated. The inferior mesenteric artery may be reimplanted into the graft.

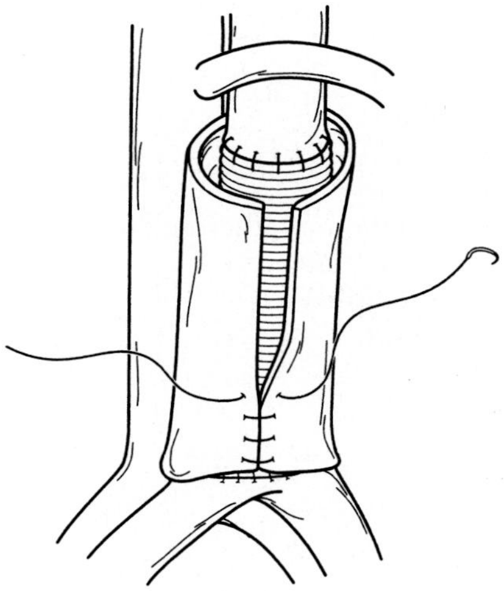

6 A cuff of the wall of the aneurysm is sewn over the graft.

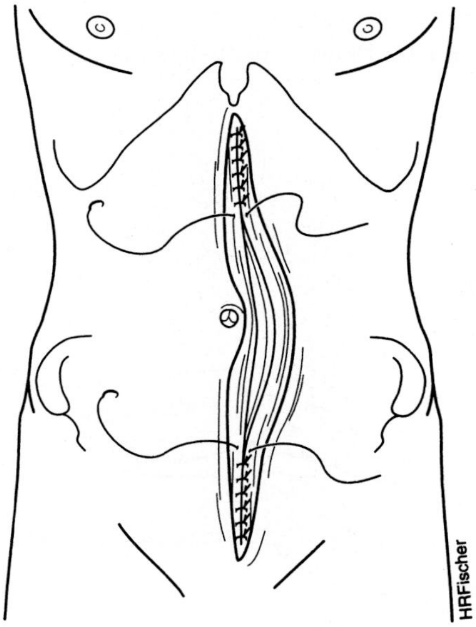

7 The abdominal cavity is irrigated and closed in a standard fashion.

Complications

Death
Renal failure
Ischemic colitis
Graft infection
Graft thrombosis
Distal embolization of atherosclerotic debris
Myocardial infarction
Aortoduodenal fistula
Pseudoaneurysm

Aortobifemoral Graft

Indications

Aortoiliac occlusive disease
Incapacitating claudication
Ischemic rest pain
Impending tissue loss

Procedure

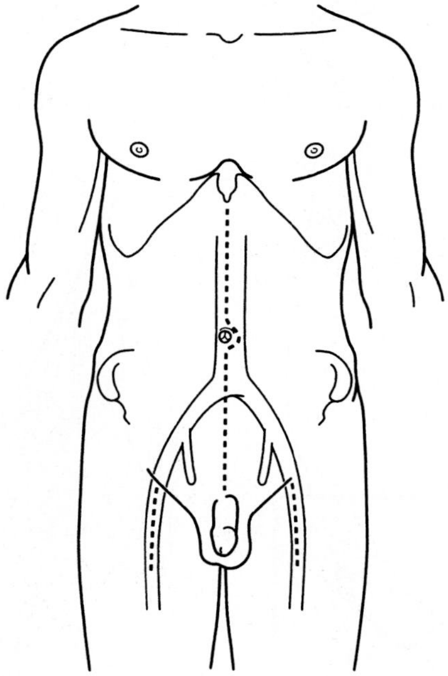

1 The aorta is approached in a similar fashion to the aneurysm repair. Both groins must be surgically prepared.

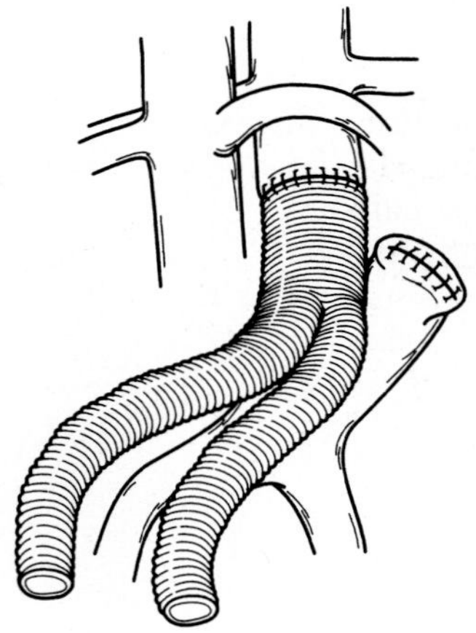

2 The proximal anastomosis is completed.

Complications
- Death
- Renal failure
- Ischemic colitis
- Graft infection
- Graft thrombosis
- Distal embolization of atherosclerotic debris
- Myocardial infarction
- Aortoduodenal fistula
- Pseudoaneurysm

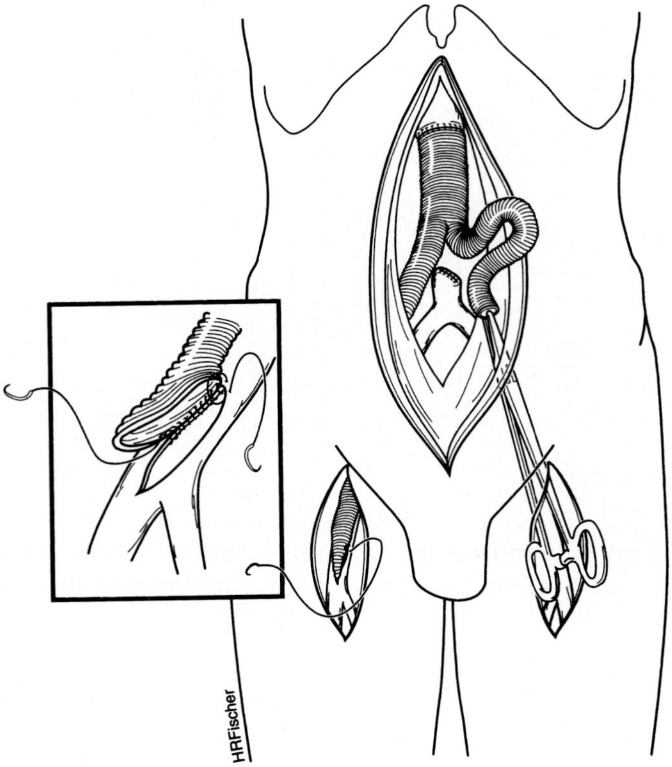

3 The femoral arteries are exposed through groin incisions. The limbs of the graft are tunneled through the retroperitoneum to lie on top of the femoral arteries.
4 Distal anastomoses are performed.
5 Abdominal closure is performed in a standard fashion. Groin wounds are closed in layers.

Femoropopliteal Bypass With Saphenous Vein

Indications
- Symptomatic femoral occlusive disease

Procedure

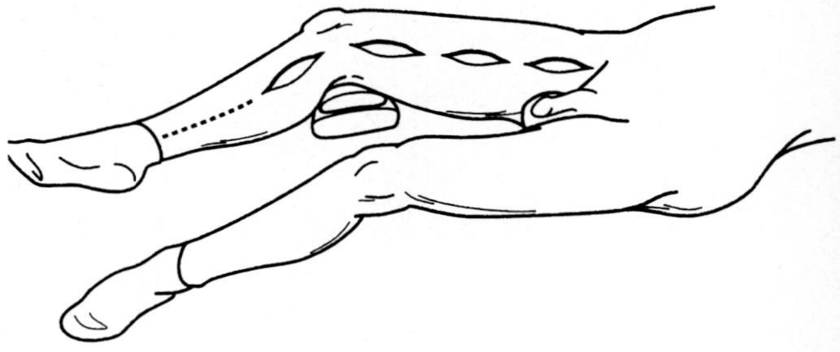

1 Both lower extremities are prepared for surgery.

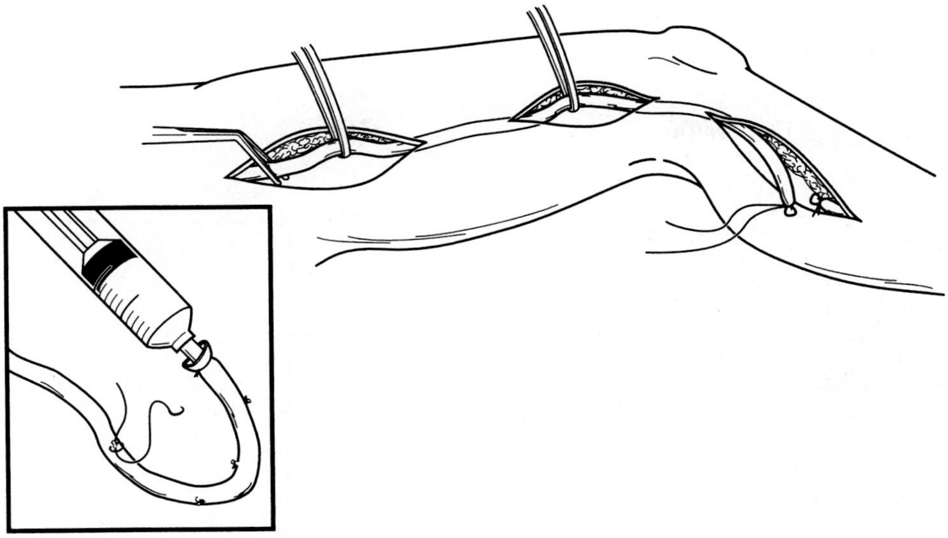

2 Saphenous vein is harvested from the ipsilateral leg. The branches are tied, and the vein is carefully dilated hydrostatically.

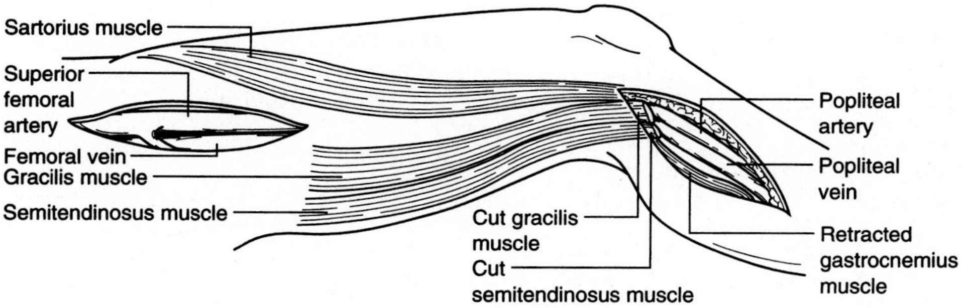

3 The femoral artery is exposed in the groin. The popliteal artery is exposed below the site of occlusion as determined by angiography.

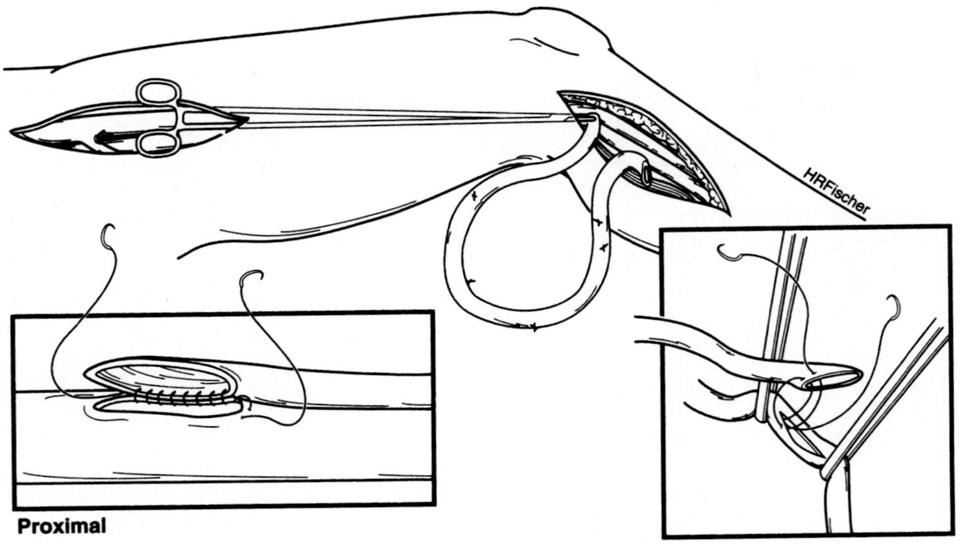

4 The vein is usually reversed, but it may be left in situ or not reversed. The valves are cut if an in situ bypass procedure is performed. The distal anastomosis is performed first, then the proximal anastomosis. Anastomoses are performed with fine monofilament permanent suture.
5 The leg incisions are closed.

Complications

Death
Renal failure
Ischemic colitis
Graft infection
Graft thrombosis
Distal embolization of atherosclerotic debris
Myocardial infarction
Aortoduodenal fistula
Pseudoaneurysm

Carotid Endarterectomy

Indications

Transient ischemic attacks
Critical carotid stenosis

Procedure

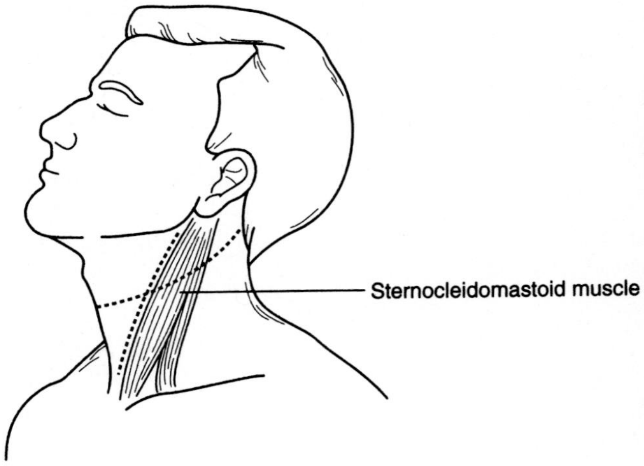

1 An incision is made over the anterior border of the sternocleidomastoid muscle. Some surgeons use a more transverse incision.
2 The carotid artery is exposed by retraction of the sternocleidomastoid muscle laterally.

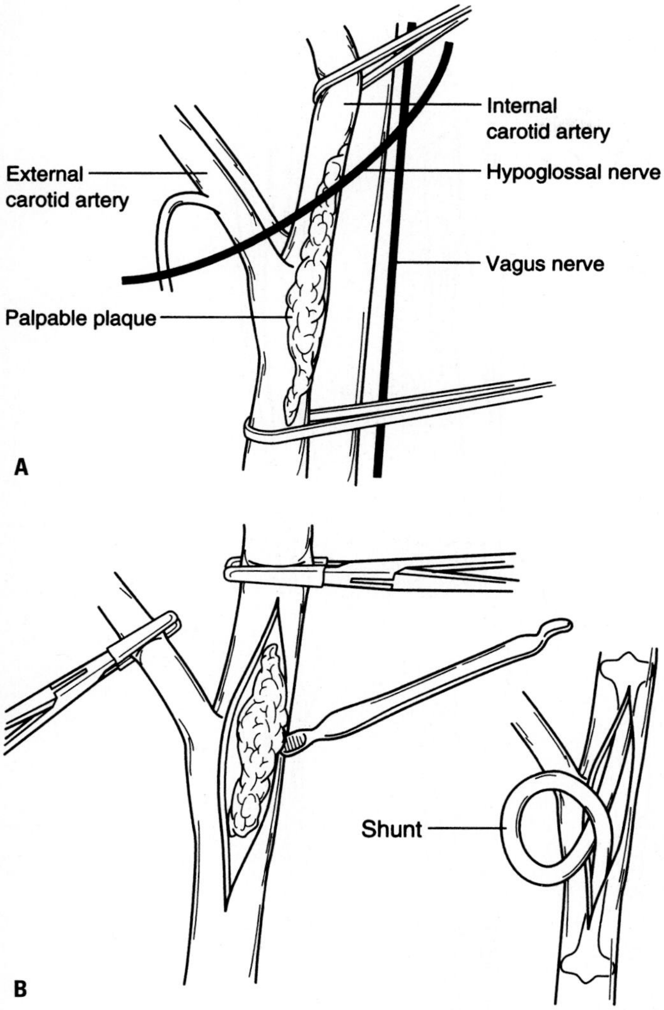

3 A, B. An arteriotomy is performed, and the plaque is exposed. It is dissected from the vessel lumen with a small periosteal elevator and removed. Some surgeons place a shunt to maintain blood flow.

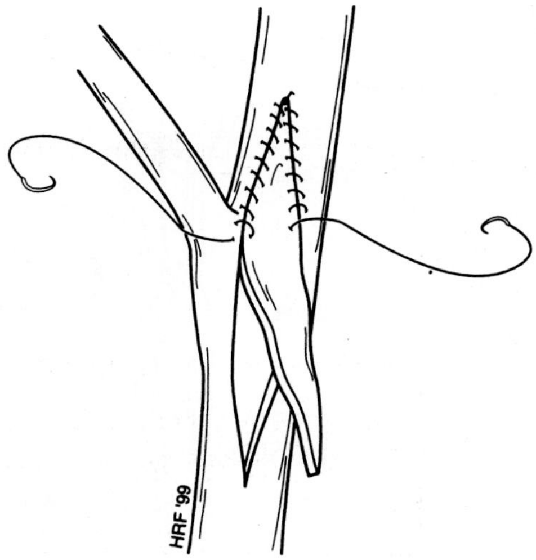

4 A vein patch is used to close the arteriotomy, or the vessel wall is reapproximated primarily. The incision is closed in layers.

Complications

Bleeding or hematoma
Stroke
Embolic event
Thrombosis
Nerve injury
- Hypoglossal
- Vagus
- Marginal mandibular
- Superior laryngeal

Vascular Access for Dialysis

Indications

Long-term hemodialysis

Procedure

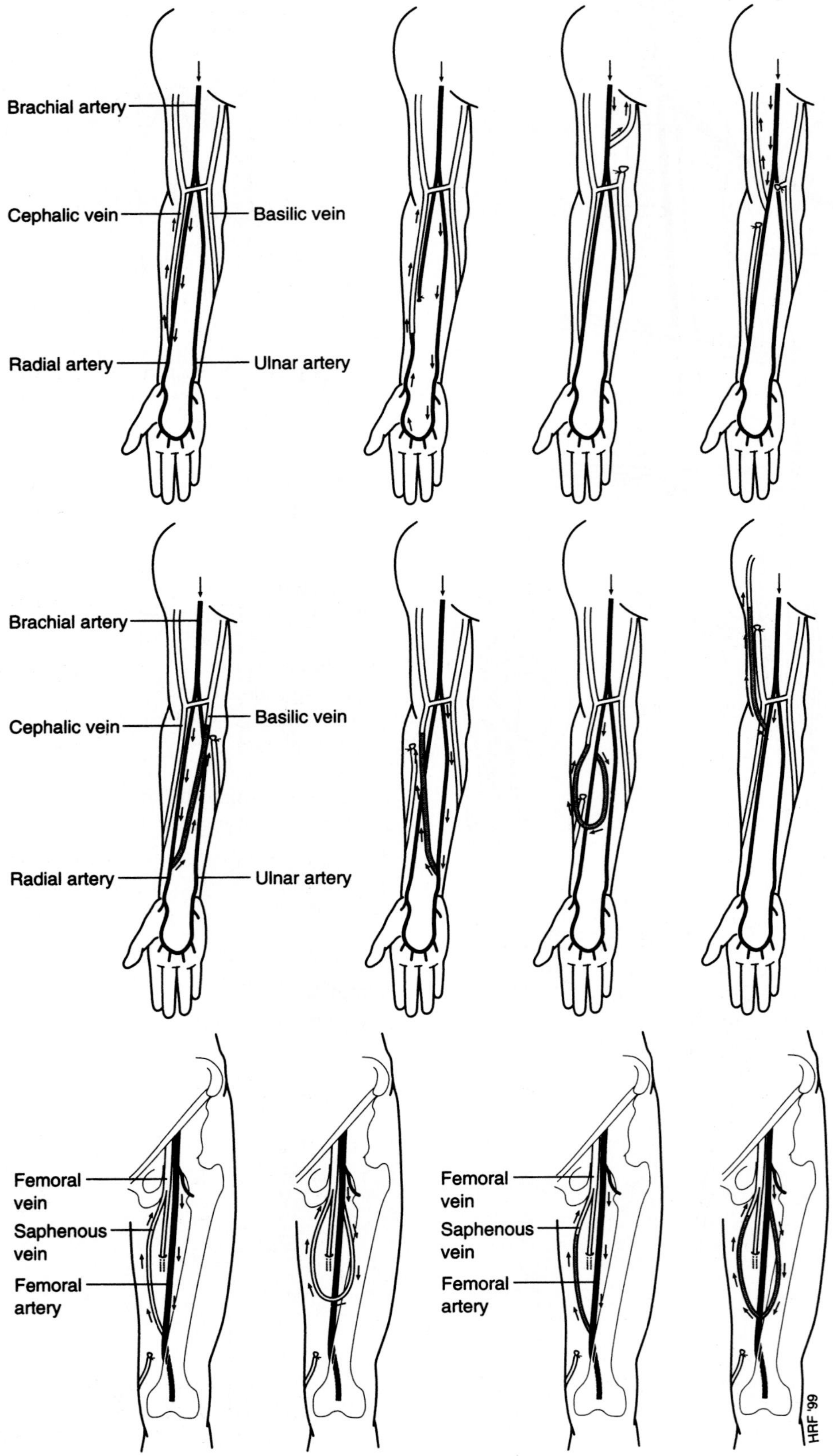
Brachial artery
Cephalic vein
Basilic vein
Radial artery
Ulnar artery
Brachial artery
Cephalic vein
Basilic vein
Radial artery
Ulnar artery
Femoral vein
Saphenous vein
Femoral artery
Femoral vein
Saphenous vein
Femoral artery
HRF '99

1 General, regional, or local anesthesia is used. After the arm is prepared, an incision is made over the artery and vein.
2 Usually, an end (of vein)-to-side (of artery) anastomosis is performed. Alternatively, a prosthetic graft is sewn between the artery and vein. These grafts are usually "looped" in the forearm.
3 If inadequate vascular structures are present in the upper extremities (usually inadequate veins), the proximal thigh vessels can be used.

Complications

Graft thrombosis
Graft infection
Erosion of graft through the skin
Pseudoaneurysm
Congestive heart failure

Central Venous Access

Indications

- Acute venous access
- Resuscitation from shock or placement of pulmonary artery catheter
- Long-term venous access
  - Chemotherapy
  - Nutritional support
  - Phlebotomy
- Dialysis

Procedure

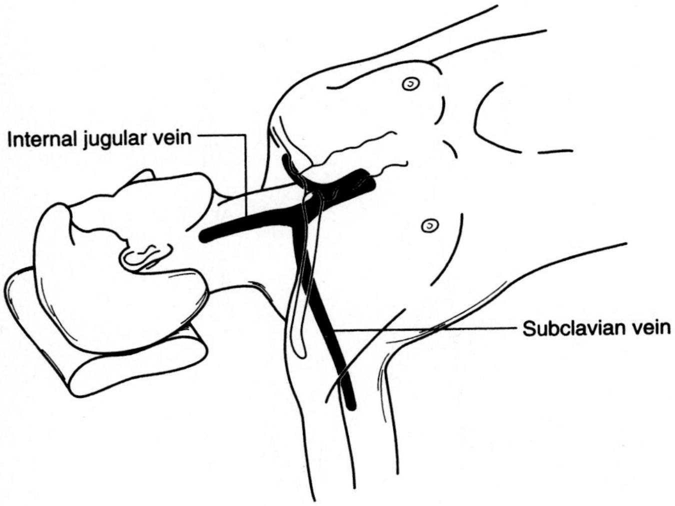

1 The subclavian or internal jugular vein is selected. The patient is placed in the Trendelenburg position, with the head turned to the opposite side.

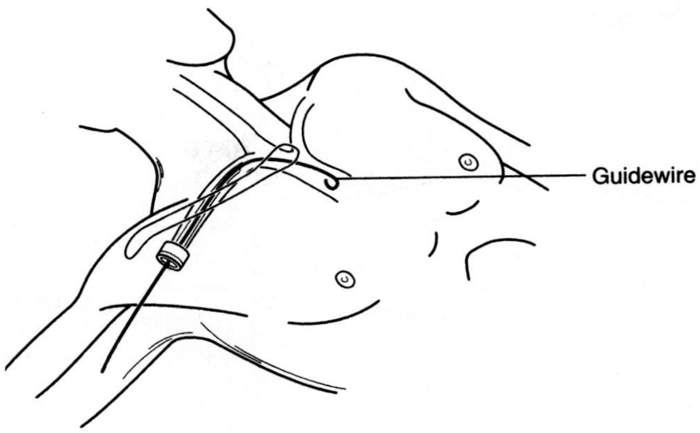

2 The vein is punctured and the guidewire inserted. The electrocardiogram monitor is observed for signs of cardiac dysrhythmia.

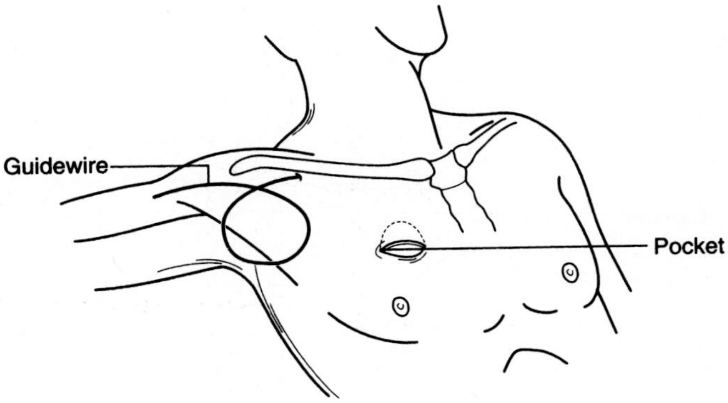

3 If a chronic port is to be inserted, local anesthesia is infiltrated along the path for the catheter tunnel. A pocket for the reservoir is made.

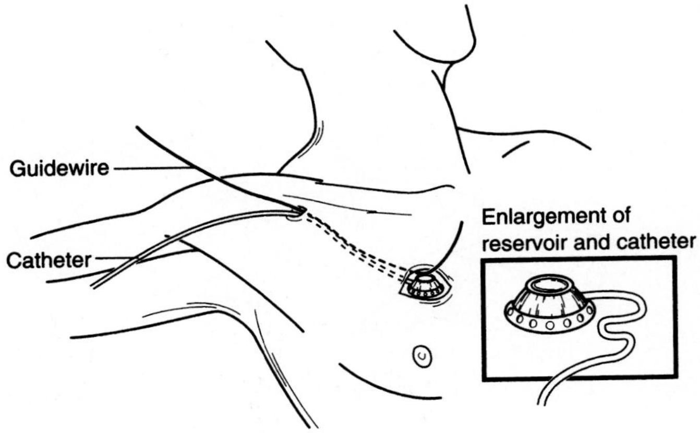

4 The device is assembled, flushed with heparinized saline, and positioned in the reservoir pocket. The catheter is brought out of the skin at the site of the guidewire.

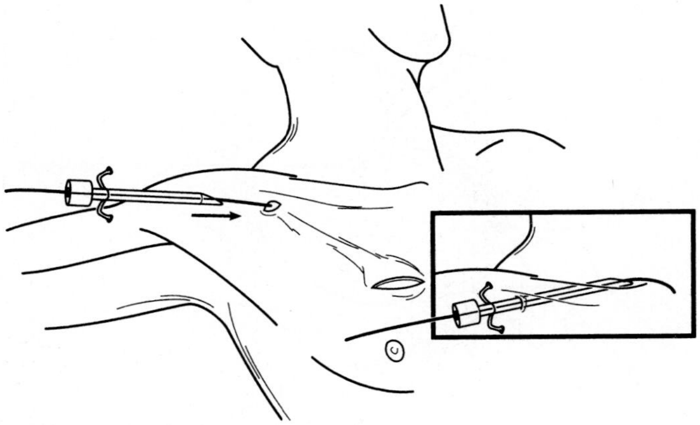

5 The final length of the catheter is measured, and the tear-away sheath over the vein dilator is inserted. The dilator and guidewire are removed.

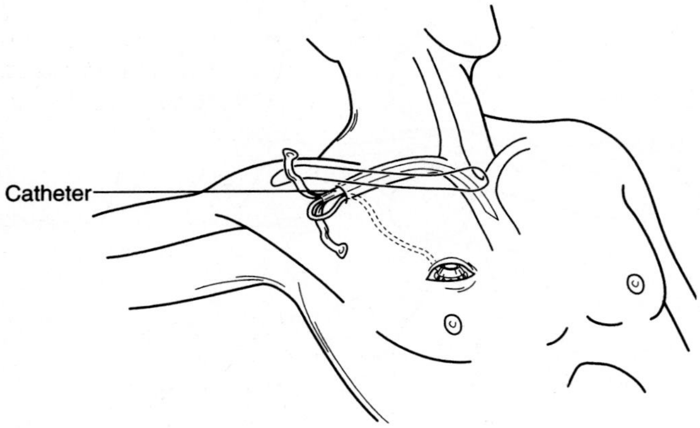

6 The catheter is inserted into the sheath, which is removed by tearing.

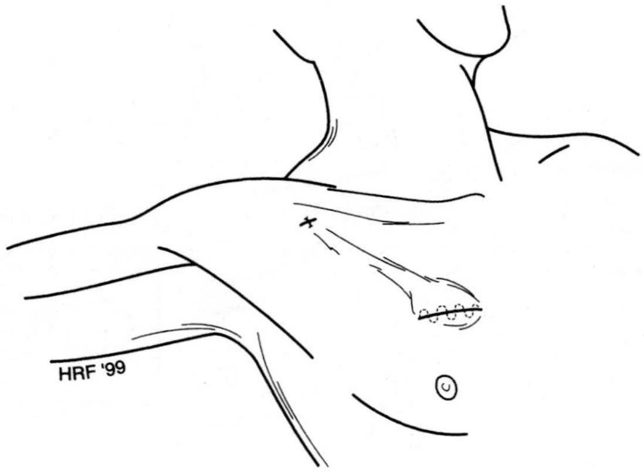

7 Wounds are closed. A chest radiograph is obtained to exclude pneumothorax and confirm proper positioning. This procedure may be performed with portable fluoroscopy.

Complications

Hemothorax or pneumothorax
Subclavian or carotid artery injury
Arrhythmia
Mediastinal hemorrhage
Venous thrombosis
Catheter malposition or malfunction
Sepsis
Skin erosion

Gastrostomy

Conventional Gastrostomy

Indications

Chronic gastric decompression
Gavage
Comfort

Procedure

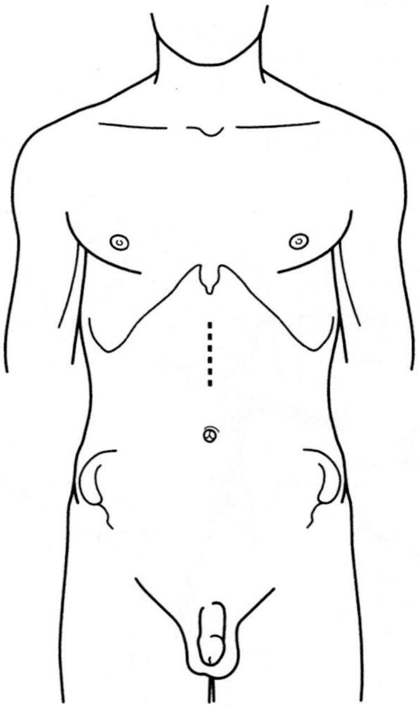

1 The abdominal cavity is entered through a small upper midline incision.

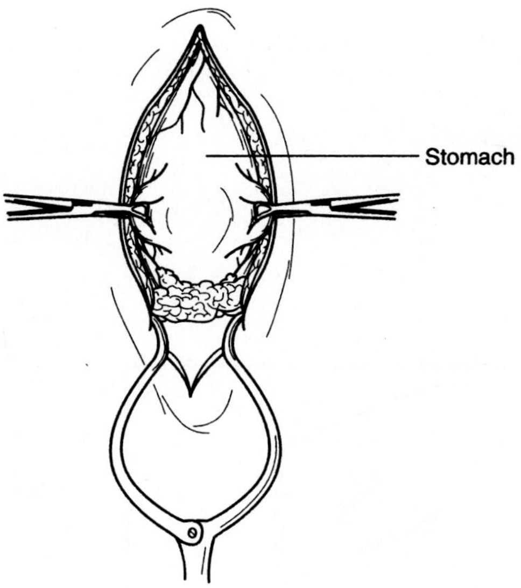

2 The stomach is mobilized into the operative wound.

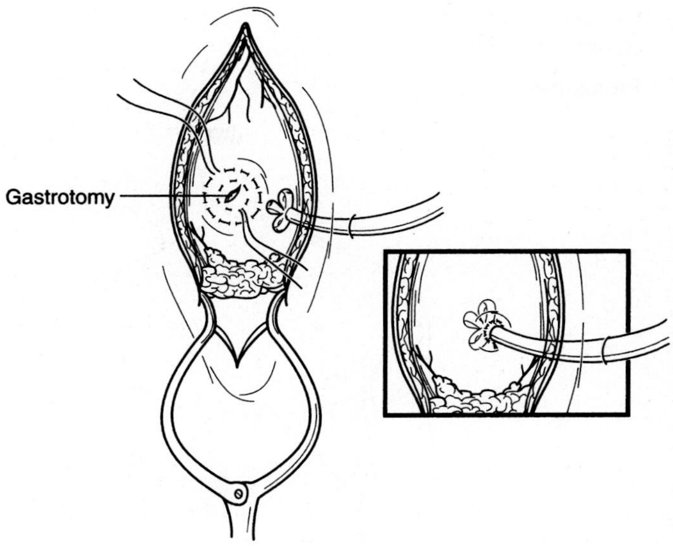

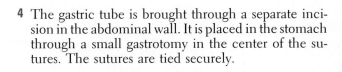

4 The gastric tube is brought through a separate incision in the abdominal wall. It is placed in the stomach through a small gastrotomy in the center of the sutures. The sutures are tied securely.

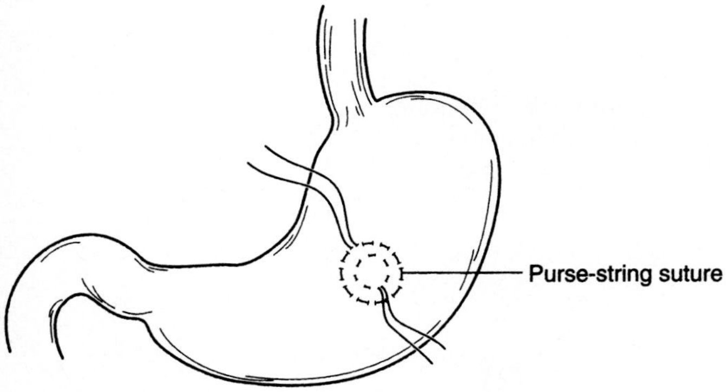

3 Two purse-string sutures are placed in the anterior wall of the stomach.

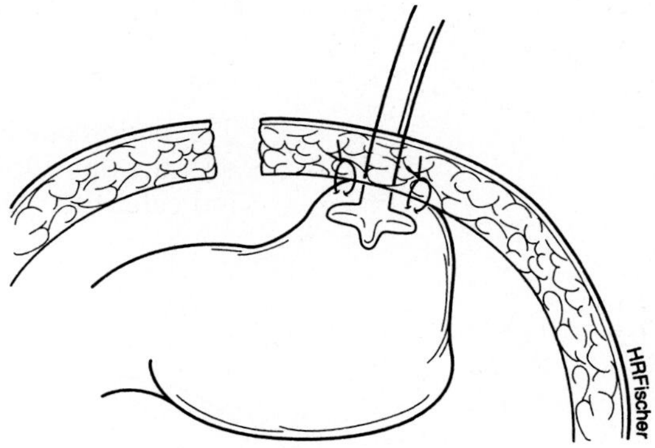

5 The stomach is tacked to the anterior abdominal wall.
6 The wound is closed.

Complications

Intraperitoneal leak
Wound infection
Tube malposition
Clogging
Inadvertent tube removal

Percutaneous Endoscopically Guided Gastrostomy

Procedure

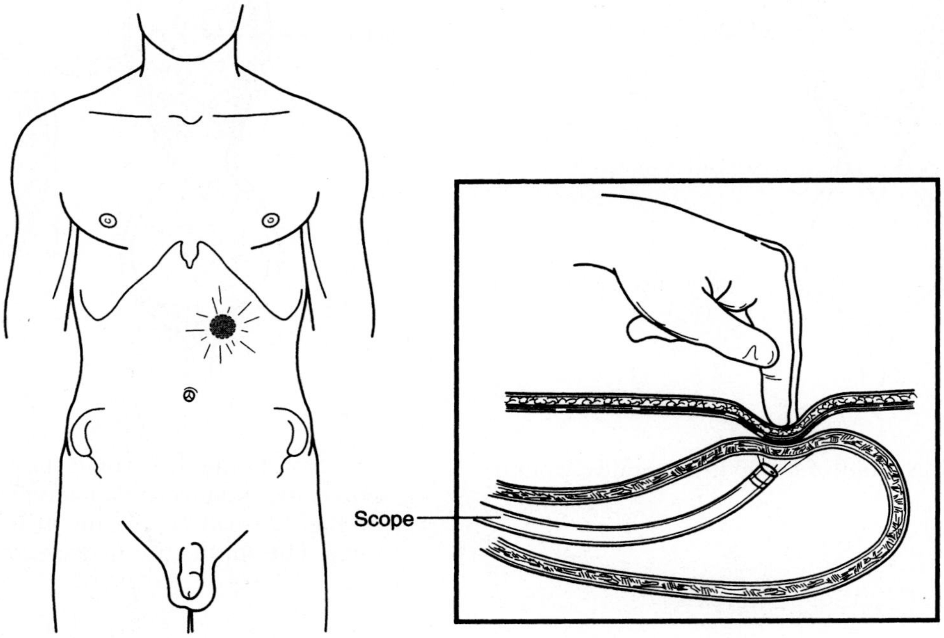

1 The endoscope is passed into the stomach. Palpation over the transilluminated spot on the abdominal wall indicates the site of percutaneous gastric puncture.

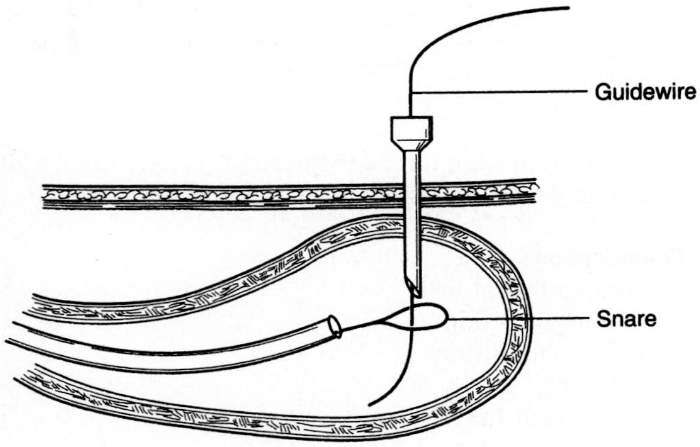

2 The stomach is punctured with a needle. A guidewire is passed into the stomach and snared while the wire is visualized through the scope.

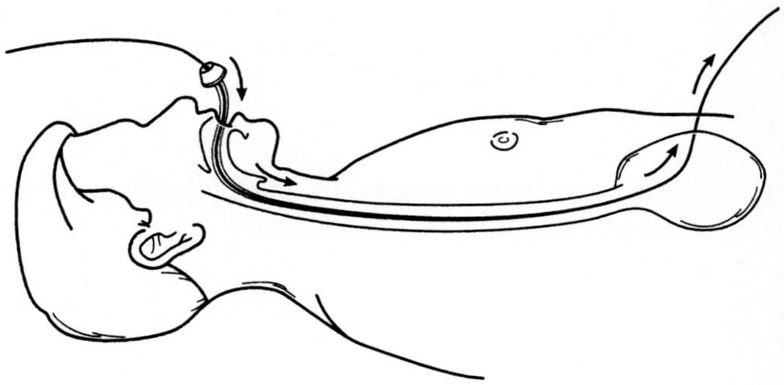

3 The scope and guidewire are removed. The gastrostomy tube is threaded over the guidewire. The tube is long and tapered, and it acts as a dilator as it passes through the anterior abdominal wall. The gastrostomy tube is drawn retrograde (i.e., from mouth to stomach).

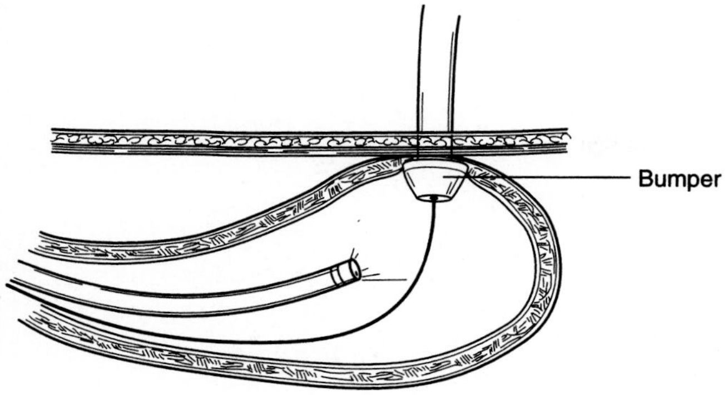

4 The bumper is positioned after the endoscope is reintroduced into the stomach.

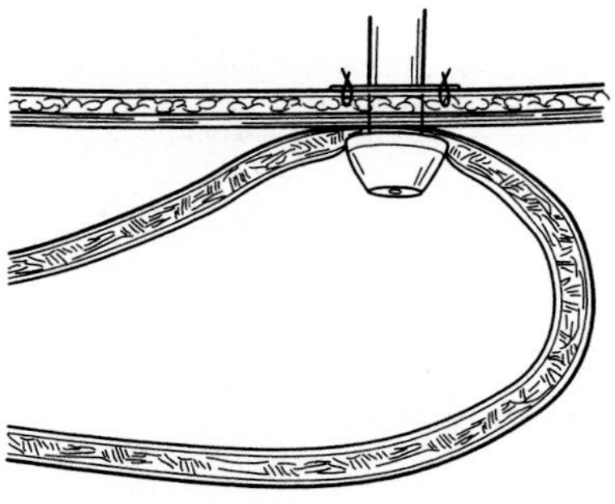

5 The guidewire is removed. The tube is fixed to the abdominal wall with a suture or with bumpers that are contained in the kit.

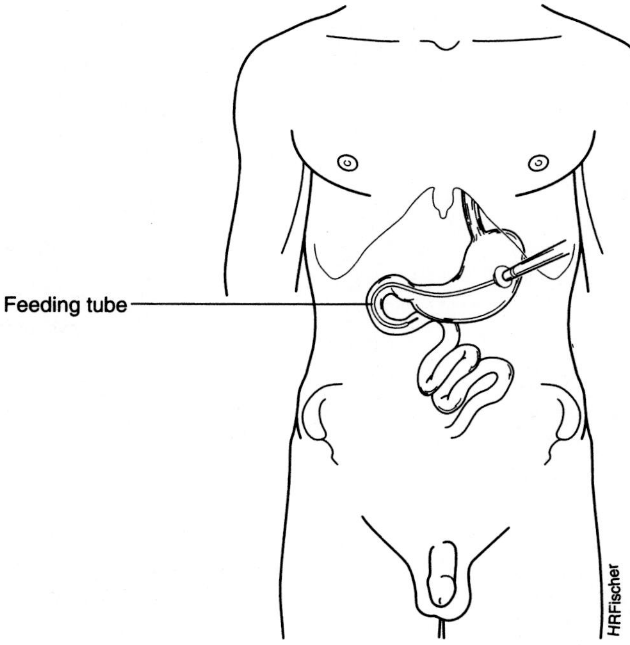

6 An enteral feeding port may be placed through the gastrostomy tube, with endoscopy assistance if necessary.

Inguinal Herniorrhaphy

Conventional Herniorrhaphy

Indications

Inguinal hernia

Procedure

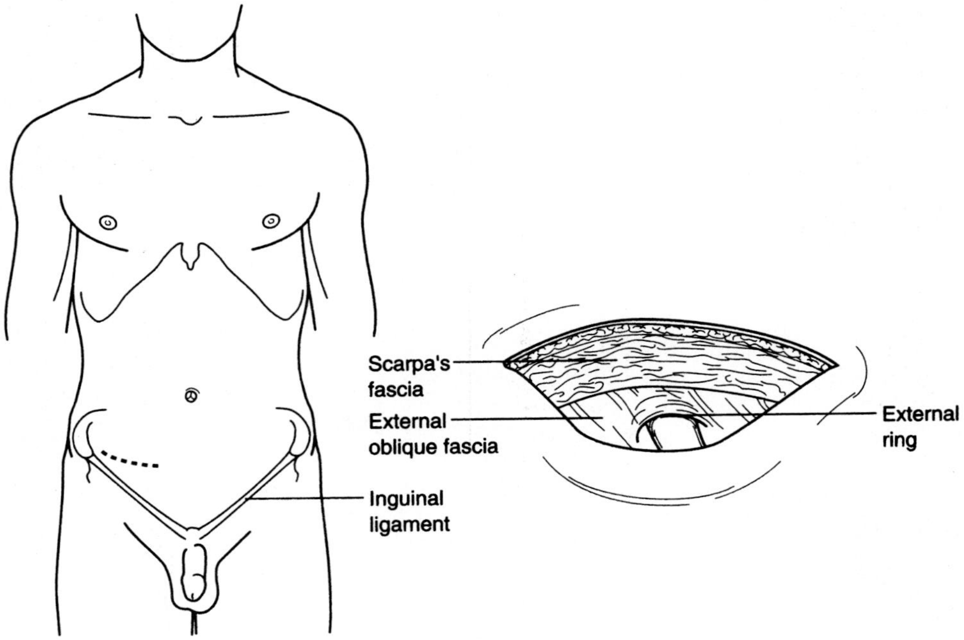

1 A transverse inguinal skinfold incision is made and carried through Scarpa's fascia to the fascia of the external oblique muscle.

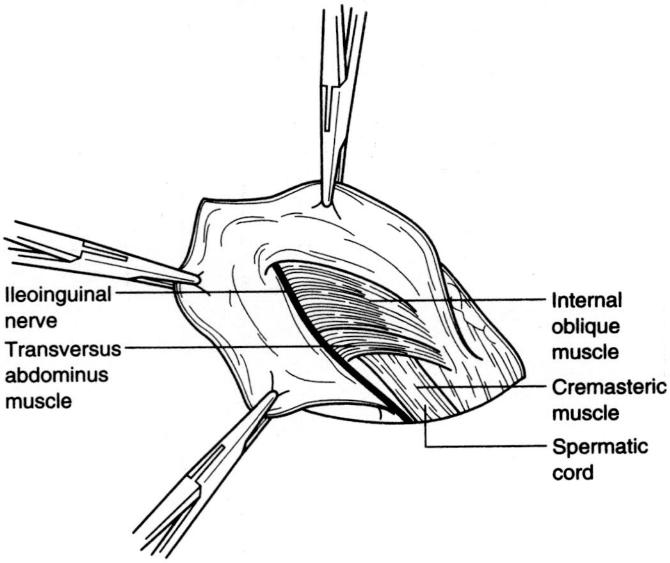

2 The external oblique fascia is opened in the direction of the fibers through the external ring, avoiding the nerves.

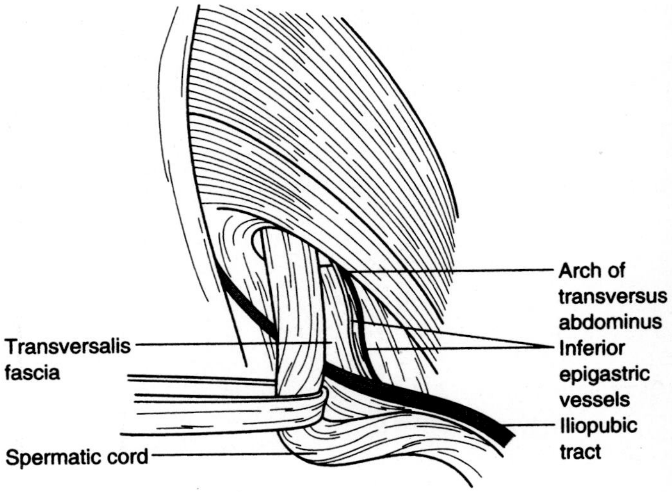

3 The spermatic cord is mobilized, and a sling is passed around the cord for traction. In women, the round ligament may be divided between ties.

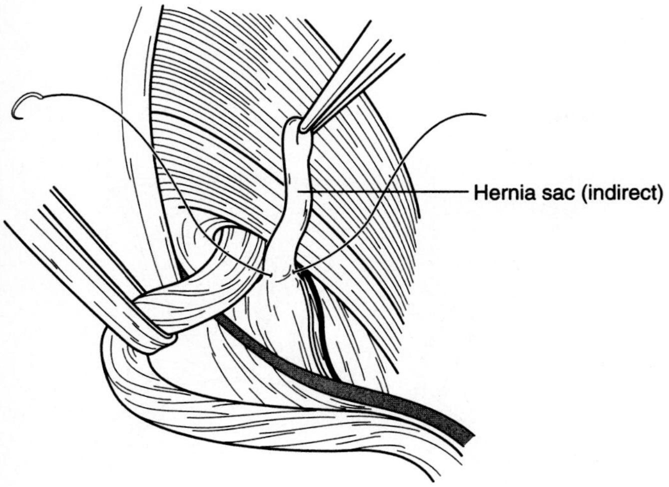

4 An indirect hernia sac is located adjacent to the cord, anteromedially, originating lateral to the inferior epigastric vessels. Direct hernias are located medially to these vessels, through a defect in the transversalis fascia. It is dissected from the cord structures and ligated at its base. It is not necessary to dissect the direct hernia sac.

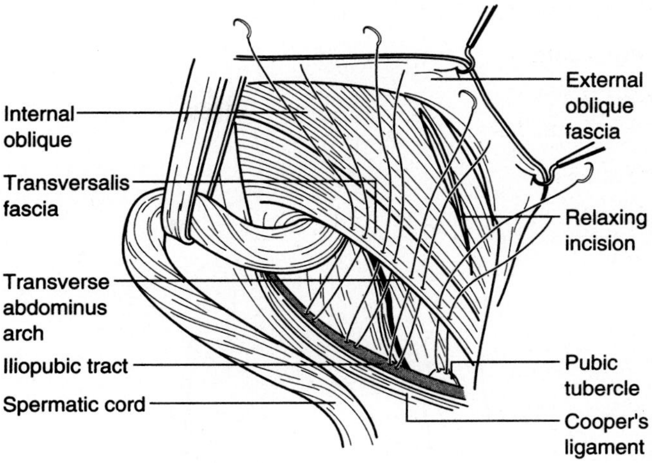

5 An anatomic repair is performed to reinforce the inguinal floor and internal ring. A relaxing incision may be required to perform the repair without tension.

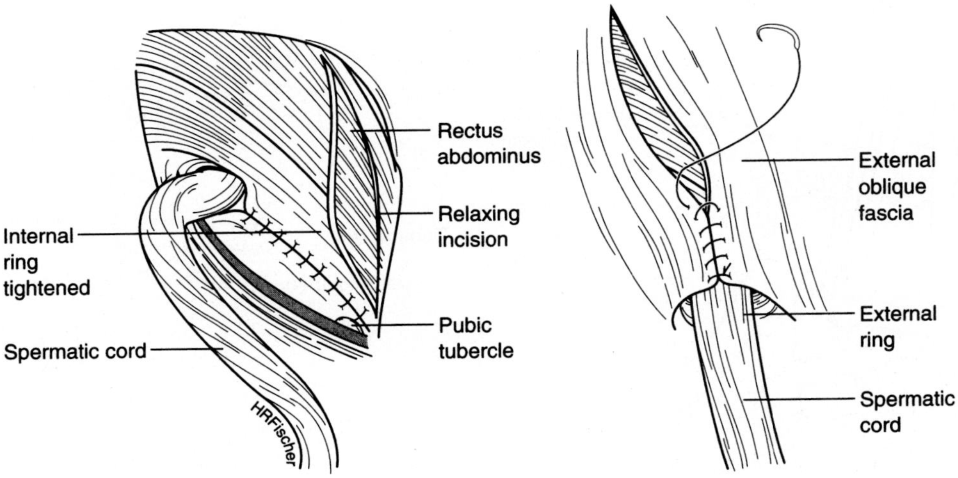

6 Closure is performed in layers.

Complications

Wound infection
Recurrence
Spermatic duct injury
Ilioinguinal nerve entrapment
Testicular swelling
Femoral vein injury

Laparoscopic Herniorrhaphy

Procedure

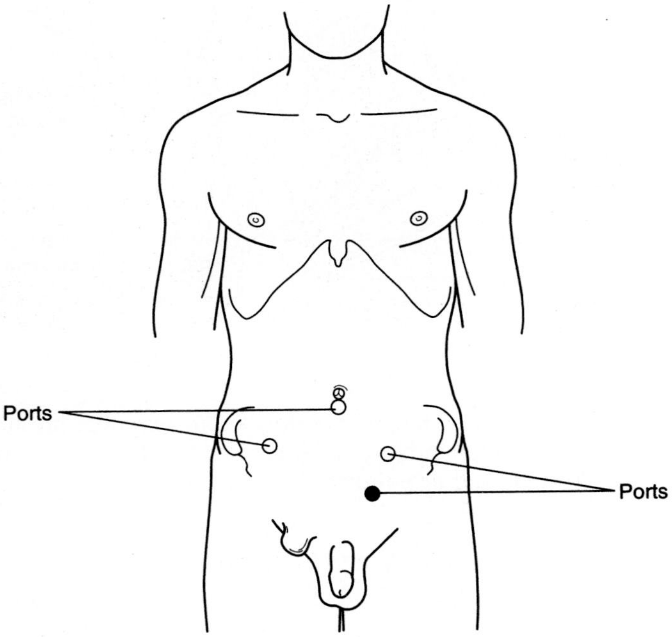

1 Operative and camera ports are placed.

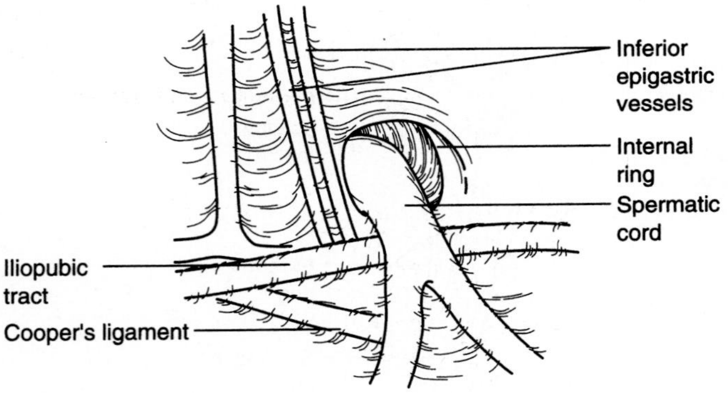

2 The anatomy of the inguinal floor is identified, and the peritoneum is opened.

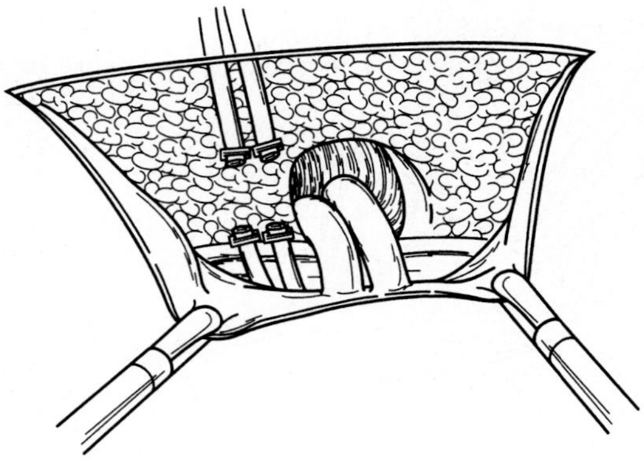

3 The indirect inguinal hernia sac is removed from the defect.

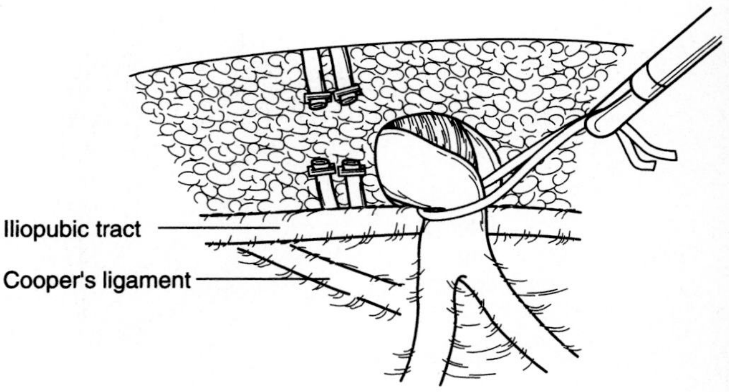

4 The inferior epigastric artery and vein may be divided. The spermatic cord is encircled with a sling.

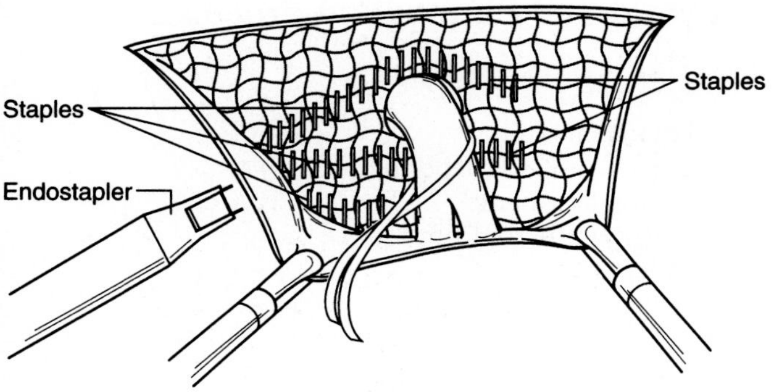

5 Polypropylene mesh is fashioned to fit around the spermatic cord and form a new inguinal floor.

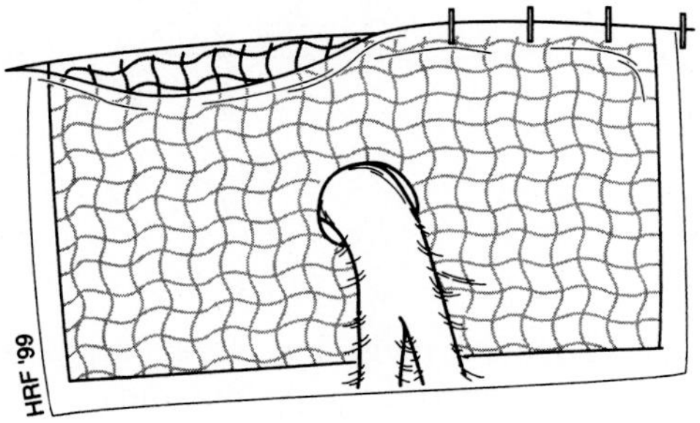

6 The peritoneum is repositioned over the mesh.
7 Ports larger than 5 mm are closed.

Anal Procedures

Indications

Infectious anal process refractory to medical management
Bleeding
Abscess
Prolapse

Procedures

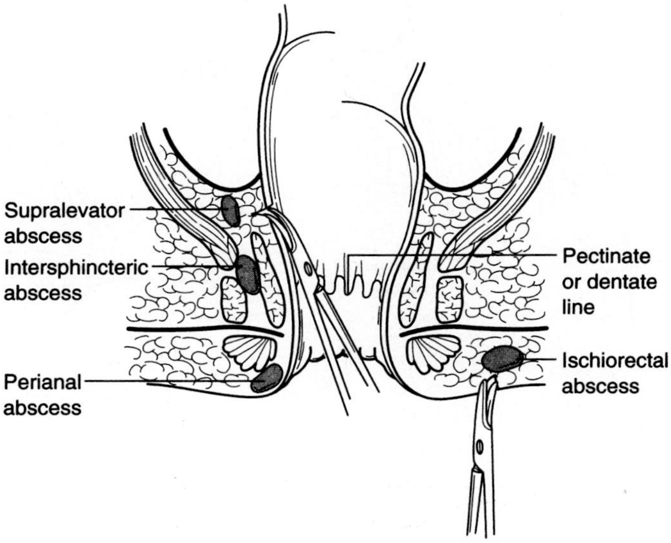

1 Incision or drainage of perirectal abscess

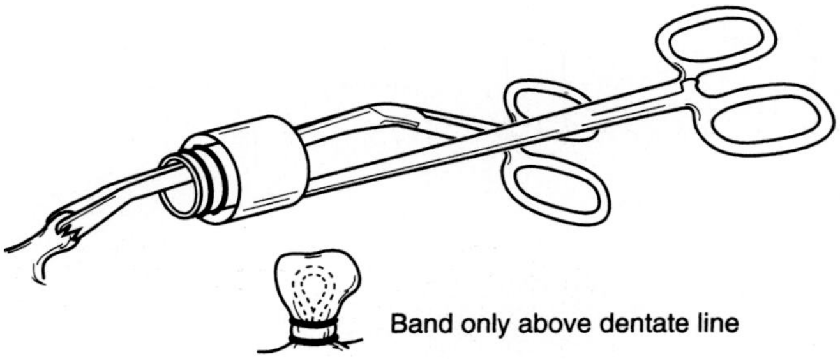

2 Rubber-band ligation of hemorrhoid

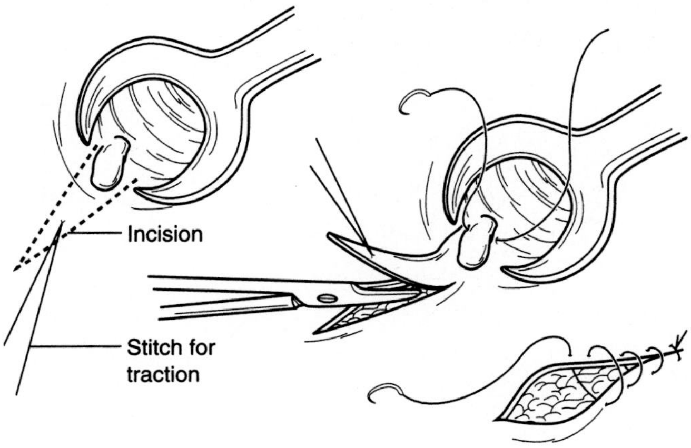

3 Hemorrhoidectomy

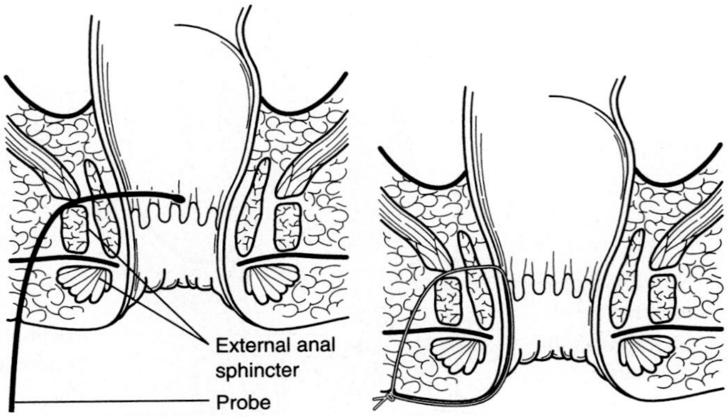

4 Placement of seton — usually a suture placed through a fistula tract to induce scarring

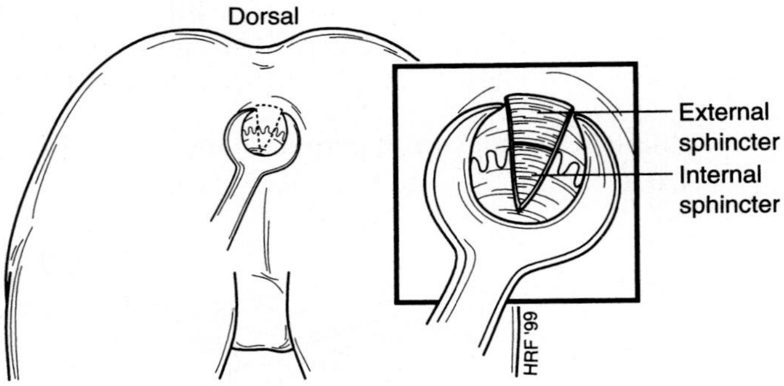

5 Internal sphincterotomy

Complications

Stenosis
Incontinence
Recurrence

Thyroid and Parathyroid Procedures

Indications

Thyroid nodule
Graves' disease (hyperthyroidism)
Metastatic disease
Hyperparathyroidism
- Adenoma
- Secondary or tertiary

Procedure

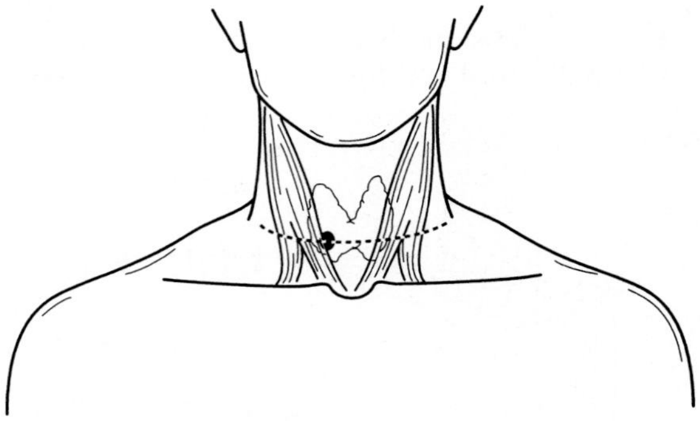

1 A transverse neck incision is made for procedures on both the thyroid and the parathyroids.

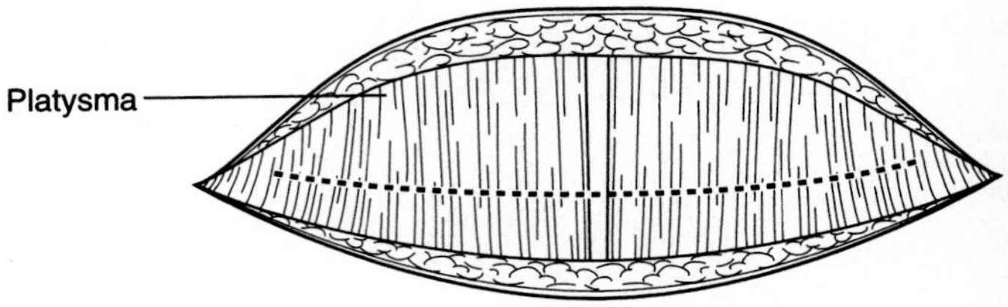

2 The platysma is transected.

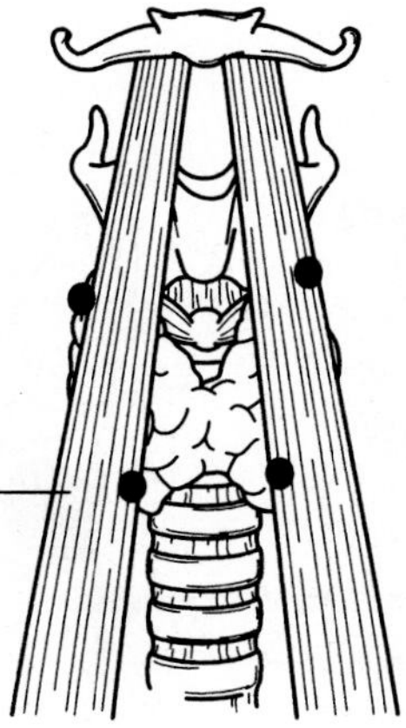

3 Strap muscles are divided in the midline.
4 The thyroid is mobilized to expose the blood supply.
5 The recurrent laryngeal nerve is identified and preserved. The position of the parathyroid glands is variable.

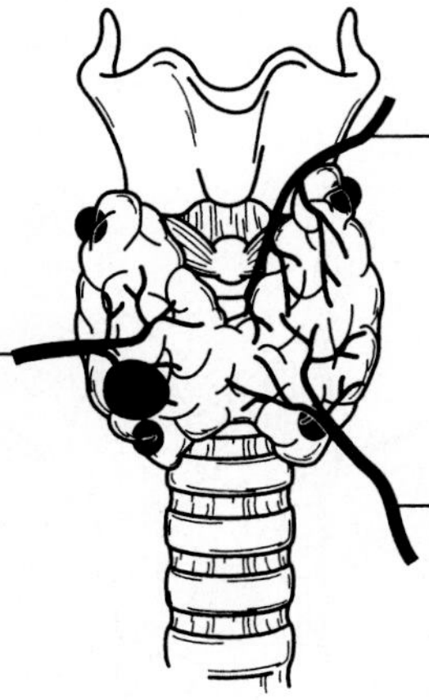

6 The inferior parathyroids are identified in proximity to the inferior thyroidal vessels. Nearly 60% of the time, they are located behind the lower third of the gland or within 1 cm of the lower pole.

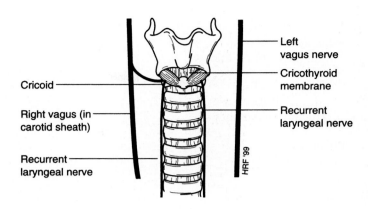

7 The superior parathyroids are found behind the middle portion of the gland (near the area where the recurrent laryngeal nerve enters the larynx) in three-fourths of cases.
8 Operations on the thyroid preserve the parathyroids with their native blood supply. If a parathyroid is devascularized, it may be minced and reimplanted in a neck muscle.
9 During operations for hyperparathyroidism, all four parathyroid glands must be identified.

Complications

Skin flap necrosis
Cellulitis
Recurrent laryngeal nerve injury
- Unilateral: hoarseness
- Bilateral: inspiratory stridor (may require tracheostomy)

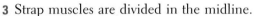

Hematoma
Hypocalcemia

Thyroidectomy

Indications

Solid thyroid nodule
Goiter
Hyperthyroidism
Graves' disease
Thyroid malignancy

Procedure

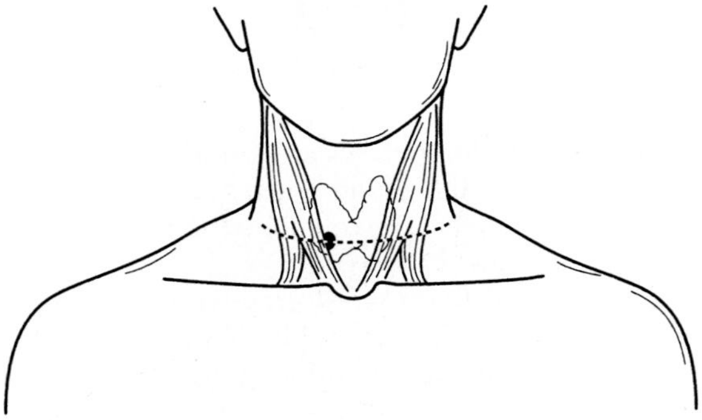

1 The neck is slightly hyperextended. An incision is made approximately two fingerbreadths above the sternal notch, usually in a natural skin crease.

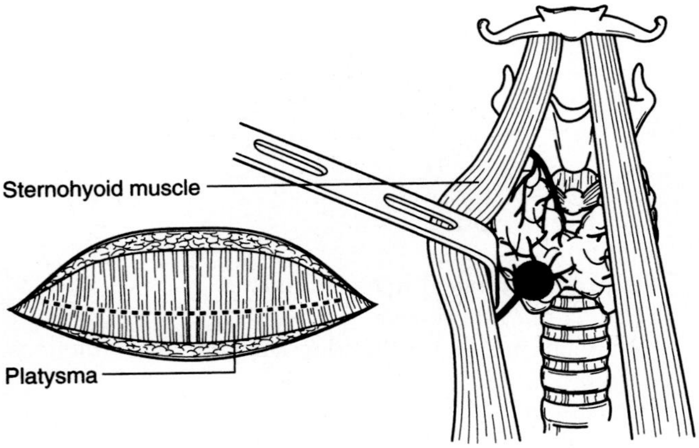

2 The platysma muscle is divided, and the strap muscles are separated in the midline. Adequate exposure is usually achieved, but the strap muscles can be divided if necessary.

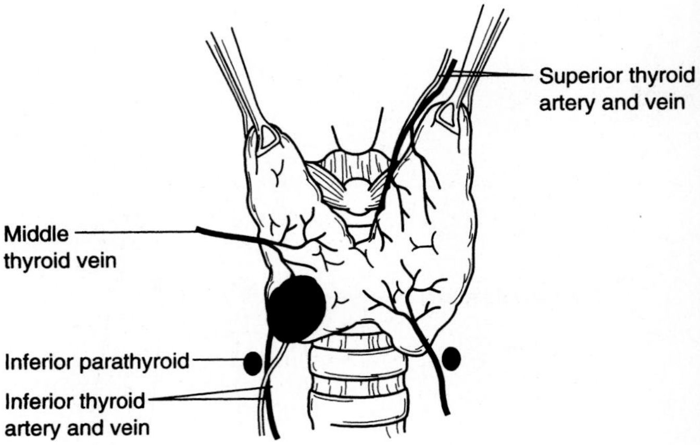

3 The thyroid gland is exposed. Dissection is usually begun inferiorly, and the inferior thyroidal artery and vein are ligated and divided. The inferior parathyroid glands are identified and preserved with their blood supply. The position of the parathyroids is variable, but 60% of the time, the inferior parathyroid glands are located behind the lower one-third of the gland or within 1 cm of the lower pole.

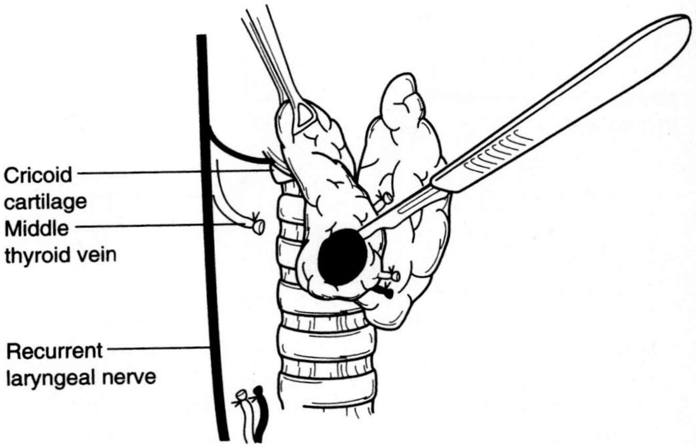

4 The middle thyroid vein is ligated and divided. The recurrent laryngeal nerve is found in the tracheo-esophageal groove and must be preserved. The superior parathyroids may be located near the middle thyroidal vein or in the area where the recurrent laryngeal nerve enters the larynx.

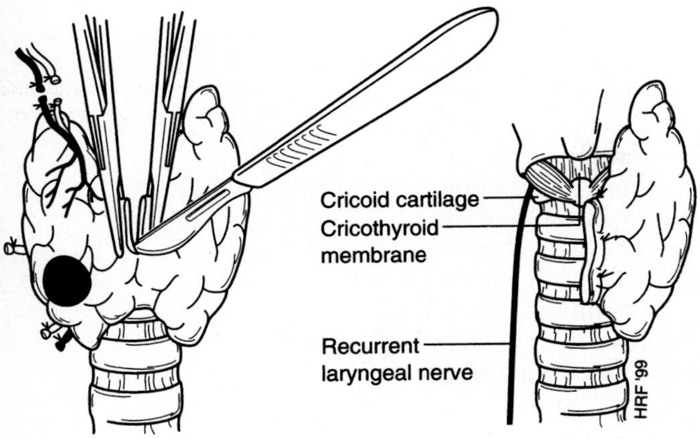

5 The superior thyroidal artery and vein are ligated. The isthmus is divided between clamps, and the remaining thyroid tissue is ligated with suture to ensure hemostasis. The lobe of the thyroid gland is bluntly dissected from the trachea. If a total thyroidectomy is planned, the procedure is completed on the opposite lobe.

Complications

Hypothyroidism
Persistent hyperthyroidism
Hypocalcemia
Recurrent laryngeal nerve injury
Superior laryngeal nerve injury (external branch)
Loss of voice quality
Hemorrhage or airway compromise

Tracheostomy

Indications

- Chronic airway access
  - Mechanical ventilation
  - Tracheal suctioning
- Proximal obstruction or stenosis
  - Laryngeal carcinoma
  - Bilateral vocal cord paralysis
  - Acute epiglottitis (children)

Procedure

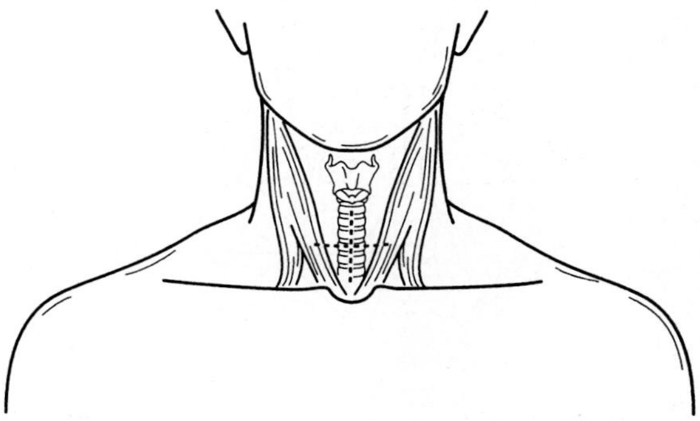

1 A transverse or vertical incision is used.

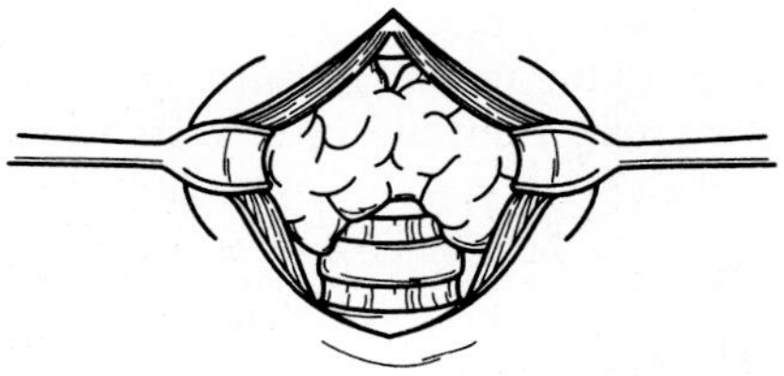

2 Strap muscles are separated in the midline.

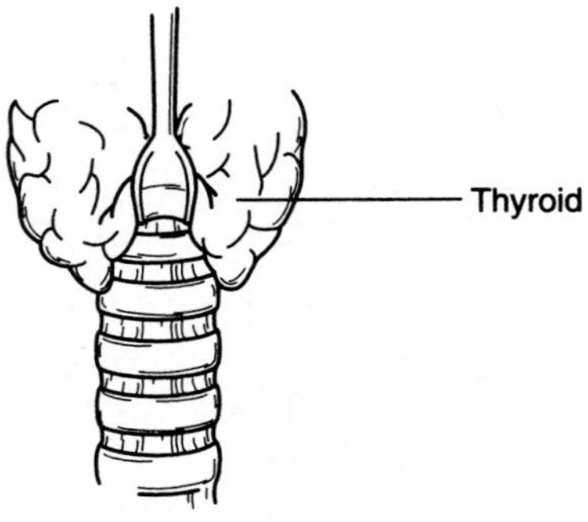

3 The thyroid isthmus is retracted or divided.

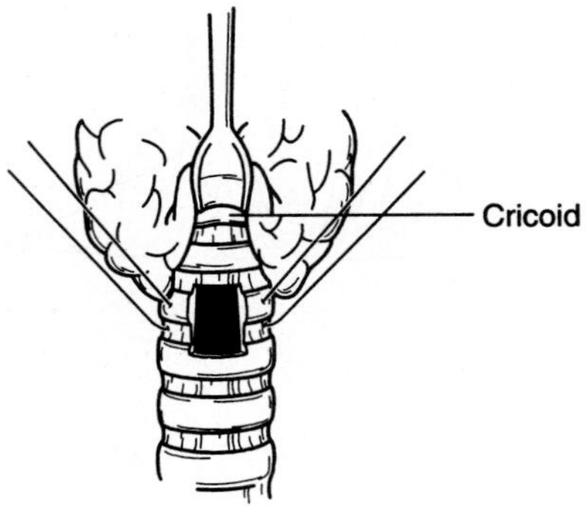

4 Traction sutures are placed laterally. A window is cut in the anterior surface of the trachea, approximately at the level of the second or third tracheal ring. Some surgeons prefer a simple vertical incision.

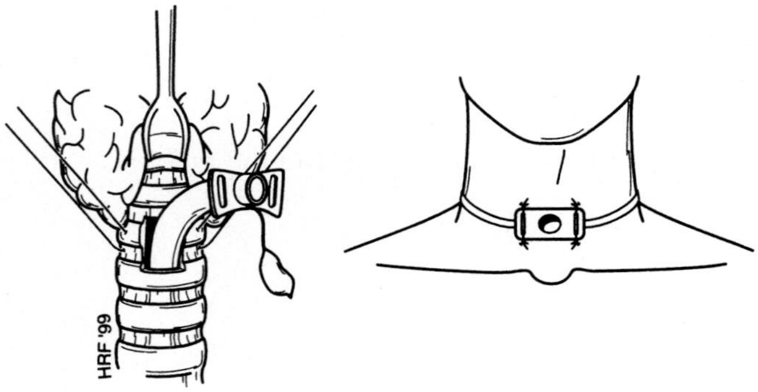

5 The tracheostomy appliance is inserted into the tracheotomy site without excessive force. It is fixed firmly to the neck to prevent dislodgement.

Complications

- Laryngeal or tracheal fracture
- Esophageal injury
- Bleeding pneumothorax
- Tracheoesophageal fistula
- Tracheoinominate artery fistula
- Tracheal stenosis
- Tracheomalacia
- Subcutaneous emphysema
- Pneumomediastinum
- Recurrent laryngeal nerve injury
- Tube displacement
- Tracheitis

Common Ward Procedures

Nasogastric Intubation

Indications

- Gastric decompression
- Gavage (feeding)
- Lavage (irrigation or dilution of the gastric contents)
- Sampling of the gastric contents for analysis

Contraindications

- Basilar skull fracture
- Facial fractures
- Obstructed nasal passage (if needed, orogastric intubation is considered)

Procedure

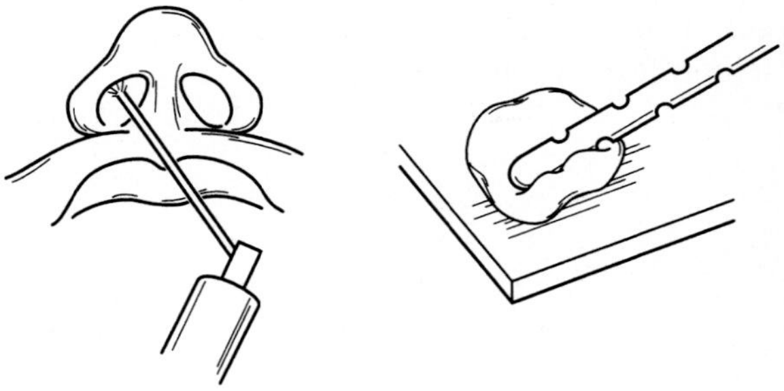

1 The nasal passage is anesthetized with a topical anesthetic. The nasogastric tube is lubricated with jelly.

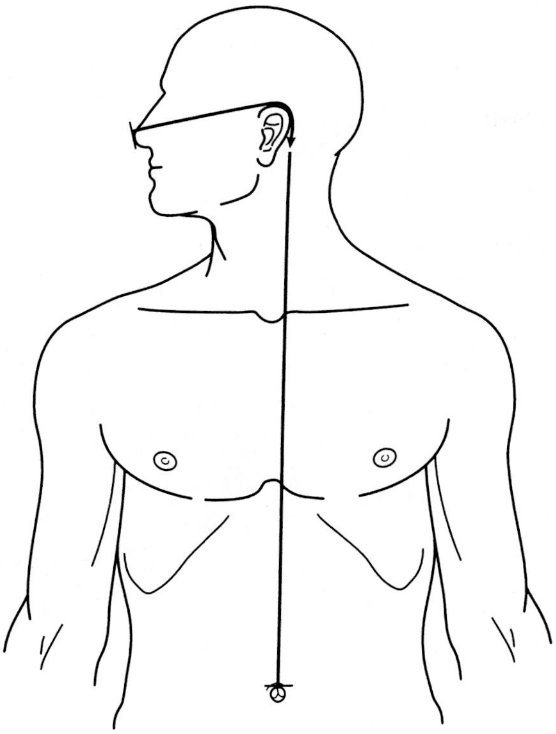

2 The length of tubing necessary to reach the stomach is estimated.

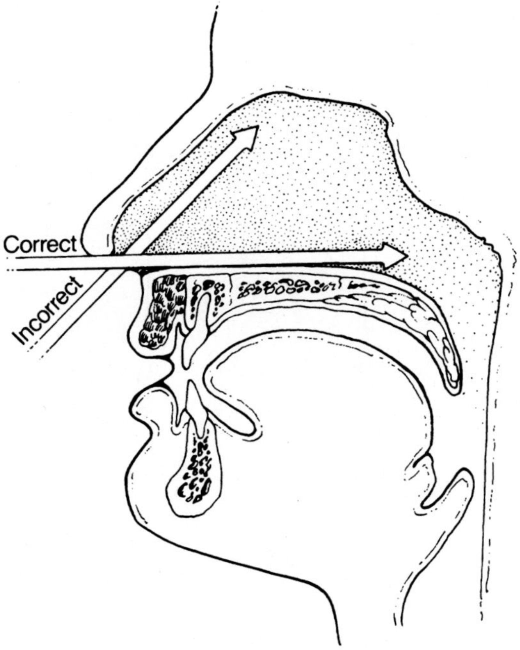

3 The tip of the tube is directed toward the hypopharynx, not toward the base of the skull. The patient is asked to swallow. Small sips of water through a straw may be helpful.

4 The tube is advanced as the patient swallows until the estimated length of tubing is inserted.

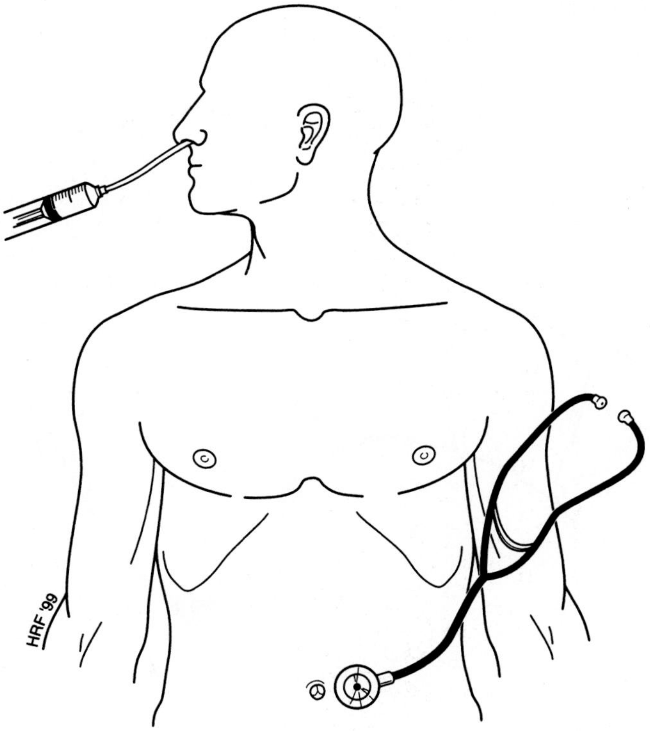

5 Auscultation over the stomach as air is injected through the tube confirms proper tube placement. The return of gastric contents or bile also confirms proper placement.

Bladder Catheterization

Indications

Bladder decompression
Measurement of urine output
Relief of obstruction
Diagnosis
Lavage

Contraindications

Suspected urethral injury
Stricture (more experience necessary)

Procedure

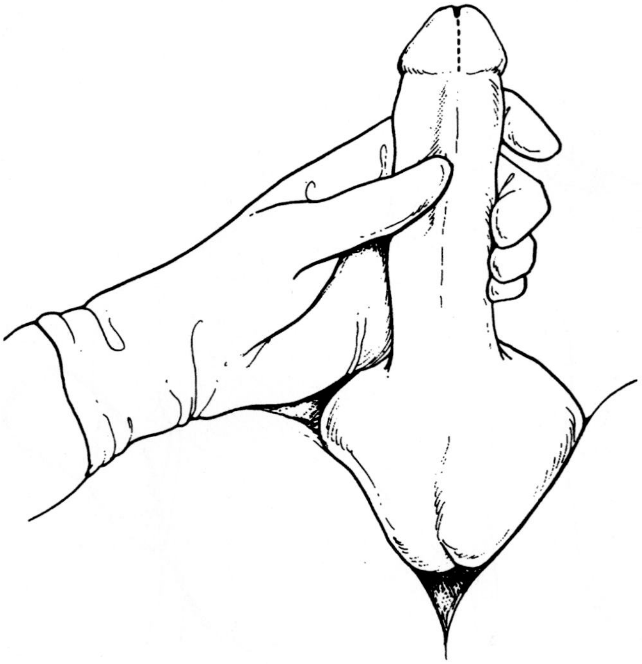

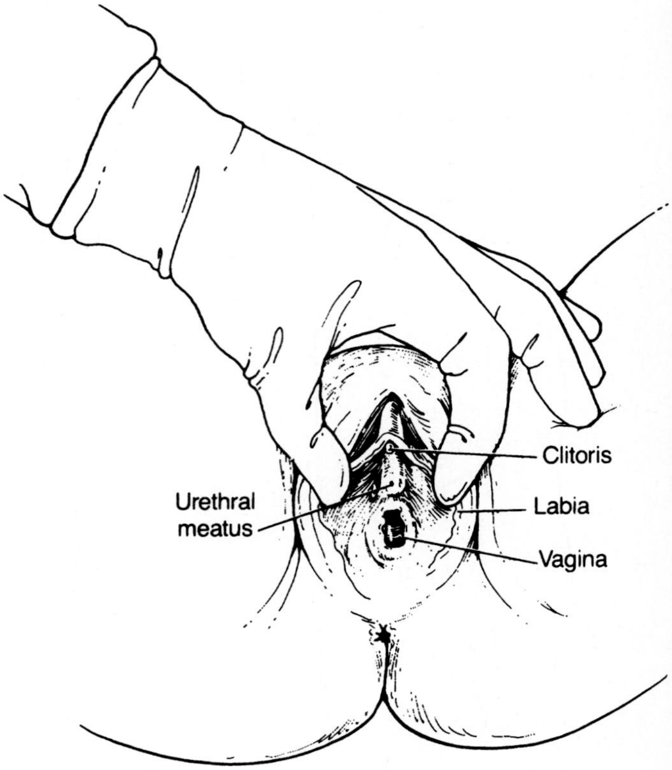

1 The meatus is cleaned with antiseptic solution.

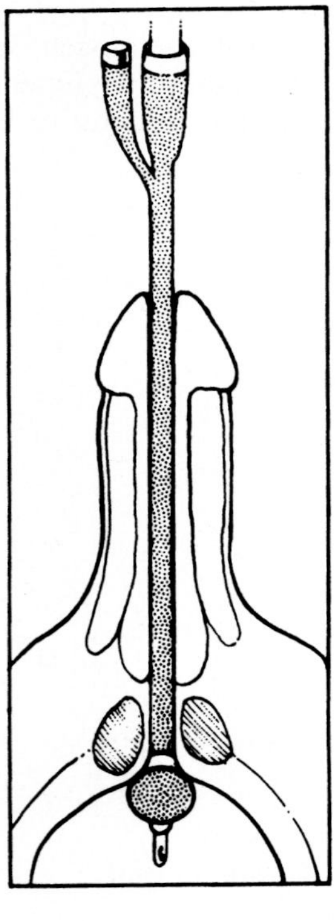

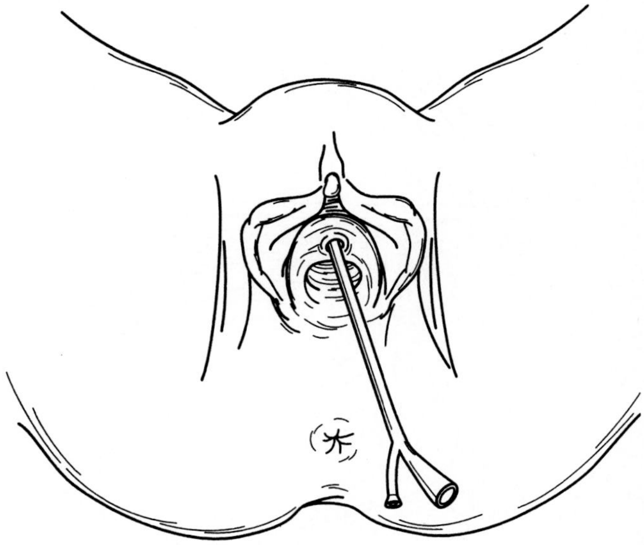

2 The penis is held upright, and the lubricated catheter is inserted into the urethra. Urine must be identified in the collection system before the balloon is inflated. In women, the labia are not allowed to reapproximate until the catheter is positioned in the bladder and the balloon is inflated.

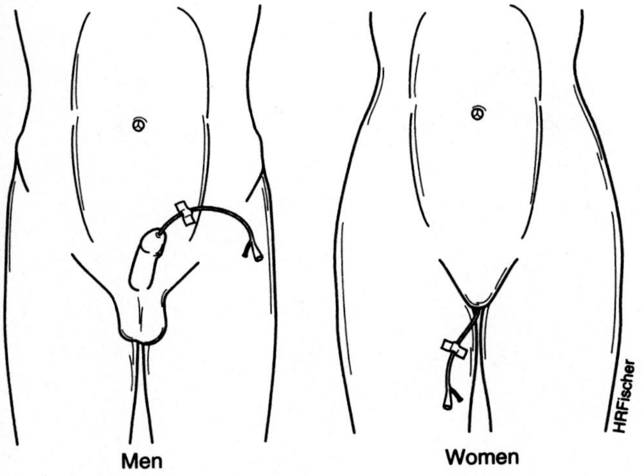

3 The catheter is taped to the lower abdomen in men and to the medial thigh in women.

Complications

False passage
Hemorrhage
Urethral disruption
Bladder spasm
Bladder contamination

Glossary

abrasion wound that has superficial loss of epithelial elements; dermis and deeper structures remain intact.

absorbable sutures surgical suture material prepared from a substance that is digested by body tissues and therefore is not permanent; available in various diameters and tensile strengths; can be treated to modify its resistance to absorption; can be impregnated with antimicrobial agents.

achalasia esophageal motility disorder characterized by failure of the circular esophageal muscle in the distal 2 cm of the esophagus to relax.

acidemia elevation of blood hydrogen ion.

acidosis primary increase in P_{CO_2} or primary decrease in HCO_3.

acral lentiginous melanoma malignant melanoma that occurs in areas with no hair follicles (e.g., palms, nail beds, soles of feet).

activated partial thromboplastin time (APTT) clotting test used to detect deficiencies in the intrinsic coagulation pathway; a prolonged APTT indicates deficiencies in factor I, II, V, VIII, IX, X, XI, or XII.

adenoma mucosal tumor of the small and large intestine; tubular, villous, and mixed cell types are seen.

adenoma, hepatic benign tumor that consists of unencapsulated sheets of hepatocytes without ductular elements; apparently hormonally responsive; risk of spontaneous rupture.

adenoma, parathyroid benign tumor of a parathyroid gland.

adenoma, toxic solitary autonomous hyperactive thyroid nodule.

adenoma, villous polyp characterized by sessile morphology; relatively high incidence of malignant degeneration.

adhesion fibrous tissue that often occurs after abdominal surgery; can lead to bowel obstruction.

adhesion, platelet sticking of platelets to surfaces other than another platelet; collagen is the common in vivo surface to which platelets adhere.

adrenal incidentaloma incidentally discovered adrenal mass that is not associated with any symptoms that overtly suggest adrenal abnormality.

adrenal insufficiency (Addisonian crisis) result of inadequate circulating glucocorticoids; common signs and symptoms are postural hypotension, dizziness, nausea, vomiting, abdominal pain, weakness, fatigability, hyperkalemia, and hyponatremia; if not treated promptly, causes complete cardiovascular collapse and death.

adrenocorticotropic hormone (ACTH) stimulation test administration of synthetic ACTH to stimulate the secretion of cortisol and evaluate the adequacy of adrenal reserve and the integrity of the hypothalamic–pituitary–adrenal axis.

advance directive a mentally capable patient's instructions regarding his or her medical care if he or she becomes incapacitated and unable to make decisions.

afterload resistance to ventricular ejection; may be increased by obstruction (i.e., aortic stenosis) or vascular constriction (i.e., increased systemic vascular resistance).

aggregation, platelet platelet-to-platelet sticking; a white clot is formed that is composed almost exclusively of platelets.

airway compromise airway obstruction; loss of airway patency from any cause.

airway, nasopharyngeal (nasal) device, usually made of rubber, designed to prevent the tongue from obstructing the nasopharynx; placed through a nostril into the nasopharynx; well tolerated in the patient with an intact gag reflex.

airway, oropharyngeal (oral) device, usually made of plastic, designed to prevent the tongue from obstructing the oropharynx; placed through the mouth and over the tongue; should not be used in a conscious patient with an intact gag reflex because it can cause gagging, vomiting, and aspiration.

aldosterone hormone produced by the zona glomerulosa in the adrenal gland; secreted as part of the renin–angiotensin system in response to decreased blood flow in the kidneys; causes sodium retention and potassium and hydrogen loss in the distal tubule.

alkalemia depression of blood hydrogen ion.

alkalosis primary decrease in P_{CO_2} or primary increase in HCO_3.

allograft (homograft) tissue transferred between genetically dissimilar members of the same species (e.g., most human transplants).

alpha$_1$-antitrypsin deficiency inherited autosomal dominant disorder that causes varying degrees of liver and lung injury over a patient's lifetime; some patients have predominantly pulmonary dysfunction; others have liver disease that leads to cirrhosis and the need for liver transplantation.

amaurosis fugax transient monocular blindness as a result of emboli to the ipsilateral ophthalmic artery; classically described as a curtain of blindness being pulled down from the superior to the inferior aspect of the affected eye.

AMPLE history mnemonic for taking a quick history: Allergies, Medications, Past illnesses, Last meal, and the Events surrounding the injury are noted.

anal fissure painful linear tear in the lining of the anal canal below the dentate line.

aneuploid having an abnormal number of chromosomes, not an exact multiple of the haploid number, in contrast to having abnormal numbers of complete haploid sets of chromosomes (e.g., diploid, triploid); prognostic factor used to estimate the risk of recurrence of breast cancer; ploidy is measured with flow cytometry, which permits analysis of DNA content per cell and allows determination of ploidy levels within a tumor cell population; diploid indicates a good prognosis; aneuploid indicates a poorer prognosis.

aneurysm dilation of an artery to greater than one and a half to two times its normal size; may be saccular (saclike bulging on one side of the artery) or fusiform (elongated, spindle-shaped diffuse dilation of the arterial wall).

angioplasty reconstruction of a blood vessel, either surgically or by balloon dilation; surgical angioplasty entails reconstruction of the artery, usually with a patch; balloon angioplasty involves percutaneous placement of an intraarterial balloon; the balloon is then inflated, thereby disrupting the arterial plaque as well as a portion of the media and consequently enlarging the artery.

ankle–brachial index comparison of the systolic blood pressure at the level of the ankle divided by the brachial arterial pressure; this ratio provides an assessment of the degree of lower extremity arterial occlusive disease, with the brachial arterial pressure used as a control.

annular pancreas ring of pancreas encircling the duodenum; caused by a failure of the embryonic primordia to unite completely; each portion has its own duct.

antibiotic resistance resistance to a previously effective antibiotic by a microbial pathogen through changes in its DNA structure.

antidiuretic hormone (vasopressin) hormone produced by the supraoptic and paraventricular nuclei of the hypothalamus; secreted in response to increased osmotic pressure and decreased effective plasma volume; also released in response to stress; regulates water balance by stimulating resorption in the distal renal tubule.

antisepsis prevention of infection by inhibiting the growth of infectious agents.

antrectomy distal gastric resection that removes the gastrin-producing cells of the stomach.

aponeurosis flat tendon; broad, fibrous sheet of tendinous fibers that provides attachment to broad muscles (e.g., oblique muscles of the abdominal wall).

appendicitis inflammation of the appendix.

asepsis absence of living pathogenic organisms; state of sterility.

asplenism complete loss of splenic function.

atherosclerosis degenerative change of the arterial wall; characterized by endothelial dysfunction, inflammatory cell adhesion, and infiltration and accumulation of cellular and acellular elements within the arterial wall; lipid deposition is associated with fibrosis and calcification and can lead to severe arterial occlusive disease.

autograft graft (e.g., skin) that consists of the patient's own tissue.

AVPU mnemonic for quickly assessing the level of consciousness in a patient with traumatic injury: Is the patient Alert, responsive to Vocal stimuli, responsive to Painful stimuli, or Unresponsive?

avulsion tearing away or forcible separation of tissue; may be partial or total.

B cells immunocytes derived from bone marrow stem cells; commonly, B cells produce circulating antibodies and are responsible for the humoral response to foreign tissues.

bacteremia presence of viable bacteria in the blood.

Ballance's sign percussion dullness of the left flank; occurs with a ruptured spleen.

Barrett's esophagus presence of columnar epithelium in the esophagus; results from a metaplastic change caused by repeated inflammation of normal squamous epithelium; small, but significant tendency toward the development of cancer.

basal cell carcinoma carcinoma of the skin that arises from the basal cells of the epidermis or hair follicles.

basal cell carcinoma, morphealike tumor with an indurated, yellow plaque with ill-defined borders; overlying skin remains intact for a long period; less common than nodular basal cell carcinoma.

basal cell carcinoma, nodular most common variant of basal cell carcinoma; characterized by a central depression and a rolled border; usually located on the head and neck.

basal cell carcinoma, pigmented similar to nodular basal cell carcinoma, except that tumors contain melanocytes; may be confused with melanoma.

Beck's triad three classic clinical signs of cardiac tamponade: (1) muffled (distant) heart sounds, (2) elevated central venous pressure (jugular venous distension), and (3) hypotension.

bezoar accumulation of a large mass of undigested material in the stomach.

biliary colic episodic epigastric or right upper quadrant abdominal pain; associated with nausea and vomiting; secondary to transient cystic duct obstruction with a gallstone; tends to occur postprandially; usually lasts 1 to 4 hours.

Billroth I procedure gastrointestinal reconstruction that creates an anastomosis between the distal end of the stomach and the duodenum (gastroduodenostomy).

Billroth II procedure gastrointestinal reconstruction that creates an anastomosis between the stomach and a loop of jejunum (gastrojejunostomy).

bleeding disorder, acquired hemostatic defect caused by a nongenetic factor (e.g., liver disease, anticoagulation therapy); more common than congenital bleeding disorders.

bleeding disorder, congenital inherited hemostatic defect (e.g., hemophilia, von Willebrand's disease); fairly uncommon.

bleeding history important part of the presurgical evaluation; a personal or familial bleeding problem is the most important predictive factor of operative and perioperative bleeding complications.

bleeding time test interval between the appearance of the first drop of blood and the removal of the last drop after incision of the forearm or puncture of the ear lobe or finger; bleeding time is prolonged in cases of thrombocytopenia, diminished prothrombin, abnormal platelet function, phosphorus or chloroform poisoning, and in some liver diseases; it is normal in hemophilia.

blood cell, red (erythrocyte) cellular portion of the blood that contains hemoglobin; responsible for carrying oxygen to the tissues.

blood cell, white (leukocyte) cellular portion of the blood that does not contain hemoglobin; classified as granular (i.e., neutrophils, eosinophils, basophils) and nongranular.

Boerhaave's syndrome full-thickness rupture of the esophagus (in contrast, Mallory-Weiss syndrome is a bleeding mucosal rupture at the same site); associated with loss of gastroesophageal contents (typically into the left side of the chest) and acute sepsis; may cause a syndrome similar to myocardial infarction.

Bowen's disease skin condition characterized by chronic scaling and occasionally a crusted, purple, or erythematous raised lesion; may become invasive squamous cell carcinoma.

brain death irreversible cessation of all brain function.

BRCA-1 gene BRCA-1 and BRCA-2 are the two major genes responsible for the inherited predisposition to breast cancer; BRCA-1 is also related to ovarian cancer; in patients who have mutations in either gene, the risk of breast cancer is approximately 80% by age 70; in contrast, the lifetime risk is approximately 12% in the general population.

Breslow system system for microstaging malignant melanomas based on the thickness of the tumor in millimeters; survival is related to tumor thickness.

bruit auscultatory sound over an artery; produced by turbulent flow.

burn center specialized care unit with facilities, personnel, and resources devoted to the care of patients with serious burn injuries.

burn, epidermal first-degree burn injury that involves only the epidermal layer of the skin; does not blister; has relatively minor physiologic effects; heals without scarring.

burn, first-degree see *burn, epidermal.*

burn, full-thickness third-degree burn injury that involves the entire epidermis and dermis; usually requires skin grafting.

burn, partial-thickness second-degree burn injury that involves some, but not all, of the dermis; variable in appearance, but because epidermal appendages are intact, heals if followed long enough; deep partial-thickness burns are usually treated with skin grafting.

burn, second-degree see *burn, partial-thickness.*

burn, third-degree see *burn, full-thickness.*

carcinoembryonic antigen antigen produced by many gastrointestinal tumors; measured in the blood; used in surveillance for cancer recurrence.

carcinoid syndrome carcinoid tumor that causes a syndrome of signs and symptoms that include cutaneous flushing, diarrhea, bronchospasm, skin lesions, and vasomotor instability.

cardiac injury, blunt myocardial injury associated with deceleration or crush injury to the anterior chest; associated with sternal or rib fractures; the anterior myocardium (right ventricle) is primarily involved; when severe, may lead to right-sided heart failure; difficult to diagnose by electrocardiogram because the weaker right ventricular electrical activity is overshadowed by the stronger left ventricular electrical activity.

cardiac output quantity of blood pumped by the heart into the pulmonary and systemic circulation each minute.

cardiac tamponade compression of the heart from accumulation of fluid or blood within the pericardial sac; ventricular filling is restricted; the increased pressure within the pericardial sac is transmitted to each cardiac chamber; results in equalization of the right atrial, right ventricular diastolic, pulmonary artery diastolic, pulmonary capillary wedge, left atrial, left ventricular diastolic, and intrapericardial pressures.

cardiogenic state decreased cardiac output from inadequate function of the heart itself, rather than deficiencies in venous return.

cerebral blood flow cerebral perfusion pressure divided by cerebrovascular resistance.

cerebrovascular accident (stroke) region of cerebral infarction secondary to arterial atheroembolism or hypoperfusion.

Charcot's triad triad of clinical findings that includes right upper quadrant abdominal pain, fever and chills, and jaundice; associated with cholangitis.

Child's classification series of five parameters (serum bilirubin, serum albumin, presence of ascites, encephalopathy, and nutrition) used to grade the status of liver disease.

chin-lift maneuver maneuver used to open the mouth so that the oral cavity can be inspected and patency assured; accomplished by placing the fingers of the left hand under the chin while the thumb is placed anteriorly below the lips; the chin is grasped and lifted forward and downward; the mouth is opened for inspection; a more secure grip on the jaw is accomplished by placing the thumb inside the mouth and behind the lower incisors.

cholangiocarcinoma adenocarcinoma that has two types: infiltrating bile duct tumor that usually arises at the level of the bile duct bifurcation and, less commonly, solid intraparenchymal tumor within the substance of the liver.

cholangiogram radiographic image of the bile ducts; obtained by injecting contrast material through a needle or catheter.

cholangiogram, percutaneous transhepatic radiologic imaging of the biliary tree; obtained by inserting a needle through the abdominal wall into the liver parenchyma and injecting contrast material directly into the intrahepatic bile ducts; used to extract stones, obtain a cytology specimen, or place a catheter.

cholangitis, acute acute infection of the bile ducts; caused by a stone, stricture, or neoplasm.

cholangitis, acute suppurative acute infection of the bile ducts; complicated by the finding of pus; requires urgent drainage.

cholecystectomy, laparoscopic removal of the gallbladder with a laparoscopic approach; preferred approach for most elective and many emergency situations.

cholecystitis, acute acute infection of the gallbladder; usually caused by calculus obstructing the cystic duct.

cholecystitis, acute acalculous acute infection of the gallbladder without underlying gallstone disease; usually occurs in patients who are being treated in intensive care units for other medical problems.

cholecystitis, acute emphysematous acute infection of the gallbladder; caused by gas-forming bacteria; characterized by air in the wall or lumen of the gallbladder or in the bile ducts;

often associated with diabetes mellitus; requires emergency cholecystectomy.

cholecystitis, acute gangrenous acute infection of the gallbladder that progresses to gangrene; requires emergency cholecystectomy.

choledocholithiasis presence of a stone or stones in the common bile duct; stones usually originate in the gallbladder and pass through the cystic duct into the common bile duct.

circulating nurse usually a registered nurse; a member of the operating room team who does not directly participate in the surgical procedure, but manages activities outside the sterile field; duties include opening sterile supplies, counting sponges, making and answering calls, delivering specimens, maintaining records, and other vital tasks.

Clark system system for microstaging malignant melanomas based on the anatomic level (I through V) of invasion of the tumor; survival is related to the depth of invasion.

claudication reproducible pain that occurs in a major muscle group; precipitated by exercise and relieved by rest; classically, pain occurs in the posterior calves after mild to moderate exercise.

closed-gloving technique method of donning surgical gloves in which the hands are not pushed fully through the cuffs of the surgical gown; usually practiced by surgical technicians as a self-gloving technique.

coagulation factor substance in the blood that is necessary for clotting; numbered with Roman numerals.

coagulation pathway, common final steps that lead to the generation of a clot; includes factors I (fibrinogen), II (prothrombin), V, and X; the end-product is fibrin.

coagulation pathway, extrinsic part of the first stage of coagulation; requires the interaction of factor VII with tissue thromboplastin to convert factor X to factor X^a.

coagulation pathway, intrinsic part of the first stage of coagulation; initiated by the interaction of factor XII with negatively charged surfaces; other coagulation factors in this pathway are factors VIII, IX, and XI; the eventual product converts factor X to factor X^a.

collagen principal structural protein of the body; its production, remodeling, and maturation define the second and third stages of wound healing.

colloid fluid for intravenous administration; consists of water, electrolytes, and protein or other molecules that are of sufficient molecular weight to exert a colloid oncotic pressure effect similar to that of endogenous albumin; packed red cells are often considered colloid, but do not meet this definition.

colonoscopy flexible diagnostic instrument that uses light-transmitting fiberoptics; allows visualization of the entire colon and terminal ileum.

colostomy surgical procedure in which the colon is divided and the proximal end is brought through a surgically created defect in the abdominal wall and sewn to the skin.

compartment syndrome elevation of the pressure within a fascial compartment of the upper or lower extremity; interstitial tissue pressure becomes higher than capillary perfusion pressure, resulting in ischemia to the muscles and nerves within the fascial compartment.

complement system of 20 or more proteins present in the serum; when activated, these proteins stimulate lymphocytes, macrophages, and reticuloendothelial cells as part of the host defense against bacterial pathogens.

contractility the force of cardiac muscle contraction under conditions of a predetermined preload or afterload.

contusion soft tissue swelling and hemorrhage without violation of the skin elements.

contusion, pulmonary injury to the lung parenchyma that causes interstitial hemorrhage, alveolar collapse, and extravasation of blood and plasma into the alveoli; causes a ventilation–perfusion mismatch that results in hypoxemia; physical examination may show blunt or penetrating injury to the chest; radiographic studies show a poorly defined infiltrate that develops over time.

Cooper's ligament strong fibrous insertion of transversus abdominus muscle on the pectineal line of the pelvis.

Courvoisier's law obstruction of the common bile duct by carcinoma of the pancreas or other malignancies of the distal common bile duct may lead to an enlarged palpable, nontender gallbladder; contrariwise, obstruction by stones in the common bile duct does not lead to a palpable, nontender gallbladder because scarring from chronic gallbladder inflammation prevents enlargement of the gallbladder.

Courvoisier's sign in a small percentage of cases, obstruction of the common bile duct by carcinoma of the pancreas causes enlargement of the gallbladder; obstruction caused by stones in the common bile duct does not cause enlargement because scarring from infection prevents the gallbladder from distending.

crepitus crackling; the sensation felt or sound heard when palpating soft tissue that contains gas or when moving fractured bones.

cricothyroidotomy incision through the skin and cricothyroid membrane through which a small tracheostomy tube is inserted to relieve airway obstruction.

Crohn's disease inflammatory process of the small intestine and colon; usually causes transmural involvement of the small intestinal wall; occasionally similar to acute appendicitis.

crossmatch in vitro process of mixing donor leukocytes with recipient serum and complement; used to determine whether the recipient produces antibodies that are cytotoxic to the leukocytes, thus predicting rejection of a potential allograft.

crystalloid fluid for intravenous administration; consists of water, electrolytes, and sometimes glucose in isotonic or hypertonic concentrations.

Cushing reflex increase in systemic blood pressure associated with bradycardia and a slowed respiratory rate; caused by increased intracranial pressure.

Cushing's disease Cushing's syndrome (see below) caused by excess production of adrenocorticotropic hormone by an adenoma of the anterior pituitary gland; first defined in 1932.

Cushing's syndrome constellation of clinical findings that result from excessive circulating glucocorticoids.

cytopenia decreased number of cells, usually hematologic cells; anemia is decreased red cell count; leukopenia is decreased white cell count; thrombocytopenia is decreased platelet count.

dead space potential or real cavity that remains after closure of a wound and is not obliterated by the operative technique.

debridement technique to remove dead skin, other nonviable tissue, and debris from a wound surface; some surgeons use this term to describe excision of burns, but it usually refers only to treatment provided at the bedside, without anesthesia.

deep-space compartment confined anatomic space; increased pressure within such a space (e.g., from edema) limits circulation and threatens tissue function and viability.

dentate line anatomic line that delineates the conversion of squamous epithelium to cuboidal and columnar epithelium in the anal canal.

dermatofibroma slowly growing benign skin nodule; poorly demarcated cellular fibrous tissue encloses collapsed capillaries, with scattered hemosiderin-pigmented and lipid macrophages.

dexamethasone suppression test dexamethasone is administered to suppress cortisol secretion; in Cushing's syndrome, this suppression does not occur.

diagnostic peritoneal lavage surgical procedure used to identify an intraperitoneal injury; under local anesthesia, a peritoneal catheter is inserted into the peritoneal cavity through a small midline incision; a syringe is attached to the catheter and aspirated; if 10 mL blood is aspirated, the test result is positive; if less than 10 mL blood is aspirated, then 1000 mL or 10 mL/kg warm lactated Ringer's or normal saline solution is infused into the peritoneal cavity; after 5 to 10 minutes, the lavage fluid is retrieved by gravity siphon technique; a 50-mL portion is sent to the laboratory for microscopic analysis, cell count, and bile and amylase analysis; the result is positive for blunt trauma if the red blood cell count is 100,000 cells/mm^3 or greater, if the white blood cell count is more than 500 cells/mm^3, if bacteria, bile, or food particles are present, or if amylase is greater than serum amylase; a negative study does not exclude retroperitoneal injury to the duodenum, pancreas, kidneys, diaphragm, aorta, or vena cava.

disseminated intravascular coagulation hemorrhagic syndrome that occurs after the uncontrolled activation of clotting factors and fibrinolytic enzymes throughout the small blood vessels; fibrin is deposited, platelets and clotting factors are consumed, and fibrin degradation products that inhibit fibrin polymerization and clot formation are created, resulting in bleeding.

Dripps-American Surgical Association Classification system of patient classification (I to IV); based on chronic health status; used to estimate perioperative risks.

duct of Santorini accessory pancreatic duct.

duct of Wirsung main pancreatic duct.

Dukes' classification staging system that correlates the prognosis in colorectal cancer with the depth of penetration of the primary tumor.

dumping syndrome complex myriad symptoms; may include crampy abdominal pain and diarrhea; secondary to ablation of the pyloric sphincter mechanism.

durable power of attorney for health care formal advance directive that names a specific person to make health care decisions for the patient if the patient becomes unable to do so.

dysphagia difficulty in swallowing.

elemental diet chemically defined enteral diet of high osmolarity and low viscosity; designed to meet specific nutritional and metabolic needs that cannot be achieved naturally.

embolism occlusion or obstruction of an artery by a transported thrombus, atherosclerotic plaque, bacterial vegetation, or foreign body.

endarterectomy surgical excision of the intima, atherosclerotic plaque, and a portion of the media of an atherosclerotic blood vessel.

endoscopic retrograde cholangiopancreatogram (ERCP) radiologic imaging of the biliary tree and pancreatic duct by retrograde injection of contrast material through a cannula placed endoscopically in the ampulla of Vater; used to extract stones, obtain a cytology specimen, or place a catheter.

eschar coating of dead skin, serum, and debris that forms on the surface of a burn wound.

escharotomy incision made through burned tissue to relieve compression caused by edema formation beneath rigid eschar.

esophageal diverticulum outpouching of all layers of the esophagus; typically located in the cervical, midthoracic, or epiphrenic region; associated with dysfunction of the cricopharyngeus muscle and lower esophageal sphincter complex; in Zenker's diverticulum, only the mucosa projects through the esophageal wall.

esophageal myotomy incision in the muscular portion of the esophagus; performed for achalasia or another esophageal motility disorder; converts the esophagus into a larger, but passive tube.

esophageal stricture stenosis of the esophagus; typically occurs from gastric acid reflux, from neglected reflux esophagitis, or after corrosive materials are swallowed.

excision, early technique of burn wound treatment; burned tissue is surgically removed before spontaneous eschar separation occurs.

excision, fascial technique of burn wound excision; the skin and subcutaneous tissue are removed to the level of the fascia.

excision, tangential technique of burn wound excision; only burned tissue is removed with a dermatome, leaving viable dermis and subcutaneous tissue behind.

extracorporeal shock wave lithotripsy (ESWL) fragmentation of gallstones with a shock wave; performed ultrasonographically; limitations include strict eligibility criteria, high failure rate, high recurrence rate, and the need for an expensive solvent (ursodeoxycholic acid) and expensive equipment.

false diverticulum diverticulum characterized by mucosal outpouching through a weakened portion of the colon wall.

familial atypical mole and melanoma (FAM-M) syndrome risk factor for hereditary melanoma; associated with mutations on chromosomes 1p and 9p.

familial medullary thyroid carcinoma autosomal dominant condition caused by a mutation of RET; associated with medullary thyroid carcinoma, but no other endocrine abnormalities.

fasciotomy incision through the fascia to relieve increased pressure; used to treat compartment syndrome.

feeding, postpyloric feeding into the gastrointestinal tract distal to the pyloric valve, usually with a nasoduodenal or gastroduodenal tube.

feeding, prepyloric feeding into the gastrointestinal tract proximal to the pylorus with a nasogastric or gastrostomy tube.

felon infection of the pulp space of the digits in the hand.

Felty's syndrome leg ulcers or chronic infection associated with splenomegaly and neutropenia in patients with rheumatoid arthritis.

fibrin essential portion of a blood clot; white, fibrous protein formed from fibrinogen by the action of thrombin.

fibrinogen factor I; globulin produced in the liver and converted to fibrin during blood clotting.

fibromuscular dysplasia idiopathic nonatherosclerotic hyperplastic and fibrosing lesion of the intima, media, or adventitia; the most common form is medial fibroplasia.

fine-needle aspiration biopsy cytology cytologic examination of cells aspirated from the thyroid; also the most commonly used technique to diagnose palpable breast masses; a small-gauge needle is used to extract three random samples of the breast mass; the contents of the needle are smeared on a glass slide using a technique similar to that used with a Pap smear.

fistula abnormal connection between two epithelial-lined structures.

fistula, aortocaval abnormal communication between the aorta and inferior vena cava.

fistula, aortoenteric abnormal communication between the abdominal aorta and the third portion of the duodenum where it overlies the aorta; usually associated with breakdown of a previous aortic bypass graft anastomosis, although primary aortoenteric fistulae occur.

fistula-in-ano abnormal communication between the anus at the level of the dentate line and the perirectal skin through the bed of a previous abscess.

flail chest result of fracture of consecutive ribs in multiple places (i.e., each rib is fractured in at least two places); the free-floating, or flail, segment of the chest wall moves paradoxically with inspiration and expiration.

follicle extracellular space within the thyroid; contains colloid; bordered by follicular cells; triiodothyronine (T_3) and thyroxine (T_4) are stored bound to thyroglobulin.

follicular cells thyroid cells that process iodine into thyroid hormone.

fulminant hepatic failure hepatic failure associated with massive hepatocyte necrosis or severe impairment; occurs within 8 to 12 weeks of the onset of symptoms; findings are not associated with chronic liver disease; unless liver transplantation is performed, may progress to coma and brainstem herniation from increased cerebral pressure.

fundoplication operation to restore competence to the esophagogastric junction as part of the treatment of sliding hiatal hernia and reflux esophagitis; the most common is the Nissen fundoplication, in which the gastric fundus is wrapped around the lower and intraabdominal segment of the esophagus to produce an acute angle of His and other functional changes.

gallstone ileus mechanical obstruction of the intestine caused by a large gallstone that erodes through the gallbladder into the duodenum; may be associated with pneumobilia; the point of obstruction is often in the distal ileum.

gas-bloat syndrome abdominal bloating associated with inability to vomit; may occur after gastric fundoplication.

gastric outlet obstruction obstruction in the pyloric area of the stomach secondary to repeated bouts of acute duodenal ulcerations with subsequent scarring.

gastrin hormone produced by the G cells of the stomach; stimulates acid secretion by the parietal cell.

gastritis diffuse erythema and disruption of the mucosa of the stomach; associated with the ingestion of irritating agents.

Glasgow Coma Scale method used to classify the severity of head injuries; eye opening score 1 to 4, verbal response score 1 to 5, and motor response score 1 to 6.

globus hystericus subjective sensation of a lump in the throat.

goiter thyroid enlargement.

graft, heterotopic graft placed at a site different from the normal anatomic position (e.g., renal transplant).

graft, orthotopic graft placed in the normal anatomic position (e.g., cardiac transplant).

granulocyte colony stimulating factor similar to erythropoietin for red cells; stimulates the maturation of white blood cells; dramatically decreases the sequelae of leukopenia after chemotherapy.

Graves' disease autoimmune thyrotoxicosis.

H_2 blockade most common modality used to treat duodenal ulcer disease; blocks the histamine receptor of the parietal cell; one-half of the total is given in the first 8 hours postburn; the rest is given over the next 16 hours.

hamartoma benign tumor; normal tissues grow rapidly compared with surrounding normal tissues.

Harris-Benedict equations pair of regression equations based on sex, age, height, and weight; used to estimate resting metabolic expenditure.

Hartmann's procedure stapling or oversewing of the distal end of a sigmoid colon resection, leaving a blind rectal stump in the peritoneal cavity.

Hashimoto's thyroiditis autoimmune thyroiditis; first described by Japanese surgeon Hakuru Hashimoto (1881–1934).

healing, primary primary adhesion of tissue after a wound is closed by direct approximation of the edges; no granulation tissue is formed.

healing, secondary closing of a wound by secondary adhesion; the wound is left open and allowed to heal spontaneously.

healing, tertiary active closing of a wound after a delay of days to weeks; an open wound is closed with sutures or sterile tape before it heals; the secondary healing process is interrupted.

Heinz bodies erythrocyte inclusions that consist of denatured hemoglobin.

Helicobacter pylori Gram-negative bacterium associated with the pathogenesis of gastritis, gastric ulcers, and duodenal ulcers.

hemangioma tumor composed primarily of blood vessels; can involve the small and large intestine and liver.

hemangioma, cavernous benign, often incidentally found, tumor; consists of endothelial vascular spaces separated by fibrous septa; spontaneous rupture is rare; most patients require no specific treatment.

hemochromatosis autosomal recessive disease; characterized by excessive absorption of iron from the intestinal tract; affects the liver, heart, pancreas, and spleen.

hemoglobinopathy abnormality in hemoglobin structure; may lead to anemia and red cell structural abnormalities.

hemolytic anemia anemia caused by destruction of red blood cells.

hemophilia, type A X-linked recessive disorder of the blood; occurs almost exclusively in men; marked by a permanent tendency to hemorrhage as a result of factor VIII deficiency; characterized by prolonged clotting time, decreased formation of thromboplastin, and diminished conversion of prothrombin to thrombin.

hemothorax blood in the pleural cavity.

hemothorax, massive rapid loss of more than 1500 mL of blood into the pleural cavity; class III or greater hemorrhage into the pleural cavity.

hepatic encephalopathy poorly understood neuropsychiatric disorder; associated with advanced liver disease and portosystemic shunting; suspected etiologies include altered amino acid levels in the systemic circulation.

hepatocellular carcinoma (hepatoma) tumor, usually in the setting of cirrhosis (70% to 80%); accounts for 90% of all primary liver malignancies; most are advanced at presentation; fewer than 20% of patients are candidates for standard surgical resection.

her-2-neu oncogene oncogene whose expression indicates a poor prognosis, particularly in patients with node-positive breast cancer.

hereditary spherocytosis inherited condition that can lead to hemolytic anemia because of rigid, abnormally shaped erythrocytes that are sequestered and destroyed in the spleen.

hernia protrusion of all or part of a structure through the tissues that normally contain it.

hernia, direct groin hernia that results from protrusion through the attenuated posterior inguinal wall.

hernia, femoral protrusion of intraabdominal structures through the femoral canal.

hernia, indirect groin hernia into a patent processus vaginalis.

hernia, Richter's hernia at any site through which only a portion of the circumference of a bowel wall, usually the jejunum, incarcerates or strangulates.

hernia, sliding hernia in which a portion of the wall of the protruding peritoneal sac is made up of some intraabdominal organ; as the sac expands, the organ is drawn out into the hernia.

hernia, umbilical protrusion of bowel or omentum through the abdominal wall under the skin at the umbilicus.

Hesselbach's triangle triangular area in the lower abdominal wall bounded by the inguinal ligament below, the border of the rectus abdominis medially, and the inferior epigastric vessels laterally; site of direct inguinal hernias.

Hodgkin's disease malignant lymphoma marked by chronic enlargement of the lymph nodes that is often local at onset and later generalized, together with enlargement of the spleen and often of the liver, no pronounced leukocytosis, and often anemia and continuous or remittent fever; associated with inflammatory infiltration of lymphocytes and eosinophilic leukocytes and fibroses.

Howell-Jolly bodies erythrocyte inclusion of nuclear remnants; usually found on peripheral blood smears after splenectomy.

human leukocyte antigens (HLA) antigens expressed by all nucleated cells; used to determine histocompatibility; the genetic loci that determine these antigens are located in the sixth human chromosome.

hyperparathyroidism, primary condition caused by excess secretion of parathyroid hormone, usually from a parathyroid adenoma.

hyperparathyroidism, secondary overactivity of the parathyroid glands in response to physiologic changes caused by chronic renal failure.

hyperparathyroidism, tertiary autonomous overactivity of the parathyroid glands; causes hypercalcemia; usually caused by chronic renal failure.

hyperplasia, atypical increased number of abnormal-appearing cells in the milk ducts; precedes ductal carcinoma in situ on the continuum from cells lining a normal milk duct, to ductal carcinoma in situ, to invasive cancer.

hyperplasia, focal nodular benign tumor that usually contains a central scar with both ductal elements and hepatocytes; spontaneous rupture is rare; most require no specific therapy.

hyperplasia, parathyroid diffuse enlargement and overactivity of the parathyroid glands.

hypersplenism excess splenic function manifested by cytopenia; may be unrelated to spleen size.

hypoperfusion inadequate blood flow to tissues.

hyposplenism diminished splenic function; usually increases susceptibility to infection, particularly with encapsulated bacteria.

hypovolemia decreased intravascular volume; causes decreased venous return.

ileoanal pullthrough operative procedure of choice for ulcerative colitis; consists of total colectomy, mucosal proctectomy, creation of a storage reservoir, and anastomosis to the dentate line; obviates a permanent ileostomy.

ileocecal valve termination of the small intestine; regulates the passage of intestinal contents into the large intestine.

immune thrombocytopenic purpura thrombocytopenia caused by antibodies directed at platelets; leads to platelet sequestration in the spleen.

incarceration confinement of a herniated structure to its protruded position.

indirect calorimetry method to measure precisely the resting metabolic rate by analysis of inspired and expired gases for O_2 and CO_2; when coupled with urine urea nitrogen, can be used to compute the proportion of protein, carbohydrate, and fat substrates being oxidized.

infection microbial phenomenon characterized by an inflammatory response to the presence of microorganisms or the invasion of normally sterile host tissue by organisms.

infection, nosocomial infection that occurs because of or during hospitalization and treatment.

infection, overwhelming postsplenectomy highly lethal infection (75% mortality rate) caused by encapsulated bacteria (*Streptococcus pneumoniae* is the most common); loss of the spleen increases susceptibility to these bacteria.

infection, polymicrobial infection that is difficult to treat because it involves multiple bacterial species.

inflammation cellular processes that are activated by a variety of cellular and tissue injuries; necessary for tissue repair and wound healing.

inflammation, severe inflammation stimulated by cellular or tissue injury; causes total body cellular or organ malfunction.

informed consent transfer of information between physician and patient that allows the patient to make a knowledgeable decision about a particular treatment.

inhalation injury injury that occurs from inhaling smoke or the products of combustion; occurs as carbon monoxide poisoning, upper-airway injury, or pulmonary parenchymal injury.

injury, reperfusion myocardial impairment, usually with arrhythmia, following the opening of arterial blockage and considered to be due to oxygen-derived free radicals.

inotropic drug agent that increases the contractility of heart muscle.

internal hemorrhoids vascular venous cushions that arise above the dentate line; often associated with swelling, bleeding, and discomfort.

iodine element concentrated and complexed exclusively by thyroid tissue.

isograft tissue transferred between genetically identical individuals (e.g., monozygotic twins).

jaw-thrust maneuver maneuver used to open the mouth so that the oral cavity can be inspected and patency assured; accomplished by standing behind the patient's head, placing the fingers behind the angle of the jaw, grasping the jaw on both sides, and then lifting it forward; the thumbs are used to open the mouth by drawing the mouth and chin downward.

Kehr's sign pain at the top of the left shoulder referred from diaphragmatic irritation (e.g., from blood from a ruptured spleen).

Kupffer cell liver-based macrophage that accounts for 80% to 90% of the body stores of fixed macrophages; responsible for hepatic clearance of toxins, including endotoxin and specific infectious organisms; also responsible for the generation of cytokines and other inflammatory mediators.

Kussmaul's sign increase in central venous pressure with inspiration; seen in severe cardiac tamponade.

laceration torn or jagged wound or accidental cut wound.

leiomyoma tumor that involves the small or large intestine or any other smooth muscle.

leiomyosarcoma malignant tumor of smooth muscle.

lentigo maligna melanoma (Hutchinson's melanotic freckle) malignant lesion of the elderly; arises in sun-damaged skin; occurs primarily on the face and neck.

ligament of Treitz area of the small intestine where the duodenum meets the jejunum; located to the left of the midline in the left upper quadrant.

lower esophageal sphincter complex of anatomic structures that acts as a sphincter and keeps gastric acid in the stomach, yet allows swallowing, belching, or vomiting.

lymphedema swelling caused by the obstruction of lymphatic vessels or lymph nodes and the accumulation of large amounts of lymph; lymphedema of the arm, one of the most disabling complications of axillary dissection, occurs in 2% to 3% of cases after a level I or level II axillary dissection; usually occurs 6 months to many years after the surgical procedure.

lymphoma lymphatic malignancy that arises in the lymphoreticular components of the reticuloendothelial system.

lymphoma, non-Hodgkin's lymphoma other than Hodgkin's disease; classified by Rappaport according to pattern (nodular or diffuse) and cell type; a working or international formulation separates lymphomas into low, intermediate, and high grades and into cytologic subtypes that reflect follicular center cell or other origin.

lyophilization process of preserving tissue by removing its water content through freezing and rewarming in a vacuum.

magnification, compression views special mammographic techniques used to evaluate an abnormal density seen on a routine two-view screening mammography; if a density is real, magnification and compression of the breast tissue make the lesion more discrete; if the lesion represents an area of breast parenchyma that is more dense than surrounding tissue, compression usually causes the area to appear normal and diminishes clinical concern.

mass contractions contraction pattern that is unique to the colon; characterized by contraction of long segments of colon and resulting in mass movement of stool.

McBurney's point point on the anterior abdominal wall; located between the middle and outer thirds of a line drawn between the anterior iliac spine and umbilicus; represents on the anterior abdominal wall the location of the appendix.

Meckel's diverticulum true diverticulum of the ileum; occurs in 1% to 3% of the population; associated with bleeding, inflammation, and bowel obstruction.

medullary thyroid carcinoma carcinoma that originates from the C-cells (calcitonin-secreting cells) of the thyroid; part of the multiple endocrine neoplasia types 2A (MEN-2A) and 2B (MEN-2B), and familial medullary thyroid carcinoma syndromes.

melanoma malignant neoplasm of the skin; derived from the cells that form melanin.

menin gene associated with multiple endocrine neoplasia type 1.

microcalcifications, mammographic breast calcifications that are classified as benign, indeterminate, or pleomorphic; benign microcalcifications are isolated, smooth, round densities that need no further evaluation; pleomorphic microcalcifications are irregularly shaped and resemble broken glass; they suggest ductal carcinoma in situ and require biopsy; microcalcifications that exhibit both benign and pleomorphic characteristics are called indeterminate; they require either biopsy or mammographic reevaluation in 6 months; if not associated with ductal carcinoma in situ, these microcalcifications are seen in fibrocystic conditions.

mitotane adrenolytic agent used to treat adrenocortical adenocarcinoma.

multiple endocrine neoplasia (MEN) familial endocrine tumor syndromes inherited as autosomal dominant conditions; three types: MEN-1, MEN-2A, and MEN-2B.

multiple endocrine neoplasia type 1 (MEN-1) autosomal dominant condition associated with primary hyperparathyroidism, pituitary adenomas, pancreatic islet cell tumors, carcinoid tumors of the thymus or bronchus, and lipomas.

multiple endocrine neoplasia type 2A (MEN-2A) autosomal dominant condition caused by a mutation of RET; associated with medullary thyroid carcinoma, pheochromocytoma, and parathyroid hyperplasia.

multiple endocrine neoplasia type 2B (MEN-2B) autosomal dominant condition caused by a mutation of RET; associated with a characteristic phenotype, medullary thyroid carcinoma, and pheochromocytoma.

multiple organ system failure altered organ function in an acutely ill patient; homeostasis cannot be maintained without intervention.

Murphy's sign sharp pain on deep inspiration during palpation in the right upper quadrant; associated with acute cholecystitis.

necrotizing fasciitis soft tissue infection that spreads along the fascia and causes necrosis; often caused by mixed aerobes and anaerobes; when the male genitalia are involved, called Fournier's disease.

Nelson syndrome development of an adrenocorticotropic hormone–producing pituitary tumor after bilateral adrenalectomy in Cushing's syndrome; causes aggressive growth and hyperpigmentation of the skin.

nevus, blue dark blue or blue-black nevus covered by smooth skin; formed by melanin-pigmented spindle cells in the lower dermis.

nevus, compound common nevus caused by nests of cells in the dermis and epidermal–dermal junction.

nevus, congenital giant hairy large, hairy congenital pigmented nevus that often involves the entire lower trunk; high risk for melanoma.

nevus, intradermal most common benign nevus in adults; caused by nests of melanocytes in the dermis.

nevus, junctional slightly raised, flat, pigmented tumor; caused by nests of nevus cells in the basal layer at the epidermal–dermal junction.

nitrogen balance nitrogen intake (g/day) minus nitrogen excretion (24-hour urine urea nitrogen plus 3 g for unmeasured nitrogen losses); crucial goal in nutritional support.

nodular melanoma most malignant melanoma tumor; grows vertically, is blue-black, has a palpable nodular component in its earliest development, and develops quickly.

normal serum laboratory values (in commonly used units and Système Internationale [SI] units)

serum	common units	SI units
K^+	3.5–5.0 mEq/L	3.5–5.0
Na^+	135–145 mEq/L	135–145
Ca^{++} (total)	8.9–10.3 mg/dL	2.23–2.57
Ca^{++} (ionized)	4.6–5.1 mg/dL	1.15–1.27
Mg^{++}	1.3–2.1 mEq/L	0.65–1.05
Cl–	97–110 mEq/L	97–110
CO_2 (serum, not Pa_{CO_2})	22–31 mEq/L	22–31
$PO_4^{=}$	2.5–4.5 mg/dL	0.81–1.45
Blood urea nitrogen	8–25 mg/dL	2.9–8.9
Creatinine	0.6–1.5 mg/dL	53–133 mmol/L
Fasting glucose	65–110 mg/dL	3.58–6.05

obturator sign clinical sign elicited during acute appendicitis by passive rotation of the flexed right thigh; an acutely inflamed appendix irritates the obturator internus.

odynophagia pain on swallowing.

oliguria in an adult, urine output of less than 500 mL/day.

omeprazole potent inhibitor of hydrochloric acid production; acts by blocking the proton pump of the parietal cell.

open-gloving technique method of donning surgical gloves when a gown is not required or when the hands have been passed fully through the cuffs of the surgical gown; usually requires an assistant because it is difficult to accomplish individually without contaminating the outside of the glove.

opsonins proteins that bind to particulate and bacterial antigens and facilitate phagocytosis.

orthostatic (postural) hypotension excessive decrease in blood pressure on assuming the erect position; usually marked by an increase in heart rate.

osmolality number of osmoles per kilogram of water; total volume is 1 L plus a relatively small volume occupied by the solute.

osmolarity number of osmoles per liter of solution; volume is less than 1 L by an amount equal to the solute volume.

pancreas divisum congenital abnormality of the pancreas; the duct of Santorini is not fused to the duct of Wirsung because of failure of the dorsal and ventral pancreatic buds to fuse during embryonic development.

pancreatic magna largest branch of the splenic arteries; supplies the body of the pancreas.

pancreaticoduodenectomy (Whipple procedure) removal of the head of the pancreas, duodenum, and distal common bile duct; performed for carcinoma of the pancreas, duodenum, or distal common bile duct, and for trauma.

pancreatitis, acute single episode of diffuse pancreatitis in a previously normal gland.

pancreatitis, acute biliary (gallstone) acute inflammation of the pancreas secondary to gallstones; usually caused by passage of small gallstones and sludge through the ampulla of Vater.

pancreatitis, chronic chronic inflammatory process in the pancreas that destroys its functional capabilities; characterized by endocrine and exocrine deficiency and constant pain.

pancreatitis, gallstone acute inflammation of the pancreas caused by gallstones occluding the ampulla of Vater.

Pappenheimer bodies iron inclusions in erythrocytes.

paradoxical aciduria aciduria in the late stages of hypokalemic metabolic alkalosis; the urine becomes acidic as the kidney, in an attempt to retain potassium, excretes hydrogen ions despite the overlying metabolic alkalosis (in which case hydrogen ions would be retained).

parafollicular cells cells of neuroendocrine origin within the thyroid that secrete calcitonin.

paraganglionoma pheochromocytoma located outside the adrenal medulla (extraadrenal pheochromocytoma).

parathyroid glands endocrine glands in the neck that secrete parathyroid hormone.

parathyroid hormone (parathormone) peptide hormone secreted by the parathyroid glands; primarily responsible for maintaining calcium homeostasis.

parenteral nutrition, peripheral 3% amino acid and 10% dextrose solution with lipid emulsion; delivered into a peripheral or central vein to satisfy the nutritional needs of a nonstressed patient.

parenteral nutrition, total high-osmolarity solution of amino acids, dextrose, and often lipid emulsion; delivered into a central vein to satisfy all of a patient's nutritional needs.

parietal cell cell found in the fundus of the stomach; produces hydrochloric acid and intrinsic factor.

Parkland formula widely used formula for resuscitation from burn shock: 4 mL lactated Ringer's solution Ñ body weight (kg) × burn (percentage of total body surface area).

paronychia local infection of the skin over the mantle of the fingernail and lateral nail folds.

PEG/PEJ percutaneous endoscopic gastrostomy, alone or with accompanying percutaneous jejunal tube placement; feeding tube placement performed in the intensive care unit or endoscopy suite rather than with laparotomy in the operating suite, which would require a general anesthetic.

pericardiocentesis needle puncture of the pericardium to aspirate fluid or blood to relieve cardiac tamponade.

peristaltic waves waves of alternate circular contraction and relaxation in the gastrointestinal tract that propel food and fluids onward.

peritonitis inflammation of the surfaces of the peritoneal cavity.

Peyer's patches aggregates of lymphoid cells in the lymph nodes in the gastrointestinal tract; concentrated in the ileum.

phase, proliferative second stage of wound healing; characterized by the laying down of collagen by fibroblasts.

phase, remodeling third stage of wound healing; characterized by the maturation of collagen and flattening of the wound scar.

phase, substrate (inflammatory, lag, exudative) first phase of wound healing; characterized by inflammation, macrophage formation, and appearance of substrates for collagen synthesis.

pheochromocytoma neoplasm of the adrenal medulla; arises from chromaffin tissue of neural crest origin; secretes excess epinephrine, norepinephrine, dopamine, or other vasoactive amine; causes a constellation of signs and symptoms as a result of catecholaminemia; associated with the familial endocrine syndromes multiple endocrine neoplasia types 2A (MEN-2A) and 2B (MEN-2B).

plasma fluid (noncellular) portion of the circulating blood; distinguished from serum, which is obtained after coagulation.

plasma, fresh frozen separated plasma, frozen within 6 hours of collection; used to replenish coagulation factor deficiencies (e.g., liver failure, excessive warfarin [Coumadin] effect).

platelet irregularly shaped disk in the blood; has granules, but no definite nucleus; approximately one-third to one-half the size of an erythrocyte; contains no hemoglobin; known chiefly for its role in hemostasis.

platelet count calculation of the number of platelets in 1 mm^3 of blood by counting the cells in an accurate volume of diluted blood; normal = 150,000 to 400,000 mL.

Plummer's disease toxic multinodular goiter.

pneumonia active infection within the lung parenchyma.

pneumoperitoneum free intraperitoneal air caused by perforation of the stomach, duodenum, or other part of the intestinal tract.

pneumothorax air or gas in the pleural cavity.

pneumothorax, open (sucking chest wound) large chest wall defect that permits equilibration of intrapleural and atmospheric pressures; leads to lung collapse; if the defect is at least two-thirds the diameter of the trachea, resistance to flow is lower through the defect than through the trachea; air moves into and out of the pleural space instead of through the trachea, and effective ventilation is prevented.

pneumothorax, tension air leaks out of the lung or bronchi into the pleural cavity and is trapped; intrapleural pressure rises and can exceed atmospheric pressure; the ipsilateral lung collapses; the mediastinum and trachea are pushed to the contralateral side, causing compression, distortion, and kinking of the superior and inferior vena cavae; venous return to the heart is significantly decreased; oxygen delivery is compromised; without rapid treatment, death ensues.

polycystic liver disease autosomal dominant disorder that causes progressive formation of multiple cysts; rarely leads to hepatic failure, but can cause significant symptoms associated with the mass effect of hepatic cysts.

polyp small mucosal excrescence that grows into the lumen of the colon and rectum.

polyp, pedunculated polyp that is rounded at the end and attached to the mucosa by a long, thin neck.

polyp, sessile flat polyp that is intimately attached to the mucosa.

polyvalent pneumococcal polysaccharide vaccines vaccines that contain polysaccharide antigens from many pneumococcal types; current vaccines contain 23 common types that cause infection in humans.

portal hypertension abnormally elevated pressure within the portal vein or its tributaries; causes gastroesophageal varices, variceal hemorrhage, and ascites.

portosystemic collateral routes multiple sites of collateralization that arise in the setting of portal hypertension; routes include the esophageal–azygos system, splenorenal system, mesenteric–hemorrhoidal system, retroperitoneal collaterals, and caput medusae at the umbilicus.

portosystemic shunts large-caliber connections between the portal and systemic circulatory systems; reduce portal pressure; effectively control varices and ascites, but may be associated with hepatic encephalopathy.

position, reverse Trendelenburg positioning of a patient so that the head is elevated and the feet are lower than the heart.

position, Trendelenburg positioning of a patient so that the head of the table is tilted at a 45° angle; the feet are elevated and the head is kept below the level of the heart.

prealbumin plasma protein with a 4-day half-life; used to reflect visceral protein status and the effectiveness of nutritional support when measured weekly.

preload magnitude of myocardial stretch; the stimulus to muscle contraction described by the Frank-Starling mechanism.

pressure, central venous blood pressure measurement taken in the superior vena cava; reflects right ventricular end-diastolic pressure (preload).

pressure, cerebral perfusion difference between mean arterial pressure and intracranial pressure.

pressure, colloid osmotic difference in pressure between intravascular and interstitial fluid; mostly caused by albumin in the plasma, but not in the interstitium.

pressure, pulmonary artery occlusion (pulmonary capillary wedge pressure, wedge pressure) left atrial pressure measured by advancing a balloon-tipped catheter into the pulmonary artery until it goes no further; normal pressure is 8 to 12 mm Hg.

primary aldosteronism (Conn's syndrome) excessive, autonomous production of aldosterone by a benign adrenocortical adenoma; rarely caused by adrenocortical carcinoma; first described in 1955 by Jerome Conn at the University of Michigan.

primary biliary cirrhosis progressive small bile duct obstruction that leads to cirrhosis, likely from cytotoxic T cells; predominantly affects middle-aged women.

primary sclerosing cholangitis idiopathic disease that causes a chronic fibrotic stricturing process; can involve both the intrahepatic and extrahepatic biliary tree; the only effective long-term treatment is liver transplantation.

prophylactic antibiotics antibiotics administered to prevent infection.

prothrombin time (PT) time required for clotting after thromboplastin and calcium are added in optimal amounts to plasma with normal fibrinogen content; if prothrombin is diminished, the clotting time increases; PT is sensitive to levels of clotting factors V, VII, and X, prothrombin, and fibrinogen.

proximal gastric vagotomy antiulcer operation; selectively denervates vagal stimulation to the parietal cells; maintains the function of the pyloric sphincter.

pseudoaneurysm dilation of the artery wall that does not contain all three layers; usually forms at areas of trauma or regions of weakened arterial graft anastomosis.

pseudocyst, pancreatic cyst (without an epithelial lining) of the pancreas or of the pancreas and adjacent structures; often the result of pancreatitis.

pseudopolyp small island of normal mucosa surrounded by deep ulceration; creates the appearance of a polyp.

psoas sign clinical sign used in acute appendicitis; elicited by extension of the right hip, which causes the inflamed appendix to irritate the iliopsoas muscle.

pulse oximetry photoelectric measurement of the oxygen saturation of capillary blood.

pulsus paradoxus decrease in systolic blood pressure, during inspiration, greater than 10 mm Hg; seen in cardiac tamponade.

pus collection of dead phagocytic cells, fibrin, and plasma proteins; densities of both dead and viable microorganisms and bacterial products that form in a closed area at the site of bacterial invasion.

pyrosis substernal pain or burning; usually associated with regurgitation of gastric juice into the esophagus.

radioactive iodine isotope (^{131}I) of iodine used to evaluate or treat thyroid disease.

radionuclide biliary scan (HIDA scan) diagnostic test in which a ^{99m}Tc-labeled derivative of iminodiacetic acid is injected intravenously; the radionuclide is excreted into the bile ducts and enters the gallbladder through the cystic duct; absence of gallbladder filling in 4 hours, along with filling of the common bile duct and passage of radionuclide into the duodenum, strongly suggests acute cholecystitis.

Ranson's criteria in patients with pancreatitis, a group of risk factors that are present on admission or within 48 hours and aid in the prediction of major complications and death.

red pulp anatomic portion of the spleen; contains the cords; site of removal of antibody-sensitized cells and particulate material.

reduced-size liver transplant use of only the left lobe or the left lateral segment of a living or cadaver liver as a transplant, especially in children.

reflux esophagitis inflammation of the lower esophagus; related to reflux of gastric acidity; contact burn related to the duration and degree of gastric acid contact.

regurgitation flow of material in the opposite direction of normal (e.g., return of undigested food from the stomach into the mouth).

rejection, accelerated acute destruction of a graft in the first few days after transplantation by a second set of anamnestic responses of preformed antibodies and lymphocytes.

rejection, acute reversible attack on a transplanted organ mediated by T-lymphocytes; causes organ dysfunction.

rejection, chronic slow, progressive immunologic destruction of a transplanted organ over years; mediated by both humoral and cellular elements.

rejection, hyperacute destruction of a graft by the recipient through preformed antibodies (e.g., ABO, HLA, or species-specific antibodies); occurs within hours of transplantation.

resection, abdominoperineal removal of the lower sigmoid colon, rectum, and anus, leaving a permanent proximal sigmoid colostomy.

resection, low anterior removal of the distal sigmoid colon and upper one-half of the rectum with primary anastomosis of the proximal sigmoid to distal rectum.

respiratory quotient (RQ) ratio of CO_2:O_2 consumption; reflects whether the patient's energy supply is inadequate ($RQ < 1$), balanced ($RQ = 1$), or excessive ($RQ > 1$).

rest pain pain in the distal extremities, especially the toes and metatarsal heads, when the extremity is elevated; elevation decreases the hydrostatic perfusion pressure of the lower extremities; they become ischemic, and pain occurs; symptoms are usually relieved with "dangling" of the affected extremities.

resting metabolic expenditure energy needed by a resting, supine person after an overnight fast.

resuscitation restoration from potential or apparent death; the airway is secured, ventilation is assured, and oxygen is administered; external blood loss is controlled with direct pressure; intravenous lines are established with a balanced electrolyte solution; Ringer's lactate is preferred in patients with traumatic injury; intravascular volume is restored; hypothermia is combated with high-flow fluid warmers; aspiration and gastric distension are reduced with the placement of a gastric tube; pulse oximetry, blood pressure, electrocardiographic readings, and urine output are monitored; in patients with traumatic injury, these measures are begun simultaneously with the primary survey.

RET proto-oncogene tyrosine kinase receptor oncogene; used as a gene marker for multiple endocrine neoplasia types 2A (MEN-2A) and 2B (MEN-2B) and familial medullary thyroid carcinoma.

Reynold's pentad right upper quadrant abdominal pain, fever and chills, jaundice, hypotension, and mental confusion; associated with acute suppurative cholangitis.

ring sign (target sign) pattern produced when a drop of bloody cerebrospinal fluid is placed on filter paper; because cerebrospinal fluid diffuses faster than blood, the blood remains in the center and one or more concentric rings of clearer (pink) fluid form around the central red spot; used to test bloody otorrhea and rhinorrhea for the presence of cerebrospinal fluid.

Rovsing's sign clinical sign of pain seen in acute appendicitis; pressure applied to the left lower quadrant of the abdomen creates pain in the right lower quadrant.

S-phase phase in the growth cycle of a cell; a finding of more than 6% or 7% of cells in the S-phase in a tissue sample, as measured by flow cytometry, suggests a rapidly growing tumor.

SCALP mnemonic for remembering the five layers of the scalp; <u>S</u>kin, sub<u>C</u>utaneous tissue, galea <u>A</u>poneurotica, <u>L</u>oose areolar tissue, and <u>P</u>eriosteum (pericranium).

scrub nurse member of the surgical team who participates directly in the surgical procedure; manages the sterile instruments and supplies; often assists with the procedure.

Seagesser's sign neck tenderness produced by manual compression over the phrenic nerve; caused by diaphragmatic irritation (e.g., by blood from a ruptured spleen).

seborrheic keratosis superficial, benign, verrucous lesion; consists of proliferating epidermal cells; usually occurs in the elderly.

secretin duodenal hormone that inhibits gastric acid secretion and gastric emptying.

selective shunts shunts that decompress gastroesophageal varices, but maintain prograde portal profusion to the liver; best known is the distal splenorenal shunt.

Sengstaken-Blakemore tube tube placed through the esophagus for balloon tamponade of gastric and esophageal varices; provides temporary occlusion.

sepsis systemic response to infection as manifested by two or more of the following conditions:

1. Temperature > 37°C or < 36°C
2. Heart rate > 90 beats/min
3. Respiratory rate > 20 breaths/min or $Paco_2$ < 32 mm Hg
4. White blood cell count > 12,000 cells/mm^3, < 4000 cells/mm^3, or > 10% immature (band) forms

sepsis, burn wound invasive infection of a burn wound; bacteria penetrate beneath the burned surface and invade viable tissue and blood vessels.

shock inadequate organ perfusion; types include anaphylactic, cardiogenic, hemorrhagic, hypoadrenal, hypovolemic, neurogenic, and septic; total body cellular metabolism is malfunctional.

shock, burn severe loss of intravascular volume caused by fluid sequestration in and beneath burn wounds.

shock, spinal neurologic condition that occurs after spinal cord injury; caused by acute loss of stimulation from higher levels; this "shock" or "stun" to the injured cord makes it appear functionless; there is complete flaccidity and areflexia instead of the predicted spasticity, hyperreflexia, and positive Babinski sign that are seen in the classic upper motor neuron lesion; not a synonym for neurogenic shock, which is inadequate organ perfusion.

silver sulfadiazene (Silvadene, SSD, Thermazene) topical antibiotic widely used in burn treatment; active against a wide range of Gram-positive and Gram-negative organisms and yeast; many other topical agents are also available.

singultus hiccup.

Sister Mary Joseph's node hard nodule at the umbilicus; associated with metastatic gastric carcinoma.

skin graft, full-thickness graft obtained by excising an ellipse of skin and subcutaneous tissue, usually from the groin or flank; donor site is closed with sutures.

skin graft, split-thickness graft obtained by excising tissue at the level of the dermis, leaving a base that heals spontaneously.

somatostatin pharmacologic agent that reduces variceal bleeding by inducing mesenteric vasoconstriction; diminishes variceal bleeding in at least 50% of patients.

splenectomy removal of the spleen.

splenic cords (of Billroth) reticular portion of the spleen in the red pulp that lacks endothelium; blood percolates slowly and comes in contact with numerous macrophages.

splenomegaly, congestive enlargement of the spleen as a result of vascular engorgement (e.g., portal hypertension).

splenomegaly, infiltrative enlargement of the spleen because of accumulation of materials within the splenic reticuloendothelial cells (e.g., Gaucher's disease with accumulation of glucocerebrosides).

spontaneous nipple discharge discharge on clothing in the absence of breast stimulation; in contrast, elicited discharge is noted after the nipple or breast is squeezed, or after vigorous mammography; only spontaneous discharge requires evaluation.

squamous cell carcinoma malignant neoplasm derived from stratified squamous epithelium; variable amounts of keratin are formed in relation to the degree of differentiation; if the keratin is not on the surface, a "keratin pearl" is formed.

sterile field operative area that is covered with sterile drapes and prepared for the use of sterile supplies and equipment; classically, includes the instrument table, Mayo stand, and operative area.

sterile technique moving, working, or functioning in a sterile environment with sterile equipment to prevent contamination of the incision site.

sterilization physical or chemical process by which all pathogenic and nonpathogenic microorganisms are destroyed.

sterilization, dry-heat killing of microorganisms through heat absorption.

sterilization, ethylene oxide gas sterilization technique used for instruments or objects that are sensitive to heat or moisture; ethylene oxide is cidal to all microorganisms, but requires a longer exposure time (3 to 6 hours) than heat sterilization.

sterilization, moist-heat sterilization technique that uses saturated steam under pressure (autoclave); easiest, fastest, and least expensive method of sterilization.

strangulation vascular compromise of an incarcerated organ.

Sturge-Weber syndrome facial hemangioma (causing a port wine stain) occupying the cutaneous distribution of the trigeminal nerve, angiomatous malformations of the brain and meninges, and occasionally pheochromocytoma.

surrogate decision-maker person empowered to make decisions for a patient who is not competent to do so.

survey, primary rapid initial evaluation of a patient with traumatic injury; involves the diagnosis and treatment of all immediately life-threatening injuries; the essence of the "ABCDEs" of trauma management; sequentially, the physician protects the cervical spine while assessing the injured patient's Airway, Breathing, Circulation, and neurologic Disability; Exposure of the patient and prevention of hypothermia are the last steps; all immediately life-threatening injuries are treated in sequence before proceeding to the next phase.

survey, secondary detailed, head-to-toe evaluation of a trauma patient; includes a history and physical examination to identify all injuries; begins after the primary survey is completed, resuscitation is initiated, and the airway, breathing, and circulation are reassessed; tubes or fingers are placed in every orifice; baseline laboratory studies are drawn if they were not drawn when the intravenous lines were started; portable radiographs are taken; special procedures (e.g., peritoneal lavage) are done during this phase.

syndrome of inappropriate secretion of antidiuretic hormone (SIADH) syndrome associated with physiologically uncontrolled production of antidiuretic hormone by malignant tumors or disturbances from intracranial injury disorders.

systemic inflammatory response syndrome syndrome that indicates systemic inflammation; caused by a variety of cellular and tissue injuries (see Chapter 6 for the criteria-based definition).

T cell thymus-derived cell; involved in the cellular response to foreign tissue; produces cytokines, recruits other cells, and differentiates into helper, suppressor, and cytotoxic cells.

target sign see *ring sign*.

tenosynovitis infection of the tendon sheath, usually of the hand.

thalassemia deficit in the synthesis of one or more subunits of hemoglobin; leads to erythrocyte abnormalities and anemia; many types are seen, but β-thalassemias are the most common.

therapy, hormone replacement therapy, often initiated after surgical or natural menopause, to prevent the perimenopausal and postmenopausal symptoms of estrogen withdrawal (e.g., hot flashes, vaginal atrophy, urogenital deterioration); also seems to significantly diminish osteoporosis and cardiac disease.

therapy, protein-sparing 3% amino acid and 5% dextrose solution delivered by peripheral veins; minimizes proteolysis in a nutritionally fit, fasting patient.

thionamides class of antithyroid drugs (e.g., propylthiouracil, methimazole); inhibit iodide organification and iodotyrosine coupling; reduce the rate of peripheral conversion of thyroxine (T_4) to triiodothyronine (T_3).

third-space fluid accumulation accumulation of extracellular and intracellular fluid in response to regional or total body cellular or tissue injury; accumulation in excess of the volume of fluid that normally occupies these regions; sequestration decreases intravascular fluid volume.

third-space fluid loss loss of intravascular or extravascular body fluid into tissue spaces or body cavities after trauma or surgery (e.g., retroperitoneal hematoma, bowel edema).

thrill palpable turbulence within an arterial vessel as a result of disturbed flow.

thrombin time time needed for a fibrin clot to form after thrombin is added to citrated plasma; prolonged thrombin time is seen in patients who are receiving heparin therapy, those who have factor I (fibrinogen) deficiency, and those with elevated levels of fibrin or fibrinogen split products.

thrombocytosis platelet count greater than $400{,}000/mm^3$.

thrombosis formation of an occlusive or nonocclusive blood clot within a blood vessel or cavity of the heart.

thrombotic thrombocytopenic purpura disease of arteries and capillaries; characterized by thrombosis and thrombocytopenia.

thrombus blood clot that forms within a blood vessel and remains in place, often causing an obstruction.

thyroglobulin molecule on which iodine is complexed to form triiodothyronine (T_3) and thyroxine (T_4).

thyroid carcinoma (papillary, follicular, medullary, or anaplastic) types of thyroid cancer; papillary and follicular carcinomas are well-differentiated carcinomas of follicular cells; medullary carcinomas are of parafollicular cell origin; anaplastic carcinomas dedifferentiate from follicular cells.

thyroid-stimulating hormone (TSH, thyrotropin) hormone secreted by the pituitary to regulate thyroxine (T_4) production and secretion by the thyroid.

thyroidectomy surgical excision of the thyroid gland.

thyrotoxicosis (hyperthyroidism) overactive thyroid.

thyroxine (T_4, tetraiodothyronine) major hormone secreted by the thyroid in response to thyroid-stimulating hormone; feeds back to regulate thyroid-stimulating hormone.

tonicity "effective" osmolality; often used to describe intravenous fluid replacement or body fluids (e.g., hypotonic, isotonic, or hypertonic solutions or fluids mean, respectively, less effective, same, or more effective osmolality).

total body water portion of body weight composed of water and fluids; in a typical 70-kg man, 60% of body weight is water and fluids; in women and the elderly, it is 50% to 55%.

toxic multinodular goiter thyroid enlargement from multiple nodules that may cause compression symptoms.

transient ischemic attack reversible changes in mentation, vision, and motor or sensory function; usually lasts seconds to minutes; completely resolves within 24 hours.

transjugular intrahepatic portacaval shunt (TIPS) radiologically placed intrahepatic shunt; connects the portal vein with the hepatic vein; bypasses the increased hepatic resistance.

triangle of Calot hepatocystic triangle bounded by the inferior margin of the liver, common hepatic duct, and cystic duct; traversed by several important normal and anomalous structures.

triiodothyronine (T_3) thyroid hormone that acts at the tissue level where it is formed by deiodinization of thyroxine (T_4).

truncal vagotomy complete transection of both vagal trunks at the gastroesophageal junction; eliminates vagal stimulation of the parietal cell.

tumor, carcinoid most common tumor of the appendix; may cause carcinoid syndrome; often malignant.

tumor, phyllodes breast tumor seen in younger women; usually a large, smooth, nontender mass; clinically similar to fibroadenoma, but larger; most are benign, but a small percentage are malignant; treatment involves wide excision.

ulcer, duodenal ulcer that usually occurs in the first portion of the duodenum as a result of acid hypersecretion.

ulcer, gastric ulcer that typically occurs on the lesser curvature of the stomach; usually secondary to mucosal breakdown of the stomach.

ulcer, Marjolin's squamous cell cancer that arises in the inflammatory scar of a nonhealing ulcer (e.g., chronic wound, fistula-in-ano, osteomyelitis).

ulcerative colitis mucosal disease of the colon; causes significant diarrhea and bleeding; tends to become malignant.

United Network for Organ Sharing (UNOS) organization of transplant centers, organ procurement agencies, and professional and patient groups; regulates organ allocation and procurement in the United States.

urine urea nitrogen 24-hour urine collection assayed for urea; used to measure nitrogen loss and calculate nitrogen balance.

vasoconstriction reduction in the caliber of blood vessels; leads to decreased blood flow.

venous return quantity of blood that returns to the right atrium from the systemic veins each minute.

volvulus rotation of a segment of the intestine on the axis formed by the mesentery; causes obstruction of the bowel.

vomiting forcible expulsion of stomach contents through the mouth.

von Hippel-Lindau disease neuroectodermal dysplasia associated with cystic cerebellar hemangioblastoma and angiomatous malformation of the retina and pheochromocytoma.

von Recklinghausen's disease common neuroectodermal dysplasia; multiple neurofibromas of peripheral nerves; associated with pheochromocytomas.

von Willebrand's disease hemorrhagic diathesis characterized by a tendency to bleed, primarily from the mucous membranes; laboratory abnormalities include prolonged bleeding time, variable deficiency of factor VIII clotting activity, prolonged activated partial thromboplastin time, reduced von Willebrand's antigen and activity, and reduced ristocetin-induced platelet aggregation; inheritance is autosomal dominant, with reduced penetrance and variable expressivity.

water brash heartburn with regurgitation of sour fluid or almost tasteless saliva into the mouth.

Wernicke-Korsakoff syndrome syndrome caused by excessive alcohol intake; bilateral sixth cranial nerve palsy, nystagmus, diplopia, disconjugate gaze, and strabismus; ataxia is typical; mental changes include generalized apathy and lack of awareness; delirium is a late manifestation.

white pulp anatomic portion of the spleen where lymphocytes and lymphatic follicles reside; probably site where soluble antigens are processed.

Wilson's disease autosomal recessive disorder caused by excess copper; causes markedly diminished copper excretion into the biliary tree; correctable with liver transplantation.

wound, clean surgical wound, made under sterile conditions, that does not enter the gastrointestinal, respiratory, or genitourinary tract; wound in which there is a break in sterile technique; wound that is not exposed to a significant bacterial population.

wound, clean-contaminated surgical wound that enters the gastrointestinal, respiratory, or genitourinary tract without significant spillage; wound in which there is a break in sterile technique; wound that is initially clean, but is exposed to endogenous colonization during the procedure.

wound, contaminated surgical wound in which extensive spillage from the gastrointestinal tract occurs; fresh traumatic wound; wound in which a major break in sterile technique occurs; wound in which gross contamination occurs during the procedure.

wound, dirty wound that contains dirt, fecal material, purulence, or other foreign material; high risk of infection.

wound, infected wound with a bacterial count of more than 10^5 organisms/g tissue.

xenograft tissue transferred between members of different species.

xeroderma pigmentosum eruption of exposed skin that occurs in childhood; characterized by numerous pigmented spots that resemble freckles; larger atrophic lesions eventually cause glossy, white thinning of the skin.

Zollinger-Ellison syndrome severe variant of duodenal ulcer disease; results from the independent production of gastrin by a tumor (gastrinoma) that arises in the pancreas or paraduodenal area.

Index

Page numbers followed by an f denote figures; those followed by a t denote tables.

C

D

Q

R